Global Maternal and Child Health: Medical, Anthropological, and Public Health Perspectives

Series Editor
David A. Schwartz
Medical College of Georgia
Augusta University
Augusta, Georgia, USA

Global Maternal and Child Health: Medical, Anthropological, and Public Health Perspectives is a series of books that will provide the most comprehensive and current sources of information on a wide range of topics related to global maternal and child health, written by a collection of international experts. The health of pregnant women and their children are among the most significant public health, medical, and humanitarian problems in the world today. Because in developing countries many people are poor, and young women are the poorest of the poor, persistent poverty exacerbates maternal and child morbidity and mortality and gender-based challenges to such basic human rights as education and access to health care and reproductive choices. Women and their children remain the most vulnerable members of our society and, as a result, are the most impacted individuals by many of the threats that are prevalent, and, in some cases, increasing throughout the world. These include emerging and re-emerging infectious diseases, natural and man-made disasters, armed conflict, religious and political turmoil, relocation as refugees, malnutrition, and, in some cases, starvation. The status of indigenous women and children is especially precarious in many regions because of ethnic, cultural, and language differences, resulting in stigmatization, poor obstetrical and neonatal outcomes, limitations of women's reproductive rights, and lack of access to family planning and education that restrict choices regarding their own futures. Because of the inaccessibility of women to contraception and elective pregnancy termination, unsafe abortion continues to result in maternal deaths, morbidity, and reproductive complications. Unfortunately, maternal deaths remain at unacceptably high levels in the majority of developing countries, as well as in some developed ones. Stillbirths and premature deliveries result in millions of deaths annually. Gender inequality persists globally as evidenced by the occurrence of female genital mutilation, obstetrical violence, human trafficking, and other forms of sexual discrimination directed at women. Many children are routinely exposed to physical, sexual, and psychological violence. Childhood and teen marriages remain at undesirably high levels in many developing countries.

Global Maternal and Child Health: Medical, Anthropological, and Public Health Perspectives is unique in combining the opinions and expertise of public health specialists, physicians, anthropologists and social scientists, epidemiologists, nurses, midwives, and representatives of governmental and non-governmental agencies to comprehensively explore the increasing challenges and potential solutions to global maternal and child health issues.

More information about this series at http://www.springer.com/series/15852

Series Editorial Advisory Board

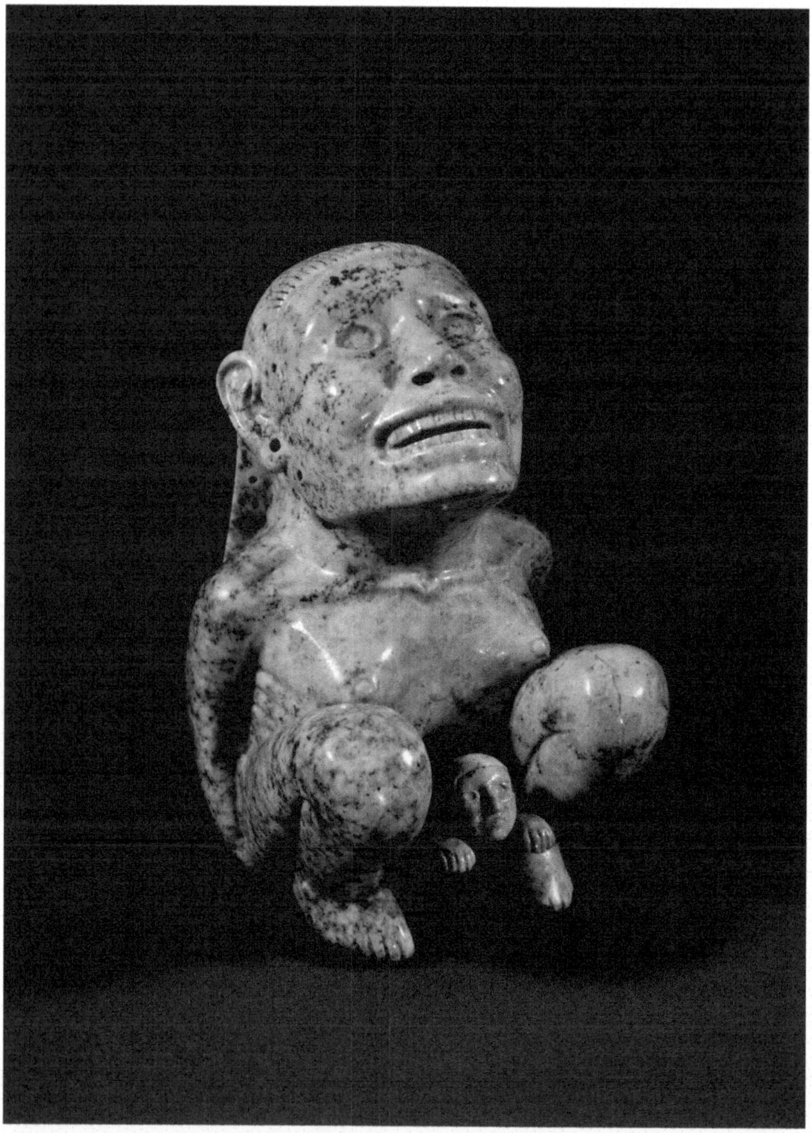

Frontispiece: Late Postclassic Aztec-style figure of a birthing woman in the squatting position. One of the most well-known images of indigenous pregnancy in the Americas, this small scapolite sculpture dramatically illustrates both the agony and ecstasy of childbirth. Often associated with the Aztec goddess *Tlazolteotl*, there is recent evidence to suggest a nineteenth-century origin for the piece. ©Dumbarton Oaks, Pre-Columbian collection, Washington, DC.

David A. Schwartz
Editor

Maternal Death and Pregnancy-Related Morbidity Among Indigenous Women of Mexico and Central America

An Anthropological, Epidemiological, and Biomedical Approach

Springer

Editor
David A. Schwartz
Medical College of Georgia
Augusta University
Augusta
Georgia
USA

ISSN 2522-8382 ISSN 2522-8390 (electronic)
Global Maternal and Child Health: Medical, Anthropological, and Public Health Perspectives
ISBN 978-3-030-10070-4 ISBN 978-3-319-71538-4 (eBook)
DOI 10.1007/978-3-319-71538-4

Printed on acid-free paper

This Springer imprint is published by the registered company Springer International Publishing AG part of Springer Nature.
The registered company address is: Gewerbestrasse 11, 6330 Cham, Switzerland

Dedicated to J. Alden Mason, Ph.D. (1885–1967) Curator, American Section, University of Pennsylvania Museum of Anthropology and Archaeology

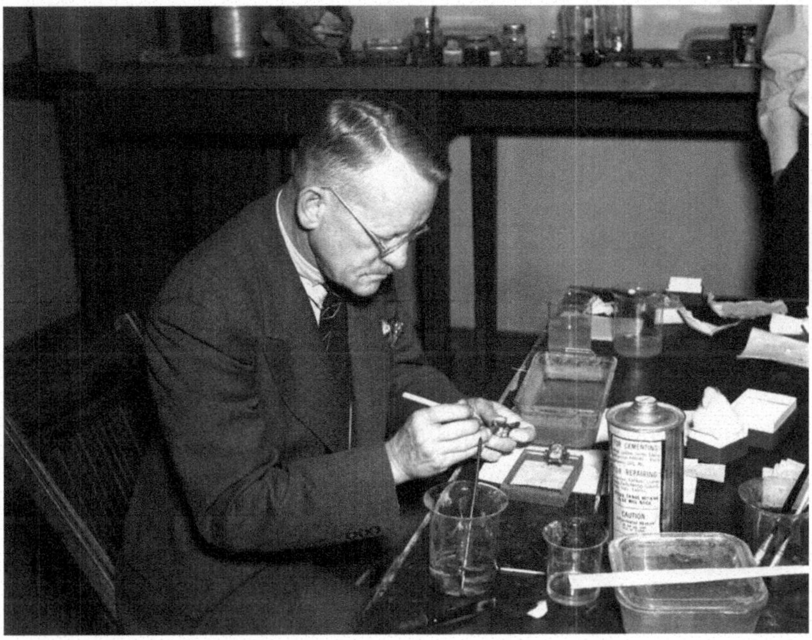

J. Alden Mason as I knew him, sitting at his desk in his office in the 1950s. Penn Museum image no. 85735

This book is dedicated to my friend and mentor, John Alden Mason, one of the last of the great generalist anthropologists of the twentieth century. Alden was raised in Philadelphia and attended the University of Pennsylvania. He graduated with a Bachelor of Arts in 1907, at the time of the origin of academic anthropology in the United States. After graduating, Alden worked as a photographer for George Byron Gordon, an archaeologist who became Director of the University of Pennsylvania Museum of Archaeology and Anthropology, excavated the Mayan site of Copán, Honduras, oversaw important excavations at Ur in Iraq and Beth Shean in Israel, and helped establish the Department of Anthropology at Penn in 1913. Alden later took graduate courses from Frank Speck, a student of Franz Boas who was an anthropological linguist and ethnologist and whose research interests included such Native American peoples as the Iroquois, Cherokee, Labrador Eskimo, and Yuchi. He also received training from Edward Sapir, an anthropologist, linguist, and former student of both Boas and

Alfred Kroeber. Following Sapir's arrival from Berkeley to the Penn Museum in 1908, Alden spent the 1909 field season with him working on the Uintah (western) Ute tribal language and culture. Alden's efforts and relationships with three of the students of Franz Boas were rewarded with a scholarship to attend the University of California at Berkeley, which was one of the preeminent centers for the emerging field of anthropology. Alden earned his doctoral degree there with the famed cultural anthropologist Alfred Kroeber, who had distinguished himself not only in anthropological linguistics but also in archaeology. Kroeber had trained under Franz Boas at Columbia University. Boas, often referred to as the "Father of American Anthropology," was a founder of the American Anthropological Association. Boas would unite the specialties of cultural anthropology, anthropological linguistics, archaeology, and physical anthropology into the modern 4-field discipline of anthropology.

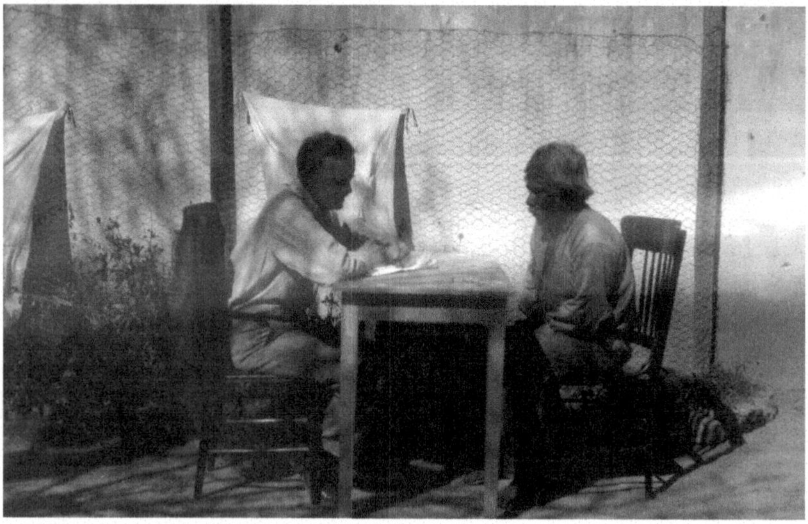

J. Alden Mason (left) with Pedro Valencia studying the Tepehuan language. Guanacevi, Durango, Mexico, 1936. Penn Museum image no. 15257

Following the defense of his dissertation, The Ethnology of the Salinan Indians, he worked as Penn's representative to the International School of American Archaeology and Ethnology in Mexico under Boas, studying the ethnography and grammar of the Tepecano people of Jalisco. Thus, even while a young anthropologist, Alden had already been a student of the pioneers of American anthropology—Boas, Kroeber, Speck, Gordon, and Sapir.

Alden spent several years in Puerto Rico conducting archaeological expeditions and studying folktales (the traditional Juan Bobo stories). He subsequently obtained his first curatorial appointment—Assistant Curator of Mexican and South American Anthropology at the Field Museum of Natural History in Chicago. Following a move in 1924 to the American Museum of Natural History as the Curator of Mexican Archaeology, Alden came to the Penn Museum as the Curator of the American section in 1926. He was to remain there as Curator until his official retirement in 1955. He directed as well as conducted archaeological excavations at two major Mesoamerican sites—Piedras Negras, a large Early and Late Classic period Mayan city in the Petén department of Guatemala, and Sitio Conte, a Pre-Columbian archaeological site and necropolis located in the Coclé province of Panama and which was used from approximately 450 to 900 A.D. He was vice president of the American Anthropological Association in 1944 and was especially proud of being editor of the American Anthropologist from 1945 to 1948. An active author, Alden wrote almost 200 titles addressing archaeology, folklore, linguistics, and ethnology. In the 46 years between 1909 and his official retirement as Curator in 1955, Alden had worked in the field 22 times, including work in Puerto Rico, Colombia, Canada, Panama, six states in Mexico, and four Eastern and five Western states in the United States. After his so-called retirement, Alden was appointed Curator Emeritus at the Penn Museum, a position which he actively maintained until his death in 1967. It was during this period that I came to both know and work with him, and when he transplanted his love of all aspects of anthropology to me as a young protégé.

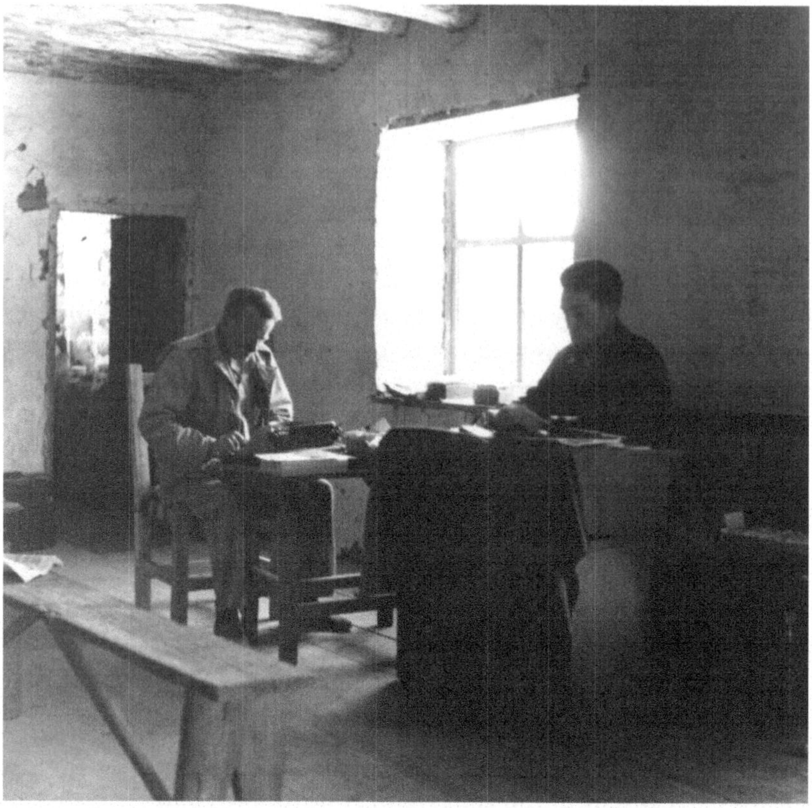

Dr. J. Alden Mason (left) and Dr. Burton "Burt" William Bascom, Jr. (right) working on North Tepecano/Tepehuan linguistic studies. Baborigame, Chihuahua, Mexico, 1951. Penn Museum image no. 85733

Working together for many years with Alden (whom we called "the chief") had a profound effect on my early life and studies, which still influences my life and career 50 years after his death. With his broad academic repertoire and expertise in all the specialties of anthropology, Alden was a true "anthropologist for all seasons"—we will never see his like again. I wish that Alden could have seen the publication of this book, which unites approaches from cultural anthropology, ethnolinguistics, epidemiology, biomedicine, public health, and archaeology into a unified approach to identify the problems and potential solutions of reproductive health and pregnancy encountered by indigenous women of Mexico and Central America. Alden loved the land and people of these countries. I think he would have enjoyed reading this book.

Foreword

The Reproductive and Maternal Health of Indigenous Women Is a Human Right

There is a common trait which is shared by almost all remaining indigenous peoples in both developed and developing countries throughout the world. They are faced with threats to their political sovereignty, economic advancement, access to education, health care, and preservation of their cultural identity, folkways, and language. Indigenous peoples are vulnerable to exploitation, marginalization, oppression, forced assimilation, and genocide by states that were formed from colonizing populations. This recognition of the limitation to basic human rights for indigenous peoples was recognized by the United Nations when they adopted the Declaration on the Rights of Indigenous Peoples (UNDRIP) in the General Assembly on September 13th, 2007. In May 2016, the Fifteenth Session of the United Nations Permanent Forum on Indigenous Issues (UNPFII) affirmed that indigenous people are distinctive groups protected in international or national legislation as having a set of specific rights based on their linguistic and historical ties to a particular territory, prior to later settlement, development, and/or occupation of a region.

Unlike many parts of the world where indigenous peoples have vanished or been markedly reduced in numbers, Mexico and some countries in Central America are fortunate to still have large populations of autochthonous peoples within their borders. With very few exceptions, however, these people have undergone tremendous stresses throughout recent history, including war, stigmatization, poverty, harsh working conditions, community-based violence, poor access to and quality of healthcare and educational opportunities, and efforts to limit or even eliminate their native languages and cultural identities.

Among the restrictions to indigenous people's human rights, the one with arguably the farthest-reaching consequences is limitation to quality health care. This has the most deleterious effect on women and their children, and especially young women of reproductive age, who are the poorest and most vulnerable members of their society. The Alma-Ata Declaration of 1978 emerged as a significant milestone of twentieth century public health when it declared that primary health care was the key to the attainment of the goal of Health for All. This was followed by the United Nations (UN) and its associated agencies addressing maternal mortality reduction following the announcement of eight Millennium Development Goals (MDGs) during the UN Millennium Summit in 2000. The aim of MDG 5a was to *reduce by three quarters,* between 1990 and 2015, the *number of maternal deaths occurring worldwide*, a goal which was especially relevant to developing countries which accounted for greater than 99% of global maternal mortality. Related to this was another goal, MDG Goal 5b—to achieve, by 2015, *universal access to reproductive health.* Although these lofty goals were achieved in a number of countries, unfortunately, for many countries in the developing world, including my own nation of Guatemala, the results fell short of meeting the substantial decrease in maternal deaths that had been hoped for.

Because indigenous people comprise a significant proportion of the populations in Mexico and some Central American countries, it would be hoped that their health concerns would be a national priority. However, indigenous peoples are typically the most marginalized ethnic community in their country, have the worst health profiles, highest rates of morbidity, shortest life expectancy, greatest maternal, neonatal, and infant mortality indices, and the least access to health services among their national populations. Typically, statistical measurements of maternal mortality, such as the maternal mortality ratio (MMR), are significantly higher among indigenous than nonindigenous women, often by severalfold, in the same geographic regions.

Here in Guatemala, indigenous peoples speaking 23 officially recognized languages (including 21 Mayan languages, *Xinca* and *Garifuna*) make up over 40% of the country's population; among our *mestizo* population, which constitute a similar proportion of our population, many if not most have partial indigenous ancestry. Following the longest civil war in the history of the Americas, which occurred in Guatemala between 1960 and 1996, the indigenous populations were left decimated, impoverished, their leaders and representatives missing, jailed, or killed, families left without fathers, mothers, sisters, and brothers, and lacking adequate infrastructure and medical care. During the civil war, healthcare reforms and improvements, especially those targeting the rural and indigenous populations, were brought to a halt. Following the signing of the Peace Accords in 1996, health care for the indigenous people was placed into the hands of the democratic government. However, even with the assistance of external agencies and nongovernmental organizations (NGOs), the healthcare system has remained insufficient to address all the healthcare needs of the Guatemalan people, and especially its indigenous population—greater than 80% currently live below the poverty line.

When I was appointed as the Minister of Health of Guatemala in July 2016, I inherited a crippled national healthcare system which was fraught with significant problems and challenges. We had only about 16,000 medical doctors for our 15.6 million people, many of whom lived in rural and remote areas. The Ministry of Health had 6218 medical doctors, and our network of health services consisted of 44 hospitals, 333 health centers, 1165 health posts, and a total of 7183 hospitals beds which is 0.44 beds per 1000 people.

At the Ministry of Public Health and Social Welfare we are aware of the need to comprehend the various ways that health and disease impact our people and the world, including their relationship with the environment, and their biological, reproductive, social, political, and economic implications. Our Guatemalan society has been organized and functions on the basis of a hegemonic model of development. As a result, there has been an unfortunate history of ideological, social, cultural, and economic divisions and antagonisms between the diverse ethnic populations—indigenous and nonindigenous—which compose the fabric of our society. At the same time, a Hegemonic Medical Model has promoted the medicalization and commodification of health to the extent that it threatens to violate our basic human right to health. We believe that health care is a public good and a fundamental right of the individual, as well as an important component of social justice and equity.

Among the problems faced by our indigenous people, women's reproductive health and complications of pregnancy and childbirth are among the most important issues that I face as our country's chief healthcare official. The young indigenous women of Guatemala, similar to those in other Latin American countries, are confronted with overwhelming challenges to their human, gender-based, and reproductive rights. These include issues related to the provision of reproductive choices, unmet need for family planning, autonomy to choose the methods of prenatal and birth care, respect and acknowledgment of traditional cultural values regarding pregnancy, child and teenage marriages, obstetric violence, language incompatibilities, pervasive lack of education, poverty, and other gender-based issues. There is a significant deficiency of clinical medical providers and nurses fluent in indigenous languages and a dramatic disparity in accessing skilled birth attendants—73% among *Ladinas* but only 36% among indigenous women. These figures highlight the barriers to access of health care among rural, indigenous populations in Guatemala.

As the large majority of Guatemalan indigenous women live in rural and impoverished areas, those problems relating to the "Three Delay" model of maternal morbidity and mortality are also significant causes of poor obstetrical outcomes. In this model, three groups of factors can delay or stop women and girls accessing the maternal healthcare they need. The first, *delay in making the decision to seek care*, occurs as a result of the low status of women, poor understanding of complications and risk factors in pregnancy and when to seek medical help, a previous poor experience with the healthcare system, a culturally determined acceptance of maternal death, and financial implications. The second delay, *a delay in reaching care*, can be due to the distance to health clinics, centers, and hospitals, availability and affordability of transportation, poor roads and infrastructure, and such geographical factors as mountainous terrain, rivers, and flooding. The third delay, *a delay in receiving adequate healthcare*, can be caused due to poor facilities and lack of medical supplies, inadequately trained and poorly motivated medical staff, inadequate referral systems, and language differences between the patient and healthcare providers. All three of these delays occur in the provision of prenatal and maternity care for indigenous Guatemalan women.

Guatemala has among the highest maternal mortality ratios (MMRs) in the Latin American region, with the departments of the west and northwest of the country having the greatest numbers of maternal deaths. These departments—Huehuetenango, Quiché, Alta Verapaz, and San Marcos-are areas in which there are large concentrations of indigenous women and in which the likelihood of a woman dying from pregnancy is up to three times greater than in the metropolitan parts of the country. With the exception of the northwest region, the regions with the highest levels of maternal mortality are also those receiving the lowest levels of total health spending per capita.

In Guatemala, as in other Latin American countries, indigenous women's reproductive options and health have been compromised by pervasive gender-based issues, including women's rights, stigmatization, education, and violence. Indigenous women, like all women, have a right to make their own choices about how they seek, obtain, and use family planning, prenatal and maternity care, health facilities, and biomedical care providers. The Right to Health is a fundamental right of people to have a better life for themselves as well as their children. In Guatemala, indigenous women, most of whom are Mayan, should have the right to "*buen vivir*," a philosophy which is rooted in a cosmovision that describes a way of doing things that is community-centric, ecologically balanced, and culturally sensitive. In addition to the indigenous Maya people of Guatemala, *buen vivir* is inspired by the worldviews of other indigenous social systems in the New World including those of *Quechua* of Peru, Bolivia, and Ecuador, the *Aymara* peoples of Bolivia, Peru, and Chile, and the *Mapuche* people of Chile and Argentina. This philosophy could incorporate aspects of traditional and culturally relevant care of pregnant women within an indigenous framework together with Western models of allopathic treatment and medicine to provide an integrated approach to maternal and reproductive health care.

To improve this situation at a national level, we have implemented the Modelo Incluyente en Salud (MIS), a long-term public health program that has four guiding principles: gender equity, intercultural equity, the right to health, and environmental stewardship. MIS is designed to improve health care via extending coverage of primary care and providing health services to all members of society without ethnic, gender, age, class, or racial distinctions. The Modelo Incluyente en Salud is organized into three phases or programmatic levels that are based on stages in the human lifecycle, and with infrastructure and human resources allocated and prioritized based on a regional assessment and sectorization process. It is of paramount importance that the decisions of indigenous peoples be respected by the State, and that the State serves a leading role in improving and guaranteeing rights to health for indigenous people within the four principles outlined in the Modelo Incluyente en Salud.

In this present book, the multitude of problems and challenges to the reproductive health of indigenous women of Central America and Mexico are addressed by a large multidisciplinary team of expert authors. The Editor of this remarkable volume is David A. Schwartz, who is a physician, medical anthropologist, epidemiologist, and researcher with many decades of experience in global maternal health and disease, especially in developing countries and among indigenous women. Dr. Schwartz has long experience at understanding and integrating the anthropological, biomedical, and public health aspects of pregnancy complications as they affect society, including women and children. The 72 authors of the 40 chapters in this book include many of the most well-respected experts in their fields—medicine, anthropology, public health, nursing, and international health. I am proud to add my voice to that of the Editor, Dr. Schwartz, and the other authors who address reproductive health and the causes and means of prevention of maternal morbidity and mortality among indigenous women in Mexico and Central America on such important issues as medical complications of pregnancy, occurrence and prevention of maternal deaths, access to obstetrical care, disparities of health care between indigenous and nonindigenous women, training and use of midwives and traditional birth attendants, risks of unsafe abortion, obstetrical violence, traditional birth practices and healing methods, teenage pregnancy, unmet need for family planning, inadequacy of epidemiological surveillance, traditional ethnomedicine, and others.

Although the authors in this book may view the problems of reproductive health, women's rights, and maternal health in Mexico and Central America through different lenses based upon their expertise, they all share one thing in common—a firm belief in the human rights of indigenous women to have a culturally relevant and successful pregnancy, and to bear healthy children. The Minister of Health of Guatemala shares their collective beliefs, and my staff and I have made a commitment to foster this process in the coming years. It is hoped that the publication of this book will motivate readers to share our dream for the future of all indigenous women.

Lucrecia Hernández Mack, M.D., M.P.H., Ph.D. (Cand.)
Minister of Health, Republic of Guatemala
Ministerio de Salud Pública y Asistencia Social
Guatemala City, Guatemala

Acknowledgments

During the production of this book, Sheila Cosminsky was always available to help both in personal meetings and via email, sharing with me her tremendous depth of knowledge and experience in the ethnological aspects of pregnancy and midwifery. Her advice was of immeasurable assistance to me. I would also like to thank Alessandro (Alex) Pezzati, Senior Archivist of the University of Pennsylvania Museum of Archaeology and Anthropology (Penn Museum), for his expert assistance with photographs. Additional assistance during the production of this book was generously provided by Edgar Kestler of CIESAR and Luis Pablo Méndez of MSPAS, both in Guatemala City. The enthusiasm, confidence, and advice of Janet Kim, Public Health Editor at Springer in New York City, were of valuable assistance to me throughout the entire production of this project. Last but not least, I would like to express my gratitude to my wife Stephanie and daughter (and future anthropologist) Jessica for their patience with me for all of the days and nights spent working on this book for 3 years.

Contents

Part II Mexico

About the Contributors and Editor

Contributors

Cristina Alonso, M.P.H., C.P.M. Mexican Midwifery Association, Mexico City, Mexico

Gabriela Alvarado, M.D., M.S.P.H. Department of Anthropology, Georgia State University, Atlanta, GA, USA

María Guadalupe Andueza-Pech, M.D., M.A.Sc. Universidad Autónoma de Yucatán, Mérida, México

Elsa María Rodríguez-Angulo, M.D., Ph.D., M.P.H. Centro de Investigaciones Regionales "Dr. Hideyo Noguchi", Universidad Autónoma de Yucatán, Mérida, México

Hilda E. Argüello Avendaño, Ph.D., M.A. Department of Anthropology, Philosophy and Social Work, Rovira i Virgili University, Tarragona, Spain

Maternal Mortality Observatory in Mexico, Chiapas, Mexico

Rodrigo Arosemena, M.D. Ministry of Health, Panama City, Panama

Shahna Arps, Ph.D. Department of Sociology and Anthropology, University of Toledo, Toledo, OH, USA

Luis Paiz Bekker, M.D., M.T.M. CIET International Guatemala (Community Information and Epidemiological Technologies), Guatemala City, Guatemala

Jorge Benavides-Rawson, M.D., M.A., Ph.D. Department of Anthropology, The George Washington University, Washington, DC, USA

Katherine E. Bliss, Ph.D. Girasol Global Policy Consulting, Dallas, TX, USA

Formerly Global Health Policy Center, Center for Strategic and International Studies, Washington, DC, USA

Angela I. Calderón, Ph.D. Department of Drug Discovery and Development, Harrison School of Pharmacy, Auburn University, Auburn, AL, USA

Arlene Calvo, Ph.D., M.P.H. Department of Community and Family Health, Global Health, and USF Panama Program at the City of Knowledge, University of South Florida, Tampa, FL, USA

Esperanza J. Carcache de Blanco, Ph.D. Pharmacy Practice and Science, Medicinal Chemistry and Pharmacognosy, Ohio State University, Columbus, OH, USA

Sobaata Chaudhry, M.S. Saving Mothers, New York City, NY, USA

Anne Marie Chomat, M.D., Ph.D., M.P.H. CIET international Guatemala (Community Information and Epidemiological Technologies), Guatemala City, Guatemala

Participatory Research at McGill (PRAM), Department of Family Medicine, McGill University, Montreal, QC, Canada

Alejandra Colom, Ph.D., M.A. Population Council in Guatemala, Guatemala City, Guatemala

Universidad del Valle de Guatemala, Guatemala City, Guatemala

Marcela Colom, M.D. Wuqu' Kawoq | Maya Health Alliance, Santiago Sacatepéquez, Guatemala

Sheila Cosminsky, Ph.D. Department of Sociology, Anthropology, and Criminal Justice, Rutgers University, Camden, NJ, USA

Alison Danch, M.S.W., M.P.H. Early Childhood Center, Indiana Institute on Disability and Community, Indiana University, Bloomington, IN, USA

Emily Dansereau, M.P.H., Ph.D. Department of Global Health, Institute for Health Metrics and Evaluation, University of Washington, Seattle, WA, USA

Brian J. Doyle, Ph.D. Departments of Biology and Biochemistry, Alma College, Alma, MI, USA

Lisette Farias, BSc(OT), MSc(OT), OT Reg, PhD Western University, London, Canada

Julia Festa, B.A. Warren Alpert Medical School, Brown University, Providence, RI, USA

Saving Mothers, New York City, NY, USA

Jennifer Foster, PhD, CNM, MPH, FACNM, NAAN Nell Hodgson Woodruff School of Nursing, Emory University, Atlanta, GA, USA

María Graciela Freyermuth-Enciso, M.D., Ph.D. Center for Research and Higher Studies in Social Anthropology-South East Unit, Chiapas, Mexico

Sistema Nacional de Investigadores, Mexico City, Mexico

Jillian De Gezelle, Ph.D. Department of Plant and Microbial Biology, North Carolina State University, Raleigh, NC, USA

Audrey Goold, M.S.W., M.P.H. George Warren Brown School of Social Work at Washington University in St. Louis, St. Louis, MO, USA

Beth Hallowell, Ph.D. American Friends Service Committee, Philadelphia, PA, USA

Gretchen A. Heinrichs, M.D., D.T.M.H., F.A.C.O.G. Department of Obstetrics and Gynecology, University of Colorado School of Medicine, Denver Health, Denver, CO, USA

Center for Global Health, Colorado School of Public Health, Denver, CO, USA

Bernardo Hernandez, Sc.D., M.S. School of Public Health, and Institute for Health Metrics and Evaluation, University of Washington, Seattle, WA, USA

Servando Z. Hinojosa, Ph.D. Department of Sociology and Anthropology, University of Texas Rio Grande Valley, Edinburg, TX, USA

Jolly Josefina Hoil-Santos, M.D., M.A.Sc. Universidad Autónoma de Yucatán, Mérida, México

April Houston, M.S.W., M.P.H. Sexual and Reproductive Health and Rights Team, CARE, Atlanta, Georgia, USA

Michaela E. Howells, Ph.D. Department of Anthropology, University of North Carolina Wilmington, Wilmington, NC, USA

Edgar Kestler, M.D., M.Sc. Epidemiologic Research Center in Sexual and Reproductive Health (CIESAR), Hospital San Juan de Dios, Guatemala City, Guatemala

Mounia El Kotni, Ph.D. Department of Anthropology, University at Albany, SUNY, Albany, NY, USA

Karen L. Kramer, Ph.D. Department of Pathology, University of Utah, Salt Lake City, UT, USA

Bry Kring, B.A. Asociación de Comadronas del Área Mam (ACAM), Concepcion Chiquirichapa, Guatemala

Jessica K. Levy, Ph.D., M.P.H. George Warren Brown School of Social Work at Washington University in St. Louis, St. Louis, MO, USA

Tracie D. Locklear, Ph.D. Outcomes Research and Assessment Group, Duke Clinical Research Institute, Duke University, Durham, NC, USA

Jenna Murray de López, Ph.D., M.A. Humanitarian Studies (Global Health/Medical Humanitarian Aid), University of Manchester, Manchester, UK

Marisol Vega Macedo, M.P.H. Alliance for Health, Food, and Nutrition (ASAN), Chiapas, Mexico

Lucrecia Hernández Mack, M.D., M.P.H., Ph.D. (Cand.) El Ministerio de Salud Pública y Asistencia Social, Guatemala City, Guatemala

Gail B. Mahady, Ph.D. College of Pharmacy, University of Illinois at Chicago, Chicago, IL, USA

Aminata Maraesa, Ph.D. Departments of Anthropology, NYU-School of Professional Studies and Fordham University, New York, NY, USA

Kelvin Nuñez Martinez, R.Ph. Universidad Nacional Autonoma de Nicaragua, Leon, Nicaragua

Jesse Alice McLeroy Department of Drug Discovery and Development, Harrison School of Pharmacy, Auburn University, Auburn, AL, USA

Jordan Alma McLeroy Department of Drug Discovery and Development, Harrison School of Pharmacy, Auburn University, Auburn, AL, USA

Joanna Michel, Ph.D. Urban Medicine Program, Department of Medical Education, University of Illinois at Chicago, College of Medicine, Chicago, IL, USA

Janneli Miller, Ph.D. Ft. Lewis College, Center of Southwest Studies, Durango, CO, USA

Ali H. Mokdad, Ph.D. School of Public Health, and Institute for Health Metrics and Evaluation, University of Washington, Seattle, WA, USA

Vinicio Mora, M.D. Epidemiologic Research Center in Sexual and Reproductive Health (CIESAR), Guatemala City, Guatemala

Wolfgang Munar, M.D., S.M. Department of Global Health, George Washington University, Washington, DC, USA

David Meléndez Navarro, M.D., M.S.M. Technical Secretary of the Promoting Committee for Safe Motherhood in Mexico, San Cristobal de Las Casas, Chiapas, Mexico

Sergio Meneses Navarro, M.D, Sc. D., M.P.H., M.S.A. Center for Research and Higher Studies in Social Anthropology, Southeast, San Cristobal de las Casas, Chiapas, Mexico

Briana Nichols, Ph.D. Department of Anthropology, University of Pennsylvania, Philadelphia, PA, USA

Ricardo Ojeda-Rodríguez, B.A. Universidad Autónoma de Yucatán, Mérida, México

Jessica Oliveira, M.S.P.A. Saving Mothers, New York City, NY, USA

Alejando Meza Palmeros, M.D., M.Ph., Ph.D. Faculty of Social Work of the Autonomous University of Nuevo León, Monterrey, Nuevo Leon, Mexico

Yolanda Oliva Peña, Ed.D., M.A.Sc. Universidad Autónoma de Yucatán, Mérida, México

Alice L. Perez, Ph.D. School of Chemistry and Natural Products Research Center, University of Costa Rica, San José, Costa Rica

Michelle M. Pieters, B.A. Department of Anthropology, University of North Carolina Wilmington, Wilmington, NC, USA

Arturo Rebollón, M.D., M.P.H., C.P.H., Dr.P.H. Department of Global Health, University of South Florida, Tampa, FL, USA

Diego Rios-Zertuche, M.P.A. Salud Mesoamerica Initiative, Inter-American Development Bank, Washington DC, USA

Maryam Rokhideh, M.A., Ph.D. Department of Anthropology, University of Notre Dame, Notre Dame, IN, USA

David A. Schwartz, M.D., M.S. Hyg., F.C.A.P. Department of Pathology, Medical College of Georgia, Augusta University, Augusta, GA, USA

Crystal Sheedy, M.A., Ph.D. Candidate Department of Anthropology, University at Albany-SUNY, Albany, NY, USA

Taraneh Shirazian, M.D., F.A.C.O.G. Department of Obstetrics and Gynecology, New York University School of Medicine and NYU Langone Medical Center, New York City, NY, USA

Saving Mothers, New York City, NY, USA

Vania Smith-Oka, Ph.D. Department of Anthropology, University of Notre Dame, Notre Dame, IN, USA

Janell Tryon, M.P.H. San Francisco Department of Health, San Francisco, CA, USA

Amanda Veile, Ph.D. Department of Anthropology, Center on Aging and the Life Course, Purdue University, West Lafayette, IN, USA

Blanca Pelcastre Villafuerte, Ph.D. National Institute of Public Health, Cuernavaca, Morelos, Mexico

Sarah A. Williams, M.A., Ph.D. Candidate Department of Anthropology, University of Toronto, Toronto, Canada

Editor

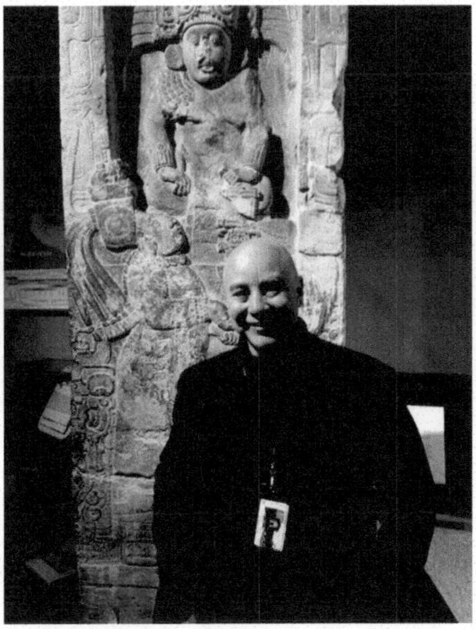

David A. Schwartz, M.D., M.S. Hyg., F.C.A.P., has an educational background in anthropology, medicine, emerging infections, maternal health, and medical epidemiology. He has professional and research interests in reproductive health, diseases of pregnancy, and maternal and infant morbidity and mortality in both resource-rich and resource-poor countries. In the field of medicine, his subspecialties include obstetric, placental and perinatal pathology as well as emerging infections. An experienced author, editor, and consultant, Dr. Schwartz has long experience investigating the anthropological, biomedical, and epidemiologic aspects of pregnancy and its complications as they affect society, in particular among indigenous populations and when they involve emerging infections. Dr. Schwartz has been a recipient of many grants, was a Pediatric

AIDS Foundation Scholar, and has organized and directed projects involving maternal health, perinatal infectious diseases, and placental pathology for such agencies as the U.S. Centers for Disease Control and Prevention, National Institutes of Health, and the United States Agency for International Development, as well as for the governments of other nations. His previous book, *Maternal Mortality: Risk Factors, Anthropological Perspectives, Prevalence in Developing Countries and Preventive Strategies for Pregnancy-Related Deaths*, was published in October 2015. Currently involved with maternal-fetal aspects of the Zika virus pandemic, Dr. Schwartz serves on the editorial boards of four international journals and is a Clinical Professor of Pathology at the Medical College of Georgia in Augusta, Georgia.

[Illustration: Dr. Schwartz standing in front of Stela 14, a Classic period (758 CE) Maya monument excavated at Piedras Negras in the Petén department of northeastern Guatemala by his mentor, anthropologist J. Alden Mason. It is displayed at the Penn Museum of Archaeology and Anthropology in Philadelphia, where Dr. Schwartz is a member of the Board of Overseers.]

Part I

Reproductive and Maternal Health Among Indigenous Women of Mexico & Central America

Introduction to Indigenous Women and Their Pregnancies: Misunderstood, Stigmatized, and at Risk

1

David A. Schwartz

1.1 Maternal Death in Developing Countries

Maternal death represents a major public health problem in most countries of the world. The United Nations (UN) and its associated agencies recognized the public health significance of maternal mortality reduction when they announced their eight Millennium Development Goals (MDGs) following the UN Millennium Summit in 2000 (United Nations 2014, 2016a). The aim of MDG 5a was to *reduce by three quarters, between 1990 and 2015, the maternal mortality ratio* (United Nations 2016b). Related to this was MDG Goal 5b—*achieve, by 2015, universal access to reproductive health.* The results showed some success—since 1990, global maternal mortality has been reduced by 45%, from an average of 380 down to 210 maternal deaths per 100,000 live births, but globally fell short of the two-thirds reduction that was hoped for (United Nations Statistics Division 2017). The 45% overall decline in maternal deaths worldwide represents a reduction from approximately 523,000 in 1990 to an estimated 289,000 in 2013. Although this annual decrease only represents a 2.6% decline per year, it has saved countless lives of women in the reproductive age group. However, this reduction in maternal death has not been equally distributed around the world. In 2013, the maternal mortality ratio (MMR) in developing nations was 230 deaths per 100,000 live births, which was 14 times higher than the ratio in developed countries of 16 per 100,000 live births. Sub-Saharan Africa has the highest regional MMR at 510 maternal deaths per 100,000 live births. Ninety-nine percent of all maternal deaths occur in resource-poor nations, averaging 800 deaths each day or 33 per hour. One study estimates that 43,684 women died as a result of complications from unsafe abortions in 2013, or approximately 15% of the global total number of maternal deaths. This figure reflects a significant decrease or no change in every region except sub-Saharan Africa, where abortion-related deaths are estimated to have increased since 1990 (Kassebaum et al. 2014). Maternal death remains the single greatest health disparity between the developed and developing nations of the world.

Looking at these statistics in a different way, the tragic loss of the RMS Titanic was the greatest maritime disaster in modern history with a loss of 1517 lives; that is equivalent to the global toll of maternal deaths occurring in only 2 days. Similarly, the crash of one large passenger aircraft may

D. A. Schwartz, M.D., M.S. Hyg., F.C.A.P.
Department of Pathology, Medical College of Georgia, Augusta University, Augusta, GA, USA

D. A. Schwartz (ed.), *Maternal Death and Pregnancy-Related Morbidity Among Indigenous Women of Mexico and Central America*, Global Maternal and Child Health: Medical, Anthropological, and Public Health Perspectives, https://doi.org/10.1007/978-3-319-71538-4_1

result in as many as 200 deaths, making world headlines for days; and yet it would take 28 of these aircraft to be lost in 1 week with no survivors to equal the number of young women lost in the equivalent amount of time from pregnancy complications in developing nations (Schwartz 2015).

Globally, the 12 countries having the highest maternal mortality ratios as of 2015, in order of their MMRs, are Sierra Leone (1360), Central African Republic (882), Chad (856), Nigeria (814), South Sudan (789), Somalia (732), Liberia (725), Burundi (712), the Gambia (706), Democratic Republic of the Congo (693), Guinea (679), and Côte d'Ivoire (645). There are only two countries outside the sub-Saharan African region that have an MMR that even approach those: Afghanistan (396) and Haiti (359) (Central Intelligence Agency n.d.). In 2013, sub-Saharan Africa had the largest total annual number of maternal deaths at 179,000 (62% of all global mother deaths), followed by Southern Asia at 69,000 (24%). Two nations account for almost one-third of all maternal deaths—India with 50,000 deaths per year and Nigeria with 40,000. Sierra Leone has the highest MMR in the world—1360 maternal deaths per 100,000 live births. Some of the nations with the highest lifetime risk for maternal death include Liberia, Mozambique, Nigeria, Somalia, Guinea, and Chad, where a woman has a 1 in 11, 1 in 11, 1 in 12, 1 in 13, 1 in 14, and 1 in 15 lifetime risk, respectively, of dying from pregnancy—in many developed countries, the lifetime risk is 1 in 12,000 and higher (World Bank 2015; World Health Organization 2014a, b). Sub-Saharan Africa accounts for 6800 (91%) of the estimated 7500 maternal deaths attributed to acquired immunodeficiency syndrome (AIDS) worldwide, while in South Africa 41.4% of all maternal deaths are due to HIV infection. There is a saying in some regions of the world which states that "Any fool can catch a baby." Unfortunately, where this saying is believed, even in the twenty-first century, there exist millions of women who must face labor and delivery without skilled assistance.

Within the regions of Mexico and Central America, maternal mortality has significantly declined since the initial year of the MDGs in 1990. In Guatemala, the maternal mortality ratio decreased from 205 in 1990 to 88 in 2015. In other Central American countries, the MMR declined from 173 in 1990 to 150 in 2015 in Nicaragua and from 272 in 1990 to 129 in 2015 in Honduras. In Mexico, the MMR declined from 90 in 1990 to 38 in 2015 (United Nations Statistics Division 2017). These data showed improvements during the 25-year period, although they failed to meet the goal of a 75% reduction of maternal mortality. However, these metrics represent countrywide statistics and, in the case of poor rural indigenous women, are somewhat misleading. The MMR data would be much higher if they were restricted to only pregnancy outcomes among indigenous women. Although seemingly low compared with some sub-Saharan countries, the lifetime risk of death due to pregnancy in Central American countries is still dangerously high—1 in 64 in Honduras, 1 in 86 in Guatemala, and 1 in 110 in Nicaragua.

Maternal deaths represent the tip of an enormous iceberg of maternal morbidity in developing nations—at least 12 million women each year survive their pregnancy but suffer severe maternal complications. Unsafe abortions are one of the three leading causes of mother death in some parts of the developing world. Among the survivors of an unsafe abortion procedure, two million to seven million women sustain long-term damage including infection and sepsis, fistula formation, incomplete abortion, rupture or tearing of the uterus, infertility, and damage to other internal organs (Guttmacher 2012; Singh 2006).

1.2 Indigenous People

Indigenous people are members of distinctive ethnic groups who are descended from and identify with the original inhabitants of a given region. This is in contrast to those ethnic groups that have settled, occupied, or colonized the area in more recent times. Groups are usually described as indigenous when they maintain traditions or other aspects of an early culture that is associated with a given region. Although there is no universally agreed-upon definition for being "indigenous," there are several characteristics that tend to be common among indigenous peoples.

Indigenous people constitute distinct populations relative to the dominant postcolonial culture of their country. They may be minority populations within the current postcolonial nation states, as occurs in Panama, El Salvador, and Nicaragua. In contrast, in Bolivia and Guatemala, indigenous people make up as much as if not greater than one-half of the population. Indigenous people usually have (or previously had) their own language, cultures, and traditions that were influenced by living relationships with their ancestral homelands. Today, from 370 to 500 million indigenous people around the world still speak greater than 4000 different traditional languages (UNESCO 2017). Indigenous people have distinctive cultural traditions that are still practiced and extend back many hundreds of years or more. Indigenous peoples may be settled in a given locale/region or exhibit a nomadic lifestyle across a large territory, have or have previously had their own lands, but are generally historically associated with a specific territory which they are tied to and depend upon. Indigenous societies are found in every inhabited climate zone and continent of the world. Indigenous people demonstrate historical continuity with precolonial and/or pre-settler societies. Indigenous people resolve to maintain and reproduce their ancestral environments and systems as distinctive peoples and communities. And finally, indigenous people identify themselves and are recognized and accepted by their community as indigenous.

The historical exposure of indigenous groups to colonizing influences has varied throughout the world. Conquest, war, enslavement of entire populations, forced relocations of ethnic and tribal groups, and destruction of whole societies and even civilizations have extended back before the written record. Within more recent historical times, it has been the European expansion that has arguably had the greatest effect on indigenous populations of the present day. Beginning in the fifteenth century, the rapid and widespread expansion of the European powers, notably Spain and England, followed by France, Belgium, Holland, Portugal, and Germany, had a profound impact on the indigenous peoples with whom they came into contact. Asia, Africa, South Asia, and notably the New World were all irrevocably altered by the exploratory and colonization efforts of these European powers. In the New World, the impact of European expansionism, colonization and suppression of indigenous cultural identities and belief systems has been most severe. This has resulted in the decline of populations as a result of conquest, enslavement, disease, malnutrition, and especially violence. Unfortunately, the impact of colonization and subjugation on the indigenous peoples of the New World continues to persist up to the present day and is clearly visible demographically by examining such statistics as life expectancy and maternal and infant mortality.

1.3 Maternal Death Among Indigenous Women in Mexico and Central America

According to the Franciscan priest and ethnographer Bernardino de Sahagún, when an Aztec woman became pregnant, she observed many taboos. She was forbidden to view an eclipse, as the sight of it could transform her unborn child into a monster or a rat, be born malformed with a harelip, or even without a nose. Seeing the eclipse could also cause an abortion. In the event that she saw even the beginning of the eclipse, she would quickly place a small obsidian knife next to her waist to protect her fetus from a potential disaster. If the pregnant Aztec woman had to go outside during the night, she placed a few small pebbles next to her waist to prevent her child from crying constantly following its birth. While she was pregnant, even her husband had to perform the same ritual, for if he went outside at night without having some pebbles and was confronted with a ghost, his infant would be born with a bad heart or another terrible disease. If her tamales stuck to the side of her cooking pan, she knew that her delivery would be difficult—like the tamales, her unborn infant would stick in her body at the time of birth. Her family and relatives warned her to avoid frightening or nauseating sights, lifting heavy objects, or taking excessively hot sweat baths, which could burn the fetus.

The strict obedience of rituals, ceremonies, and beliefs was not to be minimized—pregnancy was a dangerous time in the life of an indigenous woman, whether she was Aztec, Maya, *Tarahumara*, or *Zapotec*. For in many ethnic groups, and with the assistance of an experienced midwife—*comadronas* and *parteras* to the Maya and *tlamatlquiticitl* to the Aztec— she would observe the traditional prenatal ministrations, abdominal massage, proper foods and drinks, curing ceremonies, herbal potions, the sweat bath, physical examinations and manipulations, and the close support of her family up to the time of delivery. However, no matter how attentive was the care that she was administered, nature would frequently intervene and result in a pregnancy-related complication. Too often, this caused the death of the mother and, in many cases, the newborn.

Indigenous people compose a significant proportion of the populations of Mexico and Central America. In Mexico alone there are over 60 indigenous ethnic groups, and in Guatemala, where almost 40% of the population are indigenous, there at least 24 ethnic groups. The well-being of indigenous peoples in these countries falls far behind that of the other members of their societies—they have shorter life spans, higher rates of infant malnutrition and mortality, greater poverty, higher maternal mortality rates, and less access to education and medical care and are exposed to stigmatization, destruction of their cultural traditions, and attempts to extinguish their languages and assimilate their people into the prevailing cultures—in some cases, even genocide has occurred. The United Nations Economic and Social Council (ECOSOC 2006) succinctly summarized the status of indigenous people as follows:

> Indigenous peoples remain on the margins of society: they are poorer, less educated, die at a younger age, are much more likely to commit suicide, and are generally in worse health than the rest of the population.

Indigenous peoples throughout the world have sought recognition of their identities, ways of life, and legal rights to their traditional lands, territories, and natural resources for many years. Throughout history, and in too many cases up to the present time, their legal and human rights have repeatedly been violated. Indigenous peoples today are among the most disadvantaged and vulnerable groups of people in the world. Unfortunately, the health, illness, and death of indigenous women resulting from pregnancy in Mexico and Central America have remained persistent human rights and public health problems for many reasons. In indigenous societies, everyone is poor, women are the poorest, and young women of reproductive age are the poorest of the poor. As a result of complex social and fiscal inequalities, indigenous women can have up to several times the risk for the worst outcome possible for pregnant women—their own death—as a result of bearing children when compared with that of nonindigenous women in their own country and even in their same region.

Pregnancy is a natural physiological condition; it is not a disease. When complications occur resulting from pregnancy, they are perceived very differently by traditional birth attendants, midwives, biomedical providers such as physicians and nurses, anthropologists, and epidemiologists. Confronted with maternal morbidity in a resource-poor region, it is very difficult to intervene in such traditional societal structures as gender relations, fertility, abortion, adolescent and teenage marriage, care from traditional birth attendants, and labor and delivery practices—even when such traditional practices increase the mother's risk for poor obstetrical outcome. In fact, it may be simpler and less intrusive to focus on the access and quality of healthcare services than to attempt to change a complex system of inequalities, economics, deficiencies, and priorities in which the acutely ill pregnant woman and her baby are ultimately dependent on a few minutes to hours of lifesaving medical care (Schwartz 2015).

1.4 A Multidisciplinary Approach to Improving Maternal Survival Among Indigenous Women

In attempting to understand the causes of persistent maternal death among indigenous women in Mexico and Central America, it appears optimal to incorporate the viewpoints and experiences of individuals from a variety of areas of specialization. Often, the initial response of the biomedical community to persistently high levels of maternal mortality is by increasing the quality, distribution, and access to physician-based obstetrical care in hospitals, and minimizing the role of traditional birth attendants and midwives, as an attempt to help improve maternal survival in developing nations. However, it is evident that this cannot eliminate needless maternal deaths from occurring in developing countries. The problem of maternal death in Mexico and Central America is complex and multifactorial. It involves a complex web of cultural, physiological, sociological, spiritual, ethnological, historical, environmental, psychological, and economic factors in order to understand the myriad of root causes for the stubborn persistence of maternal death in the resource-poor regions of the world. From a global perspective, the question of maternal death involves explaining the gap between what should be done, what personnel think should be done, and sadly, what is actually done (Jaffré 2012). Modern biomedicine and the technocracy surrounding it are not equipped to comprehend these aspects of the continued prevalence of preventable pregnancy-related deaths, over 99% of which occur in the developing world. It is critically important that the human rights of indigenous people be respected when addressing such issues as reproductive and maternal healthcare, including respect for cultural traditions, norms, and mores.

Medical anthropology is a branch of sociocultural anthropology. It addresses the biological, cultural, political, economic, and gender-based aspects of human health, illness, and healing in both a historical context and the present. In contrast to contemporary biomedicine, which is based upon a diagnosis-based problem-solving approach to illness, anthropology examines how health, illness, and even death are shaped, experienced, and understood within a society itself influenced by historical, global, and political forces. It has become an increasingly valuable tool for understanding the complex interactions which affect maternal morbidity and mortality in resource-poor nations (Schwartz 2015). Most developing countries share a common bond—their indigenous people are the most stigmatized, poorest, least educated and have the highest risk for poor medical outcomes amongst their population—and this is especially true for pregnant women. By focusing on the common risk factors shared by many women of childbearing age in the developing world—in particular social exclusion, gender inequality, stigmatization, poverty, and lack of access to education— medical anthropologists have helped to understand those factors which influence health and well-being, the experience and distribution of illness, the prevention and treatment of sickness, the healing processes, the social relations of therapy management, and the cultural importance and utilization of multiple medical systems. Within the society in which they are working, medical anthropologists analyze and apportion the risks for maternal death, using the framework of the three-delay model of maternal mortality to make recommendations for improving maternal survival. Anthropologists are often able to unravel the mechanism(s) by which a pregnant woman's life may hang by a thread, even in those circumstances where they are able to reach a health facility—a woman with obstetrical bleeding dies because the blood bank staff are on their break and have taken their keys with them; a pregnant woman with severe preeclampsia and fetal distress cannot get oxygen because the hospital assistant is absent and the staff do not know how to connect the oxygen cylinder; a woman with a life-threatening infection cannot have her fever measured because the thermometer is broken; performance of a cesarean section for an adolescent with an obstructed labor is canceled because the washing machine was broken and the operating room could not be prepared, resulting in her death; a teenage girl with preeclampsia cannot have her blood pressure monitored because the blood pressure cuff is missing; there are no needles remaining for the lifesaving blood test; the list of breakdowns in the human sequence of maternal care goes on and on (Jaffré 2012; Schwartz 2015). It is the knowledge gained by anthropologists, together with anthropological research and analytical skills, that is invaluable for developing, assessing, and improving health and healthcare programs and services.

Epidemiology, a branch of public health, is another area of specialization that is necessary to reduce and eliminate unnecessary maternal deaths among indigenous women in resource-poor countries. Epidemiology is a population-based specialty, not patient-based as is biomedicine; relies on statistical methods, not medical treatment; and utilizes inclusion criteria for analysis, not empiric and differential diagnosis (Schwartz 2015). Reliable epidemiologic data regarding the rates and trends in maternal mortality are essential for resource mobilization and for planning and assessment of progress toward reduction of maternal mortality. Unfortunately, current methods for measuring maternal mortality among indigenous women have significant problems involving case-finding and diagnosis that can preclude accurate assessments of maternal disease burden, causation, and distribution in these populations. In practice, it is often impossible to determine the exact cause of death of an indigenous pregnant woman, particularly when deaths occur outside health facilities. Less than two-fifths of countries have a complete civil registration system with good attribution of cause of death, which is necessary for the accurate measurement of maternal mortality. The almost complete lack of postmortem (autopsy) examinations of indigenous women who have died from pregnancy-related complications, and the scarcity or even complete absence of physicians trained in obstetrical pathology in these regions, results in a lack of pathological confirmation of the exact cause(s) of death of pregnant indigenous mothers. The relative preponderance of maternal deaths in rural versus urban areas, where surveillance systems are most vulnerable, further degrades reliable epidemiologic analysis of indigenous mother deaths in these regions.

It is unusual for specialists in the fields of obstetrics, epidemiology, and sociocultural anthropology to share their experiences and discuss common interests in maternal death prevention from their respective areas of expertise. This is unfortunate—a significant component in understanding the continued occurrence of preventable maternal deaths among indigenous women depends not only on scientific issues involving epidemiology and biomedicine but hinges on such anthropological factors as political, social, gender, and economic issues, stigmatization, obstetrical violence, and discrimination—factors that influence and even determine maternal health and survival. The maternal mortality ratio (MMR), a fundamental measure of maternal mortality that is used in medicine, epidemiology, and public health, actually functions as an anthropological indicator of the availability, accessibility, acceptability, and utilization of a country's maternal health resources (Campbell and Graham 2006; World Health Organization 2011; Yamin 2007). As such, the MMR is a proxy measure of a nation's state of development, quality of healthcare network, economic and gender equality, and health equity.

There is a vision that "no woman should lose her life when giving birth." When a young indigenous woman in the prime of her life dies from being pregnant, she loses her life at a time when there should be great anticipation and joy of bringing new life into the world. Every mother's death is a tragedy by itself, but it also has far-reaching effects. In an indigenous community, it affects the population as a whole as well as her extended family and jeopardizes not only her surviving children's lives but also their future economic situation, education, and livelihood. Dying from a pregnancy complication such as infection, convulsions, hemorrhage, or excruciating pain from an obstructed labor is a terrible and terrifying way to die (Schwartz 2015).

Maternity is a privileged biosocial function given to women to ensure the continuation of our species. In the twenty-first century, indigenous mothers do not have to give up their lives to provide new lives to humanity—for the most part, they are not dying of conditions which we cannot treat (Schwartz 2015). It is hoped that by encouraging and providing venues for the exchange of ideas between physicians, anthropologists, nurses, midwives, public health specialists, and the individuals responsible for

Aztec Pregnancy: Archaeological and Cultural Foundations for Motherhood and Childbearing in Ancient Mesoamerica

2

David A. Schwartz

2.1 Introduction

"What's past is prologue"—uttered by Antonio in William Shakespeare's play *The Tempest*—suggests that past history sets the context for present times. This expression from a classic in English literature has relevance in both archaeology and cultural anthropology, as we try to understand modern patterns of behavior based upon historical evidence from written materials and material culture. Perhaps nowhere is this more relevant than among the indigenous peoples of the New World and, in particular, Mexico and Central America. There are estimated to be greater than 25 million indigenous people in Mexico—over 21% of the nation's population—speaking 68 officially recognized indigenous languages (INEGI 2015) and many more which are not officially recognized. In Guatemala, approximately 40% of the population is indigenous, with many more having at least part-indigenous ancestry (INE 2013). Indigenous people are also present in other Central American nations—Honduras, Belize, Costa Rica, Panama, and Nicaragua—representing in total many hundreds of ethnic and linguistic groups. These indigenous peoples, present before the initial contact with Europeans and Africans, had developed beliefs, taboos, rituals, and practices surrounding conception, pregnancy, labor, birth, and child-rearing which were characteristic of their ethnic groups. In many societies, these practices and beliefs have continued to persist as well as evolve following the initial Spanish contact, with some eventually incorporating European beliefs and customs.

This chapter will discuss various aspects of pregnancy and childbirth among precontact Mesoamerican peoples, using the Aztec, or Mexica, people of Mexico as an example, based upon material culture and historical writings. The Aztec people are highlighted because the most comprehensive and reliable information available on the birth practices of pre-Columbian indigenous peoples comes from this culture. This chapter also explores how the Aztec people dealt with such pregnancy complications as maternal death, which must have been a common event.

D. A. Schwartz, M.D., M.S. Hyg., F.C.A.P.
Department of Pathology, Medical College of Georgia, Augusta University, Augusta, GA, USA

D. A. Schwartz (ed.), *Maternal Death and Pregnancy-Related Morbidity Among Indigenous Women of Mexico and Central America*, Global Maternal and Child Health: Medical, Anthropological, and Public Health Perspectives, https://doi.org/10.1007/978-3-319-71538-4_2

2.2 The Aztecs

Believed to have originated from an ethnic group of hunter-gatherers in Northern Mexico, the Aztec were a Nahuatl-speaking group of people who flourished in the central regions of Mexico from the early fourteenth century to 1521 CE. Their arrival in South-Central Mexico occurred around the same time as the decline of *Toltecs*, who until then had been the dominant civilization in that region of Mesoamerica. The term Aztec is derived from the words *aztecatl* (singular) and *aztecah* (plural) meaning "people from Aztlan." The Aztec language, Nahuatl, had become the dominant language in Central Mexico by the 1350s. According to an ancient prophecy, the wandering Mexica tribes would locate the destined site of their future great city when they saw an eagle perched on a cactus eating a snake. The Mexica saw this on a swampy island in Lake Texcoco and began to construct their city, Tenochtitlan, which was founded in 1325 and was to become the largest and most powerful city in precontact Mesoamerica.

Together with peoples from two other city-states, the *Acolhuas* of Texcoco and the *Tepanecs* of Tlacopan, the Aztecs of Tenochtitlan under the leadership of Itzcoatl formed the Aztec Triple Alliance in 1427. After defeating the *Tepanec* people, their historic enemies, and capturing their capital of Azcapotzalco, the Aztecs extended their power by trade and conquest to adjoining territories. Controlling its client states through intermarriage between royal families and placing sympathetic rulers in local control, at the height of their power c.a. 1519, the Aztec Empire exerted its influence to Chiapas and Guatemala in the south and to both Atlantic and Pacific coasts.

After Hernán Cortéz landed on the Gulf coast in the spring of 1519, he allied himself with the confederacy of Tlaxcala, the long-standing enemy of the Aztecs and their emperor, or *tlatoani*, Moctezuma II. Hostilities erupted in 1520, resulting in the death of Moctezuma II and the massacre in the Great Temple. In 1521, the Spanish and their *Tlaxcalan* allies laid siege to Tenochtitlan, destroying it.

2.3 The Florentine Codex and Friar Bernardino de Sahagún

Bernardino de Sahagún was a Franciscan friar who was a pioneering ethnographer among the Aztec people in New Spain (Mexico) (Fig. 2.1). Following his arrival there in 1529, 8 years after the conquest of the Aztecs by Hernan Cortés, he began to investigate the indigenous cultures by using a novel methodology that is now considered to be a precursor to modern anthropological field technique. The motivation of de Sahagún to perform this research was primarily religious: he believed that to convert the natives to Christianity and eradicate their devotion to the pantheon of false gods, it was first necessary to understand those gods and their connection with the Aztec people. His corpus magnum of research was eventually published as a book, *Historia general de las cosas de nueva España* (de Sahagún 1985). As a Franciscan friar, de Sahagún was repulsed by much of their native culture, but later he came to admire many qualities of the Aztecs—he wrote, in the prologue to Book I of his work, the Mexicans "are held to be barbarians and of very little worth; in truth, however, in matters of culture and refinement, they are a step ahead of other nations that presume to be quite politic."

De Sahagún was assisted in his work by two indigenous groups—the elders (termed *principales*) of several towns in Central Mexico and also by Nahua students and former students at the College of Santa Cruz in Tlatelolco, where Sahagún worked for much of his time in Mexico. Fray de Sahagún prepared lists of questions about Aztec life, ceremonies, religion, and culture which were answered by the *principales*, and their responses were recorded in their own pictorial form of writing. The Nahua students interpreted the images and expanded upon the answers, phonetically transcribing Nahuatl using Latin letters. Following this, de Sahagún reviewed the Nahuatl text, adding his Spanish translation. The entire process of preparing the manuscript took almost 30 years to complete. The final version of *Historia general de las cosas de nueva España*, also termed the Florentine Codex, was

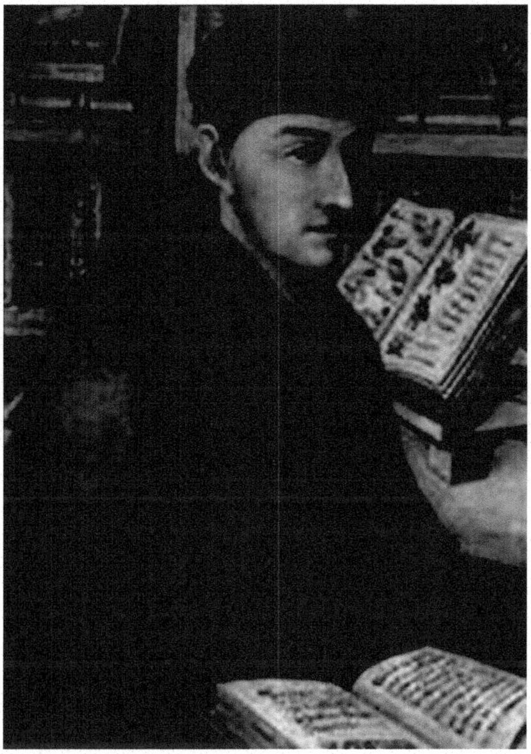

Fig. 2.1 Fray Bernardino de Sahagún. Available from: http://www.elmundo.es/ladh/numero14/sahagun.html

completed in 1569. It is a complex 2400-page document containing approximately 2500 illustrations and consisting of three integral texts—the first part in *Nahuatl*; the second part, a Spanish text; and the third part consisting of pictorials. It was taken to Spain by Fray Rodrigo de Sequera, commissary general of the Franciscans and a supporter of de Sahagún's work. Of the 12 books composing the *Historia general de las cosas de nueva España*, childbirth is described in detail in the sixth book, providing an invaluable direct source of information about the cultural and religious aspects of pregnancy.

2.4 Motherhood and Fertility Deities of the Aztecs

In the mythology of the Aztecs, there were a pantheon of goddesses associated with pregnancy, motherhood, and midwifery.

2.4.1 *Tlazolteotl*: A Goddess of Midwives

Tlazolteotl (Nahuatl pronunciation [tɬasoɬˈteotɬ]), also called *Ixcuina* or *Tlaelquani*, is a goddess of the midwives, steam bath (*temescal*), purification, and filth (sin) and a patroness of adulterers. In Nahuatl, the word *tlazolli* also refers to vice and diseases. Her other role was that of a purification deity—she forgave sins and cured diseases caused by misdeeds, particularly sexual misdeeds. *Tlazolteotl* was referred to as the "Goddess of Dirt" and the "Eater of Ordure" (*Tlaelquani*, "she who eats dirt [sin]"), with her dual role of being a goddess of purification as well as dirt. Sins were symbolized by dirt, and her dirt-eating symbolized the ingestion of the sin of those who confessed, and in doing so purified it. *Tlazolteotl* could create vicious desires, but she also could forgive and cleanse the defilement of sin. The Aztecs believed that *Tlazolteotl* and her companions could inflict disease if people indulged

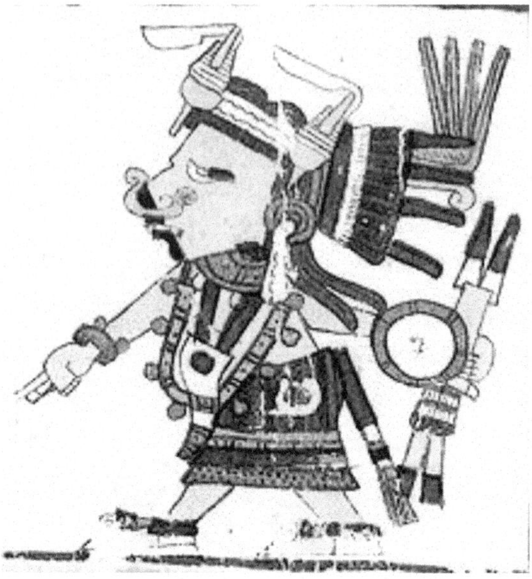

Fig. 2.2 *Tlazolteotl,* a goddess of midwives and the *temescal*. Source: Codex Borgia

themselves in forbidden love, especially sexually transmitted diseases. Uncleanliness was considered both on a physical and moral level by the Aztecs and could be cured by steam bath, a rite of purification, or calling upon *Tlazolteteo*, the goddesses of love and desires. In pregnancy, women delivering a baby were attended by a midwife who would lead prayers during the woman's labor to the goddess of childbirth. *Tlazolteotl* was depicted with ochre-colored symbols of divine excrement around her mouth and nose (Fig. 2.2). *Tlazolteotl* may have had an origin as a *Huaxtec* goddess from the Gulf Coast.

2.4.2 *Chalchiuhtlicue*: Patron Goddess of Childbirth

Chalchiuhtlicue, the goddess of the jade skirt (from the Nahuatl *chālchihuitl* [t͡ʃaːɬˈt͡ʃiwit͡ɬ] "jade" and *cuēitl* [kʷeːit͡ɬ] "skirt"), was an Aztec goddess who figured prominently in the Postclassic Aztec realm in Central America. She was the goddess of the water, storms, seas, streams, rivers, and baptism. In addition, she had a special relevance to pregnant women as she was a patroness of Aztec childbirth (Read and González 2002). As a water deity, *Chalchiuhtlicue* was depicted as a river from which grew a prickly pear cactus laden with fruit, which symbolized the human heart. She was a personification of youthful beauty and ardor. Her name in Nahuatl means "jade her skirt", but it is usually translated as "she of the jade skirt." She was the wife or, in some myths, the sister of the Aztec rain god, *Tlaloc*, and was the mother of *Tecciztecatl*, an Aztec moon god. In other myths, *Chalchiuhtlicue* was the wife of *Xiuhtecuhtli*, senior deity of the Aztec pantheon. According to Aztec myths, *Chalchiuhtlicue* at one point devoured the sun and moon. Similar to other Aztec water deities, she was often associated with serpents. *Chalchiuhtlicue's* association with both water and fertility is derived from the Aztecs' common association of the womb with waters. This dual role gave her both a life-giving and a life-ending role in Aztec mythology (Miller and Taube 1993).

As described in the Spanish codices which document the Aztec creation myth of the Five Suns, *Chalchiuhtlicue* presided over the fourth sun, or creation, as the goddess of streams and standing water. This fourth world—in the creation myth, the world preceding the current (fifth) one—was destroyed by a great flood, after which its people were transformed into fish. In her association with waters, *Chalchiuhtlicue* was known as *Acuecucyoticihuati*, the goddess of oceans, as well as the patroness of pregnant women who were in labor (de Sahagún 1970). She was also said to upset canoes and drown men; in her reign, maize was first used.

Chalchiuhtlicue is illustrated in several Mexican documents, including the *Codex Borgia*, *Florentine Codex*, *Codex Rios*, and *Codex Borbonicus*. Depictions of *Chalchiuhtlicue* show a beautiful lady with a distinctive hairdressing, whose clothing is that of a noble woman—an extravagant shawl adorned with tassels and a green skirt. She also could be seen as carrying a cross, an Aztec symbol of fertility. A stream of water, which usually included a baby of both genders, was often depicted flowing from the goddess' skirt (Figs. 2.3 and 2.4). To *Chalchiutlicue* and other deities associated with childbirth and water was dedicated a series of ceremonies called *Atlcahualo*, which lasted the all month of February.

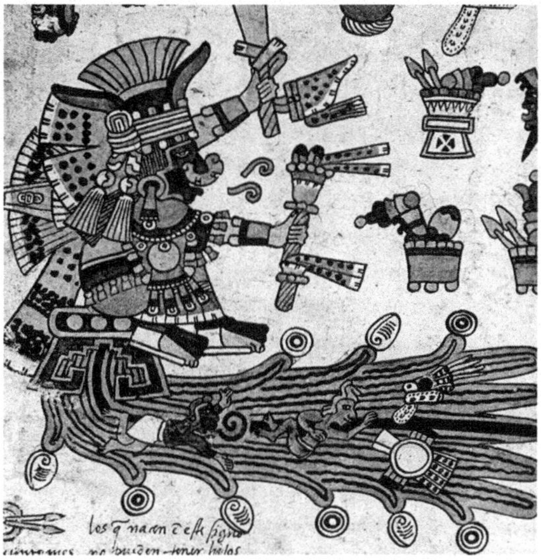

Fig. 2.3 An image of *Chalchiuhtlicue*, "she of the jade skirt," a goddess who among other roles was a patroness of childbirth

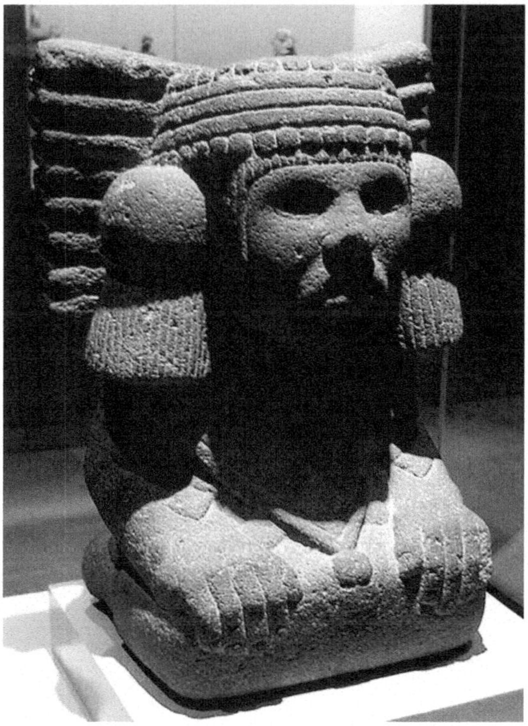

Fig. 2.4 Stone sculpture representing the goddess *Chalchiuhtlicue*. Source: Luis Garcia Zaqarbal

She was also revered by the enemies of the Aztec, the *Tlaxcalans*, who referred to her as *Matlalcueitl*, or “owner of the green skirt.”

2.4.3 *Cihuacoatl*: Goddess of Midwives and the Sweat Bath

In the Aztec pantheon, *Cihuacoatl* ([siwaˈkoːaːt͡ɬ, “snake woman”] also *Cihuacóatl* and *Quilaztli*) was one of the several goddesses of motherhood and fertility. *Cihuacoatl* was especially associated with midwives, including the sweat baths (*temazcals*) where midwives practiced. She is paired with *Quilaztli* and was considered a protectress of the *Chalmeca* people and patroness of the city of *Culhuacan*. Similar to other Aztec deities, she had multiple roles. She helped *Quetzalcoatl* create the human race by grinding up bones from the previous ages and mixing them with his blood. She is also the mother of *Mixcoatl*, whom she abandoned at a crossroads. It is believed that she often returns there to cry for her lost son, only to find a sacrificial knife (Miller and Taube 1993). *Cihuacoatl* was sometimes depicted as a young woman, similar to the goddess of pregnancy and childbirth *Xochiquetzal*, but she more frequently is depicted as a fierce skull-faced old woman carrying the spears and shield of a warrior (Fig. 2.5). The Aztecs believed that childbirth was analogous to warfare, and thus the women who died giving birth were honored as fallen warriors. Their spirits, termed the *Cihuateteo*, were depicted with skeletal faces like *Cihuacoatl* (Miller and Taube 1993; Read and Gonzalez 2002).

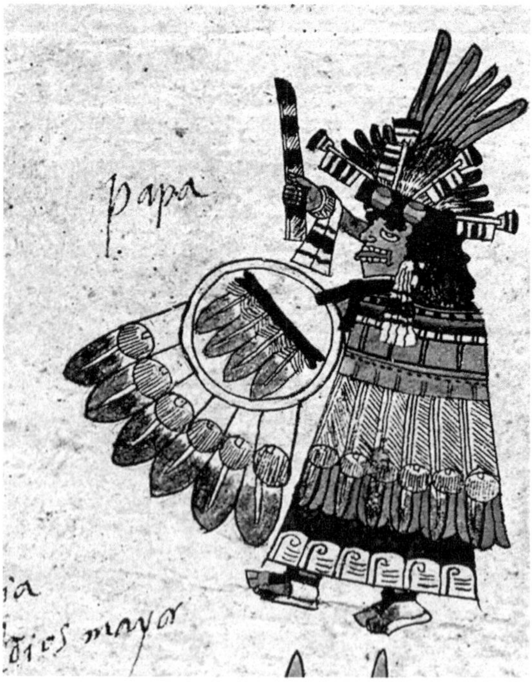

Fig. 2.5 Image of an Aztec priest wearing the costume of *Cihuacoatl*. Aztec priests dressed as deities for important religious events and ceremonies. Source: *Codex Borbonicus*

2.4.4 *Coatlicue*: Patron Goddess of Childbirth

Coatlicue (in Classical Nahuatl, *cōātl īcue*; Nahuatl pronunciation, [koːaːˈtɬíːkʷe]); "skirt of snakes"), which was also known as *Teteoh innan* (Classical Nahuatl [teːˌtéoʔ ˈíːnːaːn̥], "mother of the gods"), is the Aztec goddess who gave birth to the moon, stars, and *Huitzilopochtli*, the god of the sun and war. Other aspects of *Coatlicue* include the goddesses *Tocih* ("our grandmother") and *Cihuacoatl* ("snake woman"), the patron of women who die in childbirth, who were also seen as aspects of *Coatlicue*. *Coatlicue* was the patron goddess of childbirth and was also associated with warfare, governance, and agriculture. She was considered to be the female aspect of the primordial god *Ometeotl*. The goddess was worshipped in the spring ritual of *Tozozontli* in the rainy season and in the autumnal hunting festival of *Quecholli*, when an impersonator of the goddess was sacrificed.

Coatlicue is typically represented as a woman wearing a skirt of writhing snakes and a necklace made of human hearts, hands, and skulls. Her feet and hands are adorned with claws, and her breasts are depicted as hanging flaccid from pregnancy. Her face is formed by two facing serpents (after her head was cut off and the blood spurt forth from her neck in the form of two gigantic serpents), referring to the myth that she was sacrificed during the beginning of the present creation (Fig. 2.6).

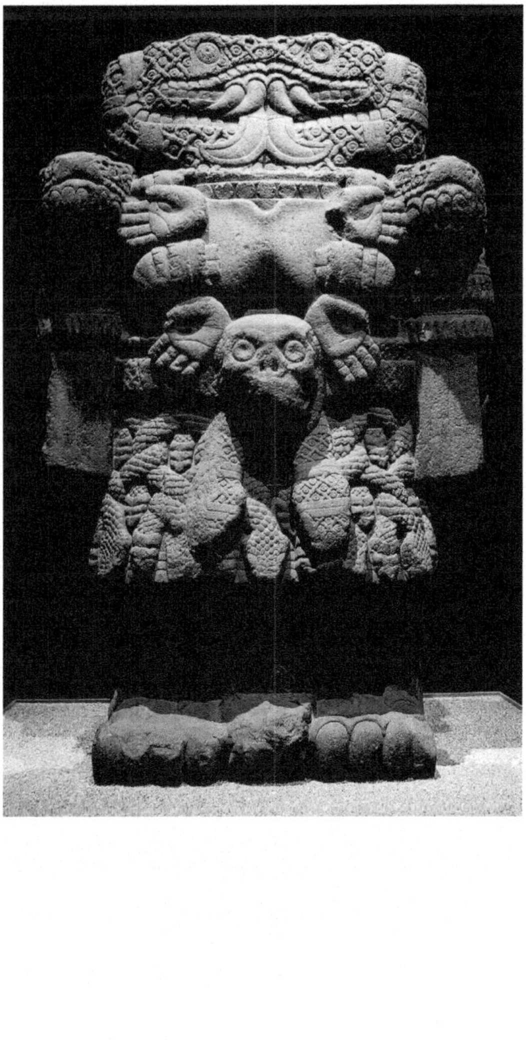

Fig. 2.6 The well-known statue of *Coatlicue* on display in the National Museum of Anthropology in Mexico City. Source: Luidger, Wikimedia

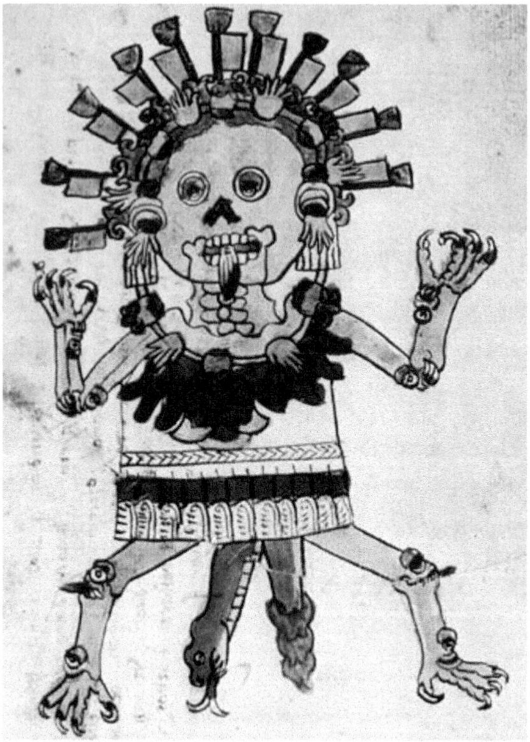

Fig. 2.7 A drawing of a *Tzitzimitl* from the *Codex Magliabechiano*. Source: https://en.wikipedia.org/wiki/Tzitzimitl#/media/File:Tzitzimitl.jpg

2.4.5 *Tzitzimitl*: Goddess of Fertility

In the Aztec pantheon and mythology, *Tzitzimitl* were female deities associated with stars. Because they were female, the *Tzitzimimeh* had a double role in Aztec religion: they were the protectresses of the feminine and progenitresses of mankind and were related to fertility. Thus, they were associated with the *Cihuateteo* and other female deities such as *Tlaltecuhtli*, *Coatlicue*, *Citlalicue*, and *Cihuacoatl* and were worshipped by midwives and parturient women. The leader of the *Tzitzimimeh* was the Goddess *Itzpapalotl*, who was the ruler of *Tamoanchan*—the paradise where the *Tzitzimimeh* resided. The *Tzitzimitl* were also powerful and dangerous deities, especially in periods of cosmic instability. The *Tzitzimimeh* were depicted as skeletal female figures wearing skirts often with skull and crossbone designs (Fig. 2.7).

2.4.6 *Ixtlilton*: God of Medicine and Healing

In Aztec mythology, *Ixtlilton* (the little black one) was the god of healing and medicine, and was associated especially with children (Shein 1986). As a gentle god in the Aztec pantheon, he was associated with dance, likely because dancing was a component of many medical cures. In his role as the god of healing and medicine, as well as being the god of games and festivals, *Ixtlilton* was also believed to be the brother of *Macuilxochitl*, the god of well-being or good luck. Based upon descriptions of appearance of the temples of *Ixtlilton*, it appears that they were derived from the tent or lodge of shamans or medicine healers. These temples contained water jars (*tlilatl*), and their contents were administered to sick children. Following the cure of the children, the grateful parents organized a feast to *Ixtlilton*, whose idol was carried to the residence of the child's father and ceremonial dances and oblations were made before it (Fig. 2.8).

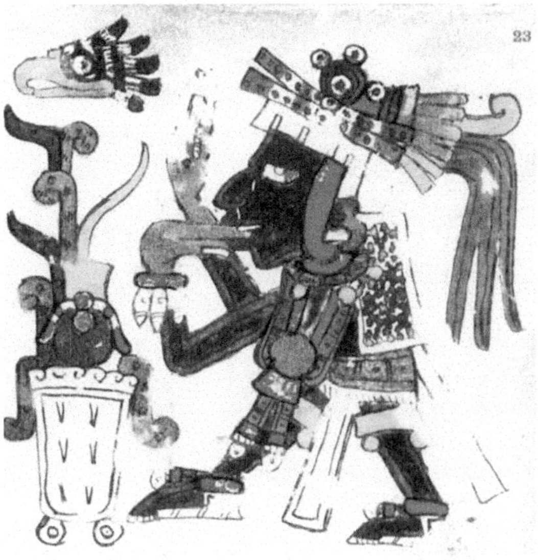

Fig. 2.8 *Ixtlilton,* the god of medicine and healing, as illustrated in the *Borgia Codex*. Source: https://es.wikipedia.org/wiki/Ixtlilton#/media/File:Ixtlilton.jpg

2.5 Aztec Pregnancy and the *Tlamatlquiticitl* (Midwife)

Marriage occurred early in Aztec society. According to León (1910), so-called women of quality were married between the ages of 14 and 16 years, while among the "common people," marriage occurred at an even earlier age (Leon 1910). The midwife was possibly one of the four old wives who carried the bride during her wedding ceremony (Guerra 1966). When the pregnancy was first announced, there were joyous and prolonged speeches made by the family members, the expectant mother, and the midwife to celebrate the occasion—if it was her first pregnancy, she was termed an *ichpuchpihua*.

Aztec adults believed in the divine supervision of childbirth and that from the moment of conception, a fetus's healthy development depended on the will of their gods. Pregnant women, regardless of wealth or social standing, were taken care of by the midwife, or *tlamatlquiticitl* (Fig. 2.9). The midwife would make frequent visits to the home, where she would monitor the pregnancy and perform physical examinations. If the midwife observed a problem, "she put the pregnant girl in a bath and pressed her belly to turn the baby if it was in the wrong position, moving it from one part to another" (Fig. 2.10).

In the case of a first-time mother (primigravida or *ichpuchpihua*), the midwife would provide instruction on the proper diet and other recommendations, including to make certain that the bath was not too hot. The *tlamatlquiticitl* would also recommend having sexual intercourse up to the seventh month; if she abstained from sex or had too much sex, the baby would be born sickly and weak (Figs. 2.11 and 2.12).

The *tlamatlquiticitl* would also prevent the future mother from lifting excess weight that could endanger the fetus and recommended to the expectant mother "to avoid sorrow, anger and surprises so as not to miscarry or damage the baby." As the birth approached, the midwife would remain in the woman's home for 4 or 5 days to prepare the future mother. Cleanliness was important—the future mother-to-be's body, hair, and the birthing room were all thoroughly cleaned. The *tlamatlquiticitl* would then prepare a steam bath in the *temazcal*—a sauna with a low roof, located just outside the home—using special smoke-free firewood and aromatic plants (Fig. 2.13). This would help the woman relax, while the midwife checked the fetus's condition. The design of the *temazcal*

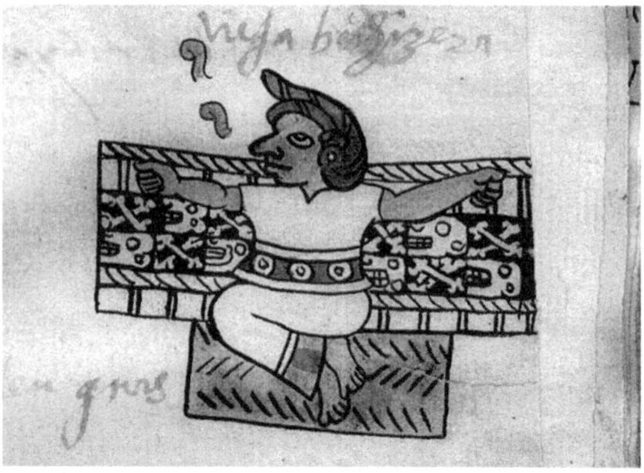

Fig. 2.9 The midwife. Source: *Codex Tudela*

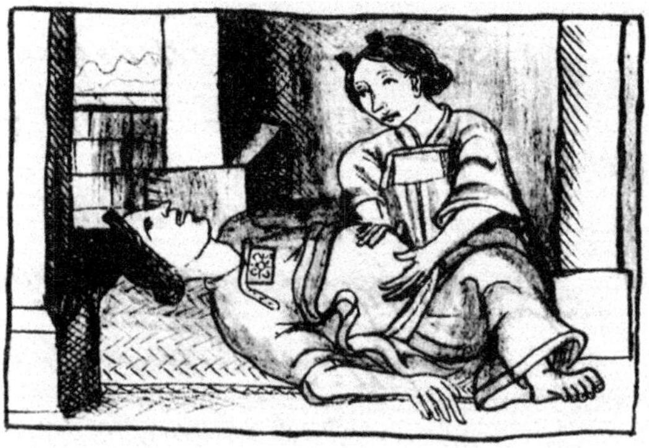

Fig. 2.10 An Aztec midwife massage the abdomen of a pregnant women. Source: *Florentine Codex*, Chapter VI

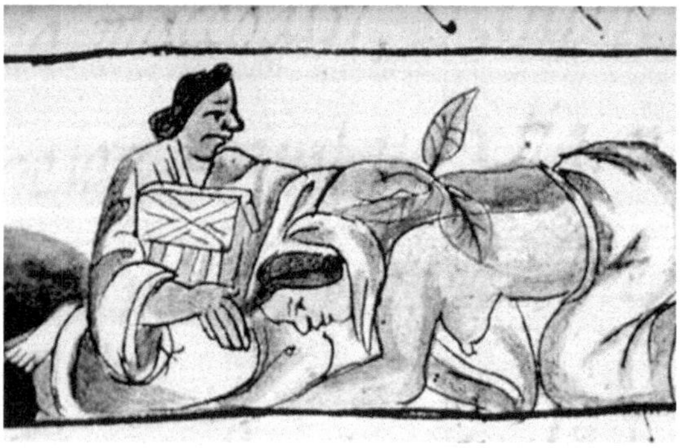

Fig. 2.11 An Aztec midwife administering herbs to a woman after childbirth. Source: *Florentine Codex*

(*or temazcalli*) was suggestive of the maternal womb - it was warm and moist, had a stone furnace the mouth of which rose to the exterior , and the junction of the furnace with the temazcal was sealed off with dry stones of either *tezontli* (a type of porous volcanic rock) or a less porous type. After the furnace was ignited and the stones began to heat, water was thrown on them to create a cloud of dense vapor that filled the upper part of the *temazcal*. Once inside the *temazcal*, the pregnant mother would recline on a mat, and the midwife would use maize leaves or herbs to direct the steam towards her. The *temazcal* was under the protection of the goddesses *Yoalticitl* and *Xochicaltzin*. It was the custom for the pregnant woman to have ritual bathing sessions at the *temazcal* at approximately 4 months's gestation and another other 2 months prior to her delivery (León 1910).

The midwife is portrayed by de Sahagún in the *Florentine Codex* as a complex woman—she is intellectually complex as well as being socioreligiously significant. This midwife, or *tictil*, was an old woman—she was "the one who brought about birth, the one delivered, the one in charge of birth." The

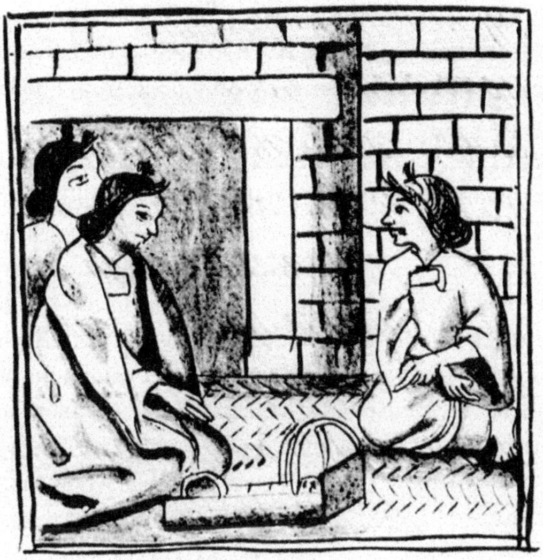

Fig. 2.12 A pregnant Aztec woman consults the midwife, or *tlamatlquiticitl*, to receive her recommendations. Source: *Florentine Codex*, Chapter VI

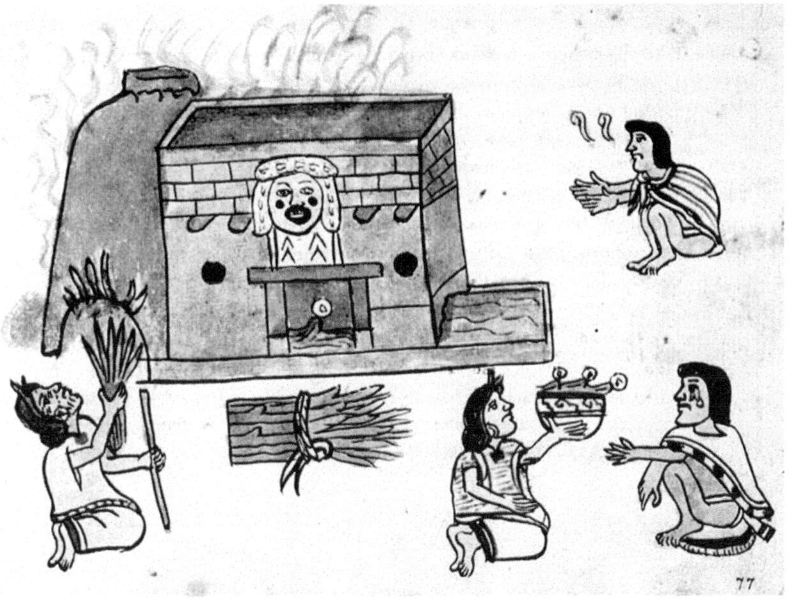

Fig. 2.13 A *temazcal*, or outdoor sweat bath used by pregnant women. From the *Codex Magliabechiano*, f.77(65)

midwife's knowledge and expertise came from the divine, and her patron deity was *Yoalticitl* (or *Toci*), who was both the mother of the gods and the midwife of darkness (Geller 2016). The midwife's skills were such that according to Bernard Ortiz de Montellano, in dealing with issues of pregnancy, the Aztec were significantly more advanced than were their Spanish conquerors (Bruhns and Stothert 1999).

Based upon de Sahagún's descriptions, Aztec midwives had methods to intervene in assisting with the expulsion of the fetus, perhaps in cases of obstructed delivery, ineffective labor contractions, or uterine atony. He describes the use of natural concoctions for ingestion in order to stimulate labor and bring about the expulsion of the fetus. In the *Florentine Codex* (VI, 159), de Sahagún describes two drinks to hasten delivery. One medicant was prepared from two fingers of ground opossum's tail (termed *tlacuatzin* in Nahua) in water - if the woman was in pain and not dilating, "they gave her half a finger of the tail of the animal called *tzlacuatzin*. Then she would give birth easily". While believed by some to represent a magical concoction, there was a laboratory report showing that a dose of opossum tail, either fresh or dried, initiated uterine contractions in rodent tissue (Bruhns and Stothert 1999). The second drink was an infusion of *ciupatili* (*cihuapatli*) root (*Montanoa tomentosa*)—contemporary practitioners have found this medication to have oxytocic properties, working to dilate the cervix and produce uterine contractions (Guerra 1966), and this tea "had the virtue of impelling or pushing the baby out". If these treatments failed to induce delivery of the infant, it was believed to be the result of sexual transgressions, and the mother would be offered the choice of confessing them or placing a little of her saliva into her vagina to deliver successfully. When childbirth was difficult, the midwife would call upon *Quilaztli-Cihuacoatl* to aid in the delivery - she was the first goddess to give birth, and her warlike aspect would assist the laboring mother to rally her strength and expel the fetus. In some cases of difficult delivery, another goddess of childbirth, *Teteoinnan-Toci*, was also summoned for help.

During an Aztec pregnancy, there were a number of taboos that had to be observed. Women should not have extensive sexual intercourse, or her infant would be born weak and sickly. The pregnant mother must not view an eclipse, or her unborn child would transform into a monster. Benign astral deities, termed *Tzitzimitl*, were visible when the sun was eclipse, but when the sun was covered they transformed into monsters. Miscarriages were also associated with an eclipse. Mothers should not eat dirt or chalk, or the infant would be born sickly or deformed. Additional things to avoid included heavy lifting, frightening sights, and excessively hot sweat baths (*temescals*) (Madsen 1960). Expectant mothers were warned not to excessively warm the abdomen by approaching too near the fire or by exposure to the sun because that could "toast" the child; napping during the day could result in deforming the infant's face or causing swollen eyelids (León 1910). The Aztec midwife would warn pregnant women to refrain from chewing chicle (a gumlike substance) because it could harden the infant's palate and gums, adversely affecting the baby's ability to suckle. Additionally, midwives suggested that pregnant women not fast during religious observances because "it would cause the baby to starve." Gazing at a red object would induce an abnormal shoulder or podalic presentation of the fetus (León 1910). Additional pregnancy risks included the mother looking at a hanged man causing strangulation of the fetus with its umbilical cord and denial of a pregnant woman's whims causing damage to the fetus (León 1910). Aztec midwives and mothers understood that during pregnancy "what the mother drank, what she ate, that also the baby absorbed; it took [substance] from her" (de Sahagún 1970).

2.6 The Birth of the Baby

When an Aztec woman realized that she was going into labor, relatives would gather in the family's home. As the woman progressed toward labor, it was common to use the previously discussed "opossum tail concoction" as a labor inducer to help stimulate her contractions. On some occasions, the midwife would administer tobacco to the laboring women to help alleviate her pain. As labor began, the *tlamatlquiticitl* would invoke her fingers, known as the five fates, together with the Earth, because the laboring woman was believed to be possessed by *Cihuacoatl*, an aspect of the Earth Mother and goddess of motherhood and midwives. Among upper-class women, it was common to have as many as three midwives with her at the time labor started. Goddesses were prayed to and medications were administered.

The traditional Aztec position of delivery was then, as it is now among indigenous women of Mesoamerica, in the squatting position—the woman squatted to give birth with the *tlamatlquiticitl* immediately behind her, holding her heels—the squatting position for delivery is also supported by archaeological evidence (see frontispiece), as well as imagery in the *Codex Nuttall* (a Mixtec codex) and the *Codex Borbonicus*. This would result in gravity assisting with some of the work of pushing the baby out, minimizing the mother's effort. De Sahagún observed admiringly that indigenous women seemed to give birth with much less effort and pain than did Spanish women and recovered so quickly that many quickly fell pregnant again soon afterward.

The day on which a woman gave birth was an exceptional day for her and for her child and a cause for great celebration because the Aztecs likened the honorable fight and pain that a woman underwent during labor to a warrior fighting on the battlefield. The *tlamatlquiticitl* handed the laboring mother a shield and toy spears with which to wage their "war" (Adelina et al. 2014):

> When the pregnant one already became aware of labor pains, when it was said her moment of death had come to pass, when already she wished to give birth, they quickly bathed her ... And when the baby had arrived on earth, then the midwife shouted; she gave war cries, which meant that the little woman had fought a good battle, had become a brave warrior, had taken a captive, had captured a baby. (Florentine Codex Book VI)

The skillful Aztec midwife understood the importance of preserving the amnion intact during labor, in order to obtain smooth and progressive dilation of the cervix and delivery while minimizing trauma. De Sahagún states that only a clumsy midwife permitted the premature breaking of the amnion (León 1910).

Following the expulsion of the newborn, the mother adopted another position for the awaited delivery of the placenta (Adelina et al. 2014). The *Codex Nuttall* illustrates a woman who has just expelled the placenta—she is resting on her right leg, and the thigh is compressing the abdomen and therefore the uterus, to facilitate the expulsion of a voluminous placenta that is observed on the floor (Fig. 2.14). Following the delivery of the baby, the midwife shouted war cries in order to honor its mother for having fought a good battle and said the following words:

> My beloved maiden, brave woman ... thou hast become as an eagle warrior, thou has become as an ocelot [jaguar] warrior; thou hast raised up, thou hast taken to the shield, the small shield.... Thou hast returned exhausted from battle, my beloved maiden, my brave woman; be welcome. Source: *Florentine Codex*, Book VI

In those cases where progression of labor was delayed or the infant had not advanced through the birth canal, the *tlamatlquiticitl* repeated *temazcal* baths during which time she palpated the progression and position of the fetus, adjusting it by external version if necessary. The midwife then waited for a day and a night, and if successful delivery still did not occur, she once again repeated the baths

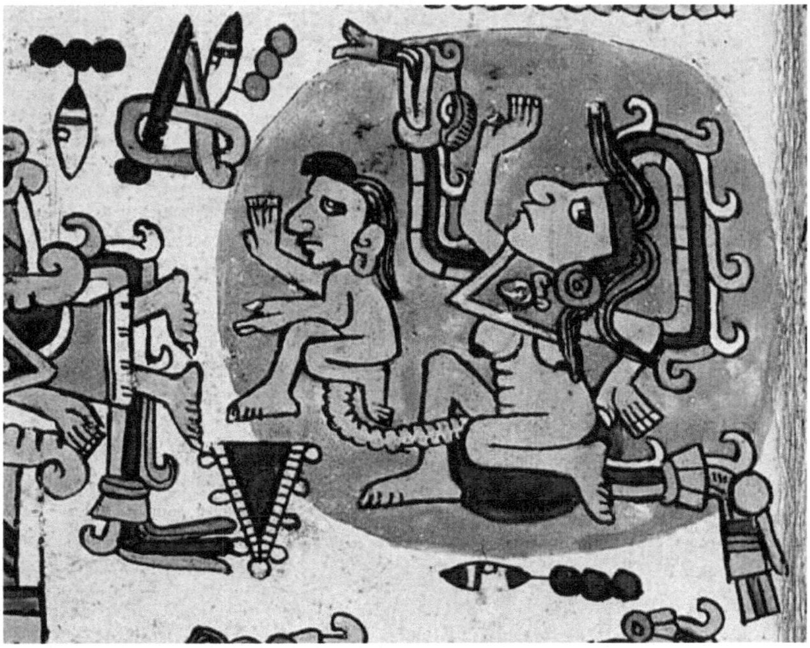

Fig. 2.14 The *Codex Nuttall*, although a Mixtec document, illustrates Lady 3 Flint giving birth, with the umbilical cord clearly illustrated. Actual birth scenes showing both the mother and newborn are very rarely illustrated in the codices. Source: *Codex Nuttall*, page 16. With permission of Mesolore, Birth Fig. 2. Available from: http://www.mesolore.org/tutorials/learn/15/Images-of-Action/155/Birth

and repeated palpating the fetal position again in the event that it had changed its position, following this with another attempt at external version. If delivery still did not occur, the *tlamatlquiticitl* shut herself together with the mother (who was at this point likely exhausted from her efforts), prayed to Aztec pantheon of gods for an eventual delivery, and kept wait on the progress.

Following delivery, the midwife cut the umbilical cord, a powerful reminder of the child's physical connection to both its mother and the source of life (Figs. 2.14 and 2.15). The midwife told the baby that it had come into a difficult life which was filled with many sorrows. The assignment of the infant's gender was begun immediately after birth - this gender would be repeatedly reinforced through infancy, childhood and adult life. A gender label was also symbolically assigned by rituals associated with its sex. If the infant was male, the umbilical cord was kept and given to an adult warrior who would bury it on a distant battlefield. Sometimes, the cord would be wrapped aro und a small shield before burial. This would ensure that the boy would have the courage he needed to become a great warrior. If the baby was a girl, the cord would be wrapped around a piece of wood, to help develop good household skills and buried under the ho use. These buried pieces of umbilical cord were termed *tonali*, meaning fate - the Aztecs believed that their fate was untimately linked with their *tonali* and the will of the gods. The ceremonial cutting of the umbilical cord was accompanied by many formal speeches describing the roles of men and women in Aztec society and encouraging the infant to work hard and to do its duty. The afterbirth, or placenta, was buried in a corner of the home (Fig. 2.16).

At the time of the baby's birth, the midwife would perform a purification ritual. She lit a fire which burned for 4 days and recited the following invocation:

> Our Lady Chalchiuhtlicue, Chalchiuhtlatonic, the tail feather, the wind feather has arrived. Receive him/her. (FC VI)

After reciting this prayer, the midwife would perform the infant's first bath (Figs. 2.17 and 2.18). Performed by the midwife, the midwife would gently immerse the newborn infant in water, instruct-

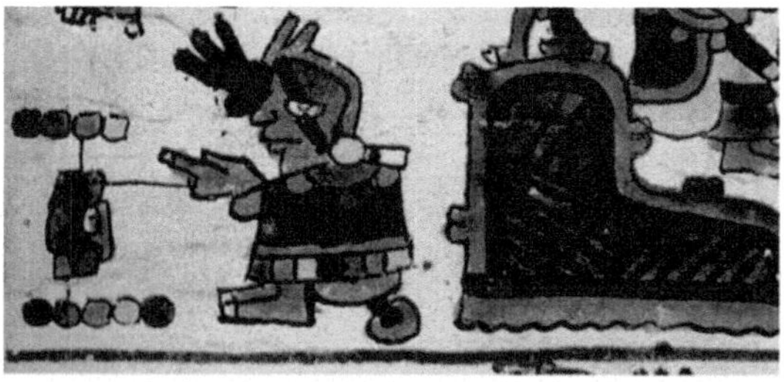

Fig. 2.15 Another Mixtec illustration of birth. Although Lord 9 Lizard appears in this image fully sized and dressed, he is squatting over his placenta, appearing gold, to which he is attached by his red umbilical cord. Source: Codex Selden, page 11. With permission of Mesolore, Birth Fig. 2. Available from: http://www.mesolore.org/tutorials/learn/15/Images-of-Action/155/Birth

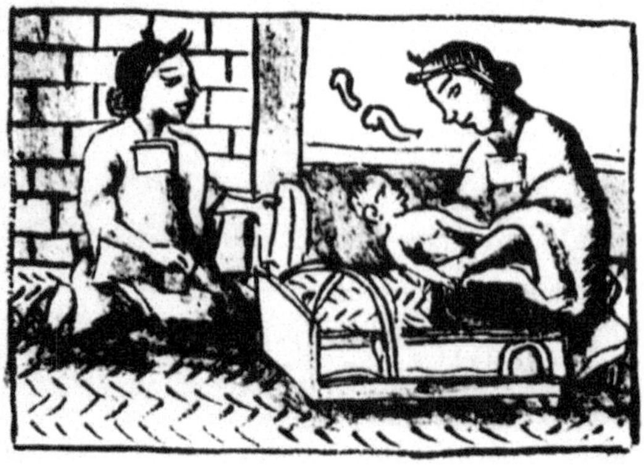

Fig. 2.16 An Aztec midwife places a newborn infant in the cradle. Source: *Florentine Codex*, Chapter VI

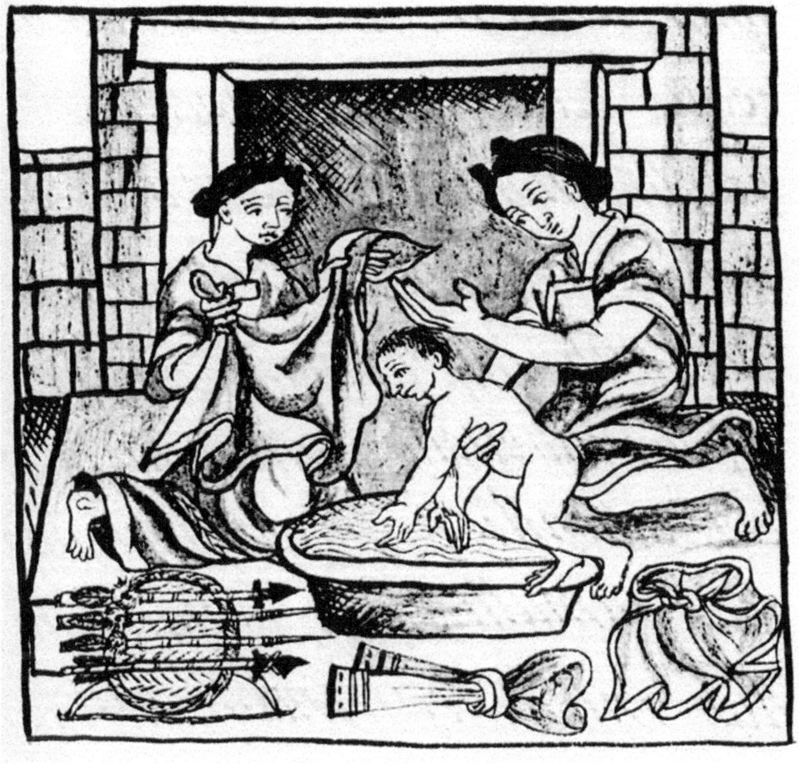

Fig. 2.17 A newborn Aztec baby boy washed in a tub. Source: *Florentine Codex*, Chapter VI

ing it to descend and be cleansed. She spoke in a low voice to the infant about *Chalchiuhtlicue,* the purifying water deity:

> Approach thy mother Chalchiuhtlicue, Chalchiuh Tlatonac! May she receive thee! May she wash thee! May she remove, may she transfer, the filthiness which thou has taken from thy mother, from thy father! May she cleanse thy heart! May she make it fine, good! May she give thee fine, good conduct! (FC VI)

> See here the very pure water that washes away all filth… I pray that it will destroy and remove from you all the evil and adversity that was given you before the beginning of the world… Now the child is born anew… Now he is purified and cleaned again. Our mother Chalchiuhtlicue has formed and conceived him again. (FC VI)

She then swaddled the infant to keep it warm and placed a jade strand around its neck. Then, the midwife spoke to the baby in a manner as she would in addressing an honored, but weary and hungry, traveler, exhorting it to rest among its parents and grandparents and describing the transitory nature of life. She commended the child to the gods, especially *Chalchiuhtlicue* (the goddess of still waters) and *Quetzalcoatl* (the feathered serpent). Following additional speeches by the midwife, she spoke with the mother and the additional guests that had arrived. Grandmothers and aunts would take their turns speaking, reverently honoring the midwife, the mother, and the child, and the midwife would reply (Townsend 2000). These speeches were an essential part of the midwife's professional training and expertise. When the childbirth occurred in the family of a wealthy merchant or nobleman, there were even more elegant speeches and visitations—these families often had more than one midwife present. The most influential and powerful families would receive visitors, including ambassadors and other noble families, from long distances for up to 20 days after the birth. The most important visitors would receive beautiful gifts of clothing from the family, including finely woven capes, shifts, and skirts, with as many as 20–40 being given. And not just the well-to-do received gifts—the humblest

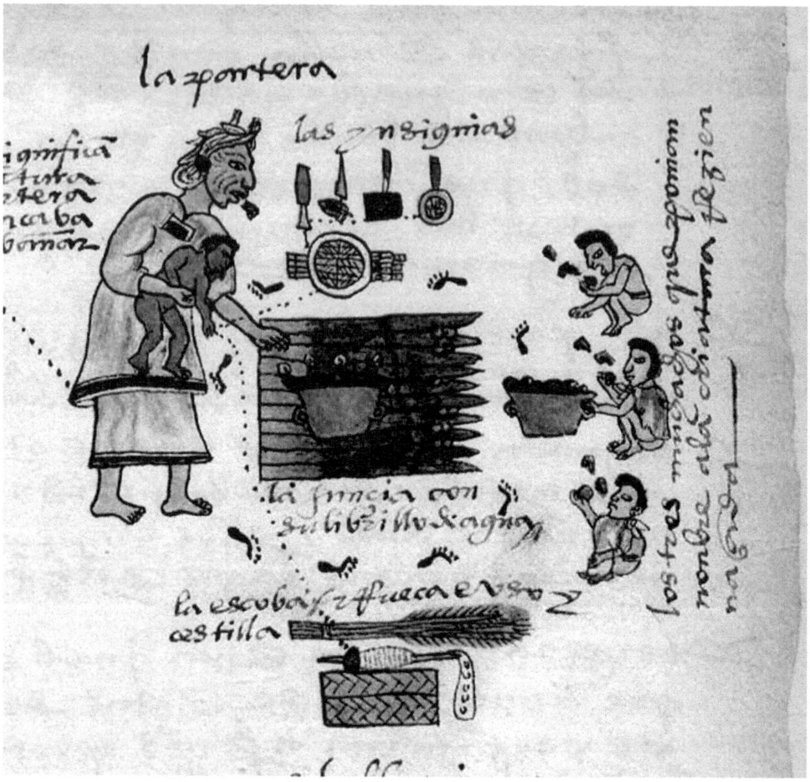

Fig. 2.18 This picture of an Aztec midwife performing the bathing and naming ceremony from the *Codex Mendoza*, written in 1535–1550. This ceremony, typically held on the fourth day following birth, was attended by the parents and relatives and conducted by the midwife (seen here holding the infant). The *tonalpouhqui*, a person knowledgeable in the Aztec sacred books, would be consulted, who would determine the sign of the child based on the moment of birth. The midwife would remove the infant from its cradle and bring him/her to a vessel filled with water, placed on a mat. As seen on the drawing, the midwife's counterclockwise-direction footprints circle around the mat, upon which two sets of sacred objects are placed. Also illustrated are five objects associated with Aztec male trades and professions: a shield with four arrows (the classic symbol for war) and tools used by a carpenter, feather worker, scribe, and goldsmith. In the lower part of the picture are three items linked to female household jobs: a broom, cotton spindle, and reed basket for storing materials. After bathing the child, the midwife, amid prayers and chants, offers the baby up to the heavens four times and then present the infant with the appropriate symbolic gifts, full of special meaning. Source: *Codex Mendoza*

visitors would be given food and drinks such as *pulque*, a slight-fermented beverage made from the fermented juice of the maguey cactus.

Following the delivery, the *tlamatlquiticitl* remained with the mother for an additional 4 days to monitor the mother's milk supply. This was an important precaution, because weaning the child would not take place until the child was 2 years or older and the Aztec had no animals whose milk could be used as a substitute. During those 4 days, many practical tasks were carried out together with reverent rituals. The mother was administered a variety of warm remedies including baths in the *temazcalli*, teas and hot foods, all of which were designed to restore her strength and speed her recovery during the puerperium. The relevant passages from the *Huehuetlatolli*, a collection of sayings, speeches, and advice from Aztec elders, were quoted soon after birth, including the words of welcome with which a midwife and grandparents should greet a newborn boy:

> Your trade and skill is war; your role is to give the sun the blood of your enemies to drink and feed the earth, Tlaltecuhtli, with the bodies of your enemies. (FC VI)

> Thou belongest out there; out there where thou has been consecrated. Thou hast been sent into warfare. War is thy desert, thy task. Thou shalt give drink, nourishment, food to (Tonatiuh) the sun, (Tlaltecuhtli) the lord of the earth. (FC VI)

If the infant child was a girl, the umbilical cord was buried next to the fireplace to make her a good wife and mother (Fig. 2.19). She was urged to "be to the home what the heart is to the body."

> Thou wilt become the heart of the home … And thou wilt become fatigued, thou wilt become tired; thou art to provide water, to grind maize, to drudge; thou art to sweat by the ashes, by the hearth. (FC VI)

After a few days, the baby was given a name. The naming ceremony was an important ritual in Aztec society. Following their birth, it was the duty of the father to inform the priests of the day and time of birth. The babies were then seen by a priest or soothsayer, called a *tonalpouhqui* (Fig. 2.18). This priest was charged by the parents with an important mission: fixing the baby's naming ceremony on a day that would bring it good luck (Fig. 2.20). The *tonalpouhqui* would consult the codices contained in almanacs to determine the most favorable dates to name the infant, initiating it to join the Aztec community. Following this, the infant would undergo a series of carefully arranged birth rituals designed to provide the infant with a soul and determine the child's destiny, establishing the link between the child and the gods. In addition to bathing and naming the infant, rituals included passing the child over a fire, reading its horoscope and presenting it to the gods, and in some cases, piercing the child and drawing a bit of its blood (Eberle 2013).

In implementing these birth rituals, priests consulted the *Tonalamatl*, a divinatory almanac used by the Aztecs, which was structured around the sacred 260-day year, the *tonalpohualli*, to identify the most appropriate name for the infant (Figs. 2.21 and 2.22). According to de Sahagún, the purpose of this "was to predict his good or ill fortune based on the qualities of the sign he was born under." An infant born under a bad sign would become a thief or a witch; a child born under a lucky sign would become a prestigious or wealthy adult, a successful warrior, or a good wife. An unlucky child could improve their chances in life by doing various tasks—making offerings to the gods and keeping vigils. Similarly, an infant born under a favorable sign could lose their advantages by such behaviors as immorality, disobedience, failure to respect the gods, and if someone carried away part of their birth fire (Madsen 1960).

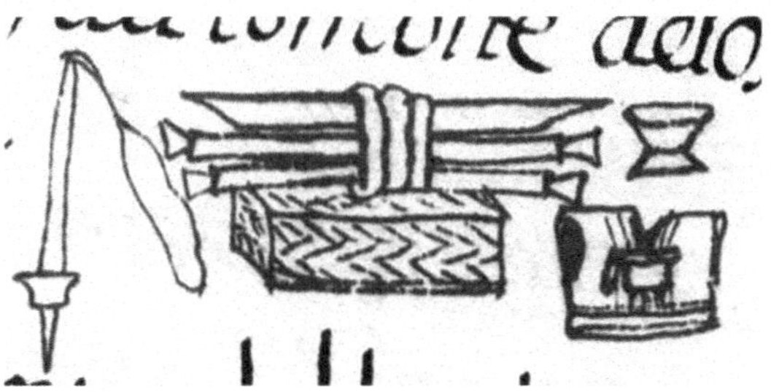

Fig. 2.19 The symbols of womanhood. Source: *Florentine Codex*, Chapter VI

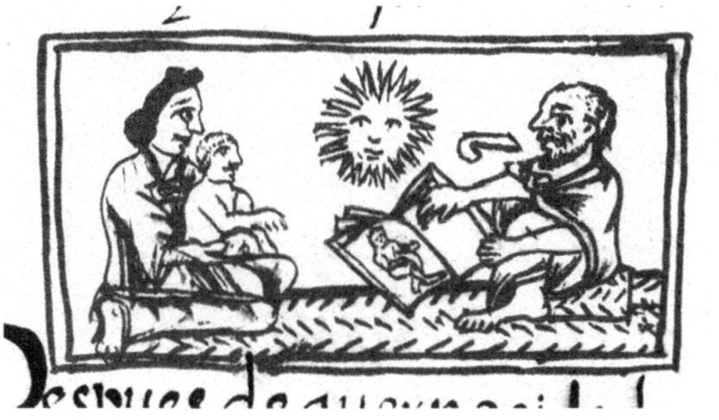

Fig. 2.20 Mother, infant, and priest (soothsayer). Source: *Florentine Codex*, Chapter VI

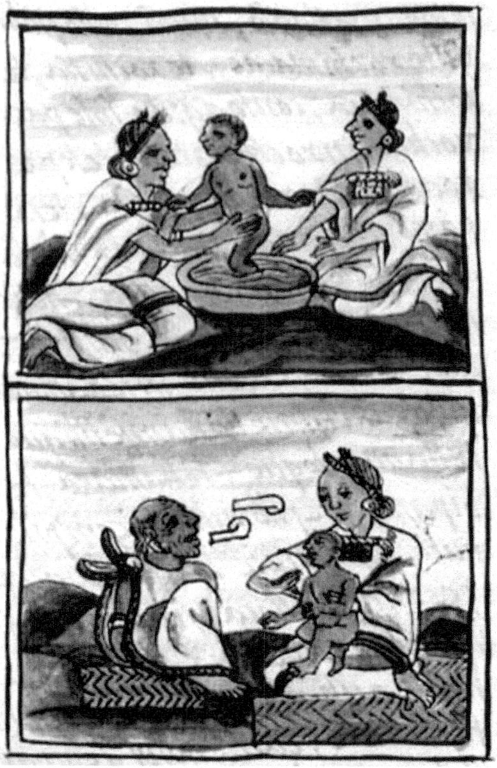

Fig. 2.21 A soothsayer, or *tonalpouhqui*, is advising the mother on the correct day to name her baby. In the lower picture, the presence of "scrolls" leaving his open mouth means that his words are important. Source: *Florentine Codex*, Chapter VI

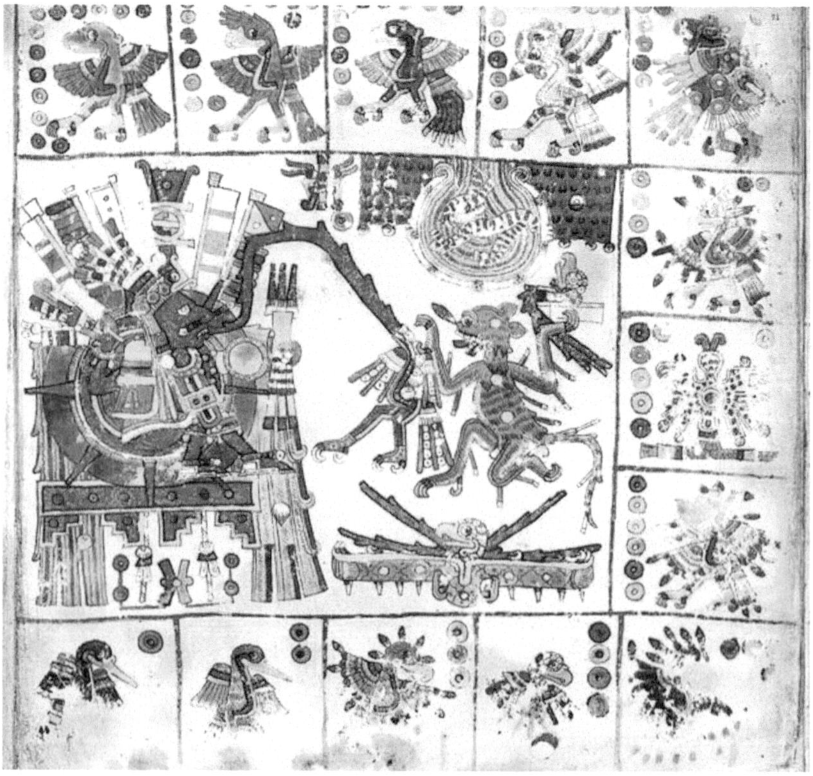

Fig. 2.22 Page 71 from the *Codex Borgia*, illustrating the sun god, *Tonatiuh*. This Codex is a *Tonalamatl* or almanac used for divinatory and ritual purposes. Source: Wikipedia, photograph in the public domain. Available from https://en.wikipedia.org/wiki/File:Codex_Borgia_page_71.jpg

Following this, the midwife placed a small amount of water in its mouth to cleanse its insides. If the infant was a boy, it received the tools of war, and if it was a girl, she received implements of weaving. The midwife then told the baby that *Chalchiuhtlicue* continually watched over it and would wash harm away with her waters.

2.7 Multiple Births

As in many indigenous societies, multiple births in the Aztec culture were feared and regarded with apprehension and mystery, foretelling ominous events. The canine Aztec deity *Xolotl* was the god of twins (*cocoua*) as well as deformities. According to Fray Bartolomé de las Casas, the sixteenth-century Dominican friar, historian, and first bishop of Chiapas (and first officially appointed "Protector of the Indians"), the occurrence of Aztec twins posed a mortal danger to their parents, as it was believed that soon after delivery, either one of the parents would die (Adelina et al. 2014). In order to avoid this, one of the twins was slain. Twins figured prominently in the creation myths of the Aztec. Quetzalcoatl, the Aztec god of wind and learning, is identified with twins, including the use of the term for twin (and snake), *coatl*, in his name.

2.8 Fetal Death and Abortion

There is little doubt that intrauterine and fetal demise and stillbirth were not uncommon complications of Aztec birth. The Franciscan friar Bernardino de Sahagún's accounts of Aztec pregnancy and midwifery are invaluable for understanding the traditions of birthing rituals during this time. Having arrived in Central Mexico in 1528, only 8 years after the Spanish conquest, his interests culminated in the production of the ethnographic research study termed the *Florentine Codex*. De Sahagún observed that the activities of Aztec midwives were not simply confined to the management of live birth but also dealt with pregnancy complications. He stated that they also used their skills with medications and herbal remedies, manual manipulative methods, and surgical techniques to deal with pregnancy cessation such as induced abortions. In cases of intrauterine fetal death, de Sahagún was impressed with the performance of embryotomies by midwives:

> Here also let something rather marvelous be told. When the baby adhered there within the mother, if the baby had died, the midwife inserted an obsidian knife within the woman. There she dismembered the baby; she drew it forth piece by piece. Thus the parent was relieved. (FC VI, 157)

After the midwife performed this procedure with an obsidian blade, termed an *itztli*, it "saved the mother from death". Given this account, it is possible that the midwife may have performed this procedure earlier during the pregnancy to cause a termination (Geller 2016). Although Aztec elders dissuaded pregnant women from having abortions, it was generally believed in Aztec doctrine that life did not begin until "the droplet of a baby is already 3 (or) 4 months formed" (Florentine Codex VI, 141 and 152]. The Aztec believed that infants who died during labor traveled to a place called *Chichiualcuauhco*, where a wet-nurse tree would feed them with its milk. They would remain there until the gods sent them back to be born of another mother, and the cycle of birth and death turned once more.

In Aztec society, the life of the mother was always placed ahead than that of the fetus. Because Cesarean sections were not performed, if natural labor was obstructed and the mother's life was at risk, the fetus was dismembered and removed.

2.9 Maternal Death

It should come as no surprise that evidence from burial sites indicates longevity during Aztec times was short, and perinatal, neonatal, and maternal mortality was very high (Sesia 2017). As has been discussed, in cases of obstructed delivery of a retained fetus, embryotomy was performed by the midwife using an obsidian knife, after obtaining the consent by the pregnant woman's parents. In his corpus, de Sahagún states:

> The midwife well experienced and knowledgeable in her craft, as soon as she realized the fetus was dead in the mother's womb because there was no movement and the mother was in great distress, readily inserted her hand through the channel of generation and with an obsidian knife cut the body of the creature and took it out in pieces. (VI Nos. 27 and 28) (Guerra 1966)

In those cases where there was no consent to perform the embryotomy and no other way to save her life, the midwife locked the woman inside her chamber to wait by herself until death came to free her from suffering and earthly life (Fig. 2.23) (de Sahagún 1970, 1985). Women who died from pregnancy or in childbirth were glorified as fallen warriors in Aztec society and thus were regarded with the same high esteem that was given to those Aztec warriors who died on the battlefield (Tovar-Rodriguez 2013). De Sahagún states that Aztec women who died during their first childbirth were considered to be *mocihuaquetzque* or "valiant women." Believed to have fought the battle between life and death with great courage, they were rewarded by joining *Huitzilopochtli* (the sun god) in its daily journey from east to west in its house, the sky, and sharing this privilege with those Aztec warriors who fought and lost their lives in battle. Immediately after dying, the bodies of the dead mothers were taken into a procession by midwives and their families. Their dead bodies were so powerful and full of magic that they had to be heavily protected in the days and nights following their death by their loved ones, including an armed party consisting of the widowed husband, all of his friends, the midwives, and old women. This determined guard remained both before and during burial—warriors would attempt to cut off their scalps or arms because they were thought to be invaluable by protecting them from falling prey to enemies in battle. Male soldiers would also try to steal their middle fingers, especially the left one, and hair, as it was believed that if these items were placed on their shields, they became braver and fiercer in battle and that these relics blinded their enemies.

Mothers who died in childbirth lived in the west, termed *Cihuatlampa*, or "in the direction of women". From there, they would emerge fully armed, and would accompany the sun as it set. After 4 years, the spirits of women dying during childbirth could then inhabit the clouds. It was at this point they were turned into *Cihuateteo* or goddesses (see below). They were then permitted to return to their earthly homes—where their former husbands sometimes saw them. Once back on earth, they would engage in women's work, looking for implements and materials so that

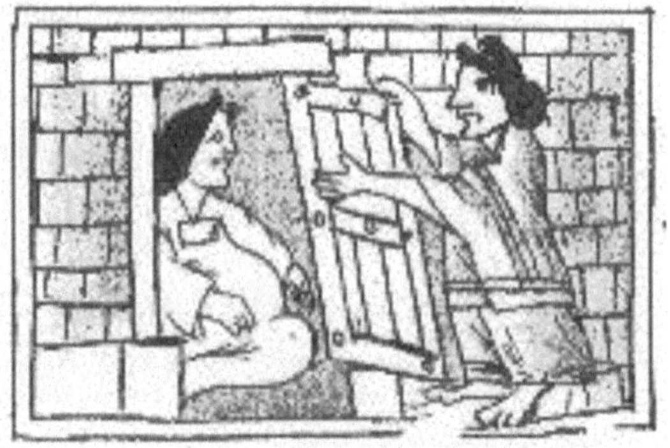

Fig. 2.23 The enclosing of an Aztec woman who died in childbirth. *Florentine Codex*, Chapter VI

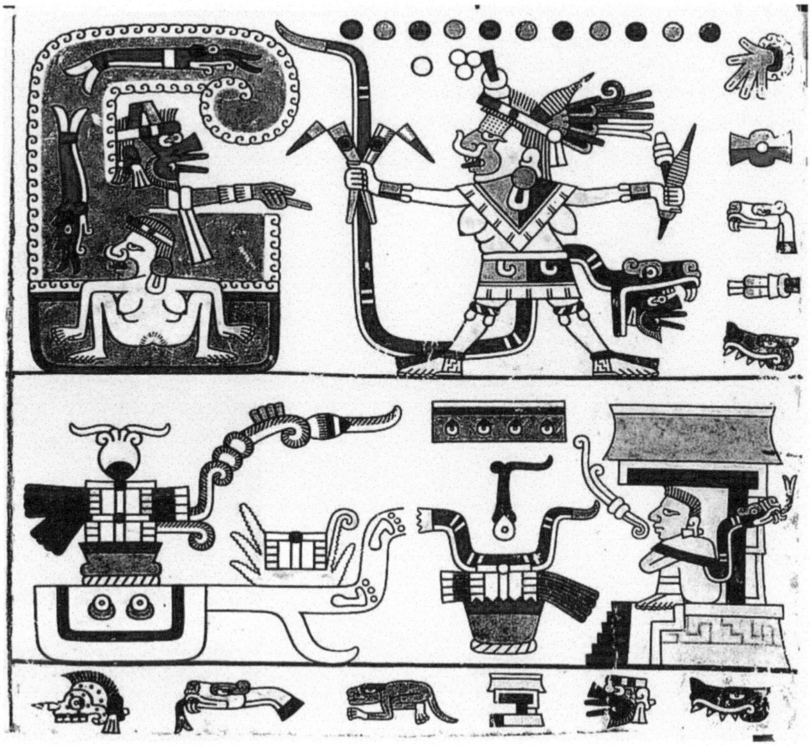

Fig. 2.24 Image of *Chimalma* (upper left) from the *Codex Laudianus*. Available from: https://en.wikipedia.org/wiki/Chimalma#/media/File:Codex_Laud_(folio_39).jpg

they could sew, spin and weave. They were also believed to cause sickness and paralysis among the living.

Maternal death also appears in Aztec mythology among the pantheon of the gods. *Chimalma* was an Aztec goddess and the mother of the Toltec god *Quetzalcoatl* (Fig. 2.24). While out hunting one day, *Mixcoatl*, the god of the hunt, saw *Chimalma* and fell in love with her. After spurning his advances, he became angry and fired five arrows at her, all of which struck her hand, hence her *Nahuatl* designation of "shield hand." Following their eventual marriage, she was unable to conceive a child. She prayed on the altar of *Quetzalcoatl*, and the priest instructed *Chimalma* to swallow a small precious stone, with the result that she became pregnant. In another version of the story, *Chimalma* became pregnant when *Mixcoatl* shot an arrow "between her legs"—on two separate occasions. This angered the brother of *Quetzalcoatl*, *Tezcatlipoca*, and he persuaded others to kill her husband *Mixcoatl*. Following her husband's death, *Chimalma* fled, returning to her native town of *Tepoztlan*. There she died giving birth to her son *Topiltzin* (Koch 2005).

2.10 *Cihuateteo*: Goddesses of Women Dying During Childbirth

Cihuateteo (also termed *Cihuapipiltin*) were the divine or noble women, the malevolent goddesses of the crossroads and spirits of women who died during childbirth (Figs. 2.25 and 2.26). The *Cihuateteo* were also associated with the spirits of warriors who had died as a result of battle—this was because a woman in labor was believed to capture the spirit of her newborn infant, similar to a warrior that had captured his enemy. *Cihuateteo* dwelled in a western region known as *Cihuatlampa*, or the "place of women," and bore the sun from its zenith at midday to its position on the western horizon at dusk. The *Cihuateteo* were characterized as "fearsome figures with clenched, claw-like fists, macabre, bared

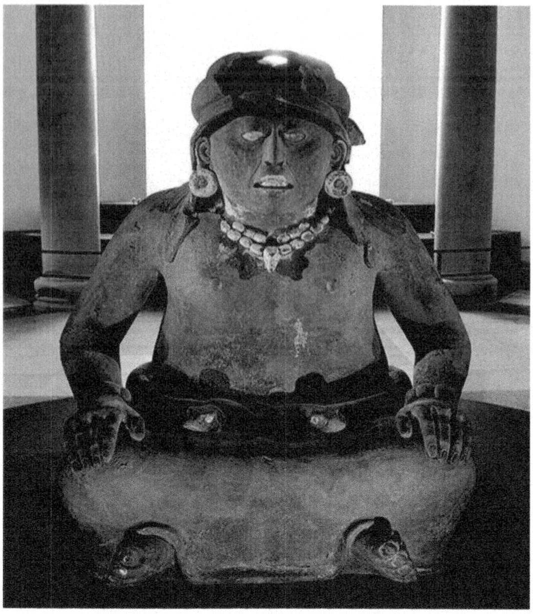

Fig. 2.25 Terra cotta statue of *Cihuateteo*, c.a. 600–900 CE, Mexico, state of Veracruz, El Zapotal style. Available from: https://en.wikipedia.org/wiki/Cihuateteo#/media/File:Cultures_pr%C3%A9colombiennes_MRAH_Cihuateotl_291211_1.jpg

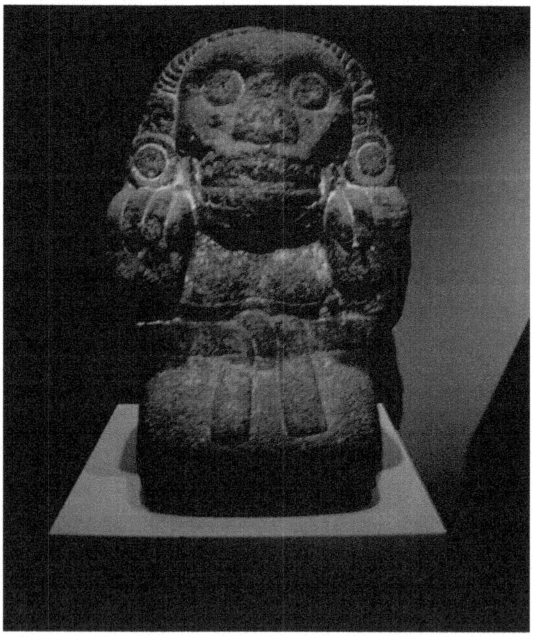

Fig. 2.26 An andesite figurine of *Cihuateteo* from the British Museum. Available from: https://pl.wikipedia.org/wiki/Cihuateteo#/media/File:Aztec_Cihuateotl_figure.JPG

teeth and gums and aggressive poses" (Moctezuma and Olguin 2003). Her appearance—taut stomach; exposed, youthful breasts; and delineated nipples serve to underscore her unrealized potential as a mother—was similar to the depiction of pregnant women in Aztec art with pendulous breasts and a stomach fold.

There were five specified days in the Aztec calendar, the *Cihuateteo* descended to Earth - 1 Eagle, 1 Monkey, 1 House, 1 Rain and 1 Deer. These five days were when they were believed "to haunt the crossroads, hoping to kidnap young children since they had been deprived of their opportunity to be mothers" (Nicholson and Quiñones-Keber 1983). The *Cihuateteo* also accompanied the sun, extinguishing it until warriors lifted it up again to the sky. The Aztecs gave the *Cihuateteo* offerings—bread or tamales shaped like butterflies or lightning—on certain feast days in order to appease them, which were left at altars or at crossroads.

References

Adelina, R. J., Méndez, O. L., Sánchez, M. S., & Castellanos, M. A. (2014). Obstetricia Azteca. Ritos y manejos desde el embarazo hasta el trabajo de parto. *Avances en Ciencia, Salud y Medicina, 2*(4), 129–136.

Bruhns, K. O., & Stothert, K. E. (1999). *Women in ancient America*. Norman: University of Oklahaoma Press. ISBN 0806131691.

Eberl, M. (2013). Nourishing gods: Birth and personhood in highland Mexican codices. Cambridge Archaeological Journal, *23*(3), 453–476.

de Sahagun, B. (1970). *Florentine Codex*. Salt Lake City: University of Utah Press. ISBN 0874800005.

de Sahagún, B. (1985). *Historia general de las cosas de Nueva España*. Prologue by Angel María Garibay, 6th edición. Mexico, D.F.: Editorial Porrúa.

Geller, P. (2016). *The bioarchaeology of socio-sexual lives*. New York City: Springer.

Guerra, F. (1966). Aztec medicine. *Medical History, 10*(4), 315–338.

Koch, P. O. (2005). *The Aztecs, the conquistadors, and the making of Mexican culture*. Jefferson, NC: McFarland & Company. ISBN: 9780786422524.

Instituto Nacional de Estadídistica y Geografía (INEGI). (2015). *Panorama sociodemográfico de México*. Retrieved January 1, 2016, from http://www.inegi.org.mx/est/contenidos/proyectos/encuestas/hogares/especiales/ei2015/doc/panorama_sociodemografico_2015.pdf.

León, N. (1910). *La obstetricia en México*. Mexico: Vda. de F., Díaz de León.

Madsen, W. (1960). *The virgin's children: Life in an Aztec village today*. Austin: University of Texas Press. ISBN 978-0292741348.

Moctezuma, E. M., & Olguin, F. S. (2003). *Aztecs*. London: Royal Academy Publications.

Miller, M., & Taube, K. (1993). *The gods and symbols of ancient Mexico and the Maya: An illustrated dictionary of Mesoamerican religion*. London: Thames & Hudson. ISBN 0-500-05068-6.

Nicholson, H. B., & Quiñones-Keber, E. (1983). *The art of Aztec Mexico: Treasures of Tenochtitlan. Catalogue of an Exhibition at the National Gallery of Art, Washington, 1983*. Washington, D.C.: National Gallery of Art.

Read, K. A., & González, J. J. (2002). *Handbook of mesoamerican mythology: A guide to the gods, heroes, rituals, and beliefs of Mexico and Central America*. Oxford: Oxford University Press. ISBN 0-19-514909-2.

Shein, M. (1986). *El niño precolombino*. Mexico City: Villicaña.

Sesia, P. (2017). Maternal death in Mexico. In: *Latin American History*. Oxford Research Encyclopedias. Retrieved from http://latinamericanhistory.oxfordre.com/view/10.1093/acrefore/9780199366439.001.0001/acrefore-9780199366439-e-50.

Tovar-Rodríguez, J. M. (2013). The religious aspects of maternal mortality at the time of the Aztecs. Cihuateteo: Dead women at first birth. *Ginecología y Obstetricia de México, 81*(9), 555–557.

Townsend, R.F. (2000). *The Aztecs*. Revised edition. New York City: Thames & Hudson.

3 Hypertensive Mothers, Obstetric Hemorrhage, and Infections: Biomedical Aspects of Maternal Death Among Indigenous Women in Mexico and Central America

David A. Schwartz

3.1 Introduction

The death of women resulting from pregnancy remains a major public health problem in many of the developing nations of the world, where greater than 99% of maternal deaths occur. It is a complicated issue that has biomedical, social, and even political issues related to its occurrence and potential solutions. A maternal death is defined as the "death of a woman while pregnant or within 42 days of termination of pregnancy, irrespective of the duration and the site of the pregnancy, from any cause related to or aggravated by the pregnancy or its management, but not from accidental or incidental causes" (CDC 2007). Globally, approximately 830 women die every day because of pregnancy or childbirth (WHO 2016, 2017). This situation was addressed as part of the Millennium Development Goals (MDGs) that were established by the United Nations following its Millennium Summit meeting, and resulted in the adoption of the United Nations Millennium Declaration in 2000. Of the eight Millennium Development Goals (MDGs), Goal 5 was to improve maternal health by the year 2015 and to reduce by three-quarters the maternal mortality ratio (MMR) by the year 2015. From 1990 to 2015, the global maternal mortality ratio, a statistical measure of maternal deaths in a population, declined by 44%—from 385 deaths to 216 deaths per 100,000 live births, according to UN interagency estimates (UNICEF 2017). This translates into an average annual rate of reduction of 2.3%. Unfortunately, in many developing and resource-poor countries of the world, these goals were unattainable.

Maternal mortality remains a significant public health problem in Mexico and Central America and, in particular, among indigenous women. Indigenous women in these countries share a common, but unfortunate, trait—they have a significantly increased risk of dying when compared with nonindigenous women as a result of becoming pregnant. What is even more disturbing is that the large majority of these maternal deaths are preventable (Schwartz 2015a). The causes of maternal death in Mexico and Central America are identical with those occurring in other parts of the developing and developed world; however, they culminate in maternal death with greater frequency among indigenous women in these countries.

D. A. Schwartz, M.D., M.S. Hyg., F.C.A.P.
Department of Pathology, Medical College of Georgia, Augusta University, Augusta, GA, USA

D. A. Schwartz (ed.), *Maternal Death and Pregnancy-Related Morbidity Among Indigenous Women of Mexico and Central America*, Global Maternal and Child Health: Medical, Anthropological, and Public Health Perspectives, https://doi.org/10.1007/978-3-319-71538-4_3

In order to understand the diverse nature of the causes of maternal death among indigenous women, it is important to have some knowledge of how and why these pregnancy-associated disorders develop. This chapter addresses three of the most frequent causes of maternal death among indigenous women of Mexico and Central America—hypertensive diseases, obstetric hemorrhage, and infection.

3.2 The Hypertensive Diseases of Pregnancy: Preeclampsia and Eclampsia

3.2.1 Epidemiology

The hypertensive disorders of pregnancy (HDP)—preeclampsia, eclampsia, gestational hypertension, and chronic hypertension—constitute a group of disorders occurring in pregnant women that all have in common the occurrence of abnormally increased blood pressure. Preeclampsia is a multisystem progressive disorder characterized by the new onset of hypertension and often proteinuria, or hypertension and end-organ dysfunction with or without proteinuria, in the last half of pregnancy (>20 week's gestation) or postpartum. Hypertension refers to the maternal blood pressure which is greater than 140 mm Hg systolic or 90 mm Hg diastolic at two separate times, more than 4 h apart, in a woman after 20 weeks of pregnancy. It can be accompanied by proteinuria (which had previously been a diagnostic criteria) and edema. Preeclampsia complicates from 2 to 8% of all pregnancies worldwide and is an important global cause of maternal death. HELLP syndrome is a life-threatening pregnancy complication usually considered to be a variant or complication of preeclampsia, resulting in hemolysis, low liver enzymes, and low platelet count. If convulsive seizures appear in a woman with preeclampsia, and in the absence of other etiologies, the syndrome is termed eclampsia (an archaic term, toxemia of pregnancy, is a misnomer and is rarely used anymore) (Osungbade and Ige 2011; Powe et al. 2011; Schwartz 2015b). Gestational hypertension (sometimes referred to as pregnancy-induced hypertension or PIH) is the development of new-onset hypertension in a pregnant woman after 20 weeks' gestation without the presence of protein in the urine or other signs and symptoms of preeclampsia. Chronic hypertension is defined as blood pressure exceeding 140/90 mmHg that existed before pregnancy or before 20 weeks' gestation. When hypertension is first identified during a woman's pregnancy and she is at less than 20 weeks' gestation, blood pressure elevations usually represent chronic hypertension. The hypertensive diseases of pregnancy remain a significant public health problem in both developed (rich) and developing (poor) countries of the world, contributing to global maternal and infant morbidity and mortality. In Mexico, Central America, and the rest of Latin America and the Caribbean nations, HDP and their complications are some of the leading causes of maternal death.

Unfortunately, the health impact and clinical outcomes of the HDP are more severe among indigenous women in developed countries than nonindigenous women for several reasons—women come to medical attention later or not at all, they are more likely to deliver in nonhospital settings, they may be assisted during birth by persons unable to care for the complications of HDP, and the availability of medications such as magnesium sulfate to treat the disorder is limited or unavailable (Ikechebelu and Okoli 2002; Onakewhor and Gharoro 2008; Onuh and Aisien 2004). Thus, the increased risk of morbidity and mortality resulting from preeclampsia and eclampsia in pregnant women, and especially indigenous women, in developing nations is intimately related to the "Three Delays": (1) delay in the decision to seek healthcare, (2) delay in reaching the health facility, and (3) delay in heath service provision (Firoz et al. 2011; Ghulmiyyah and Sibai 2012). In a report from the World Health Organization, preeclampsia was stated to occur as much as seven times more frequently in women from developing nations than pregnant women in developed countries (WHO 2005). As is the situation with other causes of maternal morbidity and mortality in developing nations, the true number of maternal deaths caused by the HDP remains mostly unknown.

3.2.2 Pathophysiology

The physiological basis of preeclampsia is generally believed to be faulty remodeling of uterine spiral arteries that supply the placenta with oxygenated maternal blood, occurring early in gestation (Nakimuli et al. 2014; Schwartz 2015b). Immunologic and genetic factors have been invoked as well as altered vascular reactivity, diffuse endothelial injury, and coagulation abnormalities. Maternal blood flow and perfusion of the placenta are reduced as a result of pathological remodeling of the maternal spiral arteries located in the decidua, thus resulting in uteroplacental malperfusion early in gestation, with the consequent production of placental ischemia. At the tissue level, renal involvement almost always occurs, and may be subclinical or clinically-evident, and contributes to maternal hypertension and proteinuria. A dreaded complication of the hypertensive disease of pregnancy is intravascular clotting, termed disseminated intravascular coagulation (DIC). It results in decreased circulating platelets (thrombocytopenia), microscopic fibrin thromboemboli in the liver, brain, and kidneys, and can cause hemorrhage as a result of a consumptive coagulopathy. Early-onset preeclampsia is an infrequent occurrence, with signs and symptoms developing at or before 32 weeks' gestation. This is associated with higher levels of morbidity and mortality. Rarely, preeclampsia may not be clinically evident until after delivery, and is termed postpartum preeclampsia. Eclampsia is a cerebrovascular disorder characterized by seizures, worsening hypertension, cerebral ischemia, and edema.

The placenta will usually have abnormalities resulting from long-term chorionic villous ischemia, decreased maternal perfusion of the intervillous space, and chronic uteroplacental malperfusion. The pathologic changes in the placenta reflect long-term reduced maternal blood flow from the uterine blood vessels to the maternal intervillous space, because in preeclampsia the spiral arteries of the uteroplacental bed never fully dilate. Early in a normal pregnancy, fetal cytotrophoblast cells extend downward, into the decidua and uterus. They invade the uterine spiral arteries and progressively replace the maternal-derived endothelium, medial elastic tissue, smooth muscle, and neural tissue. By the end of the second trimester, the normally narrow prepregnancy spiral arteries are dilated tubes lined by fetal-derived cytotrophoblast, forming a low-resistance arterial circuit that can supply the increasing oxygen and nutrient demand of the developing fetus. Defective cytotrophoblastic remodeling of the maternal uterine (spiral) arteries in early pregnancy is believed to result from abnormal expression of the adhesion molecule integrins by the fetal-derived cytotrophoblast, as well as generalized apoptosis of the cytotrophoblast. This leads to limited invasion of the decidua and spiral arteries. As a result, the spiral arteries cannot perfuse the growing fetus adequately. Resulting placental ischemia promotes release of cytokines such as tumor necrosis factor alpha (TNF-a) and interleukin-6 (IL-6).

In preeclampsia, many spiral arteries escape invasion by trophoblastic tissue and so never fully dilate. These spiral arteries commonly show fibrinoid necrosis, clusters of lipid-rich macrophages, and a perivascular infiltrate of mononuclear cells, which together are termed acute atherosis. Fibrin deposition is also seen. These vessels are often thrombosed, which result in focal placental infarcts. The combination of vasoconstriction and structural changes in spiral arteries contributes to chronic inadequate blood flow, placental ischemia, villous hypoplasia, and fetal hypoxia that can result in poor obstetrical outcomes.

Upregulation and production of such placental antiangiogenic factors as fms-related tyrosine kinase 1 (vascular endothelial growth factor) and soluble endoglin may play a role in the onset of the clinical features of preeclampsia including hypertension and proteinuria. The roles, if any, of other factors are unclear, for example, oxidative stress, antibodies (anti-endothelial cell, anti-angiotensin type I receptor agonist), increased maternal plasma homocysteine and leptin concentrations, changes of contractile proteins in maternal smooth muscle, and other mechanisms of vascular smooth muscle contraction and genetic factors.

Although the central pathogenic abnormality in preeclampsia is placental ischemia, many of the details of molecular pathogenesis remain unknown. In normal pregnancy, there are many physiologic hemodynamic and cardiovascular alterations—increased maternal cardiac output and plasma volume, reduction in total maternal vascular resistance and arterial pressure, increased renal plasma flow, and decreased pressor response and vascular reactivity to vasoconstrictive substances such as α-adrenergic agonists and angiotensin II. These changes are partially the result of physiologically enhanced endothelium-dependent vascular relaxation, as well as decreased vascular reactivity to vasoconstrictor agonists. In women developing preeclampsia, the latter beneficial vascular and hemodynamic modifications do not occur. The effectiveness of vasodilators in treating preeclampsia, including nitric oxide ($NO^{\bullet}$), prostacyclin (PGI_2), and endothelium-derived hyperpolarizing factor (EDHF), is further evidence for endothelial dysfunction in this condition (Schwartz 2015b).

3.2.3 The Placenta and Preeclampsia

The placenta is the largest organ of the fetus, and is not only directly involved in the development of the hypertensive diseases of pregnancy but also in the poor obstetric and neonatal outcomes caused by these disorders. It has long been recognized that preeclampsia is a placental disorder that results in the maternal syndrome. Interestingly, the formation of pathology abnormalities resulting from chronic ischemia, such as villous hypoplasia and other pathological changes of maternal underperfusion, in the placenta of women who will develop clinical HDP precedes the development of clinical symptoms and signs of preeclampsia by many weeks or longer. This hazardous feature of preeclampsia means that although maternal signs and symptoms of preeclampsia may have just begun, ischemic damage to the placenta and fetus may have already been remotely ongoing (Schwartz 2015b). Extensive placental infarction is seen in nearly one-third of women with severe preeclampsia, although infarction is often negligible in mild preeclampsia. Chorionic villi show signs of chronic maternal underperfusion—areas of shrunken and degenerated chorionic villi with stromal fibrosis and thickened basement membranes resulting from ischemia, termed villous hypoplasia (or uneven accelerated maturation).

Villous hypoplasia is typically present in the placentas of women who develop the hypertensive diseases of pregnancy, and results from many weeks of decreased maternal perfusion of the placenta resulting from the chronic uterine arterial disease which is the hallmark of preeclampsia. Villous hypoplasia may also be present in the placentas of mothers who have hypertension prior to pregnancy (chronic hypertension), as well as in women who smoke cigarettes during pregnancy.

Additional microscopic placental findings of maternal vascular underperfusion due to preeclampsia are often present, including villous agglutination, increased fibrin, increased placental site giant cells, syncytiotrophoblastic hyperplasia (Tenney-Parker change), and mural hypertrophy of membrane arterioles. Abnormally small placentas (less than the 10th percentile weight for gestational age) may also be seen in mothers with preeclampsia. Retroplacental hemorrhage or abruptio placentae occurs in approximately 15% of women with HDP (see Obstetric Hemorrhage below).

3.2.4 Decidua

The decidua is a term used to denote the endometrial lining of the uterus during pregnancy. Characteristic abnormalities of the decidual arteries can be present in women with HDP. Termed decidual vasculopathy and atherosis, they result from defective remodeling, or abnormal uteroplacental vascular conversion, of these vessels maternal early in pregnancy. Decidual vasculopathy cannot be identified grossly—it is a microscopic diagnosis. Decidual vasculopathy is characterized microscopically by fibrinoid necrosis, intimal and medial proliferation, and foamy macrophages (atherosis) in the decidual vessel wall. The vessel walls are thickened as a result of fibrin deposition resulting from fibrinoid necrosis. The vessels may have variable degrees of persistence of vascular muscle and elastic lamina. Small thrombi can also be present in some vessels, and lymphocytic vasculitis can occur.

3.2.5 Kidneys

The kidneys of women with hypertensive disease of pregnancy are a major target organ of the disease, and undergo glomerular changes that are termed glomerular endotheliosis. Glomerular endotheliosis is a specific variant of thrombotic microangiopathy (TMA) that only occurs in pregnancy. The glomeruli are enlarged, and the endothelial cells are swollen, forming classic "bloodless" glomeruli of preeclampsia. There is loss of endothelial fenestrae, vascular occlusion, and fibrin present between the endothelial cells and the glomerular capillary basement membrane. Mesangial cell hyperplasia is the rule. Thrombosis of glomerular capillaries is unusual. Glomerular endotheliosis occurs in approximately 70% of primiparas who develop preeclampsia, but in only 14% of multiparas who are preeclamptic. Recent evidence suggests that this renal abnormality is mediated by soluble vascular endothelial growth factor (VEGF) receptor, which acts to deprive the glomerular endothelial cells of the VEGF that they require, causing cellular injury and disruption of the cellular filtration apparatus and resulting in proteinuria. These maternal renal changes are reversible with therapy or after delivery (Karumanchi et al. 2005; Müller-Deile and Schiffer 2011; Mutter et al. 2011; Schwartz 2015b; Stillman and Karumanci 2007).

3.2.6 Liver

The liver is affected overall in approximately 10–20% of women who develop preeclampsia. However, in those women who develop eclampsia, hepatic pathology abnormalities are grossly identified in the liver of 60%, and one-third of the remaining women have microscopic abnormalities. The initial microscopic change occurs as a result of hemorrhage into the hepatic columns which is a result of dilatation of hepatic arterioles. As the disorder progresses, intense vasospasm occurs and results in ischemic changes of hepatocytes and vessels—associated findings include patchy hepatic necrosis, periportal fibrin deposits and necrosis, periportal and hepatic plate hemorrhage, and hepatic infarction. Hemorrhagic changes occur in the liver of approximately two-thirds and necrotic changes in approximately 40% of women with eclampsia—the frequency is one-half of those numbers in preeclamptic women. Involvement of the liver is especially frequent in the HELLP syndrome, a complication of preeclampsia. The occurrence of confluent hepatic necrosis may result in such infrequent but life-threatening complications as intrahepatic hematomas, subcapsular hematomas, and liver rupture with intraperitoneal hemorrhage (Creasy et al. 2014; Kenny et al. 2014; Schwartz 2015b).

3.2.7 Central Nervous System

Fatal cases of eclampsia often show cerebral hemorrhages, ranging from petechiae to large hematomas. Additional pathology findings include cerebral edema, small infarctions including perivascular infarcts, and vascular changes including fibrinoid necrosis of the blood vessel wall (Cipolla et al. 2014).

3.2.8 Hypertensive Diseases of Pregnancy in Indigenous Women in Mexico and Central America

There is scant statistical and demographic information available on the incidence of the hypertensive diseases of pregnancy among indigenous women in Central America and Mexico. However, what is known is that preeclampsia and eclampsia, together with obstetric hemorrhage, are the leading causes of maternal death among indigenous women in these countries. These two conditions—hypertensive diseases of pregnancy and obstetrical hemorrhage—although demographically listed as separate disease entities in classifications of maternal deaths, are not necessarily physiologically unrelated. Acute placental abruption (placenta abruptio) is a premature separation of the placenta from its uterine attachment which can result in life-threatening maternal hemorrhage and is highly associated with preeclampsia and eclampsia. It may be difficult to diagnose a placental abruption in the typical setting in which many indigenous women give birth, either at home, in a clinic, or a local hospital. Thus, it is likely that many maternal deaths which are recorded as being the result of "obstetric hemorrhage" are, in fact, due to placental abruption resulting from preeclampsia. Disseminated intravascular clotting, or DIC, is a feared complication of preeclampsia which can also result in a consumptive coagulopathy and uncontrolled hemorrhage.

3.2.8.1 Calcium Supplementation and Preeclampsia in Mayan Women in Guatemala

Some early observations that suggested nutrition had an effect on the development of preeclampsia were derived from observations made among the Maya in Guatemala. Investigators found an association between high dietary calcium intake and what they believed to be a low incidence of pregnancy-related hypertensive disease among Mayan women (Belizán and Villar 1980). The traditional practice of Mayan women soaking corn in lime prior to cooking was found to be associated with an unusually high calcium intake and what was believed to be low incidence of preeclampsia and eclampsia. Low calcium intake may cause hypertension by stimulating parathyroid hormone or renin release, inducing vasoconstriction, and resulting in vasoconstriction by increasing intracellular calcium in vascular smooth muscle and intensifying smooth muscle reactivity (Belizán et al. 1988). It was hypothesized that among the Maya, calcium supplementation acts on smooth muscle reactivity by reducing parathyroid hormone release and intracellular calcium. However, other studies of the role of calcium supplementation to decrease the risk of preeclampsia in different population groups have shown contradictory results.

3.2.8.2 Prepregnancy Body Mass Index and Preeclampsia in Maya-*Mestizo* Women in Mexico

Maternal obesity is a well-documented risk factor for preeclampsia. In a prospective cohort study of 642 pregnant Maya-*mestizo* women conducted in Yucatán, Mexico, who were enrolled during the first trimester, 49 developed preeclampsia (44.9% severe and 55% mild), with an incidence of 7.6%. The prepregnancy body mass index (BMI) was found to be higher in those women who developed preeclampsia when compared with those were normotensive (Canto-Cetina et al. 2017), thus confirming this association in a population of indigenous Maya-*mestizo* women.

3.2.8.3 Nitrous Oxide Synthase Genotype and Preeclampsia in Maya-*Mestizo* Women in Mexico

An essential step in the pathogenesis of preeclampsia involves endothelial dysfunction that results from impaired trophoblast invasion and spiral artery remodeling, resulting in abnormal implantation and placental underperfusion. Although some dietary, environmental, and genetic factors of preeclampsia have been identified, its mechanism is still not completely understood; therefore, its prevention remains a challenge. In addition to abnormal placental implantation, vascular remodeling and diffuse endothelial cell activation and dysfunction having important roles in the pathophysiology of preeclampsia, the susceptibility of an individual to developing preeclampsia is believed to have a genetic component.

Circulating nitric oxide (NO) is a potent vasodilator that plays a crucial role in endothelial function regulation, blood pressure control, and cardiovascular homeostasis. Nitric oxide induces vasodilatation, inhibits platelet aggregation, and prevents platelet adhesion to endothelial cells. An increment of NO production has been described in normal pregnancy; on the other hand, reduced NO formation has been implicated in the pathogenesis of preeclampsia. Endothelial nitrous oxide synthase (*eNOS*) is an enzyme that generates NO in blood vessels, regulates vascular function, and serves a protective role for endothelial cells. There are three polymorphisms in the *eNOS* gene that have been associated with preeclampsia. D'ıaz-Olgu'ın et al. (2011) investigated the role of these gene polymorphisms or their haplotypes that were associated with development of preeclampsia in a cohort of Maya-*mestizo* women in Yucatán, Mexico. In their case-control study of 127 preeclamptic women and 263 controls, they found that Maya-*mestizo* women who were homozygous for the Asp298 allele showed an association with preeclampsia. In addition, the -786C-4b-Asp298 haplotype was significantly more frequent in preeclamptic women than in controls.

3.2.8.4 Isozyme Polymorphisms and Preeclampsia in Maya-*Mestizo* Women in Mexico

The development of preeclampsia is believed to have a genetic component. To examine if isozyme polymorphisms played a role in the development of preeclampsia, a case-control study was performed in a population of Maya-*mestizo* pregnant women in Yucatán to examine whether the 5,10-methylenetetrahydrofolate reductase (MTHFR) C677T and glutathione S-transferase P1 (GSTP1) A313G polymorphisms are associated with preeclampsia in Maya-*mestizo* women. In this study, 125 preeclamptic patients and 274 healthy controls were genotyped for the MTHFR C677T and GSTP1 A313G polymorphisms by real-time PCR allelic discrimination. Allele and genotype frequencies were compared using the chi-squared tests. The MTHFR 677T allele and the 677TT genotype were significantly more frequent in the controls, suggesting an association with a decreased risk of preeclampsia (Canto et al. 2008).

3.2.8.5 Polymorphisms of Glutathione S-Transferases and Preeclampsia in Maya-*Mestizo* Women in Mexico

Glutathione S-transferases (GSTs), which were previously known as ligandins, comprise a family of metabolic isozymes that are best known for their ability to catalyze the conjugation of the reduced form of glutathione (GSH) to xenobiotic substrates for the purpose of detoxification. Deletion polymorphisms have been found in two of the genes—the GSTM1 gene (GSTM1) and in the GSTT1 gene (GSTT1). Sandoval and Carrillo (2014) investigated the relationship between the occurrence of these genetic markers and the development of preeclampsia in a population of Mexican Maya-*mestizo* pregnant women. They found an increased risk of preeclampsia in women having the GSTT1 null genotype and that a combination of deletion genotypes of the GSTM1 and GSTT1 genes conferred an even higher risk of preeclampsia in this population.

3.2.8.6 Cytokine Differences and Preeclampsia Among Mexican Maya-*Mestizo* and Mexican Women

Polymorphisms in the regulatory regions of cytokines are thought to play a potential role in the development of preeclampsia. Villalvazo and colleagues (2012) investigated the possible association between cytokine polymorphisms—rs1800896 of interleukin-10 (IL-10), rs1800795 of interleukin-6

(IL-6), and the variable number of tandem repeats (VNTR) in intron 2 of interleukin-1 receptor antagonist (IL-1Ra). They also examined gene-gene interactions between these three polymorphisms with the occurrence of preeclampsia in Mexican-*mestizo* women and one Mayan population in Mexico. Their results showed that genotypic and allelic distribution of the polymorphisms was similar, and the estimates of gene-gene interaction between the polymorphisms did not differ significantly between preeclamptic and non-preeclamptic women. However, they observed important differences in the distribution of the alleles and genotypes of the three polymorphisms between Mexican-*mestizo* women and Maya-*mestizo* women.

3.2.8.7 Polymorphisms in the *TNF*-α Promoter Gene and Preeclampsia Among Mayan *Mestizo* Women in Mexico

In order to investigate the potential relationship of genetic polymorphisms in the tumor necrosis factor-alpha (*TNF*-α) promoter gene with preeclampsia, Canto-Cetino et al. (2007) enrolled 105 Maya-*mestizo* women with preeclampsia and 200 controls who were genotyped for the G-308A and C-850T polymorphisms by restriction fragment length polymorphism (RFLP) analysis. After noting the differences in allele, genotype, and haplotype frequencies between groups that were investigated, they found that the genotypic and allelic distribution of both polymorphisms was similar between the two groups. Moreover, the estimated overall pair of loci haplotype frequencies did not differ significantly, demonstrating that there was no association between these polymorphisms and the risk for preeclampsia.

3.3 Obstetrical Hemorrhage

Obstetric hemorrhage remains an important cause of pregnancy-related death in resource-rich countries. However, in the resource-poor countries of the globe, the contribution of obstetrical hemorrhage to maternal mortality rates is even more striking (El Kady et al. 1989; Jegasothy 2002; Rahman et al. 2002). Indeed, hemorrhage is the single most important direct cause of maternal death worldwide. Obstetrical hemorrhage accounts for almost one-half of all postpartum deaths in developing countries. In the developing world, several countries have maternal mortality rates in excess of 1000 women per 100,000 live births, and World Health Organization statistics suggest that 25% of all maternal deaths are due to PPH, accounting for more than 100,000 maternal deaths per year (Smith 2016; WHO 2007). In resource-poor areas of the world including Mexico and Central America, obstetrical hemorrhage is a common pregnancy complication and is one of the leading causes of maternal death (Romero-Gutiérrez et al. 2007; Say et al. 2014).

Because postpartum hemorrhage is potentially life-threatening, rapid recognition and proper clinical management is an essential component of maternal healthcare and a necessary step in the goal to reduce worldwide maternal mortality. However, the interventions that are recommended for the identification of the causes of postpartum hemorrhage and methods for its treatment in the setting of developed countries may not be feasible in the low-resource settings characteristic of rural areas in Mexico and Central America where the majority of indigenous people reside. This is especially true when it occurs in home or clinic deliveries, and without direct and immediate access to medical interventions. Maternal deaths due to obstetrical hemorrhage occurring in indigenous women in these areas are likely to be associated with the Three Delays Model of maternal mortality. For example, in an ecological analysis of Latin American and Caribbean countries, Cruz found an inverse association between donor blood availability and both maternal mortality ratios and risk of death due to postpartum hemorrhage (Cruz 2007). Social and cultural inequalities, along with issues concerning the accessibility and comprehensiveness of healthcare, are the antecedents of maternal mortality in developing nations. Strategies that prevent and treat postpartum hemorrhage must be readily accessible, affordable, and have uncomplicated storage requirements in order to be effective in countries with limited healthcare financing and infrastructure. An urgent need for the uptake of technologies proven to work in developing countries has been identified. Furthermore, continued research into the effectiveness of postpartum hemorrhage interventions in the context of low-resource settings is required to better understand the clinical management of this potentially life-threatening obstetrical complication.

3.3.1 Causes of Obstetrical Hemorrhage

Obstetrical hemorrhage is a term that includes antepartum hemorrhage, as well as intrapartum and postpartum bleeding of a pregnant woman, and is best classified according to when in pregnancy the hemorrhage occurs. Antepartum hemorrhage (APH) is defined as bleeding from or in the genital tract occurring from the 24th week of pregnancy and prior to the birth of the newborn—it complicates from 3 to 5% of pregnancies worldwide and was, until recently, a leading cause of maternal and perinatal death due to hemorrhage in developed countries. Antepartum hemorrhage is still a major source of maternal and infant morbidity in resource-poor nations (Dolea et al. 2003). The leading causes of APH are abruptio placentae (40%) and placenta previa (20%), with the remainder unclassified. Intrapartum hemorrhage (IPH) includes excessive maternal bleeding during labor and delivery. Postpartum hemorrhage (PPH) is defined by the acute loss of greater than 500 mL of maternal blood within 24 h of a vaginal delivery. Postpartum hemorrhage is the leading cause of maternal mortality worldwide with a prevalence rate of approximately 6%; Africa has the highest prevalence rate at approximately 10.5% of all vaginal deliveries. In Africa and Asia, where the numerical majority of maternal deaths occur, PPH is responsible for greater than 30% of all mother deaths (Carroli et al. 2008; Khan et al. 2006). The most common cause of PPH is uterine atony—other causes include adherent or retained placenta (including placenta adherens and placenta accreta, increta, and percreta), traumatic injury to vessels and tissues during delivery, and coagulopathies such as the thrombophilias, fibrinolysis, and afibrinogenemia. Secondary postpartum hemorrhage can also occur, which represents a group of pathological conditions that can result in obstetrical hemorrhage varying from 24 hours up to 6 weeks following delivery. The causes include inherited coagulation disorders, postpartum endometritis, consumptive coagulopathy, retained products of conception, and trauma. An infrequent cause of secondary postpartum hemorrhage is termed subinvolution of the placental site. In this abnormality, the uterine blood vessels at the placental implantation site that had previously undergone remodeling exhibit inadequate or delayed physiological closure and sloughing, are dilated with hyaline material in their walls, and may contain thrombi. This abnormality is probably underdiagnosed, as it may require a pathologist with specialized obstetrical knowledge to make the correct diagnosis. Obstetrical hemorrhage has emerged as the major cause of severe maternal morbidity in almost all "near-miss" audits both in resource-rich and resource-poor nations.

3.3.2 Uterine Atony

Uterine atony refers to the pathological condition in which the uterus fails to contract following delivery of the fetus. Clinically, 75–80% of postpartum hemorrhages are due to uterine atony. Under normal circumstances, the uterine smooth muscle contracts during labor, compressing the uterine blood vessels and resulting in decreased blood flow to the placental implantation site, facilitating the development of coagulation and stasis of blood flow following delivery. Under normal circumstances, control of postpartum bleeding results from the contraction and retraction of interlacing myometrial fibers surrounding maternal spiral arteries of the placental bed. Myometrial contraction compresses the spiral arteries and veins, thereby obliterating their lumina. It is for this reason that these specific myometrial fibers are often referred to as "living ligatures." In addition, a contribution to postpartum hemostasis occurs by means of direct pressure as the uterine walls are forced firmly to oppose one another as a result of myometrial contraction.

Postpartum hemorrhage resulting from uterine atony occurs when the relaxed myometrium fails to constrict the blood vessels that traverse its fibers, thereby permitting blood flow and hemorrhage. As much as one-fifth of maternal cardiac output, approximately 1000 mL/min, enters the uteroplacental circulation at term, and thus uterine atony can lead to exsanguination within a short time. Failure of the uterus to contract may be associated with retained placenta or placental fragments (see below) from an abnormally adherent placenta, either as disrupted portions or, more rarely, as a succenturiate lobe of the placenta. The retained placental tissue material can physically interfere with the effective uterine contractions which are necessary to constrict placental bed vessels. In most cases, however, dysfunctional postpartum contraction is the primary reason for placental retention. It is more likely for the placenta to be retained in cases of atonic postpartum hemorrhage, and so the uterine contraction failure often becomes self-perpetuating.

In Central American countries, uterine atony has been demonstrated to be the most frequent cause of severe postpartum hemorrhage. In a study of 124,019 pregnant women in Panama, Costa Rica, Guatemala, Mexico, Nicaragua, and El Salvador having live births at 13 teaching hospitals, there were 218 patients with severe postpartum hemorrhage, 75% of which were due to uterine atony. In this multinational and multicenter study, Honduras had the highest rate of severe postpartum hemorrhage (4.18 per 1000 live births) due to uterine atony, and Guatemala has the lowest rate (0.85 per 1000 live births). There were 8 maternal deaths, for a case fatality rate (CFR) of 3.6% and a MMR of 6.45/100,000 live births (Montufar-Rueda et al. 2013).

3.3.3 Placental Abruption

An important and dreaded cause of obstetric hemorrhage is abruptio placentae or placental abruption. The term refers to the abnormal separation of the placenta from its uterine attachment after 20 weeks' gestation and prior to the birth of the infant. Abruption complicates approximately 1% of pregnancies worldwide, although the prevalence has been reported as high as from 3 to 4% in some developing nations (Nandonde 2013; Sarwar et al. 2006). Abruption is the most common pathological cause of late-pregnancy bleeding. The underlying cause of abruption is almost always the result of rupture of the maternal uterine arteries that are located at the base of the placenta in the decidua basalis. These are the vessels that supply the placenta with oxygenated maternal blood, and separation of these vessels can not only have severe life-threatening consequences for the mother in terms of hemorrhage, hypovolemia, respiratory distress, shock and coagulopathy, but also for the fetus who has been deprived of oxygen from the maternal bloodstream. Abruptio placentae and its' pathologic counterpart, retroplacental hematoma, are often the final dramatic consequences of a chronic placental disorder. This usually involves disease of the decidual and uterine blood vessels—the majority of placental abruptions are the result of preexisting maternal decidual vascular disease. Because of this, abruption is highly associated with preeclampsia, another disorder caused by maternal vascular disease.

Following the premature detachment of the placenta from its attachment to the uterine wall, or a rupture of a uterine blood vessel(s), the extravascular maternal blood can flow down the cervicovaginal tract, resulting in vaginal hemorrhage. Or, it can accumulate between the placenta and the decidua basalis, forming an area of retroplacental hemorrhage and, eventually, a blood clot (hematoma). This can create further separation (or dissection) of the placenta from the decidua basalis, extending the extent of placental separation. If the hemorrhage occurs or extends beneath the extraplacental membranes, it is termed a submembranous hemorrhage. The retroplacental hematoma formed following a placental separation may be small or may occupy the entire maternal surface of the placenta. Recent hematomas are soft, red, and easily detached from the maternal surface. Older ones are firm and brown and more adherent to the placental surface. Chronic retroplacental hematomas may indent the maternal surface of the placenta, indicative of the outline formed where they had occupied space. When a retroplacental hematoma is present for some time, overlying villous tissue will begin to show irreversible ischemic degeneration, eventually causing a placental infarct. Fetal hemorrhage within the chorionic villi, termed intravillous hemorrhage, can occur. With passage of time, hemorrhage in the hematoma and decidua will be metabolized, and a golden-yellow hemosiderin pigment will be visible, usually within macrophages. In some cases where a postpartum hysterectomy has been performed for recalcitrant uterine bleeding, it can be observed that hemorrhage had dissected into and through the uterine muscle wall, termed a Couvelaire uterus.

3.3.4 Retained Placenta

Although retained placental tissue is not a common occurrence, it has a significant maternal mortality rate in developing countries. Data on the incidence of retained placenta are limited from these parts of the world; however, it has been reported to have a higher prevalence in vaginal deliveries from developed nations (2.6–3%) as compared with resource-poor countries (0.1–1.46%) (Cheung et al. 2011; Weeks 2008). Despite the reported differences in its frequency, the maternal mortality rate of retained placenta is many magnitudes higher in developing nations, up to 10% in rural areas, as compared with the rarity of death due to this abnormality in developed countries. Retained placenta can result in maternal mortality and morbidity in several ways—postpartum hemorrhage (PPH), disseminated intravascular coagulation (DIC), and infection are the most frequent.

There are three major mechanisms for the retention of placental tissue. Placenta adherens occurs when the placenta is not spontaneously extruded as a result of failed contraction of the uterine myometrial muscle; trapped placenta develops as a result of the placenta becoming detached by subsequently trapped behind a closed cervix; and placenta accreta, in which the placenta is abnormally adhered partially or completely to the uterine wall due to faulty formation of the decidual layer between the base of the placenta and its uterine (decidual) attachment.

Placenta accreta is arguably the most dangerous of these causes of retained placenta, especially in an underdeveloped and resource-poor setting. Its incidence has been reported to be increasing in parallel with the increasing rate of cesarean section deliveries. This is because scarring of the uterus is an important risk factor for the faulty decidualization which permits the direct attachment, and in some cases invasion by, chorionic villi to the myometrium. There are three types of placenta accreta—all are based upon the definitive obstetrical pathologic evaluation of the extent of attachment and invasion of the uterus by placental tissues. Placenta accreta, the most common, is defined by the direct attachment of chorionic villi to the uterine muscle in the absence of intervening decidual tissues. In some cases, a thin layer of fibrin is present between the villi and uterine muscle, but the diagnosis of placenta accreta is still made as long as no intervening decidual layer can be identified. Placenta increta is diagnosed when chorionic villi invade into the myometrial muscle, but do not extend completely through it. The rarest of the accretas, termed placenta percreta, is diagnosed when there has been complete transmural invasion of the uterine wall by villous tissue to the serosal surface. In placenta percreta, the villous tissue can also extend beyond the uterine serosa to involve contiguous structures such as the bladder and bowel. Approximately 60% of cases of placenta accreta are associated with a low-lying placental implantation, termed placenta previa (Khong 2008; Schwartz 2015b; Tantbirojn et al. 2008).

3.3.5 Coagulopathy, Disseminated Intravascular Coagulation, and Hemorrhage

Disseminated intravascular coagulation (DIC) is a pathological process in which there is systemic activation of the intravascular clotting cascade, resulting in a coagulopathy characterized by the formation of microscopic blood clots or thromboemboli. These thromboemboli circulate in the small blood vessels of the circulatory system, where they cause tissue malperfusion, ischemia, and ultimately multiorgan damage. As the condition progresses, additional microscopic thromboemboli are formed in the blood stream, leading to the eventual consumption of circulating clotting factors, fibrin and platelets—that is why this process is often termed a consumptive coagulopathy. Because the normal clotting process is disturbed and clotting factors are consumed, bleeding can occur. Thus, the paradoxical clinicopathologic finding of thrombus formation and abnormal bleeding can be present in the same patient as a result of dysregulation of the processes of normal coagulation and fibrinolysis. DIC almost never occurs by itself—it is always the result of another pathologic process. DIC is a life-threatening condition with a poor prognosis and high mortality rate in developed nations—in poor countries it is usually fatal.

Disseminated intravascular coagulation is a common complication of many of the major causes of maternal death. In addition to such causes of obstetric bleeding as postpartum hemorrhage, preeclampsia and eclampsia, retained placenta, and HELLP syndrome, DIC can also be the results of obstetrical infections and puerperal sepsis, amniotic fluid embolism (AFE), acute fatty liver of pregnancy (AFLP), subinvolution of placental site blood vessels, uterine rupture, respiratory distress syndrome (RDS), and thromboembolic disease to name a few. Any pregnant patient developing DIC in resource-rich countries is a medical management challenge, and has a high risk for fatality. When she is a pregnant indigenous woman being cared for in a rural environment, at home or in a clinic, in a resource-poor region of the world, DIC can be an overwhelming medical problem.

3.4 Maternal Infection and Puerperal Sepsis

A wide variety of infectious diseases are associated with infection during pregnancy and maternal death in the resource-poor nations of the world. In some regions—including Mexico and Central America—these infections are indirect causes of maternal death, relating to preexisting medical conditions that may be aggravated by the physiological demands of pregnancy. These include malaria, HIV/AIDS, and viral hepatitis. Other infections are direct causes of maternal death—they are related to obstetric complications of the prenatal period, labor, delivery, and the puerperium. A major cause of maternal infections and puerperal sepsis is unsafe abortion (Schwartz 2015c).

There are numerous causes of infection relating to pregnancy—urinary tract infections, ascending cervicovaginal infections such as chorioamnionitis, breast abscesses and mastitis, catheter-related infections, necrotizing fasciitis, disturbed abscesses, episiotomy and abdominal wound infections to name a few. However, what is arguably the most serious infection of pregnancy is a bacterial infection that occurs during or after delivery, miscarriage, or abortion, termed puerperal sepsis. Puerperal sepsis accounts for approximately 15% of maternal deaths globally, with the overwhelming majority occurring in resource-poor nations. Induced abortion is illegal to varying extents in Mexico and the countries of Central America, and thus illicit and unsafe terminations of pregnancy, or “back-alley” abortions, are prevalent. In Guatemala, it has been estimated that approximately 65,000 induced abortions are performed annually, resulting in 21,600 women hospitalized for complications, many of which are infectious in nature (Singh et al. 2006). In Mexico, more than half (55%) of all pregnancies in Mexico are estimated to be unintended, making them at risk for seeking an unsafe abortion. In 2009, an estimated one million clandestine abortions were performed in Mexico, with an illegal abortion rate of an estimated 38 abortions per 1000 women ages 15–44 years. Although unsafe abortion is most prevalent in the urbanized and developed areas of Mexico, there were an estimated 26–27 abortions performed per 1000 women aged 15–44 in the two least developed regions, where indigenous women are concentrated (Guttmacher Institute 2013).

From a historical standpoint, a severe bacterial infection of the mother occurring during the perinatal period, termed puerperal sepsis or "child bed fever, was a common occurrence in the pre-antibiotic and pre-sterilization era. It occurred in epidemic proportions with the advent and popularity of birthing, or "lying-in" hospitals in the nineteenth century. During this time, puerperal sepsis was the leading cause of maternal death in Europe and America. In 1843 Oliver Wendall Holmes in the United States, and later Ignaz Semmelweis in 1847 in Europe, discovered that puerperal sepsis was contagious and that it could be transmitted from the autopsy room and from mother-to-mother by the physician's hands. They identified that hand-washing and the use of chemical agents could largely prevent maternal death from this life-threatening infection of pregnant women, and after these practices became adopted the death rate from puerperal sepsis dropped from 11% in 1846 to 3% in 1847.

Unlike the situation in developed countries where the incidence of serious maternal infections including puerperal sepsis are now rare causes of maternal death, in the resource-poor regions of the world postpartum infections remain an important and preventable cause of mother death. Unfortunately, there is no universally accepted definition of puerperal sepsis, which has led to some confusion in the diagnosis and reporting of frequency of this disease, especially in developing nations. Terms such as maternal fever, maternal sepsis, genital tract sepsis, and puerperal fever are all widely used in the literature from these nations without additional clarification, making it difficult to estimate the true incidence of puerperal sepsis in developing countries. In these regions, the diagnosis of puerperal sepsis is often based on the clinical signs, symptoms and findings of postpartum infection—in particular maternal pyrexia—but this can be caused by other conditions.

Within the context of the difficulties in case identification, confirmation, and reporting, it has been estimated that puerperal sepsis occurs in from 0.1–10% of deliveries in developing nations. Studies from sub-Saharan Africa indicate that puerperal sepsis in postpartum women has an incidence of 9% of women attending a hospital in Zambia (Lagro et al. 2003; Seale et al. 2009); another study indicates that it occurs in 19% of HIV-infected women postpartum (Sebitloane et al. 2008). Case fatality rates for puerperal sepsis in resource-poor nations are highly variable—they are reported to result in mother death in from 4% up to 50% of cases in sub-Saharan Africa (Dolea et al. 2003). A study from 2006 combined results of previous investigations to estimate the combined distribution of maternal death due to puerperal sepsis (Khan et al. 2006). In this study, it was estimated to be responsible for 11.6% of maternal deaths in Asia, 9.7% in Africa, and 7.7% in Latin America and the Caribbean. Of all major causes of maternal death, puerperal sepsis had the greatest inequality of prevalence between the developed and developing nations. Puerperal sepsis can be acquired within the health facility or externally in the community. In resource-poor nations, the incidence of puerperal sepsis acquired in the community is twice as high as health facility births. A study from Senegal demonstrated an incidence of sepsis of 8.7% for home deliveries compared to 1.9% for deliveries in health facilities (Hussein and Walker 2010).

Puerperal sepsis results from postpartum endometritis, an infection occurring during and after delivery in the endometrial lining of the uterus. Progressive bacterial invasion of the layers of the uterus, from the endometrium (decidua) into the myometrium, leads to severe inflammation, tissue ischemia and necrosis, thrombosis, and abscess formation. Eventually, there can be peritonitis, septic thromboembolism, pelvic thrombophlebitis, maternal sepsis, toxic shock, disseminated intravascular coagulation (DIC), renal failure, and adult respiratory distress syndrome (ARDS). The microbiology of puerperal sepsis usually reveals a mixed, or polymicrobial, bacterial infection, often with two to three anaerobes and aerobes from the genital tract. These may include *Streptococcus pyogenes*, *Escherichia coli*, *Bacteroides*, *Klebsiella*, *Pseudomonas*, *Proteus*, *Staphylococci*, various members of the enterobacteriaceae, and other streptococci.

If a postpartum hysterectomy is performed, the uterus should be examined for evidence of severe infection. Common findings include the presence of extensive necrosis within the endometrial cavity, with an accumulation of fibrinopurulent endometrial tissue on the surface, often most severe at the placental implantation site, with extension of necrosis down into the myometrium (endomyometritis). Thrombi may be present within the small, medium, and large vessels of the uterus. Careful examination and special Gram staining will often reveal the presence of bacteria, sometime in groups or colonies. Microscopic identification of spore-forming bacteria should alert the pathologist to the presence of a *Clostridium* necrotizing infection.

References

Belizán, J. M., & Villar, J. (1980). The relationship between calcium intake and edema-, proteinuria-, and hypertension-getosis: An hypothesis. *American Journal of Clinical Nutrition, 33*(10), 2202–2210.

Belizán, J. M., Villar, J., & Repke, J. (1988). The relationship between calcium intake and pregnancy-induced hypertension: Up-to-date evidence. *American Journal of Obstetrics and Gynecology, 158*(4), 898–902.

Canto, P., Canto-Cetina, T., Juarez-Velazquez, R., Rosas-Vargas, H., Rangel-Villalobos, H., Canizales-Quinteros, S., et al. (2008). Methylenetetrahydrofolate reductase c677t and glutathione s-transferase p1 a313g are associated with a reduced risk of preeclampsia in Maya-mestizo women. *Hypertension Research, 31*, 1015–1019.

Canto-Cetina, T., Canizales-Quinteros, S., de la Chesnaye, E., Coral-Vázquez, R., Méndez, J. P., & Canto, P. (2007). Analysis of C-850T and G-308A polymorphisms of the tumor necrosis factor-alpha gene in Maya-mestizo women with preeclampsia. *Hypertension in Pregnancy, 26*(3), 283–291.

Canto-Cetina, T., Coral-Vázquez, R. M., Rojano-Mejía, D., Godoy, S. P., Coronel, A., & Canto, P. (2017). Higher pre-pregnancy body mass index is a risk factor for developing preeclampsia in Maya-mestizo women: A cohort study. *Ethnicity & Health, 6*, 1–9. https://doi.org/10.1080/13557858.2017.1315367. [Epub ahead of print].

Carroli, G., Cuesta, C., Abalos, E., & Gulmezoglu, A. M. (2008). Epidemiology of postpartum haemorrhage: A systematic review. *Best Practice & Research Clinical Obstetrics and Gynaecology, 22*, 999–1012.

CDC. (2007). *Maternal mortality and related concepts*. Vital Health Statistics, Series 3, Number 33. February 2007.

Cheung, W. M., Hawkes, A., Ibish, S., & Weeks, A. D. (2011). The retained placenta: Historical and geographical rate variations. *Journal of Obstetrics and Gynaecology, 31*(1), 37–42. https://doi.org/10.3109/01443615.2010.531301

Cipolla, M. J., Zeeman, G. G., & Cunningham, F. G. (2014). Cerebrovascular pathophysiology in preeclampsia and eclampsia. In R. N. Taylor, J. M. Roberts, & F. G. Cunningham Lindheim (Eds.), *Chesley's hypertensive disorders in pregnancy* (4th ed., pp. 269–290). Amsterdam: Elsevier.

Creasy, R. K., Resnik, R., Iams, J. D., Lockwood, C. J., Moore, T. R., & Greene, M. F. (2014). *Creasy & Resnik's maternal-fetal medicine* (7th ed.). Philadelphia: Elsevier Saunders.

Cruz, J. R. (2007). Reduction of maternal mortality: The need for voluntary blood donors. *International Journal of Gynecology & Obstetrics, 98*, 291–293.

D'ıaz-Olgu'ın, L., Coral-V'azquez, R. M., Canto-Cetinac, T., Canizales-Quinterosd, S., Belem Ramírez-Regalado, B., et al. (2011). Endothelial nitric oxide synthase haplotypes are associated with preeclampsia in Maya mestizo women. *Disease Markers, 31*, 83–89. https://doi.org/10.3233/DMA-2011-0804

Dolea, C., AbouZahr, C., & Stein, C. (2003). *Global burden of maternal haemorrhage in the year 2000. Evidence and Information for Policy (EIP)*. Geneva: World Health Organization. Retrieved from http://www.who.int/healthinfo/statistics/bod_maternalhaemorrhage.pdf.

El Kady, A. A., Saleh, S., Gadalla, S., Fortney, J., & Bayoumi, H. (1989). Obstetric deaths in Menoufia governorate, Egypt. *British Journal of Obstetrics and Gynaecology, 96*, 9–14.

Firoz, T., Sanghvi, H., Merialdi, M., & von Dadelszen, P. (2011). Pre-eclampsia in low and middle income countries. *Best Practice & Research Clinical Obstetrics & Gynaecology, 25*(4), 537–548. https://doi.org/10.1016/j.bpobgyn.2011.04.002. Epub 2011 May 17.

Ghulmiyyah, L., & Sibai, B. (2012). Maternal mortality from preeclampsia/eclampsia. *Seminars in Perinatology, 36*(1), 56–59. https://doi.org/10.1053/j.semperi.2011.09.011

Guttmacher Institute. (2013). *Unintended pregnancy and induced abortion in Mexico*. Guttmacher Institute Fact Sheet. Retrieved from https://www.guttmacher.org/fact-sheet/unintended-pregnancy-and-induced-abortion-mexico.

Hussein, J., Walker, L. (2010). Puerperal sepsis in low- and middle-income settings. Past, present and future. In S. Kehoe, J. Neilson, J. Norman (Eds.), *Maternal and infant deaths: Chasing millennium development goals 4 and 5* (Royal College of Obstetricians and Gynaecologists Study Group, pp. 131–148). Cambridge: Cambridge University Press. doi: https://doi.org/10.1017/CBO9781107784758.011.

Ikechebelu, J. I., & Okoli, C. C. (2002). Review of eclampsia at the Nnamdi Azikiwe University teaching hospital, Nnewi (January 1996–December 2000). *Journal of Obstetrics & Gynaecology, 22*(3), 287–290.

Jegasothy, R. (2002). Sudden maternal deaths in Malaysia: A case report. *Journal of Obstetrics and Gynaecology Research, 28*(4), 186–193.

Karumanchi, S. A., Maynard, S. E., Stillman, I. E., Epstein, F. H., & Sukhatme, V. P. (2005). Preeclampsia: A renal perspective. *Kidney International, 67*(6), 2101–2113.

Kenny, L. C., McCrae, M. R., & Cunningham, F. G. (2014). Platelets, coagulation and the liver. In R. N. Taylor, J. M. Roberts, F. G. Cunningham, & M. D. Lindheimer (Eds.), *Chesley's hypertensive disorders in pregnancy* (4th ed., pp. 379–396). Amsterdam: Elsevier.

Khan, K. S., Wojdyla, D., Say, L., Gulmezoglu, A. M., & Van Look, P. F. A. (2006). WHO analysis of causes of maternal death: A systematic review. *The Lancet, 367*(9516), 1066–1074.

Khong, T. Y. (2008). The pathology of placenta accreta, a worldwide epidemic. *Journal of Clinical Pathology, 61*(12), 1243–1246. https://doi.org/10.1136/jcp.2008.055202

Lagro, M., Liche, A., Mumba, T., Ntebeka, R., & van Roosmalen, J. (2003). Postpartum health among rural Zambian women. *African Journal of Reproductive Health, 7*, 41–48.

Montufar-Rueda, C., Rodriguez, L., Jarquin, J. D., Barboza, A., Bustillo, M. C., Marin, F., et al. (2013). Severe postpartum hemorrhage from uterine atony: A multicentric study. *Journal of Pregnancy, 2013*, 525914. https://doi.org/10.1155/2013/525914

Müller-Deile, J., & Schiffer, M. (2011). Renal involvement in preeclampsia: Similarities to VEGF ablation therapy. *Journal of Pregnancy, 2011*, 176973. https://doi.org/10.1155/2011/176973. Retrieved from http://www.hindawi.com/journals/jp/2011/176973/.

Mutter, G. L., Prat, J., & Schwartz, D. A. (2011). The female reproductive system, the peritoneum and pregnancy. In R. Rubin, D. S. Strayer, & E. Rubin (Eds.), *Rubin's pathology. Clinicopathologic foundations of medicine* (6th ed., pp. 847–922). Philadelphia: Wolters Kluwer/Lippincott, Williams & Wilkins.

Nakimuli, A., Chazara, O., Byamugisha, J., Alison, M., Elliott, A. M., Kaleebu, P., Mirembe, F., et al. (2014). Pregnancy, parturition and preeclampsia in women of African ancestry. *American Journal of Obstetrics & Gynecology, 210*(6), 510–20.e1. Retrieved from http://www.ajog.org/article/S0002-9378(13)01989-3/fulltext.

Nandonde, K. (2013). *Fetal-maternal outcomes of abruptio placenta at Bugando Medical Centre*. Thesis, Master of Medicine degree in Obstetrics and Gynaecology. Catholic University of Health and Allied Sciences (CUHAS). Bugunda, Tanzania. Retrieved from http://www.bugando.ac.tz/theses/M.Sc.DissertationKEVINNANDONDE.pdf.

Onakewhor, J. U., & Gharoro, E. P. (2008). Changing trends in maternal mortality in a developing country. *Nigerian Journal of Clinical Practice, 11*(2), 111–120.

Onuh, S. O., & Aisien, A. O. (2004). Maternal and fetal outcome in eclamptic patients in Benin City, Nigeria. *Journal of Obstetrics & Gynaecology, 24*(7), 765–768.

Osungbade, K. O., & Ige, O. K. (2011). Public health perspectives of preeclampsia in developing countries: Implication for health system strengthening. *Journal of Pregnancy, 2011*, 481095. Retrieved from http://www.ncbi.nlm.nih.gov/pmc/articles/PMC3087154/.

Powe, C. E., Levine, R. J., & Karumanchi, A. (2011). Preeclampsia, a disease of the maternal endothelium. The role of antiangiogenic factors and implications for later cardiovascular disease. *Circulation, 123*, 2856–2869. Retrieved from http://circ.ahajournals.org/content/123/24/2856.full.

Rahman, M. H., Akhter, H. H., Khan Chowdhury, M. E., Yusuf, H. R., & Rochat, R. W. (2002). Obstetric deaths in Bangladesh, 1996–1997. *International Journal of Gynaecology and Obstetrics, 77*(2), 161–169.

Romero-Gutiérrez, G., Espitia-Vera, A., Ponce-Ponce de León, A. L., & Huerta-Vargas, L. F. (2007). Risk factors of maternal death in Mexico. *Birth, 34*(1), 21–25.

Sandoval-Carrillo, A., Aguilar-Duran, M., Vázquez-Alaniz, F., Castellanos-Juárez, F. X., Barraza-Salas, M., Sierra-Campos, E., et al. (2014). Polymorphisms in the GSTT1 and GSTM1 genes are associated with increased risk of preeclampsia in the Mexican mestizo population. *Genetics and Molecular Research, 13*(1), 2160–2165.

Sarwar, I., Abbasi, A. N., & Islam, A. (2006). Abruptio placentae and its complications at Ayub teaching hospital Abbottabad. *Journal of the Ayub Medical College Abbottabad, 18*(1), 27–31. Retrieved from http://ayubmed.edu.pk/JAMC/PAST/18-1/07Iram18-1.pdf.

Say, L., Chou, D., Gemmill, A., Tunçalp, Ö., Moller, A. B., & Daniels, J. (2014). Global causes of maternal death: A WHO systematic analysis. *Lancet Global Health, 2*(6), e323–e333. https://doi.org/10.1016/S2214-109X(14)70227-X

Schwartz, D. A. (2015a). Interface of epidemiology, anthropology and health care in maternal death prevention in resource-poor nations. In D. A. Schwartz (Ed.), *Maternal mortality: Risk factors, anthropological perspectives, prevalence in developing countries and preventive strategies for pregnancy-related death*. New York: Nova Science Publishers.

Schwartz, D. A. (2015b). The pathology of pregnancy. In D. S. Strayer & E. Rubin (Eds.), *Rubin's pathology. Clinicopathologic foundations of medicine* (7th ed., pp. 535–562). Philadelphia: Wolters Kluwer/Lippincott, Williams & Wilkins.

Schwartz, D. A. (2015c). Unsafe abortion: A persistent cause of maternal death and reproductive morbidity in resource-poor nations. In D. A. Schwartz (Ed.), *Maternal mortality: Risk factors, anthropological perspectives, prevalence in developing countries and preventive strategies for pregnancy-related death* (pp. 425–439). New York City: Nova Science Publishers.

Seale, A. C., Mwaniki, M., Newton, C. R., & Berkley, J. A. (2009). Maternal and early onset neonatal bacterial sepsis: Burden and strategies for prevention in sub-Saharan Africa. *Lancet Infectious Diseases, 9*(7), 248–238. https://doi.org/10.1016/S1473-3099(09)70172-0

Sebitloane, H. M., Moodley, J., & Esterhuizen, T. M. (2008). Prophylactic antibiotics for the prevention of postpartum infectious morbidity in women infected with human immunodeficiency virus: A randomized controlled trial. *American Journal of Obstetrics and Gynecology, 198*(2), 189.e1–6.

Singh, S., Prada, E., & Kestler, E. (2006). Induced abortion and unintended pregnancy in Guatemala. *International Perspectives on Sexual and Reproductive Health, 32*(3), 136–145. Retrieved from https://www.guttmacher.org/journals/ipsrh/2006/09/induced-abortion-and-unintended-pregnancy-guatemala.

Smith, J.R. Postpartum hemorrhage. (2016). *Medscape*. Retrieved March 1, 2016, from http://emedicine.medscape.com/article/275038-overview.

Stillman, I., & Karumanci, S. A. (2007). The glomerular injury of preeclampsia. *Journal of the American Society of Nephrology, 18*(8), 2281–2284. Retrieved from http://jasn.asnjournals.org/content/18/8/2281.full.

Tantbirojn, P., Crum, C. P., & Parast, M. M. (2008). Pathophysiology of placenta creta: The role of decidua and extravillous trophoblast. *Placenta, 29*(7), 639–645. https://doi.org/10.1016/j.placenta.2008.04.008

UNICEF. (2017). *Maternal mortality fell by almost half between 1990 and 2015*. Retrieved from https://data.unicef.org/topic/maternal-health/maternal-mortality/.

Valencia Villalvazo, E. Y., Canto-Cetina, T., Romero Arauz, J. F., Coral-Vázquez, R. M., Canizales-Quinteros, S., Coronel, A., et al. (2012). Analysis of polymorphisms in interleukin-10, interleukin-6, and interleukin-1 receptor antagonist in Mexican-mestizo women with pre-eclampsia. *Genetic Testing and Molecular Biomarkers, 16*(11), 1263–1269. https://doi.org/10.1089/gtmb.2012.0181

Weeks, A. D. (2008). The retained placenta. *Best Practice & Research Clinical Obstetrics & Gynaecology, 22*(6), 1103–1117. https://doi.org/10.1016/j.bpobgyn.2008.07.005. Epub 2008 Sep 14.

WHO. (2005). *The world health report 2005. Making every mother and child count*. Geneva: WHO. Retrieved from http://www.who.int/whr/2005/whr2005_en.pdf?ua=1.

WHO. (2007). *Maternal mortality in 2005: Estimates developed by WHO, UNICEF, UNFPA and the World Bank*. Geneva, Switzerland: WHO.

WHO. (2016). *Maternal mortality fact sheet*. Geneva: WHO. Retrieved from http://www.who.int/mediacentre/factsheets/fs348/en/.

WHO. (2017). *Global health observatory (GHO) data. Maternal mortality*. Geneva: WHO. Retrieved from http://www.who.int/gho/maternal_health/mortality/maternal_mortality_text/en/.

4 Speaking in Tongues: The Importance of Speaking Indigenous Languages in Maternal Health Care

Crystal Sheedy

4.1 Introduction

Speaking in tongues, academically referred to as glossolalia, references an individual that begins to speak an incomprehensible language. From an objective perspective, glossolalia is "speech-like utterances with an impoverished range of syllabic and rhythmic patterns and no systematic grammatical structure, often believed by the speaker to be a real but unknown language" (Colman 2009: 319). However, upon analysis of the speaker's utterances, the "unknown language" is unlike any natural language. Thus, to a listener that has never witnessed an individual speak in tongues, the listener may become confused and consider the speaker to be suffering from a fit of psychosis, which was a common conclusion that several scholars made on acts of glossolalia in the early- to mid-twentieth century (Goodman 1972). This conclusion has influenced outsiders' perspectives on groups of people that speak in tongues, in such that there is a stigma surrounding groups of people that engage in this practice (1972). However, from an insider perspective, to the speaker, speaking in tongues may be considered a divine language that brings an individual closer to deities or a creator that could bestow prophetic knowledge that guides the speaker and his or her community in a difficult time. Thus, there is deeper symbolic meaning attached to speaking in tongues.

I would like to begin with a metaphor, which I hope you will find fitting after you read this chapter. Acts of glossolalia can be considered similar to indigenous languages to a nonindigenous speaker. There may be sounds in an indigenous language that sound alien to a nonindigenous speaker, such as glottal stops in the Mayan languages of Mesoamerica or the "click" sounds in the Khoisan languages of Africa. To a nonspeaker, this may be disorienting and confusing, just as an outsider comes to find as he or she witnesses an act of glossolalia. Similar to speakers of glossolalia, there exists a dominant ideology that devalues indigenous languages to national languages, which influences a nonspeaker's view on indigenous peoples. Indigenous languages and cultural practices are labeled as backward, wrong, archaic, or, even worse, something that should be forgotten. Nevertheless, to indigenous peoples, just as practitioners of glossolalia, their maternal language is more than just language. This is

C. Sheedy, M.A., Ph.D.
Department of Anthropology, University at Albany-SUNY,
Albany, NY, USA

D. A. Schwartz (ed.), *Maternal Death and Pregnancy-Related Morbidity Among Indigenous Women of Mexico and Central America*, Global Maternal and Child Health: Medical, Anthropological, and Public Health Perspectives, https://doi.org/10.1007/978-3-319-71538-4_4

because intertwined to the words within indigenous languages are cultural metaphors that shed light into intricate ideologies that are full of deep symbolic meaning for native speakers.

In this chapter, I would like to speak to the importance of learning an indigenous language for workers in health care and nongovernmental organizations (NGOs) that work among populations of indigenous women within Mexico and Central America. Yet to do this, and because women's health is not an area that, as a cultural and linguistic anthropologist, I am well-versed in, I feel that I need to integrate my own experiences through ethnographic vignettes that I have had with the women that I work with in the Yucatán Peninsula of Mexico. For these vignettes, names have been changed to protect the anonymity of my participants. Furthermore, I feel that I need to first explain to you the process I underwent of learning an indigenous language to validate my stance on this issue. Second, I will provide a brief historical overview of indigenous languages throughout Mexico and Central America and their position in contemporary society using the sociolinguistic concept of markedness. Third, I will discuss the issues related to indigenous women's health care. This will lead into a final discussion about the importance of health-care workers and workers of NGOs learning indigenous languages. In this discussion, I will touch on the concept of cultural sensitivity related to indigenous women's health care, and I will explain several benefits to learning an indigenous language that not only empowers the worker or researcher but also native speakers of indigenous languages.

4.2 Learning Maya

Before I started to learn (Yucatec) Maya as an undergraduate student in 2005, my language instructor, professor, and mentor told me that if I chose to work among the Maya speakers of the Yucatán Peninsula of Mexico, I must learn their maternal language because most women are monolingual Maya speakers. He posed the question: How can an ethnographer rightfully build rapport and achieve an insider perspective of his or her participants' lives if he or she does not speak their maternal language? Convinced that I needed to learn Maya, we began our classes.

In one of my first classes, he told me that Maya, like other indigenous languages in the world, is a highly metaphorical language. Words may just be words to nonspeakers, but to native speakers, words can reveal a story. However, just understanding the word with its translation into a researcher's respective language will never reveal the full symbolic meanings within a word. In fact, as an outsider, you may never fully understand these deeper meanings, but the goal of the researcher is to try to draw this understanding for others to comprehend. Lacking the cultural knowledge and experience that my mentor had gained from years of ethnographic fieldwork, I took his word for it. However, I wondered if I would ever have a breakthrough like he experienced.

As I progressed through my language classes as an undergraduate, I never felt confident enough to speak the language to my mentor. I was afraid I was mispronouncing the glottal stops, or worse yet, I was worried that I had said one word, but meant to say another, which being a tonal language was easily done. My desire to learn and immerse myself in the language continued in my Master's degree program in 2009, where I was able to participate in the three levels of a (Yucatec) Maya language program. In the first level, I was introduced to native speakers and my field site of Xocén. I also conducted my first ethnographic fieldwork in Xocén after the program.

In my first field season, I conducted my work in Maya, and quite honestly, my fears were confirmed. I had the speaking repertoire of a toddler. I continually stumbled over proper conjugations, and I did mispronounce words. I was shocked anyone could understand me. There were days when I did not want to say anything. Although the time I spent there was fleeting, I did come to find that I bonded more closely with Maya women. These women also shared their fears of speaking Spanish to me. They were happy they could talk to me, and that I could understand them, in their maternal language.

Through the love and kindness of these women, they helped me to begin the process of learning their maternal language and teaching me how to become a Maya person.

This experience allowed me to have a second home and family to return to in my future years of ethnographic fieldwork. In the years leading up to my dissertation research, I spent many more summers in Xocén, strengthening both my connections to my female participants and language skills. However, before each trip, I was faced with the following anxiety: Did I forget Maya? Will my participants understand me? I know that I studied the language throughout the year. I even spoke to myself in Maya. Yet, I felt that I was not where I should be with the language. I still wondered if I would make the breakthrough my mentor had made all those years before me.

Then, on the eve of embarking on my journey to conduct the ethnographic fieldwork for my dissertation in 2016, I had not traveled to Xocén for a year, and I knew my language skills were rusty. Pushing fear aside, I boarded the plane to Mexico. At the end of a long day of traveling, I realized my language skills were still there. My participants understood me, but I knew I had a long way to go. As the months progressed, I saw my language skills shift. I am unsure if other language learners have this experience, but for me, I began to understand conversations more clearly. I did not merely translate into English. I started to think in Maya. Of course, this accomplishment did not come easily. Like my first field season, I started as a toddler in both the language and culture, and I grew into an adult with the guidance of my female participants. I met more women, and the initial hesitance they felt with their inadequacy in the Spanish language faded when they realized I, too, spoke and understood Maya. Their serious faces turned to smiles as language barriers were broken down, and I was invited into a world that I never dreamed I would gain access (Fig. 4.1).

I finally experienced my breakthrough with the language. In simple conversations I had or overhead women having with each other, I heard and understood the metaphors behind the words. Still a novice to both the language and culture, this allowed me to ask deeper questions about this figurative language. For example, one of my female participants, Neida, from a neighboring village was pregnant, and she had a craving to eat the cake that I had purchased for Benicio's birthday. However, he had not returned from work, and she needed to return to her village for an event. She asked her mother for a piece of the cake. Thus, her mother cut the cake and gave her a piece to satisfy this crav-

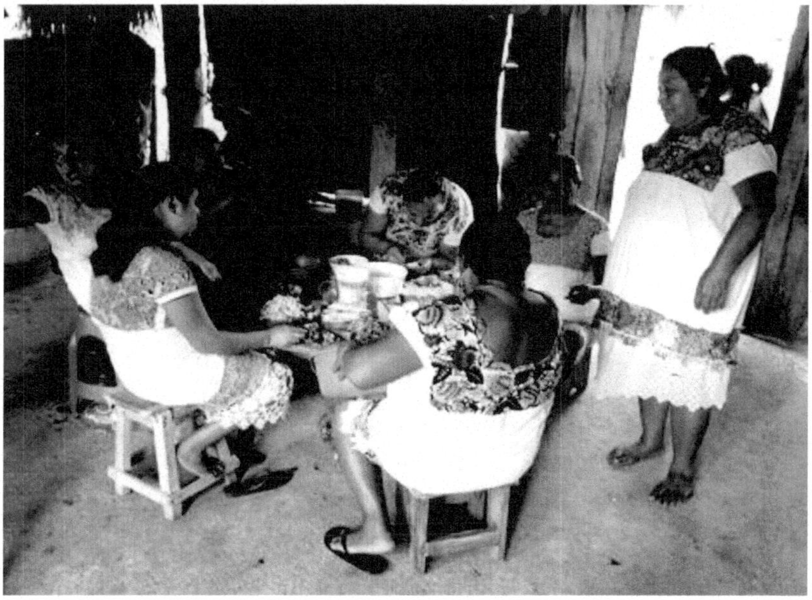

Fig. 4.1 Maya women preparing food for a ceremonial event

ing. I asked why they did not wait for Benicio to return to cut his birthday cake. Her mother replied that it is *k'eban*, or a sin, for pregnant women to not satisfy their cravings. Searching for the deeper meaning, I asked what would happen to Neida if she did not eat the cake. Her mother explained that when Neida gave birth to her child, her child's mouth would remain slightly open throughout his or her life because Neida did not eat what her child desired her to eat (i.e., her craving), when Neida was pregnant. Therefore, when a pregnant woman has a craving, it is not her craving per se. Instead, it is the craving of her unborn child. If a woman chooses to ignore her craving, her unborn child will go hungry. In this sense, after birth and through life, this child will always have his or her mouth slightly open to illustrate to everyone in the village that in the womb, his or her mother did not satisfy his or her hunger.

From my time in Xocén, I realized that my mentor had been correct. There was an entire world hidden in the words that my participants use, in which only time and perseverance with Maya allowed me to capture, an albeit incomplete, picture. As an ethnographer, I know that I will never achieve a complete insider understanding because I am not a native Maya person. I can only offer my interpretation. Thus, even after my dissertation fieldwork, I continue to hold the same inadequacies with my Maya language skills. I feel this is a burden a second language learner will always carry with them. However, I no longer consider this a hindrance, as this reminds me to be humble with the information that my participants have helped me to understand and to continue the dialogue that my participants and I have started with each other. In this sense, there are no experts, and, to quote an old adage, you never stop learning. Therefore, if an individual that seeks to help an indigenous group of peoples, whether through health care, cultural revitalization, and so forth, puts forth the time and effort into learning the respective group's maternal language, many benefits will arise, which I hope to address in the following pages. But before I do, in the next section, I will present a brief historical overview of indigenous languages throughout Mexico and Central America and their position in contemporary society.

4.3 Markedness and the Position of Indigenous Language in Society

Central America is composed of seven countries, Guatemala, Costa Rica, Nicaragua, Honduras, El Salvador, Panama, and Belize. Mexico is not generally considered to be part of Central America, although historically parts of Mexico were part of Mesoamerica. The dominant language of these countries, excluding Belize, is Spanish. In Belize, the dominant language is English because it had previously been an English colony. These countries have diverse populations within their boundaries all subsumed under a dominant language ideology that subordinates indigenous languages to the dominant language of the country. To give an example of the breadth of the linguistic diversity found within these countries, Mexico is home to 65 language families; the largest are Uto-Aztecan and Mayan (Pérez-Fernández 2011). Within these language families, there are mutually distinct languages; for instance, in the Mayan language family, there are 31 languages that span across the countries of Mexico, Belize, Honduras, and Guatemala (Coe 2005). The languages within this language family are incomprehensible to each other. A speaker of *Kaqchikel* Maya (a language within Guatemala) will not understand a speaker of (Yucatec) Maya (a language within Mexico). Furthermore, there are also dialects of the same language. For *Kaqchikel*, there are ten dialects of the language (McKenna Brown et al. 2006). Thus, although speakers of the languages within the family found within Central America and Mexico may be part of the same language family, the various language groups may not share the same cultural practices or beliefs. Yet, there is one commonality that the majority of these groups share; they are marked groups of people within the dominant discourses and ideologies of their countries. In this section, I will use markedness as a frame to deconstruct the position of indigenous peoples and their languages within Central America and Mexico.

Because indigenous populations within these countries share a history of colonization, they have been subjected to similar types of racialized discourses that mark them and work to situate them into a subordinate position in society. The concept of markedness is considered a binary opposition, in which one entity in the opposition is considered "more basic" and is utilized in "defining the nature of the opposition," while the other entity is "expressed as the absence of this defining feature[s]" (Foley 1997: 95). Markedness is inscribed on the bodies of individuals from a certain culture, and marked individuals typically have a racialized discourse ascribed to them that succinctly ties to a language ideology that positions the dominant languages of the country above the languages of indigenous populations (Urciuoli 1996). Racializing discourses are historically constructed and are "defined by a polarity between dominant and subordinate groups," where the subordinates have little control over their position (Urciuoli 1996: 15).

Although this is a gross overgeneralization, to extend across such a broad region, the unmarked groups were the colonizers. Today, they are the elites that have descended from the colonizers. In the dominant ideologies of the colonizers, they came from a position of power in the world (Escobar 2012; McMichael 2004). They believed their technology, cultural practices, religious beliefs, and languages to be superior in comparison to the primitive groups found within the world. With their power and dominance, they colonized areas and attempted to mold these regions of the world into the image of their home countries. They believed indigenous groups, or primitives, to be vestiges of the past that spoke in strange tongues, and these groups needed their souls to be saved and/or to be educated and enlightened to the proper way of life. Thus, indigenous peoples became the marked entity in this binary, where racialized discourses were attached to their bodies. If the marked persons wanted to be viewed as less marked, they would have to assimilate to the dominant culture and language, abandoning their presumably backward ways.

Although hundreds of years have passed since the time of colonization, these types of discourses are still rooted to the dominant ideologies in these countries that are perpetuated in each new generation. On a larger scale, governments still believe indigenous people's way of life as backward. Therefore, governments steadily work toward the assimilation and eradication of indigenous languages and cultures in their countries (Pérez Fernández 2011). Rooted into the dominant ideology of the country, these prejudices held against indigenous peoples seep its way into all sectors of society, in which relatively decent citizens find themselves holding these prejudices. For instance, while I was participating in the second level of the language program, I stayed with an upper-middle class family that lived in Mérida, the capital of Yucatán. Rosa, a divorced mother, lived in a house with her son and two daughters. Rosa's mother and father were of Maya descent. Rosa did not self-identify herself as *mestiza* or *maasewal*, which is an identity category typically considered of indigenous background (Loewe 2010). She identified herself as a Yucateca or, as mestizos viewed her, a *ts'ul*, which is an identity category associated with foreigners and elites (2010). She no longer spoke the Maya language, and she abandoned all cultural practices associated with Maya culture. She explained to me that as she was growing up, her parents told her that she should not speak Maya because if she did, then she would not be successful. She would be ascribed a marked identity. Thus, despite Rosa's Maya roots, she was brought up Yucateca.

This had drastic consequences for how she and her children viewed Mayas. For example, one weekend, Rosa, her daughter, and I went to a rodeo. Her daughter is part of a group of women who ride horses. They work to synchronize the movement of the horses into a dance. For this rodeo, her daughter was not selected to perform, which deeply upset her. In her place, another woman was selected. At the event, Rosa and her daughter commented on the sluggishness of one of the riders. After the rodeo, her daughter made a comment on the appearance of the slow rider. She said that she had terribly dark skin and ugly facial features. When Rosa asked if she was a Maya, her daughter responded that the woman was Maya. This sparked a racist conversation about how Mayas are inherently slow, dimwitted, and physically unappealing.

Prejudices such as these have powerful consequences to the way indigenous persons view themselves. Sadly, more often than not, indigenous persons internalize these racialized discourses, and they begin to believe the prejudices and stereotypes held against themselves, their culture, and their language. Indigenous parents desire to teach their children the dominant language because they do not feel that their native tongue will benefit them economically or socially, just as Rosa's parents. The reality is that these discourses, combined with other factors not discussed, do lead to the loss and eventual extinction of indigenous languages and cultural practices as indigenous peoples assimilate into the dominant culture. The marked bodies of indigenous peoples and these internalized racialized discourses act as a barrier for indigenous peoples to gain access to much needed resources to help support themselves and their families, such as government benefits, work, and health care. Another, more obvious, obstacle that indigenous populations confront is a language barrier. If an indigenous person speaks their maternal language or the dominant language of the country with an accent, this marks them as subordinate. Arguably, the most affected group is indigenous women because they are predominantly monolingual speakers of their native tongue (Pérez Fernández 2011). In the next section, I will discuss indigenous women's access to health care, whether state provided or by a NGO.

4.4 Indigenous Women's Access to Health Care

Imagine yourself as a monolingual speaker of an indigenous language, and an emergency comes up where you need to seek out medical care for yourself or a loved one. Traveling to the nearest city with a hospital, you are faced with a multitude of obstacles. Aside from finding the funds to pay for such a visit, the first, and most obvious barrier, is that you cannot speak the dominant language of the country. You can understand what someone says to you, but you struggle with responding to a Spanish or English speaker. However, you must find medical care. Thus, you contact a friend who owns a car or you collect the cab fare for a taxi to the city. Once in the city, you must either walk or take a collective van to the hospital. You decide to take a collective van to the hospital, but you do not know which van to take. The destinations are written on the windshield of each van, but you cannot read. You ask a few people on the sidewalk in broken Spanish or English, but you are met with stares of disgust. With perseverance, you eventually find your way to the hospital. However, once there, you ask the staff where you need to go for medical attention, and they do not understand you. You are asked to wait. You know that you may wait all day and never be seen because it's happened to you before. But if you are lucky to be admitted to see a doctor, the doctor will ask you what type of symptoms you have been experiencing. You may explain your symptoms, but the doctor seems to be more perturbed that you are speaking a broken language that is mixed with your native tongue than to actually care about finding the cure to your ailment. Thus, the doctor may make a quick diagnosis and offer you a prescription, but you know that you were prescribed the same regimen the last time you went to see the doctor, and it did not work. You try to voice your opinion, but the doctor does not want to listen to you, an indigenous person, who, they believe, is uneducated because you cannot speak the dominant language. Frustrated, you return to your village to share your experience with your friends and family, who know all too well that these are the common experiences that indigenous peoples have when faced with seeking help from the medical establishment and Spanish-speaking sources.

The experience described above happened to one of my female participants when she sought medical attention for her daughter, who was experiencing lower abdominal pain and irregular menstrual cycles. Rather than run medical tests for her daughter for this reoccurring issue, the doctor shooed her

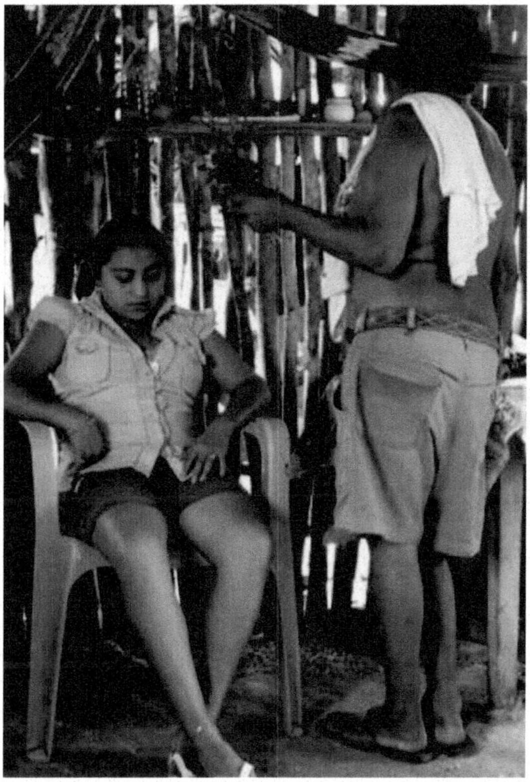

Fig. 4.2 A *jmeen* performing a ceremony on a young girl

and her daughter away by prescribing a quick fix of pain medication. This led them to seek alternative and culturally appropriate care from a *jmeen*, or male shaman (Fig. 4.2). Thankfully, the *jmeen*'s remedy worked in this situation, but similar to other indigenous groups in Central America and Mexico, this experience also fed into the cultural ideology that Western medicine and the individuals that work in health care do not understand them, do not want to understand them, and do not care about them or their well-being (Locklear et al. 2013). This section will explore indigenous women's access to health care within Central American and Mexico, whether provided by the state or a NGO.

In Central America and Mexico, indigenous women experience the most obstacles when trying to access health care. In contrast to their male counterparts, who may have received an education, speak some Spanish or English, and migrate for work, "indigenous women are often victims of extreme poverty, gender inequality, ethnic discrimination, and lack the financial resources and authority to seek prenatal and obstetric care" (Locklear et al. 2013: 38). Many indigenous women also express fear that the health-care workers will not understand them because they are monolingual. Furthermore, because of their marked identities, women believe they will be disrespected and have their opinions devalued by the workers. These beliefs can have devastating consequences. For example, similar to my female participants' experiences, they will look toward alternative medical treatments that are in congruence to their cultural belief systems from traditional specialists (Locklear et al. 2013). These treatments may never heal them. Another solution they may perceive as fit is that they will simply not get medical treatment, which ultimately could lead to a life that could have been saved if they could have accessed Western medical treatment.

Of course, not all health institutions are like this. In more recent years, organizations centered on women's health have been created to help reach the most impoverished groups of people in Central America and Mexico. For women's health, many of these types of organizations, for example, integrate traditional midwifery practices with Western medicine to provide the best possible treatment to their target populations. Groups such as *Wuqu' Kawoq*, or the Maya Health Alliance, illustrate this perfectly. *Wuqu' Kawoq* is located in Guatemala and was founded in 2007. Among many other medical services provided to their target populations, this organization's goals are to unite medicine, language, and culture as they reach some of the most impoverished populations in Guatemala. They believe that an individual "should not have to choose between [their] culture and [their] health," an individual "should be able to talk to [their] doctor in [their] own language," an individual's place of birth "should not determine if [they] live or die," an individual "should not feel locked out of [their] own health care system," and "everyone should have the highest quality health care" (wuqukawoq.org). With their expectations stated, they employ indigenous *Kaqchikel* staff and staff that knows how to speak the *Kaqchikel* language. From this, they integrate both culture and language into their outreach and services, which helps to promote pride in the language for its native speakers, as well as the preservation and revitalization of the *Kaqchikel* language (Tummons et al. 2011).

Some indigenous women are apprehensive to seek help from organizations that speak the dominant language of their respective country. *Wuqu' Kawoq* and other organizations that share similar goals that incorporate indigenous languages in their services allow these women to breathe a sigh of relief. Seeking health care from these organizations, these women know that they will be able to communicate their symptoms without a translator and be understood. An additional benefit to learning and speaking an indigenous language is that it initiates the process of workers in health care or among NGOs becoming more culturally attuned to the needs of their clientele as they begin to understand the various deeper metaphorical meanings behind the words. In the next section, I will discuss the importance of learning indigenous languages, and how this aids the worker in becoming more culturally sensitive.

4.5 The Importance of Learning an Indigenous Language

Cultural sensitivity is key when workers in health care or in a NGO try to access the most vulnerable group of the population, indigenous women. There can be many cultural mishaps performed by the best-intentioned workers. Although the first step may be learning an indigenous language to communicate with the desired population, this step leads into learning about cultural knowledge that is intertwined within the language itself. For instance, in my fieldwork, I spoke with my female participants about beliefs and practices involved in childbirth in the past versus the present. Almost unanimously the past description of childbirth took place within the home, where post-childbirth, a new mother had many restrictions placed upon her to protect both herself and her newborn. One of these restrictions included *mal de siete*, which are the first 7 days after childbirth. The deeper cultural knowledge behind these words is that it is a dangerous time for a mother and her newborn. Mother and child must be protected from *k'ak'aas iik'*, or evil wind, and a *k'ak'aas ba'al*, or a monster, that preyed upon the mother because of all the blood that had been lost in childbirth. Within the home of the new mother, a separate room was created out of *xa'an*, or a type of palm leaf, where she always had a fire lit to protect herself and her child from this evil wind and monster that wanted to kill her and her child. A deeper metaphorical meaning here lies with the use of fire—in their cultural belief system, men are considered fire, while women are considered darkness. In Xocén, it is believed that women should not sleep at night without a man present in their homes or, if they are married, in their hammocks. With a man present, there is said to have a fire lit in the darkness that monsters fear. Monsters will see this fire and run away. However, if just women were to sleep by themselves, because women are considered darkness, monsters will not be afraid, and they will attack the women. This could lead to a woman becoming sick and her eventual death, if she does not receive the proper ceremonies performed

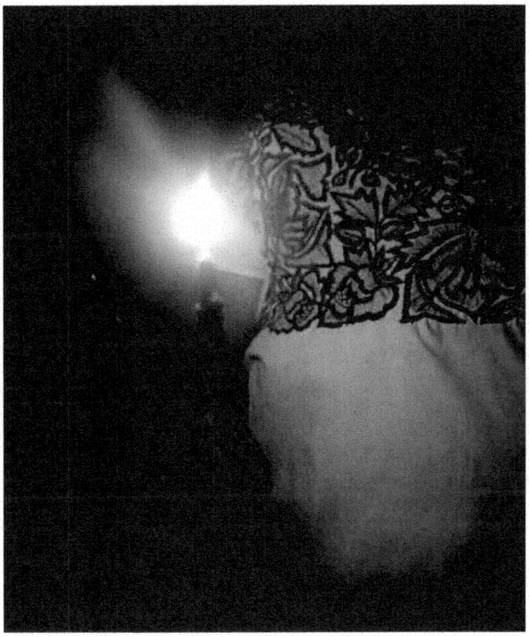

Fig. 4.3 A woman holding a candle

by a *jmeen* to heal her. Therefore, in this separately created room after childbirth, there is just mother and her child. Because of this, a fire, even if it's just a candle, must always be lit to protect her and her child from the monster (Fig. 4.3).

Younger mothers had a different experience than their mothers when they gave birth. Instead of giving birth within the home, they gave birth in a hospital. Although they had fear about giving birth in a hospital, younger mothers accept this change, now believing it to be safer and more sanitary. Nevertheless, they do not forget about the cultural restrictions that are embedded within their cultural ideology. For instance, Paloma gave birth to her children in a hospital, as did Rosaria. Both had no problems with their deliveries in the hospital. They also said that although nothing happened to them during their *mal de siete*, they, as well as other women in the village, spoke of a recent new mother that saw the monster in the hospital room. The new mother did not have a candle lit in her room with her. The hospital staff did not approve of this behavior. Paloma and Rosaria said that relatives of this woman stated she became delirious, and when she closed and opened her eyes, a black mass was standing over her. The hospital staff did not know what to do for this woman, and they would not release the new mother from the hospital. Her condition worsened, even though her family contested that she be released for a ceremony to be performed to save her life. All my female participants knew that an evil wind that could have been sent by a bad *jmeen* brought the monster. The new mother's condition was so severe that Western medicine would not heal her; she needed to have a ceremony performed by a *jmeen*. With this ceremony, her life could be saved. This woman, unfortunately, never was released from the hospital, and she passed away. They said that this woman died because of this monster, but her life could have been saved if the hospital staff understood and were culturally sensitive to their beliefs.

Much of the hospital staff in Valladolid, the closest developed city to Xocén, does not speak Maya, and even if they did have knowledge of the language, the symbolic meanings attached to certain concepts may not have been properly interpreted. The purpose of this chapter was to illustrate the importance in learning an indigenous language to help give much needed access to healthcare services to one of the most vulnerable populations in the world. With learning an indigenous language also comes cultural sensitivity. If a health-care worker takes the time to immerse himself or herself in the language and the culture of an indigenous group, this will reveal the deeper meanings behind the language. Naturally, there are always variations in cultural knowledge. For instance, my participants in Xocén share different perspectives about *mal de siete* than do individuals living in Chemax, another town in the Yucatán Peninsula, where they believe that if a baby is born at 7 months, the child will more than likely die before his or her 17th birthday because he or she did not complete the full gestational period of 9 months (M. Kanxoc Kumul, personal communication, December 10, 2016). Although there will always be these cultural nuances, the key is to try to learn the language.

Learning, speaking, and using an indigenous language not only helps bridge the gap between cultural worlds and allows the workers in health care or NGOs to do a more comprehensive job, but it also, and more importantly, empowers indigenous women. The most obvious benefit of workers speaking an indigenous language is having accessible health care and other programs with workers who can understand their target populations. This will hopefully help to minimize the number of deaths caused by treatable illnesses among indigenous women. Another benefit comes in the form of indigenous women hearing their maternal language spoken by someone in a perceived position of power. This helps indigenous women take pride in their maternal language because, being marked citizens of their countries, they have felt disenfranchised about their maternal language and culture throughout their lives. Utilizing indigenous languages within outreach, such as in videos and flyers, also helps to inspire pride in speakers of indigenous languages. This, in turn, helps to promote the preservation and revitalization of the language. In my experiences, even if a woman is illiterate, when she sees that there is literature written in her maternal language, it gives her a sense of pride. For example, one of my female participants said to fellow students in a class that was learning how to read and write in Maya for a program, *Xooknen Tin Weetel*, or Read With Me, based in Xocén and other surrounding villages in Yucatán, that having her maternal language in written form puts her maternal language on the same level as Spanish. When the instructor asked what she meant, she elaborated and said that the only language that she has ever seen in written form is Spanish, whether that is in her children's schoolbooks or on storefronts. She said having a modern writing system for Maya gives her pride in her language, and she hopes it will inspire the younger generations within indigenous communities to take pride in their language and cultural heritage. She, like the other participants in the program, does not want their maternal language to disappear.

Conclusions

Learning to speak an indigenous language is no small task for anyone. At first, you might think that you are speaking in tongues, but with hard work and perseverance, you will learn the language. After that, a new cultural world will begin to reveal itself to you. With this newly learned cultural knowledge, you will become more culturally sensitive. With this, you will be able to watch the language barriers that existed between you and the indigenous woman you are trying to help crumble as stern looks turn into smiles and sighs of relief. In time, you will achieve your own breakthrough, and you will be providing help, attention, and health-care services to individuals that need it the most. Although learning an indigenous language may only be the first step to achieving this reality, in my experiences, you must always remember to be humble with the cultural knowledge that follows and to never assume you are an expert and understand all the meanings behind the words. Never stop learning. Never stop searching for the deeper metaphorical meanings. Despite being marked citizens in their respective countries and the prejudices held against them by larger society, your most valuable teachers are the indigenous women you seek to help. They are waiting for you to start the conversation.

Acknowledgments This dissertation research was graciously funded by the Fulbright-Hays Doctoral Dissertation Research Abroad fellowship and by the Firebird Foundation for Anthropological Research.

References

Coe, M. D. (2005). *The Maya* (7th ed.). New York City: Thames and Hudson.

Colman, A. M. (2009). Glossolalia. In *Oxford dictionary of psychology* (3rd ed., p. 319). New York City: Oxford University Press.

Escboar, A. (2012). *Encountering development: The making and unmaking of the third world* (2nd ed.). Princeton, NJ: Princeton University Press.

Foley, W. A. (1997). *Anthropological linguistics: An introduction*. Malden, MA: Blackwell Publishers.

Goodman, F. D. (1972). *Speaking in tongues: A cross-cultural study of glossolalia*. Eugene, OR: Wipf and Stock Publishers.

Locklear, T. D., Perez, A., Caceres, A., & Mahady, G. B. (2013). Women's health in Central America: The complexity of issues and the need to focus on indigenous healthcare. *Current Women's Health Reviews, 9*, 30–40.

Loewe, R. (2010). *Maya or mestizo?: Nationalism, modernity, and its discontents*. Toronto: University of Toronto.

McKenna Brown, R., Maxwell, J. M., & Little, W. E. (2006). *La ütz awäch?: Introduction to Kaqchikel Maya language*. Austin, TX: University of Texas Press.

McMichael, P. (2004). *Development and social change: A global perspective*. Thousand Oaks, CA: Sage.

Pérez-Fernández, J. M. (2011). Linguistic rights of indigenous peoples in states of Latin America. *Intercultural Human Rights Literature Review, 6*, 379–425.

Tummons, E., Henderson, R., & Rohloff, P. (2011). "So that we don't lose words": Reconstructing a Kaqchikel medical lexicon. In S. M. Coronel-Molina & J. H. McDowell (Eds.), *Proceedings of the first symposium on teaching indigenous languages of Latin America* (pp. 127–135). Bloomington, IN: Center for Latin American and Caribbean Studies.

Urciuoli, B. (1996). *Exposing prejudice: Puerto Rican experiences of language, race, and class*. Boulder, CO: Westview Press.

Wuqu' Kawoq/Maya Health Alliance. (n.d.). *Who we are*. Retrieved February 10, 2017, from http://www.wuqukawoq.org/who-we-are.

5 Maternal Health in Central America: The Role of Medicinal Plants in the Pregnancy-Related Health and Well-Being of Indigenous Women in Central America

Tracie D. Locklear, Gail B. Mahady, Joanna Michel, Jillian De Gezelle, Angela I. Calderón, Jordan Alma McLeroy, Jesse Alice McLeroy, Brian J. Doyle, Esperanza J. Carcache de Blanco, Kelvin Nuñez Martinez, and Alice L. Perez

---

T. D. Locklear, Ph.D. (✉)
Outcomes Research and Assessment Group, Duke Clinical Research Institute, Duke University, Durham, NC, USA

G. B. Mahady, Ph.D.
Pharmacy Practice, College of Pharmacy, University of Illinois at Chicago, Chicago, IL, USA

J. Michel, Ph.D.
Department of Medical Education, University of Illinois at Chicago, College of Medicine, Chicago, IL, USA

J. De Gezelle, Ph.D.
Department of Plant & Microbial Biology, North Carolina State University, Raleigh, NC, USA

A. I. Calderón, Ph.D. · J. A. McLeroy · J. A. McLeroy
Department of Drug Discovery and Development, Harrison School of Pharmacy, Auburn University, Auburn, AL, USA

B. J. Doyle, Ph.D.
Departments of Biology and Biochemistry, Alma College, Alma, MI, USA

E. J. Carcache de Blanco, Ph.D.
Pharmacy Practice and Science, Medicinal Chemistry and Pharmacognosy, Ohio State University, Columbus, OH, USA

K. N. Martinez, R.Ph.
Universidad Nacional Autonoma de Nicaragua,
Leon, Nicaragua

A. L. Perez, Ph.D.
School of Chemistry and Natural Products Research Center, University of Costa Rica, San José, Costa Rica

D. A. Schwartz (ed.), *Maternal Death and Pregnancy-Related Morbidity Among Indigenous Women of Mexico and Central America*, Global Maternal and Child Health: Medical, Anthropological, and Public Health Perspectives, https://doi.org/10.1007/978-3-319-71538-4_5

5.1 Introduction

Over the past 20 years, Central America (CA) has made considerable progress in improving the health status of its populations. However, in some countries, the overall health status remains below average with poor outcomes concentrated geographically among the poor and Indigenous populations. Indigenous people make up the second largest ethnic population in CA, yet they have less access to healthcare, and funding for initiatives to improve maternal health among them is scarce. Much of the population in Central America lives below the poverty line, disproportionately concentrated among Indigenous groups (Pan American Health Organization 2012). Although Central America is experiencing economic growth and moving toward universal healthcare, inequities in healthcare are still prevalent (de Andrade et al. 2015).

The purpose of the World Health Organization's Millennial Developmental Goal (MDG) target 5.A was to reduce maternal mortality by 75% (World Health Organization 2015b). Since 1990, the maternal mortality rates for Central America have declined by approximately 33% (Pan American Health Organization 2012). Maternal care and deliveries by skilled birth attendants (SBAs) are still inequitable across rich and poor populations, with only about 60% of women in the poorest quintile receiving care by SBAs compared to nearly universal care in the wealthiest quintile (Restrepo-Mendez et al. 2015). Underlying causes of maternal mortality include the hypertensive disorders (e.g., preeclampsia, eclampsia), obstetric postpartum hemorrhages, infections, and abortive outcomes (World Health Organization 2015b). Complications from hypertension and postpartum hemorrhaging are the leading causes of maternal death in Central America (The World Bank 2016a).

Poverty, gender inequality, Indigenous status, education, and rural residence with limited access to transportation and healthcare are formidable barriers to improving maternal health outcomes and reaching the MDG 5 target (Price and Asgary 2011). These maternal health risk factors are pervasive and present even during family planning. For example, poverty is a strong determinant of contraceptive use and, by extension, the number of children a woman will bear. Women between the ages of 15 and 49 living in extreme poverty average 4.7 births over the course of their lifetimes compared to 2.7 for wealthy women (The World Bank 2006). Women from poor households are less likely to consistently use contraceptives even when they do not wish to have more children (Hall et al. 2014). Gender inequality also affects women's decisions regarding family planning (Speizer et al. 2005; Berti et al. 2015; Arps 2009).

In this chapter, we discuss the use of herbal therapies in the treatment of maternal health conditions by Indigenous, Ladino, and other groups in Central America and review supporting biological evidence for their reported use.

5.2 Methodology

A literature search was conducted during the months January through November of 2016 using the databases PubMed, Google Scholar, SciFinder, as well as gray literature (e.g., websites, books, etc.) to identify any mention of plants used for women's health in countries in Central America. Search terms included "botanicals, nutraceuticals, natural medicine, medicinal plants, herbal medicine, traditional medicine, ethnopharmacology, herbs, alternative medicine, complementary and alternative medicine" and "women's health, natural birth, midwifery, childbirth, female health, menstruation, reproductive health, postpartum, fertility, traditional birth attendants" with the terms "Latin America, Central America." All available literature was collected and reviewed. For PubMed and SciFinder searches, the conjunctions "AND" and "OR" were used with the preceding terms. For Google Scholar searches, phrases comprised of the search terms were used. PubMed, Google Scholar, SciFinder, and Napralert databases were searched to obtain biological information related to the ethnomedical uses. The plant genus and species name were used as search terms. Plantlist.org was used to validate scientific plant names.

5.3 Background and Ethnic Populations by Country

5.3.1 Belize

Located in the northeast part of Central America, Belize is bordered to the north by Mexico and on the west and south by Guatemala. By population, Belize is the smallest country in Central America, with a population estimated at approximately 353,000 with 55% under the age of 25 (Central Intelligence Agency 2016). The people of Belize are ethnically and culturally diverse, with 48.7% and 24.9% being Mestizos and Creoles, respectively (Pan American Health Organization 2012). The Indigenous Maya make up only about 10.6% and the *Garífuna* (*Garinagu*) about 6.1% of the population. Other minorities include the East Indians and some Asians (Pan American Health Organization 2012).

5.3.2 Costa Rica

Costa Rica is bordered by Nicaragua to the north, the Pacific Ocean to the west, the Caribbean Sea to the east, and Panamá to the southeast. The country is divided into 7 provinces consisting of 81 municipalities and 421 districts that are inhabited by over 4.8 million people (Instituto Nacional de Estadística y Censos de Costa Rica (INEC) 2016). Only 2.4% of Costa Rica's population identified themselves as Indigenous (Instituto Nacional de Estadística y Censos 2013). Eight Indigenous *pueblos* are found in Costa Rica: *Bribri*, *Cabécar*, *Terrabas*, *Brunca*, *Ngöbes*, *Malecu*, *Chorotega*, and *Huetar*. The groups reside in 24 Indian reservations, better known to them as territories. The higher populated territories are found in the south of the country (Instituto Nacional de Estadística y Censos de Costa Rica (INEC) 2016).

5.3.3 El Salvador

El Salvador is the smallest and most densely populated country in the Americas with an area of just over 21,000 km^2. El Salvador has 307 km of coastline on the Pacific Ocean and shares borders with Guatemala to the west and Honduras to the north. Of El Salvador's population of 6.4 million, 84% of Salvadorans are literate. Thirty-eight percent of Salvadorans live below the poverty line (Pan American Health Organization 2012). The population is comprised primarily of mestizos, 86%, and whites, 13%. Indigenous peoples of the *Nahua-Pipil*, *Lenca*, *Cacaopera* (*Kakawiru*), and *Chorti* ethnicities are reported to be between 1 and 10% of the population (United Nations 2013; Ayala 2012).

5.3.4 Guatemala

Guatemala is located in northern Central America and is bordered by Mexico to the north, the Pacific Ocean to the west, the Caribbean Sea and Belize to the east, and El Salvador and Honduras to the southeast (Villar Anleu 1998). The country is divided into 23 departments (or states) and 330 municipalities that are inhabited by over 15 million people (Central Intelligence Agency 2016; Michel et al.

2016). Guatemala is one of the poorest countries in Central America, with more than 50% of people living in poverty, 23% of which live in extreme poverty (Central Intelligence Agency 2016; Pan American Health Organization 2012). This country is the most ethnically diverse in Central America; over 20 groups of ethnolinguistic Maya origin make up near 40% of the population, majority of which are living in poverty (Central Intelligence Agency 2016; Pan American Health Organization 2012).

5.3.5 Honduras

Honduras is bordered by neighboring countries Guatemala to the northwest, Nicaragua to the southeast, El Salvador to the southwest, and otherwise surrounded by the Gulf of Fonseca and the Caribbean Sea (Central Intelligence Agency 2016). More than eight million people live in Honduras, almost equally dispersed between rural and urban areas (World Data Atlas 2015a). Honduras is the second poorest country in Central America, behind Nicaragua, with a national GDP of 20.6 billion US dollars. Over 16% of the population live on less than $1.25 US dollars a day (World Data Atlas 2015a). Rural, Indigenous people are among the poorest in Honduras, with 71% living below the poverty line (The World Bank 2016b). Women are particularly vulnerable; according to the International Fund for Agricultural Development (IFAD), households headed by females average 30% less income than male-headed households (International Fund for Agricultural Development 2014).

Although there is no official census, it is estimated that Indigenous and Afro-Honduran population make up 10% of the nation's population; the other 90% are considered Mestizo[1] (United Nation's International Children's Emergency Fund 2011). Seven Indigenous groups live in Honduras: the Maya *Chortí*, *Lenca*, *Pech*, *Tolupanes*, *Nahua*, *Miskito*, and *Tawahka* people. Additionally, there are two Afro-Honduran groups: the *Garífuna* people, on the Atlantic coast, and an English-speaking population, living in the Islas de la Bahía (United Nation's International Children's Emergency Fund 2011). Among the Indigenous groups, the *Lenca* are the largest in Honduras and 84% of the population live in poverty (The World Bank 2006; Price and Asgary 2011). Most of the Indigenous groups in Honduras rely economically on fishing, hunting, and subsistence agriculture (United Nation's International Children's Emergency Fund 2011; International Work Group for Indigenous Affairs 2015; Lentz et al. 1998; Álvarez 2015; Smith-Oka 2012; Lentz 1993). Additionally, many live in remote isolated areas such as Gracias a Dios, Olancho, and Yoro departments without all-weather roads, making travel difficult in the best of weather conditions (International Work Group for Indigenous Affairs 2015; Lentz et al. 1998; United Nation's International Children's Emergency Fund 2011; Álvarez 2015). The *Garífuna* (Black Carib) are an Afro-Amerindian population descended from African and native Carib people from the Caribbean (Merrill 1995). The *Garífuna* self-identify as Indigenous, yet their Indigenous status is contested (Álvarez 2015). A majority of the *Garífuna* live on the Atlantic coast of Honduras (United Nation's International Children's Emergency Fund 2011; Álvarez 2015). Little information is available regarding the people of Islas de la Bahia other than that they are mixed with European and African ancestry and speak a mixture of Creole and English (United Nation's International Children's Emergency Fund 2011; Álvarez 2015).

[1] Mestizo means mixed ethnicity of Indigenous and European heritage but culturally Ladino (Latino). The term Mestizo is used throughout CA, whereas the term Ladino is used mostly in Guatemala and Honduras.

5.3.6 Nicaragua

Nicaragua has a population of about six million people with over a million concentrated in the capital city, Managua (World Data Atlas 2015b). Nicaragua is the poorest country in Central America with a national GDP of 12.69 billion US dollars and 8.5% of population living on less than 1.25 US dollars a day (The World Bank 2016b; Forbes 2015). The largest population of the poor in Nicaragua live in rural areas. As of 2016, Nicaragua's age structure was distributed as follows: over 30% of the population is under the age of 15, over 60% between ages 15 and 64 years, and below 5% of the population is over 65 years (United Nations Statistics Division 2016).

The major ethnic groups in Nicaragua include Creole, *Garífuna*, *Rama*, *Mayangna*, and *Miskitu*. The *Rama*, *Mayangna*, and *Miskitu* are Indigenous peoples, while the Creole and *Garífuna* are ethnically mixed. The Indigenous populations of Nicaragua live mainly in communities on the Caribbean or Atlantic Coast. These groups are separated from the majority mestizo population in the rest of Nicaragua by a mountain range that partitions the west and the east of the country (World Directory of Minorities and Indigenous Peoples 2008).

The *Miskitu* (*Miskito*) people are the largest and arguably the most historically influential Indigenous group of Nicaragua. The rural *Miskitu* live mostly in small villages in the savannah areas between the RAAN (Región Autónoma del Atlántico Norte, or North Caribbean Coast Autonomous Region, formerly the North Atlantic Autonomous Region), an autonomous region of Nicaragua, and the Honduras border. Many live in urban areas such as Bilwi, the capital of the RAAN. The *Miskitu* have their own language, close religious ties, and leadership development programs that have enabled the emergence of a new generation of confident and more vocal *Miskitu* leaders (World Directory of Minorities and Indigenous Peoples 2008). The *Rama* mostly settled on Rama Cay, a small densely populated island in the Bay of Bluefields. Another very small group live in communities spread along the Caribbean Coast of the RAAS (World Directory of Minorities and Indigenous Peoples 2008). Their lifestyle is based on traditional knowledge of the flora, fauna, and marine life of the region (World Directory of Minorities and Indigenous Peoples 2008). The *Mayagna* people inhabit the Atlantic Coast. This group was previously known as *Sumu* because they refused to be absorbed into the then expanding *Miskito* "empire." In recent years, the group has rejected the term Sumu and has become officially referred to as *Mayagna*. They number approximately 8000 persons divided in three subgroups—the *Tawahka*, the *Panamáka*, and the *Ulwa*. All of them speak dialects of the common *Mayagna* language and live in villages along the rivers of the RAAN (World Directory of Minorities and Indigenous Peoples 2008).

The Creole population have mixed background from African and European descent who settled the Caribbean Coast beginning in the mid-seventeenth century. They are largely located in the towns of Bluefields, Corn Island, and Pearl Lagoon, though smaller communities live in the rural areas of the Monkey Point. In the RAAN, Creoles make up a small but influential minority group, particularly in Bilwi. Most Creoles in urban areas are bilingual and have high levels of education. However, Creoles in the rural communities of the RAAS towns are poor and less educated (World Directory of Minorities and Indigenous Peoples 2008). The *Garífuna* have also mixed background, although from African and Indigenous descent. This mostly bilingual group lives mainly in the Pearl Lagoon basin and Bluefields (World Directory of Minorities and Indigenous Peoples 2008).

5.3.7 Panamá

The Republic of Panamá is known for its tropical forests, ecological diversity, and, of course, the Panamá Canal. It is bordered by Costa Rica to the west, Colombia (in South America) to the southeast, the Caribbean Sea to the north, and the Pacific Ocean to the south. In 2014, the estimated population was just under four million, of which 49.8% were women (Instituto Nacional de Estadística y Censo 2016). Although accurate numbers of Indigenous women are difficult to obtain, Panamá has three *comarcas* or administrative districts whose population largely consists of Indigenous ethnic groups. The estimated population of women in the *Guna* (*Kuna*), *Emberá*, and *Ngöbe comarcas* in total as of 2014 was 124,900, about 3.2% of Panamá's total population (Instituto Nacional de Estadística y Censo 2016).

5.4 Maternal Health and Mortality in Central America

The main causes of maternal mortality include the hypertensive diseases of pregnancy (e.g., preeclampsia, eclampsia), obstetric hemorrhage, infections, and abortive outcomes (World Health Organization 2015b; The World Bank 2016a). While the prevalence for these disorders specifically in Central America is unknown, in Latin America unsafe abortions account for 17% of all maternal deaths (Grimes et al. 2006). Serious complications can arise from unsafe abortions and include incomplete abortion, hemorrhage, infection, poisoning, damage to internal organs, and maternal death (Schwartz 2015). In countries like El Salvador where all abortions regardless of the circumstance are illegal, extreme antiabortion legislation has had a negative impact on women's health, forcing women to turn to clandestine methods that are unsafe, ineffective, or both (Grimes et al. 2006; Boland and Katzive 2008). A study of physicians' perspectives on medication abortion in Latin America revealed that socioeconomic status was an important factor in determining which methods of abortion women are likely to use. Women of lower socioeconomic status were more likely to use traditional methods, such as botanicals (Espinoza et al. 2004).

5.4.1 Belize

In Belize, the maternal mortality ratio is moderately high at 41.1 per 100,000 live births, and the reported total fertility rate is three children born per each woman (Boyer et al. 2001; Pan American Health Organization and World Health Organization 2015). The Indigenous women in Belize are at a higher risk for morbidity and mortality due to poor access to modern healthcare clinics and hospitals, as well as physicians (Parham et al. 2011).

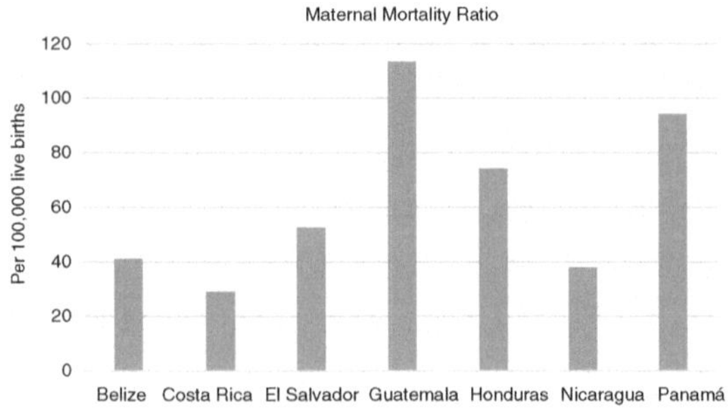

Fig. 5.1 Maternal mortality ratios across countries in Central America (Source: Data adapted from Pan American Health Organization and World Health Organization (2015) (Fig. 5.1). Health Indicators. Limited data on El Salvador and Nicaragua. Data for Belize, Costa Rica, El Salvador, Nicaragua from 2014; Honduras 2013; Panamá from 2015; and Guatemala from 2010)

5.4.2 Costa Rica

Compared to other countries in Central America, Costa Rica is a model country, insomuch as it is politically stable, has a relatively high standard of living, and promotes education to all citizens (Central Intelligence Agency 2016; Pan American Health Organization 2012). It is among the countries with the longest life expectancy in the world and has a maternal mortality ratio of 29 per 100,000 live births (Pan American Health Organization and World Health Organization 2015). Over the last two decades, the country has focused on improving healthcare, particularly reproductive health and prenatal care. In Costa Rica, social security is recognized as a constitutional right (Carro-Hernández and Espinoza-Carr 2016). The article No. 73 of the Constitution provides for the establishment of a social security system for the benefit of all workers, to protect them against illness, disabilities, maternity, old age, and death. Article 177 also establishes the universalization of social security and the protection of the family throughout sickness and maternity. An important aspect of their national regulations is the creation of the Costa Rican Social Security Fund (Caja Costarricense de Seguro Social (CCSS)), as an autonomous public office in direct coordination with the Ministry of Health and the Costa Rican central government. This institution was created in 1941. The CCSS is responsible for the administration of public health services and pension contributions and distribution. Costa Rica has one of the two most integrated health systems in the region, after Cuba, and the only one fully managed by social insurance; 85.5% of the Costa Rican population is insured. It also includes two types of protection: a "contributory" one for direct insured persons who contribute to the system, as well as for pensioners and dependents of both groups, and a "noncontributory" one for the uninsured that covers people in poverty and their families. In Costa Rica, life expectancy at birth is 78.8 years according to the World Economic Forum's Global Competitiveness Report 2016–2017 (Schwab 2016).

5.4.3 El Salvador

El Salvador is one of the few countries that has met the MDG 5 calling for a reduction in maternal mortality. The reported maternal mortality ratio in El Salvador was 52.6 per 100,000 live births in 2014, a significant drop from the estimated 157 per 100,000 live births in 1990 (Pan American Health Organization and World Health Organization 2015). Maternal deaths in El Salvador have dropped considerably over the last decade from 71.2 per 100,000 live births in 2006 to 60 per 100,000 live births in 2014 (Lozano et al. 2011; Pan American Health Organization and World Health Organization 2015). This success is likely due to several factors. The government of El Salvador has worked to reduce maternal mortality by providing geographically accessible free health services and training healthcare personnel. Contraceptive use among women has also increased, from 47% in 1988 to 73% in 2008, and fertility rates have fallen from 6.3 children per woman in the mid-1970s to 2.5 children in the period of 2003–2008. Approximately 75% of women obtained contraception from government health services. Still, 56% of pregnancies are unintended (Sedgh et al. 2014).

5.4.4 Guatemala

Maternal mortality in Guatemala is considered high at 113.4 per 100,000 live births as reported in 2013 (Pan American Health Organization and World Health Organization 2015). Guatemala has a very high individual expected birth rate as well, as less than 50% of married women use any form of contraception. Among the Indigenous Mayan women in the rural areas, maternal mortality is estimated to be more than twice the national average (Locklear et al. 2013; United Nations Population Fund 2005; World Health Organization 2005). Most Mayan populations live in remote rural areas with poor access to modern healthcare facilities or physicians (Pan American Health Organization 2004, 2012; United Nations Population Fund 2005; World Health Organization 2007). Mayan women have at least five births during their lifetime, which is the highest number of any country in Central America. The higher birth rates are influenced by religious beliefs that do not support family planning, as well as sociopolitical concerns for the survival of the Indigenous people (Hughes 2004).

Guatemala has a very active Mayan traditional medicine system, and community outreach programs have been successful in providing maternal care to the Maya women in the Guatemalan highlands, by integrating traditional Guatemalan medicine with Western medicine (World Bank 2012; Pan American Health Organization 2012; Bhatt 2012). For example, the Ministry of Health has an ongoing initiative to support the integration of traditional and conventional healing practices by forming a committee of healers representing each of the ethnolinguistic groups in Guatemala (Bhatt 2012). However, despite these new initiatives, high maternal mortality rates still persist.

5.4.5 Honduras

Between 1990 and 2015, the maternal mortality ratio in Honduras had fallen by more than half, from 272 to 74 per 100,000 live births in 2010 (Pan American Health Organization and World Health Organization 2015). Rural, Indigenous Honduran communities are impacted more heavily by maternal death than the average Honduran population. For example, in 1990, the maternal mortality ratio (MMR) in Gracias de Dios area, a predominantly Indigenous community, was 878 per 100,000 live births compared to 272 for the general population in the same year (Arps 2009; World Health Organization 2015b). Poverty, race, rural habitation, gender inequality, and education are all key contributing factors to the MMR in less advantaged, rural, Indigenous communities (Price and Asgary 2011; Arps 2009).

5.4.6 Nicaragua

According to the World Bank, 97% of pregnant women in Nicaragua receive some kind of prenatal care (World Data Atlas 2015b). However, the level of maternal mortality remains high in Nicaragua, particularly in disadvantaged groups, such as rural and Indigenous populations, the poor, adolescents, and women with low levels of schooling. In 2015, 150 maternal deaths occurred per 100,000 live births; 70% occurred in rural areas (World Data Atlas 2015b). Approximately one-third of maternal deaths in the country occur in adolescents (Foundation for Sustainable Development 2016).

5.4.7 Panamá

The maternal mortality ratio for the general population in Panamá was 94 per 100,000 live births in 2015 (World Health Organization 2015a). The Indigenous people of Panamá tend to have less favorable healthcare statistics, although data are difficult to locate. For example, maternal mortality rates were 24.9 per 100,000 live births for Panamá overall in 2010 but 246 per 100,000 in the *Kuna* population in the same year (Pan American Health Organization 2012).

5.5 Barriers to Seeking Medical Care and the Role of Midwives/Traditional Birth Attendants in Central America

Women who choose to give birth at home cite cost, location, transportation, gender inequality, and cultural reasons for their decision (Price and Asgary 2011; Arps 2009). Women in extreme poverty are two-thirds more likely to deliver at home and half as likely to have births attended by a midwife or traditional birth attendants (TBA) (The World Bank 2006). In the rural highlands of Guatemala where most of the Maya live, approximately 70% of all childbirths occur at home, around 75% of which are attended by midwives, and roughly 5% occurring without any medical assistance (Hughes 2004; Schooley et al. 2009; Bhatt 2012; United Nations Population Fund 2005). The people living in Panamá's Indigenous *comarcas* are similarly disadvantaged in terms of access to medical care. In 2009, only 61.3% of child deliveries in the *Ngöbe comarca* region received professional care versus 96% general population (Pan American Health Organization 2012).

Consistent with the three-delay model of factors which contribute to preventing women from accessing reproductive healthcare, rural isolation and transportation also pose a significant barrier to seeking medical treatment during childbirth for women throughout rural areas of Central America. Transportation to the nearest clinic may take several hours by foot or over water (Josyula et al. 2015; Cohen 1982). In such cases, families must charter a plane or motor-powered canoe and have enough money to pay for the treatment, food, and lodging for the woman and those that travel with her (Arps 2009). Once reaching the clinic, women reported having to wait in long lines, despite having traveled for hours to reach their destination; limited hours, staff, and resources; unwillingness to help in emergencies; disparaging treatment by clinic staff; high cost; refusal to come attend birth; and poor quality of care (Price and Asgary 2011; Arps 2009).

Gender inequality is another barrier to seeking treatment for some women. For example, decisions to seek medical care are often decided by the woman's family, particularly her husband, as she may not have income of her own and thus lacks economic advantage (Pan American Health Organization 2012; Arps 2009; Speizer et al. 2005). In Panamá, it has been reported that only 37% of women participate in economic activity (Pan American Health Organization 2012).

5.5.1 Traditional Birth Attendants (TBA)

In Central America, midwives or traditional birth attendants (TBAs) are referred to by various names depending on the country and source. The *Nahua* call them "paternas," while they are referred to as "comadronas" by the Maya in Guatemala (Smith-Oka 2012; Walsh 2006). A traditional birth attendant (TBA) is defined by the World Health Organization (WHO) as "a person who assists the mother during childbirth and initially acquired her skills by delivering babies herself or through apprenticeship to other Traditional Birth Attendants" (World Health Organization 1992). In general, most rural communities in Central America have at least one TBA (Montenegro and Stephens 2006; Smith-Oka 2012; Walsh 2006). Midwives or TBAs provide primary healthcare to women throughout all phases of maternity. This person, in most cases female, will visit the mother several times prior to the due date and massage her belly to position the baby and make sure the mother is following customs with regard to work, diet, etc. (Cohen 1982; Lefeber and Voorhoeve 1998). On the day of delivery, the midwife is present throughout labor, assists with delivery, and participates in neonatal and postpartum care (Lefeber and Voorhoeve 1998; Cohen 1982; Walsh 2006).

TBAs typically receive some sort of professional training or certification, but not all countries train midwives. Regardless of formal training, TBAs believe themselves to have been called to their profession and feel their gift is spiritual (Low et al. 2006; Walsh 2006). In Nicaragua, training for TBAs has been discontinued, yet roughly 55% of women in rural areas still give birth at home. The other 45% are more likely to be attended by a professional or auxiliary nurse in areas where a doctor is not available (Foundation for Sustainable Development 2016; Harvey et al. 2007). The Ministry of Health (MOH) in Belize offers a TBA training program, which consists of 6 months of midwifery instruction to women with some midwifery skills and includes program that includes the assessment of biomedically defined risk factors, and promotes the referral of high-risk pregnancies (World Health Organization 2012; Boyer et al. 2001). After the training program, the MOH recognizes these women as certified birth attendants (CBAs). CBAs are trained to assist in normal pregnancies; however, high-risk deliveries are transported to facilities that can safely manage these complicated deliveries (World Health Organization 2012). The training and certification of birth attendants began as an attempt to reduce maternal mortality rates in poor, developing countries, where childbirth outside of medical facilities is common practice. The training was started in 1957 but fell out of favor in the late 1990s. While training still exists in Belize, fewer midwives are practicing and available in the more rural areas where the majority of Indigenous women live (Boyer et al. 2001).

5.6 Traditional Medicinal Plants Used for Maternal Health in Central America

Traditional medicines, including plant medicines, are fundamental to 80% of the world's population (World Health Organization 1983). In the remote, impoverished areas of Central America, women rely heavily on the use of plant medicines for health. In Nicaragua, for example, 30–100% of Indigenous groups use herbs for different healthcare applications (Barrett 1995). Reports of medicinal plant use in Costa Rica are scarce; however, traditional medicine use is high in Honduras, Panamá, and Guatemala. In the Highlands of Guatemala, particularly, Maya women are the initial healthcare providers for their children, husbands, and other family members. They are viewed as the primary healers in their society, and as such, they assess the symptoms and determine how to proceed with medicinal plant treatments or when to seek medical help from the community healer or nearest clinic (Hughes 2004; Michel et al. 2006, 2012; Schooley et al. 2009; United Nations Population Fund 2005).

Commonly, herbal medicines are prepared as teas, decoctions, or infusions and taken orally; plants may also be steamed, smoked, or used as essential oils (Giron et al. 1991; Lentz 1993; Zamora-Martinez and de Pascual Pola 1992; Cohen 1982). After childbirth, for example, herbal baths may be employed to clean the birth canal after delivery (Lefeber and Voorhoeve 1998).

Plants reviewed in this chapter were commonly used for aiding fertility, contraception, abortion, pain associated with childbirth, preventing miscarriages and postpartum bleeding, morning sickness, inducing labor, expelling the placenta, and lactation. Table 5.1 shows the number of plants reported for each of these uses.

Table 5.1 Reported uses of medicinal plants for maternal health

Use	No. of plants reported
Pain associated with childbirth	27
Prevention of miscarriage and postpartum hemorrhage	32
Morning sickness and nausea	10
Expedite labor	20
Post-childbirth (e.g., expel the placenta)	29
Contraception/abortive	39
Lactation	10
Fertility	7
Unspecified (e.g., "childbirth")	34

Table 5.2 Plants reported used in two or more countries

Scientific name	Use	Countries reporting similar use
Hyptis verticillata Jacq.	Abortifacient	Nicaragua, Honduras
Jatropha curcas L.	Birth control	Honduras, El Salvador
Bursera simaruba (L.) Sarg.	Contraceptive; antiemetic; lactation; postpartum pain	None
Cassia grandis L.	Abortifacient; increase lactation	Costa Rica, Nicaragua
Cecropia peltata L.	Ease pain during childbirth	Guatemala, Belize, Honduras
Cedrela odorata L.	Prevent miscarriage; induce labor; stop postpartum hemorrhaging	Honduras, Nicaragua
Cinnamomum verum J.Presl.	Abortifacient; morning sickness; abdominal pain; lactation	None
Citrus aurantiifolia (Christm.) Swingle	Morning sickness; facilitate contractions during labor; expel the placenta after birth; abortifacient	None
Hibiscus rosa-sinensis L.	Postpartum hemorrhaging; infertility; speed up labor; fallen uterus; prevention of miscarriage; size of uterus	Panamá, Guatemala, Belize
Hyptis verticillata Jacq.	Conception; abortifacient; expel the placenta; amenorrhea	Guatemala, Belize, Nicaragua
Jatropha curcas L.	Abortifacient	Nicaragua, El Salvador, Honduras
Lippia graveolens Kunth.	Abortifacient; control bleeding; postpartum abdominal pain	None
Neurolaena lobata (L.) R. Br. Ex Cass	Contraception; abortifacient; labor pain; delayed menstruation; weaning; menopause	Guatemala, Belize, Costa Rica
Matricaria sp.	Facilitate and accelerate delivery	Costa Rica, Honduras
Mimosa pudica L.	Abortifacient; uterine fibroids	Guatemala, Belize, Honduras
Momordica charantia L.	Abortifacient; dysmenorrhea; amenorrhea; delayed menstruation; contraception; labor pain; postpartum treatment; menopause	Nicaragua, Honduras, Guatemala, Belize, Panamá
Ocimum campechianum Mill.	Regulate menstruation; prevent miscarriage; abdominal pain; facilitate contractions during labor; control abdominal pain postpartum	Honduras, Panamá, Guatemala, Belize
Persea americana Mill.	Postpartum hemorrhage; dysmenorrhea; contraception; emmenagogue; expel the placenta; abdominal pain	Honduras, Panamá, El Salvador, Guatemala, Belize
Pimenta dioica (L.) Merr	Abdominal pain during pregnancy; facilitate childbirth	None
Ruta chalepensis (L.)	Postpartum hemorrhage; abortifacient	None
Sida rhombifolia L.	Reduce labor pains; accelerate labor; expel the placenta; postpartum treatment; difficult childbirth	Panamá, Guatemala
Theobroma cacao L.	Facilitate childbirth; abortive before 6 months of pregnancy	None

"None" means plant species use was reported in more than one country but not used for the same or even similar purpose

Twenty-two plants were used across ethnically diverse groups in more than one country (Table 5.2). Only 15 plants were used for similar maternal health-related issues.

Table 5.3 lists a total of 166 medicinal plants used for maternal health by Central American women from various ethnic groups for contraception and during pregnancy, delivery, and postnatal care. It includes the biological activity where available. In general, most of the botanicals used in Central America for the treatment of women's reproductive health have not been systematically documented or even tested for safety and possible efficacy. Considering that a large portion of the female population, particularly in

Table 5.3 Traditional plants used across Central America for maternal health issues

Country	Scientific name	Family name	Vernacular name	Illness or use	Part of plant used	Biological activity	Ethnic group	References
Guatemala/ Belize	*Acalypha aristata* Kunth. [syn. *A. arvensis* Poepp.]	Euphorbiaceae	Yerba cancer, yerba de Cancer	Menstrual cramps, postpartum infections	Leaf	–	Q'eqchi Maya	De Gezelle (2014) and Michel et al. (2006, 2007, 2012)
Panamá	*Acalypha hispida* Burm. f.	Euphorbiaceae	Mis bonnu'guid	Facilitate childbirth	Flower	–	Kuna	Gupta et al. (1993), Onocha et al. (2011), and Ohigashi et al. (1985)
El Salvador	*Agave vivipara* var. *letonae* (F.W.Taylor ex Trel.) P.I.Forst.	Asparagaceae	Henequén	Abortifacient	Fresh leaves	–	–	González Ayala (1994)
Panamá	*Amaranthus caudatus* L.	Amaranthaceae	Ikui kinnid	Unspecified use by pregnant women	Root	–	Kuna	Gupta et al. (1993)
El Salvador	*Ambrosia peruviana* Willd.	Asteraceae	Altamisa	Abortifacient	Inflorescence	–	–	González Ayala (1994)
Panamá	*Anthurium* sp.	Araceae	Uer'uer guabin'guid dummat	Reduce size of the uterus	Flower	–	Kuna	Gupta et al. (1993) and Der Marderosian et al. (1976)
Panamá	*Aphelandra aurantiaca* (Scheidw.) Lindl.	Acanthaceae	–	Pre-birth	Whole plant	–	Ngöbe	Joly et al. (1987) and Caballero-George and Gupta (2011)
Panamá	*Aphelandra sinclairiana* Nees.	Acanthaceae	–	Antiemetic during pregnancy	Stem	–	Ngöbe	Joly et al. (1987)
Guatemala/ Belize	*Arachnothryx stachyoidea* (Donn. Sm.) Borhidi.[syn. *Rondeletia stachyoidea* Donn. Smith]	Rubiaceae	Kandel che	Reposition womb, insomnia	Leaf	Ethanol extracts of the leaves weakly bound to the serotonin receptors in vitro (Michel et al. 2007)	Q'eqchi Maya	De Gezelle (2014) and Michel et al. (2006, 2007, 2012)
Costa Rica	*Argemone mexicana* L.	Papaveraceae	Cardosanto amarillo	Postpartum hemorrhaging	Flower	–	–	Sarkis and Campos (1985)

Panamá	*Aristolochia* sp.	Aristolochiaceae	–	Female disorders, menstrual pain, contraceptive	–	Anti-inflammatory activity: *A. trilobata* leaves, chloroform extracts, 100, 300, and 1000 μg doses, reduction of croton oil-induced ear edema in mice by 52, 61, and 92% (Sosa et al. 2002). Antispasmolytic activity: *A. constricta* stems, hexane extract, 0.03 and 0.1 mg/mL, contracted guinea pig ileum by 47.1 ± 5.4% and 5.7 ± 1.5% in ECI-induced contraction (Zhang et al. 2008). Antifertility activity: *Aristolochia indica* root, 95% ethanol extract, 1.0 g dose, 3/10 rats pregnant vs. vehicle group with 9/10 rats pregnant (Che et al. 1984). Abortifacient effect: 3 chromatographic fractions of *Aristolochia indica*, chloroform extract, 40, 60, and 35 mg/kg of body weight, minimum effective doses reached 100% interceptive effect in fractions I, II, and III (Pakrashi and Chakrabarty, 1977). Analgesic effect: *Aristolochia tagala*, petroleum ether, ethanolic, and chloroform extracts, decreased reaction time to pain induced by hot plate method (Sundari et al. 2001)	–	Lans (2007), Sosa et al. (2002), Zhang et al. (2008), Nortier et al. (2000), Che et al. (1984), Pakrashi and Chakrabarty (1977), and Sundari et al. (2001)
Panamá	*Artemisia absinthium* L.	Asteraceae	–	Fertility regulator	–	–	–	Lans (2007) and Parra et al. (2000)
Honduras	*Asclepias curassavica* L.	Apocynaceae	Viborán	Morning sickness; conception; hemorrhage	Root	Latex exhibits strong thrombin-like activity (Shivaprasad et al. 2009)	Ladino (non-Indigenous)	Ticktin and Dalle (2005) and Shivaprasad et al. (2009)
Panamá	*Begonia semiovata* Liebm.	Begoniaceae	–	Women's ailments	Whole plant	–	Ngöbe	Joly et al. (1990)
Costa Rica	*Borago officinalis* L.	Boraginaceae	Borraja	Increase breast milk	Leaf	–	–	Sarkis and Campos (1985)

(continued)

Table 5.3 (continued)

Country	Scientific name	Family name	Vernacular name	Illness or use	Part of plant used	Biological activity	Ethnic group	References
Panamá	*Bursera simaruba* (L.) Sarg.	Burseraceae	Cholo pelao	Contraceptive	Stem, bark	–	Naso	Gupta et al. (2005), Centro de Investigaciones Farmacognósticas de la Flora Panameña (2004), Cepleanu et al. (1994), and Feng et al. (1962)
Honduras	*Bursera simaruba* (L.) Sarg.	Burseraceae	Indio desnudo, sorsorká, almacigo, Indian peeled, Indian skin, quiote, Indian naked, and jiñocuabe	Strengthen the blood in pregnant women; used to control vomiting and clean after childbirth; postpartum abdominal pain; lactation; swelling	Bark, sap	Oral administrations of hexane extract of *B. simaruba* (78 mg/kg) have been shown to reduce carrageenan-induced paw edema by as much as 83% after 3 h, with effects that last 7 h. This effect was comparable to the positive control phenylbutazone (80 mg/kg) (Carretero et al. 2008). Similar anti-inflammatory results were reported previously (Noguera et al. 2004). Anti-hemorrhagic activity has also been reported (Salas Estrada, 1993)	Paya/Pech, Ladino (non-Indigenous)	Ticktin and Dalle (2005), House et al. (1995), Lentz (1993), Lentz et al. (1998), Carretero et al. 2008), Noguera et al. (2004), and Salas Estrada (1993)
Costa Rica	*Bursera simaruba* (L.) Sarg.	Burseraceae	Jiñote/jiñocuave	Postpartum hemorrhage	Bark	–	–	Sarkis and Campos (1985)
Honduras	*Byrsonima crassifolia* L. Kunth.	Malpighiaceae	Nanche	Miscarriage; hemorrhage	Bark	–	Ladino (non-Indigenous)	Ticktin and Dalle (2005)
Panamá	*Carludovica palmata* Ruiz. & Pav.	Cyclanthaceae	Naiuar	Prevent complications during childbirth	Inflorescence	–	Kuna	Gupta et al. (1993)
El Salvador	*Cassia grandis* L.	Fabaceae	Carao	Abortifacient	Ripe fruit	–	–	González Ayala (1994)
Costa Rica	*Cassia grandis* L.	Fabaceae	Carao/sandal	Increase breast milk	Fruit	–	–	Sarkis and Campos (1985)
Nicaragua	*Cassia grandis* L.	Fabaceae	Bucut, canafistula, carague, and santal	Increase breast milk production	Fruit, pulp, pods	–	Not reported	Sosa-Gomez (1998)
Guatemala/Belize	*Cecropia peltata* L.	Cecropiaceae	Guarumo, aq'l, po'jor	Expel the placenta, lower womb pain, insomnia, increase labor contractions	Leaf	Ethanol extracts bound to the serotonin receptors in vitro (Michel et al. 2007) Phytochemical analysis shows the presence of chlorogenic acid and isoorientin (Costa et al. 2011; Valdes et al. 2011)	Q'eqchi Maya	De Gezelle (2014), Michel et al. (2006, 2007, 2012), Costa et al. (2011), and Valdes et al. (2011)

Honduras	*Cecropia peltata* L.	Cecropiaceae	Guarumo	Ease pain during childbirth	Flower buds	–	Paya/Pech, Ladino (non-Indigenous)	Ticktin and Dalle (2005) and Lentz (1993)
Honduras	*Cedrela odorata* L.	Meliaceae	Cedro real	Prevent miscarriage; speed contractions during labor; stop postpartum hemorrhaging; cause abortion of fetus	Bark	–	Ladino (non-Indigenous); Rama	Ticktin and Dalle (2005)
El Salvador	*Cestrum nocturnum* L.	Annonaceae	Palo hediondo	Abortifacient	Fresh leaves and flowers	–	–	González Ayala (1994)
Panamá	*Chrysothemis friedrichsthaliana* (Hanst.) H.E. Moore	Gesneriaceae	Boduö, bodo	Menstruation	Root	–	Ngöbe, Naso	Centro de Investigaciones Farmacognósticas de la Flora Panameña (2004)
Panamá	*Chrysothemis pulchella* (Donn ex Sims) Decne.	Gesneriaceae	Pirguak kinnid	Facilitate childbirth, widen birth canal	Flower	–	Kuna	Gupta et al. (1993) and Coe et al. (2012)
Honduras	*Cinnamomum verum* J. Presl	Lauraceae	Canela	Decrease swelling in legs and ankles; treat morning sickness; treat abdominal pain; calm nervousness during labor; increase lactation	Bark	–	Ladino (non-Indigenous)	Ticktin and Dalle (2005)
El Salvador	*Cinnamomum verum* J.Presl.	Lauraceae	Canela (cinnamon)	Abortifacient	Dried bark	–	–	González Ayala (1994)
Guatemala/ Belize	*Cissampelos tropaeolifolia* DC.	Menispermaceae	Bejuco de ombligo, xch'up el	Release of the placenta, induce labor, speed up prolonged labor	Leaf	Ethanol leaf extracts bound to the serotonin receptors (Michel et al. 2007); a 95% ethanol extract was antispasmodic and relaxed the uterus in rats, alkaloids such as warifteine, methyl-warifteine, berberine, hayatin, and hayatidin found in other species of the genus (Semwal et al. 2014)	Q'eqchi Maya	De Gezelle (2014), Michel et al. (2006, 2007, 2012), and Semwal et al. (2014)
El Salvador	*Citrus aurantiifolia* (Christm.) Swingle	Rutaceae	Limón (lime)	Abortifacient	Fresh root	Causes distortion and inflammation of cells in the ovaries, uterus, and vagina	Corroborated use by Rama ethnic people of Nicaragua (Coe, 2008)	González Ayala (1994) and Coe (2008)

(continued)

Table 5.3 (continued)

Country	Scientific name	Family name	Vernacular name	Illness or use	Part of plant used	Biological activity	Ethnic group	References
Honduras	*Citrus aurantium* L.	Rutaceae	Naranjo agrio	Treat morning sickness; speed contractions during labor; expel the placenta after birth; stop postpartum hemorrhaging; cause abortion of fetus	Leaf	None reported from *C. aurantium*, but the juice of *C. limon* has been shown to have an anticoagulant effect in vivo (Riaz et al. 2014)	Ladino (non-Indigenous)	Ticktin and Dalle (2005) and Riaz et al. (2014)
Honduras	*Citrus aurantiifolia (Christm.) Swingle*	Rutaceae	Limón (lime)	Treat morning sickness; speed contractions during labor; expel the placenta after birth	Root	–	Ladino (non-Indigenous)	Ticktin and Dalle (2005)
Panamá	*Clavija* sp.	Theophrastaceae	–	Women's ailments	Leaf	Antifungal (anti-yeast) activity: *Clavija nutans*, ethanol extract, 500 μg/mL, active against *Candida albicans* (Marques et al. 2013)	Ngöbe	Joly et al. (1990) and Marques et al. (2013)
Guatemala/ Belize	*Clidemia crenulata* Gleason	Melastomataceae	Teelom pim	Female contraceptive	Leaf, stem, root	–	Q'eqchi Maya	De Gezelle (2014) and Michel et al. (2006, 2007, 2012)
Guatemala/ Belize	*Clidemia petiolaris* (Schltdl. & Cham.) Schltdl. ex Triana	Melastomataceae	Xa bol q'een	Postpartum hemorrhaging, fertility regulation, blood clots	Leaf	–	Q'eqchi Maya	De Gezelle (2014) and Michel et al. (2006, 2007, 2012)
Guatemala/ Belize	*Clidemia setosa* (Triana) Gleason	Melastomataceae	Ixq q'een	Fertility regulation, promote fertility in females, male contraceptive	Leaf	–	Q'eqchi Maya	De Gezelle (2014) and Michel et al. (2006, 2007, 2012)
Panamá	*Cochliostema odoratissimum* Lem.	Commelinaceae	Tira	Regulate menstruation	Leaf	–	Ngöbe	Joly et al. (1987)
Honduras	*Cocos nucifera* L.	Arecaceae	Coco	Miscarriage; hemorrhage	Root, fruit	–	Ladino (non-Indigenous)	Ticktin and Dalle (2005)
Costa Rica	*Coffea* sp.	Rubiaceae	Café; coffee	Postpartum hemorrhaging, can cause miscarriage	Leaf	–	–	Sarkis and Campos (1985)
Honduras	*Coix lacryma-jobi* L.	Poaceae	Lágrima de San Pedro	Contractions	Seed	–	Ladino (non-Indigenous)	Ticktin and Dalle (2005)

Panamá	*Columnea sanguinolenta* (Oerst.) Hanst.	Gesneriaceae	Dakodluko	Dysmenorrhea	Stem and leaf	–	Naso	Gupta et al. (2005)
Panamá	*Costus pulverulentus* C. Presl.	Costaceae	–	Facilitate childbirth, calms post-birth pain	Stem	Antinociceptive effect (moderate): *Costus pulverulentus* stem, ethanol extract, 50, 100, and 200 mg/kg, acetic acid-induced writhing test, formalin test, hot plate test, and tail flick test in mice (Alonso-Castro et al. 2016)	Ngöbe	Centro de Investigaciones Farmacognósticas de la Flora Panameña (2004), Alonso-Castro et al. (2016), and Joly et al. (1987)
Panamá	*Costus villosissimus* Jacq.	Costaceae	Caña de mico, cañaagria	Calms post-birth pain, childbirth	Stem	–	Ngöbe, Mestizo	Joly et al. (1987) and Centro de Investigaciones Farmacognósticas de la Flora Panameña (2004)
Panamá	*Cuatresia exiguiflora* (D'Arcy) Hunz.	Solanaceae	–	Postpartum birth	Stem	–	Naso	Gupta et al. (2005)
Costa Rica	*Cupressus* sp.	Cupressaceae	Ciprés	Postpartum hemorrhaging	Seed	–	–	Sarkis and Campos (1985)
El Salvador	*Cupressus lusitanica* Mill.	Cupressaceae	Ciprés	Abortifacient	Fresh bark and stem	–	–	González Ayala (1994)
Panamá	*Cyclanthus bipartitus* Poit. ex A.Rich.	Cyclanthaceae	Nibar	Avoid enlargement of the uterus	Flower	–	Kuna	Gupta et al. (1993)
Panamá	*Cyperus luzulae* (L.) Retz.	Cyperaceae	Pina	Prevent complications during childbirth	Whole plant	–	Kuna, Mestizo	Gupta et al. (1993), Centro de Investigaciones Farmacognósticas de la Flora Panameña (2004), and Gupta et al. (1996)
Panamá	*Desmodium axillare* (Sw.) D.C.	Leguminosae	Muma	Facilitate childbirth, postpartum aid to expel the placenta	Stem	–	Ngöbe	Centro de Investigaciones Farmacognósticas de la Flora Panameña (2004 and Caballero-George and Gupta (2011)
El Salvador	*Dioscorea alata* L.	Dioscoreaceae	Ñame (yam)	Abortifacient	Fresh tuber	–	–	González Ayala (1994)
Guatemala/ Belize	*Dioscorea bartlettii* Morton	Dioscoreaceae	Cocolmeca, wild yam, xch'up ixim. k'otz	Contraceptive, infertility, prevention of miscarriage	Rhizome, stem	Extracts of the rhizome contain diosgenin and have estrogenic effects when taken orally (Hidgon et al. 2001)	Q'eqchi Maya	De Gezelle (2014), Michel et al. (2006, 2007, 2012), and Higdon et al. (2001)
Panamá	*Dracontium dressleri* Croat.	Araceae	Igar, kausis sapi, naibe naba sannuar	Facilitate childbirth	Fruit	–	Kuna	Gupta et al. (1993)

(continued)

Table 5.3 (continued)

Country	Scientific name	Family name	Vernacular name	Illness or use	Part of plant used	Biological activity	Ethnic group	References
Panamá	*Drymonia multiflora* (Oerst. Ex Hanst.) Wiehler	Gesneriaceae	–	Breast pain	Whole plant	–	Naso	Caballero-George and Gupta (2011)
El Salvador	*Dysphania ambrosioides* (L.) Mosyakin & Clemants	Amaranthaceae	Epasote	Abortifacient	Fresh whole plant	–	–	González Ayala (1994)
Panamá	*Equisetum bogotense* H.B.K.	Equisetaceae	Cola de caballo, hierba de la plata	Uterine hemostatic (stop bleeding)	Whole plant	–	Kuna, Emberá, Ngöbe	Gupta et al. (1979) and Bussmann et al. (2011)
El Salvador	*Eryngium foetidum* L.	Apiaceae	Acapate	Abortifacient	Fresh leaves	–	–	González Ayala (1994)
El Salvador	*Fernaldia pandurata* (A.DC.) Woodson	Apocynaceae	Loroco	Abortifacient	Fresh leaf and flower	–	–	González Ayala (1994)
Honduras	*Ficus insipida* Willd.	Moraceae	Higo	Used for drying the umbilical cord after childbirth	Leaf, stem, bark, latex	–	Paya/Pech	House et al. (1995) and Lentz (1993)
Panamá	*Genipa americana* L.	Rubiaceae	Sabdor	Regulate fetus growth, weakness in girls	Leaf	–	Kuna	Gupta et al. (1993) and Nakanishi et al. (1965)
Panamá	*Gnaphalium domingense* Lam.	Asteraceae	–	Menstruation		–	Mestizo	Centro de Investigaciones Farmacognósticas de la Flora Panameña (2004)
El Salvador	*Hamelia patens* Jacq.	Rubiaceae	Chichipince	Abortifacient	Fresh leaves	–	–	González Ayala (1994)
Panamá	*Hamelia patens var. glabra* Oerst.	Rubiaceae	Uvero	Postpartum relief of pain	Stem bark	Anti-inflammatory effect: *Hamelia patens* var. glabra leaves, methanol extract, chloroform extract, and hexane extract, 100.0 mcg/ear (hexane and methanol) and 300.0 mcg/ear (chloroform) doses, produced a 19% (methanol), 37% (chloroform), and 37% (hexane) edema reduction vs. croton oil-induced edema in male mice (Sosa et al. 2002). Antinociceptive activity: *Hamelia patens* var. glabra leaves, ethanol extract, 100 mcg/kg, showed antinociceptive effects with similar activity as 100 mg/kg naproxen in thermal-induced (hot plate test) and chemical-induced (acetic acid) assay in mice (Alonso-Castro et al. 2015)	Ngöbe	Joly et al. (1987), Sosa et al. (2002), and Alonso-Castro et al. (2015)

Panamá	*Heisteria macrophylla* Oerst.	Olacaceae	Hinojo	Abdominal cramps, emmenagogue	Stem, leaves	–	Ngöbe	Joly et al. (1990) and Caballero-George and Gupta (2011)
Panamá	*Heliconia platystachys* Baker.	Heliconiaceae	Taggar naku'guid	Facilitate childbirth	Fruit	–	Kuna	Gupta et al. (1993) and Centro de Investigaciones Farmacognósticas de la Flora Panameña (2004)
Costa Rica	*Heliconia tortuosa* Griseh	(Heliconiaceae)	Platanillo	Prevention of miscarriage	Root	–	–	García et al. (2004) and García-Segura (1994)
Panamá	*Heliconia vaginalis* Benth.	Heliconiaceae	Punur	Facilitate childbirth	Whole plant	–	Kuna	Centro de Investigaciones Farmacognósticas de la Flora Panameña (2004)
Panamá	*Heliocarpus americanus* L.	Tiliaceae	Lruch kua	Facilitate childbirth	Stem, bark	–	Naso	Gupta et al. (2005)
Guatemala/ Belize	*Henriettea cuneata* (Standl.) Gleason	Melastomataceae	Ixq q'een	Fertility regulation	Leaf	Ethanol extracts of the leaves bound to the serotonin receptors 5HT1A and 5 (Michel et al. 2007)	Q'eqchi Maya	De Gezelle (2014) and Michel et al. (2006, 2007, 2012)
Panamá	*Herrania purpurea* (Pittier) R.E. Schult.	Sterculiaceae	Cuin'cia	Facilitate childbirth	Fruit, stem, bark, fresh plant	–	Kuna	Centro de Investigaciones Farmacognósticas de la Flora Panameña (2004)
Guatemala/ Belize	*Hibiscus rosa-sinensis* L.	Malvaceae	Utz uj', clavel, hibiscus	Postpartum hemorrhaging, infertility, speed up labor, fallen uterus, prevention of miscarriage	Leaf, flower	Flower extracts had mild estrogenic effects in mice and rats (Murthy et al. 1997). Ethanol leaf extracts bound to the 5-HT1A and 5 receptors in vitro (Michel et al. 2007). Antioxidant effects (Chen et al. 2003). Anthocyanins, flavonoids, flavonoid glycosides, and phenolics present in the extracts (Chen et al. 2003)	Q'eqchi Maya	De Gezelle (2014), Michel et al. (2006, 2007, 2012), and Chen et al. (2003)

(continued)

Table 5.3 (continued)

Country	Scientific name	Family name	Vernacular name	Illness or use	Part of plant used	Biological activity	Ethnic group	References
Panamá	*Hibiscus rosa-sinensis* L.	Malvaceae	Panab dutu, panab dup	Controlling size of uterus	Flower	Luteotropic effect: *Hibiscus rosa-sinensis* flowers, benzene extract, 150 mg/kg dose, administered by gastric intubation to female guinea pigs (Gupta et al. 1993). Spasmolytic effect (weak): *Hibiscus rosa-sinensis* stemwood, solvent-free extract, 2.0 mg/mL concentration, in vitro electrical stimulation of guinea pig ileum (Cox et al. 1989). Estrogenic activity: *Hibiscus rosa-sinensis*, ethanol extract, 400 mg/kg, caused significant increase in uterine weight and significant uterotropic changes (diameter of the uterus and thickness of the endometrium significantly increased) in immature ovariectomized female albino mice (Vasudeva and Sharma 2008)	Kuna	Cox et al. (1989), Gupta et al. (1993), and Vasudeva and Sharma (2008)
Panamá	*Hibiscus schizopetalus* (Mast.) Hook. f.	Malvaceae	Pane'guid dutu	Facilitate childbirth	Flower	Analgesic activity: *Hibiscus schizopetalus* flowers and leaves, ethanol extract, 50, 100, and 200 mg/kg body weight concentrations, showed significant prolongation of the reaction time after 30 min when compared to control in tail flick test and dose-dependent effect in tail immersion test (Zahid et al. 2012)	Kuna	Gupta et al. (1993) and Zahid et al. (2012)

Panamá	*Hoffmannia vesiculifera* Standl.	Rubiaceae	–	Facilitate childbirth, induce childbirth	Stem	–	Naso	Gupta et al. (2005)
Guatemala/ Belize	*Hyptis verticillata* Jacq.	Lamiaceae	Verbena, cchu pim	Release the placenta, primary amenorrhea	Leaf	Anti-inflammatory activities, hormone-modulating effects (Picking et al. 2013). Leaf extracts bound to the 5HT7 receptor in vitro (Michel et al., 2007). Rosmarinic acid and sideritoflavone (Heinrich et al. 2004). Lignans, terpenes, flavonoids, and alkaloids (Picking et al. 2013)	Q'eqchi Maya	De Gezelle (2014), Michel et al. (2006, 2007, 2012), Heinrich et al. (2004), and Picking et al. (2013)
Honduras	*Hyptis verticillata* Jacq.	Lamiaceae	Barrehorno	Conception	"Cogollo"	–	Ladino (non-Indigenous)	Ticktin and Dalle (2005)
Nicaragua	*Hyptis verticillata* Jacq.	Lamiaceae	John Charles	Abortifacient	Leaf, stem, root, whole plant	None reported on this species. A similar species, *H. suaveolens*, has demonstrated antifertility effects in female albino rats at high concentrations (Garg, 1976; Attah et al. 2012)	Rama	Coe (2008), Garg (1976), and Attah et al. (2012)
El Salvador	*Jatropha curcas* L.	Euphorbiaceae	Tempate	Abortifacient	Fresh bark	–	–	González Ayala (1994)
Honduras	*Jatropha curcas* L.	Euphorbiaceae	Piñón	Control bleeding and menstrual pain; prevent miscarriage; stop postpartum hemorrhaging; control abdominal pain postpartum; birth control	Bark, stem, latex	Protein hydrolysates have demonstrated ability to inhibit platelet aggregation as well as angiotensin-converting enzyme (ACE) (Marrufo-Estrada et al. 2013)	Paya/Pech, Ladino (non-Indigenous)	Ticktin and Dalle (2005), House et al. (1995), and Marrufo-Estrada et al. (2013)
Guatemala/ Belize	*Justicia breviflora* (Nees) Rusby	Acanthaceae	Rax pim	Postpartum hemorrhage	Leaf	Leaf extracts bound strongly to the serotonin receptors in vitro (Michel et al. 2007). *J. pectoralis* had anti-inflammatory and estrogenic effects (Locklear et al. 2010). Flavones and alkaloids found in other *Justicia* species	Q'eqchi Maya	De Gezelle (2014), Michel et al. (2006, 2007, 2012), and Locklear et al. (2010)
Panamá	*Lantana hispida* Kunth.	Verbenaceae	Uu'gua	Expulsion of the placenta	Flower	–	Kuna	Gupta et al. (1993) and Caballero-George and Gupta (2011)
El Salvador	*Lippia graveolens* Kunth.	Verbenaceae	Orégano	Abortifacient	Dried leaves	–	–	González Ayala (1994)

(continued)

Table 5.3 (continued)

Country	Scientific name	Family name	Vernacular name	Illness or use	Part of plant used	Biological activity	Ethnic group	References
Honduras	*Lippia graveolens* Kunth.	Verbenaceae	Orégano	Used to control bleeding; postpartum abdominal pain	Leaf, stem	Has been shown to have a moderate spasmolytic activity on smooth muscle contractions on guinea pig ileum ($IC50 < 20$ µg/mL) likely due to high thymol and carvacrol concentrations in the oil (Rivero-Cruz et al. 2011)	Paya/Pech	Ticktin and Dalle (2005), House et al. (1995), and Rivero-Cruz et al. (2011)
Honduras	*Liquidambar styraciflua* L.	Altingiaceae	Liquidambo	Treat stomach pains during childbirth; postpartum abdominal pain; purgative	Bark, sap	Benzyl benzoate isolates reduce hypertension in vivo (Ohno et al. 2008)	Paya/Pech, Ladino (non-Indigenous)	Ticktin and Dalle (2005), Lentz (1993), and Ohno et al. (2008)
Panamá	*Lygodium venustum* Sw.	Lygodiaceae	–	Menstruation	–	–	Mestizo	Centro de Investigaciones Farmacognósticas de la Flora Panameña (2004) and Morais-Braga et al. (2013)
Panamá	*Machaerium* sp.	Leguminosae	Shren shruo	Facilitate childbirth	Bark	–	Naso	Centro de Investigaciones Farmacognósticas de la Flora Panameña (2004)
Panamá	*Malvaviscus arboreus* Cav.	Malvaceae	Papito de monte and mapola	Difficult childbirth	Branches and twigs	–	Ngöbe	Joly et al. (1987)
Guatemala/ Belize	*Maranta arundinacea* L.	Marantaceae	Kok'mox, arrow root	Infertility, menstrual cramps, heavy menstruation	Root	Anti-nausea effects and prebiotic activity (Harmayani et al. 2011)	Q'eqchi Maya	De Gezelle (2014), Michel et al. (2006, 2007, 2012), and Harmayani et al. (2011)
Costa Rica	*Matricaria sp.*	Asteraceae	Manzanilla	Facilitate and speed up delivery	Leaf	–	–	Sarkis and Campos (1985)
Honduras	*Matricaria courrantiana* DC.	Asteraceae	Manzanilla (chamomile)	Prevent miscarriage; treat morning sickness; speed contractions during labor; expel the placenta after birth; control abdominal pain postpartum; to clean womb after birth	Whole plant	–	Ladino (non-Indigenous)	Ticktin and Dalle (2005)
Panamá	*Melochia villosa* (Mill.) Fawc. & Rendl.	Sterculiaceae	Hierba de soldado	Hemostatic in uterine hemorrhage	Branches	–	Kuna, Emberá, Ngöbe	Gupta et al. (1979)

Costa Rica	*Mentha piperita* L.	Lamiaceae	Yerbabuena	Cramps	Leaf	–	–	García et al. (2004)
Guatemala/Belize	*Miconia oinochrophylla* Donn.	Melastomataceae	Xoy pim	Miscarriage prevention, frequent menstruation	Leaf	–	Q'eqchi Maya	De Gezelle (2014) and Michel et al. (2006, 2007, 2012)
Nicaragua	*Mimosa pudica* L.	Fabaceae	Sleepy bush	Abortifacient	Leaf, stem, root		Rama	Coe (2008)
Guatemala/Belize	*Mimosa pudica* L.	Fabaceae	Dormilona, dormilón, wara k'ix, sleeping prickle	Insomnia, contraception, menopause, uterine fibroids	Leaf, root	Anti-inflammatory effects in vitro and in animal models, effects due to the presence of flavanones (Patel et al. 2015). Anxiolytic effects in mice (Bum et al. 2011). Antifertility effects and prolongs the estrous cycle and disturbs the secretion of gonadotropin hormones in albino mice (Ganguly et al. 2007)	Q'eqchi Maya	De Gezelle (2014), Michel et al. (2006, 2007, 2012), Ganguly et al. (2007), and Patel et al. (2015)
Honduras	*Mimosa pudica* L.	Fabaceae	Dormilona	Used to control nerves and mitigate labor pains	Leaf, root	Ointment of a mixture of methanol and aqueous extract had significantly better wound contraction than mice treated with placebo after 8 days (Kokane et al. 2009)	Paya/Pech	House et al. (1995) and Kokane et al. (2009)
Guatemala/Belize	*Momordica charantia* L.	Cucurbitaceae	Sorosi, serosi, yamor	Dysmenorrhea, amenorrhea, delayed menstruation, contraception, abortifacient, labor pain, postpartum treatment, menopause	Leaf	Several experimental studies demonstrated abortifacient properties (Grover and Yadav 2004)	Q'eqchi Maya	De Gezelle (2014), Michel et al. (2006, 2007, 2012), and Grover and Yadav (2004)
Honduras	*Momordica charantia* L.	Cucurbitaceae	Calaica	Abortifacient, prevent conception	Leaf	Momorcharins are responsible for the abortifacient effects of the plant and act through inhibition of differentiation in the endometrium and implantation of the embryo (Law et al. 1983; Tam et al. 1984; Chan et al. 1984; Chan et al. 1985; Grover and Yadav 2004)	Ladino (non-Indigenous)	Ticktin and Dalle (2005), Law et al. (1983), Chan et al. (1984, 1985), Tam et al. (1984), and Grover and Yadav (2004)
Nicaragua	*Momordica charantia* L.	Cucurbitaceae	Sorosi	Abortifacient	Leaf, stem		Rama	Coe (2008)

(continued)

Table 5.3 (continued)

Country	Scientific name	Family name	Vernacular name	Illness or use	Part of plant used	Biological activity	Ethnic group	References
Panamá	*Momordica charantia* L.	Cucurbitaceae	Srose	Facilitate childbirth	Whole plant	–	Naso	Gupta et al. (2005)
Costa Rica	*Neurolaena lobata (L.) R. Br. Ex Cass*	Asteraceae	Jackass bitters	Postpartum care	Leaf	–	–	García et al. (2004)
Guatemala/ Belize	*Neurolaena lobata* (L.) R. Br. Ex Cass	Asteraceae	Kamank, jackass bitters, g'an mank	Contraception, abortifacient, labor pain, delayed menstruation, weaning, menopause	Leaf	Leaf extracts had analgesic and anti-inflammatory effects in rats (Gracioso et al. 1998). Leaf extracts bound to the serotonin receptor 5HT7 (Michel et al. 2007). Anti-inflammatory effects attributed to sesquiterpene lactones (McKinnon et al. 2014)	Q'eqchi Maya	De Gezelle (2014), Michel et al. (2006, 2007, 2012), Gracioso et al. (1998), and McKinnon et al. (2014)
Guatemala/ Belize	*Nopalea cochenillifera* (L.) Salm-Dyck. [syn. *Opuntia cochenillifera* (L.) Mill.]	Cactaceae	Scoggineal	Facilitate and speed up delivery	Fruit, juice, stem	–	Q'eqchi Maya	De Gezelle (2014) and Michel et al. (2006, 2007, 2012)
Costa Rica	*Ocotea* sp.	Lauraceae		Postpartum shower	Bark	–	–	García-Segura (1994)
Costa Rica	*Ocimum basilicum* L.	Lamiaceae	Albahaca	Postpartum hemorrhage, control menstruation	Leaf, fruit	–	–	Segleau Earle (2001)
Panamá	*Ocimum campechianum* Mill.	Lamiaceae	Albahaca, albahaca simarrona, albahaca silvestre	Menstruation, regulate menstruation	Branches	–	Kuna, Emberá, Ngöbe, Mestizo	Centro de Investigaciones Farmacognósticas de la Flora Panameña (2004) and Gupta et al. (1979)
Guatemala/ Belize	*Ocimum campechianum* Mill. [syn. *Ocimum micranthum* Willd.]	Lamiaceae	Obej', albahaca, b'enk	Dysmenorrhea, heavy menstruation, delayed menstruation, postpartum hemorrhage	Leaf	Contains essential oils and alkaloids (Coe and Anderson 1996). Contains flavonoids and sesquiterpene lactones (Caceres 1996)	Q'eqchi Maya	De Gezelle (2014), Michel et al. (2006, 2007, 2012), Caceres (1996), and Coe and Anderson (1996)
Honduras	*Ocimum campechianum* Mill.	Lamiaceae	Albahaca del monte	Prevent miscarriage; treat abdominal pain; speed contractions during labor; control abdominal pain postpartum	Roots, shoots	None reported on this species. A similar species, *O. basilicum* L., has also been shown to significantly reduce thermally stimulated pain in mice by as much as 52% (Venancio et al. 2011)	Ladino (non-Indigenous)	Ticktin and Dalle (2005) and Venancio et al. (2011)

Panamá	*Odontonema tubaeforme* (Bertol.) Kuntze	Acanthaceae	Kuioloym ko	Induce childbirth	Leaf, stem	–	Naso	Gupta et al. (2005)
Costa Rica	*Oryza Sativa* (*syn. Leersia oryzoides* (L.) *Sw.*)	Poaceae	Arroz, rice	Increase breast milk	Seed	–	–	Sarkis and Campos (1985)
Honduras	*Pavonia rosea* Schect syn. *Pavonia schiedeana* Steud.	Malvaceae	Titiská	Ease pain during childbirth; retained placenta; miscarriage	Leaf, stem, root	–	Paya/Pech	Ticktin and Dalle (2005) and Lentz (1993)
Panamá	*Pentagonia pinnatifida* Seem.	Rubiaceae	Kuaman dutu	Facilitate childbirth, Induce menstruation	Flower	–	Kuna	Gupta et al. (1993)
El Salvador	*Persea americana* Mill.	Lauraceae	Aguacate (avocado)	Abortifacient	Fresh seed	Molecules that stimulate uterine tissue, such as serotonin and tyramine, have been isolated from this plant (Browner and Ortiz de Montellano 1986)	Corroborated use by Rama ethnic people of Nicaragua Coe, (2008) and Q'eqchi Maya in Guatemala (Michel et al. 2006, 2007, 2012))	González Ayala (1994), Browner and Ortiz de Montellano (1986), and Michel et al. (2006, 2007, 2012)
Guatemala/ Belize	*Persea americana* Mill.	Lauraceae	Avocado, pear	Postpartum hemorrhage, dysmenorrhea, contraceptive	Seed, leaf	–	Q'eqchi Maya	De Gezelle (2014), Michel et al. (2006, 2007, 2012)
Panamá	*Persea americana* Mill.	Lauraceae	Aguacate	Menstruation, emmenagogue	Leaves	Uterine stimulant effect: *Persea americana*, 95% ethanol extract and aqueous extract, 0.33 mL/L concentration, demonstrated strong activity in mice (Feng et al. 1962). Analgesic activity: *Persea americana*, aqueous extract, 200.0 mg/kg dose, hot plate method in mice and acetic acid-induced writhing test (Adeyemi et al. 2002). Anti-inflammatory effect: *Persea americana*, aqueous extract, 800 mg/kg dose, Carrageenan-induced pedal edema in mice (Adeyemi et al. 2002)	Mestizo, Kuna, Emberá, Ngöbe	Centro de Investigaciones Farmacognósticas de la Flora Panameña (2004), Feng et al. (1962), Adeyemi et al. (2002), and Gupta et al. (1979)

(continued)

Table 5.3 (continued)

Country	Scientific name	Family name	Vernacular name	Illness or use	Part of plant used	Biological activity	Ethnic group	References
Honduras	*Persea americana* Mill.	Lauraceae	Aguacate	Expel the placenta after birth; stop postpartum hemorrhaging; control abdominal pain postpartum; birth control	Bark, seed	Anti-hemorrhagic activity was demonstrated in vivo in mice subjected to venom (Castro et al. 1999)	Ladino (non-Indigenous)	Ticktin and Dalle (2005) and Castro et al. (1999)
El Salvador	*Petroselinum crispum* (Mill.) Fuss	Apiaceae	Perejil (parsley)	Abortifacient	Fresh leaves	–	–	González Ayala (1994)
Honduras	*Pimenta dioica* (L.) Merr	Myrtaceae	Pimienta gorda	Abdominal pain during pregnancy	Seed	Extracts were estrogenic in MCF-7 cells (Doyle et al. 2009)	Ladino (non-Indigenous)	Ticktin and Dalle (2005) and Doyle et al. (2009)
Guatemala/ Belize	*Pimenta dioica* L. Merr.	Myrtaceae	Pimienta gorda	Facilitate childbirth	Seed, leaf	Extracts were estrogenic in MCF-7 cells (Doyle et al. 2009)	Q'eqchi Maya	De Gezelle (2014), Michel et al. (2006, 2007, 2012), and Doyle et al. (2009)
Nicaragua	*Pimpinella anisum* L.	Apiaceae/ Umbelliferae	Aniseed; anise, anisum; anisi fuctus	Stimulate secretion of breast milk	Seed	Secretolytic and expectorant effects discovered	Not reported	Barnes et al. (2007)
Honduras	*Piper aduncum* L.	Piperaceae	Cordoncillo; cuturo; matico	Used to control female bleeding	Fruit, leaf, stem	Contrary to traditional use, *P. aduncum* has shown antiplatelet activity in guinea pig blood when platelet aggregation was induced by adenosine diphosphate (ADP), arachidonic acid (AA), and thromboxane A2 (TXA2) agonist	Paya/Pech	House et al. (1995) and Lentz et al. (1998)
Guatemala/ Belize	*Piper auritum* H.B.K.	Piperaceae	Ob'el, cowfoot, pata de vaca	Contraceptive, dysmenorrhea, galactagogue, postpartum hemorrhage, postpartum treatment to reduce infection and pain	Leaf	Uterine stimulant effect in rats (Caceres et al. 1995). Ethanol extracts of the leaves bound to the serotonin receptors in vitro (Michel et al. 2007). Contains essential oils, sesquiterpenes, flavones, and alkaloids	Q'eqchi Maya	De Gezelle (2014), Michel et al. (2006, 2007, 2012), and Caceres et al. (1995)
Panamá	*Piper marginatum* Jacq.	Piperaceae	Hinojo	Menstruation	Leaf	Analgesic activity: 0.5 and 1.0 g/kg of aqueous extract significantly reduced the number of writhes induced by acetic acid (0.8%, intravenous injection) in mice within 30 min compared to control (D'Angelo et al. 1997)	Mestizo	Centro de Investigaciones Farmacognósticas de la Flora Panameña (2004) and D'Angelo et al. (1997)

Guatemala/ Belize	*Piper nigrum* L.	Piperaceae	Pimenta negra	Facilitate childbirth	Seed	–	Q'eqchi Maya	De Gezelle (2014) and Michel et al. (2006, 2007, 2012)
Guatemala/ Belize	*Piper pseudolindenii* C.DC.	Piperaceae	Markos q'ehen	Unspecified postpartum depression, postpartum treatment, back pain associated with pregnancy	Leaf	–	Q'eqchi Maya	De Gezelle (2014) and Michel et al. (2006, 2007, 2012)
Guatemala/ Belize	*Piper sanctum* (Miq.) Schltdl. ex C.DC. [syn. *Piper diandrum* C.DC.]	Piperaceae	Nin qui ru chaq' q'een	Body aches, reposition womb	Leaf	Essential oils, terpenes, piperolides present (Mata et al. 2004). Contains isoquinoline alkaloids, beta-sitosterol (Mata et al. 2004)	Q'eqchi Maya	De Gezelle (2014), Michel et al. (2006, 2007, 2012), and Mata et al. (2004)
Guatemala/ Belize	*Piper tuerckheimii* C. DC.	Piperaceae	Caite de diablo, kux sawi'	Inflammation, "loss of senses," eclampsia, contraceptive, heavy menstruation, menstrual cramps	Leaf	Extracts of the leaves had displacement activities in the GABA-T and GABAA-BZD bioassays (Awad et al. 2009)	Q'eqchi Maya	De Gezelle (2014), Michel et al. (2006, 2007, 2012), and Awad et al. (2009)
Guatemala/ Belize	*Pouteria sapota* (Jacq.) H.E.Moore & Stern	Sapotaceae	Mamey, rix saltul	Increase breast milk production	Bark	–	Q'eqchi Maya	De Gezelle (2014) and Michel et al. (2006, 2007, 2012)
Honduras	*Pseudelephantopus spicatus* (Juss. ex Aubl.) C.F. Baker C.F. Baker	Asteraceae	Oreja de chancho, cucuawá, San Antonio	Taken before and after childbirth to accelerate birth and control pain; Induce contractions during labor	Whole plant, roots	–	Paya/Pech, Ladino (non-Indigenous)	Ticktin and Dalle (2005), House et al. (1995), Lentz (1993), and Lentz et al. (1998)
El Salvador	*Psittacanthus calyculatus* (DC.) G.Don	Loranthaceae	Matapalo	Abortifacient	Fresh bark and leaves	–	–	González Ayala (1994)
Guatemala/ Belize	*Psychotria acuminata* Benth.	Rubiaceae	Ichaj pim, hikalit kak	Postpartum hemorrhage, heavy menstruation	Leaf	–	Q'eqchi Maya	De Gezelle (2014) and Michel et al. (2006, 2007, 2012)
Guatemala/ Belize	*Psychotria poeppigiana* Müll. Arg. [syn. *Cephaelis tomentosa* (Aubl.) Vahl.]	Rubiaceae	"Ak pere tzo," pereen pim	Postpartum hemorrhage, primary and secondary amenorrhea, hot flashes	Leaf	Ethanol extracts of the leaves bound to the serotonin receptors in vitro (Michel et al. 2007). Contains alkaloids, phenols, and flavonoids (Coe and Anderson 1996)	Q'eqchi Maya	De Gezelle (2014), Michel et al. (2006, 2007, 2012), and Coe and Anderson (1996)

(continued)

Table 5.3 (continued)

Country	Scientific name	Family name	Vernacular name	Illness or use	Part of plant used	Biological activity	Ethnic group	References
Honduras	*Quassia amara* L.	Simaroubaceae	Hombre grande	Abortifacient		Female rats treated with quassin before cohabitation with males had significantly lower estrogen levels and a reduced mean litter number and weight compared to controls (Raji et al. 2010)	Ladino (non-Indigenous)	Ticktin and Dalle (2005) and Raji et al. (2010)
El Salvador	*Rauvolfia tetraphylla* L.	Apocynaceae	Amatillo	Abortifacient	Fresh roots	–	–	González Ayala (1994)
Panamá	*Rhipsalis baccifera* (J. S. Muell) Stearn.	Cactaceae	–	Facilitate childbirth	Leaf	Spasmogenic activity: *Rhipsalis cassutha* (synonym) aqueous extract and 95% ethanol extract, 0.33 ml/L, guinea pig ileum (Feng et al. 1962)	Ngöbe	Centro de Investigaciones Farmacognósticas de la Flora Panameña (2004) and Feng et al. (1962)
Panamá	*Rhizophora mangle* L.	Rhizophoraceae	Aili	Control gender of child	Root	–	Kuna	Gupta et al. (1993)
Honduras	*Rosmarinus officinalis* L.	Lamiaceae	Romero	Speed contractions during labor; expel the placenta after birth; control abdominal pain postpartum	Whole plant	–	Ladino (non-Indigenous)	Ticktin and Dalle (2005)
Costa Rica	*Ruta chalepensis* L.	Rutaceae	Ruda, rue	Postpartum hemorrhage	Leaf, fruit	–	–	Ocampo and Maffioli (1987)
El Salvador	*Ruta chalepensis* L.	Rutaceae	Ruda	Abortifacient	Fresh stems	–	–	González Ayala (1994)
Panamá	*Ruta graveolens* L.	Rutaceae	Ruda	Contraceptive, menstruation	Leaf	Anti-implantation effect: *Ruta graveolens*, hot water extract and 95% ethanol extract, 1.0 mL/kg,40.0 mg/kg, and 80.0 mg/kg, oral administration in female rat (Guerra and Andrade 1978)	Mestizo	Guerra and Andrade (1978), Mascolo et al. (1987), Logarto Parra et al. (2001), and Centro de Investigaciones Farmacognósticas de la Flora Panameña (2004)
El Salvador	*Salix humboldtiana* Willd.	Salicaceae	Sauce	Abortifacient	Bark	–	–	González Ayala (1994)

Guatemala/ Belize	*Scoparia dulcis* L.	Scrophulariaceae	"Como escobillo"	Reduce labor pains	Leaf	Anti-inflammatory and anti-pain effects (Gupta et al. 2009). In vitro serotonin effects (Hasrat et al. 1997). Sedative effects in rats (Ahmed et al. 2001). Contains alkaloids, terpenes, phenolic compounds (Ahmed et al. 2001; Hayashi et al. 1988), as well as betulinic acid, diterpenes, and flavonoids (de Freitas et al. 2015)	Q'eqchi Maya	De Gezelle (2014), Michel et al. (2006, 2007, 2012), de Freitas et al. (2015), Hasrat et al. (1997), Ahmed et al. (2001), and Hayashi et al. (1988)
Honduras	*Senna alata* (L.) Roxb.	Fabaceae	Bruja	To clean womb after birth; birth control	Root	Alkaloids have been shown to exhibit anti-implantation activity (Yakubu and Musa 2012)	Ladino (non-Indigenous)	Ticktin and Dalle (2005) and Yakubu and Musa (2012)
Guatemala/ Belize	*Senna reticulata* (Willd.) H.S.Irwin & Barneby. [syn. *Cassia reticulata* Willd.]	Fabaceae	Barajo	Dysmenorrhea	Leaf	Phytochemical investigation (Messmer et al. 1968). The anthraquinones chrysophanol, physcion, aloe-emodin, 1,3,8-trihydroxyanthraquinone, 3-methoxy-1,6,8-trihydroxyanthraquinone, emodin, and chrysophanol-10,10'-bianthrone, the triterpenes α- and β-amyrin, the steroids β-sitosterol and stigma sterol, as well as the flavonoid, kaempferol, anthraquinones were isolated from the wood (dos Santos & Silva 2008). Aqueous extract showed antioxidant activity and high polyphenol content (Lizcano et al. 2010)	Q'eqchi Maya	De Gezelle (2014), Michel et al. (2006, 2007, 2012), Messmer et al. (1968), and Lizcano et al. (2010)
Panamá	*Sida rhombifolia* L.	Malvaceae	Kuarguo, shtoplokoglo	Difficult childbirth, facilitate childbirth	Stem	Spasmolytic activity: *Sida rhombifolia* leaves, solvent-free extract, 2.0 mg/mL, in vitro electrical stimulation of guinea pig ileum (Cox et al. 1989). Antispasmodic activity: *Sida rhombifolia* whole plant, aqueous ethanol (1:1) extract, showed activity against acetylcholine (ACH)- and histamine-induced spasms guinea pig ileum (Nakanishi et al. 1965)	Naso	Gupta et al. (2005), Centro de Investigaciones Farmacognósticas de la Flora Panameña (2004), Nakanishi et al. (1965), Dhar et al. (1968), Cox et al. (1989), and Assam et al. (2010)

(continued)

Table 5.3 (continued)

Country	Scientific name	Family name	Vernacular name	Illness or use	Part of plant used	Biological activity	Ethnic group	References
Guatemala/ Belize	*Sida rhombifolia* L.	Malvaceae	Mesb'eel	Used to reduce labor pains, speed labor, expel the placenta, postpartum treatment	Leaf	Anti-implantation activities and stimulated rat uterus (Santthawongsakul 1980). Anti-inflammatory and antioxidant effects in vivo (Narendhirakannan and Limmy 2012). Contains alkaloids, flavonols, sterols, tannins, polyphenols, and saponins (Assam et al. 2010)	Q'eqchi Maya	De Gezelle (2014), Michel et al. (2006, 2007, 2012), Santthawongsakul (1980), Assam et al. (2010), and Narendhirakannan and Limmy (2012)
Honduras	*Smilax spinosa* Mill.	Smilacaceae	Cuculmeca	Conception	Root	–	Ladino (non-Indigenous)	Ticktin and Dalle (2005)
Panamá	*Spathiphyllum friedrichsthalii* Schott.	Araceae	Ina'ulu	Facilitate childbirth, avoid enlargement of the uterus	Flower	–	Kuna	Gupta et al. (1993)
El Salvador	*Tabebuia rosea* (Bertol.) Bertero ex A.DC.	Bignoniaceae	Maquiligüe	Abortifacient	Fresh bark	–	–	González Ayala (1994)
Panamá	*Tagetes erecta* L.	Asteraceae	Rosa amarilla	Menstruation, amenorrhea, stomach colic	Flower seeds, flower	Uterine stimulant effect: *Tagetes erecta* leaves, ethanol extract, 10 mg/ml, guinea pig ileum (Mans et al. 2004). Analgesic effect: *Tagetes erecta* flowers, ethanol extract, 100 and 300 mg/kg, dose-dependent effect in writhing test in mice (Bashir and Gilani 2008). Analgesic effect: *Tagetes erecta* petal and leaf powder, ethanol or methanol extract, 40 mg/dose/week, single blind 12-week study in humans with mild hallux abducto vagus and bunion (Khan 1997)	Mestizo, Kuna, Emberá, Ngöbe	Centro de Investigaciones Farmacognósticas de la Flora Panameña (2004), Gupta et al. (1979), Khan (1997), Mans et al. (2004), and Bashir and Gilani (2008)
Honduras	*Tagetes lucida* Cav.	Asteraceae	Pericón	Entire plant consumed to speed delivery and regulate menstrual bleeding; vaginal wash	Leaf, stem	Demonstrated significant anxiolytic and sedative effect on the serotonergic and GABAergic neurotransmission in mice models (Perez-Ortega et al. 2016). Results corroborated earlier report in 1989 (Caceres and Samayoa 1989)	Paya/Pech	House et al. (1995), Caceres and Samayoa (1989), and Perez-Ortega et al. (2016)

Costa Rica	*Tanacetum parthenium* (L.) Sch. Bip.	Asteraceae	Feverfew	Tonic after giving birth	Leaf	–	–	Bernhardt (2008)
Guatemala/ Belize	*Theobroma cacao* L.	Malvaceae	Cacao	Increase breast milk	Seed	A modest daily intake of high-cocoa-content chocolate reduced blood pressure, glycemic, and liver pattern during pregnancy without affecting the weight gain (Di Renzo et al. 2012)	Q'eqchi Maya	De Gezelle (2014), Michel et al. (2006, 2007, 2012), and Di Renzo et al. (2012)
Panamá	*Theobroma cacao* L.	Sterculiaceae	Ciamachi	Facilitate childbirth, abortive before 6 months of pregnancy	Stem, bark	Platelet aggregation inhibition activity: *Theobroma cacao*, 100.0 mg/day dose, human adults (Innes et al. 2003). Abortifacient activity (inactive): *Theobroma cacao* aerial parts, aqueous ethanol extract, 200 mg/kg dose, administered by gastric intubation to pregnant rats (Gupta et al. 1993). Anti-inflammatory activity: *Theobroma cacao*, polyphenolic fraction, macrophage assay (Ramiro et al. 2005). Myorelaxant, tonic, and vasodilator activity: *Theobroma cacao*, 1–2 tsp. cocoa per cup of water and/or milk doses, in animal studies (Duke 2000)	Kuna	Gupta et al. (1993), Duke (2000), Innes et al. (2003), and Ramiro et al. (2005)
Costa Rica	*Thymus vulgaris* L.	Lamiaceae	Tomillo	Induce labor, speed up prolonged labor	Leaf	–	–	García et al. (2004)
Guatemala/ Belize	*Tococa guianensis* Aubl.	Melastomataceae	Ixq pim	Female infertility	Leaf	–	Q'eqchi Maya	De Gezelle (2014) and Michel et al. (2006, 2007, 2012)
Costa Rica	*Tradescantia zebrina* Bosse	Commelinaceae	Spiderwort	Increase breast milk, anti-inflammatory	Leaf	–	–	Segleau Earle (2001) and Ocampo and Maffioli (1987)
Costa Rica	*Triumfetta lappula* L.	Bombacaceae	Mozote	Facilitate and speed up delivery	Root	–	–	García-Segura(1994) and Quesada (2008)

(continued)

Table 5.3 (continued)

Country	Scientific name	Family name	Vernacular name	Illness or use	Part of plant used	Biological activity	Ethnic group	References
Panamá	*Vernonia* sp.	Asteraceae	Uu'sipu	Expulsion of the placenta	Flower	Analgesic effect: *Vernonia cinerea* leaves, chloroform, methanolic, and petroleum ether extracts, 100, 200, and 400 mg/kg, both chemical- and thermal-induced pain responses in mice alleviated (Iwalewa et al. 2003). Analgesic effect: *Vernonia amygdalina* leaves, aqueous extract, 50, 100, and 200 mg/kg, acetic acid-induced writhing test and formalin test in mice (Njan et al. 2008). Uterotonic effect: *Vernonia amygdalina* leaves, 95% ethanol extract, 2% concentration, in vitro virgin female rat assay (Desta 1994). Anti-implantation effect: *Vernonia amygdalina* leaves, 95% ethanol extract, 1.54 g/kg dose, in vitro virgin female rat assay (Desta 1994)	Kuna	Gupta et al. (1993), Iwalewa et al. (2003), Centro de Investigaciones Farmacognósticas de la Flora Panameña (2004), Monteiro et al. (2001), Njan et al. (2008), and Desta (1994)
Panamá	*Xanthosoma helleborifolium* (Jacq.) Schott.	Araceae	Naibe'uar, uer'uer, guabinguid bipinguad	Facilitate childbirth	Tubers	–	Kuna	Gupta et al. (1993)
Panamá	*Xanthosoma mexicanum* Liebm.	Araceae	Naibe'mor dup sipuguad	Facilitate childbirth	Fruit	–	Kuna	Gupta et al. (1993) and Jimenez et al. (2001)
Panamá	*Xiphidium caeruleum* Aubl.	Haemodoraceae	Ia, mano de dios	Facilitate childbirth, antiemetic	Stem	–	Naso	Gupta et al. (2005), Centro de Investigaciones Farmacognósticas de la Flora Panameña (2004), Joly et al. (1987), and Caballero-George and Gupta (2011)

Panamá	*Xylopia frutescens* Aubl.	Annonaceae	–	Abdominal pains	Leaves or seeds	Anti-inflammatory activity: *X. frutescens* seeds, hexane extract, 19 μg/ml concentration, 84.6% inhibition of 5-liposygenase in vitro (Braga et al. 2000). Spasmolytic activity: *X. frutescens* leaf essential oil, 729 μg/ml concentration, reduced histamine-induced contraction of guinea pig ileum by 94.6 ± 3.0% and carbachol-induced contraction by 97.2 ± 1.3% at maximum effect (Souza et al. 2015)	Ngöbe	Joly et al. (1990), Braga et al. (2000), and Souza et al. (2015)
Honduras	*Yucca guatemalensis* Baker syn. *Yucca gigantea* Lem.	Agavaceae	Izote	Contractions	Shoots	–	Ladino (non-Indigenous)	Ticktin and Dalle (2005)

rural areas, are treated with these botanical medicines and appear to prefer the use of traditional medicines and healers, there is an immediate need to document this information, collect the plant species used, and scientifically test the most commonly used plant species in a rational and systematic manner.

5.6.1 Plants Used for Contraception or to Abort the Fetus

Botanical abortifacients are a potential low-cost alternative to pharmaceutical drugs such as misoprostol. In total, 39 plants were identified as being used in Central American countries for contraception or abortion (Table 5.1). In El Salvador, alone, 21 plants were identified for use as abortifacients. Plants included are *Aristolochia* sp., *Artemisia absinthium* L., *Bursera simaruba* (L.) Sarg., *Citrus aurantifolia* (Christm.) Swingle (lime), *Mimosa pudica* L., *Persea americana* Mill. (avocado), *Quassia amara* L., and *Theobroma cacao* L. (chocolate).

5.6.2 Plant Use for Pain Associated with Childbirth

Twenty-seven plants were identified as being used in Central American countries for treating breast, abdominal, or muscle pain associated with childbirth (Table 5.1). In Honduras, it was reported that Ladino midwives prepared decoctions of *Cinnamomum verum* J. Presl (cinnamon), *Ocimum campechianum* Mill. (basil), or *Pimenta dioica* (L.) Merr. (allspice) among other herbs to treat abdominal pain (Ticktin and Dalle 2005). Fresh leaves and roots of *Mimosa pudica* L. are reportedly used to treat nerves and mitigate labor pains in Honduras (House et al. 1995). *Drymonia multiflora* (Oerst. Ex Hanst.) Wiehler was used for breast pain in Panamá (Caballero-George and Gupta 2011). The Naso and Ngöbe as well as Mestizo (Ladino) communities reported using *Costus pulverulentus* C. Presl., *Costus villosissimus* Jacq., and *Hamelia patens* var. glabra Oerst., specifically for postpartum pain (Joly et al. 1987; Sosa et al. 2002; Centro de Investigaciones Farmacognósticas de la Flora Panameña 2004). In Nicaragua, *Matricaria chamomilla* and *Bursera simaruba* were reported to be used for menstrual pain and pain associated with childbirth (Castro et al. 1999; Newall et al. 1996).

5.6.3 Plants Used to Control Bleeding and Prevent Miscarriage and Postpartum Hemorrhage

Thirty-two plants were identified as being used in Central American countries for preventing miscarriage or postpartum hemorrhaging (Table 5.1). In Honduras, the bark and latex of *Jatropha curcas* L. have been used to control bleeding. A concoction of the leaves of *Lippia graveolens* Kunth. taken several times a day was used to control bleeding in women (Fig. 5.2). The cooked leaves and flowers from *Piper aduncum* L. were used to control female bleeding when taken orally over several days. The entire plant of *Tagetes lucida* Cav. was used to regulate menstrual bleeding (House et al. 1995). Ladino midwives use the roots of *Pseudelephantopus spicatus* (Juss. ex Aubl.) C.F. Baker to induce labor (Ticktin and Dalle 2005). The use of *Persea americana* Mill. to prevent menstrual hemorrhage was corroborated by similar use in Mexico (Ortiz de Montellano and Browner 1985). *Equisetum bogotense* H.B.K. and *Melochia villosa* (Mill.) Fawc. and Rendle were used to prevent uterine bleeding by the Kuna, Emberá, and Ngöbe of Panamá (Gupta et al. 1979). In Nicaragua, *Bursera simaruba* was also reported to be used for bleeding (Castro et al. 1999).

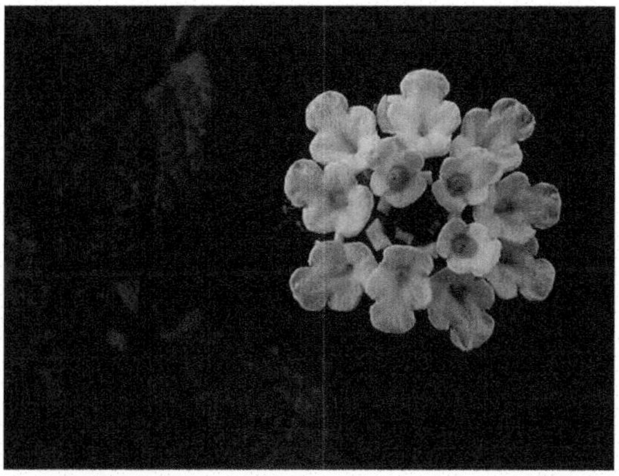

Fig. 5.2 *Lippia graveolens* Kunth. (Source: https://en.wikipedia.org/wiki/Lippia_graveolens#/media/File:Lippia_graveolens,_known_as_Mexican_Oregano_(11628265214).jpg)

5.6.4 Plants Used for Morning Sickness and Nausea

Only ten plants were identified as useful for treating morning sickness and nausea. Ladino midwives in Honduras use *Matricaria courrantiana* L., *Asclepias curassavica* L., *Cinnamomum verum* J.Presl., *Citrus aurantiifolia* (Christm.) Swingle, and *Citrus aurantium* L. to treat and prevent morning sickness and nausea during pregnancy (Ticktin and Dalle 2005). The use of *C. aurantiifolia* to control vomiting has been reported among Indigenous women in Nicaragua as well (Barrett 1994). *Bursera simaruba* L. Sarg. have been used in Honduras to prevent vomiting (House et al. 1995). Two plants (*Aphelandra sinclairiana* Nees. and *Xiphidium caeruleum* Aubl.) were used as antiemetics by the Naso in Panamá (Joly et al. 1987; Gupta et al. 2005).

5.6.5 Plants Used During Labor

Twenty medicinal plants were identified as being used by women in Central America to induce labor and expedite delivery. These include *Citrus aurantium* L., *Matricaria courrantiana* DC. (chamomile), *Pseudelephantopus spicatus* (Juss. ex Aubl.) C.F. Baker, *Ocimum campechianum* Mill., *Rosmarinus officinalis* L. (rosemary), *Persea americana* Mill., *Mimosa pudica* L., and *Tagetes lucida* Cav. (Ticktin and Dalle 2005) (Fig. 5.3). The use of some of the same or similar plants has been corroborated in the ethnobotanical literature from parts of Mexico as well. Specifically, *Mimosa albida* Willd., *Citrus aurantium* L., *Matricaria chamomilla* L., and *Tagetes lucida* Cav. are used to induce uterine contractions by Indigenous women in Mexico (Ortiz de Montellano and Browner 1985).

5.6.6 Plants Used After Childbirth and in the Puerperium

Thirty-five plants have been identified as being used after childbirth for purposes such as cleaning the womb after delivery, treating uterine prolapse, expelling the placenta, or increasing milk production. In Honduras, *Bursera simaruba* (L.) Sarg. was used by the Pech people to clean the womb after childbirth as well as to increase milk production (House et al. 1995). The bark and latex of *Ficus insipida* Willd. are used to dry the umbilical cord of the baby after childbirth (House et al. 1995). Three plants *Vernonia* sp., *Desmodium axillare* (Sw.) D.C., and *Lantana hispida* Kunth. were used for the expulsion of the placenta, with similar uses reported in Mexico as well (Gupta et al. 1993; Caballero-George and Gupta 2011; Centro de Investigaciones Farmacognósticas de la Flora Panameña 2004).

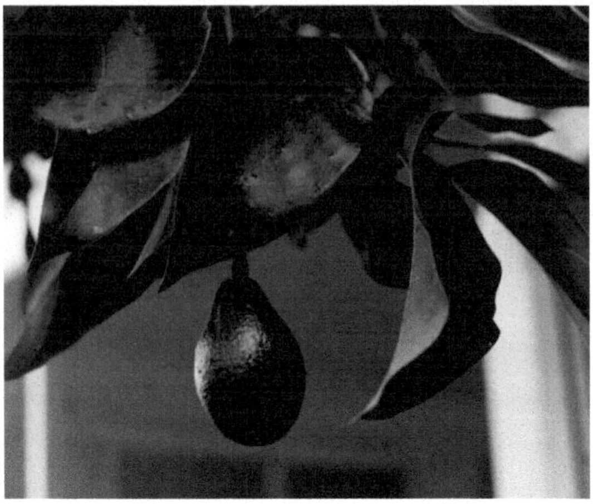

Fig. 5.3 *Persea americana* L. (Photograph by Jack Chappa)

Other maternal health uses for medicinal plants included the use of *Rhizophora mangle* L. to control the gender of the child and *Genipa americana* L. to regulate fetus growth and weakness in girls (Gupta et al. 1993; Nakanishi et al. 1965). Additionally, 34 plants were reported in the literature as used for "childbirth" or "postpartum care," but the exact use was not specified.

5.7 Scientific Evidence of Biological Activity Consistent with Reported Use

The knowledge of herbs by women in Central America and their medicinal effects has been largely ignored, and scientific evidence of safety and efficacy is lacking. As such, the body of evidence in support of the use of these medicinal plants to treat maternal health complications ranges from non-existent to very promising.

5.7.1 Anti-inflammatory Activity

Many of the plants or associated phytochemicals mentioned in this chapter as being used by TBAs or expectant mothers to treat maternal health conditions have demonstrated anti-inflammatory activity *in vitro* as well as *in vivo (*Patel et al. 2015; Patel and Bhutani 2014; Bhaskaran et al. 2010; Carretero et al. 2008; Khodabakhsh et al. 2015; Takaki et al. 2008; Noguera et al. 2004*)*. For example, the essential oil of rosemary (*R. officinalis*) has been shown to reduce carrageenan-induced paw edema in mice with a similar effect as indomethacin (5 mg/kg) at high concentrations (Takaki et al. 2008). Notably, oral administrations of hexane extract of *B. simaruba* (78 mg/kg) have been shown to reduce carrageenan-induced paw edema by as much as 83% after 3 h with effects lasting up to 7 h. The anti-inflammatory effect was comparable to the positive control phenylbutazone (80 mg/kg) (Carretero et al. 2008). The anti-inflammatory activity of *B. simaruba* has also been corroborated elsewhere (Noguera et al. 2004). Another plant, chamomile (*M. courrantiana*), has demonstrated anti-inflammatory activity, which is mediated through inhibition of cyclooxygenase-2 (COX-2) enzyme activity, and been shown to inhibit of NF-KB/ReL transcription factors which effect downstream production of inducible nitric oxide synthase (iNOS) (Bhaskaran et al. 2010).

5.7.2 Spasmodic, Antispasmodic, and Sedative Activity

In Western medicine, uterotonics stop heavy uterine bleeding and reduce the risk of postpartum hemorrhaging during labor. Some of the medicinal plants used by Indigenous and other ethnic women in Central America have a stimulating effect on smooth muscle contractions, while others are known to have sedative and antispasmodic activity. The essential oil of the aerial parts of basil (*Ocimum basilicum* L.) has been reported to have antispasmodic, sedative, as well as anti-vomiting activity (Venancio et al. 2011). An in vivo study reported that the essential oil of basil reduced acetic acid-induced muscle contractions in mice by as much as 78% (Venancio et al. 2011).

The essential oil of oregano (*Lippia graveolens* Kunth.) has been shown to have a moderate spasmolytic activity on smooth muscle contractions on guinea pig ileum ($IC_{50} < 20$ μg/mL) likely due to high thymol and carvacrol concentrations in the oil (Rivero-Cruz et al. 2011). This activity correlates with the use of the plant to reduce pain and discomfort during labor (Cohen 1982). Two studies decades apart have reported that extracts of *T. lucida* exhibit a significant anxiolytic and sedative effect on the serotonergic and GABAergic neurotransmission in mice models (Perez-Ortega et al. 2016; Caceres and Samayoa 1989; House et al. 1995). Eugenol, a common compound found in cloves, cinnamon, and basil, has been shown to modulate 5-lipoxygenase in human polymorphonuclear (PMN) cells and inhibit the formation of leukotriene C4, an inflammatory biomarker and factor in smooth muscle contractions (Raghavenra et al. 2006). Rosemary essential oil excites smooth muscle contractions at low doses yet has a spasmolytic effect on smooth muscle at higher doses as demonstrated on guinea pig stomach strips (Sagorchev et al. 2010).

5.7.3 Analgesic and Antinociceptive Activity

The essential oil of basil (50 mg/kg) has also been shown to significantly reduce thermally stimulated pain in mice by as much as 52% (Venancio et al. 2011). This response was blocked by naloxone, indicating that the biological response may involve opioid receptors. While the genus and species were not reported, a small randomized double-blind study conducted in Iran with females having dysmenorrhea found that cinnamon powder capsules were significantly better than placebo at reducing pain 8 h after ingestion. The result was less effective than that of ibuprofen (Jaafarpour et al. 2015a, b). The use of anise and chamomile to treat abdominal pain is corroborated in Arabic countries as well. A survey of herbal use in Palestinian women found that of those using herbs during pregnancy, more than half the women used anise and chamomile. The most common uses included abdominal pain, vomiting, and relaxation (Al-Ramahi et al. 2013). Aromatherapy using chamomile oil has been reported to be effective at alleviating pain during childbirth in an observational study (Burns et al. 2000). Unfortunately, the only double-blind placebo-controlled clinical trial evaluating the analgesic effects of chamomile failed to detect a significant analgesic effect over placebo for either pentazocine (opioid analgesic) or chamomile in women experiencing childbirth, so additional studies are needed (Zafar et al. 2016). Orally administered doses of anethole, a predominant constituent in anise oil, have been shown to significantly reduce swelling and produce an analgesic effect in mice (Ritter et al. 2013). Aqueous extracts of coriander may mediate analgesic response though central pain receptors (Pathan et al. 2011; Laribi et al. 2015). The medicinal use of *C. aurantium* to treat pain is supported by similar use in Iran. In one study, the active compound, neroli, was shown to inhibit acetic acid-induced writhing in rats by as much as 46% at 20 mg/kg. At 40 mg/kg, neroli delayed nociception longer than diclofenac at 30 min to 1 h, but this effect was short-lived (Khodabakhsh et al. 2015).

Rosemary is valued as an analgesic in folk medicine as well (Takaki et al. 2008). Several studies have corroborated the analgesic effects of rosemary essential oil in vivo. In one study, the essential oil was shown to have antinociceptive activity demonstrated by reducing acetic acid-induced writhing in mice at high concentrations (Takaki et al. 2008). In a separate study, the oil (20 mg/kg) had significant synergistic effect on pain response when combined with codeine, but at lower concentrations the oil diminished codeine's analgesic effect (Raskovic et al. 2015). Additionally, ethanolic fractions of rosemary administered intraperitoneally in mice demonstrated similar pain reduction at high doses (Martinez et al. 2012).

5.7.4 Antiplatelet Activity

Hypertensive disorders and thrombotic disorders are a leading cause of maternal mortality worldwide (Say et al. 2014). Anticoagulants and thrombolytics are used to prevent thromboses in pregnancy (Marino 2014). Protein hydrolysates from defatted *Jatropha curcas* flour have demonstrated ability to inhibit platelet aggregation as well as angiotensin-converting enzyme (ACE) activity which may offer some insight into its traditional use (Marrufo-Estrada et al. 2013). Similarly, *Piper aduncum* L. has shown promising antiplatelet activity in guinea pig blood when platelet aggregation was induced by adenosine diphosphate (ADP), arachidonic acid (AA), and thromboxane A_2 (TXA2) agonist (Guerrini et al. 2009). Fresh-squeezed lemon juice (*C. limon*) has been shown to have anticoagulant effect on blood coagulation in vivo. One study found that healthy rabbits intubated with lemon juice (0.4 mL/kg) had significantly longer bleeding times than placebo and had activated partial thromboplastin times very close to heparin (Riaz et al. 2014). In Chinese medicine, cinnamon is used to increase blood flow to the uterus, but literature regarding efficacy is lacking (Rao and Gan 2014). The latex of *Asclepias curassavica* L. has been shown to exhibit thrombin-like activity (Shivaprasad et al. 2009). *Persea americana* Mill. anti-hemorrhagic activity was demonstrated in vivo in mice subjected to venom (Castro et al. 1999).

5.7.5 Wound Healing

Preliminary results in mice suggest that *M. pudica* L. may have wound-healing activity. Mice treated with an ointment of a mixture of methanol and aqueous extract had significantly better wound contraction than mice treated with placebo after 8 days (Kokane et al. 2009). This activity may explain its use among Indigenous people in Mexico and Central America associated with stopping menstruation (Zamora-Martinez and de Pascual Pola 1992).

5.7.6 Anti-nausea and Anti-vomiting Activity

Very little evidence exists to support the ethnobotanical use for any of the plants discussed. However, the use of *Citrus* sp. to treat symptoms of nausea and vomiting is reported in Iran. A small randomized controlled trial (RCT) of aromatherapy with lemon oil demonstrated marginal results in reducing nausea and vomiting in pregnant women (Yavari Kia et al. 2014).

5.7.7 Contraceptive Activity

A study of the effects of a vaginal douche comprised of the juice of *C. aurantiifolia* fruit on the reproductive histomorphology of female Wistar rats showed that the douche caused distortions and

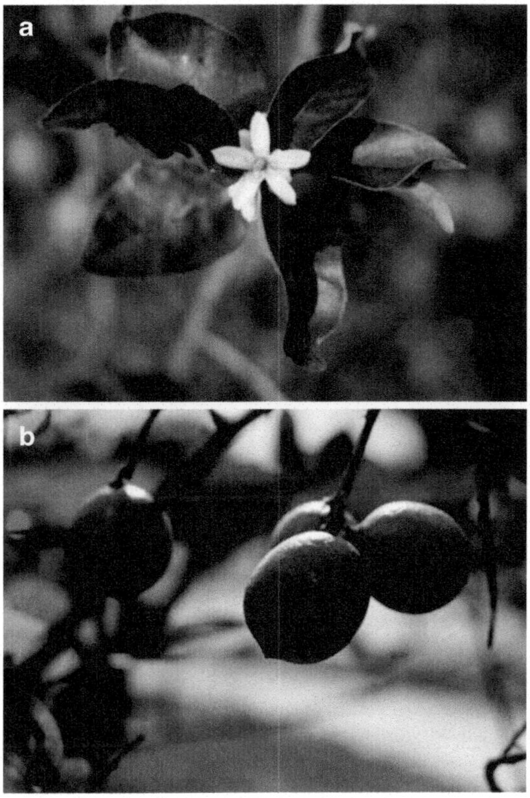

Fig. 5.4 (**a, b**) *Citrus aurantiifolia* (Christm.) Swingle (Photograph by Jack Chappa)

inflammation of cells in the ovaries, uterus, and vagina (Solomon et al. 2014) (Fig. 5.4). At higher concentrations, atrophy of fetal tissues and fibrosis (scarring) of the myometrium was observed. In another study, alcoholic extracts of the seeds of *C. limon*, a similar plant, were administered orally to female albino mice and showed a significant antifertility effect through an anti-zygotic mechanism (Kulkarni et al. 2005). *Mimosa pudica* L. has been reported to have antifertility effects and prolong the estrous cycle and disturbs the secretion of gonadotropin hormones in albino mice (Ganguly et al. 2007). Momordins (momorcharins) are active compounds from *Momordica charantia* L. and are responsible for the abortifacient effects of the plant, acting through inhibition of differentiation in the endometrium and implantation of the embryo (Chan et al. 1984, 1985; Grover and Yadav 2004; Law et al. 1983; Tam et al. 1984). Serotonin and tyramine, which are known uterine stimulants, have been isolated from *P. americana* (Browner and Ortiz de Montellano 1986).

Conclusions

Poverty, cultural stigmatization, gender inequality, and rural residence will continue to be limitations to decreasing maternal mortality in less economically advantaged countries. Women in rural, impoverished areas of Central America continue to have home births attended by local midwives or TBAs. In areas where having a skilled birth attendant at every birth is not yet achievable, the role of the TBAs should not be ignored. These women possess traditional knowledge, a wealth of experience, access to women throughout pregnancy and childbirth, and an established, trusted role within their communities. Resources directed toward formal training and integration of TBAs within the larger healthcare infrastructure may improve access to care through early identification of maternal risk and increased clinic referrals while also facilitating cultural acceptance of medical care (Price and Asgary 2011; Rodgers et al. 2004). Initiatives linking professional midwives and TBAs to the formal healthcare system have already shown some success in Guatemala (Bhatt 2012; Kestler 2014; Kestler et al. 2013).

Traditional knowledge regarding the use of medicinal plants for maternal health may not be without merit but requires additional research into the safety and efficacy of these therapies. A limited number of the plants reported here as being used medicinally to treat and prevent maternal health complications have some biological activity to support their use. These findings warrant further investigation as well as an in-depth analysis of toxicity and herb-drug interactions.

The knowledge of traditional uses of these plants to treat certain illnesses related to women's health is shrinking. The purpose of this chapter was to review the use of medicinal plants among these communities and highlight need for additional research (Montenegro and Stephens 2006; Ticktin and Dalle 2005). Many plants discussed here have had little to no scientific research conducted on them, indicating that there is further work to be done in the future to explore whether these plants can be of medicinal value. Central America's abundance of flora, the ethnomedical knowledge of Indigenous groups living there, and the Indigenous groups' dependence on natural healthcare present a unique opportunity for further research.

References

Adeyemi, O. O., Okpo, S. O., & Ogunti, O. O. (2002). Analgesic and anti-inflammatory effects of the aqueous extract of leaves of Persea americana mill (lauraceae). *Fitoterapia, 73*(5), 375–380.

Ahmed, M., Shikha, H. A., Sadhu, S. K., Rahman, M. T., & Datta, B. K. (2001). Analgesic, diuretic, and anti-inflammatory principle from Scoparia dulcis. *Pharmazie, 56*(8), 657–660.

Al-Ramahi, R., Jaradat, N., & Adawi, D. (2013). Use of herbal medicines during pregnancy in a group of Palestinian women. *Journal of Ethnopharmacology, 150*(1), 79–84. https://doi.org/10.1016/j.jep.2013.07.041

Alonso-Castro, A. J., Balleza-Ramos, S., Hernández-Morales, A., Zapata-Morales, J. R., González-Chávez, M. M., & Carranza-Álvarez, C. (2015). Toxicity and antinociceptive effects of Hamelia patens. *Revista Brasileira de Farmacognosia, 25*(2), 170–176.

Alonso-Castro, A. J., Zapata-Morales, J. R., Gonzalez-Chavez, M. M., Carranza-Alvarez, C., Hernandez-Benavides, D. M., & Hernandez-Morales, A. (2016). Pharmacological effects and toxicity of Costus pulverulentus C. Presl (Costaceae). *Journal of Ethnopharmacology, 180*, 124–130. https://doi.org/10.1016/j.jep.2016.01.011

Álvarez, R. A. C. (2015). *The Indigenous World*. International Work Group for Indigenous Affairs. p.89–96. Retrieved April 5, 2016, from http://www.iwgia.org/publications/search-pubs?publication_id=716.

Arps, S. (2009). Threats to safe motherhood in Honduran Miskito communities: local perceptions of factors that contribute to maternal mortality. *Social Science and Medicine, 69*(4), 579–586. https://doi.org/10.1016/j.socscimed.2009.06.005

Assam, A. J., Dzoyem, J. P., Pieme, C. A., & Penlap, V. B. (2010). In vitro antibacterial activity and acute toxicity studies of aqueous-methanol extract of Sida rhombifolia Linn. (Malvaceae). *BMC Complementary Alternative Medicine, 10*, 40. https://doi.org/10.1186/1472-6882-10-40

Attah, A. F., O'Brien, M., Koehbach, J., Sonibare, M. A., Moody, J. O., Smith, T. J., et al. (2012). Uterine contractility of plants used to facilitate childbirth in Nigerian ethnomedicine. *Journal of Ethnopharmacology, 143*(1), 377–382. https://doi.org/10.1016/j.jep.2012.06.042

Awad, R., Ahmed, F., Bourbonnais-Spear, N., Mullally, M., Ta, C. A., Tang, A., et al. (2009). Ethnopharmacology of Q'eqchi' Maya antiepileptic and anxiolytic plants: effects on the GABAergic system. *Journal of Ethnopharmacology, 125*(2), 257–264. https://doi.org/10.1016/j.jep.2009.06.034

Ayala, E. (2012). *Native People of El Salvador finally gain recognition*. Inter Press Service. Retrieved November 4, 2016, from http://www.ipsnews.net/2012/05/native-people-of-el-salvador-finally-gain-recognition/. Published May 14, 2012.

Barnes, J., Anderson, L. A., & Phillipson, J. D. (2007). *Herbal Medicines* (3rd ed.). Chicago: Pharmaceutical Press.

Barrett, B. (1994). Medicinal plants of Nicaragua's Atlantic coast. *Economic Botany, 48*(1), 8–20.

Barrett, B. (1995). Ethnomedical interactions: health and identity on Nicaragua's Atlantic coast. *Social Science and Medicine, 40*(12), 1611–1621. https://doi.org/10.1016/0277-9536(94)00348-W

Bashir, S., & Gilani, A. H. (2008). Studies on the antioxidant and analgesic activities of Aztec marigold (Tagetes erecta) flowers. *Phytotherapy Research, 22*(12), 1692–1694. https://doi.org/10.1002/ptr.2550

Bernhardt, E. (2008). *Medicinal plants of Costa Rica*. Costa Rica: Zona Tropical Publication.

Berti, P. R., Sohani, S., Costa, E., Klaas, N., Amendola, L., & Duron, J. (2015). An adequacy evaluation of a maternal health intervention in rural Honduras: the impact of engagement of men and empowerment of women. *Revista Panamericana de Salud Pública, 37*(2), 90–97.

Bhaskaran, N., Shukla, S., Srivastava, J. K., & Gupta, S. (2010). Chamomile: an anti-inflammatory agent inhibits inducible nitric oxide synthase expression by blocking RelA/p65 activity. *International Journal of Molecular Medicine, 26*(6), 935–940.

Bhatt, S. (2012). Health care issues facing the Maya people of the Guatemalan Highlands: The current state of care and recommendations for improvement. *Journal of Global Health Perspective,* Edition 1, *epub*. Retrieved October 2, 2016, from http://jglobalhealth.org/article/health-care-issues-facing-the-maya-people-of-the-guatemalan-highlands-the-current-state-of-care-and-recommendations-for-improvement-2/.

Boland, R., & Katzive, L. (2008). Developments in laws on induced abortion: 1998-2007. *International Family Planning Perspectives, 34*(3), 110–120. https://doi.org/10.1363/ifpp.34.110.08.

Boyer, D. B., Klima, C., & Jennrich, J. (2001). Midwifery in Northern Belize. *Journal of Midwifery and Women's Health, 46*(1), 33–39.

Braga, F. C., Wagner, H., Lombardi, J. A., & de Oliveira, A. B. (2000). Screening Brazilian plant species for in vitro inhibition of 5-lipoxygenase. *Phytomedicine, 6*(6), 447–452. https://doi.org/10.1016/s0944-7113(00)80073-2

Browner, C. H., & Ortiz de Montellano, B. R. (1986). Herbal emmenagogues used by women in Colombia and Mexico. In N. L. Etkin (Ed.), *Plants in Indigenous medicine and diet: biobehavioral approaches* (pp. 32–47). Bedford Hills, NY: Redgrave Publishing.

Bum, E. N., Soudi, S., Ayissi, E. R., Dong, C., Lakoulo, N. H., Maidawa, F., Seke, P. F., Nanga, L. D., Taiwe, G. S., Dimo, T., Njikam, N., Rakotonirina, A., Rakotonirina, S. V., & Kamanyi, A. (2011). Anxiolytic activity evaluation of four medicinal plants from Cameroon. *African Journal of Traditional, Complementary, and Alternative Medicines, 8*(5S), 130–139.

Burns, E., Blamey, C., Ersser, S. J., Lloyd, A. J., & Barnetson, L. (2000). The use of aromatherapy in intrapartum midwifery practice an observational study. *Complementary Therapies in Nursing and Midwifery, 6*(1), 33–34. https://doi.org/10.1054/ctnm.1999.0901

Bussmann, R. W., Malca, G., Glenn, A., Sharon, D., Nilsen, B., Parris, B., et al. (2011). Toxicity of medicinal plants used in traditional medicine in Northern Peru. *Journal of Ethnopharmacology, 137*(1), 121–140. https://doi.org/10.1016/j.jep.2011.04.071

Caballero-George, C., & Gupta, M. P. (2011). A quarter century of pharmacognostic research on Panamánian flora: A review. *Planta Medica, 77*(11), 1189–1202. https://doi.org/10.1055/s-0030-1271187

Caceres, A. (1996). *Plantas de Us medicinal en Guatemala*. Guatemala City, Guatemala: Editorial Universitaria: Universidad de San Carlos.

Caceres, A., Menendez, H., Mendez, E., Cohobon, E., Samayoa, B. E., Jauregui, E., et al. (1995). Antigonorrhoeal activity of plants used in Guatemala for the treatment of sexually transmitted diseases. *Journal of Ethnopharmacology, 48*(2), 85–88.

Caceres, A., & Samayoa, B. (1989). *Tamizaje de la actividad antibateriana de plantas usadas en Guatemala para el tratamiento de afecciones gastrointestinales*. Guatemala: Universidad San Carlos de Guatemala. Cited in House, P.R., Lagos-Witte, S., Ochoa, L., Torres, C., Mejia, T., Rivas, M. (1995). Plantas Medicinales Comunes de Honduras. Tegucigalpa, Honduras, CA.

Carretero, M. E., Lopez-Perez, J. L., Abad, M. J., Bermejo, P., Tillet, S., Israel, A., et al. (2008). Preliminary study of the anti-inflammatory activity of hexane extract and fractions from Bursera simaruba (Linneo) Sarg. (Burseraceae) leaves. *Journal of Ethnopharmacology, 116*(1), 11–15. https://doi.org/10.1016/j.jep.2007.10.034

Carro-Hernández, M., & Espinoza-Carr, G. (2016). La historia de la seguridad social en Costa Rica. *Revista Judicial, Costa Rica, 119*, 221–236.

Castro, O., Gutiérrez, J. M., Barrios, M., Castro, I., Romero, M., & Umaña, E. (1999). Neutralization of the hemorrhagic effect induced by venom *Bothrops asper* (Serpentes: Viperidae) venom with tropical plant extracts. *Revista de Biologia Tropical, 47*(3), 605–616.

Central Intelligence Agency (CIA). (2016). *The World Factbook*. Retrieved September 23, 2016, from https://www.cia.gov/library/publications/resources/the-world-factbook/.

Centro de Investigaciones Farmacognósticas de la Flora Panameña (CIFLORPAN). (2004). *Base de Datos de Usos Etnomédicos de Plantas Panameñas y Centroamericanas (PLANMEDIA)*. Project SEDI/AICD/106/01–04. Washington, DC, Organization of the American States. Ethnomedical database PLANMEDIA®.

Cepleanu, F., Hamburger, M., Sordat, B., Msonthi, J., Gupta, M., Saadou, M., et al. (1994). Screening of tropical medicinal plants for molluscicidal, larvicidal, fungicidal and cytotoxic activities and brine shrimp toxicity. *International Journal of Pharmacognosy, 32*(3), 294–307.

Chan, W. Y., Tam, P. P., So, K. C., & Yeung, H. W. (1985). The inhibitory effects of beta-momorcharin on endometrial cells in the mouse. *Contraception, 31*(1), 83–90.

Chan, W. Y., Tam, P. P., & Yeung, H. W. (1984). The termination of early pregnancy in the mouse by beta-momorcharin. *Contraception, 29*(1), 91–100.
Che, C. T., Ahmed, M. S., Kang, S. S., Waller, D. P., Bingel, A. S., Martin, A., et al. (1984). Studies on Aristolochia III. Isolation and biological evaluation of constituents of Aristolochia indica roots for fertility-regulating activity. *Journal of Natural Products, 47*(2), 331–341.
Chen, C. C., Hsu, J. D., Wang, S. F., Chiang, H. C., Yang, M. Y., Kao, E. S., et al. (2003). Hibiscus sabdariffa extract inhibits the development of atherosclerosis in cholesterol-fed rabbits. *Journal of Agricultural and Food Chemistry, 51*(18), 5472–5477. https://doi.org/10.1021/jf030065w
Coe, F. G. (2008). Rama midwifery in eastern Nicaragua. *Journal of Ethnopharmacology, 117*(1), 136–157. https://doi.org/10.1016/j.jep.2008.01.027
Coe, F. G., & Anderson, G. J. (1996). Screening of medicinal plants used by the Garifuna of eastern Nicaragua for bioactive compounds. *Journal of Ethnopharmacology, 53*(1), 29–50.
Coe, F. G., Parikh, D. M., Johnson, C. A., & Anderson, G. J. (2012). The good and the bad: alkaloid screening and brineshrimp bioassays of aqueous extracts of 31 medicinal plants of eastern Nicaragua. *Pharmaceutical Biology, 50*(3), 384–392. https://doi.org/10.3109/13880209.2011.608077
Cohen, F. S. (1982). Childbirth belief and practice in a Garifuna (Black-Carib) village on the North Coast of Honduras. *Western Journal of Nursing Research, 4*(2), 193–208.
Costa, G. M., Schenkel, E. P., & Reginatto, F. H. (2011). Chemical and pharmacological aspects of the genus Cecropia. *Natural Product Communications, 6*(6), 913–920.
Cox, P. A., Sperry, L. R., Tuominen, M., & Bohlin, L. (1989). Pharmacological activity of the Samoan ethnopharmacopoeia. *Economic Botany, 43*(4), 487–497.
D'Angelo, L. C., Xavier, H. S., Torres, L. M., Lapa, A. J., & Souccar, C. (1997). Pharmacology of Piper marginatum Jacq. a folk medicinal plant used as an analgesic, antiinflammatory and hemostatic. *Phytomedicine, 4*(1), 33–40. https://doi.org/10.1016/s0944-7113(97)80025-6
de Andrade, L. O., Pellegrini Filho, A., Solar, O., Rigoli, F., de Salazar, L. M., Serrate, P. C., et al. (2015). Social determinants of health, universal health coverage, and sustainable development: case studies from Latin American countries. *Lancet, 385*(9975), 1343–1351. https://doi.org/10.1016/S0140-6736(14)61494-X
de Freitas, P. L., Dias, A. C., Moreira, V. R., Monteiro, S. G., & Pereira, S. R. (2015). Antimutagenic action of the triterpene betulinic acid isolated from Scoparia dulcis (Scrophulariaceae). *Genetics and Molecular Research, 14*(3), 9745–9752. https://doi.org/10.4238/2015.August.19.7
De Gezelle, J. (2014). *Q'eqchi Maya Reprodcutive Ethnomedicine*. Cham, Switzerland: Springer International Publishing.
Der Marderosian, A. H., Giller, F. B., & Roia, F. C., Jr. (1976). Phytochemical and toxicological screening of household ornamental plants potentially toxic to humans. I. *Journal of Toxicology and Environmental Health, 1*(6), 939–953. https://doi.org/10.1080/15287397609529396
Desta, B. (1994). Ethiopian traditional herbal drugs. Part III: Anti-fertility activity of 70 medicinal plants. *Journal of Ethnopharmacology, 44*(3), 199–209.
Dhar, M., Dhar, M., Dhawan, B., Mehrotra, B., & Ray, C. (1968). Screening of Indian plants for biological activity: I. *Indian Journal of Experimental Biology, 6*(4), 232–247.
Di Renzo, G. C., Brillo, E., Romanelli, M., Porcaro, G., Capanna, F., Kanninen, T. T., et al. (2012). Potential effects of chocolate on human pregnancy: A randomized controlled trial. *Journal of Maternal-Fetal Neonatal Medicine, 25*(10), 1860–1867. https://doi.org/10.3109/14767058.2012.683085
Doyle, B. J., Frasor, J., Bellows, L. E., Locklear, T. D., Perez, A., Gomez-Laurito, J., et al. (2009). Estrogenic effects of herbal medicines from Costa Rica used for the management of menopausal symptoms. *Menopause, 16*(4), 748–755. https://doi.org/10.1097/gme.0b013e3181a4c76a
Duke, J. A. (2000). Biological activity summary for cocao (Theobroma cacao L.) *Journal of Medicinal Food, 3*(2), 115–119.
Espinoza, H., Abuabara, K., & Ellertson, C. (2004). Physicians' knowledge and opinions about medication abortion in four Latin American and Caribbean region countries. *Contraception, 70*(2), 127–133. https://doi.org/10.1016/j.contraception.2004.03.011
Feng, P. C., Haynes, L. J., Magnus, K. E., Plimmer, J. R., & Sherratt, H. S. (1962). Pharmacological screening of some West Indian medicinal plants. *Journal of Pharmacy and Pharmacology, 14*, 556–561.
Forbes. (2015). *Best Countries for Business: Nicaragua*. Retrieved October 7, 2016, from http://www.forbes.com/places/nicaragua/.
Foundation for Sustainable Development. (2016). *Child and maternal health issues in Nicaragua*. Retrieved October 7, 2016, from http://www.fsdinternational.org/country/nicaragua/healthissues.
Ganguly, M., Devi, N., Mahanta, R., & Borthakur, M. K. (2007). Effect of Mimosa pudica root extract on vaginal estrous and serum hormones for screening of antifertility activity in albino mice. *Contraception, 76*(6), 482–448. https://doi.org/10.1016/j.contraception.2007.08.008
García-Segura, A. (1994). *Plantas medicinales de la medicina bribri*. San José, Costa Rica: Universidad de Costa Rica.

García, A., Mena F., Capítulo III. (2004). *Remedios Costa Rica, Nuestra Medicina Tradicional, Libro 6 Series Culturas Populares Centroamericanas*: Coordinación Educativa Cultural Centroamericana Editores.
Garg, S. K. (1976). Antifertility screening of plants—effect of four Indigenous plants on early pregnancy in female albino rats. *Indian Journal of Medical Research, 64*(8), 1133–1135.
Giron, L. M., Freire, V., Alonzo, A., & Caceres, A. (1991). Ethnobotanical survey of the medicinal flora used by the Caribs of Guatemala. *Journal of Ethnopharmacology, 34*(2–3), 173–187.
González Ayala, J. C. (1994). *Botánica Medicinal Popular*. San Salvador, El Salvador: Cuscatlania.
Gracioso, J. S., Paulo, M. Q., Hiruma Lima, C. A., & Souza Brito, A. R. (1998). Antinociceptive effect in mice of a hydroalcoholic extract of Neurolaena lobata (L.) R. Br. and its organic fractions. *Journal of Pharmacy and Pharmacology, 50*(12), 1425–1429.
Grimes, D. A., Benson, J., Singh, S., Romero, M., Ganatra, B., Okonofua, F. E., et al. (2006). Unsafe abortion: the preventable pandemic. *Lancet, 368*(9550), 1908–1919. https://doi.org/10.1016/S0140-6736(06)69481-6
Grover, J. K., & Yadav, S. P. (2004). Pharmacological actions and potential uses of Momordica charantia: a review. *Journal of Ethnopharmacology, 93*(1), 123–132. https://doi.org/10.1016/j.jep.2004.03.035
Guerra, M. O., & Andrade, A. T. (1978). Contraceptive effects of native plants in rats. *Contraception, 18*(2), 191–199.
Guerrini, A., Sacchetti, G., Rossi, D., Paganetto, G., Muzzoli, M., Andreotti, E., et al. (2009). Bioactivities of Piper aduncum L. and Piper obliquum Ruiz & Pavon (Piperaceae) essential oils from Eastern Ecuador. *Environmental Toxicology and Pharmacology, 27*(1), 39–48. https://doi.org/10.1016/j.etap.2008.08.002
Gupta, M., Monge, A., Karikas, G., Lopez de Cerain, A., Solis, P., De Leon, E., et al. (1996). Screening of Panamánian medicinal plants for brine shrimp toxicity, crown gall tumor inhibition, cytotoxicity and DNA intercalation. *International Journal of Pharmacognosy, 34*(1), 19–27.
Gupta, M. P., Arias, T. D., Correa, M., & Lamba, S. S. (1979). Ethnopharmacognostic observations on Panamánian medicinal plants. Part I. *Quarterly Journal of Crude Drug Research, 17*(3–4), 115–130.
Gupta, M. P., Correa, M. D., Solis, P. N., Jones, A., Galdames, C., & Guionneau-Sinclair, F. (1993). Medicinal plant inventory of Kuna Indians: Part 1. *Journal of Ethnopharmacology, 40*(2), 77–109.
Gupta, M. P., Solis, P. N., Calderon, A. I., Guionneau-Sinclair, F., Correa, M., Galdames, C., et al. (2005). Medical ethnobotany of the Teribes of Bocas del Toro, Panamá. *Journal of Ethnopharmacology, 96*(3), 389–401. https://doi.org/10.1016/j.jep.2004.08.032
Hall, M. G., Garrett, J. J., & Barrington, C. (2014). La situacion economica: Social determinants of contraceptive use in rural Honduras. *Global Public Health, 9*(4), 455–468. https://doi.org/10.1080/17441692.2014.890238
Harmayani, E., Kumalasari, I. D., & Marsono, Y. (2011). Effect of arrowroot (Maranta arundinacea L.) diet on the selected bacterial population and chemical properties of caecal digesta of Sprague Dawley rats. *International Research Journal of Microbiology, 2*, 278–284.
Harvey, S. A., Blandón, Y. C. W., McCaw-binns, A., Sandino, I., Urbina, L., Rodríguez, C., et al. (2007). Are skilled birth attendants really skilled? A measurement method, some disturbing results and a potential way forward. *Bulletin of the World Health Organization, 85*(10), 783–790. https://doi.org/10.2471/BLT.
Hasrat, J. A., Pieters, L., De Backer, J. P., Vauquelin, G., & Vlietinck, A. J. (1997). Screening of medicinal plants from Suriname for 5-HT(1A) ligands: Bioactive isoquinoline alkaloids from the fruit of Annona muricata. *Phytomedicine, 4*(2), 133–140. https://doi.org/10.1016/S0944-7113(97)80059-1
Hayashi, T., Uchida, K., Hayashi, K., Niwayama, S., & Morita, N. (1988). A cytotoxic flavone from Scoparia dulcis L. *Chemical and Pharmaceutical Bulletin (Tokyo), 36*(12), 4849–4851.
Heinrich, M., Barnes, J., Gibbons, S., & Williamson, E. (2004). *Fundamentals of Pharmacognosy and Phytotherapy*. London: Churchill Livingstone.
Higdon, K., Scott, A., Tucci, M., Benghuzzi, H., Tsao, A., Puckett, A., et al. (2001). The use of estrogen, DHEA, and diosgenin in a sustained delivery setting as a novel treatment approach for osteoporosis in the ovariectomized adult rat model. *Biomedical Sciences Instrumentation, 37*, 281–286.
House, P. R., Lagos-Witte, S., Ochoa, L., Torres, C., Mejia, T., & Rivas, M. (1995). *Plantas Medicinales Comunes de Honduras*. Honduras, CA: Tegucigalpa.
Hughes, J. (2004). *Gender equity and Indigenous women's health in the Americas*. Pan American Health Organization Report. Retrieved August 10, 2016, from http://www.paho.org/hq/dmdocuments/2011/gdr-gender-equity-and-Indigenous-women-health-americas.pdf.
Innes, A. J., Kennedy, G., McLaren, M., Bancroft, A. J., & Belch, J. J. (2003). Dark chocolate inhibits platelet aggregation in healthy volunteers. *Platelets, 14*(5), 325–327.
Instituto Nacional de Estadística y Censos. (2013). *Censo Nacional de Población y VI de Vivienda: Territorios Indígenas*. San José, Costa Rica.: Instituto Nacional de Estadística y Censos.
Instituto Nacional de Estadística y Censos de Costa Rica (INEC). (2016). Retrieved November 10, 2016, from http://www.inec.go.cr.
Instituto Nacional de Estadística y Censo. (2016). *Panamá en Cifras: 2009–2013*. Retrieved October 25, 2016, from https://www.contraloria.gob.pa/inec/Publicaciones/Publicaciones.aspx?ID_SUBCATEGORIA=45&ID_PUBLICACION=622&ID_IDIOMA=1&ID_CATEGORIA=17.

International Fund for Agricultural Development (IFAD). (2014). *Rural poverty in Honduras*. Retrieved August 10, 2016, from http://www.ruralpovertyportal.org/country/home/tags/honduras.
International Work Group for Indigenous Affairs. (2015). *Indigenous peoples in Honduras*. Retrieved May 5, 2016, from http://www.iwgia.org/regions/latin-america/honduras.
Iwalewa, E. O., Iwalewa, O. J., & Adeboye, J. O. (2003). Analgesic, antipyretic, anti-inflammatory effects of methanol, chloroform and ether extracts of Vernonia cinerea less leaf. *Journal of Ethnopharmacology, 86*(2–3), 229–234.
Jaafarpour, M., Hatefi, M., Khani, A., & Khajavikhan, J. (2015a). Comparative effect of cinnamon and Ibuprofen for treatment of primary dysmenorrhea: a randomized double-blind clinical trial. *Journal of Clinical and Diagnostic Research, 9*(4), QC04–QC07. https://doi.org/10.7860/JCDR/2015/12084.5783
Jaafarpour, M., Hatefi, M., Najafi, F., Khajavikhan, J., & Khani, A. (2015b). The effect of cinnamon on menstrual bleeding and systemic symptoms with primary dysmenorrhea. *Iran Red Crescent Medical Journal, 17*(4), e27032. https://doi.org/10.5812/ircmj.17(4)2015.27032.
Jimenez, G., Hasegawa, M., Rodriguez, M., Estrada, O., Mendez, J., Castillo, A., et al. (2001). Biological screening of plants of the Venezuelan Amazons. *Journal of Ethnopharmacology, 77*(1), 77–83.
Joly, L. G., Guerra, S., Septimo, R., Solis, P. N., Correa, M., Gupta, M., et al. (1987). Ethnobotanical inventory of medicinal plants used by the Guaymi Indians in western Panamá. Part I. *Journal of Ethnopharmacology, 20*(2), 145–171.
Joly, L. G., Guerra, S., Septimo, R., Solis, P. N., Correa, M. D., Gupta, M. P., et al. (1990). Ethnobotanical inventory of medicinal plants used by the Guaymi Indians in western Panamá. Part II. *Journal of Ethnopharmacology, 28*(2), 191–206.
Josyula, S., Taylor, K. K., Murphy, B. M., Rodas, D., & Kamath-Rayne, B. D. (2015). Obstetric referrals from a rural clinic to a community hospital in Honduras. *Midwifery, 31*(11), 1054–1059. https://doi.org/10.1016/j.midw.2015.07.002
Kestler, E. (2014). Maternal Mortality in Central America: The need to accerlate efforts by 2035. *Maternal Health Task Force (MHTF) Blog*. Retrieved July 20, 2016, from https://www.mhtf.org/2014/01/23/maternal-mortality-in-central-america-the-need-to-accelerate-efforts-by-2035/.
Kestler, E., Walker, D., Bonvecchio, A., de Tejada, S. S., & Donner, A. (2013). A matched pair cluster randomized implementation trail to measure the effectiveness of an intervention package aiming to decrease perinatal mortality and increase institution-based obstetric care among Indigenous women in Guatemala: study protocol. *BMC Pregnancy and Childbirth, 13*, 73. https://doi.org/10.1186/1471-2393-13-73
Khan, M. (1997). The phytochemical study and clinical evaluation of Tagetes erecta in the treatment of hallux abducto vagus and associated condition, bunion. *Journal of Pharmacy and Pharmacology, 49*, 222–222.
Khodabakhsh, P., Shafaroodi, H., & Asgarpanah, J. (2015). Analgesic and anti-inflammatory activities of Citrus aurantium L. blossoms essential oil (neroli): involvement of the nitric oxide/cyclic-guanosine monophosphate pathway. *Journal of Natural Medicines, 69*(3), 324–331. https://doi.org/10.1007/s11418-015-0896-6
Kokane, D. D., More, R. Y., Kale, M. B., Nehete, M. N., Mehendale, P. C., & Gadgoli, C. H. (2009). Evaluation of wound healing activity of root of Mimosa pudica. *Journal of Ethnopharmacology, 124*(2), 311–315. https://doi.org/10.1016/j.jep.2009.04.038
Kulkarni, T. R., Kothekar, M. A., & Mateenuddin, M. (2005). Study of anti-fertility effect of lemon seeds (Citrus limonum) in female albino mice. *Indian Journal of Physiology and Pharmacology, 49*(3), 305–312.
Lans, C. (2007). Ethnomedicines used in Trinidad and Tobago for reproductive problems. *Journal of Ethnobiology and Ethnomedicine, 3*, 13. https://doi.org/10.1186/1746-4269-3-13
Laribi, B., Kouki, K., M'Hamdi, M., & Bettaieb, T. (2015). Coriander (Coriandrum sativum L.) and its bioactive constituents. *Fitoterapia, 103*, 9–26. https://doi.org/10.1016/j.fitote.2015.03.012
Law, L. K., Tam, P. P., & Yeung, H. W. (1983). Effects of alpha-trichosanthin and alpha-momorcharin on the development of peri-implantation mouse embryos. *Journal of Reproduction and Fertility, 69*(2), 597–604.
Lefeber, Y., & Voorhoeve, H. W. A. (1998). *Indigenous customs in childbirth and child care*. Assen, The Netherlands: Van Gorcum and Comp.
Lentz, D. (1993). Medicinal and other economic plants of hte Paya of Honduras. *Economic Botany, 47*(4), 358–370.
Lentz, D. L., Clark, A. M., Hufford, C. D., Meurer-Grimes, B., Passreiter, C. M., Cordero, J., et al. (1998). Antimicrobial properties of Honduran medicinal plants. *Journal of Ethnopharmacology, 63*(3), 253–263.
Lizcano, P. J., Bakkali, F., Ruiz-Larrea, M., & Sanz, J. I. (2010). Antioxidant activity and polyphenol content of aqueous extracts from Columbian Amazonia plants with medicinal use. *Food Chemistry, 119*, 1566–1570.
Locklear, T. D., Huang, Y., Frasor, J., Doyle, B. J., Perez, A., Gomez-Laurito, J., et al. (2010). Estrogenic and progestagenic effects of extracts of Justicia pectoralis Jacq., an herbal medicine from Costa Rica used for the treatment of menopause and PMS. *Maturitas, 66*(3), 315–322. https://doi.org/10.1016/j.maturitas.2010.04.001
Locklear, T. D., Perez, A., Caceres, A., & Mahady, G. B. (2013). Women's health in Central America: The complexity of issues and the need to focus on indigenous healthcare. *Current Women's Health Reviews, 9*(1), 30–40.
Logarto Parra, A., Silva Yhebra, R., Guerra Sardinas, I., & Iglesias Buela, L. (2001). Comparative study of the assay of Artemia salina L. and the estimate of the medium lethal dose (LD50 value) in mice, to determine oral acute toxicity of plant extracts. *Phytomedicine, 8*(5), 395–400.

Lozano, R., Wang, H., Foreman, K. J., Rajaratnam, J. K., Naghavi, M., Marcus, J. R., et al. (2011). Progress towards Millennium Development Goals 4 and 5 on maternal and child mortality: an updated systematic analysis. *Lancet, 378*(9797), 1139–1165. https://doi.org/10.1016/S0140-6736(11)61337-8

Low, L. S., Scheib, H., Bailey, J. M., & Sacks, E. (2006). Challenges for traditional birth attendants in northern rural Honduras. *Midwifery, 22*, 78–87.

Mans, D., Toelsie, J., Jagernath, Z., Ramjiawan, K., van Brussel, A., Jhanjan, N., et al. (2004). Assessment of eight popularly used plant-derived preparations for their spasmolytic potential using the isolated guinea pig ileum. *Pharmaceutical Biology, 42*(6), 422–429.

Marino, T. (2014). *Anticoagulants and Thrombolytics in Pregnancy*. Medscape. Retrieved October 2, 2016, from http://emedicine.medscape.com/article/164069-overview#a2.

Marques, M. C. S., Hamerski, L., Garcez, F. R., Tieppo, C., Vasconcelos, M., Santos, E. C. T., et al. (2013). In vitro biological screening and evaluation of free radical scavenging activities of medicinal plants from the Brazilian Cerrado. *Journal of Medicinal Plants Research, 7*(15), 957–962. https://doi.org/10.5897/JMPR12-882.

Marrufo-Estrada, D. M., Segura-Campos, M. R., Chel-Guerrero, L. A., & Betancur-Ancona, D. A. (2013). Defatted Jatropha curcas flour and protein isolate as materials for protein hydrolysates with biological activity. *Food Chemistry, 138*(1), 77–83. https://doi.org/10.1016/j.foodchem.2012.09.033

Martinez, A. L., Gonzalez-Trujano, M. E., Chavez, M., & Pellicer, F. (2012). Antinociceptive effectiveness of triterpenes from rosemary in visceral nociception. *Journal of Ethnopharmacology, 142*(1), 28–34. https://doi.org/10.1016/j.jep.2012.03.052

Mascolo, N., Capasso, F., Menghini, A., & Fasulo, M. P. (1987). Biological screening of Italian medicinal plants for anti-inflammatory activity. *Phytotherapy Research, 1*(1), 28–31.

Mata, R., Morales, I., Perez, O., Rivero-Cruz, I., Acevedo, L., Enriquez-Mendoza, I., et al. (2004). Antimycobacterial compounds from Piper sanctum. *Journal of Natural Products, 67*(12), 1961–1968. https://doi.org/10.1021/np0401260

McKinnon, R., Binder, M., Zupko, I., Afonyushkin, T., Lajter, I., Vasas, A., et al. (2014). Pharmacological insight into the anti-inflammatory activity of sesquiterpene lactones from Neurolaena lobata (L.) R.Br. ex Cass. *Phytomedicine, 21*(12), 1695–1701. https://doi.org/10.1016/j.phymed.2014.07.019

Merrill, T. (1995). *A Country Study*. Washington, DC: GPO for the Library of Congress.

Messmer, W. M., Farnsworth, N. R., Persinos, G. J., & Wilkes, J. D. (1968). Phytochemical investigation of the flowers of Cassia reticulata Willd. (Leguminosae). *Journal of Pharmaceutical Sciences, 57*(11), 1996–1998.

Michel, J., Caceres, A., Yao, P., Yuang, Y., Bolton, J., Soejarto, D. D., & Mahady, G. B. (2012). Q'eqchi May medicine for women's health: Guatemalan plants with estrogen and serotonin activities. *Acta Horticulturae, 964*, 235–250.

Michel, J., Duarte, R. E., Bolton, J. L., Huang, Y., Caceres, A., Veliz, M., et al. (2007). Medical potential of plants used by the Q'eqchi Maya of Livingston, Guatemala for the treatment of women's health complaints. *Journal of Ethnopharmacology, 114*(1), 92–101. https://doi.org/10.1016/j.jep.2007.07.033

Michel, J. L., Caceres, A., & Mahady, G. B. (2016). Ethnomedical research and review of Q'eqchi Maya women's reproductive health in the Lake Izabal region of Guatemala: Past, present and future prospects. *Journal of Ethnopharmacology, 178*, 307–322. https://doi.org/10.1016/j.jep.2015.12.006

Michel, J. L., Mahady, G. B., Veliz, M., Soejarto, D. D., & Caceres, A. (2006). Symptoms, attitudes and treatment choices surrounding menopause among the Q'eqchi Maya of Livingston, Guatemala. *Social Science and Medicine, 63*(3), 732–742. https://doi.org/10.1016/j.socscimed.2006.02.010

Minority Rights Group International. (2008). *World Directory of Minorities and Indigenous Peoples*. Nicaragua. Retrieved October 7, 2016, from http://minorityrights.org/country/nicaragua/.

Monteiro, M. H., Gomes-Carneiro, M. R., Felzenszwalb, I., Chahoud, I., & Paumgartten, F. J. (2001). Toxicological evaluation of a tea from leaves of Vernonia condensata. *Journal of Ethnopharmacology, 74*(2), 149–157.

Montenegro, R. A., & Stephens, C. (2006). Indigenous health in Latin America and the Caribbean. *Lancet, 367*(9525), 1859–1869. https://doi.org/10.1016/S0140-6736(06)68808-9

Morais-Braga, M. F., Souza, T. M., Santos, K. K., Guedes, G. M., Andrade, J. C., Vega, C., et al. (2013). Phenol composition, cytotoxic and anti-kinetoplastidae activities of Lygodium venustum SW. (Lygodiaceae). *Experimental Parasitology, 134*(2), 178–182. https://doi.org/10.1016/j.exppara.2013.03.014

Nakanishi, K., Sasaki, S., Kiang, A. K., Goh, J., Kakisawa, H., Ohashi, M., et al. (1965). Phytochemical survey of Malaysian plants preliminary chemical and pharmacological screening. *Chemical and Pharmaceutical Bulletin (Tokyo), 13*(7), 882–890.

Narendhirakannan, R. T., & Limmy, T. P. (2012). Anti-inflammatory and anti-oxidant properties of Sida rhombifolia stems and roots in adjuvant induced arthritic rats. *Immunopharmacology and Immunotoxicology, 34*(2), 326–336. https://doi.org/10.3109/08923973.2011.605142

Newall, C. A., Anderson, L. A., & Phillipson, J. D. (1996). *Herbal medicines: A guide for Health-Care Professionals*. London: Pharmaceutical Press.

Njan, A. A., Adzu, B., Agaba, A. G., Byarugaba, D., Diaz-Llera, S., & Bangsberg, D. R. (2008). The analgesic and antiplasmodial activities and toxicology of Vernonia amygdalina. *Journal of Medical Food, 11*(3), 574–581. https://doi.org/10.1089/jmf.2007.0511

Noguera, B., Diaz, E., Garcia, M. V., Feliciano, A. S., Lopez-Perez, J. L., & Israel, A. (2004). Anti-inflammatory activity of leaf extract and fractions of Bursera simaruba (L.) Sarg (Burseraceae). *Journal of Ethnopharmacology, 92*(1), 129–133. https://doi.org/10.1016/j.jep.2004.02.009

Nortier, J. L., Martinez, M. C., Schmeiser, H. H., Arlt, V. M., Bieler, C. A., Petein, M., et al. (2000). Urothelial carcinoma associated with the use of a Chinese herb (Aristolochia fangchi). *New England Journal of Medicine, 342*(23), 1686–1692. https://doi.org/10.1056/nejm200006083422301

Ocampo, R. A., & Maffioli, A. (1987). *El uso de algunas plantas medicinales en Costa Rica*. San José, Costa Rica: Litografía e Imprtenta LIL.

Ohigashi, H., Koshimizu, K., Tokuda, H., Hiramatsu, S., Jato, J., & Ito, Y. (1985). Epstein-Barr virus-inducing activity of Euphorbiaceae plants commonly grown in Cameroon. *Cancer Letters, 28*(2), 135–141.

Ohno, O., Ye, M., Koyama, T., Yazawa, K., Mura, E., Matsumoto, H., et al. (2008). Inhibitory effects of benzyl benzoate and its derivatives on angiotensin II-induced hypertension. *Bioorganic and Medicinal Chemistry, 16*(16), 7843–7852. https://doi.org/10.1016/j.bmc.2008.03.056

Onocha, P. A., Oloyede, G. K., & Bamkole, O. A. (2011). UV-visible investigation of antioxidant and toxicity activities of methanolic fractions of Acalypha hispida (Burn. f) leaves. *EuropeanJournal of Scientific Research, 49*, 322–331.

Ortiz de Montellano, B. R., & Browner, C. H. (1985). Chemical bases for medicinal plant use in Oaxaca, Mexico. *Journal of Ethnopharmacology, 13*(1), 57–88.

Pakrashi, A., & Chakrabarty, B. (1977). Biological properties of interceptive agents from Aristolochia indica Linn. *Indian Journal of Medical Research, 66*(6), 991–998.

Pan American Health Organization. (2012). *Health in the Americas: 2012 Edition. Regional Outlook and Country Profiles*. Washington, DC: PAHO. Retrieved April 15, 2016, from http://www1.paho.org/saludenlasamericas/docs/hia-2012-summary.pdf.

Pan American Health Organization. (2004). Maternal and child mortality among the Indigenous peoples of the Americas. *Bulletin of Indigenous Health, 1*, 1–3.

Pan American Health Organization and World Health Organization. (2015). *Regional Health Observatory. Health Indicators by countries and years*. Retrieved July 25, 2016, from http://www.paho.org/hq/index.php?option=com_content&view=category&layout=blog&id=2391&Itemid=2392&lang=en.

Parham, L., de Rivera, I. L., Murillo, W., Naver, L., Largaespada, N., Albert, J., et al. (2011). Short communication: high prevalence of drug resistance in HIV type 1-infected children born in Honduras and Belize 2001 to 2004. *AIDS Research and Human Retroviruses, 27*(10), 1055–1059. https://doi.org/10.1089/AID.2010.0289

Parra, Á. V., Ruiz, A. R., López, A. G., Ferrer, J. P., & González, V. P. (2000). Study genotoxic *in vitro* and *in vivo* fluid extract of *Cassia grandis* L. and gel *Aloe vera* L. *Revista Cubana de Plantas Medicinales, 5*(3), 91–96.

Patel, N. K., Bairwa, K., Gangwal, R., Jaiswal, G., Jachak, S. M., Sangamwar, A. T., et al. (2015). 2'-Hydroxy flavanone derivatives as an inhibitors of pro-inflammatory mediators: Experimental and molecular docking studies. *Bioorganic & Medicinal Chemistry Letters, 25*(9), 1952–1955. https://doi.org/10.1016/j.bmcl.2015.03.025

Patel, N. K., & Bhutani, K. K. (2014). Suppressive effects of Mimosa pudica (L.) constituents on the production of LPS-induced pro-inflammatory mediators. *Experimental and Clinical Sciences, 13*, 1011–1021.

Pathan, A. R., Kothawade, K. A., & Logade, M. N. (2011). Anxiolytic and analgesic effect of Coriander sativum Linn. *International Journal of Research in Pharmacy and Chemistry, 1*(4), 1087–1099.

Perez-Ortega, G., Gonzalez-Trujano, M. E., Angeles-Lopez, G. E., Brindis, F., Vibrans, H., & Reyes-Chilpa, R. (2016). Tagetes lucida Cav.: Ethnobotany, phytochemistry and pharmacology of its tranquilizing properties. *Journal of Ethnopharmacology, 181*, 221–228. https://doi.org/10.1016/j.jep.2016.01.040

Picking, D., Delgoda, R., Boulogne, I., & Mitchell, S. (2013). Hyptis verticillata Jacq: a review of its traditional uses, phytochemistry, pharmacology and toxicology. *Journal of Ethnopharmacology, 147*(1), 16–41. https://doi.org/10.1016/j.jep.2013.01.039

Price, J., & Asgary, R. (2011). Women's health disparities in Honduras: indicators and determinants. *Journal of Women's Health (Larchmt), 20*(12), 1931–1937. https://doi.org/10.1089/jwh.2010.2615

Quesada, A. (2008). *Plantas al servicio de la salud: Plantas medicinales de Costa Rica y Centroamérica*. San José, Costa Rica: Museo Nacional de Costa Rica.

Raghavenra, H., Diwakr, B. T., Lokesh, B. R., & Naidu, K. A. (2006). Eugenol—the active principle from cloves inhibits 5-lipoxygenase activity and leukotriene-C4 in human PMNL cells. *Prostaglandins Leukotrienes and Essential Fatty Acids, 74*(1), 23–27. https://doi.org/10.1016/j.plefa.2005.08.006

Raji, Y., Akinola, A., Oyeyipo, I. P., & Femi-Akinlosotu, O. (2010). Reproductive activities of female albino rats treated with quassin, a bioactive triterpenoid from stem bark extract of Quassia amara. *Nigerian Journal of Physiological Sciences, 25*(2), 95–102.

Ramiro, E., Franch, A., Castellote, C., Perez-Cano, F., Permanyer, J., Izquierdo-Pulido, M., et al. (2005). Flavonoids from Theobroma cacao down-regulate inflammatory mediators. *Journal of Agricultural and Food Chemistry, 53*(22), 8506–8511. https://doi.org/10.1021/jf0511042

Rao, P. V., Gan, S. H. (2014). Cinnamon: A multifaceted medicinal plant. *Evidence-Based Complementary and Alternative Medicine, 2014*, 642942. https://doi.org/10.1155/2014/642942.

Raskovic, A., Milanovic, I., Pavlovic, N., Milijasevic, B., Ubavic, M., & Mikov, M. (2015). Analgesic effects of rosemary essential oil and its interactions with codeine and paracetamol in mice. *European Review for Medical and Pharmacological Sciences, 19*(1), 165–172.
Restrepo-Mendez, M. C., Barros, A. J., Requejo, J., Duran, P., Serpa, L. A., Franca, G. V., et al. (2015). Progress in reducing inequalities in reproductive, maternal, newborn, and child health in Latin America and the Caribbean: an unfinished agenda. *Revista Panamericana de Salud Publica, 38*(1), 9–16.
Riaz, A., Khan, R. A., Mirza, T., Mustansir, T., & Ahmed, M. (2014). vitro/in vivo effect of Citrus limon (L. Burm. f.) juice on blood parameters, coagulation and anticoagulation factors in rabbits. *Pakistan Journal of Pharmaceutical Sciences, 27*(4), 907–915.
Ritter, A. M., Domiciano, T. P., Verri, W. A., Jr., Zarpelon, A. C., da Silva, L. G., Barbosa, C. P., et al. (2013). Antihypernociceptive activity of anethole in experimental inflammatory pain. *Inflammopharmacology, 21*(2), 187–197. https://doi.org/10.1007/s10787-012-0152-6
Rivero-Cruz, I., Duarte, G., Navarrete, A., Bye, R., Linares, E., & Mata, R. (2011). Chemical composition and antimicrobial and spasmolytic properties of Poliomintha longiflora and Lippia graveolens essential oils. *Journal of Food Science, 76*(2), C309–C317. https://doi.org/10.1111/j.1750-3841.2010.02022.x.
Rodgers, K. A., Little, M., & Nelson, S. (2004). Outcomes of training traditional birth attendants in rural Honduras: Comparison with a control group. *Journal of Health and Population in Developing Countries*. https://doi.org/10.12927/whp.2004.17634
Santos, R. N. D., Silva, M. G. D. V., & Braz Filho, R. (2008). Constituintes químicos do caule de Senna reticulata Willd. (Leguminoseae): Chemical constituents isolated from the wood of Senna reticulata Willd. *Química Nova, 31*(8), 1979–1981.
Santthawongsakul, S. (1980). *Studies on the uterine simulant activity of Thai medicinal plants*. Bangkok, Thailand: Chulalongkorn University.
Sagorchev, P., Lukanov, J., & Beer, A. M. (2010). Investigations into the specific effects of rosemary oil at the receptor level. *Phytomedicine, 17*(8–9), 693–697. https://doi.org/10.1016/j.phymed.2009.09.012
Salas Estrada, J. B. (1993). *Árboles de Nicaragua. Managua, Nicaragua*. Managua, Nicaragua: IRENA.
Sarkis, A., & Campos, V. M. (1985). *Cuyranderismo tradicional del costarricense*. San José, Costa Rica: Lehmann Editores.
Say, L., Chou, D., Gemmill, A., Tuncalp, O., Moller, A. B., Daniels, J., et al. (2014). Global causes of maternal death: a WHO systematic analysis. *Lancet Global Health, 2*(6), e323–e333. https://doi.org/10.1016/S2214-109X(14)70227-X
Schooley, J., Mundt, C., Wagner, P., Fullerton, J., & O'Donnell, M. (2009). Factors influencing health care-seeking behaviours among Mayan women in Guatemala. *Midwifery, 25*(4), 411–421. https://doi.org/10.1016/j.midw.2007.07.011
Schwab, K. (2016). *The global competitiveness report 2016–2017*. Geneva, Switzerland: World Economic Forum. Retrieved November 11, 2016, from https://www.weforum.org/reports/the-global-competitiveness-report-2016-2017-1.
Schwartz, D. A. (2015). Unsafe abortion: A persistent cause of maternal death and reproductive morbidity in resource-poor nations. In D. A. Schwartz (Ed.), *Maternal mortality: Risk factors, anthropological perspectives, prevalence in developing countries and preventive strategies for pregnancy-related death*. New York: Nova Science Publishers.
Sedgh, G., Singh, S., & Hussain, R. (2014). Intended and unintended pregnancies worldwide in 2012 and recent trends. *Studies in Family Planning, 45*(3), 301–314. https://doi.org/10.1111/j.1728-4465.2014.00393.x
Segleau Earle, J. (2001). *Plantas Medicinales en el Trópico Húmedo* (1st ed.). Costa Rica: Jardín Botánico Las Cusingas.
Semwal, D. K., Semwal, R. B., Vermaak, I., & Viljoen, A. (2014). From arrow poison to herbal medicine--the ethnobotanical, phytochemical and pharmacological significance of Cissampelos (Menispermaceae). *Journal of Ethnopharmacology, 155*(2), 1011–1028. https://doi.org/10.1016/j.jep.2014.06.054
Shivaprasad, H. V., Rajesh, R., Nanda, B. L., Dharmappa, K. K., & Vishwanath, B. S. (2009). Thrombin like activity of Asclepias curassavica L. latex: action of cysteine proteases. *Journal of Ethnopharmacology, 123*(1), 106–109. https://doi.org/10.1016/j.jep.2009.02.016
Smith-Oka, V. (2012). An analysis of two Indigenous reproductive health illnesses in a Nahua community in Veracruz, Mexico. *Journal of Ethnobiology and Ethnomedicine, 8*, 33. https://doi.org/10.1186/1746-4269-8-33
Solomon, I. P., Oyebadejo, S. A., Ekong, S. I., & Asuquo, I. E. (2014). Contraceptive effect of Citrus aurantifolia juice vaginal douche on reproductive histomorphology of adult female Wistar rats. *International Journal of Pharmaceutical Research and Allied Sciences, 3*(4), 16–26.
Sosa-Gomez, R. (1998). *The power of medicinal plants*. Doral, FL: Inter-American Publishing Association.
Sosa, S., Balick, M. J., Arvigo, R., Esposito, R. G., Pizza, C., Altinier, G., et al. (2002). Screening of the topical anti-inflammatory activity of some Central American plants. *Journal of Ethnopharmacology, 81*(2), 211–215.
Souza, I. L., Correia, A. C., Araujo, L. C., Vasconcelos, L. H., Silva Mda, C., Costa, V. C., et al. (2015). Essential oil from Xylopia frutescens Aubl. reduces cytosolic calcium levels on guinea pig ileum: mechanism underlying its spasmolytic potential. *BMC Complementary and Alternative Medicine, 15*, 327. https://doi.org/10.1186/s12906-015-0849-3
Speizer, I. S., Whittle, L., & Carter, M. (2005). Gender relations and reproductive decision making in Honduras. *Internatial Family Planning Perspectives, 31*(3), 131–139. https://doi.org/10.1363/ifpp.31.131.05.

Sundari, S., Valarmathi, R., Akilandeswari, S., & Ruckmani, K. (2001). Analgesic and antimicrobial activity of the dried leaves' extracts of Aristolochia tagala Cham. *Hamdard Medicus, 44*(3), 17–19.
Takaki, I., Bersani-Amado, L. E., Vendruscolo, A., Sartoretto, S. M., Diniz, S. P., Bersani-Amado, C. A., et al. (2008). Anti-inflammatory and antinociceptive effects of Rosmarinus officinalis L. essential oil in experimental animal models. *Journal of Medicinal Food, 11*(4), 741–746. https://doi.org/10.1089/jmf.2007.0524
Tam, P. P., Law, L. K., & Yeung, H. W. (1984). Effects of alpha-momorcharin on preimplantation development in the mouse. *Journal of Reproduction and Fertility, 71*(1), 33–38.
Ticktin, T., & Dalle, S. P. (2005). Medicinal plant use in the practice of midwifery in rural Honduras. *Journal of Ethnopharmacology, 96*(1–2), 233–248. https://doi.org/10.1016/j.jep.2004.09.015
United Nations. (2013). *World population prospects: The 2012 Revision*. Retrieved September 9, 2016, from http://www.un.org/en/development/desa/publications/world-population-prospects-the-2012-revision.html.
United Nation's International Children's Emergency Fund (UNICEF). (2011). *Honduras country programme document: 2012–2016*. Retrieved July 15, 2016, from https://www.unicef.org/about/execboard/files/Honduras_final_approved_2012-2016_English_20_Oct_2011.pdf.
United Nations Population Fund. (2005). *Country profiles for population and reproductive health: Policy developments and indicators. Maternal mortality statistics by region and by country*. Retrieved October 7, 2016, from http://www.prb.org/pdf05/2005unfpa_countryprofiles.pdf.
United Nations Statistics Division. (2016). *Countrymeters-Nicaragua Population*. Retrieved November 2, 2016, from http://countrymeters.info/en/Nicaragua.
Valdes, A. F., Mendiola, M. J., Acuna, R. D., Caballero, L. Y., Scull, L. R., & Gutierrez, G. Y. (2011). Antimalarial activity and cytotoxicity of hydroalcoholic extracts from six plant species used in Cuban traditional medicine. *Revista Cubana Medicina Tropical, 63*, 52–57.
Vasudeva, N., & Sharma, S. K. (2008). Post-Coital Antifertility Activity of Hibiscus rosa-sinensis Linn. roots. *Evidence-based Complementary and Alternative Medicine, 5*(1), 91–94. https://doi.org/10.1093/ecam/nem003
Venancio, A. M., Onofre, A. S., Lira, A. F., Alves, P. B., Blank, A. F., Antoniolli, A. R., et al. (2011). Chemical composition, acute toxicity, and antinociceptive activity of the essential oil of a plant breeding cultivar of basil (Ocimum basilicum L.) *Planta Medica, 77*(8), 825–829. https://doi.org/10.1055/s-0030-1250607
Villar Anleu, L. (1998). *La Flora Silvestre de Guatemala*. Guatemala City, Guatemala: Universidad de San Carlos.
Walsh, L. V. (2006). Beliefs and rituals in traditional birth attendant practice in Guatemala. *Journal of Transcultural Nursing, 17*(2), 148–154. https://doi.org/10.1177/1043659605285412
World Bank. (2006). *Honduras poverty assessment, attaining poverty reduction. Volume I: Main Report*. Retrieved October 2, 2016, from http://documents.worldbank.org/curated/en/443701468031594535/Main-report.
World Bank. (2012). *Health Systems Innovation in Central America: Lessons and impact of new approaches*. Retrieved September 9, 2016, from http://www.who.int/management/country/latinamerica_carribean/HealthSystemInnovatonsCentralAmerica.pdf.
World Bank. (2016a). *Disease control priorities: Reproductive, maternal, newborn, and child health* (Vol. 2, 3rd ed.). Washington, DC: International Bank for Reconstruction and Development/The World Bank.
World Bank. (2016b). *Honduras: Economic memorandum/poverty assessment. Poverty reduction and equity*. Retrieved June 15, 2016, from http://web.worldbank.org/WBSITE/EXTERNAL/TOPICS/EXTPOVERTY/EXTPA/0,contentMDK:20207592~menuPK:443285~pagePK:148956~piPK:216618~theSitePK:430367,00.html.
World Data Atlas. (2015a). *Honduras*. Retrieved October 7, 2016, from https://knoema.com/atlas/Honduras.
World Data Atlas. (2015b). *Nicaragua*. Retrieved October 7, 2016, from http://data.worldbank.org/indicator/SH.STA.MMRT?locations=NI.
World Health Organization. (1983). In R. H. Bannerman, J. Burton, & C. Wen-Cheih (Eds.), *Traditional medicine and health care coverage*. Geneva, Switzerland: WHO.
World Health Organization. (1992). *Traditional birth attendants. A joint WHO/UNFPA/UNICEF Statement*. Geneva, Switzerland: WHO. Retrieved July 21, 2016, from http://apps.who.int/iris/bitstream/10665/38994/1/9241561505.pdf.
World Health Organization. (2005). *Make every mother and child count. The World Health Report*. Geneva, Switzerland: WHO. Retrieved October 2, 2016, from http://www.who.int/whr/2005/whr2005_en.pdf.
World Health Organization. (2007). *Maternal mortality in 2005. Estimates developed by WHO, UNICEF, UNFPA and the World Bank*. Geneva, Switzerland: WHO. Retrieved October 2, 2016, from http://www.who.int/whosis/mme_2005.pdf.
World Health Organization. (2012). *WHO Guidelines on preventing early pregnancy and poor reproductive outcomes among adolescents in developing countries*. Geneva, Switzerland: WHO. Retrieved November 11, 2016, from http://www.who.int/immunization/hpv/target/preventing_early_pregnancy_and_poor_reproductive_outcomes_who_2006.pdf.
World Health Organization. (2015a). *Panamá key country indicators*. Geneva, Switzerland: WHO. Retrieved April 11, 2016, from http://apps.who.int/gho/data/node.cco.ki-PAN?lang=eng.

World Health Organization. (2015b). *Trends in Maternal Mortality: 1990–2015. Estimates by WHO, UNICEF, UNFPA, World Bank Group and the United Nations Population Division*. Geneva, Switzerland: WHO. Retrieved April 11, 2016, from http://apps.who.int/iris/bitstream/10665/194254/1/9789241565141_eng.pdf.

Yakubu, M. T., & Musa, I. F. (2012). Effects of Post-coital Administration of Alkaloids from Senna alata (Linn. Roxb) Leaves on some Fetal and Maternal Outcomes of Pregnant Rats. *Journal of Reproduction and Infertilility, 13*(4), 211–217.

Yavari Kia, P., Safajou, F., Shahnazi, M., & Nazemiyeh, H. (2014). The effect of lemon inhalation aromatherapy on nausea and vomiting of pregnancy: A double-blinded, randomized, controlled clinical trial. *Iran Red Crescent Medical Journal, 16*(3), e14360. https://doi.org/10.5812/ircmj.14360.

Zafar, S., Najam, Y., Arif, Z., & Hafeez, A. (2016). A randomized controlled trial comparing Pentazocine and Chamomilla recutita for labor pain relief. *Homeopathy, 105*(1), 66–70. https://doi.org/10.1016/j.homp.2015.09.003

Zahid, H., Rizwani, G. H., Shareef, H., Ahmed, M., & Hina, B. (2012). Analgesic and antipyretic activities of Hibiscus schizopetalus (Mast) Hook. *International Journal of Pharmacy and Pharmaceutical Sciences, 4*(3), 218–221.

Zamora-Martinez, M. C., & de Pascual Pola, C. N. (1992). Medicinal plants used in some rural populations of Oaxaca, Puebla and Veracruz, Mexico. *Journal of Ethnopharmacology, 35*(3), 229–257.

Zhang, G., Shimokawa, S., Mochizuki, M., Kumamoto, T., Nakanishi, W., Watanabe, T., et al. (2008). Chemical constituents of Aristolochia constricta: antispasmodic effects of its constituents in guinea-pig ileum and isolation of a diterpeno-lignan hybrid. *Journal of Natural Products, 71*(7), 1167–1172. https://doi.org/10.1021/np800041t

6 Gender and Family Planning Among Indigenous Women in Mexico and Central America: A Call to Action

Jessica K. Levy, Audrey Goold, April Houston, Diego Rios-Zertuche, and Wolfgang Munar

6.1 Introduction

The freedom to make informed decisions about one's fertility is essential to securing the autonomy and well-being of women and girls while promoting the health and development of families and communities. Modern contraceptive use is significantly correlated with decreases in unintended pregnancy, maternal and newborn mortality, and unsafe abortion (Ahmed et al. 2012). It is also positively correlated with gains in individual- and population-level education and economic prosperity (World Bank 2012; Bertrand et al. 2015).

As with the rest of Latin America and the Caribbean, the last 50 years has brought dramatic changes in fertility and contraceptive use to Central America and Mexico. In fact, at approximately 70%, this region has among the highest overall contraceptive prevalence rates (CPRs)[1] in all the developing world (United Nations 2015). Many sociocultural and economic improvements contribute to this rise in contraceptive use and subsequent fall in fertility, as have service delivery campaigns dedicated to

[1] *Contraceptive prevalence rate (CPR)* is the percentage of women who are currently using, or whose sexual partner is currently using, at least one method of contraception at a particular point in time, regardless of the method used. Unless stated otherwise, it is usually measured among married or in-union women aged 15 to 49.

J. K. Levy, Ph.D., M.P.H. (✉)
A. Goold, M.S.W., M.P.H.
George Warren Brown School of Social Work,
Washington University in St. Louis,
St. Louis, MO, USA
e-mail: Jessicaklevy@wustl.edu

A. Houston, M.S.W., M.P.H.
Sexual and Reproductive Health and Rights Team, CARE,
Atlanta, Georgia, USA

D. Rios-Zertuche, M.P.A.
Salud Mesoamerica Initiative, Inter-American
Development Bank, Washington, DC, USA

W. Munar, M.D., S.M.
Department of Global Health, George Washington
University, Washington, DC, USA

D. A. Schwartz (ed.), *Maternal Death and Pregnancy-Related Morbidity Among Indigenous Women of Mexico and Central America*, Global Maternal and Child Health: Medical, Anthropological, and Public Health Perspectives, https://doi.org/10.1007/978-3-319-71538-4_6

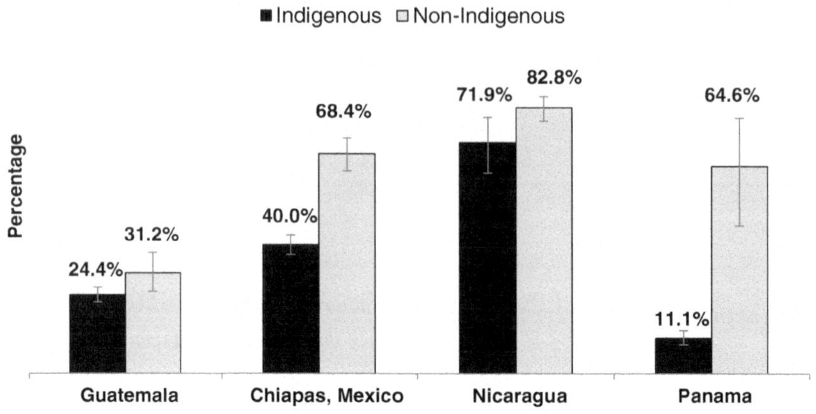

Fig. 6.1 Modern contraceptive prevalence rate by ethnicity in the poorest segments of four countries in Central America and Mexico (2011–2013). Figure uses data from Salud Mesoamerica Initiative (Rios-Zertuche et al. 2017). Values are survey-weighted and adjusted for complex survey design. Error bars show 95% confidence intervals

ensuring the availability of a mixed supply of quality contraceptives that are affordable and easy to access. Due to these successes, most big-donor funding for contraceptive commodities and family planning interventions has been phased out in Latin America, drawing attention to ongoing challenges that face countries where national-level indicators mask wide variations within subpopulations, such as those across wealth quintiles, rural/urban populations, and ethnic groups including indigenous women and their families (USAID 2012a).

Of note, recent data show that despite the overall improvement in CPR across Central America and Mexico, no country in the region has been able to bridge the gap in contraceptive use between indigenous and nonindigenous populations (Bertrand et al. 2015) (see Fig. 6.1). Indigenous women—and adolescents, in particular—are far more likely to have an unmet need for modern contraception[2] than their nonindigenous counterparts and are, therefore, at higher risk for experiencing an unintended pregnancy (Inegi 2015; Muiser et al. 2011; Bermúdez-Madriz et al. 2011; Becerril-Montekio and López-Dávila 2011). In fact, evidence shows that indigenous women continue to have, on average, more children than nonindigenous women throughout Latin America (Jaspers-Faijer and Montano 2013). For example, in Mexico, at the time of the latest census, indigenous women were having on average 3.2 children, compared to the 2.3 children born to nonindigenous Mexican women (Jaspers-Faijer and Montano 2013). Likewise, in Panama, indigenous women were having on average 5.2 children, whereas their nonindigenous counterparts were having 2.3 children (Jaspers-Faijer and Montano 2013).

These disparities are even more pronounced between indigenous and nonindigenous youth. For example, aggregate-level trends show that young adults throughout Latin America are getting married and having children later in life, in order to focus on work and education. However, when data are disaggregated by ethnicity, we do not see the same patterns among indigenous youth, many of whom lack easy access to education and employment opportunities (Jaspers-Faijer and Montano 2013). Furthermore, though there has been a recent decrease in pregnancy rates among indigenous adoles-

[2] *Unmet need* is a useful measurement for identifying and targeting women at high risk of unwanted pregnancy. It can be defined as the contraceptive needs of fecund women who want to delay or limit childbearing, yet who are still sexually active and not using contraception. Unmet need for modern contraception usually refers to the need for permanent methods (male and female sterilization), short-acting hormonal methods (pills, injectables, and vaginal ring), long-acting reversible contraception (implants and IUDs), barrier methods (male and female condoms, diaphragm, sponge), and/or emergency contraception.

cents, they are still more likely—across all countries surveyed—than their nonindigenous peers to have given birth by the age of 19. In Panama, for example, one in three indigenous girls between the ages of 15 and 19 were mothers at the time of the 2010 census (Jaspers-Faijer and Montano 2013).

To effectively limit these pockets of unmet need for modern contraception among the indigenous populations of Central America and Mexico, program planners and policy-makers must acknowledge the important role gender norms and inequalities play on family planning outcomes. Specifically, in this chapter, we assert that for any intervention to fully succeed, two things must happen: (1) gender norms and inequalities must be considered and addressed at all levels of program and policy planning, implementation, and evaluation; and (2) addressing these norms and inequalities will require integrated, crosscutting approaches. To make our argument, we first highlight the pathways through which social constructs of gender roles and expectations serve as strong predictors for family planning outcomes. Then, through an analysis of gender norms among the indigenous populations across the region, we identify areas where program implementers and policy-makers can best leverage their efforts to see positive family planning results. Building on this analysis, we conclude by making recommendations on how to integrate gender into current and future family planning initiatives and make a call for inter-sectorial action and systems-informed evaluation processes that have sufficient scope and scale to address such complex challenges.

6.2 Rationale for Considering Gender

Data from different regions of the world confirm that when women and girls have the same opportunities and access to resources as men and boys, benefits are felt at the individual, community, and national levels (World Bank 2012; Swiss et al. 2012; Kabeer and Natali 2013; Blanc 2001; Ahmed et al. 2010). Discriminatory gender norms, on the other hand, have been shown to negatively impact health and development outcomes (Taukobong et al. 2016). Within the context of family planning, social constructs of gender roles and expectations can strongly influence a woman's ability to delay childbearing, space births, and avoid unintended pregnancies. Women's control over financial resources and power, for example, is fundamental to determining who has access to family planning information, who holds the power to negotiate contraceptive use or to withhold sex, who decides on family size, and who controls the economic means to obtain family planning-related health services (Cleland et al. 2006; Taukobong et al. 2016).

Considering its fundamental and crosscutting role as either a facilitator or barrier to health and development, it is now widely accepted that failing to take discriminatory gender norms into account may not only limit positive outcomes but could also inadvertently lead to doing harm (World Bank 2012; USAID 2012b). As such, national governments are becoming increasingly responsive to gender equality mandates that have emerged from global gatherings and summits over the past several decades, including – but not limited to – The Convention on the Elimination of All Forms of Discrimination Against Women (CEDAW) (1979), the Cairo Program of Action (1994), and the Beijing Platform for Action (1995).

In addition to these well-known mandates, milestones in this process now include the internationally agreed-upon 2030 Agenda for Sustainable Development (successor to the Millennium Development Goals), in which there exists a stand-alone goal to improve gender equality and women's and girls' empowerment (GEWE). By highlighting GEWE, the United Nations is acknowledging the fact that gender equality is not only a human right but that it also plays a powerful role in promoting health and development and in reducing poverty:

> Ending all forms of discrimination against women and girls is not only a basic human right, but it is also crucial to accelerating sustainable development. It has been proven time and again, that empowering women and girls has a multiplier effect, and helps drive up economic growth and development across the board. (UNDP 2015)

Finally, as a way to manifest the vision of these mandates and reach the UN goals, bilateral and multilateral organizations, including the Pan American Health Organization (PAHO), now have policies that require integrating gender considerations into all levels of reproductive health and family planning programming and evaluation (USAID 2012b; DfID 2011; AusAid 2011; PAHO 2005).

6.3 Gender Analysis

6.3.1 Gender Terminology

There continues to be some confusion around, and often interchangeable use of, key gender terms in the literature; therefore, to minimize misunderstanding, we felt it important to clarify the gender-related vocabulary that we will be using in this chapter (see Table 6.1). First, the term "gender" is not to be confused with "sex." It is defined as a social construct that encompasses the economic, political, and sociocultural characteristics, constraints, and opportunities associated with being male or female, rather than the biological characteristics defined by chromosomes, hormones, internal reproductive organs, and genitalia. Furthermore, unlike the more immutable traits grounded in one's "sex," gender is contextual, dynamic, and open to change over time (USAID 2012b; WHO 2010).

When we refer to "gender norms," we are referring to dominant social expectations and standards related to the roles, attributes, and behaviors associated with being "male" or "female" within a given culture (Kågesten et al. 2016). Though not all gender norms are harmful, they do often assume differential structures of power and status between men and women. The more patriarchal a society is, the more it gives value to things that are stereotypically linked to masculinity and being male.

In this chapter, we are particularly interested in the gender norms that perpetuate unequal, discriminatory power relations between women and men, which can ultimately lead to poor health outcomes and reproductive health disparities. Furthermore, while the focus of this chapter is ultimately on women's and girls' empowerment, it is important to note that men and boys play a critical role in achieving gender equality and improving health outcomes and should also be considered in the design and implementation of programs and policies (as we will discuss in Sect. 6.5.3).

Table 6.1 Common definitions for gender terms (USAID 2012b; WHO 2010)

Concept	Definition
Gender equality	The equal enjoyment by women, girls, men, and boys of rights, opportunities, resources, and rewards. Equality does not mean that women and men are the same but that their choices and opportunities are not governed or limited by whether they are female or male
Gender equity	The process of being fair to women and men, which includes compensating for cumulative economic, social, and political disadvantages that prevent women and men from operating on a level playing field. *Note: gender equity strategies are the means to gender equality*
Gender gap	A difference in status of males and females. It is often measured by comparing sex-disaggregated data, including educational achievement, health outcomes, income or wealth indices, and levels of political participation
Gender-based violence	Violence that is directed at individuals based on their biological sex, gender identity, or perceived adherence to culturally defined expectations of what it means to be a woman/girl and man/boy. It includes public or private physical, sexual, and psychological abuse; threats; coercion; arbitrary inhibition of liberty; and economic deprivation
Female empowerment	When women and girls acquire the power to act freely, exercise their rights, and fulfill their potential as full and equal members of society. While empowerment often comes from within the individual, cultures, societies, and institutions create conditions that facilitate or undermine the possibilities for empowerment

6.3.2 Levers for Gender Equality and Women and Girl's Empowerment

To effectively close the gaps in modern contraceptive use and fertility outcomes within Central America and Mexico, we need programs and policies that are not only focused on traditional modes of family planning intervention (e.g., improving access to and quality of modern contraceptive supply), but that also work toward eventually transforming discriminatory gender norms that perpetuate poor health and development outcomes. To establish these "gender-transformative" interventions, we must first explore the unequal distribution of power between indigenous women and men in the region. These power differentials manifest through various gender norms and can be found in all components of the Social Ecological Model (SEM), including at the individual, interpersonal, institutional, community, and policy levels. Furthermore, both evidence and experience tell us that gender norms and inequalities are highly contextual and are often mediated by the power differentials within and between other sociodemographic factors such as age, race, place of residence, and income (Taukobong et al. 2016).

Considering the complex and even controversial nature of this topic, the literature provides various frameworks that address issues of power and gender and that attempt to systematically identify important information about the social, economic, and political realities of women and men in a given setting. No one framework can be comprehensive; each one has a different focus and is best suited to specific contexts (USAID 2013; Duban 2012; Jhpiego 2016; LINKAGES 2017). For this chapter, we have decided to concentrate on women and girls as a way to "level the playing field" in order to achieve desired outcomes. Therefore, our framework for analysis highlights particular gender components that can—either alone or in combination—be *leveraged* to increase the freedom of women and girls to reach their full potential and be able to choose whether and when to have children. These overarching and interrelated components, or GEWE "levers" as they are called, are among the variables that are repeatedly found in the literature as significant predictors of both gender equality and improved family planning outcomes (Taukobong et al. 2016). They include equitable interpersonal relationships, access to and control over assets, decision-making power, education, and mobility (see Table 6.2).

Table 6.2 Gender levers and their operationalization in practice (Taukobong et al. 2016)

Gender lever	In practice
Equitable interpersonal relationships	Roles and expectations put on women and men Attitudes about and experience with gender-based violence Intimate partner violence
Access to and control over assets	Access to tangible assets (money, seeds, land, wealth) Access to intangible assets (knowledge, information, time, social networks)
Decision-making power	Bargaining power Intra-household decision-making Community status and rights Head of household Freedom from asking permission
Education	School (traditional and nontraditional) enrollment Attainment Higher education Literacy
Mobility	Freedom of movement Autonomous mobility

6.4 Gender Norms Among Indigenous Communities

6.4.1 Overview

Although information from pre-colonial time in Latin America is limited, some scholars argue that current gender norms among indigenous populations would not exist without the influence of Spanish colonizers (Babb 2013). Prior to European involvement, women and men were considered to be complementary to each other; they shared community and household authority, and both participated in domestic labor and other activities designed to maintain and improve familial livelihoods (Kellogg 2005). When the Spanish conquistadors invaded North and Central America in the sixteenth century, they used violence, religion, and governance to impose their patriarchal beliefs onto indigenous populations (Hardin 2002; Byam 2008; Valaskakis 2009).

In recent years, Latin America has shown marked progress toward gender equality (USAID 2012a). All Latin American countries have ratified CEDAW, affirming that women and men have equal rights and that traditional, discriminatory gender roles should be challenged (UN Women 2014). There is near-gender parity in health and education, and overall rates of fertility and maternal mortality have been reduced. Additionally, several countries have made significant gains in terms of female participation in democratic governance and in the labor force (USAID 2012a). In fact, female labor force participation has increased more in Latin America over the last three decades than in any other part of the world, rising from 36% in 1980 to 53% as of 2012 (Chioda 2016); and the addition of women's income to households has reduced extreme poverty in the region by 30% (Mercer 2016).

Despite these gains, there are persistent and relative underlying gender gaps and gender-based constraints throughout the region. Indigenous women, in particular, are subject to experiencing gender inequality and discrimination because of their combined vulnerable status as being women, indigenous, and of a lower socioeconomic class (USAID 2012a). Furthermore, as compared to their male counterparts, indigenous women have less access to opportunities and resources and are more likely to experience violence and oppression (Jaspers-Faijer and Montano 2013).

Using the gender levers listed in Sect. 6.3.2, we will explore how these gender norms and inequalities relate to the family planning and fertility gaps we find between indigenous and nonindigenous women. As with all gender norms, the dominant social expectations and standards associated with being "male" and "female" within indigenous communities are influenced by cultural traditions, religious beliefs, and history. Therefore, though commonalities can be found, sweeping statements about gender norms within indigenous populations of Central America and Mexico would be irresponsible and may undermine the heterogeneity found both within and across groups.[3] For this chapter, we have sought to identify and summarize common themes under each lever that could be found in the gray and white literature while highlighting illustrative examples of gender dynamics from specific regions.

6.4.2 Equitable Interpersonal Relationships

Interpersonal relationships refer to the relationships between two or more people, whether they are based in love, friendship, business, provider-patient interactions, or some other type of social bond. These relationships are considered "equitable" if they are based on mutual respect, decency, and fair treatment. Often, interpersonal relationships are influenced by cultural and institutional belief systems

[3]For example, though lack of decision-making power and control over resources are two overarching issues that come up in the literature, in Mexico there are a few matriarchal societies, such as the indigenous Zapotec community of Juchitan in Oaxaca, where women dominate trading and decision-making (DevTech Systems, Inc. 2012).

around what it looks like to have power and, relatedly, what it means to be a man or woman in a specific society. These beliefs affect how men and women behave with one another and can dictate levels of familial and community participation, decision-making capacity, and even access to education, services, and economic opportunities.

It is impossible to discuss equitable interpersonal relationships in Latin America without acknowledging the persistence of *machismo*, an expression of masculinity that celebrates displays of hypersexuality, heteronormativity, physical strength, and aggressiveness, as well as violence, especially against women (Gibbons and Luna 2015). The superior status of men in indigenous Latin American societies is thought to come from their physical strength, which allows them to adequately protect and provide for the physically "weaker" family members (women and children). Women, on the other hand, are characterized by the term *marianismo*, a particularly chaste, virtuous, and subservient concept of femininity oftentimes based on the Catholic Virgin Mary (Gibbons and Luna 2015). Where indigenous men are usually expected to have sexual experience and knowledge of women before they marry, virginity is deeply valued among females (Hardin 2002). Indeed, women who are believed to have been sexually active before marriage have been known to be stigmatized and rejected by fellow community members (Karver et al. 2016).

Addressing the issue of machismo is relevant for tackling the linkages between gender disparity and improved family planning outcomes at various levels. For instance, the traditional masculine values associated with machismo, such as the perceived link between manhood and virility or control over women, may be fueling opposition to the use of modern contraception among indigenous women who, other things held constant, would be current users of modern methods. Also, patriarchal, discriminatory views held by healthcare providers can manifest as restricted access to health services for those who do not conform to prevailing social norms of sexual identity and/or behavior, making it difficult for women and girls to access family planning services (USAID 2012a). Likewise, issues of marianismo may lead young women or girls to not discuss, seek out, or use contraception for fear that they will be stigmatized for being promiscuous or unchaste (Faulkner 2003). In fact, due to the value placed on motherhood, some young indigenous women may not view pregnancy as a negative consequence of unprotected sex and that having a baby will result in increased devotion from the baby's father (Romo et al. 2002).

When gender norms of masculinity are combined with unemployment, alcohol, and drug use, there is an increased probability of men engaging in forms of gender-based violence (GBV) (Hindin et al. 2008). Often sustained by gender norms of femininity and the devaluation of women and girls, GBV acts as a catalyst that, if not altered, can perpetuate a cycle of violence for women, men, girls, and boys across generations. Furthermore, the acceptability and incidence of GBV are commonly linked to the presence and acceptance of violence in society and are currently complicated by the decline of positive male role models in much of Central America and Mexico because of the breakup of families due to migration, separation, or divorce, as well as male involvement in gang or other criminal activity (USAID 2012b). Regardless, experts recognize that GBV is both a cause and a consequence of gender inequality (CEPAL 2013). Men will often use physical and sexual violence to dominate, control, and punish women and "weak" men. With violence comes coerced sex and controlled decision-making regarding contraceptive use and even fertility; and data show that indigenous women are disproportionately victims (UNICEF et al. 2013).

There has been a long history of violence against indigenous women, predicated on circumstances surrounding armed conflict, militarization of traditional land, being physically uprooted from homes, the prohibition of cultural practices, state-perpetrated violence, and institutionalized racism and discrimination (Jaspers-Faijer and Montano 2013). For example, European colonizers and other armed combatant groups (including counterinsurgency forces in Guatemala and Peru in the 1980s and 1990s) used violence against indigenous women, in the form of widespread rape, as a tactic in their overall military strategy (MADRE and FIMI n.d.). Even now, law enforcement and government officials have been known to harass and violate indigenous women at Central American border crossings (Corpuz 2015). Additionally, some indigenous communities view contraception as a form of violence, fearing that it may be used as a tool for ethnic cleansing and political control (Barroso-Calderon 2004); and accusations of forced sterilization have increased distrust toward efforts to improve family planning outcomes (Santiso and Bertrand 2000).

Finally, literature sources suggest that a significant percentage of indigenous women have historically accepted certain forms of violence as being a normalized part of relationships (Vinding 1998). Though we know that indigenous men can be the perpetrators, frequently demonstrating their *machismo* or expressing their frustrations by abusing their partners (Hughes 2004), data on the current prevalence of violence against indigenous women in Latin America is controversial. For example, in Guatemala approximately 24.3% of indigenous women (e.g., measured as indigenous language speakers) stated they had experienced physical or sexual violence by an intimate partner at least once in their lives, yet only 8.6% reported having experienced violence within the last 12 months (Bott et al. 2012; CEPAL 2013). There are multiple obstacles that all women face when reporting physical or sexual violence, some of which are more pronounced for indigenous women because of their long histories with discrimination, marginalization, and state-perpetrated violence (CEPAL 2013). Some of these obstacles include whether a woman will be believed when a report is made, stigma associated with being a victim, and cultural or familial beliefs and values that may encourage a woman to remain silent (CEPAL 2013).

6.4.3 Decision-Making Power

Decision-making power is an important lever for influencing gender equality at the individual, household, and community levels. Having decision-making power at the individual or household level gives women the ability to help shape the present and future for herself and/or her family. Freedom to negotiate vital life decisions such as whether to use modern contraception (and if so, what kind), timing of first sex, and whether and when to get married can have dire short- and long-term consequences. When a woman or girl does not have a voice in making decisions about her life, she is more vulnerable to having an unintended pregnancy and experiencing violence. It also limits her chances to pursue opportunities like education and employment, making it difficult to leave the shadows of poverty. These consequences do not only affect her own health and well-being, but also that of her children and family (Greene 2013). At the community level, women leaders and decision-makers can offer a unique experience and knowledge base and can serve as excellent role models and change agents for altering stereotypes of female vulnerability, as well as laws and policies that, among other things, limit access to family planning and general reproductive health services (USAID 2012a).

Within indigenous families, adults may divide or share decision-making responsibilities, depending on the decision, whether they live in urban or rural areas, and the social norms at play (Wehr et al. 2014). In general, however, indigenous women are often known to make decisions regarding tasks for which they are directly responsible, including what foods to cook, how to care for the home and all family members, and how to best utilize scarce resources (Meentzen 2001).

According to a study by Kolodin et al. (2015), indigenous women in rural Central America and Mexico often have little or no input over decisions affecting their own health. The study indicates that such decisions depend not only on education level but also on a woman's network of influence, ethnic group, cohabitation relations with other family members, and the type of decision being made, such as where to give birth or whether to use contraception. For example, in Guatemala and Chiapas, Mexico, the couple often lives with the man's parents, so the husband and mother-in-law have strong influence over a woman's decisions; whereas, in indigenous parts of Nicaragua and Honduras, the woman and her mother have more influence. In the *mestizo* communities of Panama, young couples either live with the man's family or independently, and both husband and wife participate in decisions around contraception and family size (Kolodin et al. 2015).

In many places around the world, women and girls do not have the power to choose when and whom they will marry. In most countries in Central America, laws allow adolescents to marry before 18 years of age with parental consent or under special circumstances (UNICEF 2016). Although the girl's consent is legally required for marriage (UNICEF 2016), they are often compelled by their parents' desires and not permitted to choose freely (Meentzen 2001). Poverty often drives these decisions, and it is not uncommon for indigenous girls as young as 12 to be married to older men in exchange for payment (UNFPA 2012). In Guatemala, over 40% of Mayan girls are married by the age of 18 (Girls Not Brides 2017). Marriages are often strategic, planned by the parents of both the bride and groom, and designed to ally families and strengthen community bonds (Meentzen 2001). It is also often the groom's decision as to whether or not he will move in with his wife and her family or if she will move in with his. More frequently, an indigenous woman is expected to relocate and assume her mother-in-law's duties of caring for her now-husband, as well as the other family members in the residence (Meentzen 2001).

When it comes to community decision-making, there are increasing examples of how indigenous women are leading advocacy efforts through nongovernmental organizations and networks, serving as parliamentarians and playing other leadership roles; however, these examples vary by group and proximity to urban centers (USAID 2012a). In general, due to a combination of language skills, family responsibilities, and mobility constraints, indigenous women tend to be underrepresented in community governance. Many indigenous women have described feelings of being scared or embarrassed when speaking out in front of men (Meentzen 2001). There is also an increased tension in communities where there is a mix of both indigenous and nonindigenous residents when indigenous women participate along with members of the dominant culture (Meentzen 2001). Interestingly, there can be social pressure in indigenous communities for single women, who are often outcast for being single, to take on more visible roles when participating in community decision-making. These women are viewed as having more freedom to make their own decisions because they are not responsible for the care of a husband and/or family member (Meentzen 2001).

6.4.4 Access to and Control over Assets

Access to and control over *intangible* assets such as knowledge, information, and time, as well as *tangible* assets like income or land, can provide multiple avenues for empowerment, increased contraceptive use, and decreased or delayed fertility. Most directly, the more women know about contraceptives that are available to them, the more likely they are to find a method that meets their particular needs. And by having access and control over income/money and time, women are more likely to be able to obtain the methods of their choosing (Corroon et al. 2014; Do and Kurimoto 2012).

Among indigenous women in Central America and Mexico, misinformation and knowledge about modern methods are a real problem. According to Rios-Zertuche et al.'s (2017) pooled sample of over 7000 women in the poorest areas of Central America and Southern Mexico, more than 30% did not know any modern contraceptive method, and on average, women knew less than two modern methods (see Fig. 6.2). Furthermore, in a study of indigenous women in rural Honduras, approximately 40% of respondents reported that they learned their information about family planning through the media; however, the messages were ambiguous and did not clearly specify whether they were even pro- or anti-contraceptive use (Kolodin et al. 2015).

Even when women know about contraceptive options, they may not have control over the resources needed to obtain them. Among indigenous populations, access to and control over resources are not evenly distributed. Men are expected to work and make money, and they ultimately have control over how that money is spent, including what proportion of the money earned is used for household finan-

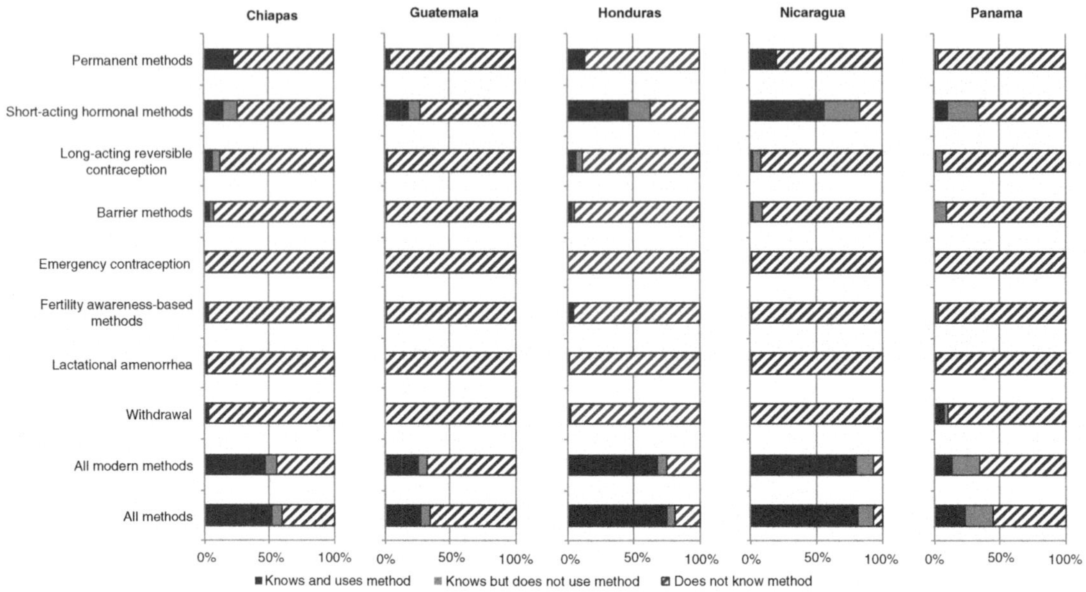

Fig. 6.2 Knowledge about and use of contraceptive methods among women in the poorest areas of Central America and Southern Mexico (2012–2013) (Rios-Zertuche et al. 2017). Survey-weighted knowledge and use of contraceptives among partnered women in need from the poorest areas. Modern methods include permanent methods (male and female sterilization), short-acting hormonal methods (pills, injectables, and vaginal ring), long-acting reversible contraception (implants and IUDs), barrier methods (male and female condoms, diaphragm, sponge), and emergency contraception. Traditional methods include fertility awareness-based methods (rhythm), lactational amenorrhea, and withdrawal

cial support or leisure activities (Meentzen 2001). On the flipside of that, indigenous women spend more time performing unpaid labor than their male counterparts (Lambert et al. 2010). In addition to keeping up the home, indigenous women—especially those living in rural areas—may also be expected to work in the fields, maintaining farms or gardens to provide food for the family (International Fund for Agricultural Development 2011). When they do earn income by making crafts, selling items at market, or otherwise participating in the local economy, they do not always have control (or decision-making power) over how that money is spent (Hughes 2004).

As for more indirect relationships, increased access to and control over tangible assets like land can also have an influence on whether or when a woman uses contraception. Land not only provides its owner with a physical place to build a home and live, but it can also be used to grow food, be borrowed against for credit, act as a means to build and transfer wealth, and serve as a sign of social status. Furthermore, a place to live or the ability to earn a livelihood can provide a safety net against crises or build the resources to leave an abusive situation. In communities of extreme economic deprivation, each of these choices increases the opportunity costs of delaying pregnancy and choosing when and if to use contraception (Diaz and Fiel 2016). Said simply, if a woman or girl does not have prospects for further employment opportunities and economic prosperity, then she does not have much to lose if she becomes pregnant.

Unfortunately, access to land (and land rights) for indigenous women is a challenge in Central America and Mexico. Land used by indigenous communities often lacks property titles or is considered to be of communal ownership (CEPAL 2013). When the land is owned communally, it is common for traditional practices, inheritance, and local leadership to set aside or devalue women's rights and participation. For those who have access to private property, indigenous men continue to hold titles more frequently than indigenous women (Corpuz 2015).

The fact that women can be named on land titles is not a widespread knowledge in many indigenous communities, nor do state institutions make efforts to educate women about the option (Meentzen 2001). Furthermore, when a family member dies and land is divided between surviving children, indigenous men frequently receive larger portions of land compared to indigenous women, restricting their access to significant land ownership and its associated resources (Meentzen 2001). As a result, the livelihoods of indigenous women tend to suffer as their options outside the home are more limited, leaving them vulnerable to poor reproductive health and family planning outcomes, as well as abuse, violence, and poverty (Corpuz 2015).

6.4.5 Education

Education is fundamental to women's empowerment and ability to choose when and if to use contraception and give birth. Quality education can expose women and girls to various ways of thinking about and understanding the world and their place in it, thereby expanding their vision of alternative lifestyles and life's decisions (Kågesten et al. 2016). In addition to being exposed to a greater range of options that she will consider for herself and her family, an educated woman or girl will be more likely to understand her rights and have the self-confidence to act on them. In that regard, education is significantly correlated to girls marrying later in life, using modern contraception, and effectively navigating institutions like health clinics, banks, and local government services (Taukobong et al. 2016). These variables enable a woman or girl to make safe and healthy decisions both for herself and those in her care.

Historically, in Latin America, men have achieved higher levels of education than women. Though there have been recent shifts in this trend, with several countries now reporting either gender parity or that more women than men are obtaining college degrees (World Bank 2012; World Economic Forum 2016), the gender gap remains in countries where there are large indigenous populations (USAID 2012a). Indigenous students complete far fewer years of education than their nonindigenous peers, and indigenous girls suffer the most. Indeed, although indigenous boys and girls may begin primary school together, young girls are disproportionately kept at home as they get older to tend to household tasks and agriculture work, while boys are expected to focus on their education for a few more years (Meentzen 2001).

Another barrier to education among indigenous populations is the fact that many groups speak a geographically specific dialect with little or no Spanish and have skills and competencies that are not necessarily aligned with the cultural requirements of formal education (CEPAL 2013). As the sole or predominant language of instruction, knowing Spanish is a requirement within the mainstream education system. Therefore, non-Spanish-speaking indigenous children either do not begin school or become discouraged enough to abandon their studies. Since indigenous females are less likely to be bilingual than their male counterparts, they are less likely to remain in school and attain higher levels of education (CEPAL 2013).

The repercussions of not knowing Spanish, coupled with the differing levels of education between indigenous women and men, further perpetuate cycles of discriminatory gender norms and gender disparities within the population. Being bilingual means more social acceptance and the ability to interact and participate in the dominant nonindigenous culture (CEPAL 2013). Therefore, in addition to the potential economic loss that comes with a lower education, indigenous women are less exposed to new ways of thinking and have a limited ability to participate in the dominant culture, lending to the stereotype that indigenous women are often more reserved and submissive in social settings and reinforcing norms around masculinity and femininity (Meentzen 2001).

6.4.6 Mobility

Reduced mobility (e.g., freedom of movement or the ability to travel and move around cities and rural areas) limits one's ability to complete schooling, participate actively in civil societies, engage in economic activity, and seek needed health services, including those related to family planning. Conversely, being able to travel within or between communities enables opportunity and influences exposure to alternative realities and new ideas that may alter important life choices about fertility and contraception. Whether it be because of limitations put on them by their partners or families, fear of crime or violence while traveling alone, or cultural/economic barriers to accessing a reliable means of transportation, a woman's mobility is often determined by gender norms and inequalities.

As the family providers, and with little expectation to participate in domestic chores or childcare responsibilities, indigenous men have the freedom to leave their homes and interact freely in public spaces, even for days at a time (CEPAL 2003). This is a luxury that is not always afforded to indigenous women and girls (Meentzen 2001). Instead, the home is generally considered to be the woman's domain, as she is responsible for managing all household chores, cooking, and childcare (Hughes 2004). Activities outside the home may be monitored and/or limited by their partners, brothers, or fathers. In Guatemala, where more than half of the population is indigenous, 80% of men and 70% of women reported that women and girls should obtain permission from male family members to leave their home, even for a short time (Guinan 2015). The combination of these factors serves to reinforce prevailing gendered social norms by positioning indigenous women to be economically and socially dependent on the men in their lives.

6.5 A Call to Action: Recommendations and Next Steps

Our analysis demonstrates only a portion of the discriminatory gender norms and inequalities that exist among indigenous populations within Central America and Mexico. Nevertheless, we know that these disparities can compound the negative effects of poverty and discrimination already associated with being indigenous and can lead to poor family planning and fertility outcomes. To simultaneously address these inequalities and improve family planning and fertility outcomes within the region, we offer a few recommendations. Though these recommendations are overarching and interrelated, we present them in a manner such that they build on one another to create a holistic approach to policy and programming advocacy.

6.5.1 Recommendation 1: Gender Integration

Decreasing the gaps in modern contraceptive use and fertility outcomes, as well as the gender inequalities between indigenous women and men that influence such outcomes, will require interventions that are—at the very least—aware and accommodating of unequal gender norms or that, at the very best, can responsibly transform such norms (see Fig. 6.3). Either way, gender must be integrated into existing and future programs and policies at all levels of planning, implementation, and evaluation. Not doing so could delay or limit outcomes and even—at worst—do unintentional harm.

Bilateral and multilateral organizations, including PAHO, have made firm commitments to gender integration and are in the process of implementing gender equality policies at the central and country levels (PAHO 2005). However, with the diminishing presence of donor funding for family planning in Latin America over the past few decades, a schism in leadership has formed at the

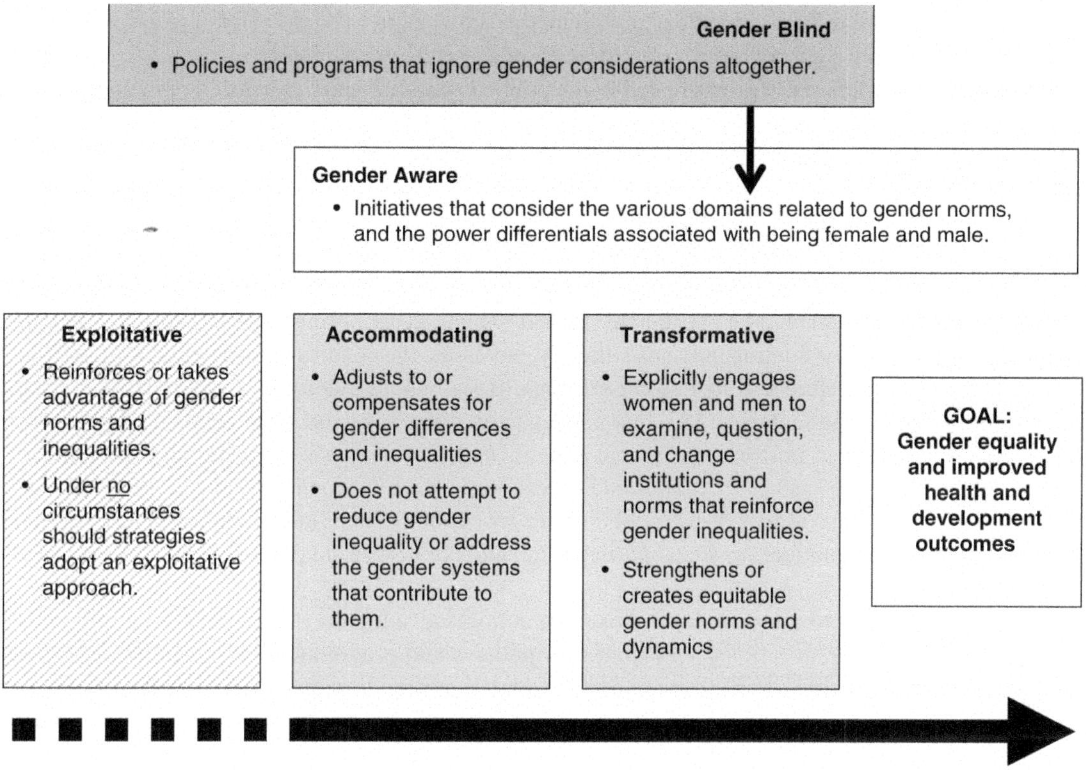

Fig. 6.3 Gender Integration Continuum (IGWG n.d.). With the goal of moving toward more gender-transformative programming, the Gender Integration Continuum serves as a diagnostic tool to assess if and how well programmatic interventions are currently identifying, examining, and addressing gender dynamics. It reflects a two-tiered process of analysis that begins with determining whether interventions are "gender blind" or "gender aware" and then considers whether they are exploitative, accommodating, or transformative

regional level. There remains a clear role for national governments and nongovernmental organizations to play in promoting gender integration in all program and policy efforts. In an ongoing basis, and at all points of program and policy planning, implementation, and evaluation, we should be asking (IGWG n.d.; Greene 2013):

1. How will the different roles and expectations of women and men affect the work to be undertaken (i.e., the achievement of sustainable family planning results)?
2. How will the program or policy influence or change relations of power between women/girls and men/boys?

6.5.2 Recommendation 2: Inter-sectorial Action and Systems-Informed Evaluation

For gender-transformative interventions to be effective, at least two major changes need to occur in the ways in which the practice of official development aid and public policy are done today. First, inter-sectorial action (ISA) would be required for social systems to be able to address the myriad mechanisms and pathways through which the outcomes of interest would occur (e.g., improved fertility outcomes and women's and girls' empowerment); and, second, conventional impact evaluation approaches would have to be complemented with methods that address complexity. Given space limitations, we will only give a brief description for each of these change domains.

ISA has been conventionally promulgated in the public health literature as a necessary condition to address the social determinants of health (Solar and Irwin 2010) and as a valid framework to design and evaluate health promotion programs (Solar et al. 2009). The concept has multiple meanings and tends to lack a generally accepted theoretical framework. However, for the purposes of this chapter, inter-sectorial action could be conceptualized as having a few basic features. First, ISA is desirable in situations where the social problem of interest is complex and multicausal. Workable solutions to these complex problems would thus require a whole-system perspective with the involvement of multiple governmental stakeholders (Cunill-Grau and Ospina 2012; Ospina and Cunill Grau 2011). That is, ISA may not target contraceptive use directly, but create the conditions which make it possible for a woman to have the freedom to choose when and if she would like to have children and/or use contraception. The second feature of ISA that is relevant to this discussion is the framing of solutions that produce measurement performance improvements and that sustain such focus on performance through time. Finally, the kind of ISA required to meet our objectives would address the limits of collective action and the weaknesses of the public sector by explicitly building the design, implementation, and evaluation of solutions on social participation and public-private partnerships (Andrews and Entwistle 2010).

The focus on inter-sectorial work that is driven by action and solutions to complex social problems is a departure from the conventional view that sees policies and programs as "interventions" to one that recognizes that the kind of problems under consideration is addressing issues of power, politics, and social conflict. It therefore follows that the approaches used to measure the effects of gender-integrated family planning solutions cannot follow conventional approaches to impact evaluation either. The complex and political nature central to the use of a gender lens to design new solutions demands a set of unique innovations in the design and implementation of measurement and learning systems.

We argue that the complex dynamics related to gender norms and inequalities demand systems-informed approaches to impact evaluation (Williams 2015; Williams and Imam 2006). Such approaches would increase the ability of the conventional measurement toolkit to address the interrelations among causal factors and pathways related to health and GEWE outcomes. They would also have to be highly competent in understanding the perspectives of social and community actors, beyond those of funders, evaluators, and governmental stakeholders, in order to provide richer insights of the effects generated by the solutions being evaluated. Finally, systems-informed evaluations ought to be able to question and critique the boundaries used by policy-makers and solution designers to conceptualize the programs or policies under analysis. Not doing so may essentially perpetuate or hide power asymmetries in the design of the solutions and would limit our ability to understand what aspects of a policy or program were considered important, relevant, or "worthy." System science methods that are well-suited for these approaches include social network analysis (Valente 2012), system dynamics (Hovmand 2014; Sterman 2006), and group model building (Black and Andersen 2012; Munar et al. 2015), among others.

6.5.3 Recommendation 3: Focus on GEWE Levers

Using ISA and systems-informed evaluation, we recommend focusing on the GEWE levers defined in this chapter to operationalize gender-transformative programs and policies. For example, understanding which social institutions and/or specific social network structures moderate and sustain the persistence of norms related to machismo could lead to the design of initiatives that—at the very least—mitigate the harmful influence of machismo by working within the constructs of such norms (i.e., taking an accommodating approach) or, at best, progressively change such norms around the cultural beliefs altogether (i.e., taking a transformative approach). These efforts should take place at the individual and community levels, as well as within institutions and national policies.

At the individual and community level, social networks to which indigenous women and men belong, such as networks of friends, neighborhood associations, community groups, or religious affiliations, should be targeted to improve the flow of information about autonomy and decision-making, thereby increasing women's and girls' ability to make or negotiate major decisions around contraceptive use, family size and/or the spacing of children. Furthermore, adopting women's empowerment as a strategic approach often requires engaging men and boys as a critical component of work at this level. Promising approaches for working with indigenous and non-indigenous men and boys as allies can include elements such as (1) structured spaces for women, girls, men, and boys to reflect on masculinity, femininity, gender, power, and privilege in their individual lives; (2) conversations with intimate partners and within families to promote more open communication, equitable relationships, nonviolence, support, and trust; (3) individual outreach and regular meetings to share testimonies and strengthen relationships among allies to build and expand social support and solidarity; and (4) reinforced linkages with advocacy efforts led by women's groups and feminist movements for social and policy change at local, regional, and national levels (CARE n.d.).

At the institutional level, entities within the health system, market, state, and the judiciary can facilitate changes in gender norms over time through several advocacy platforms and policy changes. Institutions have the power to reinforce the message of gender equality and women and girls' rights and responsibilities through their own workforce policies and training mandates. By providing the space and time for economic, political, and leadership opportunities, they can also increase possibilities for indigenous women to educate themselves and develop skills, competencies, and voice. Additionally, they can create safe spaces by developing and enforcing new and existing institutional rules/policies regarding the prevention and/or treatment of gender-based violence; and they can monitor and actively challenge discriminatory practices that prohibit indigenous women and girls from furthering their education and/or taking on male-dominated roles of leadership or entrepreneurship. Perhaps most urgently, however, institutional entities can use their capacity to disseminate information about already existing policies that promote gender equality and empower women and girls.

Finally, coordination at the regional and national level among sectors is necessary (but not sufficient) to ensure that indigenous women are entitled to "positive discrimination" policies and programs that give them priority access to tangible assets, such as property and lines of credit. The policy agenda should also consider barriers related to language and mobility, supporting adaptations for cultural integration, and include the provision of universal access to education and healthcare. Such policies will have both short-term and intergenerational effects, ensuring that indigenous women and girls are exposed to and influenced by emergent ideals about the roles and rights of women and girls, family size, age of marriage, autonomy, and overall decision-making.

Conclusions

Due to the region's macro-level success over the past few decades in modern contraceptive use and fertility, financial and political capital for family planning is paradoxically waning across Latin America. A great deal is still at stake, however, and decisions must be made about how to prioritize and invest in the challenges that need further attention. In this chapter, we call on program planners and policy-makers to be purposive in their efforts to generate measurable gains in women's and girls' empowerment, in order to close the gaps in contraceptive use and fertility among indigenous and nonindigenous populations. Moreover, we assert that addressing the complex power dynamics related to gender norms and inequalities will require gender-transformative initiatives, as well as inter-sectorial action, and systems-informed evaluation to bring efforts to scale. As outcomes improve for indigenous women and girls, the family planning and fertility gap between indigenous and nonindigenous populations will begin to close across Latin America, and macro indicators of health and well-being will prosper multiplicatively.

References

Ahmed, S., Creanga, A. A., Gillespie, D. G., & Tsui, A. O. (2010). Economic status, education and empowerment: Implications for maternal health service utilization in developing countries. *PLoS One, 5*(6), e11190. https://doi.org/10.1371/journal.pone.0011190

Ahmed, S., Li, Q., Liu, L., & Tsui, A. O. (2012). Maternal deaths averted by contraceptive use: An analysis of 172 countries. *The Lancet, 380*(9837), 111–125.

Andrews, R., & Entwistle, T. (2010). Does cross-sectoral partnership deliver? An empirical exploration of public service effectiveness, efficiency, and equity. *Journal of Public Administration Research and Theory, 20*(3), 679–701. https://doi.org/10.1093/jopart/mup045

AusAid. (2011). *Promoting opportunities for all: Gender equality and women's empowerment*. Resource Document. Australian Government. Retrieved from www.ausaid.gov.au.

Babb, F. (2013). *Gender in postcolonial Latin America*. Oxford Bibliographies in Latin American Studies. https://doi.org/10.1093/obo/9780199766581-0100.

Barroso-Calderon, C. G. (2004). La fecundidad indígena en México bis a bis la visión de los programas oficiales ¿caminos divergentes? *Estudios sobre las Culturas Contemporáneas X, 20*, 79–105.

Becerril-Montekio, V., & López-Dávila, L. (2011). Sistema de salud de Guatemala. *Salud Pública de México, 53*(2), 197–208.

Bermúdez-Madriz, J. L., Sáenz, M. d. R., Muiser, J., & Acosta, M. (2011). Sistema de salud de Honduras. *Salud Pública de México, 53*(2), 209–219.

Bertrand, J.T., Ward, V.M., Santiso-Gálvez, R. (2015). *Family planning in Latin America and the Caribbean: the achievements of 50 years*. Carolina Population Center, MEASURE Evaluation. Retrieved from https://www.measureevaluation.org/resources/publications/tr-15-101.

Black, L. J., & Andersen, D. F. (2012). Using visual representations as boundary objects to resolve conflict in collaborative model-building approaches. *Systems Research and Behavioral Science, 29*(2), 194–208. https://doi.org/10.1002/sres.2106

Blanc, A. K. (2001). The effect of power in sexual relationships on sexual and reproductive health: An examination of the evidence. *Studies in Family Planning, 32*(3), 189–213.

Bott, S., Guedes, A., Goodwin, M., & Adams-Mendoza, J. (2012). *Violence against women in Latin America and the Caribbean: A comparative analysis of population-based data from 12 countries*. Washington, DC: PAHO & CDC. Retrieved from http://www.paho.org/hq/index.php?option=com_content&view=article&id=8175%3A2013-violence-against-women-latin-america-caribbean-comparative-analysis&catid=1505%3Aviolence-against-women&lang=fr

Byam, M. (2008). The modernization of resistance: Latin American women since 1500. *Undergraduate Review, 4*(1), 145–150. Retrieved from http://vc.bridgew.edu/cgi/viewcontent.cgi?article=1096&context=undergrad_rev.

CARE. (n.d.). *Enegaging men and boys for gender equality*. Retrieved from http://gender.care2share.wikispaces.net/Engaging+Men+%26+Boys.

Comisión Económica para América Latina y el Caribe (CEPAL). (2013). Proyecciones de población. In *América Latina y El Caribe: Observatorio Demográfico*. Santiago de Chile: Naciones Unidas. Retrieved from http://repositorio.cepal.org/bitstream/handle/11362/36854/1/S1420023_mu.pdf

CEPAL. (2003). *Educacion reproductiva y paternidad responsable en el istmo Centroamericao*. Retrieved from http://www.cepal.org/es/publicaciones/2731-educacion-reproductiva-paternidad-responsable-istmo-centroamericano.

Chioda, L.(2016). *Work & family: Latin American and Caribbean women in search of a new balance*. World Bank Group, Latin American Development Forum.https://doi.org/10.1596/978-0-8213-8485-5.

Cleland, J., Bernstein, S., Ezeh, A., Faundes, A., Glasier, A., & Innis, J. (2006). Family planning: The unfinished agenda. *The Lancet, 368*(9549), 1810–1827.

Corroon, M., Speizer, I. S., Fotso, J. C., Akiode, A., Saad, A., Calhoun, L., et al. (2014). The role of gender empowerment on reproductive health outcomes in urban Nigeria. *Maternal and Child Health Journal, 18*(1), 307–315. https://doi.org/10.1007/s10995-013-1266-1

Corpuz, V.T. (2015). *Report of the special rapporteur on the rights of indigenous peoples*. (Annual Report HC) UN General Assembly, Human Rights Council, 13th Session, Agenda item 3. Retrieved from http://unsr.vtaulicorpuz.org/site/index.php/documents/annual-reports/83-report-hrc-2015.

Cunill-Grau, N., & Ospina, S. M. (2012). Performance measurement and evaluation systems: Institutionalizing accountability for governmental results in Latin America. *New Directions for Evaluation, 134*, 77–91. https://doi.org/10.1002/ev.20020

DevTech Systems, Inc. (2012). *USAID/Mexico gender assessment*. Short-term technical assistance & training task order, under Contract No. GEW-I-01-02-00019-00. Retrieved from https://pdf.usaid.gov/pdf_docs/pnadz184.pdf.

DfID (Department for International Development) and UKaid. (2011). *A new strategic vision for girls and women: Stopping poverty before it starts*. Retrieved from https://www.gov.uk/government/publications/a-new-strategic-vision-for-girls-and-women-stopping-poverty-before-it-starts.

Diaz, C. J., & Fiel, J. E. (2016). The effect(s) of teen pregnancy: Reconciling theory, methods, and findings. *Demography, 53*(1), 85–116. https://doi.org/10.1007/s13524-015-0446-6

Do, M., & Kurimoto, N. (2012). Women's empowerment and choice of contraceptive methods in selected African countries. *International Perspectives on Sexual and Reproductive Health, 38*(1), 23–33. https://doi.org/10.1363/3802312

Duban, E. (2012). *Toward gender equality in Europe and Eurasia: A toolkit for analysis*. Washington, DC: USAID.

Faulkner, S. L. (2003). Good girl or flirt girl: Latinas' definitions of sex and sexual relationships. *Hispanic Journal of Behavioral Sciences, 25*(2), 197.

Gibbons, J. L., & Luna, S. E. (2015). For men life is hard, for women life is harder: Gender roles in central America. In S. Safdar & N. Kasakowska-Berezecka (Eds.), *Psychology of gender through the lens of culture* (pp. 307–325). New York: Springer.

Girls not brides. (2017). *Child marriage around the world: Guatemala*. Retrieved from http://www.girlsnotbrides.org/child-marriage/guatemala/.

Greene, M. E. (2013). *A practical guide for managing and conducting gender assessments in the health sector*. Washington, DC: Population Reference Bureau. Retrieved from http://www.prb.org/pdf13/IGWG-GenderAssessmentGuide-2013.pdf.

Guinan, J. (2015). *Guatemala: Gender-based violence at epidemic levels*. Atlanta: CNN. Retrieved from http://www.cnn.com/2015/04/02/world/iyw-guatemala-gender-violence/index.html

Hardin, M. (2002). Altering masculinities: The Spanish conquest and the evolution of the Latin American machismo. *International Journal of Sexuality and Gender Studies, 7*(1), 1–22. https://doi.org/10.1023/A:10130508295.97

Hindin, M. J., Kishor, S., & Ansara, D. L. (2008). *Intimate partner violence among couples in 10 DHS countries: Predictors and health outcomes, DHS analytical studies no. 18*. Washington, DC: USAID. Retrieved from https://dhsprogram.com/pubs/pdf/AS18/AS18.pdf

Hovmand, P. S. (2014). *Community based system dynamics*. New York: Springer.

Hughes, J. (2004). *Gender, equity, and indigenous women's health in the Americas*. Washington, DC: Pan-American Health Organization. Retrieved from http://www.paho.org/hq/dmdocuments/2011/gdr-gender-equity-and-indigenous-women-health-americas.pdf

IGWG. (n.d.). *Gender integration continuum. Adapted from IGWG training materials*. Retrieved from https://www.igwg.org/training/programmaticguidance/.

Inegi, C. (2015). *Encuesta nacional de la dinámica demográfica ENADID 2014: Principales resultados*. Mexico: Instituto Nacional de Estadística y Geografía y Consejo Nacional de Población.

International Fund for Agricultural Development. (2011). *Enhancing the role of indigenous women in sustainable development*. Retrieved from https://www.ifad.org/documents/10180/3629656a-70f3-4c94-b58f-fd1e7ea2f4dc.

Jaspers-Faijer, D., & Montano, S. (2013). *Mujeres indigenas en America Latina: Dinámicas demográficas y sociales en el marco de los derechos humanos*. Santiago: CEPAL. Retrieved from http://repositorio.cepal.org/bitstream/handle/11362/4100/S2013792_es.pdf?sequence=1

Jhpiego (2016). *Gender analysis toolkit efor health systems*. USAID's maternal child survival program. Retrieved from http://gender.jhpiego.org/analysistoolkit/.

Kabeer, N., & Natali, L. (2013). Gender equality and economic growth: Is there a win-win? *IDS Working Papers, 2013*(417), 1–58. https://doi.org/10.1111/j.2040-0209.2013.00417.x

Kågesten, A., Gibbs, S., Blum, R. W., Moreau, C., Chandra-Mouli, V., Herbert, A., et al. (2016). Understanding factors that shape gender attitudes in early adolescence globally: A mixed-methods systematic review. *PLoS One, 11*(6), e0157805. https://doi.org/10.1371/journal.pone.0157805

Karver, T. S., Sorhaindo, A., Wilson, K. S., & Contreras, X. (2016). Exploring intergenerational changes in perceptions of gender roles and sexuality among indigenous women in Oaxaca. *Culture, Health & Sexuality, 18*(8), 845–859. https://doi.org/10.1080/13691058.2016.1144790

Kellogg, S. (2005). *Weaving the past: A history of Latin America's indigenous women from the Prehispanic period to the present*. New York: Oxford University Press.

Kolodin, S., Rodriguez, G., & Alegria-Flores, K. (2015). *Asuntos de familia: Estudio cualitativo sobre las redes sociales durante el embarazo y parto en Mesomearica Chiapas-Mexico*. Guatemala, Panama: Honduras y Nicaragua. Retrieved from http://dx.doi.org/10.18235/0000008#sthash.aHct2Cpx.dpuf.

Lambert, V., Roos, E., & Pinilla, S. (2010). *Gender assessment: USAID/Panama*. Washington, DC: USAID. Retrieved from http://pdf.usaid.gov/pdf_docs/Pdacr977.pdf

LINKAGES. (2017). *Gender analysis toolkit for key population HIV prevention, care, and treatment FHI 360*. Retrieved from https://www.fhi360.org/projects/linkages-across-continuum-hiv-services-key-populations-affected-hiv-linkages.

MADRE and FIMI. (n.d.). *Inputs for the secretary-General's study on violence against women*. New York: UN Women. Retrieved from http://www.un.org/womenwatch/daw/vaw/ngocontribute/MADRE-FIMI.pdf

Meentzen, A. (2001). *Estrategias de desarrollo culturalmente adecuadas para mujeres indígenas*. Washington, DC: Banco Interamericano de Desarrollo, Unidad de Pueblos Indígenas y Desarrollo Comunitario. Retrieved from http://www.iidh.ed.cr/comunidades/diversidades/docs/div_enlinea/EstrategiadeDesarrolloculturalparamujeresIndigenas.pdf

Mercer. (2016). *When women thrive, businesses thrive: The world's most comprehensive research on women in the workplace*. Retrieved from https://www.mercer.com/our-thinking/when-women-thrive.html.

Muiser, J., SáenzMdel, R., & Bermúdez, J. L. (2011). Sistema de salud de Nicaragua. *Salud Pública de México, 53*(2), 233–242.

Munar, W., Hovmand, P., & Darmstadt, G. L. (2015). Scaling-up impact in perinatology through systems science – Bridging the collaboration and translational divides in cross-disciplinary research and public policy. *Seminars in Perinatology, 39*, 416–423. https://doi.org/10.1053/j.semperi.2015.06.003

Ospina, S., Cunill Grau, N. (2011). *Institutionalizing accountability for governmental results: Public performance measurement and evaluation systems in Latin America*. Paper presented at the Public Management Research Association Conference.

PAHO. (2005). *Pan American Health Organization gender equality policy*. Retrieved from http://www1.paho.org/hq/dmdocuments/2009/PAHOGenderEqualityPolicy2005.pdf.

Rios-Zertuche, D., Blanco, L. C., Zuniga-Brenes, P., Palmisano, E. B., Colombara, D. V., Mokdad, A. H., et al. (2017). Contraceptive knowledge and use among women living in the poorest areas of five Mesoamerican countries. *Contraception, 95*(6), 549–557. https://doi.org/10.1016/j.contraception.2017.01.005

Romo, L. F., Lefkowitz, E. S., Sigman, M., & Au, T. K. (2002). A longitudinal study of maternal messages about dating and sexuality and their influence on Latino adolescents. *Journal of Adolescent Health, 31*, 59–69.

Santiso, R, Bertrand, J.T. (2000). *The stymied contraceptive revolution in Guatemala*. Working paper WP-00-22. Chapel Hill, NC: Measure Evaluation.

Solar, O., & Irwin, A. (2010). *A conceptual framework for action on the social determinants of health*. Geneva: WHO. Retrieved from http://apps.who.int/iris/bitstream/10665/44489/1/9789241500852_eng.pdf

Solar, O., Valentine, N., Rice, M., Albrecht, D. (2009). *Moving forward to equity in health: What kind of intersectoral action is needed? An approach to an intersectoral typology*. Paper presented at the 7th Global Conference For Health Promotion, Nairobi, Kenya.

Sterman, J. D. (2006). Learning from evidence in a complex world. *American Journal of Public Health, 96*(3), 505–514. https://doi.org/10.2105/AJPH.2005.066043

Swiss, L., Fallon, K. M., & Burgos, G. (2012). Does critical mass matter? Women's political representation and child health in developing countries. *Social Forces: a Scientific Medium of Social Study and Interpretation, 91*(2), 531–558.

Taukobong, H., Kincaid, M., Levy, J., Bloom, S., Platt, J., Henry, S. K., et al. (2016). Does addressing gender inequalities and empowering women and girls improve health and development programme outcomes? *Health Policy and Planning, 31*(10), 1492–1514. https://doi.org/10.1093/heapol/czw074

UNICEF. (2016). *Las edades mínimas legales y la realización de los derechos de los y las adolescentes*. Panama City, Panama: UNICEF Oficina Regional para América Latina y el Caribe. Retrieved from https://www.unicef.org/lac/20160406_UNICEF_Edades_Minima_Esp(1).pdf

UNICEF, UN Women, UNFPA, ILO, OSRSG/VAC. (2013). *Breaking the silence on violence against indigenous girls, adolescents and young women: A call to action based on an overview of existing evidence from Africa, Asia Pacific and Latin America*. Retrieved from https://www.unfpa.org/sites/default/files/resource-pdf/VAIWG_FINAL.pdf.

United Nations. (2015). *Department of economic and social affairs, population division: Trends in contraceptive use worldwide 2015*. Retrieved from http://www.un.org/en/development/desa/population/publications/pdf/family/trendsContraceptiveUse2015Report.pdf.

UNDP. (2015). *Sustainable development goals: 17 goals to transform our world*. Retrieved from http://www.un.org/sustainabledevelopment/sustainable-development-goals/

UNFPA. (2012). *Marrying too young: End child marriage*. New York: United Nations Population Fund. Retrieved from https://www.unfpa.org/sites/default/files/pub-pdf/MarryingTooYoung.pdf

UN Women. (2014). *UN Women Americas and the Caribbean - Results achieved in 2014*. Retrieved from http://www.unwomen.org/en/digital-library/publications/2015/8/lac-annual-report

USAID. (2012a). *United States Agency for International Development/Latin American & Caribbean (LAC) Regional Sustainable Development Office: Gender assessment*. Washington, DC: USAID. Retrieved from https://pdf.usaid.gov/pdf_docs/pnadz186.pdf

USAID. (2012b). *Gender equality and female empowerment policy*. Washington, D.C.: USAID. Retrieved from https://www.usaid.gov/sites/default/files/documents/1865/GenderEqualityPolicy_0.pdf

USAID. (2013). *ADS chapter 205: Integrating gender equality and female empowerment in USAID's program cycle*. Washington, DC: USAID. Retrieved from https://www.usaid.gov/sites/default/files/documents/1870/205.pdf

Valaskakis, G. G. (2009). *Restoring the balance: First nations women, community, and culture*. Winnipeg: University of Manitoba Press.

Valente, T. W. (2012). Network interventions. *Science, 337*(6090), 49–53.

Vinding, D. (1998). *Indigenous women: The right to a voice*. Copenhagen: International Work Group for Indigenous Affairs. Retrieved from http://www.iwgia.org/publications/search-pubs?publication_id=140

Wehr, H., Chary, A., Farley Webb, M., Rohloff, P. (2014). Implications of gender and household roles in indigenous Maya communities in Guatemala for child nutrition interventions. *International Journal of Indigenous Health, 10*(1). https://doi.org/10.18357/ijih.101201513196.

Williams, B. (2015). Prosaic or profound? The adoption of systems ideas by impact evaluation. *IDS Bulletin, 46*(1), 7–16.

Williams, B., & Imam, I. (2006). *Systems concepts in evaluation: An expert anthology*. Point Reyes, CA: EdgePress of Inverness.

World Bank. (2012). *World development report 2012: Gender equality and development*. Washington, D.C.: World Bank.

WHO. (2010). *Defining sexual health: Working definitions*. Geneva: World Health Organization. Retrieved from http://www.who.int/reproductivehealth/topics/sexual_health/sh_definitions/en

World Economic Forum. (2016). *The global gender gap report 2016*. Retrieved from http://www3.weforum.org/docs/GGGR16/WEF_Global_Gender_Gap_Report_2016.pdf.

7 Antenatal Care Among Poor and Indigenous Women in Central America and Mexico: A Cross-Country Study of Access, Utilization, and Barriers

Emily Dansereau, Bernardo Hernandez, and Ali H. Mokdad

7.1 Introduction to Antenatal Care Disparities in Central America and Mexico

Antenatal care (ANC) is widely recognized as an important health service for improving maternal, infant, and child health outcomes and is shown to reduce maternal mortality, complicated births, premature deliveries, and low-birth-weight infants (Abdal Qader et al. 2012; Aminu et al. 2014; Beeckman et al. 2013; Bhutta et al. 2014; Carroli et al. 2001). Antenatal care is essential for preventing, identifying, and treating complications during pregnancy and provides an opportunity to educate women about other health services including in-facility delivery, child vaccinations, and postpartum family planning (Dixit et al. 2013; Pervin et al. 2012). Since 2002, the World Health Organization (WHO) has recommended a minimum of four antenatal care visits during a woman's pregnancy (UNDP et al. 2002). As of November 2016, this standard was increased to a minimum of eight visits, but this chapter will use the reference point of four visits that applied for the past 15 years.

On average, 90% of pregnant women in the Latin America and Caribbean region receive at least four antenatal care visits (UNICEF 2016). However, in many countries, high national averages mask significant disparities depending on a woman's ethnicity, wealth, and education. Table 7.1 summarizes the findings of national surveys conducted since 2005 in Central America and Mexico. In each country, the proportion of women receiving four ANC visits is substantially lower for the poorest wealth quintile compared to the richest. Using the most recent survey for each country, this gap ranges from 14 percentage points in El Salvador and Guatemala to 23 percentage points in Panama. In Honduras, consecutive surveys allow us to examine changes in disparities over time and show that the gap in ANC coverage narrowed from 31 percentage points in 2005–2006 to 17 percentage points in

E. Dansereau, M.P.H., Ph.D. (✉) · B. Hernandez, D.Sc., M.S. · A. H. Mokdad, Ph.D.
Institute for Health Metrics and Evaluation and School of Public Health, University of Washington, Seattle, WA, USA
e-mail: edanse@uw.edu

D. A. Schwartz (ed.), *Maternal Death and Pregnancy-Related Morbidity Among Indigenous Women of Mexico and Central America*, Global Maternal and Child Health: Medical, Anthropological, and Public Health Perspectives, https://doi.org/10.1007/978-3-319-71538-4_7

Table 7.1 Disparities in the percentage of women receiving four ANC visits in national surveys, 2005–present

Country	Year	Proportion of women receiving four ANC visits			Gap between poorest and richest	Survey
		National average	Poorest quintile	Richest quintile		
El Salvador	2014	90%	84%	98%	14 PP	MICS 2014
Guatemala	2014–2015	86%	81%	95%	14 PP	DHS 2014–2015
Honduras	2011–2012	89%	79%	96%	17 PP	DHS 2011–2012
Honduras	2005–2006	81%	66%	97%	31 PP	DHS 2005–2006
Mexico	2012	91%	Not reported			ENSANUT 2012
Mexico	2009	86%	Not reported			ENADID 2009
Nicaragua	2011–2012	88%	Not reported			ENDESA 2011–2012
Nicaragua	2006–2007	78%	61%	92%	31 PP	DHS 2006–2007
Panama	2013	88%	74%	97%	23 PP	MICS 2013

Table 7.2 Sample for the Salud Mesoamérica Initiative Baseline Study

Country	Number of women giving birth in the 2 years prior to survey	% Indigenous
Guatemala	1757	73
Honduras	1326	0
Chiapas, Mexico	2193	70
Nicaragua	625	10
Panama	1079	97
El Salvador	1386	Not measured

Data from Dansereau et al. (2016)

2011–2012. Unfortunately, most national surveys are not designed to provide representative estimates stratified by ethnicity, and therefore do not report on coverage for indigenous and nonindigenous women. The lack of disaggregated data makes it difficult to expose, understand, and address ethnic disparities. However, there are strong overlaps between indigenous ethnicity and poverty, and economic coverage disparities can typically indicate related ethnic disparities. The following sections address in-depth an epidemiological exploration of antenatal care among women in the poorest communities.

7.2 Methods

This chapter presents and discusses information from the largest cross-country study ever conducted specifically among poor and indigenous women in Central America and Mexico (Mokdad et al. 2015a). This survey was conducted from 2011 to 2013 (Dansereau et al. 2016) to provide baseline information for the Salud Mesoamérica Initiative, a public-private results-based financing initiative to reduce maternal and child health disparities in Central America and the state of Chiapas, Mexico. For this survey, 8366 women (Table 7.2) living in the poorest regions of Guatemala, Honduras, Nicaragua, Panama, El Salvador, and Chiapas answered questions about their reproductive health knowledge, attitudes, and practices (KAP). The study sample was composed of municipalities having a high concentration of indigenous and poor women and purposefully designed to include the 20% poorest population in each country/state. The detailed methodology and results of the analysis are available online as open-access publications (Dansereau et al. 2016; Mokdad et al. 2015a).

The following results describe the landscape of ANC in these communities, including information about who receives ANC services, when, and how frequently. Unless otherwise stated, the results, statistics, and conclusions in Sect. 7.3 apply to the poor and indigenous communities that are part of the Salud Mesoamérica Initiative (SMI) baseline household survey and are based on the data from that survey. We also present and discuss the results of country-specific logistic regression analyses that serve to explore the demographic, socioeconomic, and health system risk factors associated with receiving adequate care. Unless otherwise cited, the associations discussed in Sects. 7.4 and 7.5 were found to be significant predictors of ANC outcomes in logistic regression analyses, also using data from the SMI baseline household survey. As the data will demonstrate, "poor women" are far from a homogenous group, and targeted efforts are needed to achieve universal and equitable ANC coverage.

7.3 The Landscape of Antenatal Care Access, Timing, and Continuity Among Poor and Indigenous Women in Mesoamerica

7.3.1 Initiating Antenatal Care

Most women in El Salvador, Guatemala, Honduras, Chiapas, Nicaragua, and Panama's poorest communities receive at least one antenatal care visit from any type of provider. The lowest proportions are in Guatemala (84%) and Panama (87%), while the highest are in Nicaragua (97%) and El Salvador (98%) (Fig. 7.1). However, not all women receiving ANC have contact with a "skilled provider," which WHO and most countries define as doctors, professional nurses, and skilled midwives. Under this "skilled ANC" definition, Nicaragua and El Salvador again stand out, with 95% and 94% skilled ANC coverage, respectively (Fig. 7.1). However, stark differences are seen in Guatemala, where only 31% of women receive a visit with a doctor, professional nurse, or skilled midwife compared with 84% receiving any visit. This is primarily due to Guatemalan women visiting auxiliary nurses, which

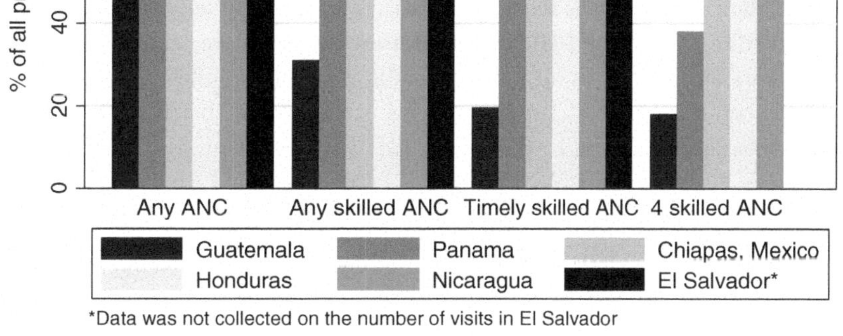

Fig. 7.1 Coverage of any, skilled, timely, and four ANC visits among the poorest populations of Guatemala, Panama, Chiapas, Honduras, Nicaragua, and El Salvador

do not meet the WHO "skilled" definition but may still be considered qualified by Guatemalan norms. Gaps between "any" and "skilled" ANC are also seen in Chiapas, a region in Mexico with a high proportion of indigenous inhabitants, where 75% of women receive a skilled visit compared to 94% receiving any visit. In Chiapas, the gap is explained largely by women visiting unskilled midwives. "Skilled ANC" coverage is also substantially lower than "any ANC" in Honduras (96% any vs. 84% skilled) and Panama (87% any vs. 78% skilled).

There is also remarkable variation within countries by geographic location, even looking only among the poorest municipalities. For example, Honduras, Chiapas, Nicaragua, and El Salvador all contain one or more municipality where all women receive at least one skilled ANC visit. However, Honduras and Chiapas (as well as Guatemala) also contain municipalities where the majority of women do not receive any skilled visits.

7.3.2 Timeliness of Antenatal Care

Antenatal care should be not only skilled but also timely. Many of the most important prenatal interventions are only possible if the complications are detected early. For instance, early detection is needed to treat anemia, avoid malaria complications, and prevent congenital syphilis (Lincetto et al. 2006). Therefore, WHO and all six countries mentioned in this chapter recommend that a woman begin receiving care in the first trimester.

However, many women wait until the second or even third trimester for their first skilled prenatal visit. In Guatemala and Panama, only 63% of women who ultimately receive a skilled visit initiate care in the first trimester. The proportion is slightly better in Nicaragua (67%), Honduras (70%), and Chiapas (76%) and highest in El Salvador (82%). However, when looking among all pregnant women, this translates to only 20% having a skilled visit in the first trimester in Guatemala, 49% in Panama, 57% in Chiapas, 59% in Honduras, 64% in Nicaragua, and 77% in El Salvador (Fig. 7.1). Encouragingly, it is uncommon for women to wait until the final trimester for their first ANC visit. This occurs most commonly in Panama, where it comprises 7% of women receiving ANC.

Intra-country variation is again apparent. Guatemala, Honduras, Chiapas, and Nicaragua all contain municipalities where every woman attends her first skilled visit in the first trimester. However, these same four countries (as well as El Salvador) also contain a municipality where less than half of women do.

7.3.3 Continuity of Antenatal Care

Once a woman has received one skilled visit, ideally in the first trimester, it is essential that she continue to receive care throughout her pregnancy. Guatemala and Nicaragua (according to WHO's recommendation, which was recently increased from four to eight visits) both have a norm of four ANC visits, while Mexico and Honduras each recommend five, and Panama recommends seven. The El Salvador survey did not collect information about the number of visits and is therefore not discussed in this section. However, some countries experience a sharp drop-off between the first and second visit. Most dramatically, in Panama, 78% of all pregnant women have a first skilled ANC visit but only 47% have a second. Women with at least one skilled ANC visit receive an average of 3.8 skilled visits in Panama, 4.3 in Guatemala, 5.5 in Chiapas, 5.6 in Nicaragua, and 5.8 in Honduras.

Despite having the highest number of nationally recommended visits, less than half (49%) of Panamanian woman who initiate skilled ANC ultimately achieve even the WHO-recommended four visits. Guatemala also has a low proportion of women completing four visits (58%), followed by Chiapas (79%), Honduras (83%), and Nicaragua (85%). Overall, among all pregnant women, this equates to only 18% of women receiving four visits in Guatemala, 38% in Panama, 59% in Chiapas, 70% in Honduras, and 81% in Nicaragua (Fig. 7.1). In Honduras and Chiapas, 61% and 52% of pregnant women meet the national guideline of five visits, respectively. In Panama, only 15% meet the nationally recommended seven visits. Still, there are pockets of success in most countries. For instance, Honduras, Chiapas, and Nicaragua all have municipalities where greater than 90% of women receive four visits. The exception is Guatemala, where less than half of women attend four skilled visits in every municipality.

7.4 Demographic Risk Factors for Inadequate Antenatal Care

7.4.1 Women's Education

Women's education is one of the most consistent predictors of receiving skilled, timely, and ongoing ANC in poor communities. In all countries but El Salvador, women with a postprimary education are significantly more likely to receive at least one skilled ANC visit as compared to women with preprimary or no education. Postprimary education also predicts receiving timely ANC and at least four skilled visits in Guatemala, Chiapas, and Nicaragua. Lack of education is a very strong risk factor in some settings—for instance, in Honduras, women with postprimary education have 4.5 times greater odds of receiving skilled ANC than do the least educated women. Even a primary education offers benefits in some cases: it increases the odds of any skilled ANC in Guatemala and Chiapas, timely care in Guatemala, and four visits in Nicaragua.

Access to education is a significant challenge for poor women in these countries. Nicaraguan women are most likely to have a postprimary education, and even there, less than half of poor women achieve this (45%). Education is lowest in Guatemala, the only country where fewer poor women have a postprimary education (18%) than preprimary or no education (30%), and also the country with the highest percentage of indigenous inhabitants in Central America.

A strong relationship between maternal education and ANC has been demonstrated in a number of low- and middle-income settings. In an analysis of 17 Demographic and Health Surveys, unschooled women were 55% less likely to use prenatal care than those with a secondary education; this association was stronger than education's impact on many other health behaviors (Jejeebhoy 1996). There are a number of hypothesized relationships between maternal education and utilization of health services including ANC (Levine and Rowe 2009). One explanation is that women living in areas with good educational opportunities also have access to better healthcare, both driven by a government commitment to social services. An alternate explanation is that education is associated with better health knowledge and health literacy. Young women may directly learn about health topics in school, develop the literacy and skills to acquire the knowledge on their own, or more generally cultivate an accepting attitude toward western medical interventions (Kilfoyle et al. 2016). Somewhat circularly, ANC is also seen as a major opportunity to improve health literacy among women (Lori et al. 2017; Renkert and Nutbeam 2001). Another potential mechanism is that school serves to modify gender roles, empowering women to make decisions about their health in their household (Ahmed et al. 2010). Women with secondary education are also less likely to marry and become pregnant at a young age, which is a risk factor for inadequate ANC. Finally, educated women are afforded more employment opportunities, reducing their economic vulnerability and reliance on their partner, and increasing their autonomy for health behavior decisions including ANC (Grown et al. 2005).

7.4.2 Indigenous Households

As described throughout this book, indigenous populations are highly marginalized across much of Mesoamerica. Over half of women in the poor communities of Guatemala, Panama, and Chiapas described in this chapter are of indigenous or mixed ethnicity. As compared to the other poor women in these communities, indigenous women are less likely to receive any skilled ANC, timely ANC, and four ANC visits in Chiapas and less likely to receive timely ANC in Nicaragua. These associations are independent of factors such as education and wealth. In Chiapas, a gradient is observed: women from households that speak both Spanish and an indigenous language are less likely to receive skilled, timely, and continuous ANC than are those from households that speak only Spanish, and those from households that speak only indigenous languages are the least likely to receive it.

There are strong intersections between indigenous ethnicity and other socioeconomic and demographic characteristics related to ANC (Locklear et al. 2013). Indigenous women are subject to a number of economic and structural barriers to care, including lower education, lower income, and greater distance from health facilities (Davy et al. 2016; Stephens et al. 2005). However, it is important to note that associations between ethnicity and ANC coverage are significant even after controlling for these factors, indicating that being indigenous is, in and of itself, associated with lower ANC coverage. The potential drivers of this association are multiple and interrelated. Many indigenous women hold strong cultural preferences for traditional medicine and midwives rather than Western medicine (Ibáñez-Cuevas et al. 2015; Pelcastre-Villafuerte et al. 2014). Indigenous communities often have their own extensive health systems that include prenatal and delivery care such as herbal remedies, sweat baths, and massage (Montenegro and Stephens 2006). Aversion to Western medicine is also driven and reinforced by exclusionary and discriminatory practices, obstetrical violence, language incompatibilities, and health caregivers' attitudes at health facilities (Bello and Alvaro-Rangel 2002). For instance, many facilities do not have any staff who speak an indigenous language, and staff can exhibit culturally insensitive behaviors, and practice stigmatization or even overt racism.

7.4.3 Poverty

As the national surveys presented in the introduction to this chapter demonstrate, wealth is a strong predictor of ANC behaviors. Most commonly, studies approach this by grouping the total population into wealth quintiles and subsequently analyze the poorest 20% of women as a single group. However, the gradient of poverty and health service utilization is also apparent *within* the poorest category. For example, looking exclusively within the poorest communities of Guatemala, Honduras, and Chiapas, women whose household expenditure is in the lowest 20% compared to other households in these communities are less likely to receive skilled ANC than those from the top 20% in the communities.

The associations between poverty and health service utilization are well-documented. Disparities within the poorest quintile are seen across a spectrum of maternal and child health services, from ANC to in-facility delivery to childhood vaccinations. In some countries, ANC is one of the least equitable interventions within poor communities. For instance, in Guatemala 35% of women in the highest expenditure quintile of poor communities receive four ANC visits compared to 19% of those in the bottom quintile (Mokdad et al. 2015b). This disparity is greater, in both absolute and relative terms, than disparities in skilled birth attendance, in-facility delivery, breastfeeding, postnatal care, postnatal contraception, and childhood vaccinations. In contrast, ANC is a relatively equitable intervention in poor Chiapan communities (42% vs. 58% for four visits). This may be affected by the presence of the conditional cash transfer program Prospera; however, but there are even greater gaps in skilled birth attendance, in-facility delivery, postnatal care, and postnatal contraception (Mokdad et al. 2015b).

7.4.4 Previous Children and Pregnancies

The average number of children per woman varies from a low of 2.5 in Nicaragua to a high of 3.5 in Panama. In Honduras, Nicaragua, and El Salvador, women are more likely to receive timely ANC for their first child compared to subsequent children, and a clear gradient exists of declining odds as the number of children increases. One possible factor underlying this association is low access to or utilization of health services leading to lack of both family planning and ANC. Additionally, resources and time are stretched in families with many children. This can present financial and logistical barriers to a woman seeking ANC; for instance, a qualitative study of Ecuadorian women found that they were restricted by the need to care for their other children (Paredes et al. 2005).

Women can also be deterred from seeking care for their second or later child by a bad experience with the health system during their first pregnancy; this may be particularly relevant for indigenous women subjected to discriminatory, stigmatizing, and culturally insensitive care (Bello and Alvaro-Rangel 2002). Another reason women may stop seeking ANC after delivery of their first child is the sense of security provided by a healthy first pregnancy (Glei et al. 2003). Following this, it is logical that complications during a past pregnancy would encourage women to seek ANC early on. Indeed, poor Honduran and Nicaraguan women who previously experienced a complicated pregnancy or delivery are more likely to begin their ANC in the first trimester. The prevalence of reported prior complications varies by country, from a low of 6% in Panama to a high of 11% in Honduras.

7.4.5 Desire for Pregnancy

In Guatemala and Nicaragua, women are significantly more likely to attend timely ANC if they had wanted to become pregnant. Unplanned pregnancies are a common occurrence; at the extreme, one-third of pregnancies in poor Nicaraguan communities are unwanted. The proportion is lowest in Guatemala (13%), and the other countries fall in between. This association demonstrates the intersection of ANC and other maternal health services, namely, family planning (Eggleston 2000). The link may be indirect, in that women without reliable access to family planning also lack prompt access to ANC services, or choose to delay or avoid both. However, there is also a plausible direct association, as women who were not planning to have a child often do not realize they are pregnant until after the first trimester. As outlined in other chapters of this book, family planning is a particularly complex issue for indigenous women, and an effective response will require crosscutting approaches that address gender norms and inequalities in indigenous populations.

7.4.6 Age and Marital Status

The Latin America and Caribbean region has the world's second highest adolescent fertility rate, at 67 births per 1000 (United Nations, Department of Economic and Social Affairs, Population

Division 2015). Indeed, a substantial proportion of births are to girls under 20 years of age in the poorest communities of Chiapas (13%), Nicaragua (15%), Panama (15%), Guatemala (16%), Honduras (16%), and El Salvador (16%). Adolescent pregnancies are associated with increased risks of low birth weight, premature birth, maternal complications, and worse economic and educational outcomes for girls (Caffe et al. 2017). Yet despite being considered high-risk pregnancies, adolescents are also less likely to receive ANC services. In Guatemala, adolescents are less likely to attend any skilled ANC; in Chiapas, they are less likely to receive care in the first trimester; and in Nicaragua, they are less likely to attend four skilled visits. Independent of age, unmarried women are also vulnerable to insufficient ANC care, specifically in terms of timeliness, in Chiapas and El Salvador.

A number of national, regional, and subregional efforts have attempted to reduce adolescent pregnancies, including COMISCA's Strategic Plan for the Prevention of Adolescent Pregnancy in Central America and the Dominican Republic (COMISCA 2014) and national plans in Mexico (Instituto Nacional de las Mujeres 2017) and Honduras (Secretaria de Salud Honduras 2012). However, they have yet to meaningfully decrease the adolescent fertility rate, and an expert meeting on adolescent pregnancy in Latin America was convened to define several actions for accelerating this process. These included collecting better data and stories about adolescent pregnancy, designing targeted interventions, empowering youth to drive the interventions, focusing on proven interventions, strengthening intersectoral collaboration, scaling up to large and sustainable programs, and creating an "enabling environment for gender equality and adolescent sexual and reproductive health and rights" (Caffe et al. 2017). While we strive for these systemic changes, countries must acknowledge adolescents as a priority group for targeted ANC outreach and support them in overcoming financial, structural, and cultural barriers to accessing care.

7.5 Health System Facilitators and Barriers to Skilled Antenatal Care

7.5.1 Distance to Health Facility

In Nicaragua and Panama, poor women living greater than an hour away from a health facility are significantly less likely to receive timely ANC than are those who live closer. This represents a substantial proportion of poor women: 30% in Nicaragua and 23% in Panama, as well as 24% in El Salvador, 22% in Honduras, 21% in Guatemala, and 15% in Chiapas. In a qualitative study conducted in Honduras, Costa Rica, and Panama, access to healthcare was described as "the most crucial problem" for dispersed, poor populations (Leon 2003); this was echoed by indigenous Guatemalans in another study (Hautecoeur et al. 2007). There are high opportunity and transportation costs associated with traveling long distances to a facility, particularly when medications may be out of stock or the doctor unavailable. Indigenous communities in Honduras and Panama also reported traveling to medical facilities by horseback, which can be difficult for pregnant women (Leon 2003).

A major intervention to address geographic barriers is increasing the provision of community-based care (Mbuagbaw et al. 2015). Nicaragua has implemented large-scale community-based delivery through a health system reform that, by 2011, had introduced nearly 4400 home-based community clinics and 33 maternity homes and trained numerous community-level health workers, including 12,700 "*brigadistas*" health volunteers, 6200 midwives, 7100 "voluntary collaborators," and 2800 health promoters (PATH 2011). El Salvador, too, is implementing reforms to develop multidisciplinary teams called Equipos Comunitarios de Salud Familiar (ECOS-F) that follow a strong community-outreach strategy to offer comprehensive primary care, as well as teams of specialists to support them (Clark 2015). Similar community-delivery initiatives have also been successfully established in Costa Rica and Brazil. While the impact of these reforms on ANC coverage has not been formally evaluated, Nicaragua and El Salvador have some of the highest levels of ANC among poor populations.

7.5.2 Health Insurance

Most (83%) women living in Chiapas' poorest communities have health insurance, almost entirely through the Seguro Popular de Salud public insurance program. Chiapas is a clear outlier compared to 11% insurance coverage in Guatemala, 8% in El Salvador, and less than 5% in Honduras, Nicaragua, and Panama. Poor Chiapan women enrolled in Seguro Popular are more likely to receive skilled ANC than those not enrolled. This corroborates the findings of a rigorous national evaluation, which found Seguro Popular coverage increased the probability of skilled ANC by 2.0 percentage points and the probability of four ANC visits by 2.7 percentage points (Serván-Mori et al. 2017). However, there is no evidence that Seguro Popular improves the timeliness of ANC nationally or among poor Chiapan women. Poor women with insurance are also more likely to receive skilled ANC in Guatemala. However, the Guatemalan health system is far more fragmented compared to Mexico's and does not have a comprehensive coverage package corresponding to Seguro Popular. The main insurance provider is the public Instituto Guatemalteco de Seguridad Social (IGSS), which covers formal sector workers; there are also a number of small private insurance providers (USAID 2015).

7.6 Recommendations

There are a number of potential levers for increasing access to and utilization of ANC for Central America and Mexico's poor and indigenous women.

The first step is ensuring high-quality and culturally sensitive ANC services. Alongside trainings to reinforce guidelines for the timing and components of ANC, providers should be taught and incentivized to respect indigenous patients' cultures. Indeed, cultural sensitivity training is a component of SMI in several countries. A complementary, longer-term solution is to train indigenous and poor individuals, particularly in rural areas, to become skilled providers and serve their own communities. Ensuring that patients are treated with respect and dignity is essential to improving the demand for ANC.

Second, countries must work to overcome geographic and financial barriers to care. Countries can learn from successful community-based models such as those in Nicaragua, which bring services directly to women in even the most remote regions. Voucher programs are another strategy to offset the cost of transportation to health facilities for women in rural areas. Targeted strategies are also needed to reach those least likely to receive care, including adolescent, indigenous, and unmarried women. Women from these target populations should play a prominent role in developing these strategies, which can also draw from existing national and regional models such as COMISCA's Strategic Plan for the Prevention of Adolescent Pregnancy.

Third, improving ANC will require strong intersectoral action (ISA)[1] (WHO 2011). Educating women, empowering women to control their fertility, and improving economic conditions for the poorest households are systemic issues with drivers and implications extending far beyond the

[1]Intersectorial action for health (ISA) refers to the inclusion of multiple sectors, in addition to the health sector, in the process of designing and implementing public policies to improve the quality of life.

health system. Rather than focusing on any one specific health issue, the current ISA agenda in Latin America is primarily focused on comprehensive poverty-reduction strategies, which are certain to benefit numerous outcomes including ANC and maternal health (PAHO 2015). ISA is not a "one size fits all" approach and will require strong regional, national, and subnational political resolve to achieve its vision.

Finally, countries must generate and use high-quality data to monitor progress toward ANC goals and guide decision-making. Surveys like those discussed in this chapter are an important tool to expose and understand disparities, particularly if they are designed to capture differences across ethnic groups and other key demographics. However, surveys must be complemented by strong health information systems that provide accurate, real-time, and locally relevant information. Most importantly, data must be continually analyzed and put to use to improve care.

Across these recommendations, inter- and intranational sharing of best practices is an important tool for achieving progress. For instance, El Salvador's community-based health reforms were based on examples from Brazil and Costa Rica. Lessons can also be learned from Cuba, where 98% of women receive four ANC visits (MINSAP and UNICEF 2014). Our study shows that within countries, too, there are nearly always municipalities that achieve high ANC coverage despite poverty and large indigenous populations. These can offer solutions to municipalities with lower coverage.

Conclusions

The health of mothers and their children depends on skilled, timely, and continuous ANC. While national averages demonstrate significant gains in ANC coverage across Mexico and Central America, these averages conceal stark disparities by ethnic and economic groups, which are especially prominent among indigenous women. In this chapter, we have explored the landscape of risk factors and challenges that prevent marginalized women from receiving essential ANC services, including lack of education, indigenous ethnicity, poverty, adolescent pregnancies, and geographic, cultural, and financial barriers. The foremost challenge for the region now is ensuring accessible, inclusionary, and culturally sensitive care for poor and indigenous women. Universal ANC is possible, and it is now a matter of political and financial commitment to bring these critical services to the most marginalized women.

References

Abdal Qader, M. A., Badilla, I., Mohd Amin, R., & Ghazi, H. F. (2012). Influence of antenatal care on birth weight: a cross sectional study in Baghdad City, Iraq. *BMC Public Health, 12*(Suppl 2), A38. https://doi.org/10.1186/1471-2458-12-S2-A38

Ahmed, S., Creanga, A. A., Gillespie, D. G., & Tsui, A. O. (2010). Economic status, education and empowerment: implications for maternal health service utilization in developing countries. *PLoS One, 5*(6), e11190. https://doi.org/10.1371/journal.pone.0011190

Aminu, M., Unkels, R., Mdegela, M., Utz, B., Adaji, S., & van den Broek, N. (2014). Causes of and factors associated with stillbirth in low- and middle-income countries: a systematic literature review. *BJOG: An International Journal of Obstetrics and Gynaecology, 121*(Suppl 4), 141–153. https://doi.org/10.1111/1471-0528.12995

Beeckman, K., Louckx, F., Downe, S., & Putman, K. (2013). The relationship between antenatal care and preterm birth: the importance of content of care. *European Journal of Public Health, 23*(3), 366–371. https://doi.org/10.1093/eurpub/cks123

Bello M., Alvaro-Rangel, M. (2002). *La equidad y la exclusión de los pueblos indígenas y afrodescendientes en América Latina y el Caribe*. Retrieved August 1, 2017, from http://repositorio.cepal.org//handle/11362/10800.

Bhutta, Z. A., Das, J. K., Bahl, R., Lawn, J. E., Salam, R. A., Paul, V. K., et al. (2014). Can available interventions end preventable deaths in mothers, newborn babies, and stillbirths, and at what cost? *Lancet, 384*(9940), 347–370. https://doi.org/10.1016/S0140-6736(14)60792-3

Caffe, S., Plesons, M., Camacho, A. V., Brumana, L., Abdool, S. N., Huaynoca, S., et al. (2017). Looking back and moving forward: can we accelerate progress on adolescent pregnancy in the Americas? *Reproductive Health, 14*, 83. https://doi.org/10.1186/s12978-017-0345-y

Carroli, G., Rooney, C., & Villar, J. (2001). How effective is antenatal care in preventing maternal mortality and serious morbidity?. An overview of the evidence. *Paediatric and Perinatal Epidemiology, 15*(Suppl 1), 1–42.

Clark, M. A. (2015). The new left and health care reform in El Salvador. *Latin American Politics and Society, 57*(4), 97–118. https://doi.org/10.1111/j.1548-2456.2015.00291.x

COMISCA. (2014). *Plan estrategico regional para la prevencion del embarazo en adolescentes de Centroamerica y el Caribe*. Retrieved from http://www.codajic.org/sites/www.codajic.org/files/FolletoPEA-CA-RD%20(2).pdf.

Dansereau, E., McNellan, C. R., Gagnier, M. C., Desai, S. S., Haakenstad, A., Johanns, C. K., et al. (2016). Coverage and timing of antenatal care among poor women in 6 Mesoamerican countries. *BMC Pregnancy and Childbirth, 16*, 234. https://doi.org/10.1186/s12884-016-1018-5

Davy, C., Harfield, S., McArthur, A., Munn, Z., & Brown, A. (2016). Access to primary health care services for Indigenous peoples: A framework synthesis. *International Journal for Equity in Health, 15*, 163. https://doi.org/10.1186/s12939-016-0450-5

Dixit, P., Dwivedi, L. K., & Ram, F. (2013). Strategies to improve child immunization via antenatal care visits in India: A propensity score matching analysis. *PLoS One, 8*(6), e66175. https://doi.org/10.1371/journal.pone.0066175

Eggleston, E. (2000). Unintended pregnancy and women's use of prenatal care in Ecuador. *Social Science & Medicine, 51*(7), 1011–1018. https://doi.org/10.1016/S0277-9536(00)00010-1

Glei, D. A., Goldman, N., & Rodríguez, G. (2003). Utilization of care during pregnancy in rural Guatemala: Does obstetrical need matter? *Social Science & Medicine, 57*(12), 2447–2463.

Grown, C., Gupta, G. R., & Pande, R. (2005). Taking action to improve women's health through gender equality and women's empowerment. *The Lancet, 365*(9458), 541–543. https://doi.org/10.1016/S0140-6736(05)17872-6

Hautecoeur, M., Zunzunegui, M. V., & Vissandjee, B. (2007). Barriers to accessing health care services for the indigenous population in Rabinal, Guatemala. *Salud Publica De Mexico, 49*(2), 86–93.

Ibáñez-Cuevas, M., Heredia-Pi, I. B., Meneses-Navarro, S., Pelcastre-Villafuerte, B., & González-Block, M. A. (2015). Labor and delivery service use: indigenous women's preference and the health sector response in the Chiapas highlands of Mexico. *International Journal for Equity in Health, 14*, 156. https://doi.org/10.1186/s12939-015-0289-1

Instituto Nacional de las Mujeres. (2017). *Estrategia Estrategia Nacional para la Prevención del Embarazo en Adolescentes*. Mexico: Instituto Nacional de las Mujeres. Retrieved from https://www.gob.mx/inmujeres/acciones-y-programas/estrategia-nacional-para-la-prevencion-del-embarazo-en-adolescentes-33454

Jejeebhoy, S. J. (1996). *Women's education, autonomy, and reproductive behaviour: Experience from developing countries*. Oxford, NY: Oxford University Press.

Kilfoyle, K. A., Vitko, M., O'Conor, R., & Bailey, S. C. (2016). Health Literacy and women's reproductive health: A systematic review. *Journal of Women's Health, 25*(12), 1237–1255. https://doi.org/10.1089/jwh.2016.5810

Leon, M. (2003). Perceptions of health care quality in Central America. *International Journal for Quality in Health Care, 15*(1), 67–071. https://doi.org/10.1093/intqhc/15.1.67

Levine, R. A., & Rowe, M. L. (2009). Maternal literacy and child health in less-developed countries: evidence, processes, and limitations. *Journal of Developmental and Behavioral Pediatrics: JDBP, 30*(4), 340–349. https://doi.org/10.1097/DBP.0b013e3181b0eeff

Lincetto, O., Mothebesoane-Anoh, S., Gomez, P., Mujanja, S. (2006). Chapter 2: Antenatal Care. In *Opportunities for Africa's Newborns* (pp. 51–62). WHO on behalf of The Partnership for Maternal Newborn and Child Health. Retrieved December 8, 2017, from www.who.int/pmnch/media/publications/oanfullreport.pdf.

Locklear, T., Perez, A., Caceres, A., & Mahandy, G. (2013). Women's health in Central America: The complexity of issues and the need to focus on indigenous healthcare. *Current Women's Health Reviews, 9*, 30–40.

Lori, J. R., Ofosu-Darkwah, H., Boyd, C. J., Banerjee, T., & Adanu, R. M. K. (2017). Improving health literacy through group antenatal care: a prospective cohort study. *BMC Pregnancy and Childbirth, 17*, 228. https://doi.org/10.1186/s12884-017-1414-5

Mbuagbaw, L., Medley, N., Darzi, A. J., Richardson, M., Habiba Garga, K., & Ongolo-Zogo, P. (2015). Health system and community level interventions for improving antenatal care coverage and health outcomes. In *Cochrane database of systematic reviews*. Hoboken: John Wiley & Sons, Ltd. https://doi.org/10.1002/14651858.CD010994.pub2

MINSAP, UNICEF. (2014). *Cuba Encuesta de Indicadores Múltiples por Conglomerados 2014*. Retrieved from https://mics-surveys-prod.s3.amazonaws.com/MICS5/Latin%20America%20and%20Caribbean/Cuba/2014/Final/Cuba%202014%20MICS_Spanish.pdf.

Mokdad, A. H., Colson, K. E., Zúñiga-Brenes, P., Ríos-Zertuche, D., Palmisano, E. B., Alfaro-Porras, E., et al. (2015a). Salud Mesoamérica 2015 Initiative: design, implementation, and baseline findings. *Population Health Metrics, 13*(1), 3. https://doi.org/10.1186/s12963-015-0034-4

Mokdad, A. H., Gagnier, M. C., Colson, K. E., Zúñiga-Brenes, P., Ríos-Zertuche, D., Haakenstad, A., et al. (2015b). Health and wealth in Mesoamerica: Findings from Salud Mesomérica 2015. *BMC Medicine, 13*, 164. https://doi.org/10.1186/s12916-015-0393-5

Montenegro, R. A., & Stephens, C. (2006). Indigenous health in Latin America and the Caribbean. *The Lancet, 367*(9525), 1859–1869. https://doi.org/10.1016/S0140-6736(06)68808-9

PAHO. (2015). *Intersectoral action and health equity in Latin America: An analytical approach*. Washington, DC. Retrieved December 8, 2017, from http://iris.paho.org/xmlui/handle/123456789/33873.

Paredes, I., Hidalgo, L., Chedraui, P., Palma, J., & Eugenio, J. (2005). Factors associated with inadequate prenatal care in Ecuadorian women. *International Journal of Gynaecology and Obstetrics, 88*(2), 168–172. https://doi.org/10.1016/j.ijgo.2004.09.024

PATH. (2011). *The Nicaraguan health system: An overview of critical challenges and opportunities*. Retrieved December 9, 2017, from: https://www.path.org/publications/files/TS-nicaragua-health-system-rpt.pdf.

Pelcastre-Villafuerte, B., Ruiz, M., Meneses, S., Amaya, C., Márquez, M., Taboada, A., & Careaga, K. (2014). Community-based health care for indigenous women in Mexico: a qualitative evaluation. *International Journal for Equity in Health, 13*, 2. https://doi.org/10.1186/1475-9276-13-2

Pervin, J., Moran, A., Rahman, M., Razzaque, A., Sibley, L., Streatfield, P. K., et al. (2012). Association of antenatal care with facility delivery and perinatal survival—a population-based study in Bangladesh. *BMC Pregnancy and Childbirth, 12*(1), 111. https://doi.org/10.1186/1471-2393-12-111

Renkert, S., & Nutbeam, D. (2001). Opportunities to improve maternal health literacy through antenatal education: An exploratory study. *Health Promotion International, 16*(4), 381–388.

Secretaria de Salud Honduras. (2012). *Estrategia nacional para la prevencion del embarazo en adolescentes de Honduras*. Tegucigalpa: Secretaria de Salud Honduras. Retrieved http://www.paho.org/hon/index.php?option=com_docman&view=download&category_slug=salud-materna-nino-y-adolescente&alias=332-estrategia-nacional-para-la-prevencion-del-embarazo-en-adolescentes-en-honduras&Itemid=211

Serván-Mori, E., Contreras-Loya, D., Gomez-Dantés, O., Nigenda, G., Sosa-Rubí, S. G., & Lozano, R. (2017). Use of performance metrics for the measurement of universal coverage for maternal care in Mexico. *Health Policy and Planning, 32*(5), 625–633. https://doi.org/10.1093/heapol/czw161

Stephens, C., Nettleton, C., Porter, J., Willis, R., & Clark, S. (2005). Indigenous peoples' health—why are they behind everyone, everywhere? *The Lancet, 366*(9479), 10–13. https://doi.org/10.1016/S0140-6736(05)66801-8

UNDP, UNFPA, WHO, World Bank Special Programme of Research, Development and Research Training in Human Reproduction. (2002). *WHO antenatal care randomized trial: Manual for the implementation of the new model*. Retrieved from http://whqlibdoc.who.int/hq/2001/WHO_RHR_01.30.pdf.

UNICEF. (2016). *Health Equity Report 2016: Analysis of reproductive, maternal, newborn, child, and adolescent health inequities in Latin America and the Caribbean to inform policymaking*. Panama City, Panama. Retrieved from http://www.apromiserenewedamericas.org/wp-content/uploads/2016/11/20160929_LACRO_APR_Health-Equity-Report-SUMMARY-8.pdf.

United Nations, Department of Economic and Social Affairs, Population Division. (2015). *World fertility patterns 2015 - Data booklet*. Retrieved from http://www.un.org/en/development/desa/population/publications/pdf/fertility/world-fertility-patterns-2015.pdf.

USAID. (2015). *Guatemala health system sssessment 2015*. Retrieved from https://www.usaid.gov/sites/default/files/documents/1862/Guatemala-HSA%20_ENG-FULL-REPORT-FINAL-APRIL-2016.pdf.

WHO. (2011). *Intersectoral action on health: A path for policy-makers to implement effective and sustainable action on health*. Kobe, Japan. Retrieved from www.who.int/kobe_centre/publications/intersectorial_action_health2011/en/.

Part II

Mexico

Structural Violence: An Important Factor of Maternal Mortality Among Indigenous Women in Chiapas, Mexico

8

Mounia El Kotni

8.1 Introduction

Located in the southeastern part of Mexico (Figs. 8.1 and 8.2), Chiapas is Mexico's poorest state: 74.7% of its population lives in poverty and extreme poverty (SEDESOL and CONEVAL 2015). The state often makes the news for its high rates of poverty and maternal deaths, yet the same cultural and economic characteristics that mark it as a marginal place are also presented as central to its identity. In February 2016, during Pope Francis' visit to the region, which centered the cameras of the world on Chiapas, the constant marginalization that indigenous peoples face on a daily basis dominated the conversation (Mandujano 2016). Similarly, development campaigns led across Chiapas use poor indigenous families as poster children for launch crusades aimed at fighting hunger, educating children, or family planning. These high-profile and newsworthy topics inevitably sideline other issues such as indigenous rights and structural violence, which are then left for local nongovernmental

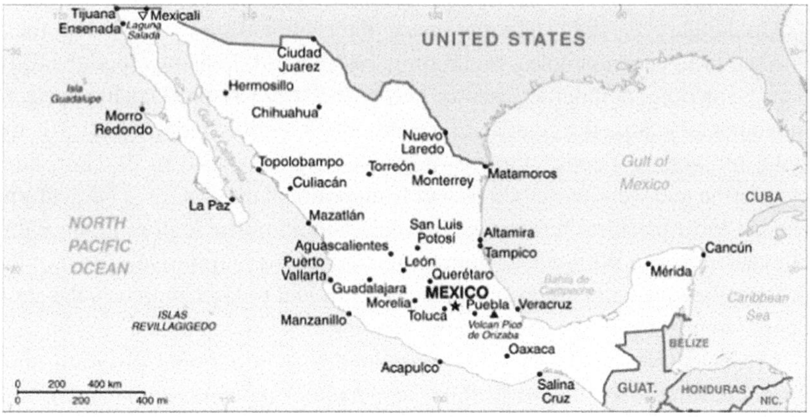

Fig. 8.1 Map of Mexico (Courtesy of Wikimedia, https://commons.wikimedia.org/w/index.php?curid=89495)

M. El Kotni, Ph.D.
Anthropology Department, University at Albany AS 237, Albany, NY, USA
e-mail: melkotni@albany.edu

D. A. Schwartz (ed.), *Maternal Death and Pregnancy-Related Morbidity Among Indigenous Women of Mexico and Central America*, Global Maternal and Child Health: Medical, Anthropological, and Public Health Perspectives, https://doi.org/10.1007/978-3-319-71538-4_8

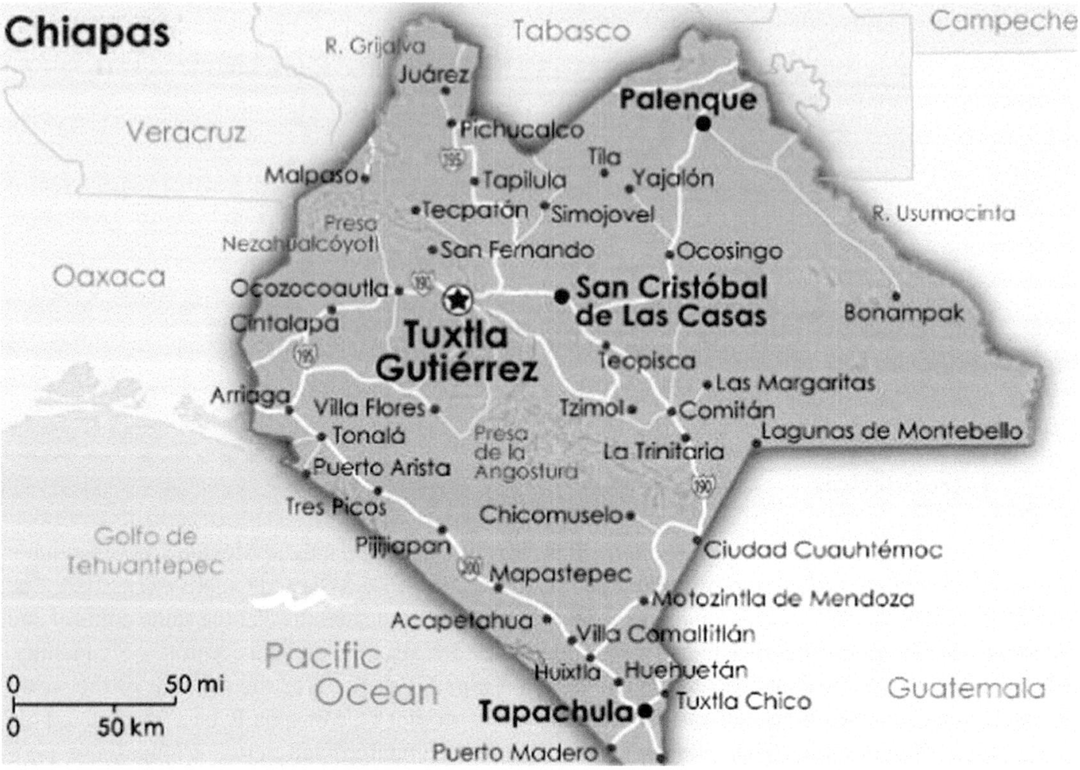

Fig. 8.2 Map of Chiapas (Courtesy of SMF)

organizations (NGOs) to care for (SIPaz 2014). Despite their marginalization (or sometimes because of it), indigenous peoples claim public spaces and create unique processes in the country.

On January 1, 1994, Chiapas made international news following the uprising of thousands of masked indigenous peoples, reclaiming "work, land, housing, food, health care, education, independence, freedom, democracy, justice and peace" (EZLN 1993). This uprising, known as the Zapatista movement, became the center of international attention and drew crowds to this 4.8 million habitants state. Indigenous people, the majority who are from Mayan descent, comprise 25% of the state's population and were until then absent from political discourses. In the aftermath of the uprising, much needed infrastructural reforms were implemented in the region, along with government programs to alleviate poverty. While these government efforts have improved some of the population's living conditions, they have not always been successful, and today Chiapas is the state with the highest rates of people living in poverty and extreme poverty.

Prospera (previously called Oportunidades) is a national program aiming to fight poverty. The program, funded by the World Bank, targets poor mothers, who need to follow a set of rules in order for their family to receive a monthly stipend. The two main branches of the program target education and health, focusing on the "co-responsibility" of mothers in complying with a set of actions. In the case of the maternal branch of the Prospera program, for example, pregnant women have to attend monthly prenatal checkups as well as monthly health workshops at their local health clinic. In addition, they are required to get ultrasounds at the nearest town's hospital (rural clinics are not equipped with such technology), which is costly in terms of both time and money. Though Prospera's goal is to improve poor families' living conditions, the maternal branch of the program aims at improving poor women's reproductive health through biomedicalization. The program is built on the premise that birthing at home with an indigenous midwife is unsafe, and so if women want to keep their stipend, they have to attend prenatal appointments at their local clinic. Policies such as Prospera thus isolate one factor accounting for maternal mortality—the lack of access to appropriate level of healthcare when needed—and generalize it to all pregnant women, eliminating women's ability to choose when and where they want to give birth.

In 2000, the United Nations' Millennium Development Goals (MDG) merged concerns for maternal health and the need for development by relying on health statistics to measure progress in universal access to reproductive health. Through MDG Goal 5.A, developing countries were urged to diminish by three quarters their rates of maternal mortality (together with the complementary MDG Goal 5.B of achieving universal access to reproductive healthcare). In Mexico, the proportion of maternal deaths (per 100,000 live births) has moved from 77 in 2002 to 54.7 in 2013 (OMM 2013), after which it increased again to 68.1 in 2014. A closer look at these numbers reveals that rural indigenous women are the ones who still die in childbirth.[1] In Chiapas, the maternal mortality rate (MMR) of women in reproductive age group (between 15 and 49 years old) has actually increased between 2010 and 2013 and that of indigenous women has almost doubled (1.7 times) over the time period (*ibid*). What factors put indigenous women at greater risk of dying in childbirth?

To answer such a question, this chapter relies on an anthropological approach to uncover the realities behind the statistics of maternal deaths. In this chapter, I argue that an anthropological approach to maternal death needs to take into account the structural factors which lead too many indigenous women to die during pregnancy and childbirth. Anthropology focuses on individual stories while replacing them in the broader context of international policies, as well as national and local settings of violence. This chapter concludes with some examples of local activists and midwives organizing to change these statistics.

8.2 An Anthropological Approach to Maternal Deaths

The research presented in this chapter stems from 13 months of ethnographic fieldwork in Chiapas, Mexico, between 2013 and 2015. All the participants in this study have given their informed consent, and the study itself has been approved by the Institutional Review Board at the University at Albany. During my stays in Chiapas, I have been in contact with indigenous and nonindigenous midwives, medical staff in public hospitals, workers of the Ministry of Health, mothers, activists, and researchers. The ethnographic research methods I used included qualitative in-depth interviews, observation (what people do), participant observation (participating in daily activities), and long-term immersion into the field (Bernard 2006). Combined, these qualitative research methods bring to the surface underlying social mechanisms and dynamics, which could not be revealed by one of these methods alone.

What is central to the discipline of anthropology is the trust building with our participants, called "rapport" in anthropological jargon. This trust building happens through seemingly non-research activities: making tortillas, attending a religious ceremony, learning how to greet strangers, chatting. As anthropologists have shown, these actions help members of the community judge the research and integrate her/him in their social network, which then leads to agreeing to share their personal story (Bernard 2006; Eber 1995; Little 2004). Medical anthropologists have highlighted the difficulty of conducting participant observation in the context of public clinics. How much participation is allowed, and what type of knowledge is accessible, varies depending on hospital and university regulations but also on very down-to-earth criteria such as the friendliness of the staff (Andaya 2014; Gálvez 2011; Howes-Mischel 2012). The long-term involvement on their field sites allows anthropologists to gain a unique access to people's personal stories, sometimes across generations and borders, like in the case of Rebecca Howes-Mischel who worked on indigenous women's reproductive care in Oaxaca, Mexico, and in the United States (2012).

[1] Those numbers reflect deaths that have been reported and registered as maternal deaths. Research has indicated a severe underreporting of such deaths, partly due to the pressure to comply with MDGs (Freyermuth Enciso and Cárdenas Elizalde 2009; Freyermuth, this volume).

The combination of various research methods, as well as the time spent alongside our informants, lies at the core of anthropological research and allows medical anthropologists to shed a light on the local consequences of global health policies.

8.3 International Health Policies

> At global, national, and regional levels, the Every Newborn Action Plan is supporting developments in health programs, for pregnant women, mothers, and their newborns. (…) Now there is good evidence that these investments in self-help groups are also paying off: as women encourage and support one another to adopt both pre and postnatal care routines. And what I'm excited about about [sic] self-help groups, is [that] we're learning how to really measure the results they are getting, and I think we're only going to get better at that as a world, and that's going to help us with the supply and demand issues that we have to get women really using the services provided. (Melinda Gates, Global Maternal Newborn Health Conference (GMNHC), Mexico City, October 19, 2015 (GMNHC 2015))

Melinda Gates' discourse, held at an international conference on maternal and child health in Mexico City, illustrates the many paradoxes of Mexico: a country where people die from poverty-related illnesses yet one that is eager to become Latin America's next leader. In order to achieve this goal, Mexico measures its progress through statistics and maternal and child health indicators in particular. As anthropologists working in the field of birth have pointed out, at the global level, these indicators serve as a scale to measure nations' economic development and their progress toward achieving modernity (Andaya 2014; Howes-Mischel 2012). Countries like Mexico invest in hospital-based birth so as to become modern and credible in the eyes of international institutions. In the United States, 99% of babies are delivered in hospitals (Gálvez 2011, p. 87). Mexico follows in these footsteps: in 1990, 76.7% of births occurred in health institutions; in 2013, it was 96.1%. The changes are even more significant in Chiapas, one of the states where a large number of women still give birth at home; in the last 25 years, numbers increased from 22.4% up to 72.9% (OMM 2013, p.28).

Poor women's reproductive choices have been on the international agenda since the 1970s; however, it is the International Conference on Population and Development meeting in Cairo, Egypt, in 1994 that framed for the first time women's reproductive health as a human right. The following year, the Fourth World Conference on Women in Beijing, China, implemented the Gender and Development approach, which tied economic empowerment to women's reproductive choices. The Gender and Development approach promotes women's empowerment through their participation in the public sphere, which is intimately connected to their reproductive behaviors. Policies created under the Gender and Development approach overlook the fact that choices are "inseparable from the economic and physical hardships [women] endure under global conditions" (Ginsburg and Rapp 1995, p. 14). The emphasis on individual choice of family planning does not necessarily lead to improving women's care or diminishing maternal mortality rates, which are never "entirely matters of private, individual, and moral concerns" (Pinto 2008, p. 221). For example, even in a context of a socialist state providing free childcare like Cuba, women struggled to balance work and family life (Andaya 2014).

International policies aiming at improving mother and child health have focused on the training of "traditional birth attendants" (TBAs) since the 1970s. From Malawi to Mexico, the stereotypical TBA targeted by these policies is an older woman who has not received formal schooling and relies on her empirical knowledge and practical experiences to help women deliver their children at home (Berer and Sundari Ravindran 2000). Launched in 1987, the Safe Motherhood Initiative (joined by Mexico in 1993) relies on a rhetoric of modernity to encourage women to give birth in hospitals and to push the TBAs to transfer their patients from home to clinics (Berry 2010). Following the Safe Motherhood Initiative, and the funding which resulted from the program, maternal mortality and maternal and child health became major concerns in every developing country (Berer and Sundari Ravindran 2000).

Anthropologists have questioned the shift in the World Health Organization's (WHO) policies regarding traditional midwives, who moved from allies in diminishing international maternal mortality rates in the 1970s and 1980s to antagonists in the 1990s after the rates did not decrease (Berry 2010; Pigg 1997). In parallel to the dismissal of TBA's knowledge, international guidelines pushed for the training of skilled birth attendants (SBAs). In contrast to TBAs, SBAs are personnel who have undergone formal training and are able to navigate the hospital environment. Still today, SBAs are seen as the key element to improving poor mothers' health (United Nations 2014), as illustrated in another part of Melinda Gates' speech:

> Quality care at facilities is one of the absolute keys to saving mothers and newborns. So we need to continue to insure that we are satisfied and that those Skilled Birth Attendants are staffed at all clinics for women. That the clinics themselves are well-supplied and well-trained, so that we can make childbirth even safer. (GMNH 2015)

Gates' quote illustrates the contemporary face of maternal mortality reduction policies. The presence of SBAs in health centers and clinics is proportionate to the absence of TBAs, who deliver babies in homes. The former are integrated in the health system and provide quality care, while the latter work outside of the system and are implicitly associated with maternal deaths. In Mexico, to comply with international development goals and diminish maternal mortality rates, indigenous midwives are trained in detecting risk factors in pregnancy and birth, while women are encouraged to give birth in hospitals. In 2000, the United Nations' Millennium Development Goals (MDG) merged concerns for maternal health and the need for development by relying on health statistics to measure progress in universal access to reproductive health. Through MDG Goal 5.A, developing countries were urged to diminish by three quarters their rates of maternal mortality. In Chiapas, the proportion of maternal deaths (per 100,000 live births) decreased from 77 in 2002 to 54.7 in 2013 (OMM 2013), before increasing again to 68.1 in 2014.[2]

8.4 Life and Death in the Highlands

8.4.1 Structural Violence as Risk Factor

As stated in the Introduction of this chapter, in Chiapas, 74.7% of the population lives in poverty and extreme poverty, compared to the national 43% rate[3] (Enciso 2014). Highlands Chiapas (Fig. 8.3) concentrate the poorest municipalities of the state. In the Highlands, 65% of the *municipios* (municipalities) are classified as having the highest rate of marginalization (CONAPO (Consejo Nacional de Población). 2010, p. 88). Ethnicity and poverty often conflate, and the indigenous population of the state is also the poorest (Nash 2001; O'Donnell 2010).

> Mayan women and their families experience tremendous economic hardship, including extreme rates of malnutrition, lack of running water and electricity—conditions which produce poverty—related illness like TB, intestinal problems due to unclean water sources, and high rates of infant and maternal mortality. (O'Donnell 2010, p. 18)

The concept of "poverty-related illnesses" demonstrates the violence of poverty: men and women live in infected environments and die of curable diseases, and indigenous women die in childbirth. Anthropologists have considered poverty as a form of violence exerted by a state on its citizen and more generally by the global social order toward poor people (Farmer 2005; Gupta 2012). Poverty adds on to the many forms of violence indigenous women face on a daily basis; "There are many forms of vio-

[2]The national goal for the country was 22.2, which Mexico did not reach (the 2015 national MMR was 38.2) (Objetivos de Desarrollo del Milenio #5 n.d.).

[3]Disparities are even stronger for extreme poverty: 38 percent for Chiapas, 7.9 percent at the national level.

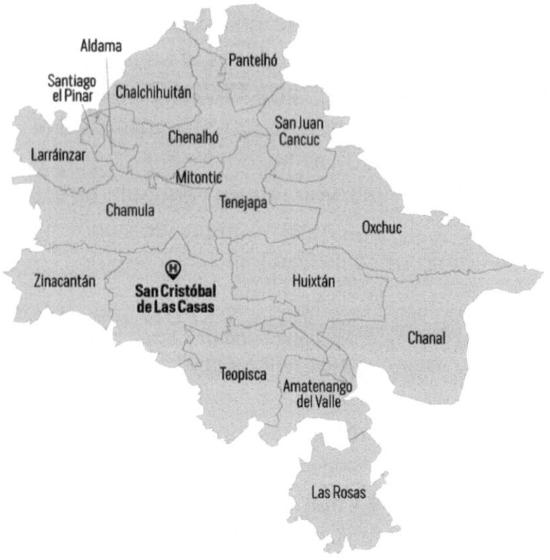

Fig. 8.3 Map of Highlands Chiapas (Courtesy of GIRE)

lence—domestic violence, sexual violence, and poverty which is violence to women's minds, hearts, and bodies, as they worry about the next day and how to get food" (O'Donnell 2010, p. 119). Out of the 18 municipalities of the Highlands jurisdiction, San Cristóbal, the cultural capital of the state, is the only one that is not considered as having "high" or "very high" marginalization. In the last national census, Chiapas had the highest fertility rate (3.07), while the national average was 2.39.[4] In this state, women have experienced the loss of 9.4% of their children—almost one out of ten (INEGI 2010).

In Chiapas, indigenous people have been living in a state of low-intensity warfare since the Zapatista uprising of 1994 and the government's violent response, which concretely and directly impacts women and their health. In the Highlands, the deployment of paramilitaries has fueled gender-based violence; indigenous women report being harassed and sexually violated by the military (Antillón Najlis 2013). Violence is the product of a multiplicity of forces that intertwine and reinforce one another and can be lethal for poor women.

> We also think of the women in Chiapas who have died for having fought for a new life, about those women who have died because of a lack of health services, who have died from domestic violence. (O'Donnell 2010, p. 210)

The combination of warfare and lack of healthcare illustrates the "absent present state," a concept developed by anthropologist Daniel Goldstein in his work in Bolivia (Goldstein 2012): a state very much present through its armed forces but desperately absent when infrastructure is needed. Similar to Bolivia, the absence presence of the Mexican state reinforces *structural violence*[5] in the lives of the poor and marginalized. In Chiapas, the state was very much present in the years following the Zapatista uprising; over 55 million pesos (about US$ 7 million at the time) were transferred from the federal to the state level between 1995 and 1997 (Freyermuth Enciso 2003, p. 349). Despite an improvement in the infrastructures and the construction of rural clinics, maternal mortality rates (although they have decreased) are still among the highest of the country (Fig. 8.4).

[4]The fertility rate is much higher in rural areas: out of the forty-four *parteras* I interviewed, half had carried over four pregnancies.

[5]Galtung (1969) identifies structural violence as violence that cannot be traced directly to an actor or institution. Structural violence is intimately linked to social injustice, which was at the heart of the Zapatista demands.

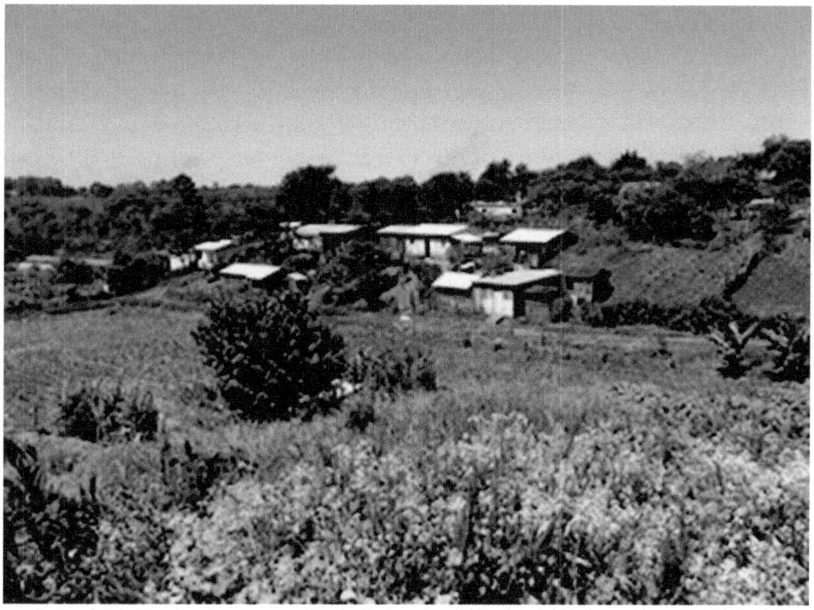

Fig. 8.4 Rural village in Chiapas. Published with kind permission of © Mounia El Kotni 2017. All Rights Reserved

Structural violence can be defined as an abstract violence that cannot be traced directly to health institutions or individuals (Galtung 1969); it is the "violence of injustice, (…) caused by social structures and processes that marginalize people and sustain social inequalities" (Rylko-Bauer et al. 2009, p.7).

When analyzing risk factors in health, medical anthropologists have included the structural conditions under which people live, such as poverty and marginalization (Farmer 2005; Rylko-Bauer et al. 2009). In Mexico as in other settings, the challenges women face in childbirth are deeply rooted in the social constructions surrounding reproduction (Andaya 2014; Jordan 1993; Murray de López 2016). When combined to structural barriers, such as the lack of access to health clinics in rural areas, policies aiming to reduce maternal mortality rates might send out the message that the bodies of poor women need to be controlled, inscribing women's access to healthcare into socio-economic hierarchies. One-size-fits-all solutions promoted by international organizations homogenize the historical, political, and social factors that underlie women's lives. *Stratified reproduction* becomes a useful tool to analyze structural and global factors constraining poor women's reproductive choices.

8.4.2 Maternal Mortality and Stratified Reproduction in Chiapas

In Mexico, historical inequalities put indigenous women more at risk of dying in childbirth (Chopel 2014; Freyermuth Enciso and Argüello Avendaño 2010). In Chiapas, indigenous women represent less than one-third of the female population (Gobierno del Estado de Chiapas 2014) but almost one-half of the overall maternal deaths (OMM 2013). Women, depending on their socioeconomic status and ethnicity, do not have the same power to make decisions over their reproductive health—what Shellee Colen coined *stratified reproduction* (Colen 1995; Ginsburg and Rapp 1995).

In her work with West Indian care providers in New York City, Colen highlights how immigrant women give up their own reproductive life, often leaving children in the hands of family networks in their home countries, to nurture the children of wealthier women in the United States (1995). *Stratified reproduction* is rooted in social inequalities and often mirrors social stratification.

The desirability of one's reproduction is tied to idea(ls) of citizenship, making reproductive futures easier for some groups and more difficult for others, and is intimately tied to hierarchies of nationality, class, and ethnicity. For Maya women in Chiapas, maternal health policies can contribute to stratified reproduction, by controlling where and how they should give birth—while wealthier women in the same region can have access to private clinics or professional midwives (El Kotni 2016a; Murray de López 2016).

Table 8.1 illustrates the maternal mortality rates of Chiapas, compared to national maternal mortality rates and the 2015 Millennium Development Goal. Although both national and state rates decreased between 2002 and 2013, the decrease is not constant, and in Chiapas there are several examples of an increase of maternal deaths from 1 year to another. As stated in the introduction, at the national level, the rate of maternal deaths (per 100,000 live births) has moved from 77 in 2002 to 54.7 in 2013 (OMM 2013), before increasing again to 68.1 in 2014. In Chiapas, the maternal mortality rate of women in reproductive age (between 15 and 49 years old) has actually increased between 2010 and 2013 and that of indigenous women has almost doubled (1.7 times) over the time period (*ibid*). Under the Millennium Development Goals, Mexico's strategy has been to train TBAs, namely, indigenous midwives, to detect risks in pregnancy and transfer to hospitals. In the next section, I discuss this strategy.

Table 8.1 Maternal mortality rates in Chiapas and Mexico (2002–2013) (Source: OMM 2013)

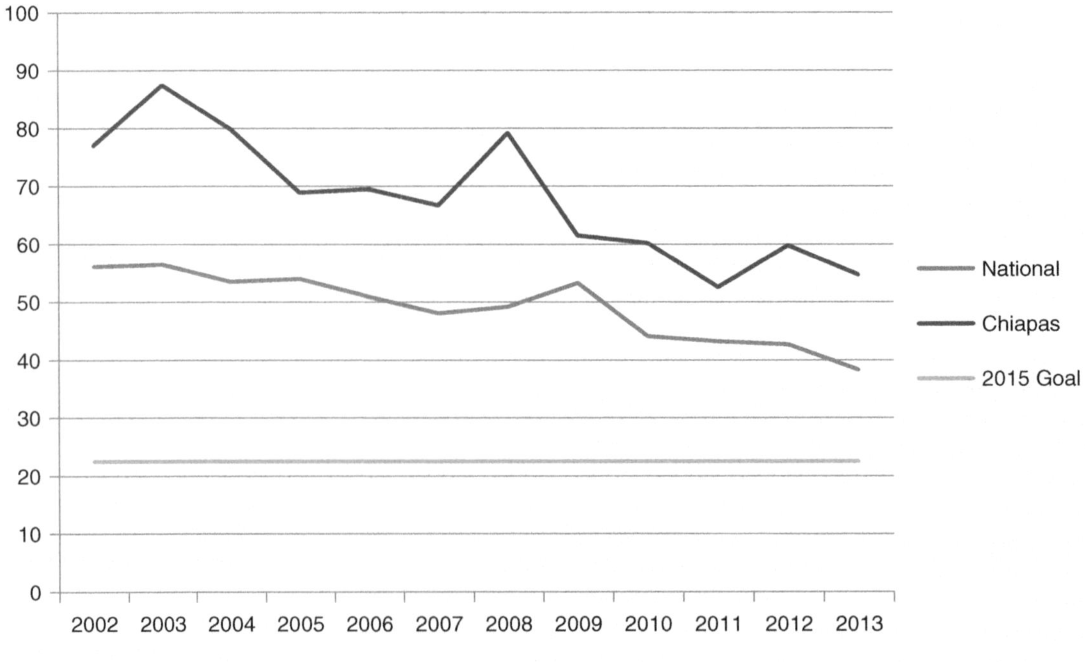

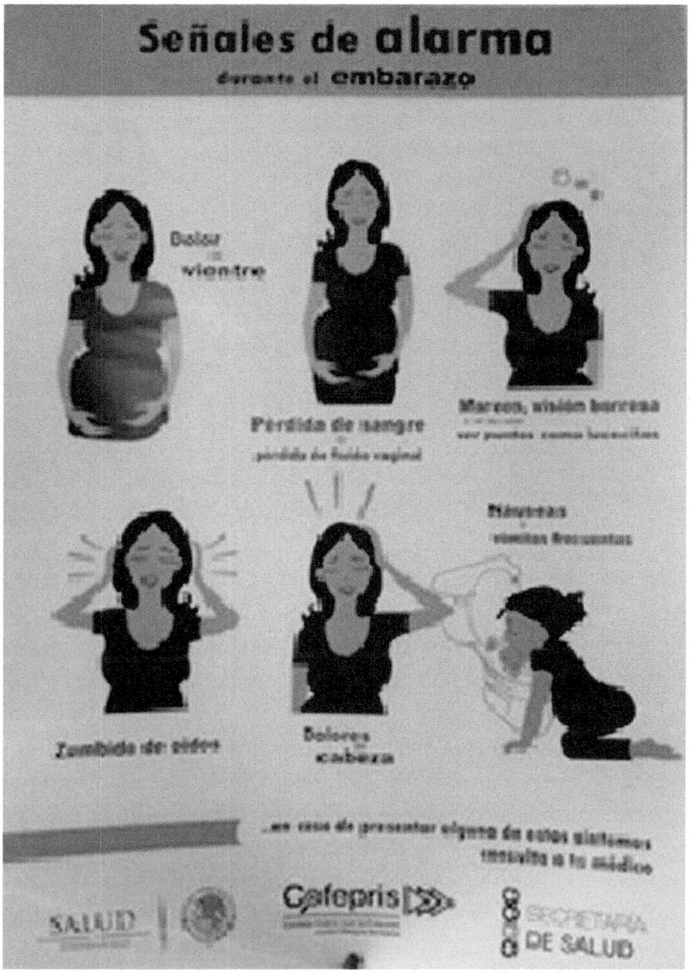

Fig. 8.5 Alarm signals in pregnancy, a poster in Spanish. Published with kind permission of © Mounia El Kotni 2017. All Rights Reserved

8.4.3 Government Campaigns Against Maternal Mortality[6]

At each consult with a pregnant woman, Doña Gabriela starts by asking: "Does your head hurt? Do you hear buzzing in your ears? Do you feel nauseous? Have you vomited? Do you see little lights?" After more than 15 years of monthly trainings at a local clinic, these questions have become part of Doña a Gabriela's routine. Doña a Gabriela knows that if the woman answers yes to one of these questions, called *señales de alarma* (danger signs) (Figs. 8.5 and 8.6), it means that she (a midwife) might not be allowed to attend the woman's birth:

> If the woman has all of these [signs], then we won't be overseeing the birth, it is better if she goes with the doctor. This way, we come out clean. This is what we learn. (…) [When we get to the hospital] we just hand the woman over and that's it. They don't allow us in. We hand her over in the emergency room, that's it. Before, they allowed us in, but now they don't anymore.

In some rural areas of Highlands Chiapas, traditional indigenous midwives like Doña Gabriela (*parteras* in Spanish[7]) attend up to 70% of births (Gómez Mena 2012). Following international guide-

[6] Partly reproduced from a post on Anthropology-News (El Kotni 2016b).

[7] *Partera* is the generic word for midwife in Spanish. It has been used to refer to indigenous midwives and professional

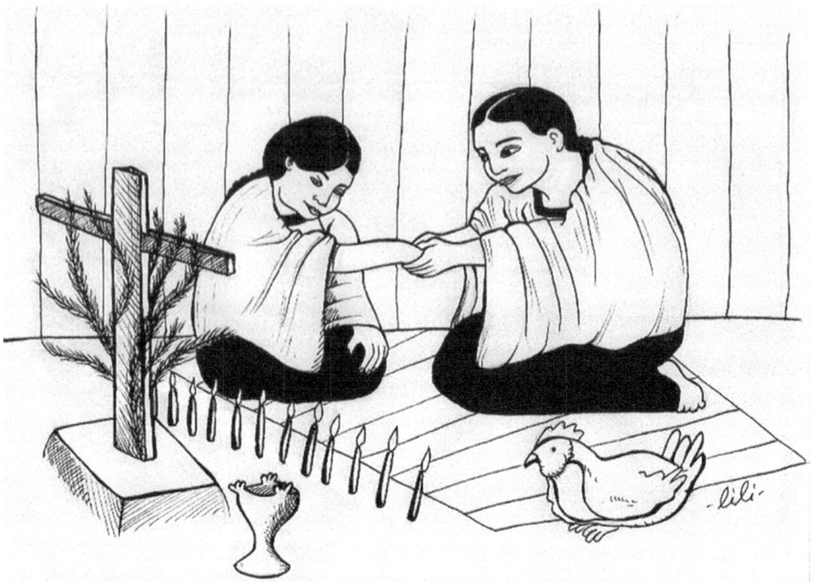

Fig. 8.6 Ritual prayer. Drawing by Alice Bafoin

lines from the WHO, the steps to diminish maternal mortality rates have focused on training these birth attendants. Mexican public health policies encourage practitioners in health centers and clinics to train the *parteras* in the detection of danger signs, while on their end, *parteras* are urged to transfer their patients to hospitals. The trainings for midwives focus on the opportune detection of alarm signals during pregnancy, birth, and postpartum. The doctors and nurses who train them insist that the *parteras* learn these signals in order to recognize them and immediately transfer women to the nearest hospital. While opportune transfers have the potential to save the lives of the mother and child, government trainings do not discuss alternatives to transfer, in a context where the distance to the nearest hospital can often be of 6 or 7 h, with patients having to pay for the cost of transportation. State policies aiming to train indigenous midwives gradually reshape their role in the healthcare system; indigenous *parteras* shift from being independent healthcare providers to becoming health auxiliaries (El Kotni 2016a).

Since the WHO's launch of the Safe Motherhood Initiative in 1987, international efforts have focused on training TBAs in hygiene (boiling instruments, washing hands) and encouraging them to refer women to hospitals. In this framework, pregnancy and childbirth are perceived as risky processes, with every pregnant woman being potentially at risk of having a complication. Anthropologists working in different cultural settings have analyzed how the medical discourse transforms a natural event into a risky one (Fordyce and Maraesa 2012). The Mexican state's particular construction of birth as a risky process, combined with monetary incentives to give birth in hospitals through conditional cash-transfer programs targeting poor women (Prospera), constrains women's reproductive choices and disrupts Mayan women's birth practices. Birth is no longer a natural event where the woman is supported by her family but becomes a risky practice performed by a technocrat, the obstetrician (Jordan 1993).

Given the cultural importance of birthing at home in Maya-speaking communities (discussed in the next section), surrounded by one's family and in-laws, and with very little intervention, the shift from home to hospital is not only a change of physical place but also of space, social environment, and language. In indigenous women's and midwives' accounts, the hospital is often described as an unfa-

midwives alike.

miliar place with foreign codes, a dangerous place in which women are reluctant to give birth (Berry 2006; El Kotni 2016a).

During their encounter with government workers and medical staff, indigenous women are exposed to a discourse built on the premise that birthing at home with a traditional midwife is unsafe and that hospitals are the best place to give birth for all women—and poor, indigenous women in particular (Smith-Oka 2009). The paradox of insisting that *parteras* transfer women to hospitals is that even when they do so in cases of labor complications, they are still blamed for the situation. *Parteras* and mothers are scolded for attempting what is considered a risky birth—that is, trying to birth outside of the hospital. Because the national policies urge midwives to send every woman to the hospital, public hospitals are saturated, and an efficient birth is a quick birth. The search for efficiency leads to routine episiotomies and skyrocketing cesarean section rates (Mexico has the second highest cesarean section rate among OECD countries[8]). Since there is a high chance women will be badly treated in hospitals, sometimes family members refuse to send women to the hospital, even if *parteras* are able to identify alarm signals. These structural factors are part of the explanation behind the rates of maternal deaths in the region.

8.4.4 Homebirth as a Cultural Practice

> The gift that the *partera* has, it has been given to her by God. It is not something easy, to care for women in childbirth; it is not for everyone. Because the most important thing is the life of the baby and of the mother. The *parteras*, they work day and night, at any time; there is always work for *parteras*, and it is now that we have to pass on this knowledge, for the benefit of the mother and her family (…) We must not lose these medicinal traditions, because they are transmitted from generation to generation. (Maya *partera*, during a meeting of the Organization of Indigenous Doctors or Chiapas in 2014)

Pioneering medical anthropologist and ethnographer Brigitte Jordan (deceased 2016) developed a biosocial framework to analyze childbirth, by highlighting that while birth is a physiologically universal event, it is also deeply culturally constructed (1993). In Mesoamerica, traditional midwives are key actors during pregnancy and childbirth. Their hands can tell when a child is due and replace it correctly if they detect an abnormal positioning (breech). *Parteras* also rely on their wide knowledge of plants and their properties, transmitted through generations, to care for women and their families. During their pregnancy, Maya women accumulate heat, an energy needed to create a new life. Childbirth, the culmination of pregnancy, is a very "hot" stage because of the accumulation of blood of the mother (from the retained menstrual blood) (Freyermuth Enciso 2003; Groark 1997; Guiteras Holmes 1961, p. 105). In the Highlands, birth is a family event: the woman labors at home, fully dressed, with the help of her husband (who sustains her while she is squatting, as in Fig. 8.7); the *partera* massages her (*sobada*), performs prayers, and catches the baby, while family and in-laws are in charge of warming the room and heating water, among others (Berry 2010; Freyermuth Enciso 2003; Jordan 1993). As women lose blood during labor, they lose heat and must be careful not to fall into a colder state. This is the reason why sources of heat such as the kitchen fire, the *temazcal*, and the various teas that a woman is given to drink are essential elements during childbirth. Some anthropologists analyze the masculine presence of the husband or father-in-law during childbirth as an element that reflects patriarchal control over women's reproductive decisions (Freyermuth Enciso 2003). However, some indigenous midwives interpret the future father's presence as an important emotional support facilitating the birthing process. In the neighboring state of Yucatán, women also express that

[8]http://www.forbes.com/sites/niallmccarthy/2016/01/12/which-countries-have-the-highest-caesarean-section-rates-infographic/#f6d56744ff86.

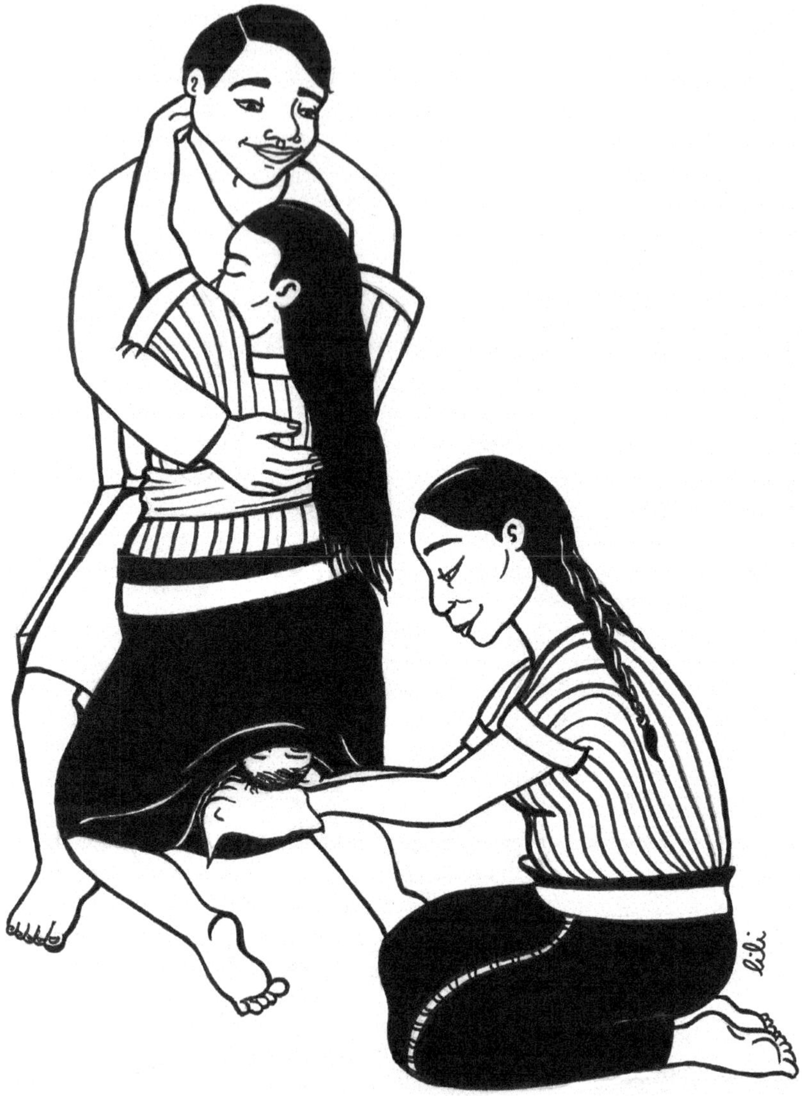

Fig. 8.7 Homebirth in the Highlands. Drawing by Alice Bafoin

the father's presence makes his bonding with the child easier (Miranda 2015). This situation is in stark contrast with what happens to women in the hospital, where the loneliness they experience is perceived by their families and *parteras* as an element of complication during childbirth—which is common across the Mayan region (Berry 2008).

During birth, the mother alternates positions, the most common being a squat with the support of the husband, seated on a chair (Fig. 8.7). Among Catholics, the midwife also provides support through prayers, candles, and chants (Fig. 8.6). During the immediate postpartum,[9] the midwife works in team with the rest of the family, making sure that both the mother and the baby are cared for. They do not cut the umbilical cord until the placenta (meaning "the mother of the baby" in Maya-*Tseltal*) is deliv-

[9]The postpartum period is divided into the first or acute phase (the first 6–12 h), the second or subacute phase (2–6 weeks), and the third or delayed postpartum period (up to 6 months) (Romano et al. 2010).

ered. Practices regarding the disposal of placenta vary throughout the region, but most of the women and *parteras* bury it (Cadenas Gordillo 2002; OMIECH 2011; Freyermuth Enciso 2003).

The various therapeutic elements used during birth—heat, plants, and prayers—as well as the presence of the family contrast with the treatment women receive in public hospitals. There, women are confronted with a staff that often does not speak an indigenous language and are left to labor alone in a cold environment. These are some of the reasons why many women and their families refuse to go to hospitals, despite the government pressures to do so.

8.4.5 Difficulties of Accessing Healthcare Structure

> The midwives are the first contact. It is important. Women, they keep having trust in the midwives. While there is a good control, there are no problems; the midwife knows it. The problem is if she does not identify the alarm symptoms, when there are risks. (Male doctor in urban health center)

Located in Highlands Chiapas, a couple of hours in public transportation from San Cristóbal, the town of Oxchuc (on Fig. 8.3) benefits from one public health center and one clinic. Twice a month, the only doctor and director of the health center meets with the midwives: the first meeting consists of a training course, and the second one is for the midwives to report their activities. "The themes of the trainings change, but always with a focus on risk." The doctor adds that in this center, out of 100 births, 60 are considered high risk, either because the woman has had more than four children or because she is a teenager. While he takes pride in the fact that thanks to this program maternal deaths have diminished, he also notices a correlative effect: "the care by midwives has decreased."

In most public health institutions, in order to lower maternal mortality rates, the staff trains indigenous midwives in the detection of alarm signals in pregnancy and childbirth. If the midwives were to encounter any of the signals, they should report the woman to their local clinic in the case of a pregnancy and transfer to the nearest hospital in the case of a birth (Fig. 8.8). The midwives affiliated with this health center comply with transferring their patients from home to the hospital if they detect an alarm symptom, but, according to the doctor, those who do not come to the trainings "attend risky births]." Moving beyond the discourse of individual blame, why do some midwives do not transfer women to the hospital? The paradox of the trainings in rural towns like those around Oxchuc is that even if/when the midwife detects a complication, she cannot transfer to the health center outside of opening hours (8 am to 4 pm, Monday to Friday); and neither the health center nor the clinic in the main town is equipped to perform a cesarean section. The woman needs to be transferred while in labor to one of the two closest hospitals (San Cristóbal de las Casas or Ocosingo), each 90 min away from this municipal center. Like in Guatemala, for this reason physicians encourage women to go to the hospital before a complication emerges (Berry 2006). However, as described in the next section, these recommendations also contribute to overcrowding in public hospitals. Women such as those that traditional midwives attend in Oxchuc (Fig. 8.9) do not have private health insurance and cannot afford to pay for a private clinic at any stage of their journey. They face economic and social barriers that impede their access to health facilities and ultimately impact their health conditions.

The strategy of sending virtually all women to give birth in hospitals in order to lower the prevalence of maternal deaths has led to the saturation of public hospitals (like in Guatemala, (Cominsky 2012)). More women also go to the hospital because of government programs such as Prospera, which aims to send them to give birth with skilled birth attendants but without the necessary infrastructures. As mentioned earlier, the need to attend to as many patients as possible contributes to the rising rates of cesarean sections in Mexico (70% in private hospitals and 40% in public hospitals at the national level (Sánchez 2010)).

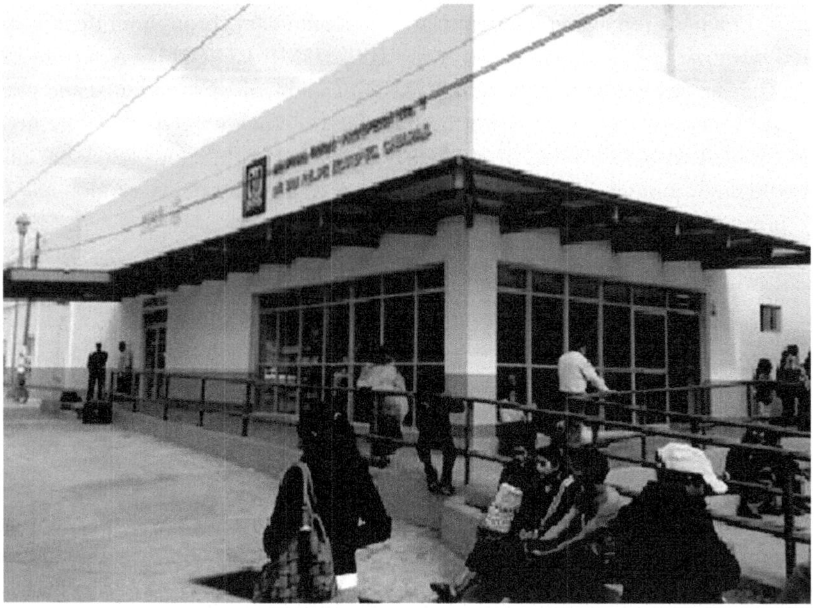

Fig. 8.8 Waiting outside an urban clinic. Published with kind permission of © Mounia El Kotni 2017. All Rights Reserved

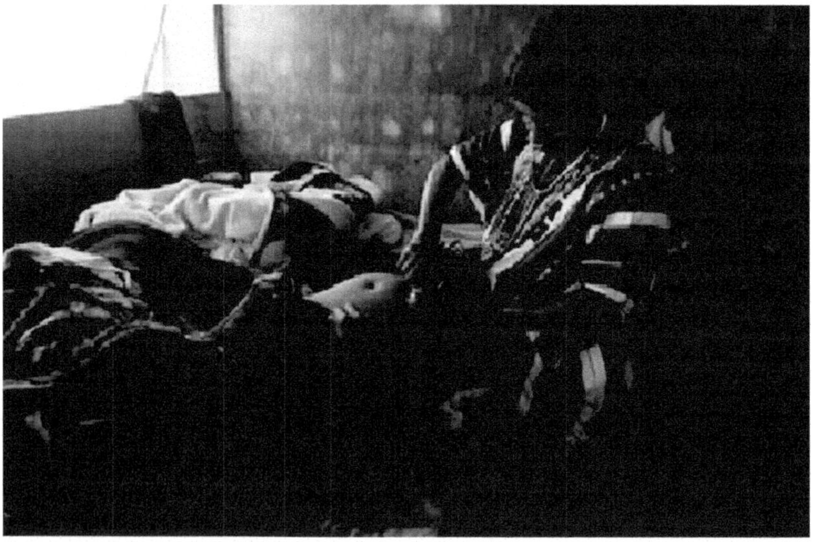

Fig. 8.9 Prenatal consult at home. Published with kind permission of © Mounia El Kotni 2017. All Rights Reserved

> This was a strategy that the government initiated, not just here in Mexico, but in many countries, that was suggested to diminish infant mortality; hospitals are saturated and a C-section is a good way of programing who comes in, when they do, and when they come out. [We have] a failed health system that does not know how to care for pregnant women—C-sections are a clear example of that—and it is not possible that we keep having a C-section rate three times higher than what is recommended by the World Health Organization. (Redacción AZ Noticias 2015)

Despite infrastructural changes in the past decades, including the construction of roads and rural clinics (Fig. 8.10), indigenous women still live at the margins of Mexican society, targeted by development programs (such as Prospera) that focus on their reproductive behaviors.

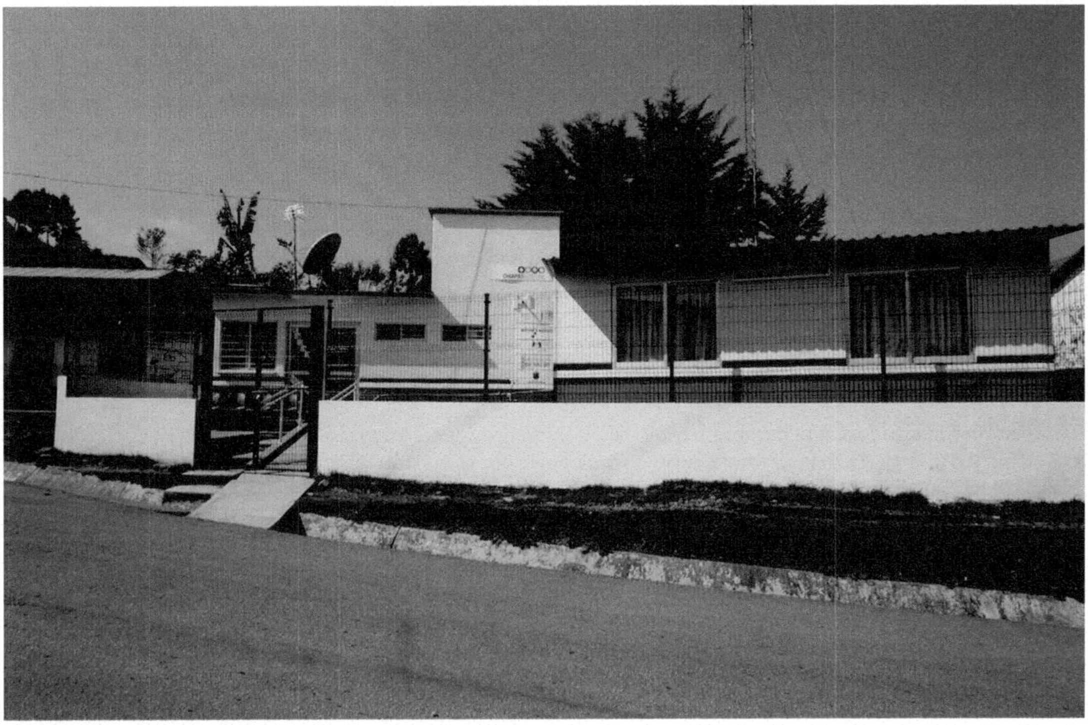

Fig. 8.10 A rural clinic in Chiapas. Published with kind permission of © Mounia El Kotni 2017. All Rights Reserved

8.5 Obstetric Violence Is Structural Violence

> Maternal mortality might be one of the most serious expressions of a series of omissions and violations of the economic, social, and cultural rights of the woman and her whole community (Arana 2002).

Framing maternal health as a matter of human rights underlines the injustice of maternal deaths, which can then be analyzed as violations of women's rights. It also highlights how blaming indigenous midwives is a violation of their rights as indigenous peoples. This blame happens in everyday discourses and is implicit during government trainings for *parteras*. In San Cristóbal de Las Casas, the Organization of Indigenous Doctors of the State of Chiapas (OMIECH) addresses the injustice of indigenous maternal deaths in a comparative perspective: why are indigenous midwives systematically blamed for maternal and child mortality when hospitals are not held accountable for routinely violating women's rights?

> They never admit that babies die, that mothers die over there [in the hospital]. They put the blame on the women, on the *parteras*, because they are indigenous… (…) [They say] that the midwife is worth nothing, that it is the pregnant woman's fault, that it's because of this, because of that…. (OMIECH founder, cited in El Kotni and Icó Bautista 2014)

For OMIECH, there is an uneven reaction to maternal mortality depending on where it occurs. Indigenous midwives are systematically blamed, while doctors are hardly ever held to account because of the social prestige their profession carries. On the other end, poverty and illiteracy make it difficult for indigenous women to navigate the medical system. In Chiapas, only 28.8% of indigenous women from 15 to 19 attend school, compared with 48.7% of nonindigenous women (INEGI 2009). Similar to other states of Mexico, indigenous women suffer:

> different kinds of institutional violence and ethnic and gender discrimination, for example when they are discriminated against in health services because of their monolingualism, when doctors fail to explain ailments or treatments to them, or when they try to make a complaint and the state authorities scold and insult them. (Sieder and Sierra 2010, p. 25)

In a national context of widespread gender-based violence, where women struggle to gain control over their own body (Arteaga Botello and Valdes Figueroa 2010), the hospital becomes a place where violence is reproduced, as women's intimate reproductive experiences are controlled by male (or masculinized) professionals. The treatment women receive in hospitals pushes them away. Such was the case for Carlita, a 20-year-old mother of indigenous descent living in San Cristóbal.

> When labor started I went to the hospital, but they wouldn't pay attention to me. Finally, a *doctora* checked me [performed a cervical exam]. She told me to go back home because I still had time. The *doctora* was nice, but I did not like how she touched me. So when I left [the hospital], I told my mother 'I don't want to give birth in this place, it's better to call my grandmother so that she can come and care for me at home.' (Interview, April 2015)[10]

When indigenous women do not comply with the government programs (of giving birth at a clinic) or expectations of modernity (of having less children), they expose themselves to scolding, coercion, and mistreatment from the health personnel. The violation of women's reproductive rights during childbirth takes the form of verbal insults (Castro and Erviti 2003), routine invasive procedures (including cervical checks (Smith-Oka 2013) and uterine revision (Zacher Dixon 2015)), and forced sterilization (Castro 2004), among others. The physical violence women experience in the maternity ward is one of the reasons some women refuse to go to the hospital (Berry 2008; Smith-Oka 2013; Zacher Dixon 2015). Women's fears stem, to some degree, from such stories of violence which are in part linked to the poor working conditions of public hospitals in Mexico and which are reinforced by the medical, gender and ethnic stratification occurring during the medical encounter.

Researchers and NGOs have been documenting obstetric violence in Mexico for more than a decade (Castro and Erviti 2003; Freyermuth Enciso 2004; Kirsch and Arana 1999). In 2013, the photograph of an indigenous Mazatec woman giving birth on the lawn of a Oaxacan hospital after being denied medical care was widely shared on the internet (Gomez Licon 2013). The picture created outrage throughout the world, with Mexican organizations urging the government to act on the topic of obstetric violence. Since then, organizations from the civil society such as the Information Group on Reproductive Choice (GIRE) have encouraged women and their families to present demands to the National Commission of Human Rights (CNDH) and lobbied for legislation on the matter. Currently, three states criminalize obstetric violence—Chiapas, Guerrero, and Veracruz—and similar legislation is underway in two others (Jalisco & Zacatecas) (GIRE 2015a).

In line with international organizations, GIRE places obstetric violence on the human rights terrain, to achieve the WHO standard of "every woman's right to the highest attainable standard of health, which includes the right to dignified, respectful health care." In particular, women of low socioeconomic status and minorities are more likely to suffer obstetric violence. In their 2015 report, GIRE analyzes how criminalizing obstetric violence is not the solution to its ending; rather the state should recognize such violence as institutional violence and act to provide women with quality care (GIRE 2015b).

In the hospital, actions of violence are not always "the product of the acts of rogue individual practitioners, but rather of a systemic failure that reinforces outdated practices" (Zacher Dixon 2015,

[10]Carlita's son was born in her home with the help of her grandmother, a recognized midwife in her community.

p. 449). The medical professionals I have met have been generally very skeptical about such laws, which are impossible to implement, "the Obstetric Violence law has a very noble purpose and very good concepts; the problem is that [politicians] they make such a law and [as a doctor] you think: 'and how am I going to implement this if I don't have any means?", (female obstetrician working in urban hospital). Another limitation of the law is the lack of legal recourse to denounce obstetric violence and the little trust Mexicans, and indigenous people in particular, have in their judicial institutions (Sieder and Sierra 2010).

8.6 Contesting Violence: Midwives Organizing

Since the Zapatista uprising in Chiapas, human rights have provided a powerful framework for NGOs and civil society to call attention to the structural violence in indigenous peoples' lives. Organizations working in the field of indigenous health rely on human rights to reframe maternal deaths not as the consequence of *partera* care but as the outcome of a series of state neglect. A human rights approach to maternal mortality allows framing maternal deaths as a violation of women's rights. It also points out to the complex entanglement between rights, culture, and blame, reinforced by government programs focusing solely on midwifery training to diminish maternal mortality rates.

The Organization of Indigenous Doctors of the State of Chiapas frames health and reproductive knowledge as a right—a right that can save lives. Although OMIECH started to form in the late 1970s, it was officially founded in 1985. The organization's headquarters are located in San Cristóbal de Las Casas, but communities from any region of Chiapas can decide to become members. The goal of the organization is to valorize indigenous medical knowledge by training health promoters and midwives in the Highlands of Chiapas through community workshops (Fig. 8.11). To date, there are 13 communities within 11 municipalities participating in the project. In the face of the stigmatization of indigenous midwives and of government incentives for women to give birth in hospitals, OMIECH members have revived indigenous plant knowledge and natural care for women, reinforcing in turn the cohesion of the community which is then better prepared to face an emergency. The organization

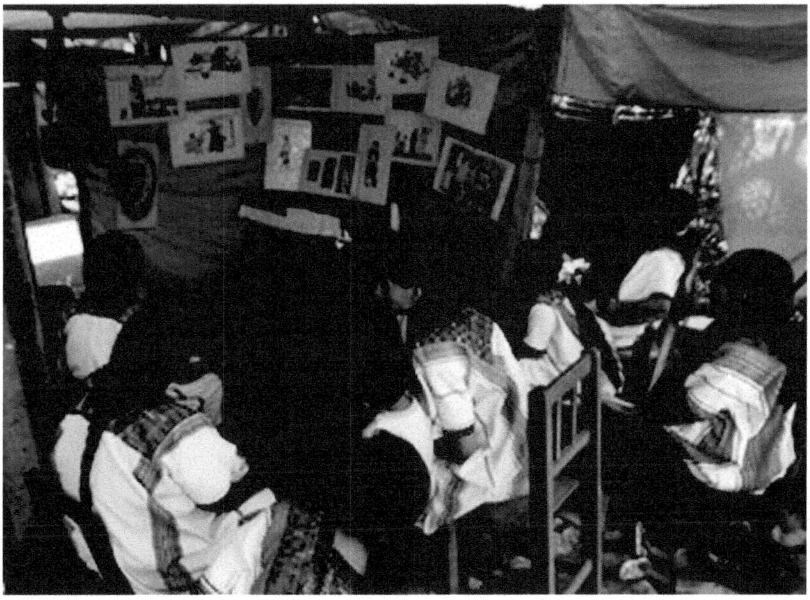

Fig. 8.11 OMIECH community workshop with women and midwives. Published with kind permission of © Mounia El Kotni 2017. All Rights Reserved

runs the Museum of Mayan Medicine in San Cristóbal and has promoted its work through partnership with organizations in France and Germany. The 50 midwives who constitute the membership of the organization also meet annually to share their knowledge about reproductive health and their concerns about changes in their communities.

In a 2005 documentary on homebirth in Mayan communities, the organization highlights the importance of the traditional knowledge of midwives, who speak the same language as the women they care for and are available at any time of the day or the night to attend a birth in the mother's home (Icó Bautista 2005). As described earlier in this chapter, indigenous midwives' role is not limited to childbirth; they also carry a variety of knowledge related to healthcare. OMIECH claims that medicine is not only Western and that indigenous medicine should not be perceived only as a replacement when the former is lacking. The simultaneous use of the two medical systems is not uncommon in Chiapas (Ayora Diaz 2000). What OMIECH argues is for Mayan men and women to be able to turn to both systems of medicine to exercise their right to health, without fearing socioeconomic punishment.

Conclusion

In this chapter, I discussed how in Southern Mexico, when it comes to the politics of birth, the sociocultural determinants to healthcare access put some women at risk more than others. In Highlands Chiapas, poor mothers, often of Maya descent, are the target of government programs aiming to diminish maternal mortality by encouraging them to give birth in medical structures rather than in their homes with an indigenous midwife. The desire to attract indigenous people into the hospital for childbirth results from Mexico's global commitments to improving their health conditions but has so far focused on training midwives in detecting alarm signals, transferring their patients, and pressuring women to give birth in hospitals. These two policies have led to overcrowding of public hospitals, which has increased both cesarean section rates and the violation of women's human rights in childbirth. By not focusing on the structural roots of maternal deaths, such as poverty, racism, and marginalization, the policies will continue failing indigenous women and their families.

References

Andaya, E. (2014). *Conceiving Cuba: Reproduction, women, and the state in the post-soviet era*. New Brunswick, N.J: Rutgers University Press.

Antillón Najlis, X. (2013). El territorio del alma. Una experiencia de acompañamiento psicosocial en la zona norte de Chiapas. In *Luchas "muy otras". Zapatsimo y autonomía en las comunidades indígenas de Chiapas* (pp. 229–316). CIESAS-Mexico D.F.: UAM-Xochimilco, UACH-San Cristobal de Las Casas.

Arana, M. (2002). El derecho a una maternidad voluntaria y sin riesgos. Apuntes para una discusión. In G. Freyermuth Enciso & M. C. Manca (Eds.), *Luna Golpeada. Morir durante la maternidad: Investigaciones, acciones y atención médica en Chiapas, y otras experiencias en torno a la Mortalidad Materna* (pp. 47–49). Tuxtla Gutiérrez: Comité por una Maternidad Voluntaria y Sin Riesgos en Chiapas, Comité Promotor por una Maternidad sin Riesgos en México.

Arteaga Botello, N., & Valdes Figueroa, J. (2010). ¿Que hay detrás de los feminicidios? Una lectura sobre sus redes socioales y culturales y la construcción de nuevas subjetividades. In N. Arteaga Botello (Ed.), *"Por eso la maté". Una aproximación sociocultural a la violencia contra las mujeres* (pp. 15–54). México, D.F.: UNAM.

Ayora Diaz, S. I. (2000). Imagining authenticity in the local medicines of Chiapas, Mexico. *Critique of Anthropology, 20*(2), 173–190.

Berer, M., & Sundari Ravindran, T. (2000). *Safe motherhood initiatives: Critical issues*. London: Blackwell Science Limited for Reproductive Health Matters.

Bernard, H. R. (2006). *Research methods in anthropology. Qualitative and quantitative approaches* (4th ed.). Lanham, New York: Altamira Press.

Berry, N. S. (2006). Kaqchikel midwives, home births, and emergency obstetric referrals in Guatemala: Contextualizing the choice to stay at home. *Social Science & Medicine, 62*, 1958–1969.

Berry, N. S. (2008). Who's judging the quality of care? Indigenous Maya and the problem of "not being attended". *Medical Anthropology, 27*(2), 164–189.

Berry, N. S. (2010). *Unsafe motherhood: Mayan maternal mortality and subjectivity in post-war guatemala*. (Reprint edition). New York: Berghahn Books.

Cadenas Gordillo, B. (2002). El trabajo de salud y la vida cotidiana de las parteras. In G. Freyermuth Enciso & M. C. Manca (Eds.), *Luna Golpeada. Morir durante la maternidad: investigaciones, acciones y atención médica en Chiapas, y otras experiencias en torno a la Mortalidad Materna* (pp. 114–124). Tuxtla Gutiérrez: Comité por una Maternidad Voluntaria y Sin Riesgos en Chiapas, Comité Promotor por una Maternidad sin Riesgos en México.

Castro, A. (2004). Contracepting at childbirth: The integration of reproductive health and population policies in Mexico. In A. Castro & M. Singer (Eds.), *Unhealthy health policy: A critical anthropological examination* (pp. 133–144). Walnut Creek, CA: Altamira Press.

Castro, R., & Erviti, J. (2003). Violations of reproductive rights during hospital births in Mexico. *Health and Human Rights, 7*(1), 90–110.

Chopel, A. M. (2014). Reproductive health in indigenous Chihuahua: Giving birth "alone like the goat". *Ethnicity & Health, 19*(3), 279–296.

Colen, S. (1995). "Like a Mother to Them": Stratified reproduction and West Indian childcare workers and employers in New York. In F. D. Ginsburg & R. Rapp (Eds.), *Conceiving the new world order: The global politics of reproduction* (pp. 78–102). Berkeley and Los Angeles: University of California Press.

Cominsky, S. (2012). Birth and blame. Guatemalan midwives and reproductive risk. In *Risk, reproduction and narratives of experience* (pp. 81–101). Nashville: Vanderbilt University Press.

CONAPO (Consejo Nacional de Población). (2010). *Índice de Maginación por entidad federativa y municipio 2010* (p. 117). Mexico, D.F.: CONAPO.

Eber, C. (1995). *Women and alcohol in a highland Maya Town: Water of hope, water of sorrow*. Austin: University of Texas Press.

EZLN (Ejercito Zapatista de Liberación Nacional). (1993). *Primera Declaración de la Selva Lacandona*. Retrieved August 25, 2015, from http://enlacezapatista.ezln.org.mx/1994/01/01/primera-declaracion-de-la-selva-lacandona/.

El Kotni, M. (2016a). *"Porque Tienen Mucho Derecho." Parteras, Biomedical Training and the Vernacularization of Human Rights in Chiapas*. (Ph.D. Dissertation). University at Albany, SUNY.

El Kotni, M. (2016b). Reforming pregnancy care and childbirth in Chiapas. *Anthropology Newsletter, 57*(2), e7–e8.

El Kotni, M., & Icó Bautista, M. (2014). *Responding to gendered structural violence: Indigenous midwives in Chiapas*. Presentation presented at the Society for Applied Anthropology Annual Meeting, Albuquerque.

Enciso, G. F. (2004). *Maternidad peligrosa: evaluación de la atención institucional a la urgencia obstétrica en los altos de Chiapas*. Mexico, D.F.: SEDESOL.

Enciso L. A. (2014). *Casi el doble que la población en general, la pobreza entre indígenas. La Jornada*. Retrieved January 7, 2016, from http://www.jornada.unam.mx/ultimas/2014/08/07/por-desventaja-social-situacion-de-rezago-de-la-poblacion-indigena-coneval-8587.html.

Farmer, P. (2005). *Pathologies of power: Health, human rights, and the new war on the poor*. Berkeley: University of California Press.

Fordyce, L., & Maraesa, A. (Eds.). (2012). *Risk, reproduction and narratives of experience*. Nashville: Vanderbilt University Press.

Freyermuth Enciso, G. (2003). *Las mujeres de humo: morir en Chenalho: género, etnia y generación, factores constitutivos del riesgo durante la maternidad*. México, D.F: CIESAS, Instituto Nacional de las Mujeres, Comité por una Maternidad Voluntaria y sin Riesgos en Chiapas.

Freyermuth Enciso, G., & Argüello Avendaño, H. (2010). La Muerte Prematura de Mujeres en los Altos de Chiapas. Un Análisis desde la Violencia. *Revista Pueblos y Fronteras Digital, 6*(10), 181–216.

Freyermuth Enciso, G., & Cárdenas Elizalde, R. (2009). Evaluación del subregistro de la mortalidad materna en Los Altos de Chiapas mediante las estrategias RAMOS y RAMOS modificada. *Salud Pública Mexicana, 51*, 450–457.

Galtung, J. (1969). Violence, peace, and peace research. *Journal of Peace Research, 6*(3), 167–191.

Gálvez, A. (2011). *Patieent citizens, immigrant mothers: Mexican women, public prenatal care, and the birth weight paradox* (1st ed.). New Brunswick, N.J: Rutgers University Press.

Ginsburg, F. D., & Rapp, R. (1995). *Conceiving the new world order: The global politics of reproduction*. Berkeley and Los Angeles: University of California Press.

Global Maternal Newborn Health Conference. (2015). *Global maternal newborn health conference*. Mexico City. Retrieved February 1, 2016, from http://www.ustream.tv/recorded/75821049.

Gobierno del Estado de Chiapas. (2014). *Instrumentos Normativos para la Formulación del Anteproyecto de Presupuesto de Egresos* (p. 15).

Goldstein, D. M. (2012). *Outlawed: Between security and rights in a Bolivian City*. Durham: Duke University Press Books.

Gomez Licon, A. (2013). *Indigenous woman gives birth on hospital lawn in Mexico after doctors denied her care*. The Huffington Post. Retrieved September 24, 2015, from http://www.huffingtonpost.com/2013/10/09/woman-gives-birth-on-hosp_n_4073416.html.

Gómez Mena, C. (2012). *Parteras atienden 70 por ciento de los nacimientos en comunidades indígenas*. La Jornada. Retrieved from http://www.jornada.unam.mx/2012/07/12/sociedad/043n1soc.

Groark, K. (1997). To warm the blood, to warm the flesh: The role of the steambath in highland Maya (tzeltal-tzotzil) ethnomedicine. *Journal of Latin American Lore, 20*(1), 3–96.

Grupo de Información en Reproducción Elegida. (2015a). *Niñas y Mujeres sin justicia. Derechos Reproductivos en México* (p. 303). México, D.F: GIRE. Retrieved March 1, 2016, from http://informe2015.gire.org.mx/#/marco-normativo-violencia-obstetrica

Grupo de Información en Reproducción Elegida. (2015b). *Niñas y Mujeres sin justicia: Violencia Obstétrica*. Retrieved September 21, 2015, from https://www.youtube.com/watch?v=P3FfspMqnfM&feature=youtu.be.

Guiteras Holmes, C. (1961). *Perils of the soul: The world view of a tzotzil Indian*. Glencoe, IL: Free Press of Glencoe.

Gupta, A. (2012). *Red tape: Bureaucracy, structural violence, and poverty in India*. Durham: Duke University Press.

Howes-Mischel, R. (2012). *Gestating subjects: Negotiating public health and pregnancy in transborder oaxaca*. (Dissertation). New York: New York University.

Icó Bautista, A. (2011) *El Parto (En comunidades indígenas maya de Chiapas, México)*. Retrieved February 6, 2015, from https://www.youtube.com/watch?v=lsT0Fok2TrI&feature=youtube_gdata_player

Icó Bautista, A. (2005). *Una experiencia en Salud Intercultural*. Chiapas: San Cristóbal de Las Casas.

Instituto Nacional de Estadística y Geografía. (2009). *Perfil sociodemográfico de la población que habla lengua indígena* (p. 204). México, D.F: INEGI.

Instituto Nacional de Estadística y Geografía. (2010). *Perfil Sociodemográfico. Estados Unidos Mexicano* (p. 168). Aguascalientes: INEGI.

Jordan, B. (1993). *Birth in four cultures: A crosscultural investigation of childbirth in Yucatan, Holland, Sweden, and the United States* (4th ed.). Prospect Heights, Ill: Waveland Pr Inc..

Kirsch, J. D., & Arana, M. (1999). Informed consent for family planning for poor women in Chiapas, Mexico. *The Lancet, 354*(9176), 419–420.

Little, W. E. (2004). Mayas in the marketplace. In *Tourism, globalization, and cultural identity*. Austin: University of Texas Press.

Mandujano, I. (2016 15). *Papa Francisco reivindica la defensa de los pueblos indígenas con su visita a Chiapas*. Proceso. Retrieved April 6, 2016, from http://www.proceso.com.mx/430083/papa-francisco-reivindica-la-defensa-los-pueblos-indigenas-visita-a-chiapas.

Miranda, V. (2015). Lingering discourses from Yucatan's past: Political ecologies of birth in rural Yucatan. In J. Shaw (Ed.), *The maya of the Cochuah region: Archaeological and ethnographic perspectives on the northern lowlands* (pp. 235–256). Albuquerque: University of New Mexico Press.

Murray de López, J. (2016). *Becoming (M)other: Political economy and maternal transition in urban Chiapas*. (Ph.D Dissertation). Manchester: The University of Manchester.

Nash, J. C. (2001). *Mayan visions: The quest for autonomy in an age of globalization* (1st ed.). New York: Routledge.

Objetivos de Desarrollo del Milenio #5. (n.d.). Retrieved from http://www.objetivosdedesarrollodelmilenio.org.mx/cgi-win/odm.exe/OBJODM0050,E.

OMIECH. (2011) *El Parto (En comunidades indígenas maya de Chiapas, México)*. Retrieved February 6, 2015, from https://www.youtube.com/watch?v=lsT0Fok2TrI&feature=youtube_gdata_player.

OMM (Observatorio de Mortalidad Materna en México). (2013). *Indicadores 2013. Objetivo de Desarrollo del Milenio 5: Avances en México* (p. 105). México, D.F y San Cristóbal de Las Casas, Chiapas: Observatorio de la Mortalidad Materna en México. Retrieved from http://www.omm.org.mx/omm/images/stories/Documentos%20grandes/INDICADORES%202013%20OPS.pdf

O'Donnell, K. (2010). *Weaving transnational solidarity: From the catskills to Chiapas and beyond*. Leiden, Boston: Brill.

Pigg, S. L. (1997). Authority in translation. Finding, knowing, naming, and training "Traditional birth attendants" in Nepal. In *Childbirth and authoritative knowledge: Cross-cultural perspectives* (pp. 233–262). Los Angeles: University of California Press.

Pinto, S. (2008). *Where there is no midwife: Birth and loss in rural India*. New York: Berghahn Books.

Redacción AZ Noticias. (2015). *Anuncian falla en sistema de salud en México por exceso de cesáreas*. AZ Noticias. Retrieved June 30, 2015, from http://www.aznoticias.mx/index.php/mexico-movil/14958-anuncian-falla-en-sistema-de-salud-en-mexico-por-exceso-de-cesareas.

Romano, M., Cacciatore, A., Giordano, R., & La Rosa, B. (2010). Postpartum period: Three distinct but continuous phases. *Journal of Prenatal Medicine, 4*(2), 22–25.

Rylko-Bauer, B., Whiteford, L., & Farmer, P. (Eds.). (2009). *Global health in times of violence*. Santa Fe: School for Advanced Research Press.

Sánchez, C. (2010). *En México, uno de cada dos niños hoy nace por cesárea*. El Universal. Retrieved August 25, 2015, from http://archivo.eluniversal.com.mx/cultura/63403.html.

SEDESOL & CONEVAL (Secretaría de Desarrollo Social, & Consejo Nacional de Evaluación de la Política de Desarrollo Social). (2015). *Informe Anual sobre la Situación de Pobreza y Rezago Social 2015* (p. 2). Retrieved from http://www.sedesol.gob.mx/work/models/SEDESOL/Informes_pobreza/2015/Estados/Chiapas.pdf.

SIPaz (Servicio Internacional para la Paz). (2014). Derechos Humanos en México: "Retroceso", "simulaciòn" e "impunidad" afriman organizaciones civiles. *SiPaz Informe, XIX*(3), 1–6.

Sieder, R., & Sierra, M. T. (2010). *Indigenous women's access to justice in Latin America.*

Smith-Oka, V. (2009). Unintended consequences: Exploring the tensions between development programs and indigenous women in Mexico in the context of reproductive health. *Social Science & Medicine, 68*(11), 2069–2077.

Smith-Oka, V. (2013). Managing labor and delivery among impoverished populations in Mexico: Cervical examinations as bureaucratic practice. *American Anthropologist, 115*(4), 595–607.

United Nations. (2014). *State of the world's midwifery 2014. Universal Pathway*. A Woman's RIghts to Health. UNFPA.

Zacher Dixon, L. (2015). Obstetrics in a time of violence: Mexican midwives critique routine hospital practices. *Medical Anthropology Quarterly, 39*(3), 437–454.

9 Maternal Mortality and the Coverage, Availability of Resources, and Access to Women's Health Services in Three Indigenous Regions of Mexico: Guerrero Mountains, Tarahumara Sierra, and Nayar

Sergio Meneses Navarro,
Blanca Pelcastre Villafuerte,
and Marisol Vega Macedo

9.1 Introduction

Studying indigenous people gives us the opportunity to analyze those unnecessary and preventable gaps and inequities that divide these populations from the rest of the country's inhabitants, including those factors that result and exacerbate such differences. Some of the most pertinent health indicators used in understanding these differences are life expectancy at birth (LEB), maternal mortality (MM), and infant mortality (IM). These statistics provide a window on the state of health conditions, inequality, and the guarantee of human rights that ultimately determine the length and quality of life for minority individuals and social groups. They also are useful in evaluating the prevalence of premature death that results from preventable causes occurring in mothers during pregnancy, labor and delivery, the postpartum period, as well as their infants. In addition to the circumstances in which people are born, develop, work, and age, an important determinant of health for these populations is the health system's response to caring for these individuals.

In this chapter, we analyze the cases of three indigenous regions where the poorest indicators for LEB, MM, and IM are concentrated: the Guerrero Mountains, the Tarahumara Sierra, and the Nayar municipality of Nayarit (Figs. 9.1, 9.2, and 9.3). We focus our analysis on several elements

S. M. Navarro, M.D., Sc.D. (✉)
CIESAS Sureste-CONACYT, Carretera a Chamula Km 3.5,
San Cristóbal de Las Casas, 29247 Chiapas, Mexico

B. P. Villafuerte, Ph.D.
National Institute of Public Health,
Cuernavaca, Mexico

M. V. Macedo, M.P.H.
Alliance for Health, Food, and Nutrition (ASAN), Chiapas, Mexico

D. A. Schwartz (ed.), *Maternal Death and Pregnancy-Related Morbidity Among Indigenous Women of Mexico and Central America*, Global Maternal and Child Health: Medical, Anthropological, and Public Health Perspectives, https://doi.org/10.1007/978-3-319-71538-4_9

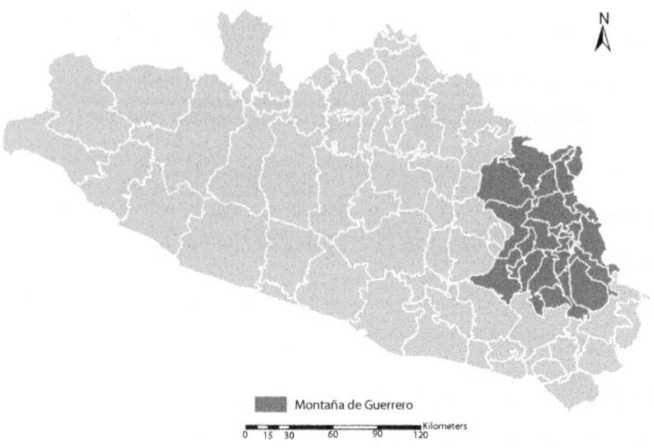

Fig. 9.1 Map of the Guerrero Mountain region

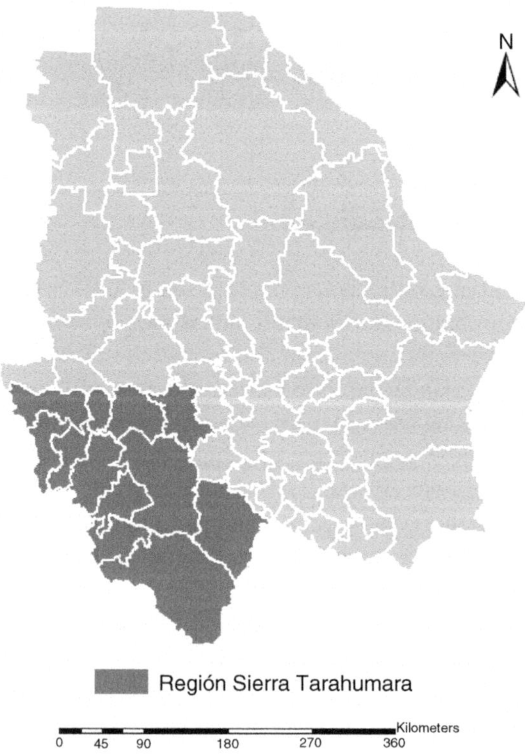

Fig. 9.2 Map of the Tarahumara Sierra region, Chihuahua. Source: Freyermuth and Gómez, 2016, based on the INEGI, 2010

of the health system necessary to guarantee the right to heath protection for indigenous women: health coverage, availability of resources, access to services, and quality of obstetric care. We emphasize indigenous women's health because they experience greater barriers to access services given gender inequality, as well as other social inequalities such as ethnic and class-based ones. We would like to also highlight the MM indicator, given that it exemplifies the social determinants of health, inequities, and the guaranteed ability to exercise the right to health. Finally, the performance of unnecessary cesarean section deliveries is an indicator that may serve as proxy for problems related to quality of care for indigenous women, including the right to respectful care. In the following section, we also present the background information describing the regions included in the study.

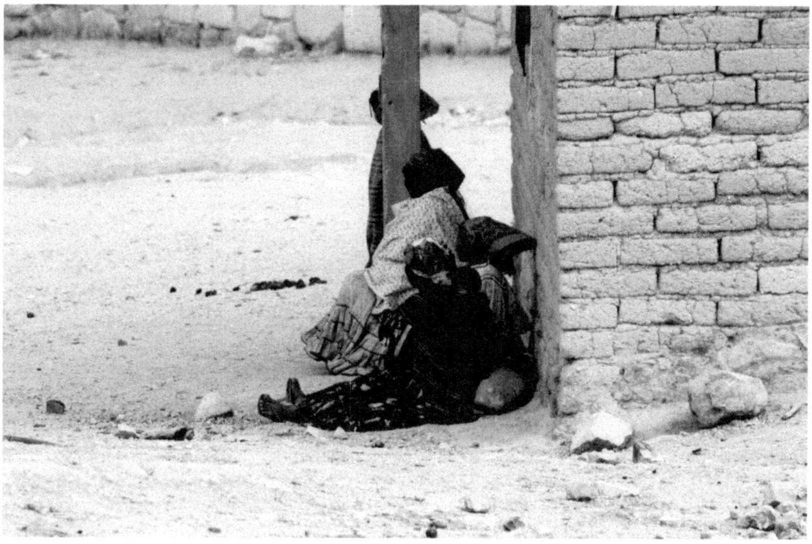

Fig. 9.3 Indigenous women from the Tarahumara Sierra region. Photograph from Mauricio Andrada, 2015

9.2 Background

9.2.1 Guerrero Mountain Region

Guerrero is located on the Pacific Coast of Mexico (Fig. 9.1). In 2015, the state had the second lowest average LEB in the country at 72.89 years of age (only surpassed by the state of Chiapas), 4 years lower than the state with the highest LEB, Nuevo León, at 76.37 years of age. In 2013 Guerrero had the third highest average MM with a rate of 59.4 women who died due to a cause related to childbirth per 100,000 live births. This was in dramatic comparison to the state with the best outcome, Nuevo León, at 14.8 deaths per 100,000 live births and the national outcome of 38.2 deaths per 100,000 live births. That same year, Guerrero was in the fourth place in infant mortality with 14.7 recorded deaths per 1000 children under the age of 1. This represented a fivefold difference compared to the state of Nuevo León (9.4/1000) (INEGI 2016).

The state of Guerrero has 81 municipalities, 19 of which are located in the Mountain Region on the extreme eastern side of the state, where the south of Puebla, the Mixteca region of Oaxaca, and the Costa Chica of Guerrero meet (Fig. 9.1). The 19 municipalities that make up the Mountain Region are Alcozauca de Guerrero, Alpoyeca, Atlamajalcingo del Monte, Atlixtac, Copanatoyac, Cualác, Huamuxtitlán, Malinaltepec, Metlatónoc, Olinalá, Tlacoapa, Tlalixtaquilla de Maldonado, Tlapa de Comonfort, Xalpatláhuac, Xochihuehuetlán, Zapotitán Tablas, Acatepec, Cochoapa el Grande, and Iliatenco.

There are 3,533,251 residents in the state, 10.46% of these (369,821) are in the Mountain Region. Of the total of 498,510 residing in Guerrero, approximately 15% speak an indigenous language; most are concentrated in the Mountain Region, where 7 out of every 10 residents speak an indigenous language. Of the 19 municipalities in Guerrero, 15 are considered indigenous, while 14 of them are designated as extremely marginalized and 3 as highly marginalized (Table 9.1). As such, the Mountain Region is simultaneously one of the primary indigenous territories in the country and one of the poorest and most marginalized.

Another distinctive indicator of social inequity is literacy. In 2015, 14.7% of men and 16.24% of women older than 12 years of age in Guerrero did not know how to read or write. However, 26.9% of

Table 9.1 Sociodemographic data for the state of Guerrero and Mountain Region, 2015

Municipalities		State of Guerrero		Mountain Region		Rest of the state	
		Number	%	Number	%	Number	%
		81	100	19	23.46	62	76.54
Reported level of marginalization	Extremely high	43	53	14	73.68	29	46.77
	High	18	22	3	15.79	15	24.19
	Medium	16	20	2	10.53	14	22.58
	Low	4	5	0	0.00	4	6.45
Classification by the Commission of Indigenous Development[a]	Indigenous	24	29.63	15	78.95	9	14.52
	Presence of indigenous population	9	11.11	0	0.00	9	14.52
	Dispersed indigenous population	48	59.26	4	21.05	44	70.97
Population	Total	3,533,251	100	369,821	10.46	3,163,430	89.53
	Men	1,699,059	48.08	177,132	47.1	1,521,927	48.2
	Women	1,834,192	51.9	196,528	52.9	1,637,664	51.8
	Indigenous language	498,510	15.32	338,957	70.76	159,553	7.7
Illiteracy (15 years of age and older)	Overall	341,517	13.61	63,394	27.95	278,123	12.2
	Women	210,340	16.24	40,806	33.00	169,534	13.7

Source: Vega and Meneses based on the 2015 Inter-Census Survey, INEGI http://www.inegi.org.mx/est/contenidos/proyectos/encuestas/hogares/especiales/ei2015/default.aspx (consulted August 23, 2016)

[a]The Commission of Indigenous Development classifies municipalities as indigenous if 40% or more of the population speaks an indigenous language, describes themselves as indigenous, or lives in a home where the head of the household is indigenous. The municipalities with the presence of indigenous population are those municipalities where less than 40% of the population meets the aforementioned criteria but where there are at least 5000 indigenous individuals. The municipalities with a dispersed indigenous population are those municipalities where the indigenous population is less than 40% and less than 5000 individuals, but there is an indigenous presence

men and 33% of women in the Mountain Region were illiterate; one in every four men and one in every three women did not know how to read or write. These data show the deep social inequities and exclusion experienced in the region, particularly by women (Table 9.1).

9.2.2 Tarahumara Sierra of Chihuahua

Located in the north of the country, Chihuahua is geographically the largest state in Mexico (Fig. 9.2). The total state population is 3,556,574, of which 2.67% speaks an indigenous language. The primary indigenous languages are *tarahumara* or *rarámuri*, *tepehuano* or *ódami*, *guarojío* or *makurawe*, and *pima* or *o'oba* (Table 9.2).

Chihuahua is made up of 67 municipalities. Approximately one-fourth of these are classified as high or extremely high marginalization with an indigenous presence. Twelve of these municipalities are in the southern part of the state, intersecting with Durango, Sinaloa, and Sonora, in the region known as the Tarahumara Sierra: Balleza, Batopilas, Bocoyna, Carichí, Chínipas, Guachochi, Guadalupe y Calvo, Guazapares, Maguarichi, Morelos, and Urique y Uruachi (Fig. 9.2). According to the data from the 2015 Inter-Census Survey, the Tarahumara Sierra is home to 218,268 individuals, most of whom live in poverty. A comparison of the literacy indicators between the Tarahumara population and the rest of the state of Chihuahua exemplifies the social inequities: while only 2.6% of the residents of Chihuahua are illiterate, 16.14% of the Tarahumara population over 12 years of age do not know ,how to read or write, representing an 8 to 1 ratio (Table 9.2).

Table 9.2 Sociodemographic data for the states of Chihuahua and Tarahumara Sierra, 2015

Municipalities		State of Chihuahua		Tarahumara Sierra		Rest of the state	
		Number	%	Number	%	Number	%
		67	100	12	17.91	55	82.09
Reported level of marginalization	Extremely high	11	16.4	11	91.7	0	0.00
	High	3	4.5	0	0.00	3	5.45
	Medium	12	17.9	1	8.33	11	20.00
	Low	41	61.2	0	0.00	41	74.55
Classification by the Commission of Indigenous Development[1]	Indigenous	5	7.5	5	41.7	0	0.00
	Presence of indigenous population	9	13.4	4	33.3	5	9.1
	Dispersed indigenous population	53	79.1	3	25	50	90.9
Population	Total	3,556,574	100	218,268	6.13	3,338,306	93.87
	Men	1,752,275	49.26	108,323	49.62	1,643,952	49.24
	Women	1,804,299	50.74	109,945	50.37	1,694,354	50.75
	Indigenous language	900,175	2.67	175,321	29.75	724,824	20.0
Illiteracy (15 years of age and older)	Overall	664,197	2.60	23,210	16.14	640,987	2.1
	Women	131,020	2.9	11,779	16.01	119,241	1.6

Source: Vega and Meneses based on the 2015 Inter-Census Survey, INEGI http://www.inegi.org.mx/est/contenidos/proyectos/encuestas/hogares/especiales/ei2015/default.aspx (consulted August 23, 2016)

9.2.3 Nayar Region

The state of Nayarit is located on the west coast of Mexico, sharing its northern border with Durango and Sinaloa, Jalisco to the southeast, and the Pacific Ocean to the west. In pre-Hispanic times, Nayarit was the territory of such indigenous groups such as the *Cora*, *Huichol*, *Tepehuanos*, and *Mexicaneros*, who currently reside in the mountainous region known as El Nayar in the Western Sierra Madre mountain region (Fig. 9.4).

The population is distributed into 1908 locales organized into 20 municipalities across the state. The majority of the population is concentrated in the capital city of Tepic as well as the cities of Tuxpan, Santiago Ixcuintla, Tecuala, Acaponeta, Ixtlán del Río, and Compostela. The Nayar region is in the northeast part of the state. It is the largest municipality at 5264 kilometers and extends across the cañons and mountains of the Sierra Madre. It is the ancestral land of the *Cora* and *Huichol* people and, to a lesser degree, the *Tepehuanos* and *Mexicaneros*. Their settlements in the mountains made access to these ethnic groups quite difficult, preserving their independence and geographic isolation from the dominant *mestizo* society in the rest of the state and country, as well as being the source of constant friction, throughout the nineteenth century.

The predominant languages are *Cora* and *Huichol*. Approximately 78% of the region's population speaks one of these two languages, with a lesser percentage speaking the indigenous languages of *Tepehuano*, *Nahuatl*, and *Mazahua*. The municipality of Nayar has a total of 525 communities, none of which have a population greater than 2500. All are considered rural and exemplify the dispersed population that characterizes the municipality. The community with the largest population is the municipal center, Jesus María, which in 2015 had a population of 2390.

The cultural region of the great Nayar is made up of municipalities from other states as well (Zacatecas, Durango, and Jalisco, in addition to Nayarit). The state of Nayarit has 1,181,050 residents, 3.59% of these (42,514) are located in the Nayar region. In the state of Nayarit, 5.41% of the population (61,460 individuals) speak an indigenous language, with most being concentrated in the Nayar region, where 88.07% of the population speaks an indigenous language. The Nayar region is

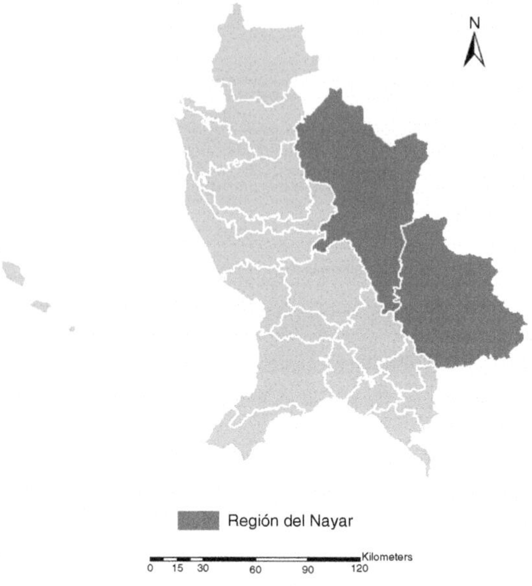

Fig. 9.4 Map of the Nayar region, Nayarit. Source: Freyermuth and Gómez, 2016, based on the INEGI, 2010

Table 9.3 Sociodemographic data for the state of Nayarit and the Nayar region, 2015

		State of Nayarit		Nayar region		Rest of the state	
Municipalities		Number	%	Number	%	Number	%
		20	100	1	5	19	95
Según grado de marginación	Extremely high	3	15	1	100	2	10.5
	High	0	0	0	0	0	0
	Medium	8	40	0	0	8	42.1
	Low	5	25	0	0	5	26.3
	Very low	4	20	0	0	4	21.05
Classification by the Commission of Indigenous Development[1]	Indigenous	2	10	1	100	1	5.3
	Presence of indigenous population	1	5	0	0	1	5.3
	Dispersed indigenous population	17	85	0	0	17	89.5
Population	Total	1,181,050	100	42,514	3.59	1,138,536	96.4
	Men	586,000	49.61	21,219	49.91	564,781	49.6
	Women	595,050	50.38	21,295	50.08	573,755	50.39
	Indigenous language	61,460	5.41	33,640	88.07	27,820	2.44
Illiteracy (15 years of age and older)	Overall	42,220	5.04	6833	29.9	35,387	3.2
	Women	21,532	5.8	7150	30.1	14,382	4.1

Source: Vega and Meneses based on the 2015 Inter-Census Survey, INEGI http://www.inegi.org.mx/est/contenidos/proyectos/encuestas/hogares/especiales/ei2015/default.aspx (consulted August 23, 2016)

considered an indigenous municipality and is also classified as extremely high in terms of marginalization (Table 9.3). The region represents one of the primary traditional indigenous regions in the western part of the country (Fig. 9.5).

Once again, the literacy indicator provides strong insights into the social inequities that exist between the indigenous population in the region and the rest of the state's population. In 2015, 5.04%

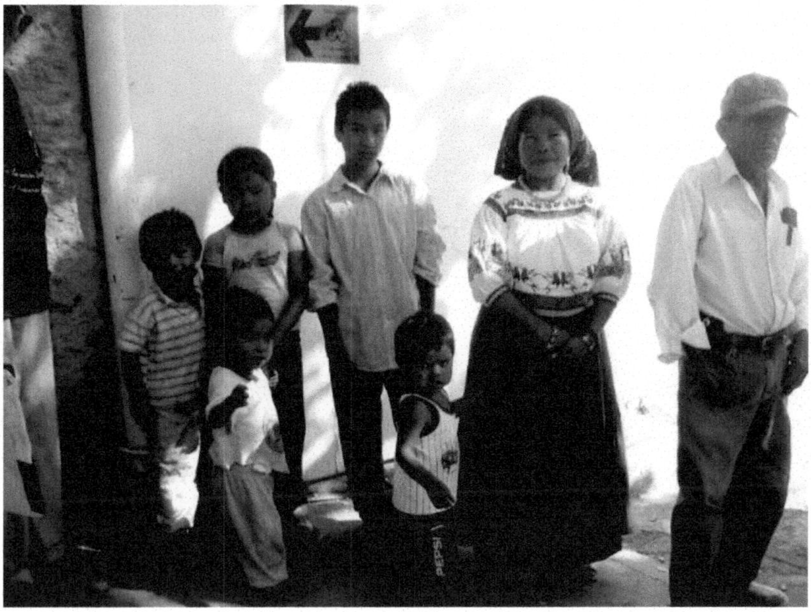

Fig. 9.5 *Huichol* family waiting at the hospital. Photograph from Gabriela Gil, 2015

of the general population and 5.8% of women over 12 years of age in the state of Nayarit did not know how to read or write. However, 29.9% of the general population and 30.1% of women in the Nayar region were illiterate (Table 9.3).

9.3 Poverty and Income

Across the three indigenous regions we analyzed, poverty is an important and widespread characteristic. Table 9.4 presents the percentages of the populations living in poverty and the income per capita for the general population, as well as for men, women, and indigenous language speakers and non-speakers across the three regions for the year 2010.[1]

Although the entire state of Guerrero is characterized by poverty—67.5% of Guerrero residents are living in this condition—the situation is most severe in the Mountain Region, where nine of every ten inhabitants live in poverty. This high level of poverty among indigenous people is comparable in the Tarahumara Sierra and the Nayar region, 85.5% and 91.6%, respectively. The indicator for extreme poverty reveals the depth of social inequities; 55.8% of individuals in the Guerrero Mountains, 43.3% in the Tarahumara Sierra, and 61.6% in the Nayar region are living below the limit of minimum well-being, which means that they do not have the means available to access even the basic nutrients necessary to live a healthy life. Comparing the prevalence of extreme poverty to the state average also reveals inequity; for example, in the state of Chihuahua, extreme poverty in the Tarahumara Sierra is seven times that of the state average (Table 9.4).

In all three indigenous regions, the monthly income per capita is considerably lower than the state average, even more so for women and the indigenous language-speaking population. In Guerrero, the poorest state of the three, monthly income per capita is $1157.14 pesos (the $ sign is the symbol for

[1]These data have not been updated with data from the 2015 INEGI Inter-Census Survey by the National Committee for the Evaluation of Social Development Policy (CONEVAL by its Spanish acronym), and as such, the information from the 2010 Census is the most updated data.

Table 9.4 Poverty and monthly income per capita in the Guerrero Mountains, the Tarahumara Sierra, and the Nayar region, 2010

Poverty and income		Guerrero	Mountains	Chihuahua	Tarahumara	Nayarit	Nayar
Population living in poverty		67.56%	86.45%	39.19%	85.51%	41.3%	91.6%
Population living in extreme poverty		31.58%	55.82%	6.62%	43.3%	8.2%	61.6%
Monthly income per capita[1]	General	$1157.14	$825.24	$1965	$890	$1940	$657
	Men	$1163.76	$830.52	$1978	$895	$1957	$662
	Women	$1151.89	$821.51	$1951	$886	$1923	$653
	Indigenous language[a]	$812.87	$699.57	$1189	$602	$615	$616
	No indigenous language[b]	$1304.90	$1192.74	$2041	$1102	$2004	$1010

Source: Vega and Meneses based on the data from the 2010 CONEVAL, 2010 poverty by states and municipalities, and 2010 mean income by age and ethnicity in Mexican municipalities (consulted August 12, 2016)
[a]In pesos August 2010. The $ sign is the symbol for the Mexican peso
[b]Indigenous language speakers

the Mexican peso). However, in the Mountain Region, it decreases to $825.24 and decreases again for women ($821.51) and indigenous language speakers ($699.57), indicative of systematic inequity associated with gender and ethnicity (Table 9.4).

Chihuahua and Nayarit are states that are classified as having a high level of development. Their monthly income per capita is similar: $1965 and $1940, respectively. Nonetheless, the inequity in income for the indigenous and female population is notable. In Chihuahua, the difference between the monthly average incomes is a little less than one-half than that of the indigenous Tarahumara Sierra population, when compared to the state average: $890 versus $1965 pesos. In the Nayar region, the difference is greater: $657 for inhabitants in the region versus the state average of $1940. In both regions, women, and, above all, indigenous women, have lower incomes: $602 pesos per month in the Tarahumara Sierra and $616 pesos in the Nayar region (Table 9.4).

9.4 Data Sources and Analyses

Data for population, ethnicity, and health coverage that were used to prepare the descriptive tables and this chapter's analysis are from the 2015 INEGI survey. We also added information regarding the municipalities in the three indigenous regions identified in the background section in this chapter. Information about poverty and income per capita in Table 9.4 of the background section is derived from the 2010 CONEVAL, where data are analyzed for the municipal level and by ethnicity. There are no more recent data available for analysis.

Maternal death data are from the database on deaths overseen by the Administration for Health Information in the Secretariat of Health. This information is only available for confirmation from 2002 to 2014 (the 2015 data were not included in the present analysis, as it could not be confirmed). For the MMR, we used the number of maternal deaths as the numerator and the number of registered live births as the denominator for each of the years under analysis multiplied by 100,000 live births. The MMR data were derived from the National Birth Registry (SINAC in Spanish).

The information in Table 9.8 is derived from the National Health Information System (SINAIS in Spanish) database, which collects data on the resources held by the health section, including data from the Health Ministry, state-level entities, social security institutions (IMSS, ISSSTE, etc.), and the private sector. Meanwhile, the Subsystem for Information on Equipment, Human Resources and Infrastructure for Health (SINERHIAS in Spanish) provides information from the federal Secretariat of Health and State Health Services (SESA in Spanish), with the most recent information being from 2014. To analyze the rate of health resources per 100,000 residents, we used the denominator of estimated population for each entity and indigenous region, based on the 2015 Inter-Census Survey.

In Table 9.9, we present the rate of health service per 100,000 women provided in a primary care setting. The information comes from the Health Information System (SIS in Spanish) from 2014, which is the most recent data available. The SIS only monitors the productivity of the federal Secretariat of Health and State Health Services but does not include IMSS, ISSSTE, or IMSS-Prospera. To produce the rate that we used, the 2014 gross productivity as the numerator and the total estimated female population from the 2015 Inter-Census Survey were multiplied by 1000. As with the previous rates, the data were analyzed for state and indigenous region.

Finally, the hospital discharge data presented in Tables 9.10, 9.11, and 9.12 are derived from the Automated System of Hospital Discharges (SAEH in Spanish), part of the General Administration for Health Information in the Secretariat of Health. The numerator represents the number of discharges for the municipality of residence for users, and the denominator is composed of the total number of women in the municipality, analyzed by indigenous region and state, with the rate given per 1000 women.

9.5 Results

9.5.1 Health Coverage

Health insurance coverage facilitates individuals receiving the care they need in a timely and financially accessible manner. In the case of public insurance, the insurance coverage is tied to public resources, and this mechanism has the objective of financially protecting individuals and families against the economic threat of loss of health.

In Mexico, there are three primary public insurance programs that individuals and families can be affiliated with. There are the employment-related social security programs: the Mexican Social Security Institute (IMSS in Spanish) for workers in the private sector and the Institute for Social Security and Services for State Workers (ISSSTE in Spanish) for government employees. As of 2004, there exists a public health insurance option, Seguro Popular (Popular Health Insurance SPS in Spanish), for citizens who are not affiliated with one of the other social security options. Although in some aspects Mexico has improved in terms of securing coverage among the population, there are still coverage gaps among those persons with the greatest need, as exemplified in the case of indigenous people in the three regions analyzed in this chapter.

The 2015 Inter-Census Survey data indicate that 9.54% of the inhabitants of the Guerrero Mountain region, 11.81% in the Tarahumara Sierra, and 27.08% in the Nayar region did not have any affiliation with any of the public insurance schema that effectively protects their right to health, as well as functioning for financial protection. However, the gaps in coverage between indigenous regions and the rest of the state have been trending toward decreasing. This is the case for Chihuahua, where in the Tarahumara Sierra as well as in the rest of the state lack of coverage hovers around 11%, or the case for Guerrero, where they have had a notable advance in coverage in the Mountain Region population, the fastest growing in the state. Nonetheless, the case for the Nayar region is a wide and important gap in coverage between the indigenous population and the state population (Table 9.5).

Another revealing indicator is the low rate of employee-based (social security) coverage in indigenous regions. In the case of the Guerrero Mountains, less than 1% of the population is affiliated with IMSS and less than 3% with ISSSTE; in the Tarahumara Sierra, less than 10% have coverage with IMSS and less than 3% with ISSSTE; and in the Nayar region, 8.6% are affiliated with IMSS and

Table 9.5 Public health insurance coverage in the Guerrero Mountains, the Tarahumara Sierra, and the Nayar region, 2015

Institution		Guerrero	Mountain region	Chihuahua	Tarahumara sierra	Nayarit	Nayar region
Health insurance coverage	IMSS	13.71%	0.55%	56.58%	9.03%	38.94%	8.64%
	ISSSTE	8.48%	2.14%	7.11%	2.85%	12.26%	2.43%
	Seguro Popular	77.29%	97.56%	31.76%	74,16%	51.37%	92.39%
No coverage as of 2015		19.48%	9.54%	11.15%	11.81%	16.08%	27.08%

Source: Vega and Meneses based on the 2015 Inter-Census Survey, INEGI http://www.inegi.org.mx/est/contenidos/proyectos/encuestas/hogares/especiales/ei2015/default.aspx (consulted August 23, 2016)

2.4% with ISSSTE. These data, along with the data on income per capita, indicate that the lack of salaried jobs in indigenous regions contributes to perpetuating poverty and its consequences on the health of indigenous people. In addition, other emerging and related social issues such as migration and family and community separation foment illegal activity such as drug trafficking and diverse forms of violence. It appears clear that low levels of social security affiliation point to the need to develop strategies that promote larger and better economic conditions for inhabitants in these regions.

9.5.2 Maternal Mortality

The overwhelming majority of deaths among women during pregnancy, birth, or the postpartum period are preventable with medical interventions that are low cost and have been scientifically tested for several decades (Campbell and Graham 2006; Schwartz 2015). The systematic occurrence of maternal death exemplifies structural and social inequity that, however persistent they may be, can be modified through public policy.

However, year after year, the indigenous regions of the Guerrero Mountains, the Tarahumara Sierra, and the Nayar report the highest incidences of maternal death, with rates that are well above the state and national averages. Table 9.6 presents the chronology of maternal death rates in the three states and their respective indigenous regions. As can be seen from these data, the MMR is systematically more elevated in the indigenous regions, where it doubles or even quadruples the state average.

Although specific interventions to reduce maternal death in Mexico, with a special emphasis on indigenous regions and including the interventions analyzed in this chapter, have been implemented since the beginning of the 2000s, we must recognize that the results have been insufficient, as evidenced by the MMR data. While we can identify a great reduction and consistent decrease in MMR in the Nayar region, particularly between 2005 and 2006 when air travel was established for obstetric emergencies, the other indigenous regions have improved in a much more modest way (Fig. 9.4).

The mean MMR in the state of Nayarit decreased from 72.2 deaths per 100,000 live births in 2002 to 50.2 in 2013, a reduction of 22 maternal deaths per 100,000 live births in 12 years. For the same time period in the Nayar region, the MMR decreased from 490.5 to 138.8. The state of Guerrero also boasted a dramatic decrease in maternal deaths from 80.3 in 2007 to 47.17 in 2013. During that same period of time, the Mountain Region had a decrease of 72 in its MMR. However, in analyzing the trend by year in the Mountain Region, we observed that the volume of maternal deaths was consistently high, which leads us to question whether the 2013 data was truly associated with the efforts to reduce maternal death, specifically those led by the health system in the region (Fig. 9.6).

In Chihuahua, the prevalence of maternal deaths has plateaued. In 2002 MMR was 61.35, and in 2013, it was 64.39. In this state, maternal deaths primarily occur in the Tarahumara Sierra. Between

Table 9.6 Evolution in MMR in the Guerrero Mountains, the Tarahumara Sierra, and the Nayar region, 2002–2014

States and regions	2002	2003	2004	2005	2006	2007	2008	2009	2010	2011	2012	2013	2014
Guerrero	80.29	87.32	70.26	86.32	85.31	65.24	63.23	72.27	55.20	75.28	61.22	47.17	44.16
Mountain Region	144.10	122.49	108.08	129.69	165.72	100.87	115.28	115.28	115.28	136.90	136.90	72.05	57.64
Chihuahua	61.35	43.47	48.34	74.15	58.39	62.54	48.23	76.73	60.31	73.08	49.92	64.39	70.37
Tarahumara Sierra	161.04	95.65	79.49	235.34	130.03	190.68	166.02	245.21	193.38	138.27	134.16	283.10	299.75
Nayarit	72.2	71.3	48.8	92.6	31.5	31.6	44.9	57.4	35.1	44.3	43.0	50.2	31.96
Nayar region	490.5	230.4	345.3	508.9	152.1	227.5	63.5	176.9	0.0	240.5	146.5	138.8	92.54

Source: Vega and Meneses based on the INEGI/SS maternal mortality database, 2002–2014 http://pda.salud.gob.mx/cubos/cmaternas.html and SINAC births, 2002–2014, http://www.dgis.salud.gob.mx/contenidos/basesdedatos/bdc_nacimientos.html (consulted August 15, 2016)

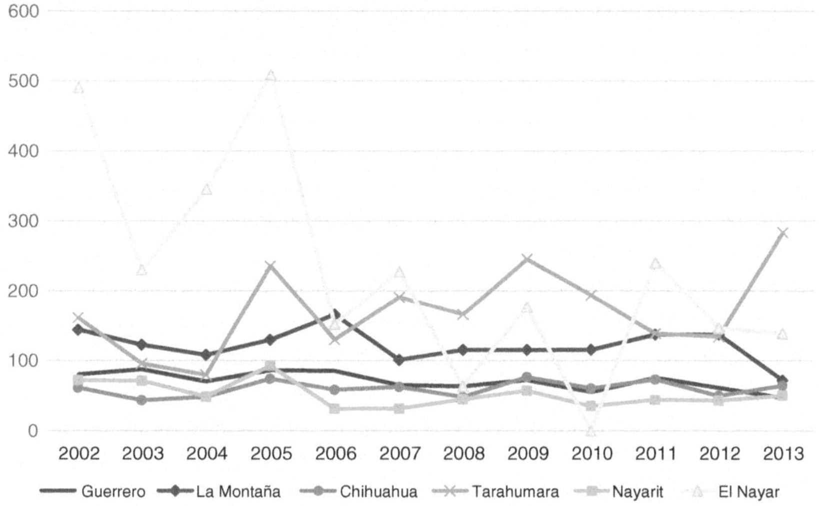

Fig. 9.6 Chronology of MMR (per 100,000 live births registered) in the Guerrero Mountains, the Tarahumara Sierra, and the Nayar region, 2002–2013. Source: Vega and Meneses based on the INEGI/SS 2002–2013 maternal death database http://pda.salud.gob.mx/cubos/cmaternas.html and births registered in 2002–2013, SINAC, http://www.dgis.salud.gob.mx/contenidos/basesdedatos/bdc_nacimientos.html (Consulted August 15, 2016)

2002 and 2013, there were 542 reported deaths in the state, and 198 were in the Tarahumara Sierra. This equate to a rate of 166.75 for the entire time period. Furthermore, 27% of these maternal deaths occurred without medical care (versus the state average was 12.7%), and one in three cases occurred in the home (versus two of ten at the state level). As such, if we focus our analysis on this indigenous region, it appears clear that maternal death has actually increased (Table 9.6, Fig. 9.6). It is worth asking the question of why, following three decades of policies and interventions specifically designed to reduce maternal mortality in the indigenous region of the Tarahumara Sierra, there has been no decrease in maternal deaths.

Specific research projects can contribute to answering this question. During our own field research in the municipalities and communities in the Tarahumara Sierra, health personnel in both administrative and operational positions commented assiduously that since the mid-2000s to the present (2014) time, one of the factors that impeded the functionality of the health system network was the growing threat of organized crime in the region. As such some health centers and mobile health units were inactive and unstaffed for weeks or even months. Nonetheless, although this was reiterated many times as being linked to the high prevalence of maternal death, the phenomenon requires deeper analysis.

Between 2002 and 2013, there were 845 maternal deaths in the state of Guerrero, with an average MMR of 65.7 deaths per 100,000 live births, 24% of these where in the Mountain Region (despite being only 10.7% of the state's population) where the MMR was 112.7 per 100,000 live births. One in every four maternal deaths in Guerrero during this time period received no medical care, while in the Mountain Region, this statistic was one of every three (34.4%). It is very probable that these maternal deaths could have been prevented with the type of timely medical care that every woman is entitled to receive, as stated by Mexico's laws including the Constitution. Moreover, during the same time period, 35% of maternal deaths in the state and nearly half in the Mountain Region occurred at home or in a public place, with no contact with the health system (Table 9.7). It is highly probable that the death of these 294 women could also have been prevented if there had existed the opportunity to access health service settings where critical obstetric care was provided. These data are evidence of the need to increase efforts to guarantee effective access to obstetric services for all women in general and indigenous women in particular, given that they face great economic, geographic, and cultural barriers.

During the same time period (2002–2013) in Nayarit, there were 138 maternal deaths, 35% of these occurring in the Nayar region (48 deaths) where only 3.2% of the state's population resides. This is compelling evidence of the high concentration of maternal deaths in this indigenous region. One in every four maternal deaths in the state during this time period did not receive medical care, and one of every three maternal deaths occurred in the home or public place; in the Nayar region, one of every two women who died did not have medical care, and 56% of deaths occurred in the home. These data once again illustrate the significant gaps in access to medical care between these two population groups. After recognition of these circumstances, and in part determined by the rough terrain in the Nayar's Sierra region, at the close of the 2000s, the state government established air transport for medical emergencies, primarily obstetric emergencies. This was an important proposal to specifically improve access for indigenous women to obtain obstetric emergency services that would prevent maternal deaths during the perinatal period. Based on the results, there have been significant advances (Fig. 9.7).

Table 9.7 Maternal mortality (2002–2013), including the number, MMR[a], and percentage of those who receive medical attention and passed away at home or in a public place, in the Guerrero Mountains, Tarahumara Sierra, and Nayar region

Maternal mortality	Guerrero	Mountain region	Chihuahua	Tarahumara sierra	Nayarit	Nayar region
Number	845	203	542	198	138	48
Rate[a]	65.73	112.71	59.86	166.75	51.58	209.17
No medical attention	25.09%	34.48%	12.73%	27.27%	26.1%	47.9%
Occurred at home or in a public place	34.79%	45.32%	19.19%	32.83%	29.7%	56.3%

Source: Vega and Meneses based on the INEGI/SS 2002–2013 maternal death database http://pda.salud.gob.mx/cubos/cmaternas.html and births registered in 2002–2013, SINAC, http://www.dgis.salud.gob.mx/contenidos/basesdedatos/bdc_nacimientos.html (Consulted August 15, 2016)

[a]Per 100,000 live birth registered in SINAC database

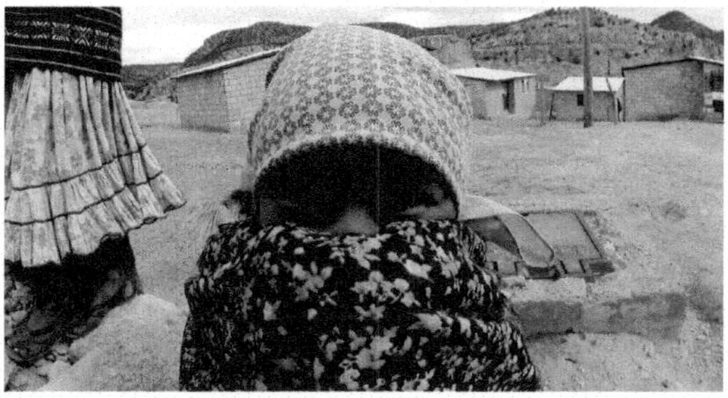

Fig. 9.7 Girl in a village of the Tarahumara Sierra region. Photograph from Mauricio Andrada, 2015

9.5.3 Resources

Table 9.9 presents data on the availability of some health system resources in the indigenous regions of interest. These data correspond with the total number of clinical consult rooms (Table 9.8), as well as those that are part of the social security systems and the services offered by the state-level Health Ministry. Also presented in Table 9.8 are data concerning hospital beds and medical and nursing personnel in contact with patients. It is evident from these data that social security resources are practically nonexistent in the Guerrero Mountains. Meanwhile, there is greater availability of health services in the Tarahumara Sierra and Nayar region in spite of the trend discussed previously that these regions do not have a high volume of individuals affiliated with social security. This effect may be explained by the presence of the IMSS-Prospera[2] program operating in Chihuahua and Nayarit, but not in Guerrero.

Guerrero has 2400 clinical consult rooms, 1864 hospital beds, 4986 primary care doctors and specialists, and 7322 nurses in contact with patients. The majority of these resources correspond to the state health services, and as previously mentioned, social security resources are nil. In the Mountains, social security resources include 20 doctors, but not a single hospital bed. As such, the primary healthcare resources in the region are provided by the state Secretariat of Health, with numbers of clinical consult rooms, hospitals beds, and providers that aim to close the gap in terms of availability of resources between the indigenous residents and the rest of the state's population. We also note efforts to concentrate on improving the availability and access to health resources for the indigenous population of the Mountain Region in Guerrero. In that region, the Health Ministry has 7 clinical consult rooms per 10,000 inhabitants, compared with 5 at the state level, 3.6 hospital beds versus 3.25 at the state level (this is due to the building of the Maternal-Child Indigenous Hospital of Tlapa in 2006), and 20.13 nurses per 10,000 inhabitants versus the state average of 14.8.

In the state of Chihuahua, it is estimated that for the year 2014, there were 2008 clinical consult rooms (5.89 rooms per 10,000 inhabitants) and 41 hospitals with a total of 2800 beds (8.22 per 10,000 inhabitants). Registered medical personnel rose to 4112 (12.07 per 10,000 inhabitants) and nursing personnel to 9173 (26.93 per 10,000 inhabitants). In the case of the Tarahumara Sierra, health coverage has been particularly difficult. This is due, in great part, to the geographic factors previously mentioned. Steep mountains and deep canyons make access and transit difficult, as well as poor infrastructure such as few paved roads for vehicles, and this has contributed to the limited coverage despite

[2]Originally known as IMSS-Coplamar between 1978 and 1988, then "Solidaridad" between 1988 and 1994, then "Progresa" from 1994 to 2000, and "Oportunidades" from 2000 to 2012

Table 9.8 Health system resources per 10,000 inhabitants in the Guerrero Mountains, Tarahumara Sierra, and Nayar region, 2014

Health system resources	Guerrero		Mountains	Chihuahua	Tarahumara	Nayarit	Nayar
Clinical consult room	Social security	1.99	0.55	3.51	5.24	3.62	4
	Secretariat of Health	5.09	7.08	2.38	4.23	5.27	10.2
	Total	7.08	7.63	5.89	9.47	8.89	14.29
Hospital beds	Social security	2.25	0.00	5.20	3.14	3.27	0
	Secretariat of Health	3.25	3.62	3.02	1.14	2.92	3.5
	Total	5.50	3.62	8.22	4.28	6.19	3.5
Primary care providers and specialists	Social security	4.20	0.55	7.13	2.88	7.71	5.8
	Secretariat of Health	10.52	10.20	4.94	5.81	8.52	16.62
	Total	14.71	10.76	12.07	8.69	16.23	22.45
Nurses	Social security	6.73	0.39	14.17	11.31	13.52	9.33
	Secretariat of Health	14.88	20.13	12.76	9.47	13.18	20.12
	Total	21.61	20.52	26.93	20.78	26.70	29.45

Source: Meneses based on the Human, Physical, Material, and Financial Resources database for the Secretariat of Health and State Health Services (SINERHIAS) 2001–2015, http://www.dgis.salud.gob.mx/contenidos/basesdedatos/bdc_recursos.html (consulted August 23, 2016)

the many efforts that have been made to provide care in this region. As Pintado Cortina (2004) states, terrain must be a key consideration in any type of program that is developed for the Tarahumara Sierra, as the cultural and territorial aspects of a particular region must be taken into account. Territorial issues may be defined in terms of environmental characteristics and the natural surroundings, which often times present an obstacle to implementing strategies from the health sector. Both elements, cultural and environmental, converge in the Tarahumara Sierra, resulting in insufficient resources for meeting the health-care needs of the population, particularly in indigenous regions.

In the indigenous communities we visited during a project entitled "Identification of a model of health care of older adults in indigenous regions" (Pelcastre et al. 2009), there were no permanently stationed health-care providers in the region; those that provided services made regular visits to the community, varying from 5 to 15 days between each visit. Moreover, doctors that arrived in the community, in addition to not visiting frequently, rarely spoke the Rarámuri language, making it difficult to communicate with the population.

The IMSS-Prospera program, which was responsible for health coverage in indigenous communities, reported in 2010 that there was an infrastructure of 144 rural medical units that have the capacity to serve 15% of the Chihuahuan population spread across 4500 communities (equaling approximately a half-million individuals) (SAGARPA 2010); the reported number of medical personnel serving these units in 2011 was 222. Nonetheless, in 2014 the Secretariat of Health reported that in the Tarahumara Sierra, there were 217 clinical consult rooms (9.47 per 10,000 inhabitants, higher than the rest of the state), 98 hospital beds (4.28 per 10,000 inhabitants, one-half of what is reported for the rest of the state), 119 doctors (8.69 per 10,000 inhabitants, 4 less than the state average), and 476 nurses (20.78 per 10,000 inhabitants, 7 less than the state average).

In the Nayar, we also identified the trend of the health system to be narrowing the gap and thus correcting the inequities between the indigenous population in the region and the rest of the state. The distribution of primary care resources indicates a major effort to reach indigenous inhabitants, with the Nayar region having more clinical consult rooms per 10,000 inhabitants (14.2 vs. 8.9), as well as more doctors (22.4 vs. 16.2) and nurses (29.4 vs. 26.7) (Fig. 9.8).

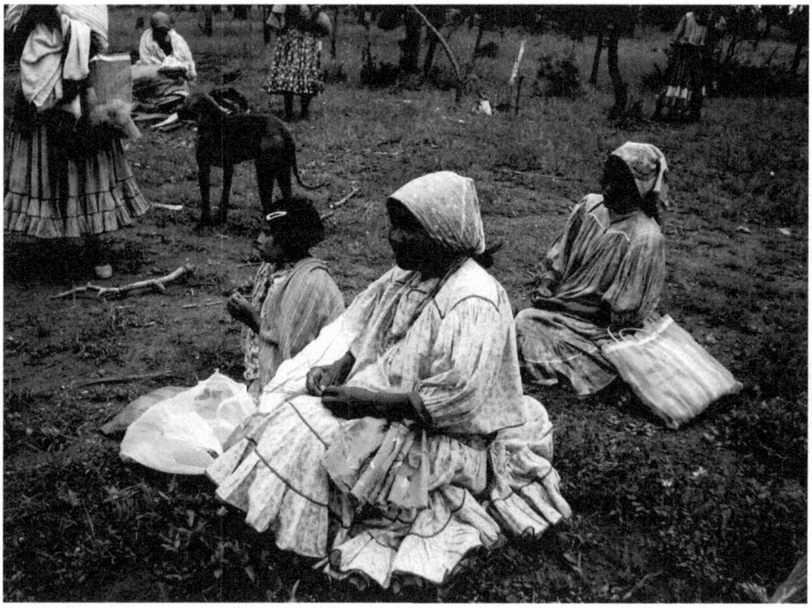

Fig. 9.8 Women and girls in the Tarahumara Sierra region. Photograph from Arturo Milán, 2015

9.5.4 Health Services Targeting Women

Table 9.9 illustrates some of the health services delivered to women at the primary care level in the three indigenous regions. It is noteworthy that in the Guerrero Mountains, the rate of services provided for menopause, sexually transmitted infections (STIs), and cancer is less that for the rest of the state; in the case of menopause services, the rate is nearly four times less in the indigenous region. However, the case of care provided for violence stands out, where the rate in the Mountain Region is nearly six times the rest of the state. This exemplifies the context of violence that affects women in this region at a much higher rate than their counterparts in the rest of the state or in the states of Chihuahua and Nayarit.

Moreover, in the three indigenous regions included in the study, the rates of services provided for family planning consults, family planning methods delivered, and primary care consults for obstetric emergencies stand out. In each of the regions, there is a greater availability of these services as compared with the rest of the inhabitants in their respective states. In the Guerrero Mountains, for example, there are 1.45 greater family planning consults, 1.13 greater contraceptive methods delivered, and 2.2 more obstetric emergency consults in primary care settings than the rest of the state of Guerrero. In the Tarahumara Sierra, there are 2.1 times greater family planning consults, 2.47 times more contraceptive methods delivered, and 10.6 times greater obstetric emergency consults in primary care settings than in the rest of the state of Chihuahua. In the Nayar region, there are 3.5 greater family planning consults, 2.66 times more contraceptive methods delivered, and 17 times more obstetric emergency consults in primary care settings than the rest of the state of Nayarit. Without additional qualitative information about the delivery of family planning and contraceptive services in the three indigenous regions analyzed, these data may lead to two distinctly different interpretations. On the one hand, findings suggest greater efforts to extend and guarantee the right to sexual and reproductive health in indigenous communities; on the other hand, they may be the result of population control policy developed based upon the belief that indigenous populations are quickly growing and need to be controlled.

Table 9.9 Rate of health services per 1000 women delivered in a primary care facility in the Guerrero Mountains, Tarahumara Sierra, and Nayar region, 2014

	Guerrero	Mountains	Chihuahua	Tarahumara	Nayarit	Nayar
Care provided for menopause	19.57	6.44	7.40	12.55	6.0	9.9
Care provided for STIs	1436.56	1262.93	544.77	1597.99	1228.3	2385.6
Care provided for violence	33.60	125.88	53.73	22.52	58.0	45.4
Women's cancer consults	8.38	7.86	9.83	1.95	19.4	0.8
Family planning consults	299.14	435.83	113.03	245.22	170.8	598.2
Family planning methods delivered	869.41	988.90	237.67	589.27	346.3	922.5
Obstetric emergency care provided in external units	1.31	2.91	0.41	4.21	0.2	3.5

Source: Vega and Meneses, based on services provided and substantive programs 2000–2014, Public Health Services http://www.dgis.salud.gob.mx/contenidos/basesdedatos/bdc_serviciossis.html (consulted August 20, 2016)

There are no doubts that either interpretation would need to be grounded in evidence and further research specifically on this topic. However, whatever is the basis for the underlying causes of the data, they can be interpreted as a direct effect of three decades of political prioritization of decreasing maternal mortality. The fact that there are 2.2 times the level of services delivered for obstetric emergencies in primary care settings in the Guerrero Mountains, 10.6 in the Tarahumara Sierra, and 17.5 in the Nayar region as compared to their respective states demonstrates the focused efforts on decreasing gaps and inequities.

9.5.5 Utilization of Hospital Services Among Women

Another indicator of service utilization is the rate of hospital discharges per 1000 women. Table 9.10 presents the evolution in the hospital discharge rate among the three states and their respective indigenous regions. In general, it is evident that access to and utilization of hospital services have improved among women across all states and regions. However, the largest increase is notable between 2004 and 2006, which corresponds to the initiation of the public insurance program, Seguro Popular. In the case of Guerrero, it can be seen that the gaps in hospital service utilization between indigenous women in the Mountain Region and the rest of the state begin to narrow during the first decade of the twenty-first century. The initial gap was nine times the state rate and by the end of that period was nearly zero. Women in Nayarit experienced a similar situation: in the year 2000, the gap in hospital services was seven times that of the rest of the state. However, by 2009 the gap has nearly been closed, and between 2011 and 2014, the rate for access and utilization of hospital services was more favorable for the indigenous regions than the rest of the state. The case of Chihuahua has been quite different—the gap has not only not been closed, but instead it has widened. We found that those who benefit from policies designed to improve access to hospital services are primarily non-indigenous women, for whom the rate of utilization of services is 24, while *rarámuri* women's rate is 16.

A similar situation occurs in the case of access and utilization of hospital gynecologic-obstetric care, as demonstrated in Table 9.11. In the indigenous regions of the Guerrero Mountains and the Nayar in Nayarit, the initial gaps for indigenous women have tended toward narrowing. In the case of the Mountains, the rate has moved from 6 in 2000 to be in indigenous women's favor in 2014. In the Nayar region, there was a gap and rate of four in 2000, which was reversed, and the indigenous women's rate surpassed the state average. Again, in Chihuahua, the gaps have become greater. The average increase of hospital gynecologic-obstetric care increased by 14 units during this time, while care for *rarámuri* women increased a little more than 12. As mentioned earlier, the emphasis on reducing maternal

Table 9.10 Rates for female hospital discharges per 1000 inhabitants in the Guerrero Mountains, Tarahumara Sierra, and Nayar region 2000–2014

Region	2000	2001	2002	2003	2004	2005	2006	2007	2008	2009	2011	2012	2013	2014
Guerrero	19.42	19.45	20.60	21.15	21.69	21.86	24.55	26.55	31.06	34.89	36.79	39.02	40.42	42.86
Mountains	10.56	11.83	12.83	14.09	14.25	15.20	33.74	29.31	31.69	34.55	36.75	38.93	42.21	42.85
Chihuahua	6.00	6.93	12.90	14.22	17.31	16.51	22.47	22.89	25.89	27.12	30.93	31.49	31.02	30.23
Tarahumara	12.12	10.64	14.74	16.51	18.92	20.88	23.17	24.07	23.17	20.72	28.74	26.19	25.69	28.15
Nayarit	25.18	24.94	28.19	28.91	30.58	33.03	35.43	37.02	41.61	45.93	41.08	40.23	41.20	38.49
Nayar	18.08	18.26	18.14	15.68	20.49	14.68	30.24	36.05	45.15	45.74	69.04	82.72	86.83	77.44

The year 2010 is excluded because that year there was a significant amount of unregistered data on hospital services. Source: Vega and Meneses, SAEH, SSA, 2000–2014 http://www.dgis.salud.gob.mx/contenidos/basesdedatos/bdc_egresoshosp.html (consulted August 23, 2016)

Table 9.11 Rate of hospital discharges for obstetrics-gynecology care per 1000 women in the Guerrero Mountains, the Tarahumara Sierra, and Nayar region, 2000–2014

Region	2000	2001	2002	2003	2004	2005	2006	2007	2008	2009	2011	2012	2013	2014
Guerrero	13.56	13.58	14.13	14.57	14.69	14.62	17.23	18.51	22.16	25.68	27.5	29.3	29.8	31.77
Mountains	7.65	8.14	8.95	9.63	10.16	10.82	27.78	22.59	23.88	26.20	28.6	31.1	32.9	33.72
Chihuahua	3.10	3.39	6.86	8.42	10.41	9.81	14.32	14.74	16.66	17.83	19.4	19.4	18.6	17.32
Tarahumara	5.87	5.13	7.35	8.87	10.44	11.17	14.61	15.02	15.38	14.20	19.4	17.1	16.5	17.74
Nayarit	16.49	16.42	18.02	18.98	20.41	22.20	23.64	26.41	28.76	30.49	29.3	27.9	26.6	25.61
Nayar	12.04	14.44	13.97	11.63	16.73	12.86	24.07	26.30	28.53	32.06	52.9	60.53	63.58	59.9

The year 2010 was excluded because that year there was a significant amount of unregistered data on hospital services. Source: Vega and Meneses, SAEH, SSA, 2000–2014 http://www.dgis.salud.gob.mx/contenidos/basesdedatos/bdc_egresoshosp.html (Consulted August 23, 2016)

mortality and the advent of Seguro Popular public health insurance may explain the increased use of hospital services by women, particularly in the second half of the first decade of the twenty-first century. However, to be able to more precisely explain the factors that have contributed to the diminished gaps in hospital service utilization in the indigenous regions of the Guerrero Mountains and the Nayar region of Nayarit, but not in Tarahumara Sierra of Chihuahua, more research studies are needed.

9.5.6 Cesarean Delivery as a Quality of Care Indicator: The Case of Guerrero

When justified from a biomedical perspective, performance of a cesarean section delivery can be an effective technique for preventing both maternal and neonatal morbidity and mortality. However, there is no demonstrated benefit for women or newborns for performing this procedure unnecessarily. To the contrary, unnecessary cesarean sections constitute an important public health problem and are associated with short- and long-term risks that can compromise the life and health of women and newborns and result in complications in future pregnancies (OMS 2015). Nonetheless, in the past three decades, there has been a documented sustained increase in the number of unnecessary cesarean sections in the majority of countries, including Mexico. As such, the frequency of cesarean operations has become an indicator for the overall quality of obstetric care.

According to the World Health Organization (Organización Mundial de la Salud or OMS), only 10–15% of births should result in a cesarean section due to obstetric complication (OMS 2015). However, the use of this procedure has consistently increased in the state of Guerrero during the first decade of the twenty-first century, increasing from 29.7% in 2000 to 48.63% in 2014, a 19% increase that may represent a decrease in the quality of obstetric care. In the Mountain Region, the percentage of cesarean section deliveries increased from 19.32 to 38.91% during this same period of time—a nearly 20% increase with no statistically significant differences from the rest of the state. However, the increased performance of cesarean section procedures in the Mountain Region is notable and coincides with the opening of Guerrero's Maternal-Child Indigenous Hospital in 2006. The opening of the hospital not only increased access and utilization of hospital obstetric services for women in the region; it also increased their vulnerability toward poor medical practice (Table 9.12). However, we cannot establish with clarity, based on these data alone, whether cesarean section deliveries were conducted based on technical and practical criteria or, on the contrary, are a reflection of iatrogenic medical practice and poor quality of care. This is an important issue that requires further attention in the form of state- and region-level studies (Fig. 9.9).

Table 9.12 Percentage of birth by cesarean section delivery[a] in the Guerrero Mountains and the rest of the state, 2000–2014

Region	2000	2001	2002	2003	2004	2005	2006	2007	2008	2009	2011	2012	2013	2014
Guerrero	29.70	31.37	32.13	33.86	34.27	35.26	35.85	35.96	35.34	37.35	40.92	46.24	47.27	48.63
Mountains	19.32	20.65	21.03	22.54	25.34	27.23	31.26	29.77	26.93	29.52	29.94	34.60	38.25	38.91
Rest of the state	30.39	32.15	33.02	34.80	35.03	35.98	36.86	36.92	36.46	38.31	42.14	47.51	48.18	49.63

The year 2010 was excluded due to that year having limited documentation available about hospital services. Source: Vega and Meneses, SAEH, SSA, 2000–2014 http://www.dgis.salud.gob.mx/contenidos/basesdedatos/bdc_egresoshosp.html (consulted August 23,2016)

[a]This is the percentage of births by cesarean out of all births in a determined year

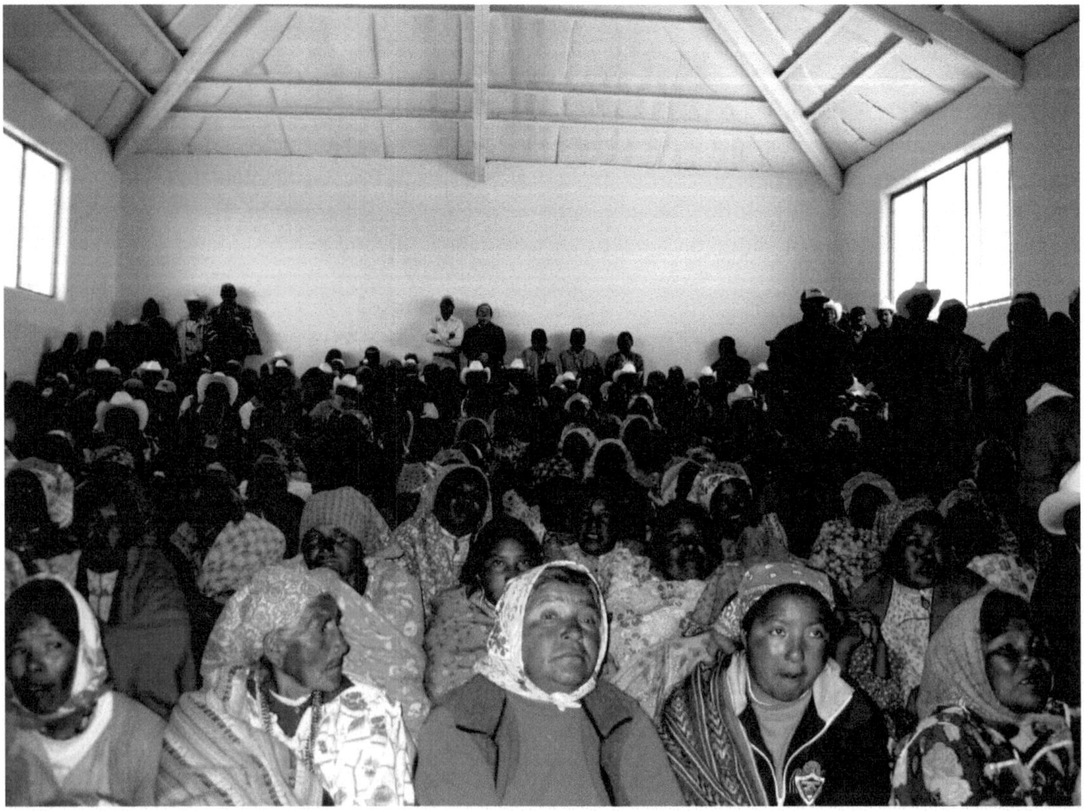

Fig. 9.9 *Rarámuri* women at the community assembly in Tarahumara region. Photograph from Arturo Milán, 2015

Conclusions

The data analyzed in this chapter provide evidence of the persistent gaps in the availability of resources, access, and utilization of health services for indigenous women in three of the country's primary indigenous regions: the Guerrero Mountains, the Tarahumara Sierra, and the Nayar region. Without any doubts, these issues have serious implications for human rights to health, as well as the protection of individuals' integrity and dignity, particularly for indigenous women.

The present analysis demonstrates an existing mechanism of systematic exclusion (and discrimination) for indigenous women that affects their income, welfare, and basic health conditions, especially involving reproductive health. This study points to the urgent need to develop measures that contribute to improving income and decreasing poverty in the country's indigenous regions, with a target population of indigenous women and youth. Although beyond the scope of this chapter, we believe that these regions and people represent the ideal space to implement pilot testing for economic programs, such as universal basic income, microcredits (for indigenous women specifically), scholarships for advanced education (again, for indigenous women specifically), and the fostering of formal employment tied to the environment, such as park rangers.

Moreover, these data also demonstrate that using specific interventions and political efforts, it is possible to close gaps and improve health outcomes when we focus on the most marginalized indigenous regions of the country. One example of this is the sustained increase in public health insurance (although inequities continue to exist) and the utilization of hospital services among indigenous women in the Guerrero Mountains and Nayar region of Nayarit. This occurred during the first decade of the twenty-first century, possibly a direct outcome of the implementation of Seguro Population, which has been demonstrated to be an effective resource for increasing access to hospital service and financial protection for the indigenous population.

In the case of the Tarahumara Sierra, it is critically important that we identify and analyze the reasons why maternal mortality has not decreased despite 15 years of policy focused on that specific issue in the region. This points to the context of violence and insecurity that has hindered health system functions and prevented access to care for indigenous women, specifically for obstetric emergencies. Furthermore, we should analyze what factors have been useful in producing decreased rates of maternal death in the Guerrero Mountains and the Nayar, both regions having difficult access in the Western Sierra Madre mountain range. In the case of the Nayar in Nayarit, one intervention that appears to have contributed to improved maternal survival outcomes is the establishment of air transport between the Nayar communities and area hospitals. This experience should be systematically analyzed, with lessons learned and best practices shared with other contexts that share similar characteristics in terms of geographic access, such as the Guerrero Mountains or the Tarahumara Sierra, as well as the vast region that includes Oaxaca, Chiapas, Puebla, and Veracruz where there is also a high documented incidence of maternal death.

It is both noteworthy and admirable how much effort and prioritization there has been to provide services that improve maternal and newborn health, such as the emergency obstetric care (EmOC) and focused contraceptive coverage, that is evident in the three indigenous regions analyzed. However, there is still a need to clarify the characteristics of the interventions that have led to the increased productivity in contraceptive and family planning services in these indigenous regions and, specifically, whether or not such services were provided with appropriate consideration to culture, gender, and reproductive rights.

Furthermore, the determinants and specific circumstances surrounding the increase in the performance of cesarean section deliveries in the state of Guerrero and the Mountain Region should be analyzed as soon as possible, given that rates have surpassed WHO's recommendations for best practice. The fact that nearly 50% of births in the state and 40% of those in the Mountain Region are cesarean births may be indicative of a problem with inadequate medical practice and low quality of obstetric care that increase risk for women as well as newborns. This is a pertinent matter that requires comprehensive investigation, with particular attention to assessing the intercultural situation in the indigenous region of the Guerrero Mountains.

Based upon our research, the authors can recommend strengthening of regional hospitals' capacity for obstetric and newborn emergencies in the three indigenous regions in this study by assuring that the presence of qualified personnel is available 24 hours a day and 365 days of the year.

We also recommend the development of a maternal-newborn safety plan with a transportation system to be used in case of emergency that connects the community to the regional hospital, as well as a referral system from the regional hospital to a specialized facility in the event that a higher level of care is needed. The transportation and referral system should include the possibility of air transport, such as the system in the Nayar, which has been proven to be effective.

References

Campbell, O., & Graham, W. J. (2006). Strategies for reducing maternal mortality: Getting on with what works. *The Lancet, 368*(9543), 1284–1299. Retrieved April 27, 2016, from http://www.thelancet.com/journals/lancet/article/PIIS0140-6736(06)69381-1/abstract

INEGI. (2016). *México en cifras. Información nacional, por entidad federativa y municipios*. Aguascalientes: Instituto Nacional de Estadística y Geografía. Retrieved April 27, 2016, from http://www3.inegi.org.mx/sistemas/mexicocifras/default.aspx?e=12

OMS. (2015). *Declaración de la OMS sobre tasas de cesáreas*. Ginebra: Organización Mundial de la Salud. Retrieved April 27, 2016, from http://apps.who.int/iris/bitstream/10665/161444/1/WHO_RHR_15.02_spa.pdf?ua=1

Pelcastre, B., Meneses, S., Ruelas, G., Reyes, H. (2009). *Proyecto: Identificación de un modelo de atención a la salud para adultos mayores en zonas indígenas*. México: Fondo Sectorial IMSS/ISSSTE/CONACyT-087123.

Pintado Cortina, A.P. (2004). *Tarahumaras. Pueblos Indígenas de México Contemporáneo*. Comision Nacional para el Desarrollo de los Pueblos Indígenas, Programa de las Naciones Unidas para el Desarrollo. Mexico City: CDI, PNUD.

SAGARPA. (2010). *Síntesis del Diagnóstico prospectivo del sector rural del estado de Chihuahua*. México: SAGARPA. Retrieved from http://www.sagarpa.gob.mx/Delegaciones/chihuahua/Documents/EVALUACIONES%20EXTERNAS/2009/SINTESIS%20DIAGNOSTICO%20PROSPECTIVO%20DEL%20SECTOR%20RURAL%20DEL%20EDO%20DE%20CHIHUAHUA.pdf.

Schwartz, D. A. (2015). Interface of epidemiology, anthropology and health care in maternal death prevention in resource-poor nations. In D. A. Schwartz (Ed.), *Maternal mortality: Risk factors, anthropological perspectives, prevalence in developing countries and preventive strategies for pregnancy-related death*. New York: Nova Science Publishers.

10 Reconquista: Obstetric Violence and Underreporting of Obstetric Complications in Yucatán and Quintana Roo

Sarah A. Williams

10.1 Introduction

In a hospital in southern Quintana Roo, the Mexican state that hosts Cancún and lies along the Caribbean coastline, a young Maya woman named Natividad arrived to give birth to her first baby. She wasn't from the small city she had to travel to during the early stages of her labor, but her own town did not at that time have the facilities to manage a birth requiring surgery or other interventions. As Natividad described, upon arriving at the hospital, she was placed on a bed in a room with other laboring women and told to lay on her back and not to move or make noise during her labor. After a few hours of quiet labor, a nurse approached and announced that she was to receive an epidural, per the doctor's orders. Natividad protested, saying that she didn't need an epidural and did not want one. "Shut up!" the nurse responded and flipped her over onto her side to administer the epidural anyway. A short time later, the doctor came in and realized that she had been given an epidural. "What did you do?" he yelled at the nurse. "The woman across the room is having a Cesarean section (C-section) and needed the epidural." So, Natividad had to have her baby with an epidural that was neither medically necessary nor consented to. A few hours later, when she was attempting to push despite the numbness caused by the epidural, her nurses screamed at her and called her lazy. As her baby was crowning, the doctor cut an episiotomy without informing her but applied too much force and cut all the way down into her anus. The doctor then sutured her to correct this but missed something fundamental, and when she began defecating from her vagina a few days later, she had to return to the hospital to have the sutures replaced.

This experience of birthing in a public hospital in Quintana Roo demonstrates several violations of Natividad's fundamental human and legal rights during childbirth, violations that fall under a legal umbrella increasingly known as "obstetric violence" in a few Latin American countries, including Mexico. When her nurse administered an epidural without Natividad's consent and, indeed, against her direct wishes, she violated Natividad's right to informed consent and bodily autonomy. When the

S. A. Williams, M.A.
Department of Anthropology, University of Toronto,
Toronto, Canada
e-mail: sarah.williams@mail.utoronto.ca

D. A. Schwartz (ed.), *Maternal Death and Pregnancy-Related Morbidity Among Indigenous Women of Mexico and Central America*, Global Maternal and Child Health: Medical, Anthropological, and Public Health Perspectives, https://doi.org/10.1007/978-3-319-71538-4_10

nurse screamed at her during her labor, Natividad's right to be treated with respect and dignity by her healthcare practitioners was violated. When her doctor used a scalpel to cut her perineum without soliciting her consent or even informing her first, Natividad's rights to informed consent and bodily autonomy were again ignored. While Natividad was in the hospital, she witnessed similar violations of other laboring and birthing women's rights, as well as gross professional misconduct and abuse. She also observed hospital staff threaten women who experienced negative outcomes such as losing their babies or suffering medical malpractice or abuse, saying that if the women told anyone what had happened, no one would believe them because they were "dirty Indians" and their medical records would show that the women were at fault for negative outcomes or that the negative outcomes had never occurred. Years later, when she relayed her story, Natividad expressed how traumatized and helpless she had felt at the time, knowing that there was nothing she could do to complain or report the mistreatment she experienced and witnessed. Natividad's experience, and those of other women in Yucatán and Quintana Roo, demonstrates that the lack of access to biomedical healthcare is not the only barrier to safe, equitable maternal healthcare for women in Mexico and that statistical outcomes such as maternal mortality rates are not the only measure of quality medical care.

By providing ethnographic examples of some of the ways that obstetric violence is manifested during labor, birth, and the postpartum period, this chapter explores the context and practice of obstetric violence in Quintana Roo and Yucatán and its relationship to racism and broader patterns of violence and marginalization of women. It also examines the role of documentation and record-keeping as a means of obscuring the practice of obstetric violence and how this may contribute to skewed and inaccurate maternal and infant mortality rates (Fig. 10.1).

10.2 Obstetric Violence

Obstetric violence is a relatively recent term coined to describe a class of abuses enacted against women during pregnancy, labor, and the immediate postpartum period. First recognized politically in Venezuela's "Organic Law on the Right of Women to a Life Free of Violence" in Article 15, obstetric violence is defined as:

> ...the appropriation of the body and reproductive processes of women by health personnel, which is expressed as dehumanized treatment, an abuse of medication, and to convert the natural processes [of labor] into pathological ones, bringing with it loss of autonomy and the ability to decide freely about their bodies and sexuality, negatively impacting the quality of life of women. (D'Gregorio 2010)

Since its legal recognition in Venezuela in 2007, obstetric violence has become a means of articulating the intersections of hypermedicalization, structural violence, and gendered violence experienced by women in Latin America during the birth year (Dixon 2015). As Dixon asserts, the value of the term "obstetric violence" lies in its ability to move beyond a critique of medical practices, instead offering a means to connect abuses within the medical establishment to patterns of violence and discrimination within society and political systems at large (Dixon 2015). Obstetric violence as a concept allows for intersectionalities of race, socioeconomic class, gender, sexuality, and education to become apparent and recognizable within discussions of childbirth and illuminates the ways in which these categories may not only determine whether a woman has access to obstetric care but also directly influence the quality and comfort of the care she manages to achieve.

Recent studies of maternal health and birthing practices in Mexico have largely focused on manifestations of obstetric violence and the reactions of women, activists, and other health practitioners to this rather recently named problem (Smith-Oka 2015; Dixon 2015; Sesia 2013). As demonstrated by the emerging scholarship on this topic, obstetric violence is more than just individual instances of

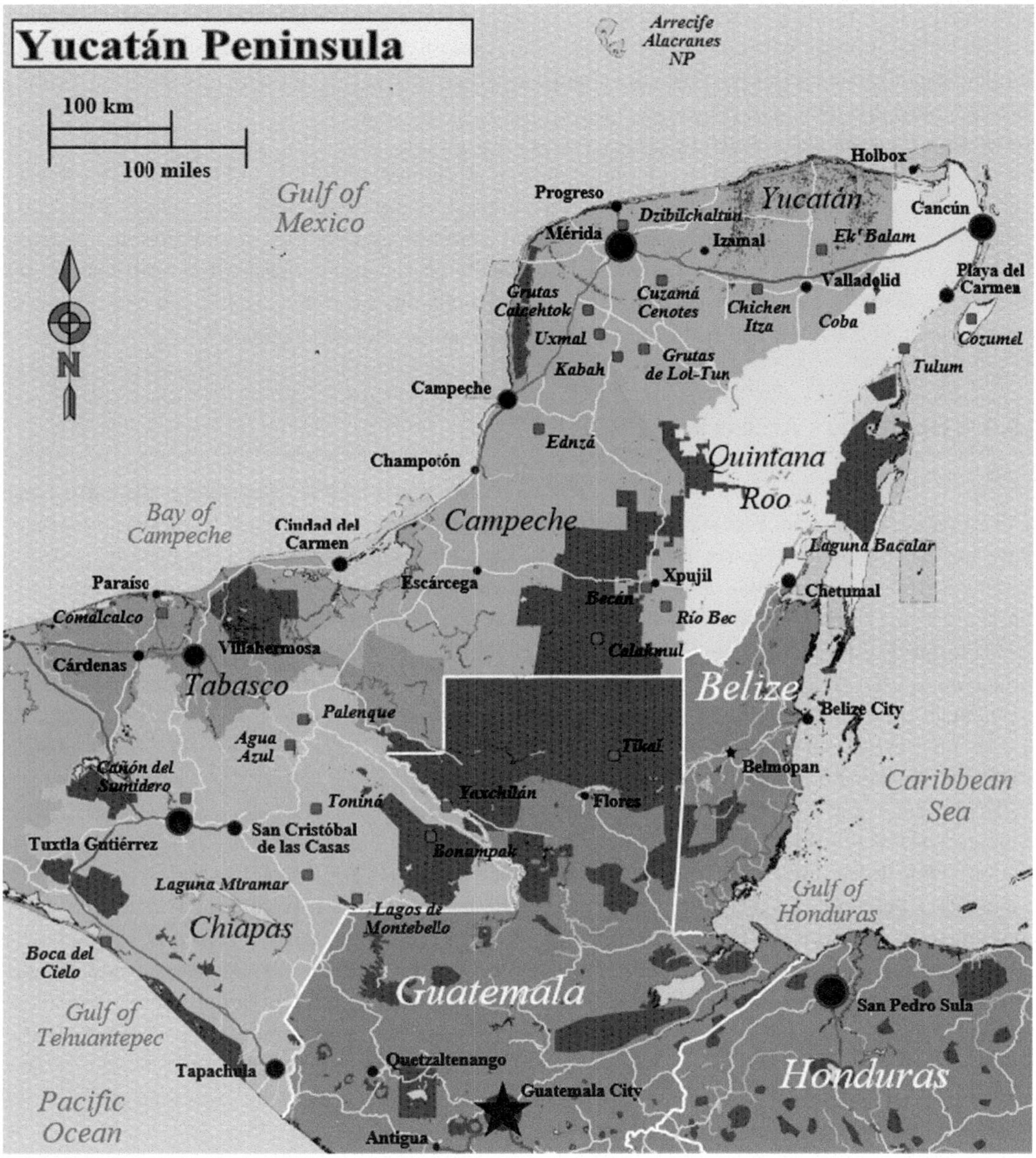

Fig. 10.1 Map of the Yucatán peninsula. By Peter Fitzgerald, OpenStreetMap (File:Yucatán_Peninsula_map.svg) [CC BY-SA 2.0 (http://creativecommons.org/licenses/by-sa/2.0) or ODbL (http://opendatacommons.org/licenses/odbl/1.0/)], via Wikimedia Commons

mistreatment or abuse and has been connected to broader patterns of discrimination, misogyny, racism, and disenfranchisement (Dixon 2015; Smith-Oka 2015). Activists and researchers have drawn attention to the disparities in maternal healthcare experienced by indigenous and rural women in Central America, such as the lack of access to quality obstetric care (Pintado et al. 2015), the high incidences of obstetric violence they endure when they do access care (Smith-Oka 2015), and the struggles faced by women in these populations as they attempt to adhere to traditional or culturally appropriate birth practices (Berry 2006; Berry 2010; Davis-Floyd 2001; Sesia 1996). As these studies have highlighted, birthing in a hospital with a medical doctor is not automatically a more "progressive" or safer option for women than birthing at home or with midwives or traditional birth attendants. Indigenous, racialized, or impoverished women are particularly at risk of being mistreated by healthcare personnel and, due to structural violence and inequalities, are least able to defend themselves or seek justice later, though obstetric violence is certainly not practiced solely against these populations nor is it solely a phenomenon of developing countries (Bohren et al. 2015). In Mexico, obstetric violence has been taken up by women's right groups, midwifery advocates, and the media as public critiques of obstetric practices in Mexico become more common and find newer and more mainstream platforms from which to promote humanized birth—the presented alternative to a birth marked by obstetric violence. Some states have enacted laws asserting women's rights to a life free from obstetric violence, and, at least politically, the concept has gained some ground (Braine 2008).

10.3 Healthcare Access in Mexico

In general, the Mexican healthcare system has three different branches: approximately half of the population accesses healthcare through social security institutions that provide coverage to workers in the formal employment sector, the largest of which is the Mexican Social Security Institute (IMSS); roughly 3–10% of the population has private insurance purchased through their employers or on the market; and the remaining ~40% of the population officially relies on the public healthcare system (SHS) formerly administered by the Ministry of Health but now largely under the domains of individual states after defederalization. Additionally, as many as 50% of the total Mexican population supplement their healthcare with services from the private system due to a combination of lack of access, mistrust of public services, and a perception of superior care in the private sector (OECD 2005; Napolitano and Flores 2003).

This rather complicated, multi-tiered, multi-siloed approach has consisted of, essentially, three separate systems of primary healthcare, emergency care, and specialty services serving different populations with little formal overlap in between (Schneider 2010:31). The system(s) serve different populations, but not necessarily different needs, and thus duplicate or triplicate each other's services, resulting in considerable waste of resources and gaps in services, particularly in rural areas. Drawbacks to this system include inequity and inequality of access to care, as public health services are chronically underfunded compared to IMSS institutions, lack of oversight and regulation of private medical services and personnel, and a dearth of consistent medical provisions in rural areas, particularly in the southern states (OCED 2005). Reports have noted that there is a strong perception of low-quality care in the SHS and that low funding has limited the system's capacity to serve the poor, thus contributing to inequalities of access between insured and non-insured populations and, ultimately, non-indigenous and indigenous citizens (OECD 2005:15).

Various plans to reform the healthcare system to increase quality and efficiency have been under way for over 20 years, beginning with the decentralization of Ministry of Health services and continuing through a variety of programs to increase insurance coverage for the poor, such as *Seguro Popular*, *Oportunidades*, and *PROGRESA* (Schneider 2010; Frenk et al. 2003; Birn 1999). In contrast to the ambitious goals of decentralization, researchers have found that decentralization in Mexico, like other neoliberal reforms, has often resulted in increased privatization of health services, which, given the lack of regulation and high costs in the private sector (Homedes and Ugalde 2009), may be considered contradictory to the reform's promises of increased quality and accessibility (Birn 1999) (Fig. 10.2).

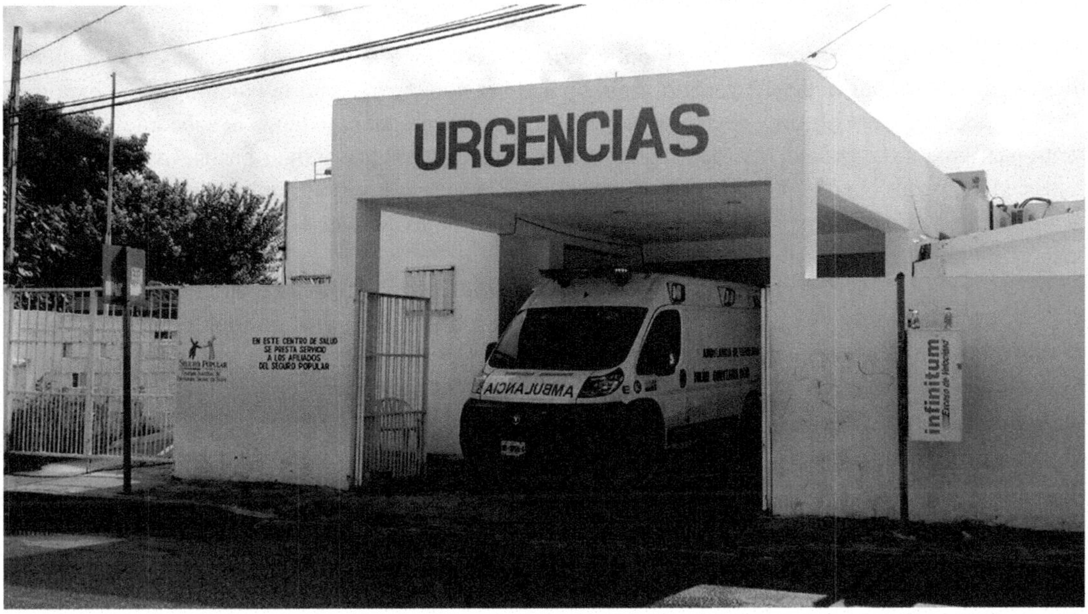

Fig. 10.2 The emergency entrance and outdoor waiting room of Tulum's *Centro de Salud*, a public health system clinic

An important facet of Mexico's plan to reduce its maternal mortality ratio (MMR) and more generally improve its standing in women's health has been the implementation of a series of welfare programs[1] predicated on a cash-for-participation model, a component of which is pregnant women's attendance at health lectures and regular prenatal appointments with doctors (Secretaria de Salud 1995; de López 2011). In exchange for completing the program's requirements, women receive cash benefits directly. The explicit underlying goal of the programs—to increase the percentage of Mexican women, particularly rural and indigenous women, who give birth in a hospital overseen by a medical doctor—was promoted as a method of rapidly improving Mexico's MMR and related statistics and, indeed, has been extremely successful in enticing women to attend regular prenatal appointments, nutrition, and exercise lectures and to birth in hospital (Secretaria de Salud 2007; Torres and Mujica 2004). Furthermore, such programs, particularly *Seguro Popular*, which offers free prenatal care and free birth, have made attendance by medical personnel during labor and birth nearly orthodox.

Researchers have critiqued these programs for numerous reasons, including the somewhat false assertion of enhancing women's empowerment and security (de López 2011), while public health studies have noted that the programs' practices may have increased cesarean section rates without a concomitant increase in skilled birth attendance or quality of care (Barber 2009; Urquieta et al. 2008). In Yucatán and Quintana Roo, the majority of the women who rely on the funds in return for their participation are very poor, often living in rural pueblos with limited access to the wage economy and, thus, to money. In such places, the nearest clinic may be in another town or city, or, if they have a *Centro de Salud*[2] in their pueblo, it may only be open for limited hours on particular days, as usually doctors prefer to live in larger cities or may be contracted to travel between multiple rural health

[1] Such as *Progresa*, *Oportunidades*, and *Prospera*.

[2] A public health clinic. While in cities they may be capable of hosting surgeries, in rural areas, they are usually quite small, underfunded, and understaffed.

outposts. Mexico's service requirement for newly graduated doctors means that generally rural citizens do have some access to care, even if only during specific days of the week, but the doctors attending them are fresh out of their 2 years of training and are not experienced in handling more exotic or serious concerns. This leads some doctors to encourage their pregnant patients to schedule a cesarean section as a matter of course, in order to guarantee a doctor's presence at their births. Even when such a procedure is not overtly planned, in order to fulfill the program requirement that they birth in a health center or hospital many rural women find themselves taking bus, taxi, or *colectivo* rides of an hour or longer during their labor.

In a country that is often criticized for having the second highest cesarean section rates in the world and very high rates of episiotomy (Niino 2011; Betrán et al. 2007), programming that increases obstetric intervention rates should be carefully evaluated. Furthermore, a 2012 study conducted by the Council for the Evaluation of Social Policies (CONEVAL) found that increased contact with the public health system was not correlated with improved maternal mortality rates (Coneval 2012; Schiavon et al. 2012). Nevertheless, the perceived and oft-touted connection between hospital birth and improved birth outcomes persists, and, as researchers have highlighted, this perception takes precedence over potential alternative means of charting the quality of the maternal healthcare system, such as through the subjective and affective experiences of women (Berry 2006, 2008; Smith-Oka 2015; Mills 2015). While countries and the World Health Organization (WHO) focus extensively on numerical outcomes of births—such as maternal and infant mortality rates—considerably less attention is dedicated to the affective experience of giving birth and whether the event was perceived by the woman as traumatic or positive. As post-traumatic stress disorder (PTSD), postpartum depression (PPD), anxiety, and stress are all known to have very strong negative effects on health and capacity, traumatic birth experiences, like obstetric violence, may have a very real effect on birth outcomes and health of the mother and baby.

10.4 Non-consensual Medical Interventions

One of the most common forms of obstetric violence is the use of non-consensual and unnecessary medical interventions and procedures on pregnant and laboring women. These interventions may include the administration of Pitocin and other pharmaceutical drugs, episiotomies, enemas and shaving, the continuous use of a fetal heart rate monitor, strapping or tying a woman to her hospital bed, and cesarean sections. Though some of these interventions are becoming less common in many countries as research has shown that such interventions often do not improve fetal or maternal outcomes, women in Yucatán and Quintana Roo report that many of these practices are routine in hospitals and health clinics. A common theme in ethnographic data gathered from Mexican women in Yucatán and Quintana Roo is a critique of the obstetric tendency toward more interventions throughout the birthing process, particularly without consent. While much of the literature on reproductive health focuses on women's access to biomedical healthcare, and rightly so, the universal application of surgical interventions in labor and delivery is also a site for the examination of inequitable healthcare allocations. The following sections examine some of the most common birth and postpartum interventions in Mexico through the dual lenses of public health-recommended "best practices" and ethnographic vignettes that situate these birth interventions in the context of the Yucatán peninsula. Many studies have highlighted the negative implications of unnecessary birth interventions in urban, Western contexts, but these implications may take on a radically different character in rural, indigenous contexts. As these are the regions where the push to "modernize" is often the strongest, it is important to consider the impact of these practices in the unique contexts where they are to be applied and how they intersect with infrastructural issues.

10.5 Cesarean Sections

In a survey of women living in the oldest Maya neighborhood in Tulum conducted in 2014, 53% of the participants reported that during one or more of their births in a hospital, clinic, or *Centro de Salud*, their doctors or nurses performed a medical intervention on their body without consent. The majority of those interventions were cesarean sections, followed closely by episiotomies. None of the respondents reported being told or having it indicated to them that there was fetal distress or that the operations were medically necessary. Though any procedure performed on a woman's body without her knowledge and consent is a violation of her human rights, non-consensual cesarean sections are particularly egregious, as a cesarean section is a major surgery requiring weeks or even months of recovery time and potential need for blood transfusions (which families in Mexico must pay for or pre-donate) and presents considerable risk to a woman's health. Added to this risk is the continued prevalence of vertical incisions, which sever the abdominal muscles and result in increased recovery time and significant scar tissue, despite the emergence of horizontal incisions as the new standard of care.

Cesarean sections that are medically necessary are quite obviously an important and critical facet of maternal healthcare, and they are a medical intervention that should be available as an option to any woman who has a need of one. Studies conducted by the WHO on overuse of C-sections have identified countries, such as Pakistan, Nigeria, and India, where C-sections are underutilized to such an extent that maternal and infant mortality outcomes are negatively affected. Mexico is not one of those countries.

Mexico is notable for its exceptionally high rates of C-sections, which reached a pinnacle as the second highest in the world in 2010. In urban areas, the rates are even higher than the national statistics. A 2012 National Institute of Public Health survey found that between 2007 and 2012, 46% of the births in Mexico for which there were records were delivered via C-section, a statistic that is more than double the recommended rates set by the Official Mexican Standards, which are themselves higher than the international standards set by the World Health Organization. In large cities, where there are typically multiple private hospitals and an urban population with insurance, C-section rates have been recorded at over 80%. Women's health advocates and the country's public health researchers have called this trend "alarming" and released numerous reports urging a decline in delivery by C-section, citing WHO guidelines which state that "There is no justification for any region to have rates higher than 10-15 percent," and declaring that consistent rates above the guideline are symptomatic of serious problems with the health system as a whole (Althabe and Belizán 2006:1472).

Overuse of C-sections has considerable implications both on a structural and individual level. A 2010 study conducted by the WHO found that medically unnecessary C-sections account for a disproportionate share of global health funds and may serve as a barrier to the equitable provision of necessary universal health services (Gibbons et al. 2010:3). Generally, C-sections are more expensive than natural, nonsurgical births and may thus serve as a source of revenue generation for independent doctors and private hospitals while shortening labor times and enabling doctors to perform more operations per day. Conversely, in the case of publicly-funded hospitals, C-sections are a drain on revenue and may further stress an already overburdened health system, though the lessened labor times may reduce the strains on the limited number of obstetricians who serve large populations with limited resources (Gibbons et al. 2010:6). For individuals, C-sections are associated with increased health risks, such as infection and infertility, and a study conducted by Althabe and Belizan found that the nearly 1.5 million unnecessary C-sections performed in Latin America every year were directly implicated as causes of maternal deaths as well as infant morbidity and mortality (2006).

In some places in Yucatán, particularly along the Riviera Maya, the C-section has become synonymous with hospital birth—locally, it is expected that a trip to the hospital by a pregnant woman will inevitably result in a C-section. Thus, women who choose to go to a hospital to deliver generally do so with the knowledge that they will be having an operation, regardless of how their own labor may actually be progressing. In interviews with pregnant Maya women, a common theme seemed to be that once in the hospital, their birth was out of their hands and whichever doctor was on shift that day would be directing the birth and making decisions. In contrast to research studies and media interviews of urban Mexican women, many Maya women emphasized that their preference was for natural childbirth, with nonsurgical interventions, if any. Many women's fears about their birth had mainly to do with complications resulting directly from hospital interventions, rather than concern about the pain of a natural childbirth. The "ideal" childbirth was one that progressed relatively smoothly, with little to no need for intervention, and, crucially, allowed for a speedy recovery and resumption of daily activities and household duties.

While married Maya women in rural areas do not normally join their husbands in working for wages outside of the home, they are usually responsible for growing and harvesting food from family gardens, animal husbandry, cooking, cleaning, child care, and supporting other members of the family in their wage labor. If a woman is unable to work and, as is becoming more common in Quintana Roo and Yucatán as families move to follow work opportunities, does not have family nearby to assist, her household may be seriously crippled while she is recuperating. Recovery from a C-section may take as long as 6 weeks, even without complications or infection. For many Maya women, most of whom do not live a middle-class lifestyle, going without working, picking up children, or otherwise caring for their families is not a possibility.

These recuperative difficulties may be partly responsible for high levels of postpartum infections in Maya women. Nearly every woman I spoke to who had given birth in the hospital referenced at least one postpartum infection as a result of a medical intervention during her labor, most commonly following a C-section or episiotomy. An infrastructural factor that likely exacerbates this is the nature of water procurement in the Yucatán peninsula. Like many other parts of Mexico, potable water must be purchased and delivered or carried to the household. Families that cannot afford this expense or who live too remotely to bother with it drink unpurified water—a factor in the high rates of diarrheal disease and communicable illnesses that plague rural populations. Water for washing and bathing must also be purchased and delivered to a reservoir in the household, unless a family has access to a cenote (from the Yucatec Maya word *ts'onot*, a natural pit exposing groundwater). During periods of drought or intense household poverty when families cannot afford to refill their reservoirs, water must be used sparingly. While this is fairly typical for rural or indigenous areas and indeed, nationally, 69% of indigenous households with children in Mexico do not have access to piped-in water, it makes a minimum level of wound care following surgery extremely difficult.

10.6 Impediments to Breastfeeding

While clinic walls often host posters singing the praises of breastfeeding, hospital staff and procedures do not always allow for it and may even actively prevent it. An example of this from a non-indigenous woman laboring in a Cancún hospital demonstrates the difficulties that a woman may face even after she has made the decision to breastfeed and communicated it to hospital staff:

> Once my son had come out, they immediately cut the cord. The put him on my chest for about 10 seconds but then they were stitching up my episiotomy and they took him away. I didn't know why or to where. Even despite the episiotomy, I was feeling wonderful and strong. I was smiling the whole labour. [My friend] and I went looking for him, and when we found him they were just about to give him a bottle! I was so angry! I had told them I wanted to breastfeed, and they ignored me! I had to sign all sorts of paperwork just to have him in the room with me, and they still insisted that they had to give him the bottle before he could be with me.

While this example certainly exhibits a disregard for the wishes of the laboring mother and family on the part of the hospital staff, it is also apparent that the mother's own ability to speak Spanish, read and understand the complicated hospital paperwork, and forcefully defend her interests and the interests of her child enabled her to prevent an unwanted outcome. Indigenous Maya women do not often have those same tools at their disposal, and this lack of power may manifest in more obviously traumatic experiences, as this experience, relayed by the woman's sister, indicates:

> Maria had her baby in a [city in Quintana Roo] hospital. The nurses there don't let the women breastfeed, and they take them away immediately. But they don't have the patience to give them the bottle, so they feed them with a syringe instead, because it takes less time. But it choked her baby! He died, and she was so upset and was crying and she said 'You killed my baby!' and the doctor said, 'No! You! You killed your baby because you don't know how to breastfeed, and you killed your baby and if you go out and say anything we'll put you in jail!.' She never filed anything against the hospital. She was so traumatized and it was horrible.

In this incident, the intervention of health practitioners led directly, according to Maria, to the death of her newborn. But instead of the hospital staff attempting to figure out what went wrong and take responsibility, Maria describes a doctor threatening her with jail to ensure that she does not file a formal complaint or attempt to launch an investigation. In this instance, the hospital seems to close ranks to protect its own and obscure the progression of events that led to the death of Maria's baby (Fig. 10.3).

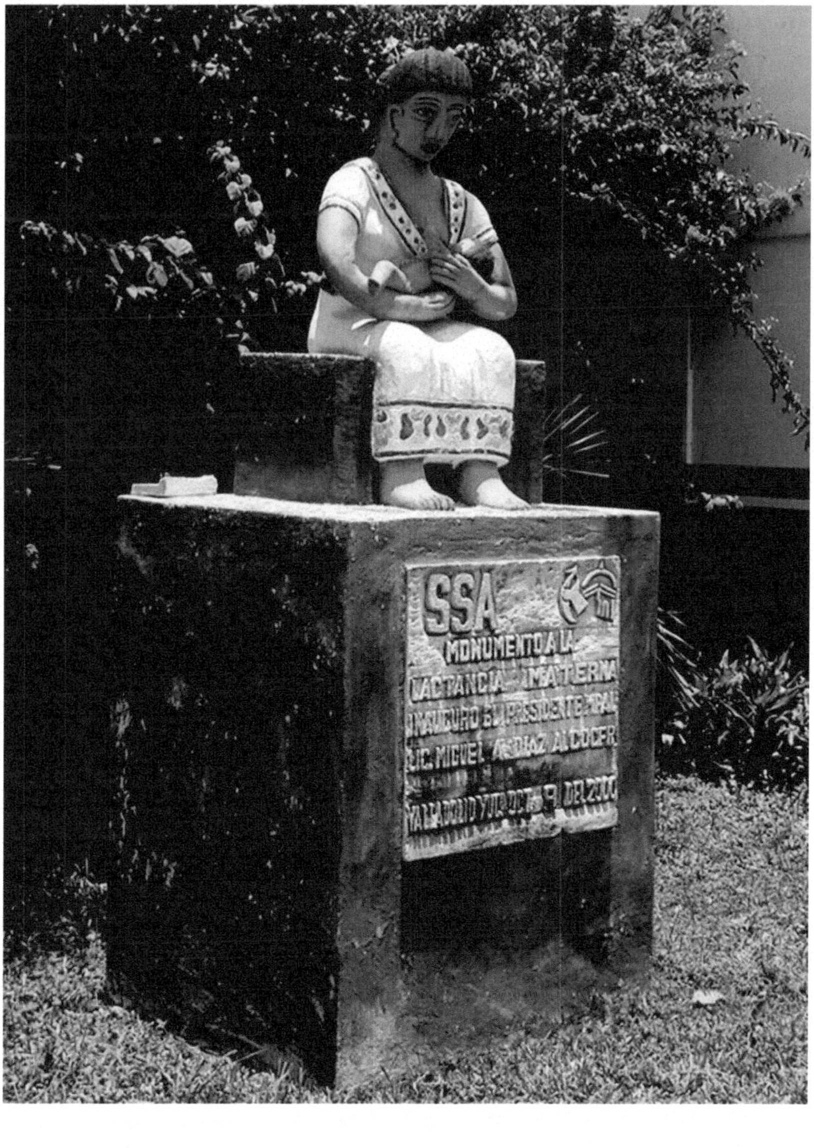

Fig. 10.3 Statue celebrating "maternity" in Valladolid, Yucatán

In the United States or Canada, the decision not to breastfeed will rarely have serious consequences for the infant. Though research has demonstrated that breastfeeding has many important benefits for infant development, in comparatively wealthy Western contexts, the inability or choice not to breastfeed does not necessarily constitute a critical loss for the child (Roberts et al. 2013). For mothers in Yucatán, the inability to breastfeed may have much more serious consequences for their children. Infant formula is a costly purchase in Quintana Roo and Yucatán, for indigenous families often prohibitively so. In rural pueblos, mothers who are unable to breastfeed and cannot afford or access formula will often feed their infants pozole, a thick drink made of watered down corn flour and sugar, which provides calories but not many nutrients. Families may also encounter problems if they cannot access or purchase purified water to mix with formula powder and may instead unknowingly expose their children to contaminated water via the bottle. In any case, the prevention or cessation of breastfeeding due to unnecessary birth interventions or the actions of healthcare personnel adds a significant expense to households that may not be capable of meeting it, and these situations place infants at risk of malnutrition, infectious waterborne illnesses, and death.

10.7 Episiotomy

Another common surgical intervention during birth is the episiotomy, a vertical surgical incision used to widen the vaginal opening if the infant's head is too large to fit, which by 2003 had been reported to be used in as many as 90% of hospital births in the United States and Mexico (Davis-Floyd 2004:57). While historically the medical community has advocated episiotomies for women considered at risk of tearing during childbirth, as surgical cuts were thought to heal neater and faster with less scarring than tearing, more recent research demonstrating that the opposite is usually the case has led most of the medical community to revise its standards (Carroli and Mignini 2009). The OECD recommendations for decreasing obstetric trauma have noted that episiotomies not only do not prevent tearing but are strongly associated with third- or fourth-degree lacerations (Hornemann et al. 2010). Because of this and associated complications and risks from the procedure, medical experts have recommended that episiotomy rates be severely curtailed and only performed after individual evaluations on a patient-by-patient basis (Gurol-Urganci et al. 2013).

While episiotomies are not tracked as closely as C-sections in Mexico, academic and media investigations have found the procedure to be extremely common. Indeed, it has been decried as an emerging ritual aspect of a hospital birth, nearly universally implemented on the bodies of women birthing vaginally regardless of their individual wishes or likelihood of tearing.

Graciela, originally from Guerrero, gave birth to her first child in a Cancún hospital. At the time of the birth, she was in her early 30s and in excellent health and had been combining midwifery and medical prenatal care. Graciela is not indigenous and is university-educated, as is her husband Jorge. While she had become friends with several midwives in Tulum, a small town 2-hours south of Cancún, her family and husband insisted that she give birth in a hospital, and she herself was nervous about giving birth in a town without a hospital. Despite choosing a hospital birth, Graciela was hopeful about avoiding unnecessary interventions and did everything she could to prepare for a healthy, happy labor. A confident, graceful woman, she had read studies about the complications associated with both C-sections and episiotomies and communicated her aversion to her doctor. In order to avoid being caught in the "snowballing effect," a chain of medical interventions starting with the lithotomic position and Pitocin and eventually requiring a C-section, Graciela labored at home in the bath until she was at 7 cm dilation and reached 9 cm during the car ride to the hospital in Tulum. By the time she arrived at the hospital, she was actively pushing, and it seemed to her that an unassisted birth was not only achievable but inevitable. However, as she described to me:

> I pushed once, and then…I felt it. It was burning already and I could feel [my son] coming. Then they cut me. During all the prenatal visits, I begged [the doctor] to allow me [to not be cut]. I know my body. I'm really, really flexible. I knew that if my yoni was as flexible as my body I could handle birth without breaking. I told him that every visit and he would say, 'No way!' He told me all this nonsense that if I tore it would be that much harder to sew up, and that I would never be the same and my poor husband would never have pleasure anymore. It was all stories like that. And [when I was giving birth] I heard something, some noise, and then [my sister] told me I'd been cut.

Graciela's experience was disappointing to her, as she felt that her body had been violated against her explicit and direct wishes, but she was quick to emphasize that in spite of everything she experienced in the hospital, overall her birth was beautiful and her son perfect. However, she was adamant that she would never give birth with a doctor again, and indeed her two subsequent children were born attended by two midwives in her own home. Graciela's birth, though not to her ideal and problematic from an ethical and medical perspective, was nonetheless a fairly benign example of the routine nature of episiotomies in many hospitals. Additionally, her experience is mediated by her and her husband's relatively privileged positions—they are financially well-off, non-indigenous, and university-educated. In a country where 32% of indigenous people over 15 are illiterate and the illiteracy rate for indigenous women is as much as double or triple that of indigenous men, the ability to read and understand hospital paperwork and attempt to negotiate it is a significant advantage (Pan American Health Organization 2012). Birth stories relayed by Maya women contain many of the same themes, but their experiences tend to be more explicitly violent and highlight patterns of treatment that go far beyond outdated medical practice.

Sofia, a Chiapanecan Maya woman whose family rented a small hut in another family's compound in a small town along the Riviera Maya, shared her experience giving birth in the *Centro de Salud*, a small government health clinic with a rudimentarily equipped operating room. Sofia went to the *Centro de Salud* fairly early in her labor and was immediately put into the lithotomy position on the table in the operating room. Her labor progressed normally, but, according to Sofia:

> The baby came so fast! I was barely on the table before my daughter was coming out. She came out so quickly and easily that I didn't tear or anything. She was born, and then the doctor cut me after she came out. He cut me after she was born, and then he had to sew me up again.

Discounting the extremely unlikely possibility that a doctor would intentionally injure a patient, what seems most probable is that episiotomies have become so routine that the doctor was in the habit of automatically performing episiotomies with every birth that wasn't a C-section. This suggests that episiotomies are being performed irrespective of two critical factors: the patient's consent and the actual medical needs of the patient. In Sofia's case, her medical chart did not note her doctor's error or the fact that her vagina was cut open without consent after her baby had already passed through the birth canal and been born. Not only was Sofia subjected to a painful and unnecessary medical procedure, but the presence of a stitched laceration also placed her at risk for a postpartum infection in the weeks following.

The experiences of Maya women within hospitals that were relayed in this study index the uncomfortable and unequal relationship that the indigenous Maya have with the Mexican state, vis-à-vis one of Mexico's largest bureaucratic systems and one of its main symbols of Western modernity and progress—the healthcare system. Within the experiences relayed here, there is a clear disparity in the treatment and reactions to that treatment reported by non-indigenous women and the experiences that indigenous women report, though the overarching themes are similar. While both groups of women find themselves at a disadvantage in navigating the hierarchies in the hospital to obtain the results they want, non-indigenous women generally reported the ability to push back against hospital protocol (whether official or merely a habit) with a strong sense of entitlement for their rights as patients and people, though not always successfully. On the contrary, the experiences reported by indigenous Maya women tend to reference a sense of helplessness and bewilderment once in the hospital and emphasize things done to them by doctors and nurses. The violence they experience during birth and the lack of attention paid to their desires and needs are experienced as traumatic and upsetting, but not necessarily surprising. For many Maya communities in the Yucatán peninsula, ill-treatment in medical institutions is an injustice with deep roots in the peninsula's colonial history that extend forward with the public health projects of the eighteenth and nineteenth centuries (McCrea 2011). Further, mistreatment, verbal abuse, and violations of bodily autonomy during birth are also experienced within a context where violence against women is, if not normalized, extremely common.

10.8 Violence Against Women

Obstetric violence, though increasingly a term with its own legal definitions, is but one category within a plethora of abuses faced by women in Mexico, particularly indigenous women. The emotional, psychological, and physical abuse of women and negation of their bodily autonomy during the vulnerable time, that is, pregnancy and childbirth, are not, for many women, out of the ordinary realm of treatment in their daily lives. In Mexico, according to a report produced by the Mexican Institute for Women in 2009, 67 out of every 100 women over the age of 15 have experienced some kind of violence, with approximately 40% of those acts taking place within the home at the hands of a spouse or family member. Further, 20% of murdered girls and women are under the age of 5, and often sexual abuse and assault are associated with the cause of death (Fregoso and Bejarano 2010).

Cartels are strongly linked to feminicide and the rape, murder, and torture of women, but so are federal police and the military, particularly in indigenous communities where both groups, illegal and legitimate, treat women's bodies as a means of demonstrating power, threatening and coercing communities into submission, and rewarding male soldiers and members. These mutilations, rapes, and murders occur within a contradictory legal climate. On the one hand, Mexico has some of the most progressive and sweeping laws against gendered violence in the world and passed *La Ley General de Acceso de las Mujeres a Una Vida libre de Violencia* (in English, the General Law of Women's Access to a Life Free of Violence) in 2006. Legally, these new juridical processes shifted women's positions as victims of violence from juridical objects to juridical subjects and made crimes of violence against women crimes against her personhood in the eyes of the law, rather than crimes against her honor or her family. Functionally, however, Mexico has very low rates of compliance with these laws, and their enforcement is very low. This even more the case in rural or peripheral regions of Mexico, where crimes against women are often still treated as crimes against juridical objects, best dealt with privately within families (Fregoso and Bejarano 2010).

This disconnect between the law and actual practice was highlighted during a meeting with 20 Maya women in southern Quintana Roo. The women ranged in ages from 19 to 60 and were from about eight different villages and towns in the same area. Discussions of obstetric violence within the group inevitably shifted to include other examples of violence that women in their communities faced. The two topics weren't seen as two topics at all, rather two faces of the same coin, particularly as many pregnant women face abuse from their spouses, in-laws, and other family members as well as mistreatment from healthcare practitioners. A story shared by an older participant, whose details were supported by others from her town, seemed to capture many elements found in other accounts of violence and precarity women face. An older participant reminded the group of a particular incidence within their own community:

> Remember that poor girl? The one who lived by the bakery? Her father died when she was young and her mother remarried. After a few years, she became pregnant at thirteen. Her stepfather had been violating her, possibly the whole time. Her mother was furious, and beat her in the street, then threw her out. She slept on the streets. She was starving. No one would help her. What could they do? Her mother didn't want her. She eventually gave birth in the *Centro de Salud*. Of course it was a hard labor—she was so young. Two weeks later, the baby died. I don't know where she is now. And her baby died. It happens all the time. The girls are violated and then thrown out of the house, and often they die or their babies die. Because they're on the streets, other men hurt them more.

Responding to a query about whether the *Secretaria de Salud* had identified intervening in these types of situations as a way to improve maternal and infant mortality rates in the region, another participant who works closely with the *Secretaria* scoffed:

> They stop considering infant deaths after 8 days. It isn't supposed to be that way, but that's what they do in these small places. Maternal [mortality] rates are low for the same reason—the deaths of pregnant and post-partum women and girls who are abused and vulnerable and have been abandoned are not investigated, accounted for, or considered. No one wants to look too deeply into it.

Even in urban areas thought to be much more tightly policed, violence against women can be ignored and swept under a rug by individuals, the community, and law enforcement and medical personnel, as this example from a suburb on the Riviera Maya demonstrates:

> I woke up from my nap and I heard screaming coming from outside. It sounded horrible, a woman was in terrible pain. I dressed and rushed out to try to help with my baby in my arms, and in the courtyard of my apartment building my neighbor was beating his pregnant wife with what looked like a piece of metal pipe. She was on the ground trying to crawl away, and he kept hitting her head and stomach. There was blood everywhere. Other people were rushing to help, following the screams, but when they saw that it was a domestic dispute, they didn't do anything, they walked away! I called down from the stairs for him to stop, but he threatened me too, and I had my baby with me. I called the police and an ambulance, but by then she had stopped moving. The police came but they didn't arrest him. She died in the ambulance but the baby lived, and now his mother is caring for the child.

These scenarios highlight the disconnect between high-level judicial laws and standards and their actual (or lack of) implementation in places where the representatives of the legal system—police and other government agents—follow the codes that are socially mandated within their towns and villages, that is, treating abuse and violence against women as a private, familial matter and, relatedly, not delving too deeply into the cause of death of pregnant or recently pregnant girls and women when it may be socially or politically inconvenient or difficult (Rodriguez et al. 2005).

10.9 Underreporting of Obstetric Complications, MMR, and IMR

As these ethnographic examples have shown, obstetric violence is extremely widespread in Yucatán and Quintana Roo. Though abuses can range from such "benign" or non-malicious actions such as impeding the start of breastfeeding by separating the mother and baby to performing major, nonmedically necessary surgeries on women without consent and against their explicit wishes, a common theme emerges in this study of doctors and hospital staff using records and record-keeping as a means of covering up instances of obstetric violence and poor outcomes. Not only this, but the reports from indigenous women indicating that hospital staff used their structural privilege to threaten women with reprisals such as jail time for reporting malpractice and mistreatment highlight institutional comfort and confidence in manipulating official channels—such as documentation and paths to investigation—in order to obscure realities of abuse. Women report requesting their medical records following negative experiences, medical mistakes, and poor outcomes and subsequently find that the records do not reflect their experiences—in one case, a woman's severe allergic reaction to an unwanted epidural caused her to have an emergency C-section, which was parsed in her medical records as a planned C-section that she had requested weeks in advance. In such an environment of institutional malfeasance, it is difficult to say just how accurate are Mexico's steadily improving MMR and infant mortality rates (IMR). The pressure on public health officials, doctors, and hospital staff to contribute to improved outcomes is immense, but underfunding and overcrowding of hospitals and maternity wards do not set the stage for conscientious and careful care. Further, medical practices that emphasize a one-size-fits-all approach to surgical interventions regardless of patient need, interest, or desire place women at risk of grave violations to their bodies and rights. Truly accurate measures of maternal and infant outcomes depend on a medical infrastructure and environment that allows for women to be treated respectfully and without violence—then there will be nothing to hide.

References

Althabe, F., & Belizán, J. M. (2006). Caesarean section: The paradox. *Lancet, 368*(9546), 1472–1473.

Barber, S. L. (2009). Mexico's conditional cash transfer programme increases cesarean section rates among the rural poor. *European Journal of Public Health, 20*(4), 383–388. https://doi.org/10.1093/eurpub/ckp184

Berry, N. S. (2006). Kaqchikel midwives, home births, and emergency obstetric referrals in Guatemala: Contextualizing the choice to stay at home. *Social Science & Medicine, 62*(8), 1958–1969. https://doi.org/10.1016/j.socscimed.2005.09.005

Berry, N. S. (2008). Who's judging the quality of care? Indigenous Maya and the problem of "not being attended". *Medical Anthropology, 27*(2), 164–189. https://doi.org/10.1080/01459740802017413

Berry, N. S. (2010). *Unsafe motherhood: Mayan maternal mortality and subjectivity in post-war Guatemala*. New York, NY: Berghahn Books.

Betrán, A. P., Merialdi, M., Lauer, J. A., Bing-Shun, W., Thomas, J., Van Look, P., et al. (2007). Rates of caesarean section: Analysis of global, regional and national estimates. *Paediatric and Perinatal Epidemiology, 21*(2), 98–113. https://doi.org/10.1111/j.1365-3016.2007.00786.x

Birn, A.-E. (1999). Federalist flirtations: The politics and execution of health services decentralization for the uninsured population in Mexico, 1985-1995. *Journal of Public Health Policy, 20*(1), 81–108. https://doi.org/10.2307/3343260

Bohren, M. A., Vogel, J. P., Hunter, E. C., Lutsiv, O., Makh, S. K., Souza, J. P., et al. (2015). The mistreatment of women during childbirth in health facilities globally: A mixed-methods systematic review. *PLoS Medicine, 12*(6). https://doi.org/10.1371/journal.pmed.1001847

Braine, T. (2008). Mexico's midwives enter the mainstream. *Bulletin of the World Health Organization, 86*(4), 244–245. https://doi.org/10.2471/blt.08.010408

Carroli, G., & Mignini, L. (2009). Episiotomy for vaginal birth. *Cochrane Database of Systematic Reviews, 1*(1), CD000081. https://doi.org/10.1002/14651858.CD000081.pub2

Coneval. (2012). *Evaluacion estrategica sobre mortalidad materna en Mexico 2010: Caractensticas sociodemograficas que obstaculizan a las mujeres embarazadas su acceso efectivo a instituciones de salud*. Mexico, DF: Consejo Nacional de Evaluacion de la Poltica de Desarrollo Social.

Davis-Floyd, R. E. (2001). La partera profesional: Articulating identity and cultural space for a new kind of midwife in Mexico. *Medical Anthropology, 20*(2-3), 185–243. https://doi.org/10.1080/01459740.2001.9966194

Davis-Floyd, R. E. (2004). *Birth as an American rite of passage: With a new preface*. Oakland, California: University of California Press.

D'Gregorio, R. P. (2010). Obstetric violence: A new legal term introduced in Venezuela. *International Journal of Gynecology & Obstetrics, 111*(3), 201–202.

de López, J.M. (2011). *Rural-urban migration in Chiapas, Mexico: Antenatal violence and the disappearing of the midwife*. Paper presented at The International Conference on Gendered Violence, University of Bristol, UK. 23-25 November 2011.

Dixon, L. Z. (2015). Obstetrics in a time of violence: Mexican midwives critique routine hospital practices. *Medical Anthropology Quarterly, 29*(4), 437–454. https://doi.org/10.1111/maq.12174

Fregoso, R. L., & Bejarano, C. L. (2010). *Terrorizing women: Feminicide in the Americas*. Durham, North Carolina: Duke University Press.

Frenk, J., Sepúlveda, J., Gómez-Dantés, O., & Knaul, F. (2003). Evidence-based health policy: Three generations of reform in Mexico. *Lancet, 362*(9396), 1667–1671. https://doi.org/10.1016/s0140-6736(03)14803-9

Gibbons, L., Belizán, J. M., Lauer, J. A., Betrán, A. P., Merialdi, M., & Althabe, F. (2010). The global numbers and costs of additionally needed and unnecessary caesarean sections performed per year: Overuse as a barrier to universal coverage. *World Health Report Background Paper, 30*, 1–31.
Gurol-Urganci, I., Cromwell, D. A., Edozien, L. C., Mahmood, T. A., Adams, E. J., Richmond, D. H., et al. (2013). Third- and fourth-degree perineal tears among primiparous women in England between 2000 and 2012: Time trends and risk factors. *British Journal of Obstetrics and Gynaecology, 120*(12), 1516–1525.
Homedes, N., & Ugalde, A. (2009). Twenty-five years of convoluted health reforms in Mexico. *PLoS Medicine, 6*(8), e1000124. https://doi.org/10.1371/journal.pmed.1000124
Hornemann, A., Kamischke, A., Luedders, D. W., Beyer, D. A., Diedrich, K., & Bohlmann, M. K. (2010). Advanced age is a risk factor for higher grade perineal lacerations during delivery in nulliparous women. *Archives of Gynecology and Obstetrics, 281*(1), 59–64.
McCrea, H. (2011). *Diseased relations: Epidemics, public health, and state-building in Yucatán, Mexico, 1847-1924*. Albuquerque: University of New Mexico Press.
Mills, L. (2015). Accounting for blame: The paradoxical consequences of measuring maternal death in Mexico. *Social Politics: International Studies in Gender, State & Society, 22*(3), 411–431.
Napolitano, V., & Flores, G. M. (2003). Complementary medicine: Cosmopolitan and popular knowledge, and transcultural translations-cases from urban Mexico. *Theory, Culture & Society, 20*(4), 79–95.
Niino, Y. (2011). The increasing caesarean rate globally and what we can do about it. *Bioscience Trends, 5*(4), 139–150. https://doi.org/10.5582/bst.2011.v5.4.139
OECD. (2005). *OECD reviews of health systems: Mexico 2005*. Paris: OECD Publishing. https://doi.org/10.1787/9789264008939-en
Pan American Health Organization. (2012). *Health in the Americas: Regional outlook and country profiles*. Washington, DC: PAHO.
Pintado, A., Sachse, M., & Lastra, Z. (2015). Maternal care during pregnancy, childbirth, and the postpartum period in primary care units, Oaxaca, Mexico. *Social Medicine, 9*(1), 29–35.
Roberts, T., Emily Carnahan, E., & Gakidou, E. (2013). Burden attributable to suboptimal breastfeeding: A cross-country analysis of country-specific trends and their relation to child health inequalities. *Lancet, 381*, S126. https://doi.org/10.1016/S0140-6736(13)61380-X
Rodríguez, E., Andueza, G., Montero, L., & Hoil, J. (2005). Subregistro de muertes maternas en Mérida, Yucatán (1997-2001). *Ginecologia y Obstetricia de México, 73*(7), 347–354.
Schiavon, R., Troncoso, E., & Polo, G. (2012). Analysis of maternal and abortion-related mortality in Mexico over the last two decades, 1990–2008. *International Journal of Gynecology & Obstetrics, 118*(Suppl 2), S78–S86. https://doi.org/10.1016/S0020-7292(12)60004-6
Schneider, S. D. (2010). *Mexican community health and the politics of health reform*. Albuquerque, New Mexico: University of New Mexico Press.
Secretaria de Salud. (2007). *Programa Nacional de Salud 2007-2012*. Mexico City: Secretaria de Salud, Mexico.
Secretaría de Salud. (1995). *Programa de salud reproductiva y planificación familiar 1995–2000*. Mexico City: Secretaría de Salud, Mexico.
Sesia, P. M. (1996). "Women come here on their own when they need to": Prenatal care, authoritative knowledge, and maternal health in Oaxaca. *Medical Anthropology Quarterly, 10*(2), 121–140.
Sesia, P. (2013). Derechos humanos, salud y muerte materna: Características, potencial y retos de un nuevo enfoque para lograr la maternidad seguro en México. *Revista Andaluza de Antropología, 5*, 66–90.
Smith-Oka, V. (2015). Microaggressions and the reproduction of social inequalities in medical encounters in Mexico. *Social Science & Medicine, 143*, 9–16. https://doi.org/10.1016/j.socscimed.2015.08.039
Torres, C., & Mújica, O. J. (2004). Salud, equidad y los objetivos de desarrollo del milenio. *Revista Panamericana de Salúd Publica [Pan American Journal of Public Health], 15*(6), 430–439.
Urquieta, J., Angeles, G., Mroz, T., Lamadrid-Figueroa, H., Hernández, B. (2008). *Impact of oportunidades on skilled attendance at delivery in rural areas*. Working Paper no. WP-08-105, MEASURE Evaluation, University of North Carolina at Chapel Hill.

11 Pregnancy, Birth, and Babies: Motherhood and Modernization in a Yucatec Village

Amanda Veile and Karen L. Kramer

11.1 Introduction

Birth is a major life history event and represents a human universal that is shaped by evolutionary, biological, and social factors (Abrams and Rutherford 2011; Davis-Floyd and Sargent 1997; Dunsworth et al. 2012; Stone 2016; Trevathan 2011). A notable characteristic of human birth is that it nearly always unfolds in a social context; assisted birth may indeed be an important part of the evolved human life history (Rosenberg and Trevathan 1995; Trevathan 1996). In the most modern of settings, birth attendants are often medical professionals, whereas in traditional societies, women may rely on their husbands, female kin, or recognized midwives (Stone 2016). One particularly well-documented system of traditional midwifery is practiced by Maya farmers in Guatemala and Mexico, where researchers have documented how these birthing practices are affected by encroaching biomedical obstetric systems (Berry 2013; Cosminsky 1982; Jordan and Davis-Floyd 1993).

Traditional Maya midwifery differs in a number of ways from biomedical obstetrics practices, which have been described by Jordan and Davis-Floyd (1993). Midwives supported, but rarely interfered with, the birthing process, though they did perform external cephalic versions (a procedure that turns a breech or transverse fetus into a head-down position before labor begins), and sometimes used herbal teas to increase the speed of mothers' contractions. Maya women would labor in a variety of positions, often giving birth while squatting or lying in a hammock. Postpartum practices would facilitate mother-infant bonding and the establishment of lactation. Mothers and infants were placed together, skin to skin, and allowed to rest together for several weeks.

Under the biomedical obstetric model, births occur in the hospital and are characterized by increased reliance on technology and interventions such as episiotomies and the use of synthetic oxytocin, epidurals,

A. Veile, Ph.D. (✉)
Department of Anthropology, Center on Aging and the Life Course, Purdue University, West Lafayette, IN, USA
e-mail: aveile@purdue.edu

K. L. Kramer, Ph.D.
Department of Anthropology, University of Utah, Salt Lake City, UT, USA

D. A. Schwartz (ed.), *Maternal Death and Pregnancy-Related Morbidity Among Indigenous Women of Mexico and Central America*, Global Maternal and Child Health: Medical, Anthropological, and Public Health Perspectives, https://doi.org/10.1007/978-3-319-71538-4_11

and cesarean sections. Women are only permitted to give birth in the lithotomy position (supine on a table with feet in the air). Postpartum practices may facilitate mother-infant bonding and breastfeeding in a hospital setting, but mothers and infants may be separated following delivery for many reasons, such as maternal or infant medical complications or because the mother is sedated. Mother-infant separation is especially prevalent following a cesarean section delivery, which interrupts mother-infant bonding and reduces early breastfeeding (Dewey et al. 2003; Veile and Kramer 2015).

Birthing practices are transitioning to the biomedical obstetric model throughout Mexico, where the national cesarean section rate is nearly 50% (Vogel et al. 2015). Though cesarean birth rates are rapidly rising among the rural poor (Barber 2010), midwifery is still practiced in some regions. As of 2012, 35,000 midwives were registered in Mexico, with the majority practicing in the states of Chiapas and Oaxaca (Torri 2012). In the Yucatan Peninsula, midwifery is still practiced, although hospital births and cesarean section rates are rising. For example, birth has become increasingly medicalized in the Yucatec Maya community of Xculoc since the late 1990s (Veile and Kramer 2015). This is in part due to the initiation of poverty-alleviation programs that provide affordable medical care; at the same time, improvements in road conditions and access to transportation have made it easier to travel to hospitals. In our previous research, we have shown that medicalization may lead to unintended consequences for maternal-infant health. In particular, cesarean births are associated with decreased breastfeeding duration and increased child body mass (Veile and Kramer 2015, 2016).

This chapter draws on longitudinal research in the Yucatec Maya community of Xculoc. We describe the experiences of three cohorts of mothers to illustrate how pregnancy, birth, and babies have changed over a 65-year period (1950–2014) as the community became increasingly modernized. Although we touch on many aspects of the maternal experience, we are particularly interested in how Maya birthing practices have changed. We consider how ongoing shifts in energetic and epidemiologic conditions, and from traditional midwifery to highly medicalized births, shape birthing and postpartum practices, pregnancy complications, fertility rates, and infant nutrition and health outcomes.

11.2 Methods

We draw from ethnographic interviews with Yucatec Maya of Xculoc (hereafter referred to as the Yucatec Maya), focusing on 56 mothers who were ages 21–85 in 2014. These women represent a subset of the village population (nearly 60% of parous women ages 21–85). The interviews included a series of target questions regarding maternal age and parity (number of live births), maternal age at first birth, the range of health-care options available to mothers throughout their reproductive careers, the location and mode (vaginal/cesarean) of each birth, and the number of infant deaths (<1 year of age) each woman had experienced. For each woman's youngest child only, the mothers were also asked a series of questions about pregnancy complications, their birthing and breastfeeding practices, infant nutrition, who was present to assist them throughout labor and birth, their postpartum rest period, and participation in ritual postpartum practices. All demographic data were cross-checked with ongoing demographic databases collected and maintained by one of the authors (KK) since 1992.

For this chapter, we stratify the 56 mothers into 3 cohorts based on the year that they began their reproductive careers: Cohort 1 women gave birth to their first child from 1950 to 1976 (n = 12); Cohort 2 women had their first birth from 1978 to 1999 (n = 22); and Cohort 3 women had their first birth from 2000 to 2015 (n = 22). For each cohort, we calculated the mean maternal age and parity, the average number of hospital and cesarean births per mother, and the average number of infant deaths per mother. For each mother's last birth, we calculated the year of birth, the average duration of their postpartum rest period, and the average timing of breastfeeding initiation and breastfeeding duration. After testing the data for normality and performing Welch's test for equal variances, we performed a one-way ANOVA in SPSS using the Games-Howell post hoc test to compare these variables across maternal cohorts.

We compared the following count variables across cohorts: maternal support during labor and birth (number of women reporting that their husbands, their mother-in-law, and their own mothers were present, respectively) and the number of mothers reporting ever having a cesarean birth. For the last birth only, we considered the following variables across cohorts: the number of mothers who had birth complications, episiotomies, and tubal ligation. We also compared the number of women who participated in ritual bandaging and the number of women who breastfed their infants, provided colostrum to their infants, and provided infant formula to their infants, respectively. These variables were compared using a chi-square test in SPSS.

11.2.1 The Study Community

The study community is located in a remote and sparsely populated area of the Puuc region in the interior of the Yucatan Peninsula, Campeche, Mexico. The indigenous Maya who inhabit this rural area live in small villages of subsistence maize farmers and in a few market and administrative towns. Longitudinal economic, demographic, subsistence, and social data have been collected in this community by the second author since the early 1990s (Kramer 2005; Kramer and Boone 2002; Kramer and McMillan 2006; Lee and Kramer 2002). The reproductive and daily lives of this Yucatec Maya community prior to the 1990s and systematic data collection have been well described during interviews with villagers over the past 25 years. Here we discuss those factors that have changed over time and that directly affect changes in pregnancy and birth and the lives of mothers and infants across three cohorts of women (Fig. 11.1).

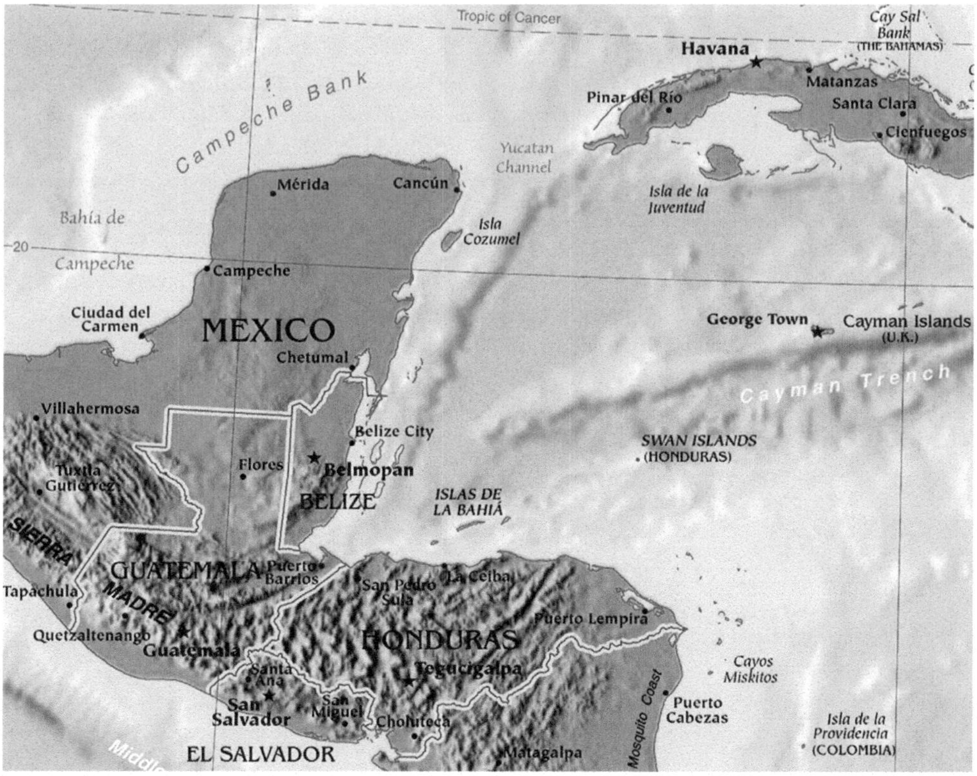

Fig. 11.1 Map of the Yucatan with surrounding countries. Map from Wikimedia Commons, https://commons.wikimedia.org/wiki/File:Bay_of_Honduras.jpg#filehistory

11.3 Cohort 1, 1950–1977: The Traditional Setting

The study community was founded in its present location by a few families in the first decades of the twentieth century. Throughout this time period, villagers lived in traditional wattle and daub, dirt floor houses and made their living as swidden subsistence farmers. By the 1950s, following the upheaval of the Mexican Revolution, the *ejido* land tenure system (consisting of collectively held village, agricultural, and forest lands) was instituted throughout rural Yucatan. This system holds particular significance for Maya women, as it ensures collective ownership of agricultural lands, guaranteeing all women within a community relatively equal and adequate access to food and other resources necessary to support reproduction and children. The study community's *ejido* allotment has been large enough to support this small but growing population for the past 65 years (Kramer 2005).

During the time period wherein the women of Cohort 1 gave birth, each family grew its own food; the majority of calories came from maize (80–90%) and to a lesser extent from beans, squash, peanuts, other fruits and vegetables, and hunted game. Domesticated turkeys, pigs, and chickens were raised for occasional domestic consumption; otherwise no livestock were kept. Forest plants were gathered primarily for medicinal purposes, except in years of extreme drought when *ramon* (breadfruit) was traditionally collected. The village had no running water or electricity. Women cooked food over an open fire and made their own clothing, the traditional white embroidered *huipil* (Fig. 11.2). Household goods were few and consisted mainly of handcrafted items (ceramic and gourd water containers, hammocks, stools, and *comals* (a smooth, flat griddle used in Mexico for cooking)).

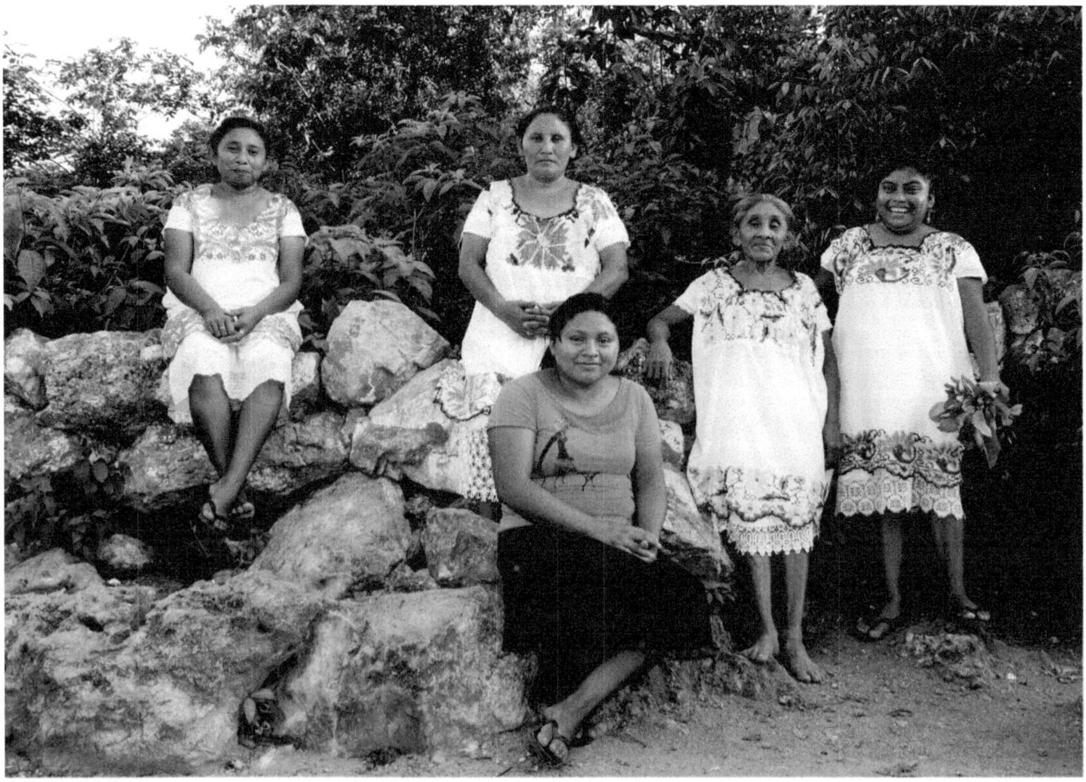

Fig. 11.2 Maya women in traditional and modern dress (Photo by Karen Kramer)

About 20 km away from the village, a road connects the states of Campeche and Yucatan and links the study community to a few market and administrative towns. Although sections of this road were paved from 1935 to 1948, those adjoining the path into Xculoc were likely not fully paved until the 1960s. Because of the long distances to market towns and the lack of roads and vehicles, villagers participated nominally in wage labor, cash cropping, or market exchange and had little access to education or health care. While a dedicated school building was not built until the end of this time period, teachers occasionally visited Xculoc. Women born before 1960 report attending school for an average of 1.5 years ($SD = 1.4$; $n = 24$). Children grew up speaking Maya as their first language, and few adults spoke Spanish. Both adults and children used Maya (and still do) when speaking to each other. Children lived and worked in their parents' household until they married in their late teens to early 20s. This was a natural fertility population, and a child was usually born within a year of marriage.

Women's lives were energetically demanding. There is no running surface water in this area of the Yucatan Peninsula. Prior to the village's founding, the Maya lived in small family units near *sartenejas*, small natural pools of water that collect in natural limestone basins. After the village was established around the abandoned hacienda, women retrieved water from its 50-m-deep well into the underlying aquifer by running out long ropes and drawing up individual containers of water, a time-consuming and energetically demanding task. Ground corn, which comprises the majority of the diet, was ground by hand with a *metate* (a flat or slightly hollowed oblong stone for hand grinding) and then with hand-cranked grinders likely introduced in the 1940s. Both are arduous activities, and villagers in the 1990s talked about their mothers and grandmothers working long hours and sleeping 5 h a night before the mid-1970s. Despite these hardships, total fertility of mothers who initiated childbearing during this cohort was high (mean = 7.4, SD = 1.6, $n = 24$; total surviving fertility mean = 6.7; SD = 1.5), and infant mortality was fairly low, for reasons discussed in section 11.7.1 (Tables 11.1 and 11.2).

Table 11.1 Descriptive statistics (mean ± SD, range) for continuous variables. Mothers in Cohorts 1, 2, and 3 are shown separately, along with results from the ANOVA comparisons

	Cohort 1 1950–1977	Cohort 2 1978–1999	Cohort 3 2000–2015	Total	*F*-value	*p*-value
N	12	22	22	56		
Maternal age	71.04 ± 8.53 (54.32–85.84)	46.74 ± 6.11 (32.55–55.26)	29.81 ± 6.39 (21.25–47.65)	45.29 ± 16.906 (21.25–85.84)	144.066	<0.001
Age of first birth	19.30 ± 3.79 (13.88–27.47)	21.11 ± 3.51 (15.71–31.74)	22.04 ± 4.73 (16.20–35.12)	21.09 ± 4.15 (13.88–35.12)	1.740	0.185
Parity (total live births)	7.08 ± 1.62 (5.00–10.00)	6.14 ± 2.77 (2.00–11.00)	2.32 ± 1.13 (1.00–4.00)	4.84 ± 2.87 (1.00–11.00)	29.072	<0.001
Hospital births per mother	0.083 ± 0.289 (0.00–1.00)	1.73 ± 1.42 (0.00–5.00)	1.64 ± 0.79 (0.00–3.00)	1.34 ± 1.21 (0.00–5.00)	11.368	0.001
Cesarean births per mother	0.00 ± 0.00 (0.00–0.00)	0.55 ± 0.86 (0.00–3.00)	0.50 ± 0.74 (0.00–2.00)	0.41 ± 0.73 (0.00–3.00)	2.555	0.087
Infant deaths per mother	0.42 ± 0.51 (0.00–1.00)	0.23 ± 0.61 (0.00–2.00)	0.91 ± 0.29 (0.00–1.00)	0.21 ± 0.49 (0.00–2.00)	1.746	0.184
Age youngest child	34.75 ± 9.85 (22.00–55.00)	12.14 ± 6.72 (0.67–25.00)	3.97 ± 3.10 (0.166–12.00)	13.78 ± 13.26 (0.17–55.00)	88.986	<0.001
Postpartum rest Period[a]	09.92 ± 3.09 (8.00–15.00)	59.91 ± 72.40 (3.00–180.00)	69.91 ± 89.13 (1.00–365.00)	53.13 ± 74.67 (1.00–356.00)	2.833	0.068
Timing of breastfeeding Initiation[a]	2.00 ± 6.93 (0.00–24.00)	7.55 ± 20.88 (0.00–72.00)	38.23 ± 153.04 (0.00–720.00)	18.41 ± 96.86 (0.00–720.00)	0.764	0.471
Weaning age[a]	31.00 ± 11.95 (12.00–48.00)	29.55 ± 18.73 (06.00–72.00)	18.76 ± 15.75 (0.033–48.00)[a]	26.32 ± 16.85 (0.03–72.00)[a]	2.609	0.085

[a]Last child only

Table 11.2 Post hoc comparison (Games-Howell) for selected variables

	Cohort	Comparison	Mean difference	Standard error	p-value
Hospital births per mother	1.0	2.0	−1.64	0.31	0.00
		3.0	−1.55	0.19	0.00
	2.0	1.0	1.64	0.31	0.00
		3.0	0.09	0.35	0.96
	3.0	1.0	1.55	0.19	0.00
		2.0	−0.09	0.35	0.96
Cesarean births per mother	1.0	2.0	−0.55	0.18	0.02
		3.0	−0.50	0.16	0.01
	2.0	1.0	0.55	0.18	0.02
		3.0	0.05	0.24	0.98
	3.0	1.0	0.50	0.16	0.01
		2.0	−0.05	0.24	0.98
Infant deaths per mother	1.0	2.0	0.19	0.20	0.61
		3.0	0.33	0.16	0.14
	2.0	1.0	−0.19	0.20	0.61
		3.0	0.14	0.14	0.62
	3.0	1.0	−0.33	0.16	0.14
		2.0	−0.14	0.14	0.62
Postpartum rest period[a]	1.0	2.0	−49.99	15.46	0.01
		3.0	−59.99	19.02	0.01
	2.0	1.0	49.99	15.46	0.01
		3.0	−10.00	24.48	0.91
	3.0	1.0	59.99	19.02	0.01
		2.0	10.00	24.48	0.91
Weaning age[a]	1.0	2.0	1.45	5.43	0.96
		3.0	12.24	5.24	0.07
	2.0	1.0	−1.45	5.43	0.96
		3.0	10.79	5.75	0.16
	3.0	1.0	−12.24	5.24	0.07
		2.0	−10.79	5.75	0.16

[a]Last child only

11.3.1 Cohort 1: Pregnancy, Birth, and Babies

We interviewed 12 mothers from Cohort 1 (50% of all village women whose first birth fell within this range), and in this section, we report on this subsample of women only. The 12 mothers were born in years ranging from 1928 to 1950 and had their first birth between 1950 and 1978. They represent the oldest women in the interview sample (aged 64–85 at time of interview). Although there are many differences between the oldest and youngest women within Cohort 1, we group them together because they began their reproductive careers in the time before major technological advances and epidemiologic change came to the community.

Over one-half (58%) of mothers reported that they had never accessed Western biomedical care for themselves or for their children, whereas 43% had visited clinics in nearby cities or towns for emergency care when their children were sick. The five mothers who had accessed health care were younger than the six who had not (mean age = 66.98 vs. 73.94, respectively, one-tailed $t = 1.86$, $p = 0.06$), suggesting that health-care access improved over time. Still, many services were limited. For example, Cohort 1 women unanimously reported that they did not visit doctors for prenatal care

Fig. 11.3 Maya midwife (Photo by Amanda Veile)

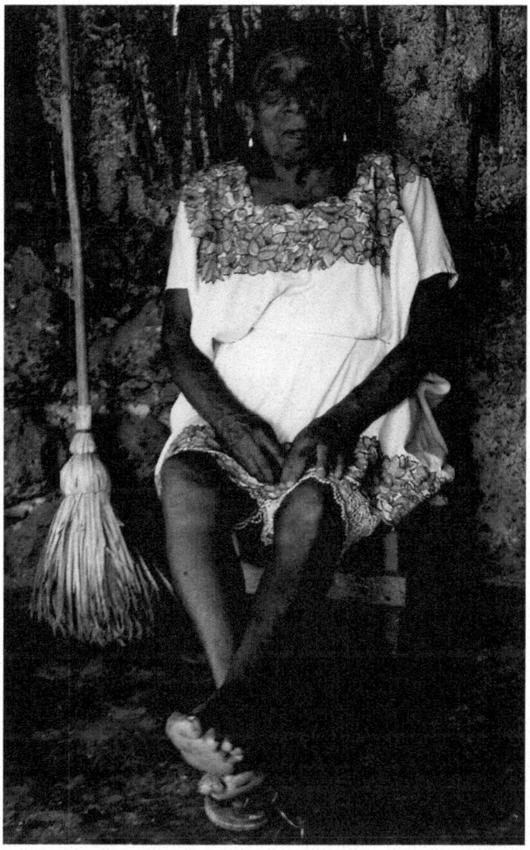

during any of their pregnancies. Recent interviews also have revealed that three maternal deaths occurred during this time period. One mother died following a prolonged period in which her placenta was retained. Two died following labors that failed to progress.

The pregnancies and births of Cohort 1 mothers were attended by respected midwives who lived in Xculoc or neighboring villages (Fig. 11.3). Their prenatal care practices resemble those reported for other Maya midwives, who would visit several times throughout the pregnancy and perform a *sobada* (massage) (Jordan and Davis-Floyd 1993). Palpation of the pregnant woman's stomach allowed the midwives to estimate the infant's gestational age and determine its position in the weeks leading up to the birth.

Mothers in this cohort reported that until the day they gave birth, they continued to cook, clean, sew, wash clothes, harvest and grind maize in a hand grinder, and haul water from the well. Several mothers mentioned that hauling water helped to move the baby into position for the birth, because the movement involved rotating their stomach and hips. Some elderly mothers suggested that their high activity levels and water-hauling prepared them for birth. They believe that birth was easier back then, and cesarean sections were therefore not needed.

The 12 women sampled in Cohort 1 collectively had 85 live births (mean = 7.08, SD = 1.62; range 5–10) (Table 11.3). Only one of these births occurred in a hospital, and none of the women had a cesarean birth (Tables 11.2 and 11.3). Women in Cohort 1 experienced an infant mortality rate of 47/1000 births (for all live births). All of the Cohort 1 mothers reported a strong preference for home births and vaginal births. The reason most commonly given is because they did not want to leave their other children behind. Among their final births, older women reported having family support at the

Table 11.3 Descriptive data (count and percent) for all count variables. Mothers in Cohorts 1, 2, and 3 are shown separately, along with results from the Pearson chi-square test. These data are drawn from maternal descriptions of their last birth only

	Cohort 1 (1950–1977)	Cohort 2 (1978–1999)	Cohort 3 (2000–2015)	Total	Pearson chi-square	*p*-value
N	12	22	22	56		
Husband present	9 (75%)	6 (27%)	3 (14%)	18 (32%)	13.799	0.001
Mother-in-law present	5 (42%)	2 (9%)	1 (4.5%)	8 (14%)	9.537	0.008
Mother present	4 (33%)	3 (14%)	0 (0%)	7 (13)	7.931	0.019
Cesarean birth (ever)	0 (0%)	8 (36%)	8 (36%)	16 (29%)	6.109	0.047
Birth complications	3 (25%)	11 (50%)	10 (45%)	24 (43%)	2.081	0.353
Episiotomy	0 (0%)	3 (14%)	13 (59%)	16 (29%)	17.245	<0.001
Tubal ligation	0 (0%)	12 (55%)	7 (32%)	19 (34%)	10.377	0.006
Bandages	12 (100%)	12 (55%)	15 (68%)	39 (70%)	9.581	0.048
Breastfeed	12 (100%)	22 (100%)	22 (100%)	56 (100%)	N/A	N/A
Colostrum	12 (100%)	22 (100%)	22 (100%)	56 (100%)	N/A	N/A
Formula	0 (0%)	9 (41%)	17 (77%)	26 (46%)	19.084	<0.001

time of birth: 75% had their husband present, 42% had their mother-in-law present, and 33% had their mother present at their last birth. However, one woman reported accidentally giving birth alone, with no complications.

Some Cohort 1 mothers (25%) reported having birth complications. One mother's baby was in the transverse position (Table 11.3). The midwife treated her with herbal teas and then performed a successful external cephalic version. Another mother reported an extremely long labor duration (7 days) that culminated in a live birth. During her long labor, the midwife did not leave her side and tried to accelerate the labor using herbal remedies. A third mother reported that she was not having contractions and therefore traveled to the hospital (in 1977). No doctor was working because it was Sunday, but a nurse gave her an injection to induce the contractions, and she eventually had a vaginal birth.

Three days after their last birth, all of the Cohort 1 mothers took a very hot bath with leaves of guava and orange trees, to help close the uterus and to make their breast milk come in. They rested in the house with the newborn on average for 10 days' post-birth before resuming their normal workloads (Tables 11.1 and 11.2). All of the Cohort 1 mothers participated in ritual binding with the midwife, in which cloths are tied around the woman's stomach to squeeze air out of the uterus. None of the Cohort 1 mothers had tubal ligation, and all reported having passed through menopause (Table 11.3).

All mothers in Cohort 1 reported breastfeeding immediately following the birth (Table 11.3). None used infant formula or nonhuman milks as an infant food, and many commented that they did not know that breast milk substitutes existed. They continued breastfeeding their lastborn children for 1–4 years (Tables 11.1 and 11.2). Common weaning foods used by mothers in this cohort were tortillas, chicken, and beans.

11.4 Cohort 2, 1978–1999: Laborsaving Technology and Energetic Transitions

The second time period is marked by the introduction of laborsaving technology, which affects women by reducing maternal work effort, with a consequent increase in fertility and rapid population growth (Kramer and McMillan 1999). As in many rural indigenous communities worldwide, one of the first modernizations to occur was the introduction of basic mechanized technology. In the late 1970s, a gas-powered mill (*molino*) and water pump were built in the village that markedly increased the efficiency with which maize could be ground and water collected. Water and ground maize are both crucial to daily Maya life and are produced exclusively by women. When using the laborsaving technologies, women worked on the order of two and a half fewer hours a day, a daily savings of an estimated 325 calories (Kramer and McMillan 1998, 1999). This savings is sufficient, for example, to satisfy the increase in energy expenditure required during the luteal phase of the menstrual cycle (Strassmann 1996).

Following the introduction of the pump and mill, age-at-first-birth among women who became mothers significantly declined from 21.2 to 19.5 years (Kramer and McMillan 1998, 1999). This decrease was linked to physiological and behavioral factors that affected the age at which young women reached maturity, left home, and married. A follow-up study showed that women in this cohort who started childbearing earlier went on to have larger families as compared to women who spent most of their childbearing years before the laborsaving technology was introduced (Kramer and McMillan 2006). Across this cohort, women who were 45 years and older and gave birth to their first child from 1978 to 2000 had an average completed fertility of 7.0 children (SD = 2.9 $n = 29$; surviving fertility mean = 6.8; SD = 2.6) (Table 11.1). In the decade between 1990 and 2000, the average annual growth rate was 3.1%, which compares to the fastest-growing regions of the world.

Besides the introduction of laborsaving technology, over the next 20 years, little else changed. Because of the long distances to commercial centers and the lack of vehicles, villagers still made their living as subsistence farmers and remained removed from much involvement in wage labor or the regional market economy. Of adults 18 years and older in 1992 ($n = 150$), only one was a full-time wage laborer. Women born between 1961 and 1982 who would have become first-time mothers during this cohort had on average 4.0 years of education (SD = 1.9, $n = 49$), a doubling of the previous cohort. Still, most of their adult lives were spent engaged in domestic tasks (Fig. 11.4).

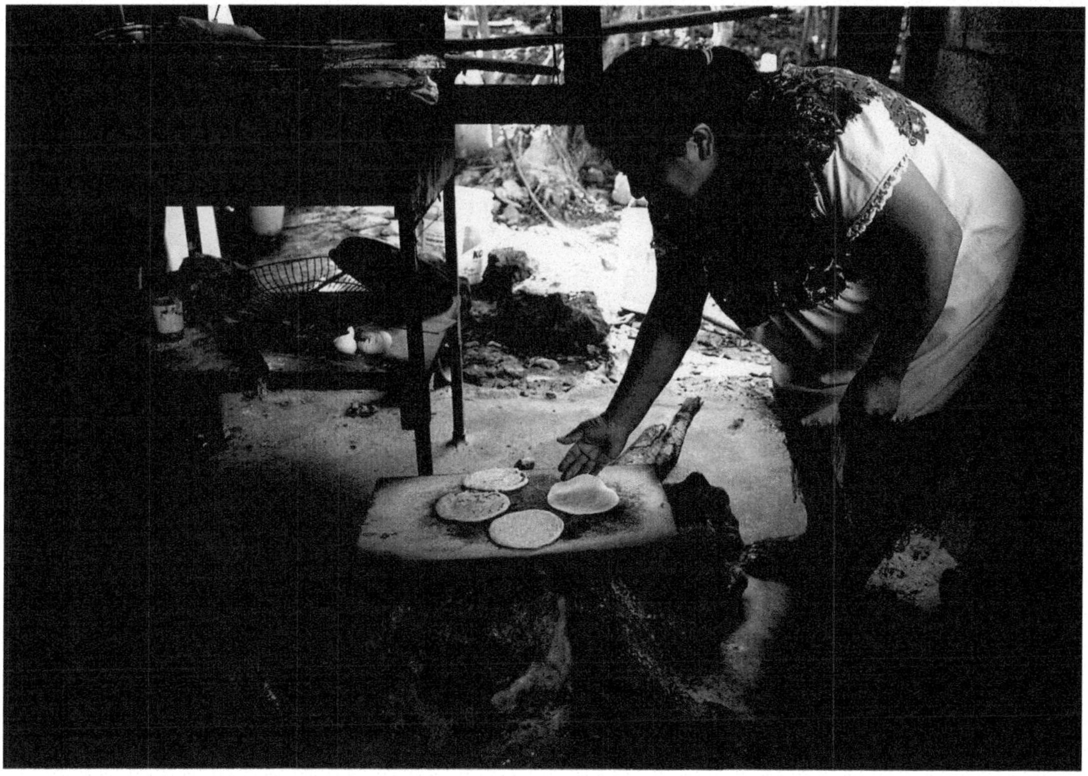

Fig. 11.4 A Maya woman cooks handmade tortillas (Photo by Rosy Garibay)

Each household grew most of the food that it consumed. Cash purchases of a few basic nonlocal goods (vegetable oil, candles, cloth, medicine, and metal tools) were made from the sale of honey or small quantities of maize. Otherwise, no cash crops were grown. Because vehicle access was rare, medical intervention was uncommon, though health-care providers did begin visiting the village sporadically in the 1980s to vaccinate children and were vigilant with cholera outbreaks (Sepulveda et al. 2006).

In 1998, electric lines were built connecting the village to a source of electric power. This provided illumination to every house, but additional laborsaving devices were not introduced until a decade later. A school with grades 1–9 was constructed in 1995. A rudimentary health clinic was built in the late 1990s, although it was not staffed with a health promoter until 2003.

11.4.1 Cohort 2: Pregnancy, Birth, and Babies

We interviewed 22 mothers from Cohort 2 (49% of all village women whose first birth fell between 1978 and 2000), and in this section, we report on this subsample of women only. The 22 mothers were born in years ranging from 1958 to 1982 (ages 32–56 in 2014). We group them into the same cohort because they had their first births between 1978 and 1999, when laborsaving technology was first introduced to the village.

Medical care access increased over time for mothers in this cohort. Some older mothers (14%) reported that they had never accessed health care for their children, and 23% reported that they took their children to a hospital or clinic in a nearby town or city when they were sick. A slightly younger group of mothers (27%) had some children who were born after the village health clinic was built in 1997. These mothers reported taking their children there; in addition, they visited hospitals or clinics in nearby towns or cities when their children were sick. Another group of women (27%) reported that they had taken their children to the village health clinic only. Despite these improvements, prenatal care became available to many Cohort 2 women only late in their reproductive careers, after the clinic was established. Recent interviews revealed that one maternal death occurred during this time period, while a mother pregnant with twins was being carried to the hospital. Neither child survived.

The Cohort 2 mothers in this sample collectively had 135 live births, a mean of 6.14 births per women (±2.77, range 2–11). Over a quarter of these births occurred in a hospital (28%) and 9% were by cesarean delivery (31% of hospital births were cesarean sections) (Tables 11.1 and 11.2). Nine mothers in this cohort reported a preference for hospital births (41%), because they perceived them to be safer. All mothers reported a preference for vaginal births. Women in this cohort experienced an infant mortality rate (IMR) of 37/1000 across their reproductive careers.

Among their final births, 73% occurred in a hospital, 23% occurred at home with a midwife, and one occurred in a truck on the way to the hospital. Some Cohort 2 mothers had no social support at the time of their last birth: 27% of mothers had their husband with them, 14% had their mother with them, and 9% had their mother-in-law with them (Table 11.3). Of the women who had family support at birth, five had homebirths and only one had a hospital birth.

Just under half of the Cohort 2 mothers (45%) reported having complications during their final birth (Table 11.3). Two had babies who were breech, and one resulted in a cesarean delivery. The other mother delivered vaginally after the doctor performed an external cephalic version. Another mother experienced postpartum hemorrhage following a hospital birth and underwent emergency surgery. Another mother experienced a cord prolapse, and following the birth, her infant was hospitalized for a long duration. Two mothers had infants with a transverse presentation, and one of the mothers also had high blood pressure. Both of these mothers subsequently had cesarean sections. Two mothers reported having no contractions. They were both injected with synthetic oxytocin to induce uterine contractions and eventually had vaginal births. One woman scheduled a cesarean delivery because she was past her due date, and another scheduled a cesarean delivery because she had had two cesarean sections previously.

Three days after their final births, 36% of Cohort 2 mothers participated in ritual postpartum bathing, and 64% participated in a postpartum massage and ritual binding under the care of a midwife. They reported resting in the house with the newborn on average for 60 days post-birth before resuming their normal workloads (Table 11.2). Over one-half of Cohort 2 women (55%) had tubal ligation following their last birth, while 27% reported having passed through menopause (Table 11.3).

All mothers in Cohort 2 reported breastfeeding following their last birth (Table 11.3). Timing of breastfeeding initiation was on average 7.6 h, with a range of 0–72 h. Two women delayed initiation for 3 days, one due to medical complications (following a cesarean delivery) and one because her milk had not yet come in. Several mothers reported providing formula to their infants (41%), but it was always used to augment, rather than replace, breast milk. Cohort 2 women breastfed their lastborn children for 1–3 years (Tables 11.1 and 11.2). Popular weaning foods among this cohort were *atole* (maize gruel), tortilla, chicken, beans, and crackers.

11.5 Cohort 3, 2000–2014: Increasing Modernization and Epidemiologic Transition

The third time period is marked by the construction of a paved road into the community in 2005, rapid epidemiologic changes, and further energetic changes. Downstream effects of the road on women's lives include increased access to contraception, medicalized birth, health care, government aid, education, and a further reduction in female energy expenditure due to mechanized farming. These changes expanded the potential for households to pursue different and new subsistence, education, and wage labor options, and economic inequality had become evident for the first time.

Shortly after the arrival of electricity, water lines were extended from the central pump to each house, further diminishing the time and energy women spent hauling water. Because many aspects of farming have become mechanized since 2001, women spend less time away from the village in fieldwork than previously (Cashdan et al. 2016). The most pronounced change in diet has been the increased consumption of soda, primarily by adults. Adult female (ages 20–40) BMI has increased from 24.8 (SD = 3.3, $n = 45$ in 1992) to 27.7 (SD = 3.9, $n = 55$ in 2010) in the past 20 years.

Women who were born between 1983 and 1997 and would have become first-time mothers during this cohort spent twice as long in school as the previous cohort (mean = 8.2 years, SD = 2.2, $n = 36$). Prior to the 2000s, female activities were exclusively centered in their homes and fields, and women and children were not involved in wage labor or any other income-producing enterprise. In 2002, following the devastation of Hurricane Isidora and the almost complete loss of crops, young women began working in wage labor for the first time, traveling 4 h each day to and from a *maquiladora* (a factory in Mexico, usually run by a foreign company) in the regional capital. Although some unmarried women may leave the village to work in wage labor jobs, mothers do not.

Women also began organizing into a number of cooperatives through bank and government loans. Some of these collectives have been successful; others have failed. In 2013, the first female craft cooperative operated at a profit. Wage labor has doubled in the last 20 years (from 3% to 6.2% of adults over the age of 18) but remains limited because of distances needed to travel to market towns and the perceived low monetary returns. Despite these changes, most households today still subsist on small-scale maize cultivation, growing most of the food they consume, and selling small quantities of corn and honey to purchase basic household goods. While many of the traditional thatched houses have been replaced by cinder block houses, the social structure of the community remains the same.

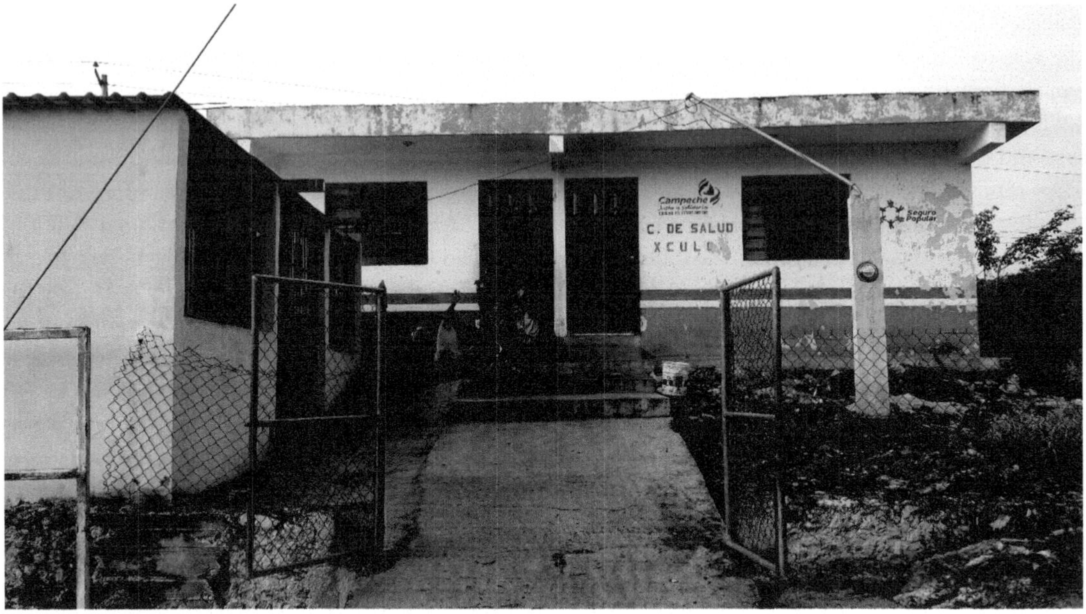

Fig. 11.5 The village clinic, ca. 2014 (Photo by Amanda Veile)

Families live in compounds that designate a commensal unit. As the Maya often say, "Those that sleep together, eat together and work together." Although women's lives are easier in many ways, all cooking is still done on hearths, often in groups enjoying the social company that it affords.

Women in this cohort had much greater access to government assistance programs, including Progresa (which was implemented in 1997 in some regions and replaced by Oportunidades in 2002). At the time of interview, 72% of Yucatec Maya families received Oportunidades benefits, which provide low-cost health care for pregnant women and children, health monitoring and education programs, and monthly cash stipends for Mexico's poorest families. The health clinic is now staffed by a local health promoter and a physician who visits bimonthly; however, it lacks basic equipment and often is not supplied with medicine and bandages (Fig. 11.5).

Birth has become increasingly medicalized among the Yucatec Maya. Although many women now opt to give birth in hospitals, one elderly midwife continues to work in the village (Veile and Kramer 2015). She participates in government-sponsored training sessions and reports her activities to the doctor. Many women still visit the midwife for prenatal massages. Birth control was introduced around 1997, most commonly as the tubal ligations performed after a hospitalized birth. By 2010, 24% (n = 104) of married women utilized fertility control.

11.5.1 Cohort 3: Pregnancy, Birth, and Babies

We interviewed 22 mothers from Cohort 3 (61% of all village women whose first birth occurred from 2001 to 2015), and in this section, we report on this subsample of women only. The 22 mothers were born in years ranging from 1966 to 1993 and had their first births between 2000 and 2015. In contrast to the mothers in Cohorts 1 and 2, their reproductive careers transpired during a period of epidemiologic transition (Figs. 11.6 and 11.7).

All of the mothers in Cohort 3 reported having access to health care when their children were sick. Several mothers (36%) reported that they only visited the village health clinic, 55% took

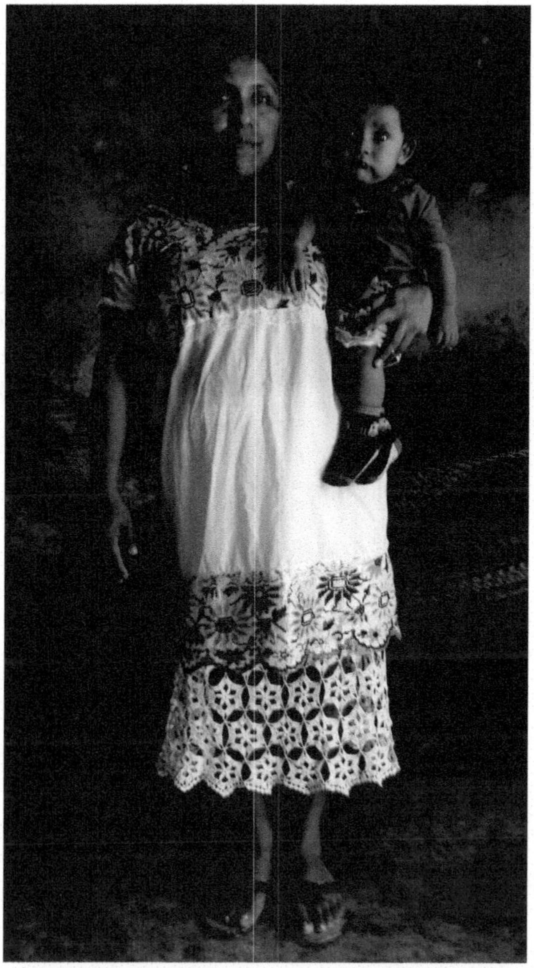

Fig. 11.6 Maya mother in traditional dress with infant (Photo by Amanda Veile)

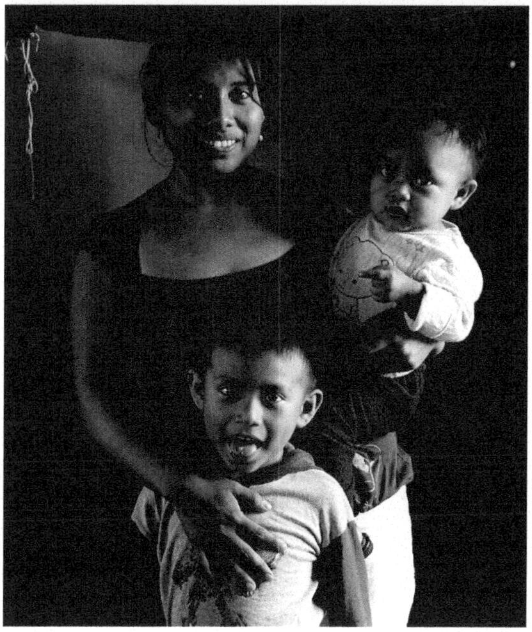

Fig. 11.7 Maya mother in modern dress, with young children (Photo by Rosy Garibay)

advantage of health-care services both in and out of the village, and only 9% of mothers reported not having accessed health care for their children. We have documented no maternal deaths from this time period.

Most of the Cohort 3 mothers benefited from prenatal care services that were (and continue to be) available at little or no cost from government health providers. Women are recommended to have five prenatal visits throughout the course of their pregnancy. For uncomplicated pregnancies, prenatal care visits occur in the village health clinic. When complications are detected, women are sent to nearby towns or cities for ultrasounds and tests.

Cohort 3 women collectively had 51 live births, 28% of which occurred in a hospital. For hospital births only, the cesarean section rate was 31% (Tables 11.1 and 11.2). Most mothers in this cohort (82%) reported a preference for hospital births, which they perceived to be safer. All mothers reported a preference for vaginal births. Women in this cohort experienced an infant mortality rate (IMR) of 39/1000 across their reproductive careers. We do not report on their total fertility here, because they are still in the midst of their reproductive careers.

Among their final births (n = 22), 91% occurred in a hospital and 9% occurred at home with a midwife (Table 11.1). The majority of Cohort 2 mothers reported having no social support at the time of their last birth. Only three mothers had their husband present, none had their mother present, and one had her mother-in-law present. Of the women who had family support at birth, one had a hospital birth and two had homebirths.

Nearly half of the Cohort 3 women (45%) reported having health complications associated with their last pregnancy or birth (Table 11.3). All of the complicated births occurred in a hospital setting. One mother had a baby who was in the breech position, which resulted in a cesarean delivery. Three mothers reported that their labors did not progress, all of these resulted in cesarean sections. One mother was diagnosed with gestational diabetes, but she was able to deliver vaginally. Three mothers were diagnosed with high blood pressure; one resulted in a cesarean delivery, while the other two delivered vaginally. One mother was hospitalized for a week postpartum due to a retained placenta. Another mother was hospitalized for a prolonged period when her episiotomy became infected.

Three days after their final births, only 18% of Cohort 3 mothers participated in ritual postpartum bathing, and 68% participated in a postpartum massage and ritual binding under the care of a midwife. They reported resting on average for 70 days post-birth before resuming their normal workloads (Tables 11.1 and 11.2). Nearly one-third of Cohort 3 women (32%) had a tubal ligation, and none had yet passed through menopause (Table 11.3).

All mothers in Cohort 3 reported breastfeeding following their last birth, though many reported having breastfeeding complications (Table 11.3). Timing of breastfeeding initiation was on average 38.2 h, with a range of 1 h to 4 months. Two mothers reported unusual breastfeeding complications. After being hospitalized due to her infected episiotomy, one lost her milk supply, and she was unable to breastfeed her infant beyond 2 days. The other mother was separated from her infant for 4 months when he was hospitalized after swallowing meconium. Using an herbal remedy (earthworm ground in *atole*), she reports being able to successfully initiate breastfeeding 4 months after birth.

Most mothers (77%) in Cohort 3 reported providing formula to their infants (Table 11.3). With one exception (as we described, a mother who could not breastfeed beyond 2 days), infant formula was used to augment, rather than replace, breast milk. Cohort 3 women report breastfeeding their lastborn children from 1 to 6 years (Tables 11.1 and 11.2). Popular weaning foods among this cohort were *atole*, tortilla, chicken, beans, crackers, and applesauce.

11.6 Pregnancy, Birth, and Babies in Transition: Changes over Time

We have documented a number of changes in birthing practices in Xculoc over the last 65 years. Based on interviews with 56 women, we find that the average number of hospital births per mother increased across the three cohorts, with statistically significant differences between Cohort 1 and the two later cohorts. We see a non-statistically significant but compelling increase in reported last birth complications (25% from 1950 to 1977 to nearly 50% from 1978 to 2014), with subsequent increases in episiotomies, tubal ligations, and postpartum rest periods.

Birth complications and interventions may increase following the shift from upright laboring (while squatting or while sitting in a hammock as per traditional Maya homebirth practices) to the hospital-dictated lithotomy position. Supine positions like the lithotomy compress female pelvic bony dimensions, which may unnecessarily complicate labor and delivery (De Jonge et al. 2004; Michel et al. 2002). Birth complications may also increase as the intrapartum social environment changes. When mothers give birth at home, husbands and female kin are often nearby and provide social support at the time of the birth. In contrast, we find that family members are typically not permitted to accompany the laboring mother in hospital settings. As suggested by other studies, Maya hospital birth outcomes might improve if laboring mothers had family members or hospital-appointed doulas to support them (Klaus et al. 1986; Langer et al. 1998).

We have documented a trend toward longer postpartum rest periods, with statistically significant differences between Cohort 1 and the two later cohorts. Younger women may report an inflated period of rest, especially after a cesarean birth, to some extent. Doctors recommend a 6-month rest period for mothers following a cesarean section, and this was the rest period that many reported. We do not know the extent to which mothers in fact adhered to this recommendation. Still, a number of women reported being unable to do heavy work for 6 months to a year following a cesarean section.

This trend exemplifies a broader suite of shifting beliefs and perceptions regarding pregnancy and birth. In general, older Yucatec Maya women report having "easy births" and fairly short postpartum rest periods. The oldest women are considered to have been stronger (during their childbearing years) than reproductive-aged women are now, because they engaged in heavy agricultural and domestic labor across the duration of their pregnancies. Villagers believe that young mothers today are not as strong and fit for pregnancy as were their grandmothers. As a result, many villagers (including young mothers) believe that today's reproductive-aged women require extensive rest while pregnant and during the postpartum period. Many villagers even believe that Maya mothers today *require* assistance while giving birth, in the form of medical interventions such as episiotomies, synthetic oxytocin, and cesarean sections.

11.6.1 The Resilience of Some Traditional Practices

Despite the many changes associated with the medicalization of birth, Yucatec Maya women still adhere to many traditional practices. For example, a number of women still visit the village midwife for prenatal and postnatal care. All mothers report a strong preference for vaginal births, even though elective cesarean sections have become fashionable in some parts of the country (Gonzalez-Perez et al. 2001). Although adherence to postpartum rituals has fluctuated over the last 65 years, we find that many younger women still participated in bathing and binding following their most recent births. Not surprisingly, mothers who gave birth since 1978 (Cohorts 2 and 3) are less likely to engage in these practices following a highly complicated, medicalized birth or cesarean section delivery.

One important finding is that Yucatec Maya mothers largely adhere to traditional breastfeeding and weaning practices, despite broader trends toward decreased breastfeeding among indigenous women across Mexico (de Cossío et al. 2013). All Yucatec Maya mothers recognize the benefits of colostrum and breast milk, and all 56 mothers breastfed for some duration. All mothers initiated breastfeeding immediately after birth if they were able, and many continued to breastfeed for 1–2 years or more. Except for the recent introduction of formula (~12 years ago), weaning foods remained fairly traditional and consistent over the last 65 years.

Though increasing numbers of women do report feeding their infants formula, it occurs under limited circumstances and most commonly within the hospital setting. For example, infants may be fed formula in the hospital if the mother and infant are separated due to medical complications or if the mother's milk has not come in. In general, infant formula augments rather than replaces breast milk. Mothers who are capable of breastfeeding report formula feeding for very short periods of time (sometimes at a doctor's recommendation). Many mothers claim that the cost of formula is prohibitive; others report that their infants had a strong preference for breast milk.

Even when they experienced birth and breastfeeding complications, the Yucatec Maya mothers were determined to breastfeed. To illustrate this, we will describe the experience of a mother using the pseudonym Maria, who gave birth in 2005. Maria could not breastfeed her baby for 4 months while the baby was hospitalized. Still, Maria resolved to maintain her milk supply and received a traditional remedy (earthworms ground in *atole*) from her mother. Even though 4 months had passed, Maria was able to breastfeed when she was reunited with her infant. She credits her mother with providing her the remedy and is grateful because she recognizes the benefits of breastfeeding for infant health. Maria is also thankful that her mother saved her from the expense from having to purchase formula and powdered milks for 2 years.

11.7 Maternal-Infant Mortality Trends Across Cohorts

11.7.1 Infant Mortality

Despite the recent medicalization of birthing practices, we find that the rate of infant mortality has not significantly changed in the last 65 years. This is unexpected because hospital births are introduced with the goal of improving mother-infant health outcomes. Furthermore, Mexico's national infant mortality declined during that time and was just 12.5/1000 in 2013. Despite these trends, and despite having more access to biomedical obstetrical care than the previous two cohorts, we find that infant mortality for Cohort 3 women (first birth from 2000 to 2014) was 39/1000. This IMR is comparable to the Mexican national rate of 3.7% in 1990, before several health care initiatives were launched.

Although the current mortality rate is over three times higher than the Mexican national rate, this may not have always been the case. From 1950 to 1974, Mexico's national IMR averaged 92/1000, whereas during the same time period, Cohort 1 women had an IMR of 47/1000. From 1975 to 1999, Mexico's national IMR averaged 44/1000, compared to Cohort 2's IMR of 37/1000. From 2000 to 2015, Mexico's national IMR averaged 20/1000, compared to Cohort 3's IMR of 39/1000. This suggests that the infant mortality rate in Xculoc was actually lower than the Mexican national IMR until recently. The recent shift may be due to advanced and specialized medical care that is more accessible to mothers in densely populated urban centers.

We emphasize that the Yucatec Maya IMRs we report from 1950 to 2015 are quite low in comparison to many other traditional farming and foraging societies worldwide (Volk and Atkinson 2013), even before biomedical care became available. Though we are currently analyzing just a subset of Yucatec Maya mothers, our ongoing demographic research suggests that infant mortality has historically been low for a number of reasons. We now consider these in turn.

First, we consider the Maya practice of midwifery. As we (and others) have described, a designated midwife would provide comprehensive prenatal and postnatal care in addition to assistance with the birth itself. Mothers also had the support of family members (husbands, mothers, and mothers-in-law) throughout the birthing process. Although traditional midwives did not receive formal medical training (until recently) and generally do not use medical equipment, they are often reported to have been quite capable and successfully managed all but the most complicated of births. For example, in our interviews of Yucatec Maya women, we find that midwives successfully performed external cephalic versions and accelerated stalled labors using traditional remedies.

In stark contrast to the traditional Maya midwifery practices, hospital births are isolating and stressful. Mothers report that hospital births are associated with more complications and interventions. In our interviews, interventions were associated with reduced breastfeeding success and poor mother-infant health outcomes, such as prolonged hospitalizations due to infections. While some interventions are undoubtedly medically necessary, there is growing concern that cesareans and episiotomies may be performed in excess in vMexico (Farland 2009; Gonzalez-Perez et al. 2001; Yam et al. 2007).

The second point we make is that breastfeeding practices have changed little over time, which has had a positive influence on infant health. During the first 6 months of a child's life, Yucatec Maya infants are breastfed on demand, and mothers and babies are nearly inseparable. Although some mothers do formula feed, as described, they do so in limited contexts. Babies are fed complementary foods by 4–6 months of age, and on average, they are fully weaned at age two and a half (Veile et al. 2014). The Maya practice of prolonged and intensive breastfeeding undoubtedly buffers young infants from infectious disease. Furthermore, the Yucatan region has a strong indigenous medical tradition of *curanderismo* (Gubler 2011; Huber and Sandstrom 2010). A *curandero* lived in the community until the 1980s, and many villagers continue to be well informed about the medicinal uses of forest plants.

A final point we make is that clean drinking water is available and protects young children from many otherwise common sources of health insults. As there are no rivers or other running surface water in most of Yucatan, drinking water historically was drawn from natural limestone basins. For the past century, drinking water was procured from a closed well in the Yucatec Maya study community. The risk of contaminated water and gastrointestinal disease is therefore attenuated in this area of the Yucatan. Furthermore, contagious diseases are rare because the community is geographically remote and the Puuc region has a low population density. Cholera affected Mexico in the 1990s, but southern Yucatan was not affected, and there have been no cases in the Yucatan Peninsula since 2002 (Sepulveda et al. 2006). Although child mortality may have been relatively low in the Yucatan for some time, immunization programs began in the 1980s and have no doubt produced further gains in infant and child survival.

11.7.2 Maternal Mortality

Extensive demographic interviews with villagers, and conversations with the elderly midwife, have yielded a very small number of maternal deaths in the Yucatec Maya community over the last 65 years. It appears that maternal mortality rates have dropped since birth became increasingly medicalized, which is consistent with declines at the national level (Hogan et al. 2010). However, some women in Cohorts 2 and 3 have not yet completed their reproductive careers and cannot be included in an analysis. The sample of maternal deaths we report ($n = 3$ from 1950 to 1977, $n = 1$ from 1978 to 1999, $n = 0$ from 2000 to 2014) is not large or complete enough to analyze statistically in its current form. Despite these caveats and limitations, we suspect that maternal mortality has been fairly low in this Yucatec Maya community for some time, for several of the reasons we described above.

Conclusions

Mexico and several other Latin American countries have developed innovative programs to support and improve population health, even in their poorest communities (Atun et al. 2015; Frenk 2015). While largely beneficial, one consequence of these programs is the increasing medicalization of birth. In one Yucatec Maya community, we find that maternal birth experiences have changed dramatically as traditional midwifery has been gradually replaced by the biomedical obstetric model. This is accompanied by a transformation in Maya beliefs and practices regarding pregnancy, birth, and babies. It is crucial to support the maintenance of beneficial traditional birthing and breastfeeding practices in rural, indigenous communities while at the same time considering the potentially detrimental effects of unnecessary medical interventions. Systematic documentation of birthing practices is therefore needed as the global medicalization of birth proceeds.

References

Abrams, E. T., & Rutherford, J. N. (2011). Framing postpartum hemorrhage as a consequence of human placental biology: an evolutionary and comparative perspective. *American Anthropologist, 113*(3), 417–430.

Atun, R., De Andrade, L. O. M., Almeida, G., Cotlear, D., Dmytraczenko, T., Frenz, P., et al. (2015). Health-system reform and universal health coverage in Latin America. *Lancet, 385*(9974), 1230–1247.

Barber, S. L. (2010). Mexico's conditional cash transfer programme increases cesarean section rates among the rural poor. *European Journal of Public Health, 20*(4), 383–388.

Berry, N. S. (2013). *Unsafe motherhood: Mayan maternal mortality and subjectivity in post-war Guatemala*. New York: Berghahn.

Cashdan, E., Kramer, K. L., Davis, H. E., Padilla, L., & Greaves, R. D. (2016). Mobility and navigation among the Yucatec Maya. *Human Nature, 27*(1), 35–50.

Cosminsky, S. (1982). Childbirth and change: a Guatemalan study. In C. P. MacCormack (Ed.), *Ethnography of fertility and birth (205–229)*. New York: Academic Press.

Davis-Floyd, R. E., & Sargent, C. (1997). *Childbirth and authoritative knowledge: Cross-cultural perspectives*. Berkeley: University of California Press.

de Cossío, T. G., Escobar-Zaragoza, L., González-Castell, D., Reyes-Vázquez, H., & Rivera-Dommarco, J. A. (2013). Breastfeeding in Mexico was stable, on average, but deteriorated among the poor, whereas complementary feeding improved: results from the 1999 to 2006 National Health and Nutrition Surveys. *Journal of Nutrition, 143*(5), 664–671.

De Jonge, A., Teunissen, T., & Lagro-Janssen, A. (2004). Supine position compared to other positions during the second stage of labor: a meta-analytic review. *Journal of Psychosomatic Obstetrics and Gynecology, 25*(1), 35–45.

Dewey, K. G., Nommsen-Rivers, L. A., Heinig, M. J., & Cohen, R. J. (2003). Risk factors for suboptimal infant breastfeeding behavior, delayed onset of lactation, and excess neonatal weight loss. *Pediatrics, 112*(3), 607–619.

Dunsworth, H. M., Warrener, A. G., Deacon, T., Ellison, P. T., & Pontzer, H. (2012). Metabolic hypothesis for human altriciality. *Proceedings of the National Academy of Sciences, 109*(38), 15212–15216.

Farland, L. (2009). The use and overuse of cesarean sections in Mexico. *TuftScope, 9*(1), 30–33.

Frenk, J. (2015). Leading the way towards universal health coverage: a call to action. *Lancet, 385*(9975), 1352–1358.

Gonzalez-Perez, G. J., Vega-Lopez, M. G., Cabrera-Pivaral, C., Muñoz, A., & Valle, A. (2001). Caesarean sections in Mexico: are there too many? *Health Policy and Planning, 16*(1), 62–67.

Gubler, R. (2011). La medicina tradicional en Yucatán: elementos y entes sagrados que intervienen en la curación. *Itinerarios, 14*, 185–211.

Hogan, M. C., Foreman, K. J., Naghavi, M., Ahn, S. Y., Wang, M., Makela, S. M., et al. (2010). Maternal mortality for 181 countries, 1980–2008: a systematic analysis of progress towards Millennium Development Goal 5. *Lancet, 375*(9726), 1609–1623.

Huber, B. R., & Sandstrom, A. R. (2010). *Mesoamerican healers*. Austin: University of Texas Press.

Jordan, B., & Davis-Floyd, R. (1993). *Birth in Four Cultures: A Crosscultural Investigation of Childbirth in Yucatan, Holland, Sweden, and the United States*. Long Grove, IL: Waveland Press.

Klaus, M. H., Kennell, J. H., Robertson, S. S., & Sosa, R. (1986). Effects of social support during parturition on maternal and infant morbidity. *British Medical Journal (Clin Res Ed), 293*(6547), 585–587.

Kramer, K. (2005). *Maya Children: Helpers at the Farm*. Cambridge, MA: Harvard University Press.

Kramer, K., & Boone, J. (2002). Why intensive agriculturalists have higher fertility: a household energy budget approach. *Current Anthropology, 43*(3), 511–517.

Kramer, K., & McMillan, G. (2006). The effect of labor-saving technology on longitudinal fertility changes. *Current Anthropology, 47*(1), 165–172.

Kramer, K. L., & McMillan, G. P. (1998). How Maya women respond to changing technology. *Human Nature, 9*(2), 205–223.

Kramer, K. L., & McMillan, G. P. (1999). Women's labor, fertility, and the introduction of modern technology in a rural Maya village. *Journal of Anthropological Research, 55*(4), 499–520.

Langer, A., Campero, L., Garcia, C., & Reynoso, S. (1998). Effects of psychosocial support during labour and childbirth on breastfeeding, medical interventions, and mothers' wellbeing in a Mexican public hospital: a randomised clinical trial. *British Journal of Obstetrics & Gynecology, 105*(10), 1056–1063.

Lee, R. D., & Kramer, K. L. (2002). Children's economic roles in the Maya family life cycle: Cain, Caldwell, and Chayanov revisited. *Population and Development Review, 28*(3), 475–499.

Michel, S. C., Rake, A., Treiber, K., Seifert, B., Chaoui, R., Huch, R., et al. (2002). MR obstetric pelvimetry: effect of birthing position on pelvic bony dimensions. *American Journal of Roentgenology, 179*(4), 1063–1067.

Rosenberg, K., & Trevathan, W. (1995). Bipedalism and human birth: The obstetrical dilemma revisited. *Evolutionary Anthropology: Issues, News, and Reviews, 4*(5), 161–168.

Sepulveda, J., Valdespino, J. L., & Garcia-Garcia, L. (2006). Cholera in Mexico: the paradoxical benefits of the last pandemic. *International Journal of Infectious Diseases, 10*(1), 4–13.

Stone, P. K. (2016). Biocultural perspectives on maternal mortality and obstetrical death from the past to the present. *American Journal of Physical Anthropology, 159*(S61), S150–S171.

Strassmann, B. I. (1996). The evolution of endometrial cycles and menstruation. *QUARTERLY REVIEW OF BIOLOGY, 71*(2), 181–220.

Torri, M. C. (2012). Traditional midwives in Tamaulipas: The difficult negotiation between traditional child-birth knowledge & the biomedical system in Mexico. *Women's Health and Urban Life, 11*(2), 42–63.

Trevathan, W. R. (1996). The evolution of bipedalism and assisted birth. *Medical Anthropology Quarterly, 10*(2), 287–290.

Trevathan, W. R. (2011). *Human birth: An evolutionary perspective: Piscataway*. NJ: Transaction Publishers.

Veile, A., & Kramer, K. (2015). Birth and breastfeeding dynamics in a modernizing indigenous community. *Journal of Human Lactation, 31*(1), 145–155.

Veile, A., & Kramer, K. L. (2016). Childhood body mass is positively associated with cesarean birth in Yucatec Maya subsistence farmers. *American Journal of Human Biology., 29*(2). https://doi.org/10.1002/ajhb.22920

Veile, A. J., Kramer, K. L., & Otarola-Castillo, E. R. (2014). *Early childhood in Yucatec Maya subsistence agriculturalists* (pp. 260–260). Hoboken, NJ: Wiley-Blackwell.

Vogel, J. P., Betrán, A. P., Vindevoghel, N., Souza, J. P., Torloni, M. R., Zhang, J., et al. (2015). Use of the Robson classification to assess caesarean section trends in 21 countries: a secondary analysis of two WHO multicountry surveys. *Lancet Global Health, 3*(5), e260–e270.

Volk, A. A., & Atkinson, J. A. (2013). Infant and child death in the human environment of evolutionary adaptation. *Evolution and Human Behavior, 34*(3), 182–192.

Yam, E. A., Grossman, A. A., Goldman, L. A., & García, S. G. (2007). Introducing birth plans in Mexico: an exploratory study in a hospital serving low income Mexicans. *Birth, 34*(1), 42–48.

Social Support and Social Suffering: Uterine Health and *Isihuayo* Among Indigenous Women in Mexico

12

Vania Smith-Oka and Maryam Rokhideh

12.1 Introduction

In this chapter we discuss the ethnomedical condition of displaced uterus (*isihuayo*), which shares many elements with the biomedical condition of prolapsed uterus.[1] *Isihuayo* contains local elements and interpretations that extend beyond the physical nature of the body. For the Nahua women whose stories we share here, *isihuayo* is a symptom of broader destabilization within their lives, expressed bodily in their uterus. This illness has shaped women's identities and how they interact with their changing world, reflecting their complicated relationship with the broader political, economic, and social forces of the Mexican state.

The lives of indigenous women in Mexico are marked by perceptions of vulnerability and weakness as well as real corporeal hardship. Among the rural Nahua of eastern Mexico, women's bodies are perceived to be vulnerable (like the Andean *debilidad*), which is attributed to the physical makeup of a woman's body, especially in regard to her reproductive system. Local perceptions view the reproductive life cycle as physically draining and wreaking havoc on a woman's body, greatly affecting her *fuerza*—her strength or bodily vigor (see also Tapias 2006). The repeated loss of menstrual blood, pregnancy, childbirth, breastfeeding, and childcare are perceived causes of this weakness (see Larme 1998 and Oths 1999 for examples in the Andes). Bodily equilibrium, a balance between hot and cold states, is also central to the Nahua understanding of female body health. Women are perceived to lose heat through blood loss during menstruation and childbirth, weakening their body and making them vulnerable to other conditions (Santos-Torres and Vásquez-Garibay 2003; Groark 2005). Our findings show that older women are especially vulnerable and more likely to experience *isihuayo* than younger women, oftentimes due to differing degrees of social support they receive as they deal with the various hardships they experience.

The women of this study have bodies that must be able to withstand hard physical labor due to a lifestyle of exertion that is common to rural, agricultural communities; yet they must also fit into a

[1]Much of the data for this chapter has appeared previously in the following article: Fallen Uterus: Social Suffering, Bodily Vigor, and Social Support Among Women in Rural Mexico. *Medical Anthropology Quarterly*, 28(1), 105–121.

V. Smith-Oka, Ph.D. (✉) • M. Rokhideh, M.A.
Department of Anthropology, University of Notre Dame, Notre Dame, IN, USA
e-mail: vsmithok@nd.edu

D. A. Schwartz (ed.), *Maternal Death and Pregnancy-Related Morbidity Among Indigenous Women of Mexico and Central America*, Global Maternal and Child Health: Medical, Anthropological, and Public Health Perspectives, https://doi.org/10.1007/978-3-319-71538-4_12

mold that is yielding to state directives—in their various social, political, or medical forms. Caught in a system intent on the development of indigenous populations, the older women have an uneasy relationship with larger Mexico. Most are enrolled in a state-sponsored conditional cash transfer program called *Prospera* (formerly Oportunidades) that requires them to participate actively in biomedical health-care centers (Smith-Oka 2013).

Prospera is the largest social program Mexico has ever run, enrolling almost one-third of the country's population, specifically targeting those who are the most impoverished. The federal government disburses money every 2 months to enrolled mothers for their children's health, nutrition, and education. The amount families receive depends on the age and sex of the child (girls and older school age children receive more). This can sometimes constitute more than 60% of the family's income (Smith-Oka 2013). However, as part of the conditions of the program, women and their families are required to receive health care from clinicians at the medical centers (Gil-García 2015). Within this biomedical system, clinicians are authorized to supervise women's compliance with the program's conditions while simultaneously extending their medical viewpoints and agendas upon their patients, leaving little room for alternatives such as traditional birth attendants (TBAs) or other forms of reproductive care. If women do not comply with *Prospera*, they risk being removed from the program, thus risking the substantial monetary benefits that come with it. By granting clinicians significant power over their patients' lives (medically and economically), this arrangement places women in a precarious position where their welfare is tied to the demands of the state (Smith-Oka 2013).

Prospera elucidates much on the political, institutional, and economic forces that shape the everyday lives of indigenous people. Applying a social suffering framework demonstrates how institutional and state pressures like *Prospera* shape the everyday lives of women, causing and exacerbating problems they face. In this chapter, we focus on the ways that older Nahua women (above the age of 45) bodily experience these transformations. We extend the arguments made by other scholars (Rock 2003; Tapias 2006) who have illustrated the effect of larger political and economic forces on people's biologies, anxieties, and fears. We show that social suffering is a bodily expression of people's experiences with macroforces; such suffering goes beyond a straightforward epidemiological disease and becomes an expression of larger issues that shape and constrain already marginalized people's health. Building on these dialogues, we argue that for indigenous Nahua women, *isihuayo* is not simply synonymous with prolapse but a lived expression of their social suffering historically and socially manifest as extensive labor, a culmination of life stressors, and dwindling degrees of social support.

The Nahua women in this study must therefore manage and adapt to a changing world both at the macrolevel (institutional pressures) and the microlevel (a lack of social support) and the in-between, what is referred to as failed sociality (Tapias 2006). We show in this chapter that failed sociality connects the social suffering and social support literature. It thus becomes central to any study that examines the interplay between local biologies (Lock 1993) and broader sociopolitical and economic worlds.

12.2 The Nahua People

Mexico usually enumerates populations by the languages they speak, not by self-identification. In 2006, 10 years before the writing of this chapter, Mexico had slightly over 10 million indigenous people nationwide, which was, at that time, approximately 10% of the population (CDI 2006a). By 2016 the percentage had dropped to approximately 6.5%, which accounted for the portion of the population who spoke an indigenous language (INEGI 2016). Yet, curiously, the same 2016 data states that approximately 24.4% of Mexico's population self-identifies as indigenous, which is three times as many as those who speak the language. In 2010, the state of Veracruz (where this research took place) had about 356,000 people who spoke Nahuatl, which is just over 50 percent of the indigenous population of the state (INEGI 2010). This rate has remained quite steady over the past decade and a half.

It is well known that in Mexico, indigenous people's access to educational, political, and health institutions is lower than that of the mainstream population. A national demographic survey estimated that on average indigenous women married younger (18 years), had a lower rate of contraceptive use (59%), and had a higher fecundity rate (2.98) than mestizo women (20 years, 73%, and 2.17, respectively) (INEGI 2016).

The Nahua are the largest indigenous group in Mexico, making up approximately a quarter of the indigenous population (INEGI 2016). They inhabit a wide swath across the central Mexican states from the Gulf coast to the Pacific coast. They are the linguistic descendants of the Aztecs and speak Nahuatl. Nahuatl belongs to the Uto-Aztecan language family, one of the largest language families in the Americas, which includes languages such as Hopi, Ute, and Comanche among US Native Americans (among others) and Tarahumara and Huichol among indigenous Mexicans (among others). A vast majority of towns and villages as well as rivers and mountains across central Mexico have Nahuatl (and Nahuatl-inspired) names, such as Citlaltepetl (Mexico's highest volcano, meaning "starry mountain"), Chapultepec (Mexico City's largest park, meaning "grasshopper hill"), Mazatlán and Acapulco (beaches on the Pacific coast, meaning "place of the deer" and "place where the reeds were destroyed," respectively), and Xochimilco (the Aztec floating gardens in Mexico City, meaning "field of flowers"), among many others.

The Aztecs ruled central Mexico until the arrival of the Spaniards in 1519. This colonization destroyed the existing culture, decimated the population, and radically shifted the loci of power away from the hands of the native populations to those of the European outsiders. This power dynamic has not changed since the Spanish conquest and is the primary structural factor that has shaped the educational, economic, and linguistic capital of indigenous communities across Mexico. The indigenous population has historically been viewed as a stumbling block to development and modernization. The Mexican state thus sought to find ways to integrate and eradicate indigeneity for the perceived "racial welfare" of the nation. The primary goal became to integrate the indigenous populations into the national ethos and make them part of the modernizing state. The indigenous problem was thus viewed as a national problem (see Smith-Oka 2013 for more detailed information on this topic).

There are different variations of Nahua customs across Mexico. The population is spread across central Mexico into small, distinct pockets surrounded by mainstream, mestizo Mexico. In the Huasteca region, where this research took place, there are more shared customs and social mores, which includes cosmology, the making and eating of *zacahuil* (a very large tamal used for feasts), as well as a musical style called the *son huasteco* that combines fiddle and guitar. There has been a remarkable preservation of ancient forms of medicine in this area, which is reflected in widely shared cultural patterns that cross both ethnic and language barriers. The use of ancient forms of healing and religious rites shows the long withstanding cultural roots that can be traced to pre-Hispanic times. For instance, some of the rituals witnessed today are similar to the Tlazolteotl cult of the fifteenth-century Mexico (Alan R. Sandstrom, personal communication 2005). The Huasteca region has been characterized by religious and healing rituals to the spirits of the pantheon, which are used to effect cures. Spirits were considered the cause of illness and other unfortunate events in people's lives, and they had to be appeased (Sandstrom 1991). The cutting of paper into the anthropomorphic shapes of these spirits was one of the elements of these rituals. By appeasing the spirits with offerings of food, drink, tobacco, and blood from chickens or turkeys, the spirits would leave the person alone and that person would eventually regain his or her health and well-being. A ritual specialist called a *curandero* ("healer") in Spanish or a *tlamatiquetl* ("person of knowledge") in Nahuatl would carry out these rituals, (Sandstrom 1991). Many of the female *tlamatiquetls* also serve as midwives, attending to the female population we discuss in this chapter.

12.3 *Isihuayo*: A Condition of Uterine Displacement

Juana was a garrulous and fast-talking woman whose voice often shifted into a high falsetto when she became animated. During one long conversation in her home, she spoke about her last pregnancy and the troubles she had experienced:

> I was just walking back [from the clinic]. I did not fall or hit myself or anything. But as we carry so many heavy things. [...] It was very hot [...] and I felt I was dying. We were walking up the hill and I felt my uterus fall. I could feel the blood come out and it hurt a lot. That is why I went to [the *partera*[2]] over there to cure it. She gave me herbs and thank God I was cured and did not miscarry.

Juana was referring to a condition that the Nahua call *isihuayo*. *Isihuayo* is the Nahuatl term used in this region to describe the "female part." The *isihuayo* is an organ situated in the lower torso of a woman and is believed to have roots radiating out from it. *Isihuayo* was historically used to describe a specific part of the woman's body (López Austin 1988). However, over the last few years in this region—especially with the increasing contact the women have had with biomedicine—*isihuayo* is frequently synonymous with two other thoracic organs: *matriz* (uterus) and *vejiga* (bladder).

Isihuayo is an ethnomedical category of illness with local cultural and biological characteristics.[3] It is an illness of organ displacement (see Castañeda et al. 1996; Fuller and Jordan 1981; Hinojosa 2008). In this illness category, specific organs or parts of the body shift from their original position and cause health problems. It shares many of the latter characteristics with the biomedical condition of prolapsed uterus (Doshani et al. 2007). The biomedical symptoms for prolapsed uterus include discomfort while urinating, urinary incontinence, constipation, backache, and a lump that projects outside of the vagina (Doshani et al. 2007). One nurse stated, "[Women] have [prolapse] from having too many children; the ligaments begin to come away with so many pregnancies... There is no pain. They feel that something has fallen [inside], or they sometimes feel they cannot urinate or [have] a urinary infection." While prolapsed uterus is a condition identified and treated by biomedicine, *isihuayo* differs from prolapse in its etiology and treatment.

Abdominal and navel pain are central symptoms of *isihuayo*—primarily caused by the roots radiating out of the thoracic region (see López Austin 1988:167), which cause pain to envelop the lower body. One woman, Enriqueta, stated, "It fell a lot when I was pregnant with this [second child]. I could feel it when I moved. I came to Lourdes so she could massage me. That's how it was." Refugio, a very sought-after TBA, confirmed the etiology of *isihuayo*. She said about one of her patients, "They say she carries too many buckets and containers of water. And she came to me and said she has pain here [belly] and that is why I massaged her."

The women spoke of various treatments for the illness, from massages by a TBA to medicinal plants and to the use of biomedical techniques (medications or surgery). Altagracia, who had experienced such a severe case of *isihuayo* that she underwent a hysterectomy in Mexico City, commented:

> [Juana] said that [...] just by taking a plant she got better. [...] But that plant is far away and none grow near here. It is difficult to go for it. Her husband helped her [to get it]. [...] She said that just with that she got better, that the [uterus] lifted back [into place]. But the doctor says that nothing will cure it; that neither massages nor plants work. [He says] only surgery works.

---

[2] *Partera* is the Spanish name for traditional birth attendant.

[3] This particular illness is known in other parts of Mesoamerica as caída de matriz, baja de matriz, or caída de vejiga (Cosminsky 2001).

In the next few sections, we discuss the factors that shaped women's experiences with uterine ill health, particularly highlighting the effects of bodily vigor and social support. The former was often considered an underlying factor of *isihuayo*, while the latter was a contributing force in its prolongation.

12.4 Northern Veracruz: The Village of Amatlán

Amatlán is located in the northern region of the Mexican state of Veracruz (see Map, Fig. 12.1). This is a beautiful region of lush rolling hills that have been primarily used for cornfields and small cattle pastures. These agricultural forms are slowly giving way to orange groves that increasingly dot the landscape. During orange harvest, large trucks travel along the pothole-filled highways, taking this cash crop to weighing stations for sale to markets across the nation (Fig. 12.2).

Many rivers flow from the Sierra Madre mountains toward the Gulf of Mexico, providing water to the area during the wet season. The abundant rain comes from the warm, moist Gulf winds that drop rain as they cool over the sierras. The majority of this rain falls in the form of strong thunderstorms in the wet season from July to November. Only about a third of the precipitation falls during the rest of the year, the dry season. The precipitation during the dry season is due to the *nortes* or cold winds from the north that envelop the mountains in clouds, providing very little moisture to the ground. The end of the dry season, usually in May, can bring droughts that can severely affect these populations entirely dependent on agriculture.

Northern Veracruz is very complex and diverse, both in its physical characteristics as well as the populations that live there. It sits within a region known as the Huasteca, which is known for its high proportion of indigenous populations. Approximately 80% of the municipalities in the Huasteca are classified as indigenous (CDI 2006b). The main indigenous groups in this region are the Nahua, Huasteco, Otomí, and Tepehua. Mexico enumerates its indigenous population primarily based on people's ability to speak an indigenous language.[4] The Nahua are the most numerous indigenous group in Mexico with approximately 1.3 million speakers across the nation, followed by the Maya with just over 3 quarters of a million speakers (INALI 2010).

This region has some of the highest rates of illiteracy in the country and a marked lack of services, communications, schools, and jobs. These features are mostly found within the rural, indigenous, and peasant populations rather than in the more politically powerful segments of the population. The latter group, though small, has a high socioeconomic standard of living due to the export of citric fruits and cattle to other parts of Mexico and the United States (Ruvalcaba 1998). This area also sees very high rates of human rights violations, economic exploitation, and oppression by the wealthy landowners who control much of the community and local government as well as discrimination against indigenous peoples that dates back to Colonial times (Sandstrom 1991). Ariel De Vidas (2007:4) describes the many social inequities suffered by the indigenous populations of the region as emerging from the quotidian "racist, exploitative, and paternalistic" interactions between *mestizo* and indigenous populations. Indeed, land tenure remains one of the fundamental problems in this region (Ruvalcaba 1998). In a seemingly contradictory manner, it is also an area where independent indigenous/peasant organizations have acquired (or are striving to acquire) the political strength to peacefully confront the oppression they are facing (Ruvalcaba 1998) (Fig. 12.3).

The village of Amatlán is a small Nahua indigenous village of approximately 600 people. This population has remained surprisingly stable over the past two decades (Sandstrom 1991). The village is picturesque, surrounded on three sides by a small stream that is used by the villagers for bathing and

[4]Other markers of ethnicity are used as well (dress, religion, customs) to enumerate population but to a lesser extent than language.

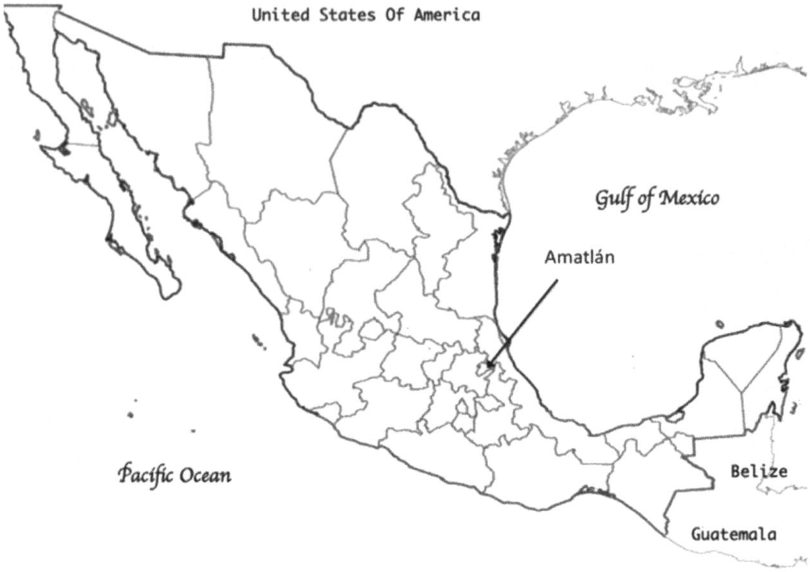

Fig. 12.1 Map of Mexico showing Amatlán in the state of Veracruz

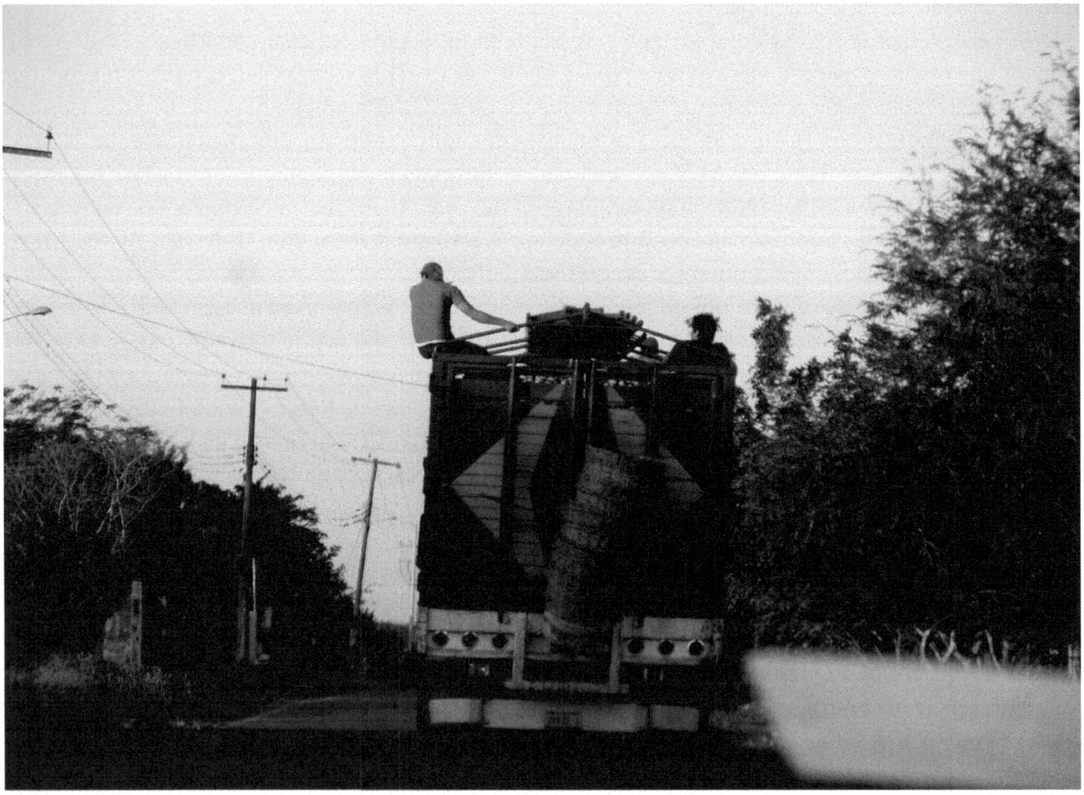

Fig. 12.2 A truck carrying oranges to the market

washing clothes. Toward the back of the village are a series of low hills that have been used for cornfields, cattle pastures, and, most recently, oranges. Households frequently consist of multiple generations, from aging grandparents who wear the traditional dress to youngsters who buy cards for Internet

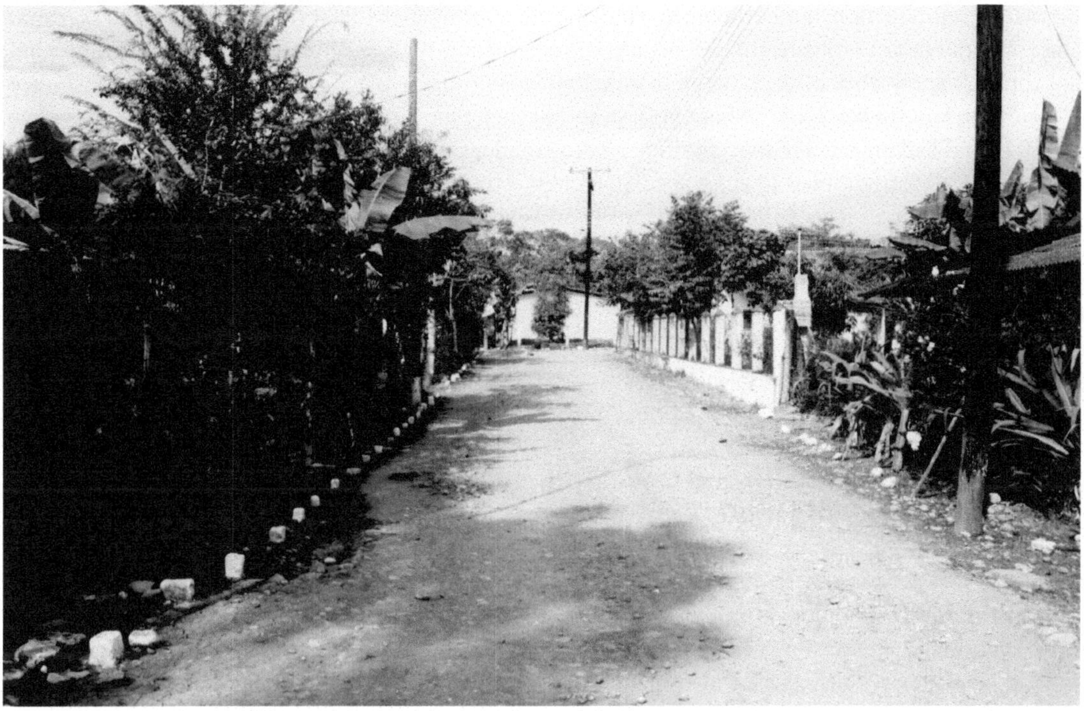

Fig. 12.3 The village of Amatlán: A view of one of the roads

access from the local store. The village is rarely silent. Roosters crow and dogs bark all night, *banda* music blares from stereos in several homes, and people call out greetings as they walk by taking children to school or going to visit relatives. Cars and trucks drive in and out of the village ferrying passengers to local markets or taking students to high school or college in nearby towns.

12.5 Ethnographic Fieldwork

One of the authors (VSO) conducted the ethnographic fieldwork for this study over the course of 11 months during 2004, 2005, and 2007, with brief visits in 2012, 2013, and 2016. She lived in the home of Esperanza and Ildefonso, where she was treated as a member of the family. Esperanza was a shy and quiet woman blessed with an incredible sense of humor and a remarkable ability to haggle with street vendors. She worked hard in caring for her household, whose composition changed over the years—sometimes it was only herself, Ildefonso, and Tito (their disabled grandson); sometimes their son lived with them too; at other times they were joined by daughters and their children. Regardless of whom lived at home, Esperanza managed the domestic sphere, cooking all the daily meals, washing the clothes with water drawn from a well (and later a spigot), or feeding her many chickens and turkeys. Ildefonso was a kind and gentle man who labored daily in the cornfields, weeding, spraying pesticides, or harvesting the corn. He never had a harsh word for anyone and supported his family as best he could as he aged and saw his health slowly decline.

We carried out participant observation as well as semi-structured and unstructured interviews with 53 women of reproductive and post-reproductive age (ranging in ages from 18 to 73 years)[5]. Interviews

[5] All interviews were confidential, and we have used pseudonyms for people and communities.

focused on reproduction, motherhood, and health care. During many interviews, the women expressed concern about their uterine health, especially *isihuayo*. *Isihuayo* was a relatively common complaint, and approximately 20% of the women in Amatlán of reproductive age and above had it at least once in their life (Smith-Oka 2008). About 90% of the women who suffered this condition were above the age of 45 and had on average five children. These are the women we focus on in this chapter. We also interviewed all 9 traditional healing specialists about their practices and carried out structured and semi-structured interviews with 11 clinicians (nurses and physicians) at 3 regional health centers.

We analyzed the data collected during this fieldwork using open coding, focused coding to gain a more nuanced understanding of the data, as well as pile sorts of relevant statements and events. We grouped data into existing patterns (health concerns, social support, anxiety and fear, labor and weakness, etc.) and then combined and catalogued the related patterns into subthemes that inductively emerged from the data.

12.6 Navigating Health and Development Within the State-Indigenous Context

When this research was carried out, there were nine traditional healing specialists in Amatlán—consisting of *parteras* (traditional birth attendants, TBAs), *curanderos* (ritual specialists), and *sobadores* (bone setters) (see Sandstrom 1991 for a deeper examination of healing specialists in the region). Two of these healers have since passed away, and all the others are now over the age of 60. So far, none of the young people have apprenticed these skills nor have acquired a healing ability (believed to be furnished by the gods). These practices are thus aging and dying along with their practitioners (Fig. 12.4).

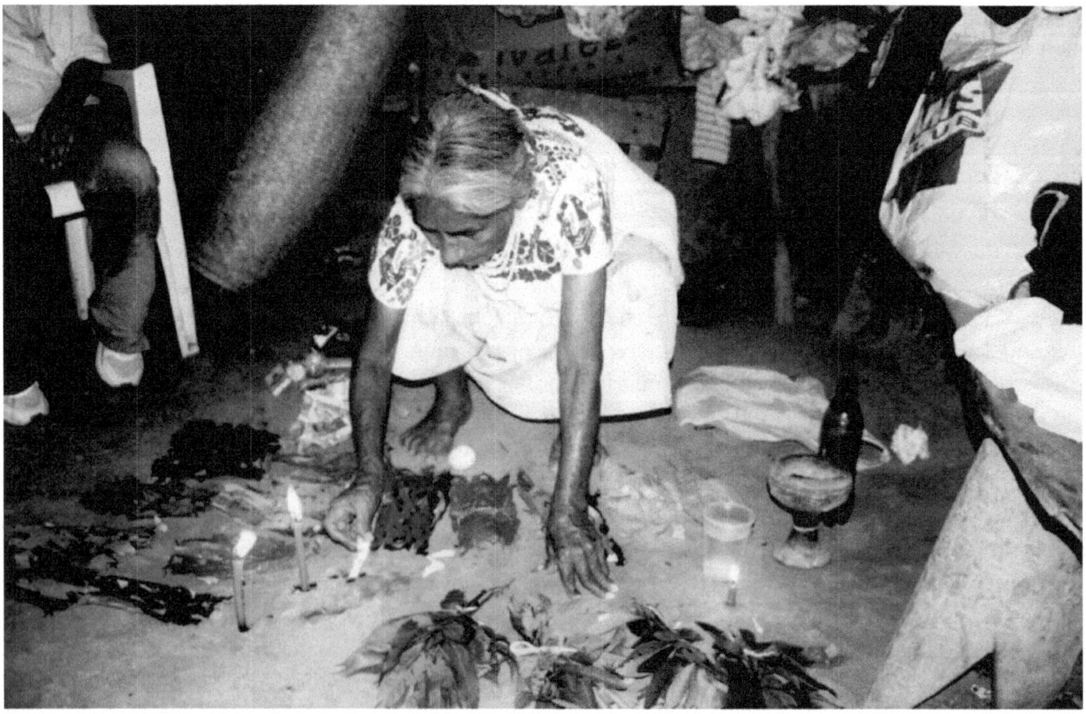

Fig. 12.4 Older traditional healing specialist setting up her altar

Besides care from traditional healers, villagers have access to free biomedical care at publicly funded clinics and hospitals in nearby towns. These hospitals are primary care centers that are staffed with nurses and primary care physicians (obstetricians/gynecologists, general practitioners, and pediatricians). Any health case requiring more complex care is referred to a regional tertiary care hospital, such as in the cities of Poza Rica or Chicontepec. From there some cases might also be sent to hospitals in Mexico City.

When we did this research, almost all the families were enrolled in *Prospera*, the conditional cash transfer program we described at the beginning of this chapter. *Prospera's* objectives are closely tied to Mexico's concern with maternal health and maternal mortality. Hence, nowadays almost all the births in this region take place in the clinics and hospitals, as the Ministry of Health has increasingly encouraged women to receive prenatal and birth care from clinicians as opposed to TBAs. The village TBAs have thus seen their client base decrease over the years as more women go to clinics for healthcare needs. Some of these *parteras* shifted their care to more gynecological problems, such as the *isihuayo* we discuss in this chapter.

The interaction between the *parteras* and their patients tend to be quite egalitarian because in such a small village almost everyone is somehow related, in actual or fictive-kin ties. Thus, the *parteras* can provide emotional support to their female patients as well as health support during moments with health issues. This support plays an important role for women and their health experiences (Fig. 12.5).

Most villagers had an ambivalent relationship with the government-sponsored institutions—such as *Prospera* or the clinicians at health centers. They appreciated the health benefits from vaccines against childhood diseases and the opportunity for regular care from physicians and nurses. They also felt the great benefits from having the steady and sizeable income from *Prospera*, which allowed them occasional liquidity and the ability to educate their children. The lack of *Prospera* often hampered people's abilities to get an education. Alicia, for instance, shared how her eldest daughter left the village to work in Mexico City:

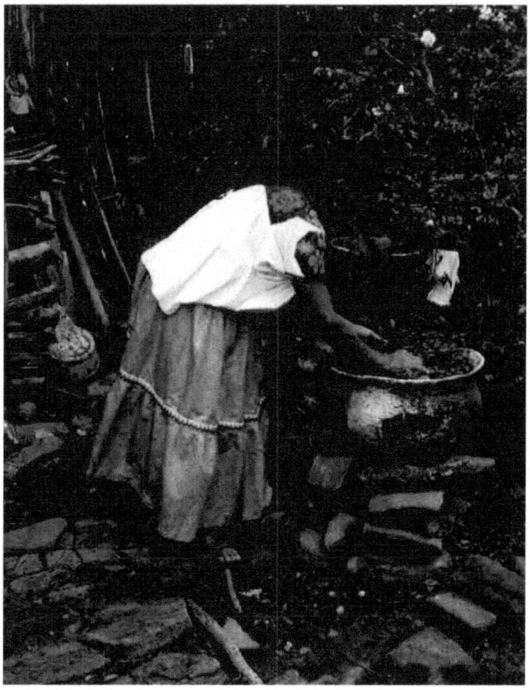

Fig. 12.5 Traditional birth attendant tending her medicinal plants

> She was twelve! After elementary school she left because she was angry since we didn't let her go to school any longer because at that time they didn't give us [*Prospera*]. And, well, my husband asked what was the point of sending her [to school], 'as she's a woman and women don't like to study; they only marry.' […] And now she is married and because she's still very young she doesn't know [anything] and she did not take care (use contraception) and so she's pregnant.

Most people's comments about the economic and health programs were negative, however, and reflected their dissatisfaction with the system (see Smith-Oka 2013 for an in-depth analysis of this dissatisfaction). Although both programs (*Prospera* and health care) were officially managed by two separate government ministries, within the clinical space, they came together to shape the health and well-being of the enrolled populations. The nurses and physicians checked that enrolled mothers and children met the conditions of *Prospera* and were tasked with dropping delinquent participants from the program. The persistent sentiment about both institutions was one of coercion and fear—coercion from the state to participate in clinic demands and fear of losing their income. Esperanza voiced the concerns of many women when they were asked to walk several kilometers to the clinic so the clinicians could talk with them, "But if we don't go they tell us that they will take our [financial] support, our [*Prospera*] away. But the doctor doesn't even come here. [He says] he doesn't want to. […]. All of us [women] have to go there. But it's not easy."

12.7 Social Suffering and Failed Sociality

Social suffering places the individual and their health within the larger social context by pointing to the ways in which social, political, and economic forces shape not only health problems but also people's responses to them (Kleinman et al. 1997). Kleinman (2010) suggests that the artificial boundaries between a health problem and a societal problem collapse when analyzed through the lens of social suffering. A focus on social suffering is thus useful to highlight how individuals deal with and move through constantly changing social, political, and economic spaces. Other scholars add to this notion of individual and collective suffering (Rock 2003) by showing how the experience of giving and receiving care and the ways these roles are perceived are shaped by collective frames of reference (Barg et al. 2014). The framework of social suffering can thus explain the connection between the indigenous women's bodily fragility and vulnerability, their changing levels of social support, and their entanglements with the web of the global political economy.

Indigenous Mexican women enrolled in large-scale neoliberal economic programs such as *Prospera* can experience increased anxieties about their autonomy and their obligations to the state. These embodied manifestations of distress are caused by everyday forms of social suffering and are linked to social conflict, economic scarcity, and failed sociality (Tapias 2006:402)—when certain relationships are no longer tenable or when one is unable to meet certain societal expectations. Failed sociality captures the shifts in both the relationships women traditionally relied on and having to conform to social, political, and economic pressures.

Failed sociality was illustrated through women's perceptions of what *isihuayo* meant and the feelings of shame that surrounded it. The women we spoke with frequently mentioned how *isihuayo* was an embarrassing condition; thus many women avoided treating it until it became painful because they were mortified at the thought of members of their family knowing, especially their husbands. As Rosario said, "A woman I know had [*isihuayo*] with her first baby. [The female part] came out. But she was embarrassed and didn't say anything. And it can't be fixed anymore." Cristina added, "The [treatment] works if you are attended to right away. Some keep silent because they are embarrassed. And only eventually they might call someone to massage them."

Altagracia's problem with *isihuayo* began when she gave birth to her last child 23 years prior to our interview; she felt her uterus fall but was too embarrassed to tell anyone. She suffered pain for many years by the time the physician at the clinic diagnosed her with prolapsed uterus and referred her to physicians in Mexico City to undergo a hysterectomy. She said, "I didn't want to go but I did, because I had *caída de matriz*. But they did not open my belly; they did it from below. It hurt a lot." Despite no longer having a uterus, by 2005, she had just begun to experience pain again and had once more diagnosed her condition as *isihuayo*. As far as we know, she was the only woman to experience this condition in this manner (without a uterus). And yet, despite being an exception, her story is important to illustrate how much of *isihuayo* is about larger factors such as support and strength and less about physiological factors. The women's feeling of shame often stemmed from a sense of somehow failing—not having children or support to rely on was somehow a reflection of their inability to keep their family together as well as failing society or a "failed sociality" (Fig. 12.6).

We show in this chapter that social relations clearly shape, and are reflected in, women's health. While social support is important for people's experiences with other illnesses, it takes on a much more significant role in shaping the course of *isihuayo*. *Isihuayo* is not simply a physiological condition but also a reflection of individual, local, and national changes they face as indigenous, marginalized, and impoverished women. Our work, therefore, provides an important contribution to the discussion on the ways that marginalized populations cope with a changing world. By looking at *isihuayo* as a local manifestation of the disenfranchisement faced by peasant societies across the world, one can then ask, in how many other societies across the world are some of these bodily expressions of disenfranchisement simply ascribed to local, culturalist explanations rather than to expressions of broader structural socioeconomic forces?

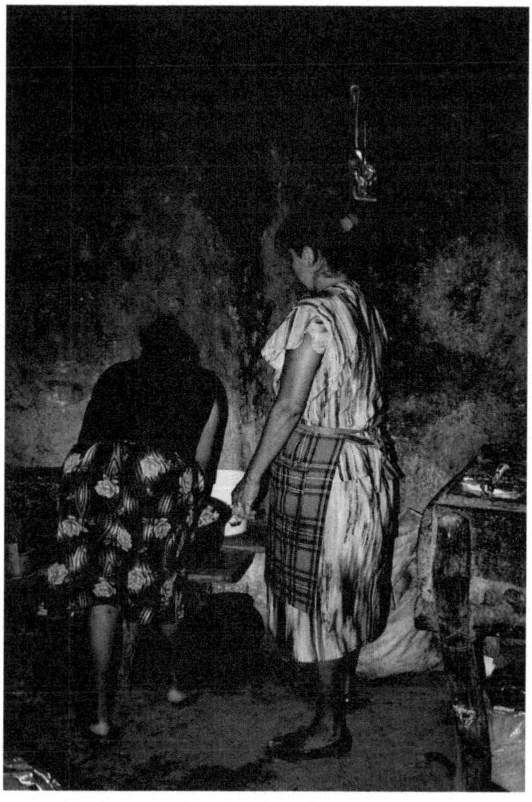

Fig. 12.6 Sisters-in-law cooking together

We suggest that the women in this study cope with social suffering not via governmental institutions, such as *Prospera*, but via their own social networks. Tapias (2006) points out that when social relations are problematic, they become reflected bodily. As indigenous women, the participants of our study feel constant pressure from state institutions to conform to mainstream notions of motherhood, family, and health. The women know that if they do not conform to these expectations, they risk losing their monetary support and income from *Prospera*. As the political economic forces reform the family structure through urbanization and employment by leading young people to search for jobs to cities and abroad, feelings of social exclusion become expressed in health outcomes (Spangler 2011). Thus, the women's experience of failed sociality becomes an expression of their bodily weakness—through reproductive malaise—as they must cope with both hard physical labor in order to survive as well as a changing social world. The women's social disharmony becomes reflected in bodily internalities through uterine displacement.

12.8 Enduring Too Much: Perceptions of Weakness

Clinicians at regional health centers stated that local women who had prolapse developed it because of having many children and because, as one nurse said, "They do not allow [their uterus] to rest; they are constantly using it." The village women disagreed with this etiology. Rosario, an energetic woman in her late 30s, scoffed, "They say in the clinic that [it is caused] because they have lots of children one after another, but I don't believe that because my mother had 14 and her [uterus] never fell." Other women, such as Paz, said uncertainly, "Who knows? People think that it is maybe because of having lots of children, or because of lifting heavy things. [Or] chopping wood, [or carrying] water. I have not had that."

Benita, who was in her 40s when we spoke, was a woman who gave birth to four boys. She described the fear and pain she felt in her first birth but tempered it by describing the joy she felt at her eldest son's achievements in school. She confided that her husband had wanted a girl and had been angered by the series of male children. The anger prompted him to force Benita to receive a tubal ligation. She softly recounted the *isihuayo* her mother experienced many years before, "[She had it] because of all the *fuerza*—effort—women make. And she endured all that. She had six children."

One of the first women who discussed *isihuayo* was Juana. By 2004 she had experienced this condition twice. The first time she was 6 months pregnant with her seventh and last child. The second time occurred a few months later when she tripped and fell while walking in the fields. Both times she went for treatment with a TBA, who massaged her and prescribed medicinal plants. She did not go to a biomedical clinic because, "Those doctors only write up papers [for you] to be operated, they just operate you and take your uterus; [your body] is no longer the same. The doctor wanted to operate me; he asked me questions about how I became better." Her words directly reflect tensions with the biomedical approach to care.

Juana was not originally from Amatlán, having moved there years ago after her marriage to Hilario, an itinerant musician with no rights to agricultural land (a vital source of income and subsistence). Because her oldest children were unmarried boys when she had *isihuayo*, she could not rely on them for help around the house. Once her children grew, however, Juana's health improved as not only did her younger daughters help around the house, but also a daughter-in-law moved in who became a very important source of social support. She said, "Now I will look after myself; my children will look after me." In 2016 she was still healthy, though her family's situation had changed in many ways. While her daughter-in-law still lived there, Juana also had to care for a son who had become blind due to alcohol-induced diabetes.

For women such as Juana or Benita, they perceived the number of children they had as a blessing but knew that having children was also a means for their bodies to weaken over time. The women's reproduction—having as many children "[as there are] ants" as Altagracia mentioned—contributes to the excessive weakening of a woman's body. With each pregnancy and birth, women's bodies lose strength (Groark 2005)—through loss of blood—and, as one woman stated, "Any little thing will make [the uterus] fall."

Daughters were important sources of help from very young, while sons became increasingly important as adults, as on marriage they brought in daughters-in-law who provided valuable help with daily work and household chores. Such was the contradictory nature of having many children and the paradox of caregiving—though some women had many mouths to feed while the children were younger, all of them expected that as their children grew they would be able to rely on them for help.

12.9 "Send Me Someone to Help Me Out": Lack of Social Support

Increasingly, the role and importance of social support has been recognized as a significant factor in influencing positive health outcomes (Seeman 1996, Uchino 2006). Social support refers to the resources—instrumental, emotional, and informational—an individual receives from their network of relationships (Cohen 2004). These resources help form healthy behavioral coping strategies that include a wide range of benefits from assistance with daily tasks to a sense of community and identification with one's social roles (Cohen 2004). Studies that examine the mechanisms that link social support and health have shown that the structure and function of social networks, support, and care from others (Brissette et al. 2000), the quality and quantity of social interactions (Kiecolt-Glaser and Newton 2001), and feelings of isolation and loneliness (Cacioppo et al. 2002) are reliable predictors of ill health. As a predictor of physical and psychological health, social integration and support have proven to limit the intensity and duration of stressful states, increase motivation to care for oneself, and boost neuroendocrine, immune, and cardiovascular functions (Uchino et al. 1996). Having a wide range of relationship and social network ties also provides multiple sources of knowledge and information that influence healthy-promoting behaviors and use of health services (Cohen 2004). All of these factors can be reflected in the experiences shared by the women of Amatlán.

Social support is integral to people's experience with illness. Ribera and Hausmann-Muela (2011) suggest that support is a means by which kin and family in a person's social network can advise and help during times of need. Uchino et al. (1996) emphasize emotional factors, stating that the process of social support is when one feels cared for and loved. They show that such support has stress-buffering effects that positively impact health. Clark's (1993) work among Anglo and Mexican-American women's experiences with health issues shows that Mexican women were more likely to rely on female kin for support than on their partners. Relations with male partners can be extremely complex; sometimes men can hamper women's reproductive choices (possibly making them more vulnerable to illness), while at other times they may positively influence a woman's health status, allowing her to quickly regain health (Browner 2000) (Fig. 12.7).

All of the women in the village frequently spoke about their support from kin and friends or the lack thereof. Esperanza was a woman in her 50s who had experienced the pain of losing two children—one in infancy to neonatal tetanus and one adult son, many years later. She said, "I dreamed the other day that my [dead] mother came to me. She holds me and tells me, 'you will die here because you work too much, while up there [in heaven] it is so nice'." Esperanza paused a second and then laughed, "But [...] I scold her and tell her not to take me and instead to send me someone to help me out."

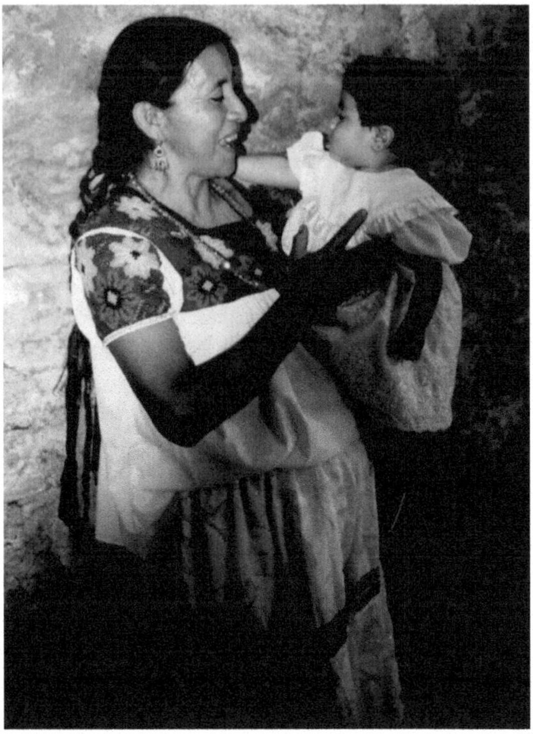

Fig. 12.7 Grandmother and grandchild

Ribera and Hausmann-Muela (2011) discuss the importance of mutual support in reducing people's vulnerability to illness. Factors such as a woman's social support and how much physical labor she had exerted over the course of her life were often integral to her illness experience. A woman who was taken care of by her family after giving birth, who had children to help around the house, and who had help in doing heavy manual housework (such as fetching wood and carrying water) was less likely to suffer from *isihuayo* than one who did not have support. She was less vulnerable. For Cristina, the mother of five children, "the reason [for getting *isihuayo*] is not taking care, we have no one to look after us."

Esperanza over the years took care of between one and four grandchildren because her children had migrated to other cities to work. She had suffered *isihuayo* twice. The first time occurred when she was carrying cement in a wheelbarrow when she and her husband were fixing their home. She began to experience lower back pain during this time. Her second experience with *isihuayo* began mildly in May 2004. It came about from daily carrying heavy containers of water from the nearby well on her head.

On both occasions, she treated it by traditional birth attendant massages and medicinal plants. Refugio, a TBA, stated, "[She] told me that water was coming out and I told her it was the uterus that was coming out." While the home remedies worked for a while, Esperanza was told at the clinic that she had prolapse and had to receive surgery. Esperanza could not agree to surgery, however, as this meant no one to take care of her or her family while she was convalescing. Her primary means of social and emotional support came from her *comadre*[6] Altagracia, who lived across the street. Though Esperanza began to pay someone to carry water for her, with no other women at home all the

[6] *Comadre* is the Spanish term for fictive kinswoman.

housework fell to her. By 2016, the government had installed water spigots in most homes, thus greatly decreasing the women's literal load of carrying water.

Cristina, who had a relatively comfortable income from managing the village's only phone for many years, described women's lives the most bluntly. She stated:

> It's just that as women we have to do everything, get pregnant and be nauseated for the first few months and when everything makes you feel sick. And [cleaning] the pigsty made me feel so sick. And then in the last [months] it is difficult to stand up and do everything. It is so much trouble. And then the pain of the birth, and to breastfeed, and to get up to change the baby in the middle of the night. Your husband is happily asleep but not you. [...] We [women] have to do everything. There is only the condom and the vasectomy for men, but they don't want them. We have to do it if we don't want to get pregnant. And well, one has to satisfy the husband and also not have so many children.

Many of the women who suffered from *isihuayo* expressed a similar overwhelming sense of lack of support from parents, children, husbands, or other kinsmen.

In Juana's case, it was the lack of her mother-in-law that contributed to her experiencing *isihuayo*. Her mother-in-law—a traditional source of help for married women—worked in Mexico City as a maid and was rarely around. Thus Juana lacked the usual female support network available to women in this community, one that she could draw on and rely upon during times of illness or crisis. For Lourdes, her daughter-in-law Ofelia was excellent support, particularly in helping her with cooking. But Ofelia also had her own family of four children to feed and look after. Lourdes's sons provided her with some income, especially those working in the city, but she spent much of her time worrying about her youngest son, Samuel, who was still in university—an expensive enterprise. Esperanza felt that her primary health problems stemmed from her children—through their presence or lack thereof—and the lack of helping hands at home. She described how her eldest son's lackluster interest in work brought her much grief, stating, "He is no use to me here. He should go away to work but he doesn't want to. I don't know what to do with him. [...] When he is far away I don't worry. My head can rest."

Many women considered that *isihuayo* emerged from stress associated with social suffering and lack of care during sensitive reproductive years. Altagracia gave birth to seven children during her reproductive years. She believed that *isihuayo* came about from, "Not looking after ourselves when we are pregnant. We carry many heavy things, because we carry corn and wood, and if the husband is not there then we do it and it harms us." Altagracia and her husband, Aparicio, had no children at home. All of them migrated to the cities to work. Aparicio additionally had no rights to farmland. His brother conceded him some land to farm on, but it was not his officially. He had been an alcoholic for many years and would beat Altagracia, but he had converted to Pentecostalism two decades prior and had become a strict teetotaler. Altagracia had a hard upbringing—her father was abusive and, until he died and she became an orphan, she lived in very wretched conditions. She confided that to this day she still struggled to consider that her home with Aparicio was her own.

Because of her lack of social support from female kin or from her spouse, Altagracia had no time to rest after birthing her children. She said that a woman is expected to rest at least a week after giving birth, to be taken care of, and to receive a postpartum bath to return their strength and counteract the loss of blood (Smith-Oka 2008; see also Groark 2005). She stated, "[I should have] rested for eight days. But I could not rest and by four days I was cooking tortillas. With my first three children [I rested] a week. Afterwards no more. I began to work in the kitchen." Esperanza had a similar experience, stating, "Some women [rest] eight days, others fifteen or a month. But by the next day I was working, as I have no one to help me. [...] My mother-in-law could not help. I could barely make tortillas. And I became sick. I felt no hunger and my body began to waste away. My hands were [as thin as] fingers." Her statement follows the empirical evidence that confirms the important link between social support and health (Uchino 2006).

Gender relations are another lens through which to analyze the relationship between social support and women's health. Support primarily derived from female relatives (daughters or mothers-in-law) and from fictive kin (neighbors, friends). Male kin, especially husbands, also played an important role in support—financial, structural, or emotional. All the women in this study were married; many of them had companionate marriages. Though the gender domains were quite strict—men in public (fields, politics) and women in private (household)—there was relative gender equality, where the responsibilities and contributions of each gender were equally valued. This relative equality did not mean, however, that women felt entirely supported by their male kin, as they often complained about how much work they had. Men supported their wives during ill health, either financially or by accompanying them to the clinic/hospital if needed. For instance, Juana's husband, though an alcoholic, was supportive in finding medicinal plants for her. Esperanza's and Lourdes's husbands also supported them emotionally when they were told that they needed surgery. Rarely, however, would a man help his wife with domestic duties (childcare, laundry, or cooking) if she were ill. That role fell upon the female kin. Thus, Cristina's statement that women had to do everything was true, as women needed support from other women in order to protect from body vulnerability and illness.

The strength of women's social support also derived from their connection to the village (whether they were born there or had married in), their children's ages and their abilities to help with domestic chores, the presence of a mother-in-law, and the presence of daughters and daughters-in-law. There is strong evidence for the role of familial social support on people's improved health (Uchino et al. 1996; Ribera and Hausmann-Muela 2011). For Juana, her support network, or lack thereof, was central in her experience of the illness. Her husband's lack of land and, frequently, any income meant that the majority of her family's income came from *Prospera* money as well as money her older children sent from Mexico City. As a result, support was important in shaping her health, especially when her children were younger and she had to take care of them because of her mother-in-law's absence. Though Esperanza was urged by the physicians to have surgery (likely a hysterectomy), she chose not to because of lack of female support and care, which would make her convalescing and recovery period almost impossible. She had heard Altagracia's stories of struggle after her hysterectomy and was loath to undergo the same. Altagracia lacked the support of her children when she experienced *isihuayo* for the second time. This was not the case in the previous episode, during which she stayed with her children while she convalesced. As seen from these various women's lives, it is not only the presence of social support that is central to their experience of illness but also the presence of close emotional ties to these sources of support in dealing with day-to-day activities as well as larger changes and stressors (income, land, children leaving, etc.) (Uchino et al. 1996). Ribera and Hausmann-Muela (2011:108) consider such "rich in people" ties as indispensable to the experience of illness.

12.10 Living a Labor-Intensive Life

The participants in our study cited perceptions of female vulnerability and bodily capacity, coupled with the social suffering they faced, as underlying factors for their reproductive malaise. As mentioned before, a widely accepted cultural conception in the region is that women are weaker than men—mostly due to their workload and their reproductive lives. If a woman fell or was physically hurt, energy was believed to travel into her body dislodging her uterus. Lourdes, a hardworking 58-year-old *partera* and traditional healer, said, "You see, women are more delicate than men and so any little bump hurts us. [...] It's just that we all have a small bone here (touches area underneath the uterus), and if the legs open like this (opens arms wide) after a fall, it will separate and the bladder falls." The uterus is believed to fall through the space and hang down, causing it to become tired and begin to hurt. Jordan (1992:43) also noted in her research among the Maya the idea of "bones that [open] during childbirth," which might be a similar etiology to the one experienced by the Nahua women of this region. One of the TBAs stated that if a weakened woman continued with hard physical labor, the uterus would likely remain in this state.

Lourdes worked very hard tending her home garden, collecting firewood and carrying water, shucking corn, and walking to nearby villages to attend to patients. A few years before 2004, she was walking back from another village and cut across a cow pasture; one of the cows chased her and she tripped and fell, which caused *isihuayo*. She said that when she fell she developed *espanto* (magical fright), which was the underlying cause of her *isihuayo*.

Lourdes was ill for several years and was anxious to find a cure. She said, sadly, "I lack *fuerza* (strength); I lack vitamins. With so much work one gets tired. I need medicine, a treatment." Lourdes was also a diabetic. Because of the diabetes and the lack of *fuerza*, she was more prone to weakness and thus was frequently ill. Her low strength also came from the high amount of energy she expended in her healing practice—walking to other villages (sometimes a day and a half's sojourn) and in the treatments themselves, many of which required her to carry out complex religious rituals that sapped her strength. Her energy and health had declined over the years, which were possibly contributing factors to her suffering from *isihuayo* later in life.

Carrying heavy loads was believed to weaken a woman's uterus over time—especially during pregnancy and early postpartum. Adela, one of Lourdes's daughters, stated about *isihuayo* in general, "Because women have a month-old baby and they lift something heavy and [the uterus] falls [...] and only a month has passed since they gave birth." Floriana, one of the oldest women in the village, who sadly admitted she gave birth to only one child, concurred that women's work was often the cause of ill health. She stated:

> Some women's uterus falls. It is dangerous. Because they pick up heavy things. They also push really hard (*hacen mucha fuerza*) when their baby is being born. [...] The uterus can fall very easily. [...] My daughter-in-law had that. [I told her], 'Don't lift heavy things. Just chop a bit of wood. If not your uterus will fall. If not, what will we do? [We'll have to go] all the way to Chicón.[7]' I tell her that every day.

Rosario's experience mirrored Floriana's comments, as she suffered from *isihuayo* after the birth of her first child. She said:

> I also had that. [...] It was because I exerted a lot of *fuerza* to push out the placenta, that's why. But I was not ashamed and I told my husband that something had come out and that I could feel it hanging. And we asked a *partera* to come and she massaged and massaged me and put in some hot oil. And it was very hot, and she would put it on her hands and warm the area. And like that she put [the uterus] back. And it did not happen again. It is not because of having many [children]. It is because [women] do not look after themselves and they carry heavy things.

The clinicians emphasized to us that women need rest during postpartum, though one of the nurses expressed concern that the women did not follow *cuarentena*—40 days of rest. Among the Mapuche of Chile, for instance, the *cuarentena* is considered a period of fragility during which the woman must maintain bodily equilibrium, abstain from sex, and refrain from arduous physical labor (Alarcón and Nahuelcheo 2008). Not taking care of one's self thus leads to a continued weakening of the body.

Some of the village women developed *necaxantle*—"the weakening disease"—something postpartum women are believed to develop because of lack of rest. *Necaxantle* was caused by a general lack of care postpartum (especially a lack of social support) and a bodily imbalance leading to weakness. Its symptoms included body pain, weight loss, lack of interest in food, chills, and a feeling of

[7]Chicón is short for Chicontepec, a town about 3-h drive north of the village. It has a hospital that many patients are sent to when the local hospital cannot handle their condition.

weakness. Its treatment included rest from physical labor, the avoidance of sexual relations, and the use of certain medicinal plants (Smith-Oka 2008). *Necaxantle* not only expresses similar manifestations associated with the need for rest and social support as *isihuayo,* but it also reflects preferences or ways of dealing with ill health through medicinal plants rather than biomedical practices.

Additionally, Altagracia lost a child to *tentsocopale*—infant tetanus. *Tentsocopale* was a significant cause of infant death before vaccinations became prevalent in the 1980s. Almost all of the older women had lost a child this way. Altagracia said sadly, "One of my [babies] died with that illness that came. If it gets ill, it does not get better and it dies." Refugio, the TBA, also had lost a child. She described the illness: "when their little mouth curls up and they cannot suckle or suck … My boy died [when he was] seven days old because I was still too young and did not know about remedies. He cried, foam came out of his little mouth, and he could not suckle. Now the doctors and the clinics inject them." Altagracia also credited the doctors with preventing infant death, stating, "Now they are born into the hands of doctors" (Fig. 12.8).

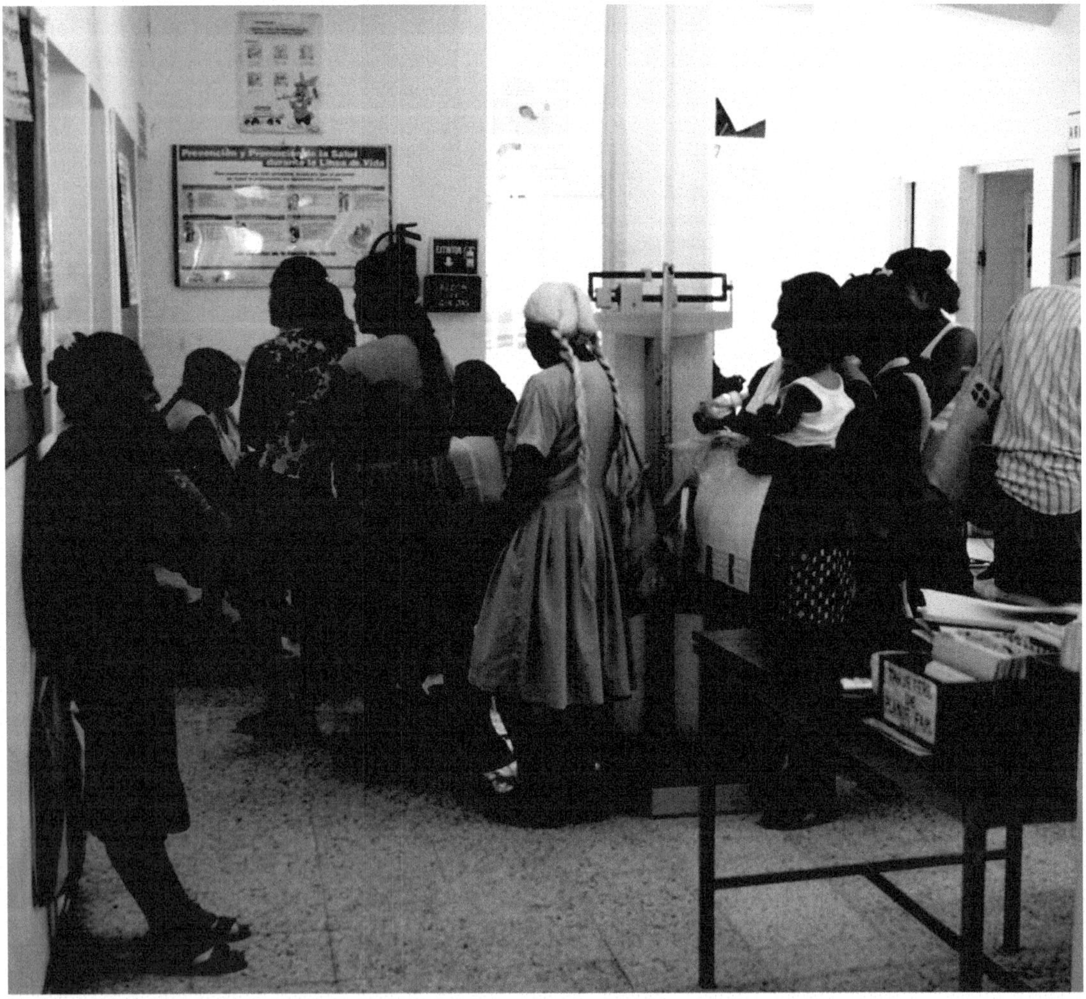

Fig. 12.8 Women lined up at the clinic

Scholars who have done research in the Andes have shown that weakness can be an underlying condition that may lead to illness, similar to stress in the West (Larme 1998:1009). Tapias shows that the underlying constitution of a person can reflect their "past histories of distress and illness" (2006:407). The Amatlán women's past histories of distress certainly play a role in their health and emotional well-being. They feel worry and stress from their own lives—the lack of money or lack of land; but they also worry about their children's lives. The multifactorial nature of prolapse is also evident in *isihuayo*—though in the latter case these factors are both physical and emotional. While physical factors might make a woman more at risk for *isihuayo*, it is the underlying emotional factors that can turn it into a chronic, debilitating condition. This reflects how social suffering becomes embodied as illness.

The women who have suffered *isihuayo* have a labor-intensive life—in all senses of the word. Not only have they given birth various times, but they also work very hard in their domestic chores. Their "techniques of the body" (Mauss 1973:70)—the ways that they use their bodies—create certain physiques and relationships between their tangible, bodily selves and their emotional selves. They, and their bodies, are physically exhausted. Over the years of knowing Lourdes, we saw her weaken and diminish from a strong, vital, and energetic woman to a woman whose physical strength dissipated, leading to a series of small accidents—a hot oil burn, a deep cut—that cumulatively added to her heightened sense of weakness. Because of her lack of strength, she was predisposed to suffering from other ailments. This suffering is what Tapias (2006:408) refers to as a "circularity of influence" wherein each bout of illness leaves the sufferer weaker than before, thus more vulnerable to additional health concerns.

Scholars have shown that illnesses of this sort are exacerbated during times of crisis, conflict, or hardship (Henry 2006; Tapias 2006). Signaling "tensions in the social landscape," *isihuayo* could additionally point to the root causes of the "materiality of poverty" on the women's lives (Tapias 2006:411). Rents in the social fabric for the Amatlán women emerge from the social and economic disparity between them and the larger institutions that place conditions over their reproductive bodies. Fleuriet's work (2007:177) among indigenous people in northern Baja California demonstrates the links between the local construction and experience of illness and the larger historical and economic contexts that shape the "experience of being sick, poor, female, and indigenous in Mexico." She adds that physical suffering is frequently tied to cultural identity in an "environment of disparity." Similarly, the women of Amatlán live in such an environment of disparity, where they often bear the brunt of social, economic, and political policies that have historically excluded (or forcibly included) them from participation in the larger mainstream culture (Smith-Oka 2009).

A connection exists between women's health and shifting ideas of women's roles in society (Larme 1998). The older, more traditional women who followed local motherhood ideas were likely to experience *isihuayo*. The younger women, who had fewer children and frequently worked for wages in other regions of Mexico, were less likely to develop the condition. This was not simply because they were younger and their uteruses had not yet had the "opportunity" to be hurt, as many of the older women suffered *isihuayo* when they were younger. Younger women, significantly, received social support from older women—their mothers, sisters, or mothers-in-law—who provided help in childcare and life in general. Esperanza's daughters often left their own children with her for months or even years at a time, while they worked in *maquilas* on the border. This "socially meaningful strategy" (Leinaweaver 2007:175) of fosterage permitted younger women to earn money while ensuring that their children grew up and developed under the guidance of their own mothers. It also, unintentionally, allowed the younger women to protect their bodies from reproductive harm.

12.11 Conclusions for Moving Forward

This chapter not only builds upon but also connects two related areas of research that have yet to be connected thus far—social suffering and social support—by illustrating the role of social support on women's experiences with uterine distress. Additionally, we suggest that the concept of failed sociality is a key bridge that reflects both the struggles of coping with dwindling and changing networks of support and the inability to meet the institutional pressures placed on them. As we stated above, failed sociality encapsulates the multiple ways that the women's lives are shifting from under them—they are getting older and their bodies are weakening, they see their social roles changing as their children grow and leave the village or return with children of their own, and they see their identities of motherhood and indigeneity challenged by mainstream Mexico. All of these pressures and stressors contribute to a decrease in health and to a symbolic and bodily displacement of their female-ness. *Isihuayo* is an ethnomedical issue yet reflects these broader issues that Nahua women must face every day. In contrast to illnesses with a primarily emotional basis, *isihuayo* has both physical and emotional causes expressed physically in a woman's uterus. This multifactorial, biological, emotional, and social condition is "rooted in the experiences of rural, indigenous communities" (Fleuriet 2007:157). It also illustrates the ways by which marginalized populations cope with their changing world. Our work thus deepens the discussion of the role of social conditions on women's health (Rock 2003; Tapias 2006; Fleuriet 2007; Spangler 2011) by empirically showing how illness becomes a lived expression of marginalized people's social suffering due to external pressures and differing degrees of social support.

For most of these older indigenous women, the larger social, political, and economic pressures such as Spanish language, dress, manners, and bodily concepts are uneasy and foreign. Although they all participate in state development and health-care programs, such as *Prospera*, *Seguro Popular*, etc., this interaction is not comfortable. In addition, many have seen their children leave the village to find jobs elsewhere, leaving them to care for grandchildren and the many household duties on their own. They see their children leave the community not only to a different place but to an entirely different life. Contact between them is often left to the impersonal remittances sent home. The fragility of their bodies and their changing social relations result in what Tapias (2006:400) calls "embodied manifestations of distress." Furthermore, for some of these women, the lack of social support from kin (Ribera and Hausmann-Muela 2011) and the suffering of living in a society as marginal and alienated (Pylypa 2007) can become expressed in bodily form in a woman's uterus.

Pylypa (2007:362) states that local discourses on illness can serve two functions: one is a resistance to biomedical hegemony, while the second is a way to "express dissatisfaction with a health care system that is oftentimes disempowering." For the women of this study, biomedical care was disempowering because their perceptions about their bodies and their health were frequently disparaged by clinicians. The participants had little to no agency in the clinical setting and thus the action of going to the clinic meant a loss of dignity and personal autonomy. *Isihuayo* in Amatlán appears to serve similar functions as described by Pylypa (2007), whereby women who have suffered this condition express their concerns about the illness while simultaneously scorning biomedical care. The women felt that their bodies were shaped by larger institutional forces and as such were no longer their own. Juana's words above, "They just operate you and take your uterus; [your body] is no longer the same," illustrates a dual concern—reduced choice over one's own body and its dismemberment and disappearance by others.

Regardless of whether the women were diagnosed biomedically with prolapse, what they suffered from was *isihuayo*. This illness embedded many more aspects than simply the physical displacement. The women lived *isihuayo* as an example of their broader issues, as a culmination of social, economic, and political stressors, not just a biomedical category. This is evidenced by the fact that

Altagracia suffered from *isihuayo* even after she had a hysterectomy, thus lacking a uterus. Statistics and biomedical models assume that one prolapse is fundamentally like another. But this abstract concept ignores the lived experience of the women. *Isihuayo* for the women was symptomatic of larger social problems in their lives—lack of support, their poverty, their labor-intensive life, and even their shame at their family dissolution. Thus, illness cannot be removed from the social context nor should people's experience with illness be separated from collective frames of reference (Rock 2003). And, similarly to Rock's research on diabetes among Canada's Cree, our argument demonstrates how distress and duress accompany the falling of a uterus. Within such a system of disenfranchisement, it is thus inevitable that *isihuayo* would become an expression of a woman's internal lack of strength *compounded* by an external set of forces that intentionally or unintentionally shape uterine health.

12.12 Coda: Precariousness and Vulnerability

Life is precarious for indigenous, impoverished, and marginalized populations where unexpected problems can radically shift their well-being and health. Imelda's life exemplified this precariousness. She had five children, though only her youngest lived at home. Her husband Felipe was a very enterprising man who, over the years, innovated and diversified his small-scale agricultural land into a series of economic successes. He converted his maize fields first into cattle pastures and subsequently to orange groves. He built a successful small storefront in his home, where he and Imelda sold basic necessities, as well as coffee, sugar, candies, yogurt, ice creams, and toiletries, to the villagers. It was the largest and most successful store in the village and was a regular meeting place for various people in town. He made enough money to be able to buy two pickup trucks that he used to transport passengers and goods to other villages and towns, earning a comfortable income. He installed large water barrels on his roof, filling them with water. His family was the first in the village to have "running" water. He was a successful man and well-liked by everyone in the village. But he died suddenly and tragically in 2013 when he fell out of a tree.

Imelda's life radically changed. Unable to drive, she could no longer go to town to buy the goods to sell at her store. She had to sell various belongings, including both trucks, to make ends meet. And she began to consider enrolling in a government-sponsored micro-loan program despite its high default fees because she could no longer maintain her household. By 2016, while she still owned the store, it could not compete with others and only sold small amounts of basic goods. She had visibly aged and spoke about feeling tired and weaker. Her youngest son was a few weeks from leaving home to live with his older siblings in the city of Guadalajara where he hoped to make a different life for himself. Imelda and Felipe had been fervent followers of Pentecostalism, which created a fissure between her and her traditional healer father as well as with her Catholic siblings. Thus at Felipe's death and the departure of her son, Imelda would have little remaining social support in the village, except that provided by female neighbors and kin. While she did not speak about *isihuayo* in our conversations, we include her story as an illustration of just how precarious the life of an impoverished population can be and how this precariousness is embodied in their daily lives.

The implications of our study extend beyond the issues of reproduction or the illness of *isihuayo*, given that it answers questions about a seemingly straightforward medical condition and places it in a broader discussion about change, social support, and delivery of health care. The data from this research links to broader social processes that explain how people view illnesses and how social factors shape them. The tensions in the social landscape are lived by these women through their uteruses, connecting their lack of support to a resonance with their broader disenfranchisement. An anthropological framework encourages one to view ill health as something that is not simply biological but that is, instead, always shaped by larger social contexts. We thus offer the following suggestions for researchers and practitioners.

First, one needs to be aware that vulnerable populations will often be affected by broader political and socioeconomic processes and that the effects and outcomes of these processes might not always be straightforward, as we have shown here. Second, it is important to understand the role that a person's social support plays in their good or bad health. Good social support, where a sick person is cared for and fed, will ensure a faster recovery from illness than poor social support. Significantly, at times social support comes from unexpected sources (such as Juana's alcoholic, itinerant musician husband), which are important to identify and not dismiss. Third, it is important to recognize that family structures and gender roles are factors that can either exacerbate or improve a woman's health; it is thus necessary to identify some of the rules of behavior and gender norms when providing care to a community. And fourth, as we have shown in this article, illnesses are best understood within their social context; thus people's experience with illness cannot be separated from local frames of reference.

References

Alarcón, A. M., & Nahuelcheo, Y. (2008). Creencias sobre el embarazo, parto y puerperio en la mujer mapuche: conversaciones privadas. *Chungará (Arica), 40*(2), 193–202.

Ariel De Vidas, A. (2007). *Una piedrita en los zapatos de los caciques: ecos y repercusiones de las políticas de desarrollo rural en la huasteca veracruzana*. Wellington:Nuevo Mundo. Retrieved September 24, 2016, from http://nuevomundo.revues.org/index3343.html.

Barg, F. K., Keddem, S., Cohen, W. S., & Henderson, R. (2014). An anthropology of caregiving. In R. C. Talley & S. S. Travis (Eds.), *Multidisciplinary coordinated caregiving* (pp. 177–194). New York, NY: Springer.

Browner, C. H. (2000). Situating women's reproductive activities. *American Anthropologist, 102*(4), 773–788.

Brissette, I., Cohen, S., & Seeman, T. E. (2000). Measuring social integration and social networks. In S. Cohen, L. G. Underwood, & B. H. Gottlieb (Eds.), *Social support measurement and intervention: A guide for health and social scientists* (pp. 53–85). Oxford, UK: Oxford University Press.

Cacioppo, J. T., Hawkley, L. C., Crawford, L. E., Ernst, J. M., Burleson, M. H., Kowalewski, R. B., et al. (2002). Loneliness and health: Potential mechanisms. *Psychosomatic Medicine, 64*(3), 407–417.

Castañeda, X., García, C., & Langer, A. (1996). Ethnography of fertility and menstruation in rural Mexico. *Social Science & Medicine, 42*(1), 133–140.

Clark, L. (1993). Gender and generation in poor women's household health production experiences. *Medical Anthropology Quarterly, 7*(4), 386–402.

Cohen, S. (2004). Social relationships and health. *American Psychologist, 59*(8), 676.

Comisión Nacional para el Desarrollo de los Pueblos Indígenas (CDI). (2006a). *Regiones indígenas de México*. Retrieved September 16, 2016, from http://www.cdi.gob.mx/regiones/regiones_indigenas_cdi.pdf.

CDI. (2006b). *Indicadores socioeconómicos: Los números*. Retrieved March 7, 2006, from http://www.cdi.gob.mx/index.php?id_seccion=399.

Cosminsky, S. (2001). Maya midwives of southern Mexico and Guatemala. In B. R. Huber & A. R. Sandstrom (Eds.), *Mesoamerican healers* (pp. 179–210). Austin, TX: University of Texas Press.

Doshani, A., Teo, R. E., Mayne, C. J., & Tincello, D. G. (2007). Uterine prolapse. *British Medical Journal, 335*(7624), 819–823.

Fleuriet, K. J. (2007). Articulating distress on multiple levels: Illness, history, and culture among the Kumiai of Baja California, Mexico. *Mexican Studies/Estudios Mexicanos, 23*(1), 155–180.

Fuller, N., & Jordan, B. (1981). Maya women and the end of the birthing period: Postpartum massage and binding in Yucatan, Mexico. *Medical Anthropology, 5*(1), 35–50.

Gil-García, Ó. F. (2015). Gender equality, community divisions, and autonomy: The *Prospera* conditional cash transfer program in Chiapas, Mexico. *Current Sociology, 64*(3), 447–469.

Groark, K. P. (2005). Vital warmth and well-being: Steambathing as household therapy among the Tzeltal and Tzotzil Maya of highland Chiapas, Mexico. *Social Science & Medicine, 61*(4), 785–795.

Henry, D. (2006). Violence and the body: Somatic expressions of trauma and vulnerability during war. *Medical Anthropology Quarterly, 20*(3), 379–398.

Hinojosa, S. (2008). The Mexican American sobador, convergent disease discourse, and pain validation in south Texas. *Human Organization, 67*(2), 194–206.

Instituto Nacional de Estadística y Geografía (INEGI). (2010). *Diversidad*. Retrieved March 10, 2017, from http://www.cuentame.inegi.org.mx/monografias/informacion/ver/poblacion/diversidad.aspx?tema=me&e=30.

Instituto Nacional de Estadística y Geografía (INEGI). (2016). *Estadísticas A propósito Del Día Internacional De Los Pueblos Indígenas (9 De Agosto). Datos Nacionales*. Retrieved March 17, 2017, from http://www.inegi.org.mx/saladeprensa/aproposito/2016/indigenas2016_0.pdf.

Instituto Nacional de Lenguas Indígenas (INALI). (2010). *Programa de revitalizacion, fortalecimiento y desarrollo de las lenguas indigenas nacionales 2008–2012, PINALI*. Retrieved July 2, 2016, from http://site.inali.gob.mx/pdf/02_JUL_PINALI-2008-2012.pdf.

Jordan, B. (1992). *Birth in four cultures: A crosscultural investigation of childbirth in Yucatan, Holland, Sweden, and the United States*. Long Grove, IL: Waveland Press.

Kiecolt-Glaser, J. K., & Newton, T. L. (2001). Marriage and health: His and hers. *Psychological Bulletin, 127*(4), 472–503.

Kleinman, A. (2010). Four social theories for global health. *The Lancet, 375*(9725), 1518–1519.

Kleinman, A., Das, V., & Lock, M. M. (1997). *Social suffering*. Berkeley, CA: University of California Press.

Larme, A. C. (1998). Environment, vulnerability, and gender in Andean ethnomedicine. *Social Science & Medicine, 47*(8), 1005–1015.

Leinaweaver, J. B. (2007). On moving children: The social implications of Andean child circulation. *American Ethnologist, 34*(1), 163–180.

Lock, M., 1993. Cultivating the body: Anthropology and epistemologies of bodily practice and knowledge. Annual Review of Anthropology, *22*(1), 133–155.

López Austin, A. (1988). The human body and ideology: Concepts of the ancient Nahuas, Vol. 1. Thelma Ortiz de Montellano and Bernardo Ortiz de Montellano (Trans.), Salt Lake City:University of Utah Press.

Mauss, M. (1973). Techniques of the body. *Economy and Society, 2*(1), 70–88.

Oths, K. S. (1999). Debilidad: A biocultural assessment of an embodied Andean illness. *Medical Anthropology Quarterly, 13*(3), 286–315.

Pylypa, J. (2007). Healing herbs and dangerous doctors: "Fruit fever" and community conflicts with biomedical care in northeast Thailand. *Medical Anthropology Quarterly, 21*(4), 349–368.

Ribera, J. M., & Hausmann Muela, S. (2011). The straw that breaks the camel's back redirecting health seeking behavior studies on malaria and vulnerability. *Medical Anthropology Quarterly, 25*(1), 103–121.

Rock, M. (2003). Sweet blood and social suffering: Rethinking cause-effect relationships in diabetes, distress, and duress. *Medical Anthropology, 22*(2), 131–174.

Ruvalcaba, J. (1998). Presentación. In J. Ruvalcaba Mercado (Ed.), *Nuevos aportes al conocimiento de la Huasteca* (pp. 11–26). Mexico City: CIESAS.

Sandstrom, A. R. (1991). *Corn is our blood: Culture and ethnic identity in a contemporary Aztec Village*. Norman, OK: University of Oklahoma Press.

Santos-Torres, M. I., & Vásquez-Garibay, E. (2003). Food taboos among nursing mothers of Mexico. *Journal of Health, Population and Nutrition, 21*(2), 142–149.

Seeman, T. E. (1996). Social ties and health: The benefits of social integration. *Annals of Epidemiology, 6*(5), 442–451.

Smith-Oka, V. (2008). Plants used for reproductive health by Nahua women in northern Veracruz, Mexico. *Economic Botany, 62*(4), 604–614.

Smith-Oka, V. (2009). Unintended consequences: Exploring the tensions between development programs and indigenous women in Mexico in the context of reproductive health. *Social Science & Medicine, 68*(11), 2069–2077.

Smith-Oka, V. (2013). *Shaping the motherhood of Indigenous Mexico*. Nashville, TN: Vanderbilt University Press.

Spangler, S. A. (2011). "To open oneself is a poor woman's trouble": Embodied inequality and childbirth in south–central Tanzania. *Medical Anthropology Quarterly, 25*(4), 479–498.

Tapias, M. (2006). Emotions and the intergenerational embodiment of social suffering in rural Bolivia. *Medical Anthropology Quarterly, 20*(3), 399–415.

Uchino, B. N. (2006). Social support and health: A review of physiological processes potentially underlying links to disease outcomes. *Journal of Behavioral Medicine, 29*(4), 377–387.

Uchino, B. N., Cacioppo, J. T., & Kiecolt-Glaser, J. K. (1996). The relationship between social support and physiological processes: A review with emphasis on underlying mechanisms and implications for health. *Psychological Bulletin, 119*(3), 488–531.

Characteristics of Maternal Death Among Mayan Women in Yucatan, Mexico

13

Elsa María Rodríguez Angulo,
María Guadalupe Andueza-Pech,
and Yolanda Oliva Peña

13.1 Introduction

At present, it is unfortunate that preventable deaths of women during pregnancy, delivery, and the puerperium still take place (Schwartz 2015; WHO 2015). According to estimates by the World Bank, these deaths take place overwhelmingly in developing countries. In other words, the poorest countries are the ones with the highest numbers of deaths, with maternal mortality ratios (MMRs) that show the disparity between resource-poor and resource-rich countries (Schwartz 2015). For example, Sierra Leone has the highest maternal mortality ratio (MMR) at 1360 maternal deaths per 100,000 children born alive (BA), while Iceland and Poland have the lowest ratios of 7 and 3 maternal deaths per 100,000 live-born children, respectively. In the Americas, the highest level of deaths occurs in Haiti, with 359 maternal deaths per 100,000 live-born children, while Canada displays the lowest levels, having only 7 maternal deaths per live-born 100,000 children (World Bank 2016).

Mexico is classified as a developing country. Although it has succeeded in reducing maternal mortality (MM) since 1990, the rate of reduction is not what had been hoped for according to estimates made by the World Health Organization (WHO). This is illustrated by the maternal mortality data since the close of 2015. In 1990, the MMR of Mexico was 88.7, with a goal set for reduction of the MMR to 22.3 by 2015. However, this was not achieved, and at the close of 2015, the MMR was 38.9 (ODM-Mexico 2015).

The definition of a maternal death is the death of a woman during pregnancy, delivery, or puerperium, i.e., within 42 days after pregnancy, as a consequence of an obstetric complication from any cause related to or aggravated by the pregnancy but not from accidental or incidental causes. The clinical causes that unfold during pregnancy, delivery, or puerperium are known as maternal complications. They are well known and referred to in the International Classification of Diseases, Tenth Revision (ICD-10) (PAHO 1995).

E. M. R. Angulo, M.D., Ph.D., M.P.H. (✉) • M. G. Andueza-Pech, M.D., M.A.Sc.
Y. O. Peña, Ed.D., M.A.Sc.
Centro de Investigaciones Regionales
"Dr. Hideyo Noguchi", Universidad Autónoma de Yucatán, Mérida, Mexico
e-mail: rangulo@correo.uady.mx

D. A. Schwartz (ed.), *Maternal Death and Pregnancy-Related Morbidity Among Indigenous Women of Mexico and Central America*, Global Maternal and Child Health: Medical, Anthropological, and Public Health Perspectives, https://doi.org/10.1007/978-3-319-71538-4_13

Obstetric deaths can be direct or indirect. The former result from obstetric complications of gravidity (pregnancy, labor, and puerperium), interventions, omissions, incorrect treatment, or the chain of events leading to any of the aforementioned. The latter are a consequence of a previously existent disease or a disease that appeared during pregnancy, not due to direct obstetric causes but aggravated by the physiological effects inherent to pregnancy.

The major maternal complications occurring worldwide are the hypertensive diseases of pregnancy (preeclampsia, eclampsia, and HELLP syndrome), hemorrhage, and abortion, although the order of prevalence varies between specific countries and regions. In developed countries, complications from preeclampsia are the most common, but in most poor countries, hemorrhage prevails as the leading cause of maternal death (Bonnet et al. 2011; Oliveira et al. 2009; Veloz et al. 2010; Rodríguez et al. 2007). Maternal deaths caused by these conditions are related to the quality and the access to care that women have when the complication arises.

However, there are other non-clinical causes tied to social determinants that limit the care of obstetric complications (Karlsen et al. 2011). In other words, mortality derived from maternal complications is not only due to clinical causes, but there are also other factors that have to be taken into account because they contribute to a pregnant women not receiving timely or appropriate care in order to prevent her death. The social determinants for maternal death include poverty, poor education, and lack of income and nutrition, as well as women's inequality regarding development opportunities and decision-making, which leaves them in a socially vulnerable position. Thus, a maternal death is not only another number on the list of national statistics but has implications which extend far beyond the clinical causes that led to the death of the woman. These include prevailing conditions of the social and cultural context existing before the onset of the complication that ultimately contribute to a fatal pregnancy outcome.

In Mexico, there are important regional differences in the prevalence of maternal deaths. For example, in 2015, states such as Nayarit (central Mexico) (Fig. 13.1), as well as Tabasco, Guerrero, Oaxaca,

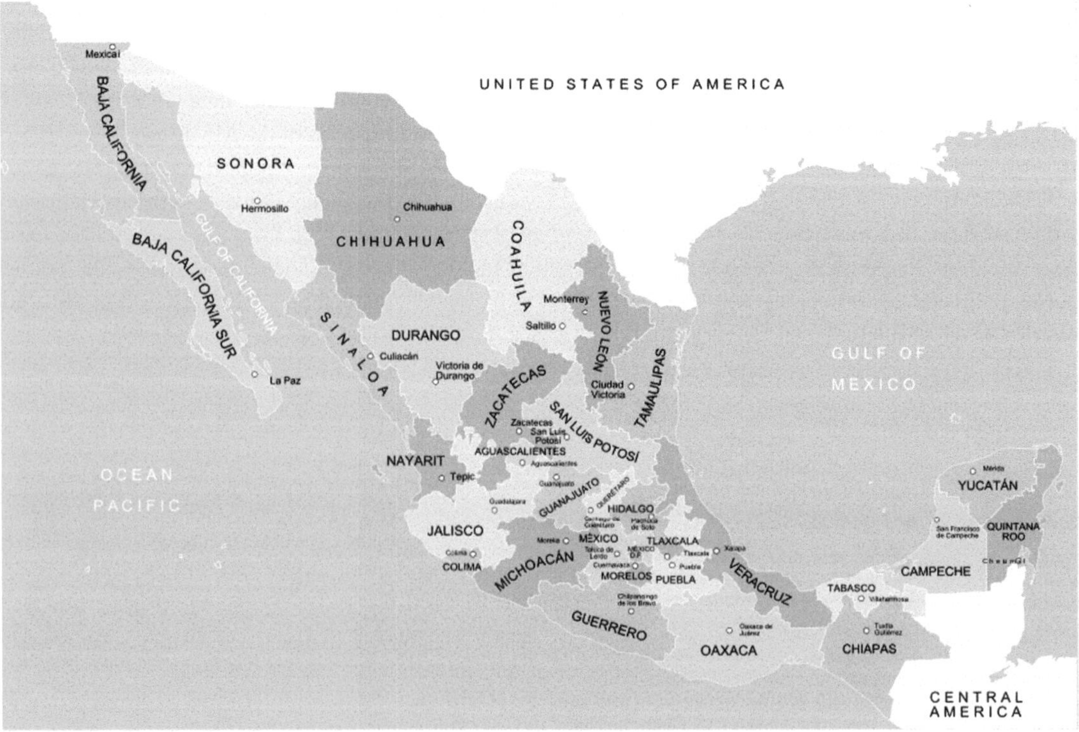

Fig. 13.1 The states of Mexico

and Yucatan (south-southeast Mexico), reported the highest MMRs, while in the northern states, like Sinaloa and Sonora, maternal mortality was lower (MMRs of 40–50 vs. 10) (Sistema Nacional de Vigilancia Epidemiológica–SINAVE 2015). The state of Yucatan has been classified as a state with an intermediate MMR, which has decreased from 69.4 in 1990 to 42.4 in 2014 (SINAVE 2015).

From the standpoint of official statistics, the issue of maternal mortality is not as serious in Yucatan as it is in other states in Mexico. However, it is far from overtaking those states in Mexico that have a low MMR. Furthermore, it has been shown that under-registration of maternal death cases masks the real magnitude of the problem (Rodríguez et al. 2005).

Although there are geographic differences in the number of maternal deaths, the sociocultural, sociodemographic, and individual aspects of the deceased women have been well-studied. In the state of Yucatan, it is the indigenous Mayan women in particular that have the highest risk of dying when a maternal complication arises. In previous studies, it has been determined that this risk is six times higher among women living in highly marginalized regions (Rodríguez and Ordóñez 2006).

The objective of this chapter is to describe the characteristics of the maternal deaths, as well as the maternal health-related needs, knowledge, and practice in Mayan women from the state of Yucatan, Mexico.

13.2 The Land and People of the Yucatan

The state of Yucatan, located in southeast Mexico, has a population of 2,097,175 inhabitants, of which 1,069,627 are women (51.0%) and 1,027,548 are men (49.0%). The Yucatecan territory represents 2.02% of the total size of Mexico and is made up of 106 municipalities, of which 84% are in urban areas and 16% in rural areas. Almost 9% (8.8%) of the population has attended the second year of high school, and 30% of the population speak an indigenous language, most commonly Yucatec Maya. The major activity in the Yucatan is the textile and fishing trade, with a contribution of 1.5% to the national gross domestic product (GDP) (INEGI 2016).

Poverty exists in 48.5% of municipalities, with 11.7% having extreme poverty; the educational gap is 24.6%, with 22.4% of the population lacking access to health services, 56.8% lacking access to social security, and 45.3% lacking economic well-being (CONEVAL 2012).

In the state of Yucatan, the simultaneous presence and consequent interaction of biomedical (allopathic) and "traditional" models of reproductive healthcare are a reality in many rural communities that make up the state. To completely understand this situation, a deep and complete look at the historical, social, economic, educational, ethnographic, and medical aspects of pregnancy among indigenous women in this area is required. The complex process of pregnancy, childbirth, and puerperium should not be understood and treated only for its physiological aspects but also in its social and cultural dimensions, indispensable for therapeutic efficacy to be integral. This means not only considering demographic, geographic, and economic variables but also understanding the practices, conceptions, and values within a context where they are legitimized and explained. For this reason, the ways of dealing with pregnancy and childbirth vary according to the history, the socioeconomic context, and the geographical location. Pregnancy itself and the proximity of childbirth constitute a risk of death, because for a Mayan woman to become pregnant may also mean dying. As a consequence, Mayan women and their culture have historically built a set of representations and cultural practices to face this potential hazard. Its knowledge is dynamic; it transforms and appropriates the knowledge that biomedicine has put at its disposal through its representatives, since it solves some of the health problems that afflict the population. Mayan women and men recognize that women who formerly would have died during pregnancy or childbirth are now likely to survive, especially if health facilities are within their reach. However, an obstacle to adequate access for indigenous people to health services is the poor communication between medical personnel, midwives, and women of reproductive age, mainly as a result of language and social differences. Indigenous women would prefer that staff doctors and nurses communicate with them in Maya. In addition, the discomfort of being attended by male doctors as well as the lack of knowledge of health personnel about the prenatal and postnatal practices of the indigenous population (eating and behavioral practices) further compromises the care of pregnant indigenous women (Rodríguez et al. 2006; Quattrocchi 2007).

13.3 Methods

13.3.1 Study Design

The data come from five descriptive, cross-sectional, retrospective, mixed-method studies that combined qualitative and quantitative research on the characteristics of maternal deaths in women that had complications during pregnancy, delivery, or the puerperium.

13.3.2 Population and Samples

The total number of maternal deaths which occurred during the study period between 2007 and 2010 was 335. The inclusion criteria for this study were based upon examination of the death certificates of women between 15 and 49 years of age, native to communities of the state of Yucatan, in whose certificates an obstetric complication was stated as the basic, intermediate, or direct cause of death. These maternal deaths corresponded to women living in 44 of the106 municipalities of the state of Yucatan. Interviews with close relatives of the deceased (verbal autopsies) were carried out. Women of childbearing age that survived an obstetric complication, health personnel, and community leaders were also interviewed in order to gather information on maternal healthcare-related knowledge, practices, and needs.

13.3.3 Methods of Data Collection

Data collection was performed in two ways: through the examination of death certificates and by means of interviews carried out with relatives, women of childbearing age, health personnel, and community leaders regarding clinical and sociodemographic variables, as well as variables related to the access and availability of maternal health services. Information was first extracted from the death certificates, and the missing data were completed by means of a questionnaire. The clinical variables associated with the maternal deaths, including direct and indirect obstetrical conditions, were classified according to ICD-10 codes O00–O99. Other variables, such as the number of pregnancies and abortions, use of contraception, prenatal monitoring, and care during delivery and obstetric events, were also analyzed. The sociodemographic variables analyzed together with the information on the death certificates included the maternal age, civil status, occupation, religion, level of education, and place of residence. Religious practices, language, and knowledge of the risk of death during pregnancy, delivery, or puerperium were also studied. Finally, the relatives' perceptions on the causes of death were also explored.

The variables related to the access to and availability of the health services included the approximate time between initiation of the search for assistance and the administration of care during delivery and between the onset of the medical complication and the initiation of care. These periods were estimated according to the relatives' comments on the type and availability of transportation used to transfer the women; this was corroborated by touring the different municipalities where the women

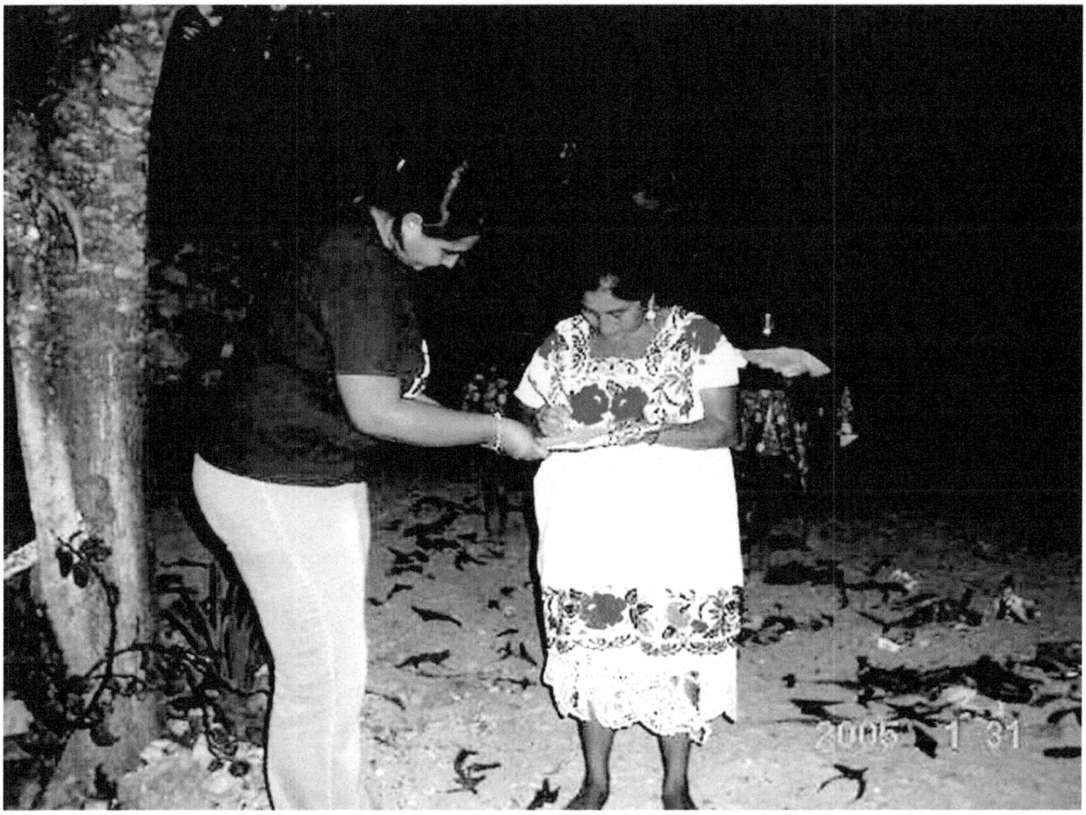

Fig. 13.2 Mayan pregnancy woman signing the informed consent

resided. To collect the information from the women's relatives, the informant had to be aware of the deceased woman's reproductive history and had to have lived the process of pregnancy, delivery, and puerperium closely. The questionnaire included 15 questions on the aforementioned variables. Before applying it, the relatives' informed consent was obtained (Fig. 13.2).

13.3.4 Data Processing and Analysis

Data were entered into a database produced using the EPI-Info 6.04 software, and the frequencies of every quantitative variable were calculated. Regarding the qualitative information, a discourse analysis of each participant's answers was prepared. The arguments selected were the ones related to the two analysis axes of the study (maternal health needs and knowledge and practice of maternal health) that were most frequently repeated. Information was presented in a tabular format.

13.3.5 Instrument

The questionnaire was tested for validity in ten women of the communities where the deceased women resided. Two researchers with experience in interviewing Mayan women examined the statements and the answers to the questionnaires. Where the lack of clarity of the questions led to confusion, the researcher was allowed to rephrase the interview to enhance clarity.

13.4 Ethical Considerations

A letter stating the project's objective and ensuring confidentiality of the information was given to each participant for voluntary signing. In cases of illiteracy, the interviewer read the letter verbally. A Mayan interpreter was available when needed. The study protocol was submitted and approved by the "Dr. Hideyo Noguchi" Center of Regional Investigations at the Autonomous University of Yucatan.

13.5 Results

The results correspond to studies carried out regarding 335 maternal deaths occurring between 1997 and 2010 in the state of Yucatan. In terms of their location, they corresponded to areas of both low and high marginalization.

We observed that the maternal deaths occurred among young women whose ages varied from 20 to 29 years (40.70%); most of them were married (90.60%); they were engaged in housework (95.30%); their level of schooling was low (illiterate, incomplete elementary education) (65.70%); and they were Catholic (81.80%) and native speakers of Mayan, although they understood Spanish (84.40%) (Table 13.1).

In terms of their reproductive health background, the registered data showed that the pregnancies occurred among primiparous women (11.50%), women in their second to third pregnancies (44.70%), and women with multiple (4 or more) pregnancies (43.80%). The majority did not use contraception (95.50%), and prenatal monitoring during the last pregnancy was irregular (88.89%) (Table 13.2).

Table 13.1 Social and demographic features of the women in this study

Characteristics		Frequency $n = 335$	Percentage
Age (years)	10–14	9	2.80
	15–19	21	6.40
	20–24	105	31.30
	25–29	32	9.40
	30–34	32	9.40
	35–39	94	28.20
	40–44	42	12.5
Civil status	Married	303	90.60
	Single	11	3.10
	Free union	21	6.30
Occupation	Home duties	319	95.30
	Others	16	4.70
Education	Illiterate	115	34.40
	Incomplete primary school	105	31.30
	Completed primary school	52	15.60
	Secondary school	52	15.60
	Unknown	11	3.10
Religion	Catholic	274	81.80
	Other	61	18.20
Language	Only Maya	283	84.40
	Maya and Spanish	52	15.60

Table 13.2 Obstetrical and reproductive health characteristics of the maternal deaths in this study

	Characteristics	Number (n = 335)	Percentage
Pregnancies	First pregnancy	39	11.50
	Two to three pregnancies	150	44.70
	Four or more pregnancies	146	43.80
Abortions	None	209	62.50
	One	73	21.90
	Two or more	53	15.60
Contraception	None	320	95.50
	Yes	15	4.50
Prenatal monitoring	None	38	11.11
	Yes (irregular)	297	88.89

The most frequent direct obstetric causes of death included hemorrhage (34.60%), sepsis (21.90%), and the hypertensive diseases of pregnancy including preeclampsia and eclampsia (15.60%). It is noteworthy that indirect obstetric deaths, including arteriovenous malformations, aneurysm of the left frontal-parietal hemisphere, liver cancer, anemia, grade III (severe) malnutrition, renal failure, and cardiomyopathy, were also identified. Our data indicated that maternal healthcare during delivery was in most cases provided by a physician, and the places of death were mainly public hospitals or the households.

The estimated time between the search for medical assistance and the initiation of care during delivery varied from between 10 min and 2 h in the case of home deliveries. For those deliveries which were cared for in hospitals, the range was between 1 h and 2 h. The time elapsed between the onset of the complication and the initiation of care for it varied from between 1 h and 2 h in the cases of hemorrhage, approximately 5 h in the case of eclampsia, and between 3 and 5 days in the case of sepsis.

13.6 Maternal Healthcare Needs

Within the communities studied, people's outlook on maternal health needs, the way in which gender relationships are conducted, and the care that they received from the health services was variable. However, their opinions on the maternal healthcare needs revolved around the lack of permanent medical staff, of a health center in the community, and the issue of infrastructure. Some of the communities are hours away from the municipal seat and the roads are unpaved, with the result that pregnant women approaching their date of delivery would leave their houses up to 2 weeks in advance and travel to a place closer to the municipal seat in order to prevent the risks of a preterm complicated delivery.

Discourses also point to the need for women to be very interested in their health and nutrition. Some of the women's husbands acknowledge the scarce or absent participation of men during informative talks on the reproductive process and, above all, during prenatal consultations. In general terms, husbands do not worry much about their wives' health and few are aware of these issues, although some leaders demand that husbands pay more attention to their wives and join them in the programs promoted by the health sector. The fact that women are subjected to violence on the part of their husbands also appears in the accounts.

Other aspects observed in the interviews point to the treatment that people are given when seeking a medical consultation and the limited relationship established between women and the personnel at the clinics. However, this attitude came up regarding not only hospital care but also the assistance given by traditional midwives (*parteras*).

Some women of childbearing age count on their experiences during previous pregnancies to be able to recognize aspects that might endanger their lives. In other cases, they take into account the distance between their communities and a hospital or a clinic where they could seek care during delivery. They are also aware of other factors such as nutrition, hard work, the presence of other endangering diseases, extremes of age, and exposure to cold weather.

Thus, in the state of Yucatan, the trend of rural populations (primarily indigenous women) having fewer opportunities and less access to health services is still persistent. In these communities, both men and women perceive the lack of specialized medical equipment, medicines, and sufficient infrastructure to fulfill the needs of women during the reproductive process (Table 13.3) (Fig. 13.3).

Table 13.3 Maternal healthcare needs according to relatives and women in childbearing age

Permanent physician in the communities, infrastructure, and medicines	"That doctors be sent to take care of women when they have their children; medicines; a place where the woman can have her baby and can recover inside the clinic. That beds be sent, or at least ambulances that can transfer those women that need to be taken elsewhere (husband)" "A hospital with a doctor's office is needed, with everything that can be useful when women can die; and, well, I feel that an ambulance is needed for any health problem that cannot be resolved here in Xcan (father)" "I think that we should have our own clinic and that the road to leave should be in better conditions, since that's a problem because it's very bad and it takes a long time to get there; even though it's not a big distance, but due to the type of road, it takes one a long time (mother)" "A room where pregnant women can be operated, medicines and specialists are needed, so we don't have to move to other places and run the risk of something happening on the way, because while we are taken, there's a one-way freight charge of 300 pesos to Tizimín and when you are discharged it's another 300 (woman)" "Here, who is going to take care of them? They have to go to 'Colonia Yucatan' so they're taken care of, because otherwise, they can go through what my aunt lived: she died because she bled out; the midwife did not take good care of her and her husband did nothing to take her to another place (niece)"
Diet for the pregnant woman	"They need to eat well, to get nourished, that their husbands take good care of them, that they have all they need at home. I, when I remember how my daughter lived, I can't take it, I start crying (mother)" "So the ladies don't die, they should make an effort to get checked every month, have their pressure taken and be mindful of what they eat [...]. In the 'Oportunidades' (Opportunities) program, by law, they have to attend their talks (sister-in-law and sisters)" "Those that are in risk of dying are the malnourished ones, those that don't eat well, those that are not well nourished, don't take their vitamins and sometimes don't go to the doctor (woman)"
Husband's participation	"I think it would be better if we had our own health center and, as the doctor says, husbands should be interested and not falling asleep (husband)" "There still is the influence that husbands exert on their wives so they don't undergo analyses or tests such as the Papanicolaou. It is necessary that the men be given learning talks as the ladies are, and more so the husbands who belong to the 'Oportunidades' (Opportunities) program. They should go so they can have their analyses carried out too and, at the same time, keep their wives company and thus not get upset. Furthermore, there's also the influence of the beating that the husbands give their wives so they have a miscarriage, and they don't say anything to the family, out of shame or out of fear of being beaten up again (sister-in-law and sisters)"
Dignified treatment	"I don't know what's going on; sometimes you go pick up your card and they don't give it to you. It's the nurse's fault. I think it's because there's no doctor. Pregnant women are treated a bit better (mother)" "A relative should be present when the midwife is in charge, because I don't know what my mother died of; the midwife wouldn't let us in (daughter)" "That they be honest; I was deceived. Honesty towards the family and towards them, that they be informed about their condition (husband)" "In the urban health center there isn't everything that's needed to take care of a delivery and you're sent to a hospital and nobody pays attention to you, the nurses don't look after you, they are talking or just putting make-up on. There's a preference for rich people, and the poor ones are pushed aside (mother)"

Table 13.3 (continued)

Material and equipment	"My wife was nine-months pregnant. One morning, she said she was in some pain and wanted me to take her to the doctor so he could see her. I took her to the doctor at the health center, and when we arrived she couldn't stand it anymore and she felt she couldn't breathe. The doctor checked her and said it would be better to take her to the hospital. There, they said the delivery was normal. They asked me to buy a blade, scissors, talc, soap and diapers for the baby because they had none of that. I bought what they asked for and when I got to the hospital I was told my wife was going to be operated on because things had complicated. The girl was born all right, but when I went in to see my wife after the operation, she was not looking well; she looked pale and didn't talk. The doctor told me it was better to take her to another hospital because there wasn't enough equipment where we were. My wife was taken to another hospital. There I was told that they needed to give her blood and I had to donate it, but that her body wouldn't take it, that in the same way they gave it to her, it came out. My wife remained like that for 8 days until she died. I was told that her death was due to the fact that she was wrongly operated, that two veins had been cut (husband)"

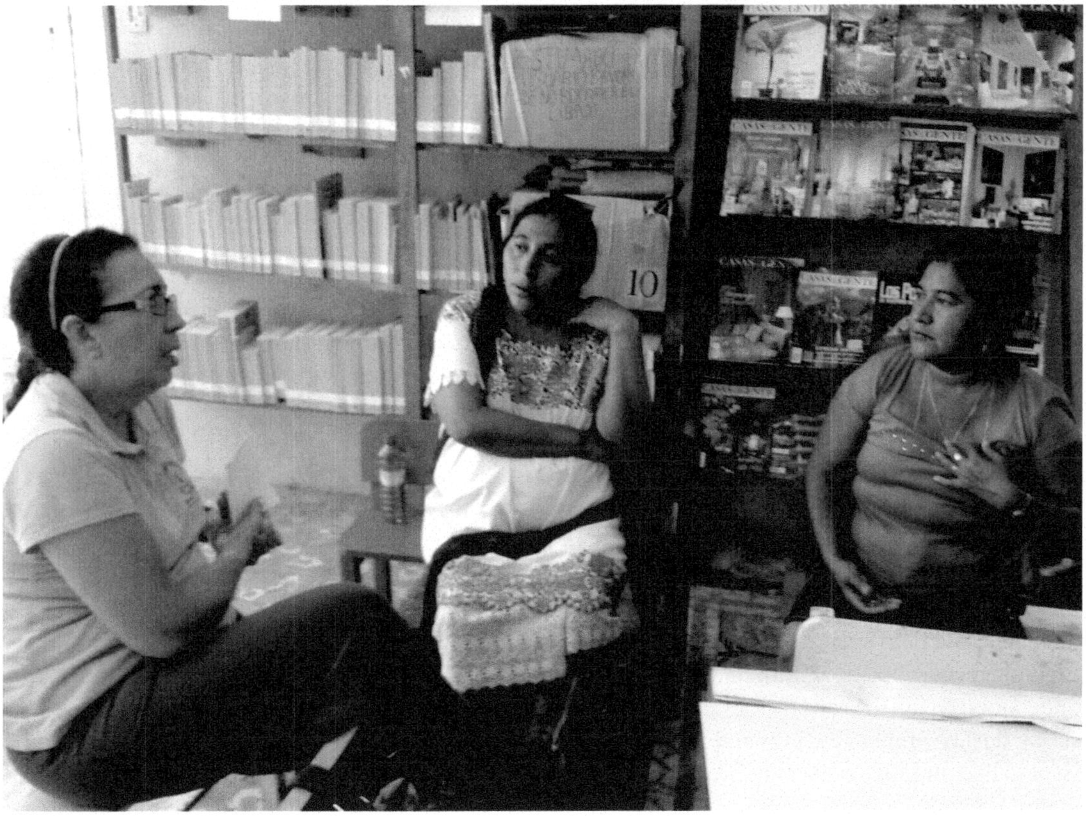

Fig. 13.3 Pregnant Mayan woman with the Mayan language translator and interviewer

Table 13.3 shows the discourses of both men and women regarding their perception of the health-care needs of women in their communities, such as having specialists, better infrastructure, feeding, greater participation of the male, and better relationship of the community by health personnel.

At the health center, where women go for prenatal monitoring but deliveries are not performed there, members of the clinic staff were interviewed. When asked what was needed to improve reproductive health services and thereby reduce the risk of maternal death in the locality, they pointed to the need for specialized medical personnel, and they also mentioned the women's lack of information, the conditions in which they live, and the manner in which they are given medical information

Table 13.4 Maternal healthcare needs according to health personnel

Specialized medical personnel	"A delivery room and an emergency room; a specialist so the pregnant woman isn't transferred to another place and so the risk of something happening to her on the way is prevented (physician)" "In case the woman is 9 months pregnant, the clinic doesn't have all the necessary instruments, so she is sent to a hospital. I almost begged the husband that if he didn't take her, she would die. A lot of things are needed, like medical personnel and medicines (physician)"
Information for the pregnant woman	"That women be more aware of the risks they run when they get pregnant younger than 19 or older than 35; the environment where they develop; their ignorance in terms of information; their religion; 'machismo' (male chauvinism), their being traditional; their lack of responsibility as a father or mother (nurse)" "Women still have a lot of prejudices and men are the ones that tell them what they're going to do. Women between 14 and 15 years of age are more aware, they ask us about their doubts and all that is related to family planning, unlike the ones that are 24–25 years old, which think that they will have all the children that God sends to them (nurse)"
Transmission of information	"Education is lacking, not training, because it is 'untraining': some days you give them talks and that's it; they don't even know if they did things as they should; they never come to see if they really understood; this should begin in school, in elementary school [...], knowing how to educate the boys and the girls. We can't do anything. See what things are like here, a super small place, we don't have space to move, we have about 30 or 40 consultations... and the truth is that when a patient is sent for an ultrasound, she goes to the second level [of care] and she comes back and it has not been performed; the truth is that there are deficiencies and they have the patient going around in circles and her problem is not solved (consultant physician)"

(Table 13.4). Table 13.4 shows what health personnel consider to be the maternal health needs. These include the need for better infrastructure and medical specialists so that deliveries can be attended in the same communities, improving knowledge about risks by women, and also the way information is transmitted between health personnel and women on cultural issues.

The community leaders who were interviewed consisted of the midwives (*parteras*) in the communities and a Catholic priest. The midwives are important actors during all stages of pregnancy, delivery, and in the postpartum period, when they apply the knowledge that has been transmitted to them generationally. During pregnancy, women avoid both temperature changes as well as eating certain foods which are considered dangerous. During the postpartum period, they do not seek care by a doctor, but only the midwife's and their relatives' support, in spite of the established procedures to warrant a safe delivery and postpartum period (NOM-007 2016) (Fig. 13.4).

With respect to the comments made by the midwives, most of whom spoke Mayan but also understood Spanish well, the actions to improve women's health are focused on nutritional counseling during pregnancy, prenatal monitoring, vitamin intake, and similar maternal health-related issues. The plurality regarding the care of pregnant women and the legitimacy of their practice and that of doctors is clearly seen in their accounts through which they establish meeting points in the process of pregnancy. On the other hand, the priest emphasized the need to offer information on care during pregnancy (Table 13.5). In Table 13.5 we illustrate topics that community leaders such as midwives and the catholic priest emphasized regarding maternal health needs—the midwives' discourse focused on feeding during pregnancy and prenatal care including the provision of vitamins to women, while the priest discussed the lack of information about care during pregnancy.

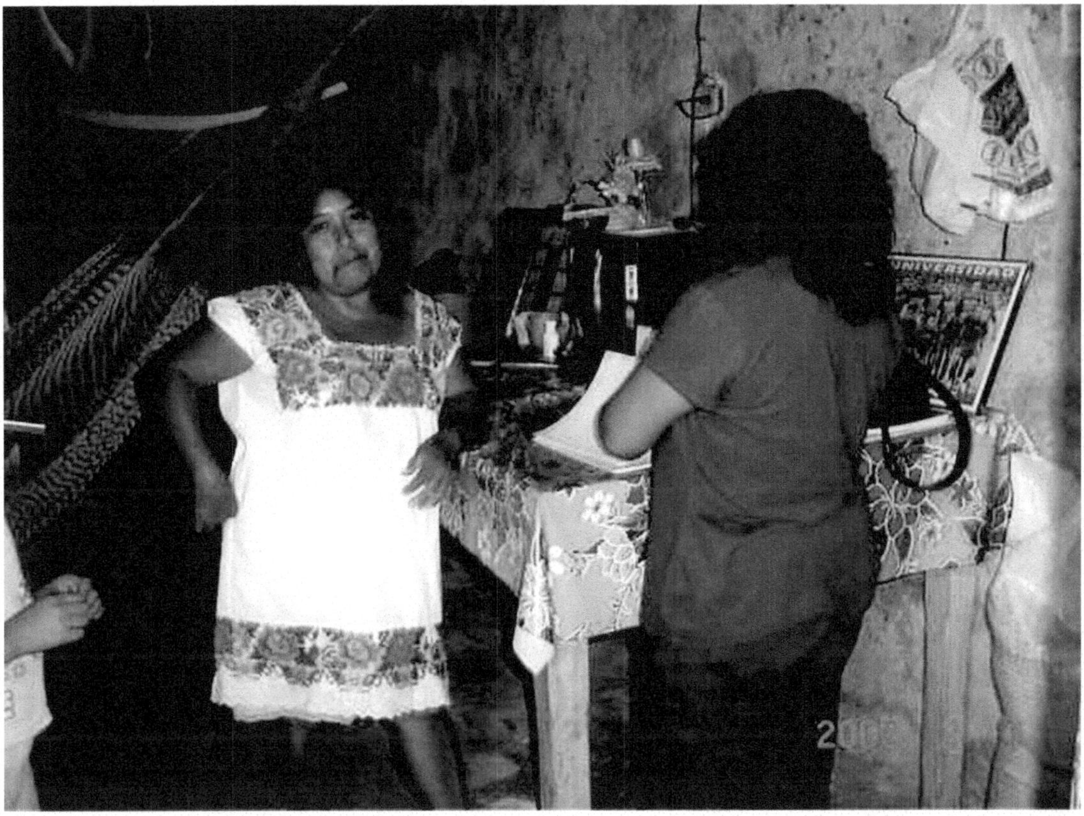

Fig. 13.4 Midwife conducting an interview in the Mayan language

Table 13.5 Maternal health care needs according to midwives and a priest

Nutrition during pregnancy	"Women should eat properly and according to their possibilities; say something when they aren't feeling well, not remain silent. That they be taken care of at home and that they take what they're told, because they are taking care of their child. During delivery, to do what they are told, help their body so [the delivery] is easier. And during quarantine, having good personal hygiene and speaking up if they don't feel well (midwife with 41 years of experience)" "Those who come from the mountain don't seek care at the beginning, they wait until they feel very bad and then they come; their nutrition is poor and they are not taken care of at their homes (midwife)"
Prenatal monitoring	"That she be monitored at the hospital, because they are given vitamins and that she take care of herself during the pregnancy, so at the time of delivery, neither she nor the baby are in danger; and during recovery, that she be at rest, so she recovers soon (midwife)"
Information and specialist physicians	"A little more information on how to take care of a pregnancy is needed. More physicians are needed; efforts should be made to create more health centers. There is a need for more professional personnel, specialists, gynecologists, etcetera (priest)"

13.6.1 Knowledge and Practices on Maternal Health

In terms of the family environment and reproductive practices, women's knowledge and practices during the three stages of the reproductive process (pregnancy, delivery, and the postpartum period) were explored. The information obtained from the relatives and from women of childbearing age demonstrated knowledge about their bodies for a healthy delivery, the desirable age to have a child, the risk of suffering from other diseases, and the lack of interest in self-care as factors that can lead to higher risk during pregnancy (Fig. 13.5). With respect to the practices, it was observed that during the reproductive process, some women still consult only with the midwife (*partera*) for pregnancy care, while others follow complementary practices by attending two health systems. On the one hand, they go to the midwife to confirm if they are pregnant, to find out the baby's position, and for a *sobada* (rubbing or massage) (Quattrocchi 2007); but on the other, they are taken care of by the physician who on occasion visits communities far away from the municipal seat and where there is no health center.

Indigenous women of childbearing age frequently visit both the traditional midwife (*partera*) and the physician during their pregnancy—the midwife performs massages (*sobada*) and recommends their diet, and the physician performs checkups of the mother and baby and administers

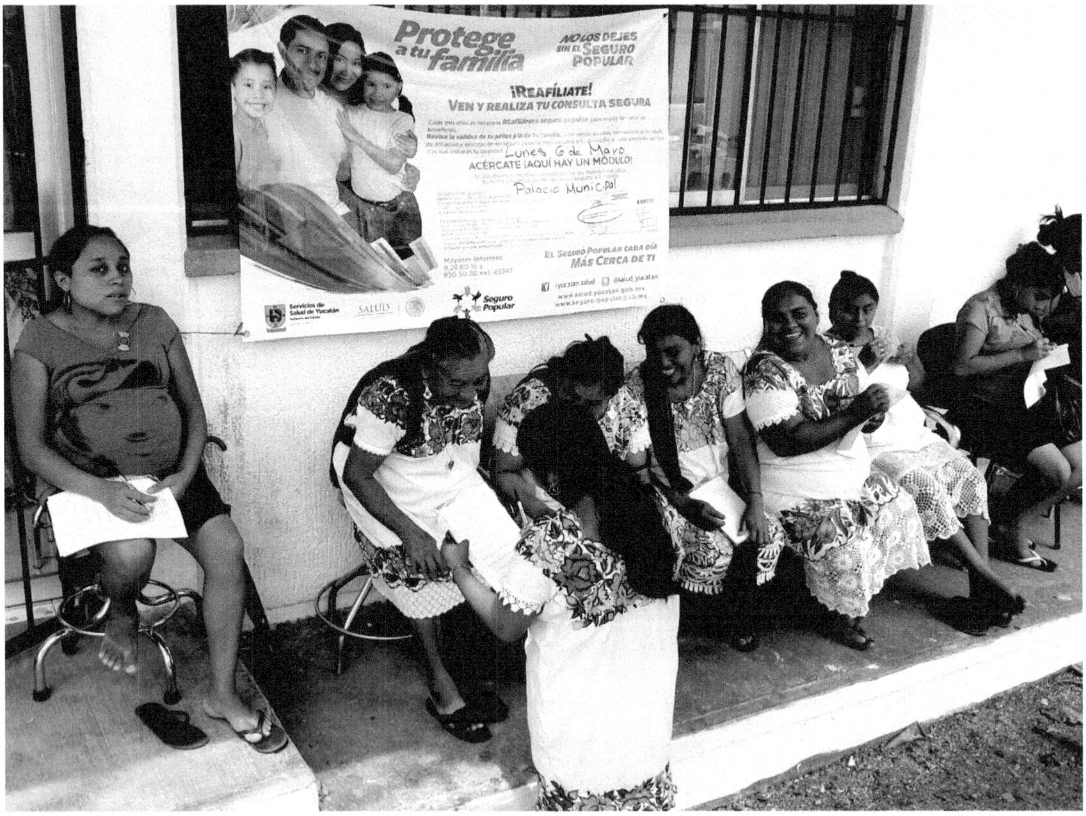

Fig. 13.5 Pregnant Mayan women, a midwife, and grandmother discussing knowledge and practices on maternal health

prenatal vitamins. The diversity of indigenous women's answers regarding various aspects of maternal care and pregnancy, and even the antagonism between some of the discourses, reflects important changes in the way of perceiving and understanding the reproductive process within the community. This may partly be a consequence of the fact that they have modified their way of living and, in particular, their way of taking care of themselves during pregnancy, delivery, and postpartum. Following delivery, some women closely abide by the care strategies recommended by the midwife, who takes care both of the mother and the child and recommends that her nutrition be based on beans, egg, vegetables, and chicken and beef broth, which they complement with the vitamins prescribed by the physician at the health center. During the 40 days after delivery, women pay close attention to nutrition, rest, and exposure to cold. During this period, the help they receive from their mothers and mothers-in-law, and even from the midwives, who bathe the child in the first days and do laundry so the new mother can rest adequately, is essential. The beliefs centering around the reproductive process and care during delivery held by indigenous women in the communities are no less important. For instance, the death of a young woman named Rudencina is attributed to the bad attitude and behavior of another young woman, considered inadmissible and banned by the population. The death of another woman was attributed to luck (Table 13.6). The following (Table 13.6) describes knowledge, beliefs, and practices on maternal health from the perspective of family members and women in the childbearing age, which relate to the woman's body, the age of the pregnant woman and the diseases that can accompany pregnancy and put it at risk, and their experiences related to attitudes and beliefs to which they attribute death.

Health personnel were asked about their perception of the health of women of childbearing age within the community, as well as the ideas they shared about recognizing the customs and beliefs of the Mayan culture. Regarding the perception by healthcare personnel of maternal risk, they attributed it to the delay in seeking medical care and the lack of vehicles for transfer. However, maternal deaths are seen as a matter of numbers, without social relevance, by the health personnel (Table 13.7) (Fig. 13.6). Table 13.7 shows the maternal health knowledge and practices according to the healthcare personnel, including their perceptions on the number of births, maternal care, care by midwives, care-seeking behavior, and maternal deaths.

Midwives were asked about the nature of the care that they offered to women when their assistance was sought. Their response indicates their knowledge of the woman's body regarding maternal health and its relationship with cold and heat, not only in order to become pregnant but also after delivery to prevent complications. The recognition of these cultural elements and their connection to the body show an integration of the body in its individual and social dimension. The midwives also made reference to the pregnant woman's nutrition, delays when they or their relatives ask for help, as well as to the latter's maneuvers (abdominal massages or tightening the abdomen with the belt) to assist with the birth.

The priest was asked if he gave the women advice on healthcare during pregnancy, delivery, and the postpartum, and he answered that his job was the guidance of women. However, regarding risk, he made reference to the problem of adolescent pregnancies, pregnancy outside of marriage, the changes with respect to the expectations of marriage by the church, and the inequities of some communities compared to others in terms of access to prenatal monitoring (Table 13.8). The following table describes the main knowledge and practices of midwives and religious representatives, who addressed the advice and remedies they give to pregnant women, delays in seeking care, and some maneuvers they utilize to assist in delivery. They also mention the lack of information to prevent teenage pregnancies.

Table 13.6 Maternal health knowledge, beliefs and practices according to relatives and women in childbearing age

The body	"The woman should be slim to have a good pregnancy (mother)" "She should have ample hips so it's not a C-section; she should not be chubby; it is said she should not be too short (woman)" "I don't think so. She should look healthy, that the woman looks fine is important, that she doesn't look sick. What good is a pretty body if she is pale or sick? Her body won't help her (sister)" "It has to do with it because sometimes if you are very chubby, it's difficult when we get pregnant; and those who are too skinny and are always dieting and don't eat well, when they get pregnant, they start having problems and diseases (woman)" "No, because sometimes fat women have a baby with no problem, but the doctor says that one should not exceed because you accumulate a lot of fat (woman)" "She should be chubby so she doesn't get hurt (mother)"
Age and diseases	"I think that the ones that are in a greater risk are those between 30 and 35 years of age, since their blood pressure can be high or because they are older (woman)" "She would be in greater risk if she is sick and she gets pregnant" (daughter) "There are many who have blood pressure problems, so if they want to get pregnant they have to go for a check-up, so they are doing fine. The same for those who don't eat well, and if your sugar level is high, it's dangerous to get pregnant" (mother) "Older women—it's not the same for a girl to get pregnant than for a lady. The lady can have blood pressure issues, her pressure can rise; if she has had many children, doctors say that one's womb gets tired" (mother) "Young women, because their body isn't fully developed yet, and they begin giving life to another human being and their body doesn't finish developing" (woman)
Practices with the midwife	"During pregnancy, women here keep doing the same thing, I keep doing the same thing, I don't quit doing anything: picking up things, washing, cooking. My mother tells me that I shouldn't lie down so the baby is born fine, because if you lie down, you slacken; that is why many girls that lie down have to be operated on" (woman) "When I have my children, I prefer to go with the midwife because I trust her more and I know her" (woman) "I almost never go to the doctor, because I don't like it; I'm scared and ashamed. I have always gone to the midwife; she would rub me every other week when I was pregnant. I went because when I picked up things, I felt how the child went down; 1 h later, she helped me and rubbed me again" (woman) "She would go to the midwife to be rubbed, for back pain and to adjust the baby. She would go to her prenatal monitoring appointments, vaccines, analyses and talks and they supposedly measured her blood pressure. Why was she never told it rose?" (husband) "She would go to the health center or to the midwife, who is her child's godmother; she preferred going to the midwife because at the San Carlos Hospital, they offer care, but only for the most serious cases" (husband) "Besides going to the clinic, I would go to the midwife to have a rub every month. And at the time of delivery, the midwife is the one who receives my children; they go get her and they bring her home. Then, she waits for the pain to be more intense and she prepares to receive your baby, and when I had my babies, my husband and my mother were always by my side. After my baby is born, she cleans me and 'ties me up' to prevent complications, headaches. She also tells me that during the next 40 days I should not go out into the evening moisture ('sereno') or be close to the smoke, because a woman's milk dries out" (woman)
Attitude and practices about risk and death	"The baby was born at Rudencina's home, with the help of the midwife. Five days after the delivery, both were doing fine. Then, her sister went to visit, but she was pregnant, and she asked why she had come to visit, since in the town it is said that pregnant women shouldn't visit those who have just given birth. When her sister left, she started having a strong headache and went to a herbalist. This man sent her a white powder that she had to mix with alcohol and spread it on her head, because that was the area that hurt. They followed the indications; but some time later, she felt a pain in her chest and that was when she began to experience shortness of breath and couldn't breathe well. Soon after, she died" (woman) "They don't die if it's not their time. I think that's the way it was supposed to be. One of my children's mothers-in-law has lost two daughters during delivery; it's her luck" (woman)

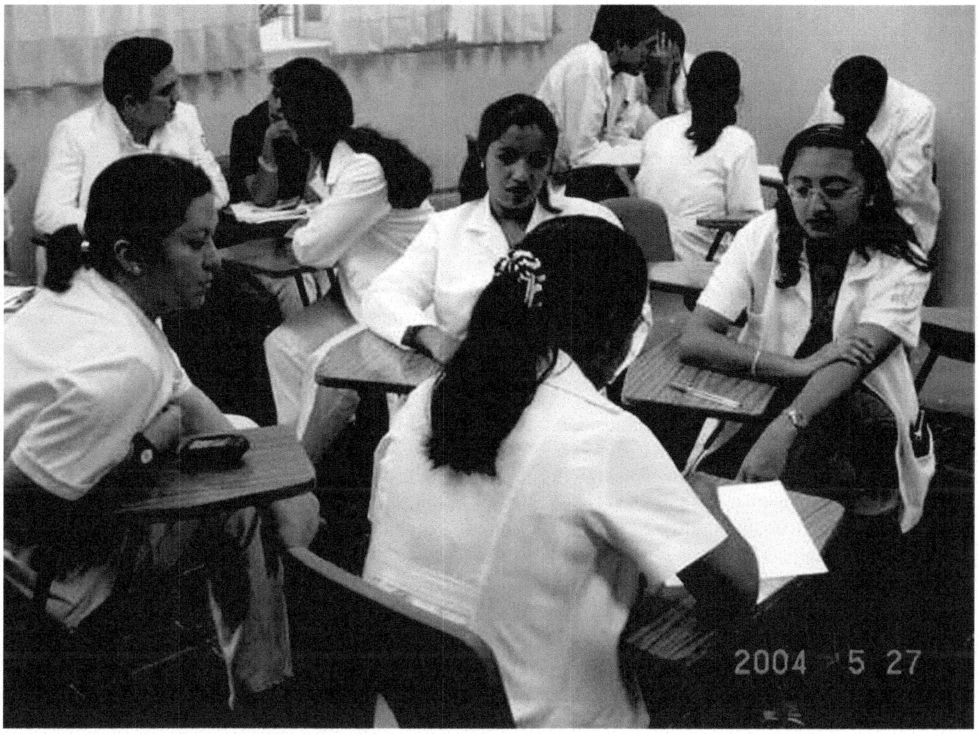

Fig. 13.6 Health personnel discussing a case of maternal death

Table 13.7 Maternal health knowledge and practices according to the health personnel

Number of births	"Women's health is good because I notice that there are many births and that means it's fine. Women live their sexuality freely, whether they are well off or not. In Tizimín, the average number of children among women in all families is five. One should consider that women's education plays an important, regardless of their socio-economical level" (male nurse)
Maternal care	"Pregnant women are mostly underage. Women (not all of them) are not interested in taking care of their health; some of them don't go to prenatal monitoring. In general, women's health is average, due to their ignorance" (female nurse) "Women's health is much neglected, totally; women are very irresponsible" (physician) "Here, women don't take care of themselves because they see the pregnancy process as something natural. I recommend that they reduce their burden of work, that they have a good nutrition, that they reduce their sexual relations. They only come to prenatal monitoring due to the 'Oportunidades' (Opportunities) Program" (physician, nurse and health promoter)
Care by midwives	"The mother dies because they go first to the midwife and the cases are difficult, and the midwife manipulates her patient a lot. In the olden days, they would give the patient a shot, but not anymore; before they would force the patient, even if she was not completely dilated, and the uterus would rupture. This provoked the death of the lady; then, the midwife referred the lady when there was nothing to be done" (male nurse) "They keep on with their custom of being taken care of by the midwife. It's the people's culture; they think the midwives are chosen by God. At the time of delivery, the midwife goes to the pregnant woman's house, sometime they give her an oxytocin shot, because the woman is taking too long to give birth to the baby, and that's when things go wrong and they take them to the clinic, but sometimes their condition is already very serious. The problem is when they have already been manipulated by midwives, and they have uterine ruptures or vulvar edemas" (physician)
Seeking care	"I remember a case of preeclampsia 3 years ago: The patient came, it was detected, she was told she had to be admitted, she didn't want to at the time, but said she would do it. She was told it was urgent; instead of doing it, she went to pick her daughter up at the kindergarten and went to get admitted until the evening. That lady died, that's why a vehicle exclusively for these cases is important" (physician)
Maternal deaths	"There are few maternal deaths compared to the number of women in childbearing age. Just because God is so great, nothing happens to them" (physician)

Table 13.8 Maternal health knowledge and practices according to midwives and a priest

Words of advice and remedies	"So when some of them don't get their period, I regularize it with a preparation they must take. When they are already pregnant, keeping an eye on them so they take the vitamins and pills prescribed by the doctor. Their nutrition is important, that they be clean; I rub them, I touch to feel how the baby is doing. If the baby is lying in transverse position, I place it correctly so the delivery is normal. When the time is come, I go with them if they go to the clinic, or I take care of them at the time of birth. I tell them it's natural, that their body already knows what to do, to be calm. Afterwards, I recommend that they take care of themselves for a while, so their body recovers. I advise them no to lie with their husband during 3–4 months, although not all of them wait that long, also to use [contraceptive] pills" (midwife) "If the woman doesn't feel well because she has been married for 2–3 years and hasn't been able to get pregnant, I rub them three times every week, during 3 weeks and I prepare their medicine with liquor. I use *x'tabentún* (traditional local drink) with herbs, and this beverage causes the woman's blood to get cleaned because in most women that have not been able to get pregnant it is because they are stunned, their blood is no good because they eat things with chili, or they bathe in cold water and that's why the babies don't stick. Therefore, first we have to clean the blood, so she can then get pregnant" (midwife) "During pregnancy they come to get rubbed and to see if they are pregnant. Many come to have the baby adjusted so there are no complications at the time of delivery and everything proceeds normally. When the time of delivery has come, I go to their houses and they decide where they want the baby to be born, on the bed or the hammock, where they feel comfortable. Once the baby is born, they wait for 2 h before they can eat hen broth without spices" (midwife) "The best advice is to guide them towards the person who can help them with their process, to go to the physician, to put them back on track" (priest)
Delays and maneuvers during delivery	"Years ago, a woman was about to have her child; my mother-in-law, who's (also) a midwife, took care of her. The woman's husband wrapped her with a big belt and squeezed her belly because she started to feel bad. She had contractions and by squeezing her belly, he forced the baby to be born. Four days later, she had an infection with fever. She died 6 days later. The relatives said that a piece of placenta was left inside, but my mother-in-law said that it was complete when it was buried next to the tray, that everything started when the font (bag with amniotic fluid) broke and they didn't take her to the doctor, and also because the husband forced her and hurt her when he squeezed her belly" (midwife)
Adolescent pregnancy	"Their [sexual] activity is very noticeable in all the children I baptize and in the teenage pregnancies as a worldwide phenomenon. They get pregnant without getting married; they are girls between 14 and 17 years of age. In the middle class, some get married and others not; most get married civilly […]; others prefer to wait and see how things develop; the same happens when they are poor or from an upper class. There's little culture with respect to prenatal monitoring; people don't know they should get checked regularly to have a good outcome. A culture of knowledge is being created, but it's not the same in the marginalized areas where they don't have this opportunity" (priest)

13.7 Obstetrical Death in the Yucatan

The profile of Mayan women who die from obstetrical causes in the state of Yucatan is similar to that of women who die due to the same causes and conditions in other regions in Mexico, as well as in other developing countries (WHO 2015). In Yucatan, there remains a widespread contribution to maternal morbidity from sociocultural factors, as well as additional problems related to both the access to and quality of medical care, and which play an important role in the fatal outcome in cases of obstetrical complications. According to the information collected, the highest risk for maternal death was in young women, most of whom were married and were unaware of the obstetric risks.

In spite of the efforts carried out by the health sector in Yucatan to prevent maternal deaths, the population's inability to recognize the warning signs of pregnancy complications was noted. These signs should be detected during the prenatal monitoring appointments, when the pregnant woman goes to the physician or the midwife for a checkup; in addition, with proper prenatal education, the pregnant woman should be able to recognize them herself in order to seek timely assistance. The inability to recognize them is directly related to the prevalence of the signs among pregnant women, such that if they are common in the region, then they are considered to be normal and nonthreatening. For instance, a multicenter study based in hospitals in Africa showed that 13% of the population reports fever, pallor, and vertigo as normal signs among pregnant women (Thonneau et al. 2004). The same situation has been reported in other countries such as India and Jordan (Shah et al. 2009; Hynes et al. 2012; Okour et al. 2012; Combs et al. 2012); in Latin America, it has been studied in Argentina, Venezuela, and Colombia (Rosestein et al. 2008; Mazza et al. 2012; Amaya et al. 2010).

In Yucatan in 2008, educational strategies to improve the knowledge of pregnancy-related warning signs among Mayan women were assessed through the design of a community intervention trial to test their effect, which was funded by the National Council for Science and Technology (Rodríguez et al. 2012a). The success of the strategy has allowed additional funding from such international sources such as the Kellogg's Foundation in order to develop educational materials and distribute them among communities. Additional foundations, such as Population Council and Save the Children, have requested these materials for reproduction. Nevertheless, resources are still insufficient to make the strategy permanent and available in all regions of the state.

13.8 Prevention of Maternal Mortality in the Yucatan

The cultural heritage of the Mayan women considered in this study has been transmitted from one generation to the next. The culture of a society and its ensuing implications greatly influence the reproductive process. This is especially true regarding the role of midwives, who in spite of their valuable knowledge and experience lack the training, knowledge, equipment, and medicines to take care of obstetrical emergencies. Comprehensive emergency obstetric care (CEmOC) is one of the recommendations to reduce maternal mortality (WHO 2015). It has been tested in developing countries, and even in such resource-limited countries such as Bangladesh, the number of maternal deaths have decreased following its implementation. As part of this program, training midwives has been important for the timely care of obstetrical emergencies, together with the financial support of non-governmental organizations (NGOs) and other sectors of society, which have participated by donating emergency equipment and facilities (Naimul 2012; World Bank 2016).

In Yucatan there remains much to be accomplished in terms of access to obstetric emergency care. Those localities that only have health centers available, that is, units that offer care of general ailments but without care for even mild risk deliveries, lack the basic equipment to treat obstetric emergencies, such as oxygen, parenteral solutions, or medicines to treat seizures and hypertensive diseases of pregnancy, among others (Rodríguez et al. 2012b). Through meetings with community leaders, the necessity to supply health centers with basic CEmOC equipment has been shown, and commitments from middle management levels (jurisdictional heads) of the health system for financial resources within municipal budgets to buy the equipment have been made (Rodríguez et al. 2015). However, in additional to providing financial resources, implementation of training for all levels of human resources, including the community midwives, in the management of obstetrical emergencies will be crucial (Rodríguez 2016).

Educating the indigenous population on their essential reproductive rights in order to ensure safe maternity is a core activity in order for women and their family to follow the necessary care during pregnancy and to promptly seek help if a complication arises. Excessive physical work during pregnancy can increase the risk of preterm delivery, which can endanger the well-being and even the life of both mother and infant. This is why pregnant women should take a rest and have their choices respected in the face of the risks for such losses. Conditions of women in the rural context are at best precarious, especially when compared to those living in urban areas. The former have to tackle the tough work of household chores without enough services and economic resources or the support of other people to deal with these adverse situations. This limits their free time to rest and their chances to care for themselves, even though they might have received warnings during prenatal monitoring appointments or when talking to their peers in the waiting rooms at the health center.

Moreover, the social conditions of Mayan women compared to those of men are disadvantageous. Because of their gender, women have been entrusted with the care of both their health and their children's. This gender-based conception of mother and child health has underrated the role that the husband should play in taking care of the woman's health during pregnancy, delivery, and postpartum. This is evident in the discourse of the women that have had to go by themselves to their prenatal monitoring appointments or among those who were asked (or told) to engage in sexual relations regardless of their own health status. Currently, promoting male participation in taking care of the wife's health is an issue that has been increasingly explored. This is especially timely because gender perspective is no longer limited to the woman's role, but it also pursues equality between men and women and encourages social support for the pregnant woman, not only from the husband but also from other relatives (Figueroa 1993).

Mayan women from the communities are limited in terms of decision-making when labor begins, which is even more evident when a maternal complication arises. They are generally not prepared for such an event, nor do they have an emergency plan in place that takes into account expenses, care for their children, obtaining transportation to a health care facility, etc. In other words, the event arises unexpectedly, leaving the woman at both high maternal and social risk in the face of several circumstances—she must seek help to take care of her family; the husband is not there to pay for the transfer to the hospital; she has to go to the doctor or to the midwife to be taken care of; she has to be transferred to another clinic because emergencies cannot be handled in her locality; there are no ambulances nor drivers for the transfer; the clinics or hospitals are many hours away; inclimate weather can make travel difficult; and when she arrives there, she must wait because demand of care is extremely high. All of these factors combine to create an environment of great vulnerability which exposes both the mother and her infant to a high risk of morbidity and, in too many cases, mortality. The limited decision-making capacity of women in these circumstances, in a context of poverty, is an all-too-common expression of the inequity that indigenous women face in terms of health care. This needs to be further studied in order to determine the factors that condition it and, hence be able to plan, develop and implement interventions focused in empowering women and adolescents to reduce the health-related gender gaps (Toukobong et al. 2016; Vidler et al. 2016; Ismayilova 2015).

Access to quality health services for indigenous women during pregnancy, delivery, and the puerperium is far from reaching the minimal international standards. In Mexico, quality care for women and children has been encouraged through initiatives and programs derived from the NOM-007 2016, so they can have the same healthcare opportunities. However, in the poorest areas of the country, the lack of resolutive capacity when handling complicated deliveries is still an unfulfilled need and an important factor related to maternal deaths. Even in those communities where there are specialized medical services for handling complicated deliveries, maternal deaths continue to occur among women who live several kilometers away from the municipal seat. Most communities lack permanent and reliable transportation, and although a mobile health unit may visit them regularly, it is not enough to solve an acute obstetric complication. The "Three Delays" Model of maternal death was originally developed in the 1990s to understand how maternal deaths occur in resource-poor countries: (1) delay in recognizing the complication and seeking help, (2) delay in the transfer to a medical service, and

(3) delay in the care, diagnosis, and timely treatment (Thaddeus and Maine 1994; Reyes 1994; Rodríguez et al. 2012c). In the state of Yucatan, the global risk of maternal death when the three types of delays are combined is 54% (Rodríguez 2016).

13.9 Maternal Health Knowledge, Beliefs, and Practices

It could be said that women adopt a plural vision, mixing knowledge of the reproductive process acquired at talks offered at the health center with popular knowledge passed down from mothers and grandmothers to daughters and granddaughters. Medical advice from these sources occurs more frequently during pregnancy because sometimes women attend prenatal monitoring appointments and to get vitamins. Midwives not only play an important role during the pregnancy but also during delivery and the postpartum period, when the knowledge carefully passed down from generation to generation becomes more evident. It is during that period that women avoid eating certain foods considered dangerous and being exposed to temperature changes. During the postpartum period, the presence of physicians is not evident; instead, the midwife's and the relatives' support is essential, even though there are procedures established to ensure safe delivery and postpartum (SEGOB Mexico 1993; SEGOB Mexico 2016b).

The practices that Mayan women carried out during their reproductive stage consist of negotiations to incorporate both allopathic (biomedical) and traditional medicine in order to support their welfare and that of their baby's (Ortega 1999). They also respond to constitutive risk factors that are product of the social situation of women in marginalized areas (Rodríguez et al. 2006) and serve as elements to know and understand a therapeutic practice performed in Yucatan: the *sobada* (rubbing) to adjust the baby (Quattrocchi 2007). On the other hand, although procedures have been established to guarantee a safe delivery and puerperium, the deaths of women during the latter stage of pregnancy are more frequent. Even though mothers are aware that dangerous situations can arise during the postpartum period, they do not seek medical support because care is focused on the newborn, and maternal care is neglected. This is reflected in the low attendance of postpartum consultations at the healthcare centers and the diminished importance given to maternal care—this evidenced in some of the deceased women who were forced to resume their everyday chores 2 days after having given birth, without the right to rest.

What Mayan women know about maternal risk is what they basically associate with the dangers of becoming pregnant in the extremes of life. However, they have not adopted this knowledge as their own and, in fact, what we see are very young women getting pregnant, and continuing doing so when they are 40 years old. They are still far from being empowered to decide about care at the time of delivery in cases of a complication. The lack of social support—a conditioning factor of poor maternal health that has been discussed in several studies (Villar et al. 1992)—points to the fact that maternity and all that happens around it still remain a female responsibility only, although in the discourse, male participation is acknowledged as necessary to prevent maternal deaths. The husband plays an important role during delivery because he is the one who takes the woman to the midwife or to the doctor, or it is he who goes for the midwife to bring her home to take care of the delivery. This is when the economic factor becomes particularly relevant. However, what men actually know about caring for the pregnant woman comes from their interactions with other men, but not from the information provided by the health services or the midwife; they are unaware of the signs of a complication (Rodríguez et al. 2012d).

The lack of access to quality maternity care can still be observed in communities far away from the municipal seat, where the health services try to prevent premature pregnancies. The interviewees' comments with respect to the bodily risks were related to women's moods and feelings, more than to their physical constitution. Thus, the social representation of the body linked to the mind, with a strong emotional burden and a structure of its own (Wagner et al. 1994), was shared by the people interviewed.

Conclusions

Maternal deaths of Mayan women in Yucatan reflect their lack of access to health services in order to receive quality care during pregnancy, delivery, and the postpartum period. Greater attention should be paid to those communities located distant from the municipal seat because they have the most vulnerable women with an increased risk of dying due to lack of resources and of prenatal monitoring. Care units having communication systems with hospitals that can manage obstetric emergencies until a hospital is reached have to be located at strategic sites near the remote communities. Thus, in case of an obstetric emergency, women can depend upon support and counseling from specialists who can manage the situation while she is transferred to a higher level of care. Some hospitals have begun the implementation of immediate-response equipment (IRE) that is connected to health centers and clinics by means of cell phones. Nevertheless, greater efforts should be focused in investing more resources for programs to improve maternal health, taking into account the characteristics of Mayan women in order to reduce maternal deaths in Yucatan. This should be implemented in the context of respect toward the indigenous traditions and beliefs related to the reproductive process. Recently, an intercultural transdisciplinary model involving the interaction of different actors has been proposed. Its objective is to develop strategies that are suitable to the Mayan culture in order to reduce maternal mortality in Yucatan. This project includes the participation of gynecologists, obstetricians and public health specialists, pregnant women and women of childbearing age, representatives of community groups including midwives and transport workers, as well as specialists from several disciplines such as economics, psychology, nutrition, and anthropology (Rodríguez 2016).

References

Amaya, A., Boleros, A., Cuevas, A., & Díaz, D. (2010). Factores asociados con la mortalidad materna en las afiliadas a una EPS del régimen subsidiado, durante el año 2008. *Cuadernos latinoamericanos de administración, 7*(10), 103–118.

Bonnet, M. P., Deneux-Tharaux, C., & Bouvier-Colle, M. H. (2011). Critical care and transfusion management in maternal deaths from postpartum haemorrhage. *European Journal of Obstetrics & Gynecology and Reproductive Biology, 158*, 183–188. https://doi.org/10.1016/j.ejogrb.2011.04.042

Combs, V., Sundby, J., & Malata, A. (2012). Piecing together the maternal death puzzle through narratives: The three delays model revisited. *PLoS One, 7*(12), e52090. https://doi.org/10.1371/journal.pone.0052090

Consejo Nacional de Evaluación de la Política de Desarrollo Social. (2012). Informe de pobreza y evaluación del estado de Yucatán. Retrieved February 8, 2017, from http://www.coneval.org.mx/coordinacion/entidades/Documents/Informes%20de%20pobreza%20y%20evaluaci%C3%B3n%2020102012_Documentos/Informe%20de%20pobreza%20y%20evaluaci%C3%B3n%202012_Yucat%C3%A1n.pdf.

Figueroa, J. (1993). El enfoque de género y la representación de la sexualidad: algunas reflexiones. *Cuadernos de Capacitación en Investigación sobre Planificación Familiar*, Dirección General de Planificación Familiar. Secretaría de Salud. México, p. 201–244.

Hynes, M., Sakani, O., Spiegel, P., & Cornier, N. (2012). A study of refugee maternal mortality in 10 countries, 2008–2010. *International Perspectives on Sexology and Reproductive Health, 38*, 205–213. https://doi.org/10.1363/3820512

Instituto Nacional de Estadística, Geografía e Informática (INEGI). (2016). *Número de habitantes. Yucatán-Cuéntame INEGI (2016).* Retrieved January 18, 2017, from http://www.cuentame.inegi.org.mx/monografias/informacion/yuc/poblacion/default.aspx?tema=me&e=31.

Ismayilova, L. (2015). Spousal violence in 5 transitional countries: A population-based multilevel analysis of individual and contextual factors. *American Journal of Public Health, 105*(11), e12–e22. https://doi.org/10.2105/AJPH.2015.302779

Karlsen, S., Say, L., Souza, J. P., Hogue, C. J., Calles, D. L., Gülmezoglu, A. M., et al. (2011). The relationship between maternal education and mortality among women giving birth in health care institutions: Analysis of the cross sectional WHO global survey on maternal and perinatal health. *BMC Public Health, 11*, 606. https://doi.org/10.1186/1471-2458-11-606

Mazza, M., Vallejo, C., & González, B. M. (2012). Mortalidad materna: análisis de las tres demoras. *Revista de Obstetricia y Ginecología Venezolana, 72*(4), 233–248.

Naimul, H. (2012). *Capacitan a parteras para atender mujeres rurales. Bangladesh se esfuerza en reducir muerte materna*. CIMAC/IPS Noticias. Retrieved August 9, 2016, from http://www.cimacnoticias.com.mx/node/60684.

Okour, A. M., Khader, Y., Amarin, Z., Jaddou, H., & Gharaibeh, M. (2012). Maternal mortality in Jordan: Role of substandard care and delays. *Eastern Mediterraneum Health Journal, 18*(5), 426–431.

Oliveira, A. F., Papinelli, M. A., Cecatti, J. G., Souza, U. P., & Souza, M. H. (2009). Factors associated with maternal death in women admitted to an intensive care unit with severe maternal morbidity. *International Journal of Gynaecology and Obstetrics, 105*, 252–256. https://doi.org/10.1016/j.ijgo.2009.01.025

Organización Mundial de la Salud. (2015). *Mortalidad materna. Nota descriptiva Núm.* p. 348. Retrieved June 13, 2016, from http://www.who.int/mediacentre/factsheets/fs348/es/.

Organización Panamericana de la Salud. (1995). *Clasificación estadística internacional de enfermedades y problemas relacionados con la salud, 10ª revisión*. Retrieved August 9, 2016, from http://www.sssalud.gov.ar/hospitales/archivos/cie_10_revi.pdf.

Ortega, J. (1999). *Proceso reproductivo femenino: saberes, géneros y generaciones en una comunidad maya de Yucatán.* Tesis doctoral. México 1999.

Quattrocchi, P. (2007). ¿Qué es la sobada? Elementos para conocer y entender una práctica terapéutica en Yucatán. In P. Quattrocchi & M. Guemez (Eds.), *Salud reproductiva e interculturalidad en el Yucatán de hoy* (p. 86). México: Peninsular Editorial Company S.A de C.V.

Reyes, S. (1994). Resultados. Subestimación de la mortalidad materna en el Distrito Federal. In G. Borrego, N. Treviño, O. Muñoz, & H. Guiscafré (Eds.), *Mortalidad materna en México* (pp. 15–220). IMSS: México.

Rodríguez, E. (2016). *Modelo preventivo de demoras en la atención de la embarazada con complicación obstétrica.* Tesis doctoral, México 2016.

Rodríguez, E., Aguilar, P., Montero, L., Hoil, J., & Andueza, G. (2012a). Demoras en la atención de complicaciones maternas asociadas a fallecimientos en municipios del sur de Yucatán, Mexico. *Revista Biomedica, 23*(1), 23–32.

Rodríguez, E., Andueza, G., & Kú, L. (2006). Cuidados, hábitos y riesgos de las mujeres de Chemax, Yucatán, durante el proceso reproductivo. *Temas antropológicos. Revista Científica de Investigaciones Regionales, 28*(1), 69–98.

Rodríguez, E., Andueza, G., & Montero, L. (2012b). Un abordaje cualitativo de las defunciones maternas en Tizimín, Yucatán, México. *Alteridades, 22*(43), 145–158.

Rodríguez, E., Andueza, G., Montero, L., & Hoil, J. (2005). Subregistro de muertes maternas en Mérida, Yuc. México (1997–2001). *Ginecología y Obstetricia de México, 73*(7), 347–354.

Rodríguez, E., Andueza, G., Rosado, L., Ortiz, E., & Hernández, B. (2012c). Effect of a community-based intervention to improve the knowledge on the warning signs of maternal complications among Mayan women from Yucatan randomized controlled trial. *Revista de Investigación Clínica, 64*(2), 154–163.

Rodríguez, E., Montero, L., Andueza, G., & Manrique, W. (2007). Características médico-sociales de las muertes maternas en una comunidad Maya de Yucatán, Méx. *Ginecología y Obstetricia de México, 75*(2), 79–85.

Rodríguez, E., Santana, A., Andueza, M., & Hoil, J. (2012d). Conocimientos de los hombres sobre tres complicaciones maternas en una comunidad maya de Yucatán, México. In M. Briseño & F. Ruiz (Eds.), *Género y Cultura* (pp. 239–248). México: Universidad Autónoma "Benito Juárez" de Oaxaca.

Rodríguez, E., Urtecho, C., Andueza, G., Hoil, J., Santana, A., Odóñez, M., et al. (2015). Prevención intercultural de la muerte materna y perinatal en tres comunidades mayas de Yucatán. In R. Canto & M. Zarco (Eds.), *Extensión y responsabilidad social. Los proyectos sociales en comunidades de aprendizaje implementados en la Universidad Autónoma de Yucatán* (pp. 437–460). México: Universidad Autónoma de Yucatán. Mérida, Yucatan, Mexico.

Rosestein, M., Romero, M., & Ramos, S. (2008). Maternal mortality in Argentina: A closer look at women who die outside of the health system. *Maternal and Child Health Journal, 12*, 519–524. https://doi.org/10.1007/s10995-007-0268-2

Schwartz, D. A. (2015). Interface of epidemiology, anthropology and health care in maternal death prevention in resource-poor nations. In D. A. Schwartz (Ed.), *Maternal mortality: Risk factors, anthropological perspectives, prevalence in developing countries and preventive strategies for pregnancy-related death* (pp. ix–xiv). New York: Nova Science Publishers.

SEGOB México. (2016a). *Objetivos de desarrollo del milenio de México. ¿Cómo va México?* Retrieved March 29, 2016, from http://www.objetivosdedesarrollodelmilenio.org.mx.

SEGOB México. (2016b). *Norma Oficial Mexicana NOM-007-SSA2-2016, Para la atención de la mujer durante el embarazo, parto y puerperio y de la persona recién nacida*. Retrieved May 24, 2016, from https://drive.google.com/file/d/0B_Wsl17nCOpWNGtjd1dYSTZXYzQ/view.

SEGOB México. (1993). NOM Vigentes. Información importante. Norma Oficial Mexicana NOM-SSA2-1993. Retrieved November 10, 2015, from http://www.spps.gob.mx/marco-juridico/normas-oficiales.html.

Shah, N., Hossain, N., Shoaib, R., Hussain, A., Gillani, R., & Khan, N. (2009). Socio-demographic characteristics and the three delays of maternal mortality. *Journal of the College of Physicians and Surgeons-Pakistan, 19*(2), 95–98. doi: 02.2009/JCPSP.9598.

Sistema Nacional de Vigilancia Epidemiológica. (2015). *Dirección General de Epidemiología. Razón de mortalidad materna real e ideal por entidad federativa.* Retrieved August 9, 2016, from http://www.omm.org.mx/imagenes/stories/Documentos%20grandes/BOLETIN_52_2015_COMPLETO.pdf.

Taukobong, H., Kincaid, M., Levy, J., Bloom, S., Platt, J., Henry, S., et al. (2016). Does addressing gender inequalities and empowering women and girls improve health and development programme outcomes? *Health Policy and Planning, 31*(10), 1492–1514. https://doi.org/10.1093/heapol/czw074

Thaddeus, S., & Maine, D. (1994). Too far to walk: Maternal mortality in context. *Social Science and Medicine, 38*(8), 1091–1110.

The World Bank. (2016). *Tasa de mortalidad materna estimado mediante modelo, por cada 100,000 nacidos vivos.* Retrieved July 14, 2016, from http://datos.bancomundial.org/indicador/SH.STA.MMRT.

Thonneau, P. F., Matsudai, T., Alihonou, E., De Souza, J., Faye, O., Moreau, J., et al. (2004). Distribution of causes of maternal mortality during delivery and post-partum: Results of an African multicenter hospital-based study. *European Journal of Obstetrics & Gynecology and Reproductive Biology, 114*, 150–154. https://doi.org/10.1016/j.ejogrb.2003.12.004

Veloz, M. G., Martínez, O. A., Ahumada, E., Puello, E. R., Amezcua, F. J., & Hernández, M. (2010). Eclampsia, obstetric hemorrhage and heart disease as a cause of maternal mortality in 15 years of analysis. *Ginecología y Obstetricia de México, 78*(4), 215–218.

Vidler, M., Ramadurg, U., Charantimath, U., Katageri, G., Karadiguddi, C., Sawchuck, D., et al. (2016). Utilization of maternal health care services and their determinants in Karnataka state, India. *Reproductive Health, 13*(Suppl 1), 37. https://doi.org/10.1186/s12978-016-0138-8

Villar, J., Farnot, U., Barros, F., Victoria, C., Langer, A., & Balizan, J. (1992). A randomized trial of psychosocial support during high-risk pregnancies. *The New England Journal of Medicine, 327*, 1266–1271. https://doi.org/10.1056/NEJM199210293271803

Wagner, W., Elejabarrieta, F., & Valencia, J. (1994). Estabilidad en las representaciones sociales de paz y de guerra en dos países. *Revista de Psicología Social y Personalidad, 10*(2), 123–143.

Rodríguez, E., & Ordóñez, M. (2006). Maternal mortality and marginality in the State of Yucatán. Rev Biomed, 17, 237–42.

14 Contraceptive Counseling and Family Planning Services in the Chiapas Highlands: Challenges and Opportunities for Improving Access for the Indigenous Population

Sergio Meneses-Navarro, David Meléndez-Navarro, and Alejandro Meza-Palmeros

14.1 Introduction

The ability to control fertility—to decide whether or not to have children, as well as the appropriate moment to have them if desired—is a human right. To make this human right possible and available, it is necessary to assure access to comprehensive contraceptive and family planning (CFP) services. When all members of a population group have the information and means to control their reproduction, social benefits follow: reduction in maternal mortality, prevention of undesired pregnancy, decreased school dropout rates and an increase in education, and strengthening of women's autonomy, among other benefits (Campbell and Graham 2006; OPS 2012; SSA 2014). These outcomes highlight the importance of guaranteeing access to CFP services for all individuals, particularly those in the most vulnerable conditions.

This chapter analyzes the perceptions and practices of contraceptive counseling among public health service providers who serve the indigenous population of the Chiapas Highlands in Mexico (Fig. 14.1). Our objective is to describe and analyze how contraceptive counseling targeting the indigenous population is delivered, and what perceptions exist about delivery among the public health professionals involved, with an emphasis on the cultural relevance of their services and whether it fits within a human rights framework. The first section of this chapter describes the background and

S. Meneses-Navarro, M.D, Sc.D., M.P.H., M.S.A. (✉)
CONACYT/Center for Research and Higher Studies in Social Anthropology, Southeast (CIESAS-Sureste), San Cristobal de Las Casas, Chiapas, Mexico

D. Meléndez-Navarro, M.D., M.S.M.
Promoting Committee for Safe Motherhood in Mexico, San Cristobal de Las Casas, Chiapas, Mexico

A. Meza-Palmeros, M.D., M.Ph., Ph.D.
Faculty of Social Work of the Autonomous University of Nuevo León, Monterrey, Nuevo Leon, Mexico

D. A. Schwartz (ed.), *Maternal Death and Pregnancy-Related Morbidity Among Indigenous Women of Mexico and Central America*, Global Maternal and Child Health: Medical, Anthropological, and Public Health Perspectives, https://doi.org/10.1007/978-3-319-71538-4_14

Fig. 14.1 Chiapas Highlands, Mexico

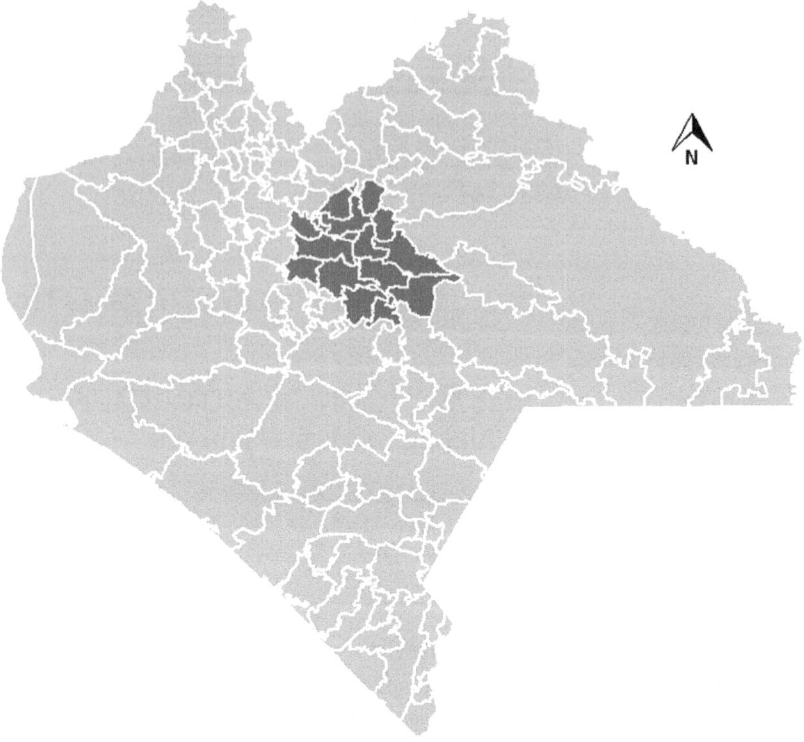

conceptual reference that guide our analysis: the legal framework for CFP; the statistical landscape of contraceptive use in Mexico, Chiapas, and among the indigenous population; the definition and scope of contraceptive counseling; and what factors determine utilization of CFP services among the indigenous population. Following this, we describe the study design, methods, our results, and discussion. The chapter concludes by identifying windows of opportunity to implement intercultural adaptations and specific recommendations to improve access to and coverage of CFP services among the indigenous population of the Chiapas Highlands.

14.2 Background and Framework

14.2.1 The People and Culture of Chiapas

The state of Chiapas is located at southeast of Mexico, bordering Guatemala. It is one of the poorest entities in the country and, at the same time, has the greater concentration of indigenous populations. According to the National Institute of Statistics and Geography of Mexico (INEGI 2015), in 2015 Chiapas had 5,217,908 peoples, 36.1% of whom self-registered as indigenous. Almost 2,700,000 people are in the reproductive age (15–49 years), of whom 1,404,361 are women. Greater than 75% of the population lives in poverty, and 31.8% are in extreme poverty (CONEVAL 2014). Some statistical data illustrate the lack of social progress of the inhabitants of Chiapas. The maternal mortality ratio is among the highest in the country (68.1 maternal deaths per 100,000 live births), 15% of the population above 15 years of age is illiterate, more than 10.6% of households have a dirt floor, and 11.2% of adults report that they have stopped eating some food due to their lack of money (INEGI, Ibid).

Although the official language is Spanish, in the state of Chiapas, there are more than 15 indigenous languages, mainly of Mayan origin (related to the language of the ancient Mayan people of the Yucatan peninsula) or *mixe-zoque-popoluca* (related to the ancient Olmec people, one of the first cultures of the American continent). The indigenous languages with the most speakers in the state of Chiapas are the *Tseltal*, *Tzotsil*, *Tojolabal*, *Chol*, *Zoque*, and *Lacandon*.

There are about 400,000 *Tzotsil* speakers and 500,000 *Tseltal* speakers who live mainly in the Chiapas Highlands. Both languages are of Mayan origin with a deep rootedness among the indigenous inhabitants of the region, who preserve traditional customs and forms of life that give sustenance to their identity. The linguistic difference is a very important aspect for access to education and health services, as 22.6% of men and 35.7% of indigenous women speak only their mother language and do not speak Spanish. However, most public services, including health and education, are provided in the Spanish language.

The Chiapas Highlands has a great cultural, religious, political, and ethnic diversity. At the same time, it is a region that registers high levels of poverty and marginalization, as well as lags and gaps in health and education, mainly among indigenous peoples. The economic activity of the indigenous population is mainly self-consumption agriculture, but it also registers high levels of internal and international migration.

The Chiapas Highlands is characterized by mountains, valleys, forests, and jungle areas, which are sometimes difficult to access and where people live in small communities of less than thousands. These factors can make it difficult and expensive to provide such basic services of well-being such as water, electricity, health, and education (Fig. 14.2).

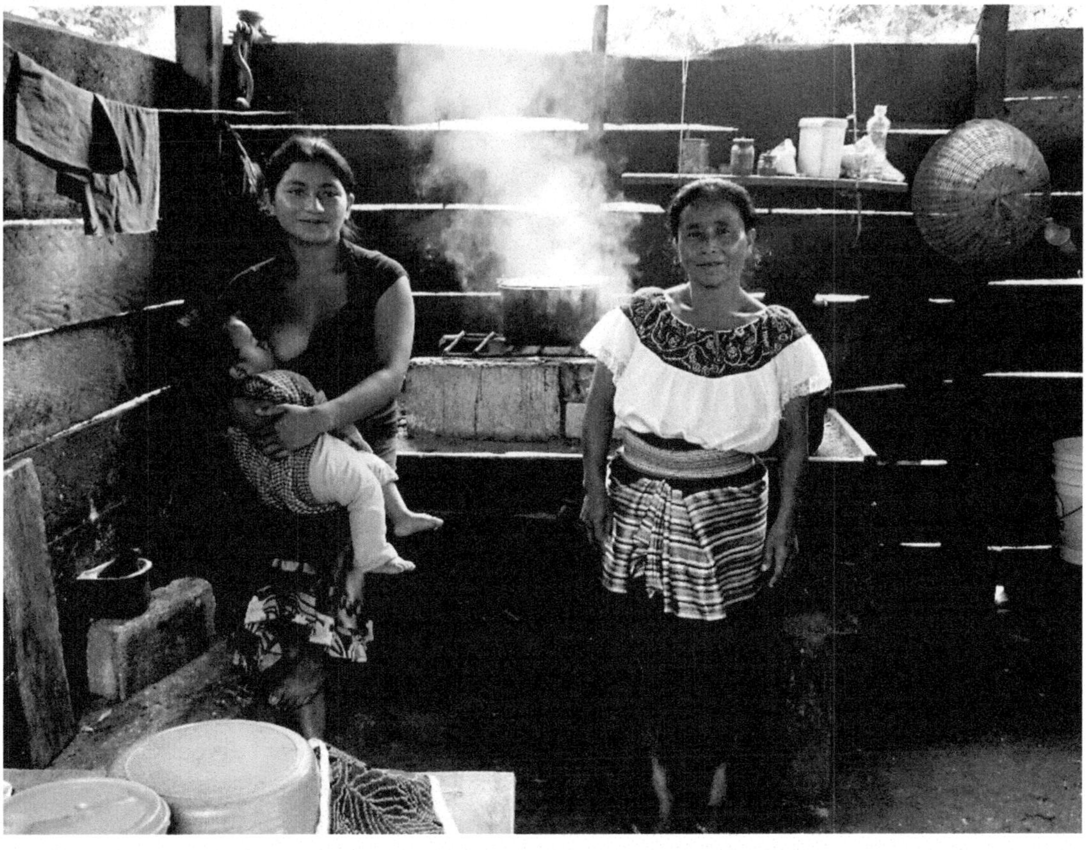

Fig. 14.2 Indigenous women cooking in a wood stove, Bachajón, Chiapas, Mexico. Photo by Álvaro Abadía

14.2.2 Legal Framework

Article 4 of the Mexican Constitution establishes that all individuals have the right to make informed and responsible decisions of their own free will regarding the number and spacing of their children. Given the high priority of this right, Article 3 of the General Health Law defines family planning as a basic health issue (Ley General de Salud, 2016). To make this right possible, it is critical to have educational and CFP services available. Chapter VI of the General Health Law (Articles 67–71) is dedicated to this topic. Among its primary precepts, Article 67 affirms that family planning is a priority and should include educational and orienting information for adolescents and youth regarding contraceptive care that is opportune, effective, and comprehensive. These services are the medium by which the right to make informed and responsible decisions of their own free will regarding the number and spacing of their children is made possible, and Article 67 emphatically states that services should be delivered with dignity. Later, the same article proclaims that those who practice sterilization without consent, or pressure patients to undergo the procedure, will be sanctioned under the law, independent of any penal repercussions incurred.

In light of delivering these services to indigenous populations, the article specifies that activities related to educational and orienting information in indigenous communities should be conducted in Spanish as well as the indigenous language(s) used in the region or community at hand (Article 67). Within this article it is worth highlighting the emphasis placed on information oriented toward adolescents and youth, with dignity (which includes respect for their autonomy, values, preferences, and expectations) and, in the case of the indigenous population, in their mother tongue. Also, it is relevant the punishable mark that makes the law for those who practice any form of coercion so that some person utilizes contraception or apply contraceptive methods without consent or in a forced manner.

Article 68 indicates the elements that constitute family planning services, including the promotion of development of health communication and education programs about family planning services and sexual education. The same law establishes that the Secretariat of Health shall coordinate the activities of the different entities of the health sector to lead and operate the actions tied to the national family planning program formulated by the National Population Council, in alignment with the General Population Law (Article 70), as well as provide consultation for the development of educational programs about family planning services and sexual education as required by the national education system. The regulation regarding service provision and medical attention in the General Health Law establishes that the private and public sectors are obligated to provide free informational contraceptive services:

> It is the obligation of public sector, social, and private institutions to provide, free of charge and within their facilities the services that include information, orientation and motivation regarding family planning, according to the Technical Standards emitted by the Secretariat (Article 118)

It is also a requirement to obtain informed consent from individuals interested in an irreversible contraceptive method:

> To conduct a tubal ligation or vasectomy it is required to obtain clearly expressed and written authorization from the individual, as well as provide information about the nature and consequence of the intervention (Article 119)

The Secretariat of Health, in their leading role for the sector, has defined the Program for Specific Action for Family Planning and Contraceptives 2013–2018[1] which establishes the strategies, actions,

[1] The specific action programs are defined as "the guiding instruments that have been developed through consensus, with strategies based on best practice and scientific evidence available, to define the direction that all institutions and levels of government should follow to move forward collectively and harmoniously towards confronting the primary health

and specific goals for the present administration. There are three objectives: *(1) increase effective access to services and improve the quality of CFP care*; *(2) address the specific CFP needs of the population, particularly in groups belonging to the lower social strata*; *and (3) incentive active and chosen fatherhood and men's responsibility in CFP* (SSA 2014:53). A crosscutting thread for achieving these objectives are informational and contraceptive counseling services.

Furthermore, access to CFP has been defined as a priority at the international policy level. The Millennium Development Goals (MDGs) initiated by the World Health Organization (WHO) in 2000 included in their goals indicators for contraceptive prevalence rate (indicator 5.3), adolescent birth rate (indicator 5.4), and unmet need for family planning (indicator 5.6) (PNUD 2010). The third Sustainable Development Goal (SDG), *ensure healthy lives and promote well-being for all at all ages*, includes within its objectives ensuring universal access to sexual and reproductive health-care services, including for family planning, information, and education, by 2030 (ONU 2015). As such, there is a solid legal framework that protects the rights of individuals to access CFP and a legal mandate from the state to guarantee access to comprehensive CFP services.

14.2.3 Statistical Landscape

The total fertility rate (TFT)[2] in Mexico has decreased in recent years from 2.29 births per woman in 2009 to 2.26 in 2014 (INEGI 2014). Nonetheless, recent data reveal two worrisome trends. First is the increase in fertility rates among adolescents 15–19 years of age; in 2009 this age group was reported to have 70.9 births per 1000 adolescents, but in 2014 this increased to 77 per 1000. This situation is even more relevant when considering the current demographics of Mexico where the youth population is the highest in the history of the country: 21 million people between 12 and 24 years of age (INEGI 2010). Several factors associated with increased fertility rates include rural location and low educational levels: rural women have a TFT of 2.81, while urban women have 2.04 births on average; women with low levels of education have 3.3 births on average, while higher educated women have nearly half that rate: 1.79 births per woman (INEGI 2014).

Secondly, recent information reveals important heterogeneity in access to FP services across the country. For example, women in Chiapas—the state with the weakest outcomes in the topic at hand—have nearly doubled the rate (2.90 births per woman) as in Mexico City (1.47 births per woman). Although the national TFT decreased between 2009 and 2014 (from 2.29 to 2.26), in Chiapas the TFT increased (from 2.84 to 2.90). This provides evidence not only of the magnitude of the gap in TFT but also the trend of increasing TFT. Despite Chiapas having the highest TFT[3] of the country, it simultaneously reports the lowest age for sexual initiation for women and the lowest percentage of contraceptive use[4] and extreme lack of knowledge about family planning (FP)[5]. Given these realities, it is clear why Chiapas is the state with the lowest contraceptive use

challenges" (SSA 2008:7).

[2]Total fertility rate (TFT) refers to the total number of children who would be born per woman (or per 1000 women) if she/they were to pass through the childbearing years bearing children according to a current schedule of age-specific fertility rates.

[3]In 2014 the TFT in Chiapas was 2.90 births per women, while the national average was 2.26, and the lowest rate, Mexico City, was 1.47 (INEGI 2014).

[4]In 2014, 40.4% of women from Chiapas reported using FP, while the national average was 51.6%, and the highest rate of FP, Chihuahua, was 59.3% (INEGI 2014).

[5]In Chiapas, 10% of women of reproductive age had no knowledge of FP. At the national level only 1.3% of women of reproductive age had no knowledge of contraception, and in locales such as the state of Sonora, only 0.3% had no knowledge (INEGI 2014).

at first sexual encounter[6] and the state with the highest number of women who have never used any contraceptive method (INEGI 2014).

However, it is paradoxical that in indigenous municipalities with the lowest levels of maternal health, the highest incidence of undesired pregnancy and maternal and child death, highest rates of illiteracy, and lowest rates of education among women also report the highest percentage of unmet need for FP. In support of this, a survey was conducted in 2013 by the Institute for Health Metrics and Evaluation at the University of Washington which collected data from over 24,000 homes in 30 municipalities in Chiapas[7] as part of the 2015 Mesoamerican Health Initiative. This study identified that among women who had given birth in the previous 2 years, 11% of pregnancies were undesired or occurred sooner than desired, and 5.3% did not want any more children; of women who were pregnant at the time of the survey, 15.7% of pregnancies were undesired or occurred sooner than desired, and 9% did not want any more children (BID 2013:67). At the same time, 52.7% of women of reproductive age reported unmet need for FP[8] (Ibíd 78).

14.2.4 What Are Contraceptive Counseling and Family Planning?

Counseling refers to providing information and orientation about contraception to facilitate the decision-making process (SSA 2008). Through contraceptive counseling, information and orientation are provided to individuals and couples about the biology of reproduction and contraceptive methods, the benefits of birth spacing, and different aspects of sexuality and reproduction. The goal is that with this information, individuals can identify their needs and expectations in order to consciously and voluntarily plan and make informed decisions about their sexual and reproductive life. A central function of counseling is to explain how contraceptive methods work and to clarify any doubts about instructions, efficacy, security, usage, and undesired side effects (SSA 2008:52).

As the Culturally Relevant Contraceptive Counseling Guide (ISECH 2014:6–7) suggests, counseling should be:

> Delivered in a comprehensive manner, with high quality technical expertise and interpersonal skills, as well as cultural relevance. Comprehensive because other aspects relevant to sexual and reproductive health can be addressed, such as the prevention of sexually transmitted infections, maternal-child health, preconception risk or timely identification of cervical or breast cancer, depending on the life stage of users. Technical expertise because information should be based on the best evidence available regarding contraceptive methods. Quality interpersonal skills because counseling should include respectful care and respect for the privacy, autonomy and decisions of all people. Cultural relevance because it is critical to recognize and respect the world view, values, and beliefs, as well as the native language of users. As such, contraceptive counseling should be systematically offered to all individuals of reproductive age that seek out health services, independent of their initial motivation for care-seeking, especially women and their partners living in vulnerable social conditions.

[6]In Chiapas 14.7% of women of reproductive age utilized some form of contraception during their first sexual encounter, while the national average was 34%, and the state with the highest use of contraceptive methods at first sexual encounter for women was the Federal District (Mexico City) at 48.2% (INEGI 2014).

[7]Aldama, Amatenango del Valle, Chalchihuitán, Chanal, Chenalhó, Huixtán, Larraínzar, Mitontic, Oxchuc, Pantelhó, San Cristóbal de Las Casas, San Juan Cancuc, San Juan Chamula, Santiago El Pinar, Tenejapa, Teopisca, Zinacantán, Amatán, El Bosque, Huitiupán, Pueblo Nuevo Solistahuacán, Simojovel, San Andrés Duraznal, Sabanilla, Salto de Agua, Tila, Tumbalá, Yajalón, Chilón y Sitalá

[8]Unmet need consisted of the number of married or partnered women of reproductive age who wished to limit of space out births and were not using any kind of contraceptive method out of the total number of women of reproductive age.

14.2.5 Determinants of CFP Service Utilization Among the Indigenous Population of Chiapas

Determinants of health service utilization include characteristics of resources and services, as well as characteristics of the target population. The driver of utilization is the recognition of lack of recognition of a health condition in need of medical care (Donabedian 1988). Recognizing a need leads to the desire for care, which may or may not lead to care-seeking. Seeking care is mediated by availability and access to the appropriate resources. If such resources are not available of inaccessible, the service cannot be provided and the seeking out of such a service is halted. However, if the resources that result in service provision are available and accessible, the seeking of care will continue until satisfied. As such, the analysis of service utilization must consider aspects related to the supply of services, as well as aspects related to the population that demands them (Frenk 1994).

Moreover, geographic, financial, and organizational factors may act as barriers or facilitators for the analysis of access and utilization of public health services by indigenous populations; cultural aspects must also be considered such as language and worldview when it comes to health/disease processes and care for these, as well as myriad discrimination, including racism (Meneses 2004). The following table (Table 14.1) shows key findings from the literature regarding determinants of utilization of contraceptive services among the indigenous population in general and Chiapas in particular.

Table 14.1 Determinants of utilization of contraceptive and family planning (CFP) services among the indigenous population in Chiapas (Source: created by author, based on literature review using the following databases: LILACS, EBSCO, OVID, BEME Collaboration, SCIELO Y COCHRANE)

Recognition of need	Desire for care	Care-seeking	Availability of resources and services	Accessibility		Quality of care
				Financial	Cultural	
Lack of acknowledge of the need for CFP Social expectation of large families Representations of motherhood Little autonomy over women's own body Value assigned to children	Perceptions about forced sterilization Segmentation of population by government health insurance New generations express greater desire for CFP	Distrust of the medical establishment Mix of "traditional" (indigenous knowledge and biomedical knowledge facilitate the use of CFP in the private sector New generations, with increased education or history of migration, express growing interest in CFP	The availability of CFP in primary care setting is insufficient and unreliable	40% of indigenous women CFP users pay out of pocket	Language Lack of adequate explanation Perception that the promotion of CFP is tied to discrimination of racism toward indigenous women and families	Mistreatment Lack of clear, complete, and understandable explanations

14.2.6 Recognition of Need

In reproduction and motherhood are social expectations held by family and the community at large about the role of indigenous women (Castro 2000; Freyermuth 2003). Based on the literature, contraceptive use is not recognized as a need given the high value assigned to motherhood, particularly in the most traditional families. In Castro's (2000) view, the experience of reproduction among indigenous women is often in response to the social and familial expectation (within a patriarchal framework), but women narrate their experience as suffering and deference. This is related to the factor of women possessing little autonomy to be decision-makers about their body, their health, and medical care, including reproductive decisions (Nazar et al. 2011; Freyermuth 2003).

Moreover, in a study conducted with the rural population in the state of Morelos, Castro (2000) found that men viewed their sexuality as a natural force, frequently uncontrollable. This directly contrasts with the case of women, whose sexuality can be controlled by men, given their role of servitude to their partners, including the realm of sexuality. As such, reproductive decision-making is led by males, without women's participation. Men as well as women recognize that men are responsible for deciding how many children are to be had, strengthening male power. That is why, Castro purports that women become pregnant and give birth in service to their partners. The woman is there to serve men, in both sexual and reproductive aspects (Castro 2000).

Further, the value assigned to children is also a determining factor in why the need to limit reproduction is not recognized. Children hold great value for the support they provide in domestic activities, productivity, and economic support for the family, whether it be with the father in agriculture or trade—as is typically the case with male children—or with domestic activities, childcare of younger siblings, or "women's work," as is typically the case with female children (Palma and Suarez 1994). At the same time, several researchers have suggested that the establishment of these types of asymmetric gender-defined relationships may be reinforced by public policy when there is not adequate consideration of how gender relations function in a certain time and place. One example cited is Mexico's Oportunidades program (now called Prospera) which has contributed to reinforcing the economic value assigned to children: families who are affiliated with the program (based on low socio economic status) receive cash transfers for each of their children to attend school. This has been argued to disincentivize contraception, given that school-age children represent an investment that can contribute to increasing household income (Loewenberg 2010; Sesia 2009).

Political factors also present a barrier to recognizing birth control as a necessary component of public health. Within some indigenous populations, there is active resistance to governmental intervention. For example, the Zapatista Army of National Liberation rejects some of the institutional health services—particularly contraceptive methods—attributing their use as an intentional effort to annihilate indigenous populations (Declaración de Moisés Gandhi 1997). Finally, another aspect that contributes to CFP not being recognized as a critical need is the explicit opposition expressed by many religious organizations.

14.2.7 Desire and Care-Seeking

As described above, some key voices have expressed the opinion that hidden behind CFP promotion targeting the indigenous populations is the intention of population control with the ultimate goal of making them disappear (Declaración de Moisés Gandhi 1997). In line with this negative perception, in the state of Chiapas among the indigenous population, there have been documented cases of forced sterilization, IUD insertion without informed consent, or coercion into the acceptance of FP methods (Kirsch and Arana 1999; PHR 1999; Ibañez et al. 2015). While the state has the lowest percentage of active CFP users, Chiapas also has the greatest percentage of users who opted for an irreversible surgical method (60.2%) (INEGI 2010). It is also revealing that surgical sterilization is more widely used by indigenous women (especially those with low level of education) than non-indigenous women (Ibid). Data from the 2014 ENADID indicate that 3.4% of users in Chiapas received sterilization without their consent, with the majority being indigenous women (INEGI 2014). In fact, the method used among 23% of indigenous women is surgical (Ibid). As such, some authors have concluded that indigenous men and women harbor beliefs of being the constant victims of exploitation and abuse by the social sector, particularly medical professionals and health systems. Moreover, there is the self-perception of being "on the last rung" of the social ladder, which translates to a permanent perception of uncertainly based on precarious social position, internalized gender inequity, and social and structural violence, often perpetrated by the state (Castro 2000). The latter acts as a deterrent to the desire and act of care-seeking CFP services, even among individuals and couples that wish to plan their family.

Additional research indicates that when women and their family are not beneficiaries of Oportunidades, they believe they do not have the right to seek prenatal care, labor, and delivery services or CFP at public health institutions, resulting in distancing themselves from the services (PHR 1999; Sesia 2009). On the other hand, beneficiaries of Oportunidades report being threatened with losing their benefits if they refused to obtain their Pap smear, to have an intrauterine device (IUD) inserted, and even surgical sterilization (Kirsch and Arana 1999; PHR 1999; Declaraci6n de Moisés Gandhi 1997).

14.2.8 Availability and Barriers to Access

The primary barrier to accessing CFP services is language and, above all, lack of an understandable explanation about contraceptive methods and how they function (Ibañez et al. 2015). It is important to also mention supply shortages and the unavailability of contraceptive methods and financial barriers to accessing them as well (INEGI 2014).

14.2.9 Initiation and Continuity of Care

One of the primary prohibitive factors for continuity of care is the perception of violence practices perpetrated by health professionals, termed obstetric violence. Some indigenous women indicate that they are scolded by providers for having too many children (Castro 2000). Moreover, users perceive that the provider, not the woman, is ultimately in control of the decision about the use of CFP; this is due to unclear information and not being addressed in their native language regarding the specifications of the methods. Finally, several researchers have documented the use of CFP being instituted too late in life, given the young age that many users marry, which translates to limited results in terms of fertility (Nazar et al. 1996).

14.3 Methodology

We conducted a qualitative analysis of the CFP practices delivered by public health service providers to the indigenous population in the Chiapas Highlands, as well as the perceptions providers have about their practices, within this context. We employed three data collection techniques: (1) participant observation (of users and simulated users), (2) semistructured interviews, and (3) discussion-based workshops with service providers.

14.3.1 Observation of CFP Practices Using Simulated Users

A group of nine indigenous collaborators (four women and five men between 17 and 36 years of age) acted as simulated users (Figs. 14.3, 14.4, and 14.5). They were sexual and reproductive health promoters from various municipalities in the region and members of the NGO *Sakil Nichim*. Prior to applying the simulation methodology, the simulated users were trained. The technique consisted of personification of a user who was starting the search for contraceptive counseling in a public health facility, based on hypothetical cases. The first case was a young indigenous woman who had unprotected sexual intercourse with her partner the day before and did not want to become pregnant. In this case, it was expected that the service provider would provide the user with information regarding emergency contraception, as well as provide counseling so that the patient could select a method according to her needs and preferences. The second case was a young woman in search of information to help her plan for sexual activity without becoming pregnant. In this case, it was expected that service providers would provide counseling and supply the selected method. The third case was a male user who wanted condoms. In his case, it was also expected that service providers would provide counseling and supply the selected method.

During the training workshop, the collaborators were familiarized with the hypothetical cases, the expected behavior of service providers, and the participant observation data collection instruments. Several scenarios were rehearsed to practice the technique and identify relevant issues that would need special attention during the observation of real counseling. Afterward, each of the

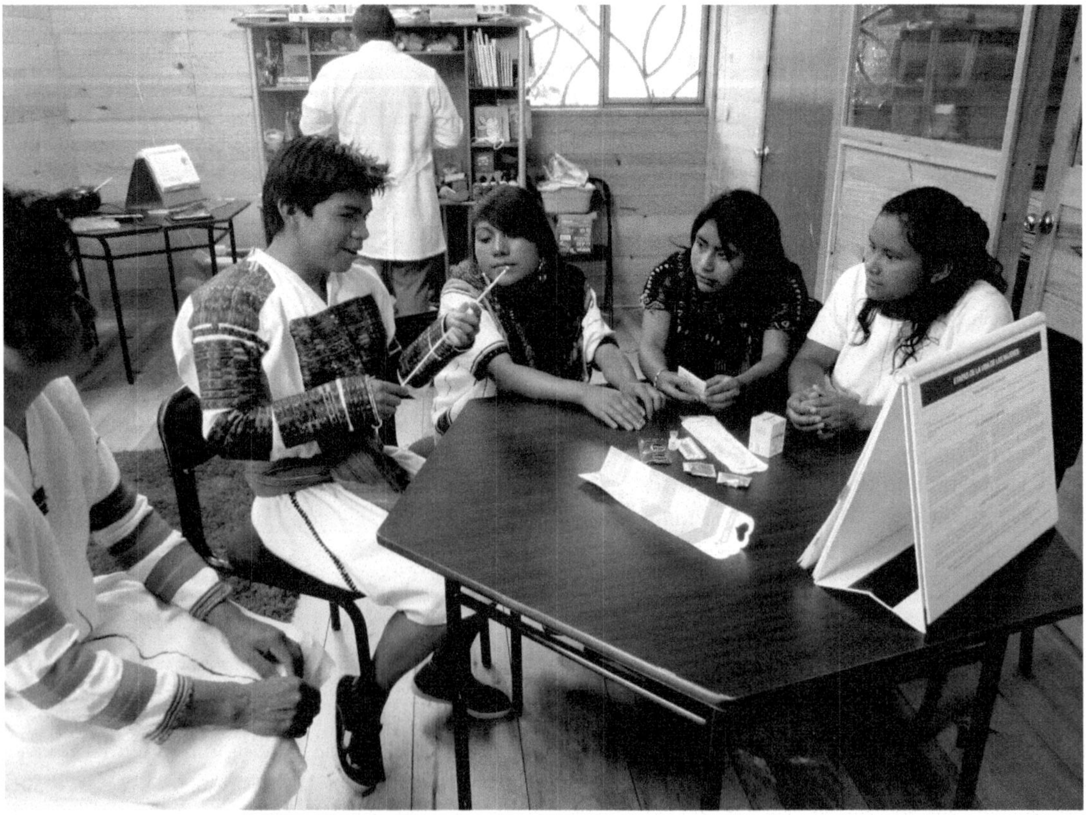

Fig. 14.3 Training workshop with the indigenous collaborators who acted as simulated users. Photo by Ivette Cerecero

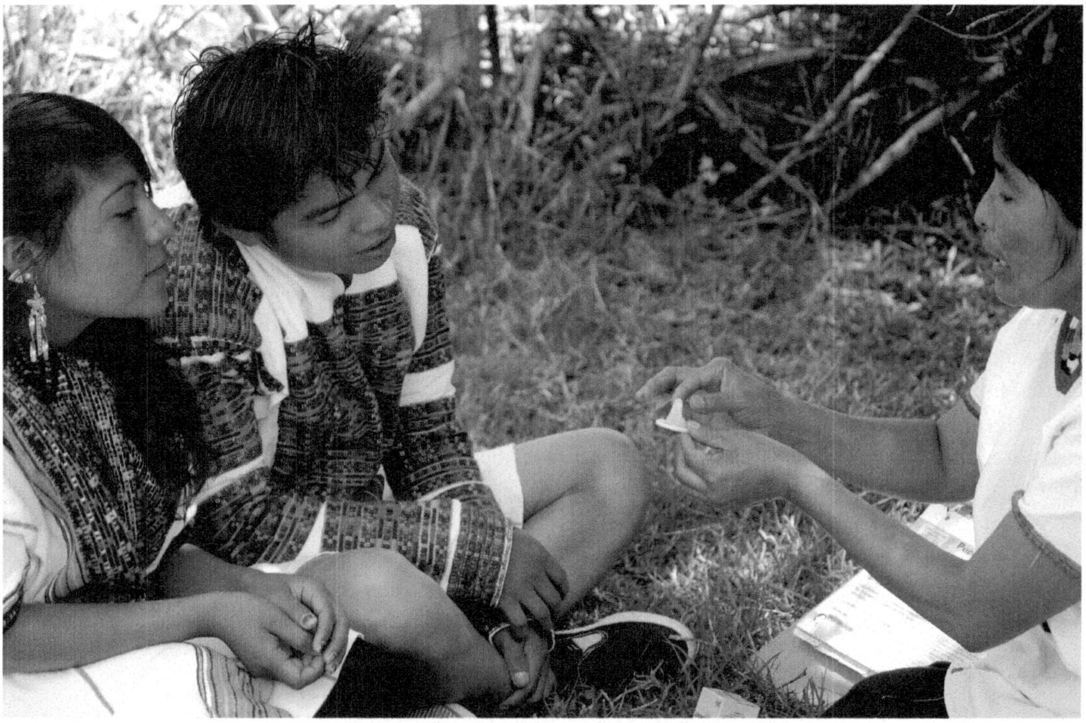

Fig. 14.4 Training workshop with the indigenous collaborators who acted as simulated users. Photo by Ivette Cerecero

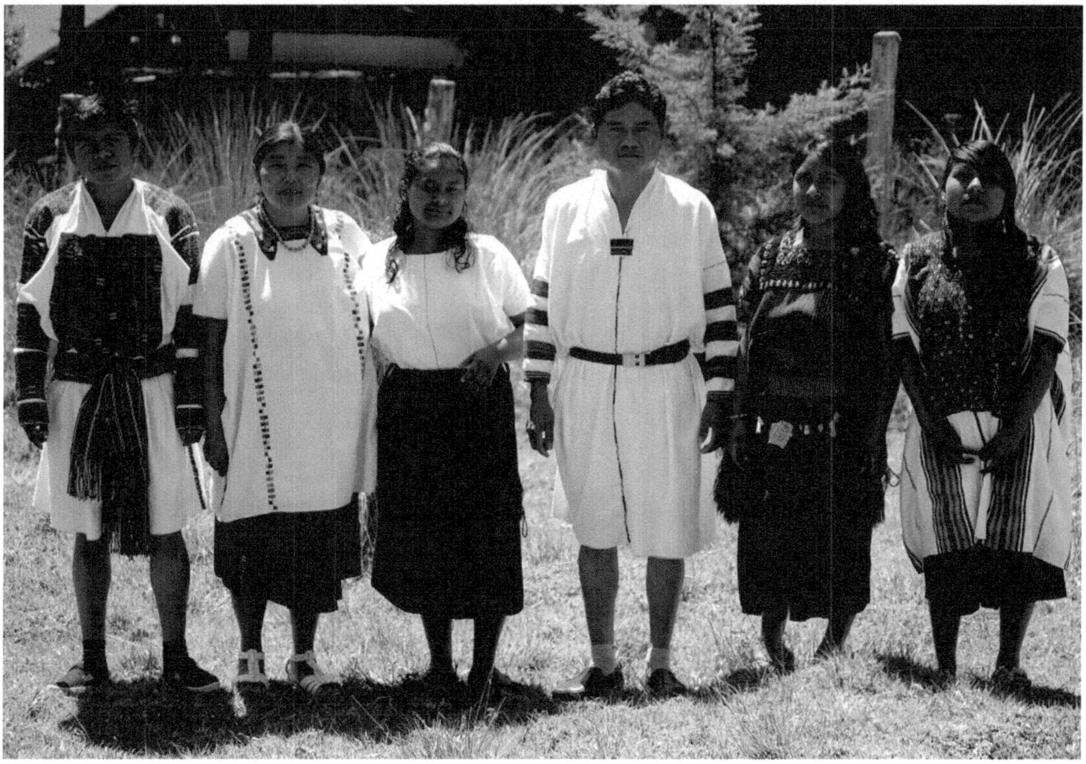

Fig. 14.5 Some of the indigenous collaborators who acted as simulated users. Photo by Ivette Cerecero

collaborators conducted a pilot test in a health center and discussed their experience at a follow-up workshop in order to fine-tune methodological details before beginning forma data collection. After the fieldwork and data collection was completed, there was another meeting to analyze and discuss findings.

Key information was recorded from the observation guide and detailed documentation provided by each of the users: location[9] and municipality, affiliated institution, time of access and care, wait time, barriers to access, reason for care, location where counseling was provided, provider attitudes, demonstration of contraceptive methods, explanation of each method, information about sexually transmitted infections (STIs), clarification of any doubts, use of native language, whether the indicated CFP methods were provided, and satisfaction of the user with the care provided. To document the relevant information, simulated users were given an observation guide in checklist format and a fieldwork journal for a more in-depth description of their observations. The data collected through the checklist observation guide were organized in a database using Microsoft Access software, and the data from the journals were transcribed into Microsoft Word for organization and analysis.

We selected primary care units for the study based on convenience sampling in 12 of the 18 municipalities of the Chiapas Highlands. All of them had over 95% indigenous population and were classified as highly marginalized.[10] We excluded the municipalities with lower percentages of indigenous population and lower levels of marginalization.[11]

14.3.2 Discussion Workshops and Semistructured Interviews

We conducted discussion workshops with providers (medical, nursing, and technical staff) and administrators (in charge of CFP, sexual and reproductive health, or maternal health programs at the time of the study) to analyze and discuss the practices and perceptions about CFP (Fig. 14.6). All of the participants had work experience in the selected municipalities. During the discussion workshops, participants identified key stakeholders who were then invited for in-depth interviews to more deeply explore the content from the workshops. Participation in the workshops and interviews was voluntary, with an informed consent process and guarantee of confidentiality.

The workshops and interviews were audio-recorded, transcribed, and systematically organized and analyzed. Table 14.2 summarizes the number of workshops and interviews conducted, as well as the geographic distribution of the participants' workplace. The data yielded the following themes: perceptions about CFP programs; service supply; availability of resources; determinant of utilization for the indigenous population; provider practices, competencies, and skill in delivering counseling; availability of the tools needed for decision-making; perceptions about users and nonusers of CFP services; and service demand from the indigenous population.

[9] In the manuscript we do not list the specific locations so as to preserve confidentiality.

[10] Aldama, Chalchihuitán, Chamula, Chenalhó, Mitontic, Oxchuc, Pantelhó, San Andrés Larrainzar, San Juan Cancuc, Santiago el Pinar, Tenejapa, and Zinacantan. We did not work in Chanal or Amatenango del Valle given that we did not have collaborators or local contacts in these municipalities.

[11] Altamirano, Las Rosas, San Cristóbal de Las Casas, and Teopisca

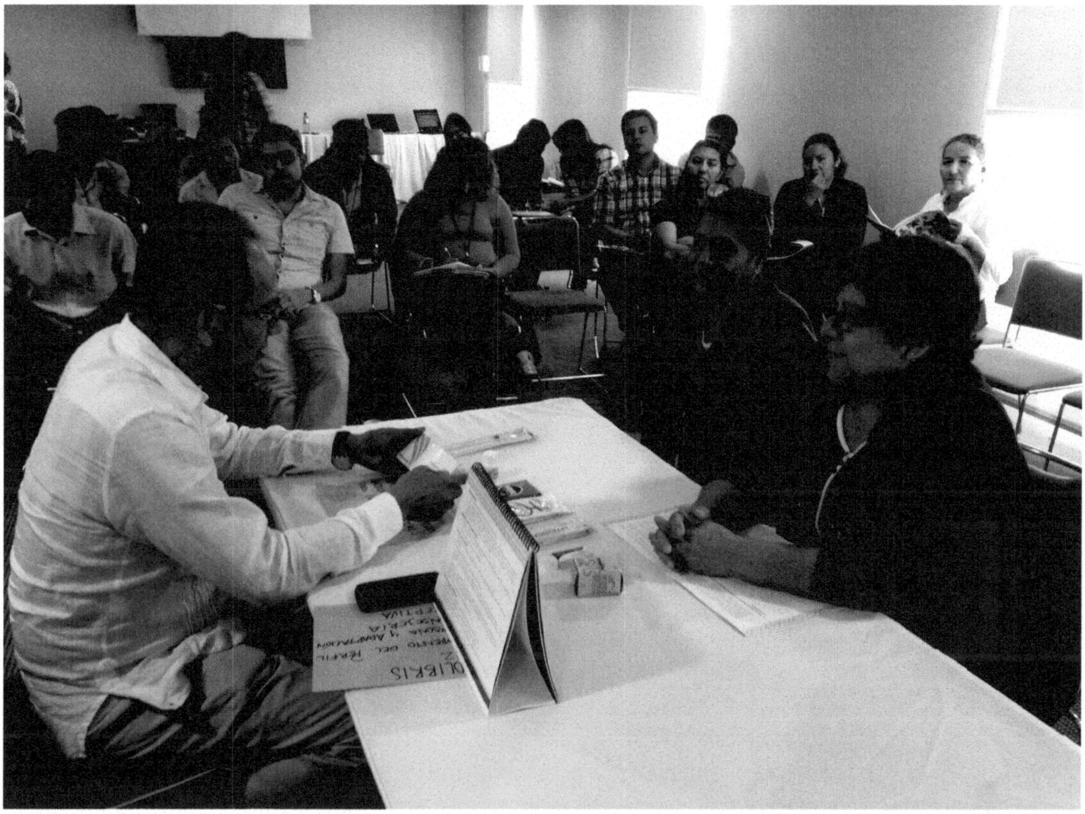

Fig. 14.6 Workshops with providers and administrators. Photo by Alvaro Abadía

Table 14.2 Workshops and interviews with providers and the municipalities where they work

	Participants	Municipality
Workshops (3)	36	Aldama, Chalchihuitán, Chamula, Chanal, Chenalhó, Larrainzar, Mitontic, Pantelhó, Las Rosas, San Cristóbal, Tenejapa, Santiago el Pinar
Interviews	5	San Andrés Larráinzar, San Cristóbal

14.4 Results

14.4.1 Simulated Users

We evaluated a total of 32 cases with simulated users. Each case was conducted in a different healthcare setting; 18 were with men and 14 with women. The majority of the simulated users (18/32) were not able to obtain the contraceptive method that they needed. Table 14.3 presents the distribution of simulated users by gender, age, and whether they obtained the contraceptive method.

Among female simulated users, only 4 of the 14 cases obtained the method requested. Men had greater success; 10 of 18 of those who requested condoms received them (Table 14.3). These data

Table 14.3 Simulated users by gender, age, and method obtained

Gender	Age	CFP obtained?	Gender	Age	CFP obtained?
Female	17	No	Male	19	Yes
	21	No		19	No
	21	Yes		19	Yes
	21	No		19	No
	17	Yes		19	Yes
	37	No		21	No
	37	No		21	Yes
	21	No		21	Yes
	21	No		35	No
	21	No		35	No
	17	No		35	No
	37	No		35	No
	37	Yes		22	Yes
	37	Yes		22	Yes
				22	Yes
				19	Yes
				19	No
				19	Yes
Total	14	4		18	10

Source: Prepared by the authors

indicate possible gender discrimination in accessing contraceptive methods, where being female is associated with greater barriers to access CFP. This finding would need to be corroborated with a more representative sample. Of the 7 cases of simulated users who needed emergency contraceptives, only 2 received them (17 and 21 years of age). This finding is relevant given the context where 20% of pregnancies occur in women younger than 20 years of age, and 36% of youth report an unmet need for CFP. The health system must develop and implement a precise strategy that guarantees that any woman who needs emergency contraceptives, particularly adolescents and indigenous women, can receive them in a timely manner.

Among male simulated users, 12 of the 25 men who requested condoms received them. In the case of women who requested condoms, only two of five cases received them. However, it is important to note that the woman who successfully received the condoms (in two different health facilities) was 37 years old; the rest of the female simulated users were young women who did not receive their requested method. Again, it must be noted that this finding points to possible age discrimination of users, as well as whether or not to provide condoms. Moreover, only one-fourth of the cases were given information about STIs and their prevention.

In the majority of the cases (20/32), the simulated users initially reported that they did not experience barriers to accessing health services. Later, several cases were analyzed, and we did discover barriers to access. In three of every ten cases, service providers used samples of the contraceptive methods to explain the characteristics, advantages, and disadvantages to each. This exemplifies a weakness in service provision, but also an opportunity for improvement; this could be an indicator for infrastructure (availability of samples), processes (systematic use of counseling), and outcomes (user knowledge/adoption of method) in the practice of contraceptive counseling.

In 11 of the 32 cases, information was provided in the simulated users' native language (*tzeltal* or *tsotsil*). Use of native language was greater when the user was female (6 out of 14 cases versus 5 out of 18 cases for males), corresponding directly to the greater percentage of monolingual females. In the following section, we describe and analyze several representative cases from the simulated users.

14.4.1.1 Case 1

María, a 17-year-old adolescent female, sought out care in one of the busiest health centers in the Chiapas Highlands, located in a rural, indigenous municipality. She arrived at 10:25 in the morning, went into the waiting room where other women were waiting, and noticed the stares and whispers about not recognizing her as one of their neighbors. She sat down. Nobody asked her what she was there for. She saw a few nurses taking notes while they hurriedly walked through the waiting room. They saw her, but did not ask her anything. Fifteen minutes later María asked the cleaning woman where she could find the medical provider in charge; the woman said the doctor was busy at the moment, but maybe another doctor would see her. A very serious man asked María for her insurance paperwork and what she was there for, without greeting her first or introducing himself. After explaining to him that she was there regarding contraceptive methods and did not have the paperwork with her, he confirmed that they would help her but after the other appointments were done and all the other patients had been seen. Two and a half hours later, María saw the doctor, who asked her if she spoke Spanish. María shared that she did not and the doctor called the *tsotsil* language interpreter. María describes the following dialogue:

> The doctor asked me, 'what can I help you with?' I told her that the night before I had sexual intercourse and did not want to become pregnant. The interpreter translated what I said. The doctor stopped to think, I thought she wouldn't understand my situation, that she didn't understand what the interpreter told her. So I asked the interpreter to ask me more about my situation and whether I was married or just had a boyfriend. After she understood my situation, the doctor told me that the ideal medication for this moment was called 'Post Day,' but that they didn't have any right now. She said I could take other medications, but she didn't remember the names or how to take them. She stopped to think some more, and told me it was best if I went and bought 'Post Day' and came back to her so she could read the box and she would tell me how to take it. She was about to give me the prescription, when she asked me to wait a minute in the waiting room because she wanted to verify that they didn't have any at the health center pharmacy. 10 min passed, she came back and stood by the desk in the waiting room and in front of all the people in the room she said there wasn't any, and read the prescription out loud and told me I had to go buy them because they didn't have any there. She told the interpreter to translate what she said. Some of the people in the waiting room gave me funny looks. The assistant toll me to the doctor's consult room and explained how I was going to take the pills. The doctor did not say goodbye, or anything else. She just left the prescription and left.

Analysis

Although there were no barriers to accessing the facility, María encountered a problem when she was asked for her insurance paperwork. We want to highlight that when the intake staff realized that María did not have the proper document and was seeking contraceptive care, they put her on the bottom of the list despite her arriving before other patients. Moreover, they agreed to "help" her, ignoring that this is a right and that adolescents are a priority group for addressing this issue.

When the doctor saw María after an extensive (greater than 2 h) wait time, she offered her the method pertinent to the case: emergency contraceptives. However, it appeared that the doctor was unfamiliar with how to administer the medication, and it was also unavailable. Although the correct method was recommended, there was insufficient information given. The simulated user's native language was used via an interpreter, but they did not cover all components of contraceptive counseling: contraindications and precautions, duration of protection, safety, side effects, follow-up, and evaluation of the contraceptive method. No other information about other contraceptive methods were provided. We also want to emphasize that what caught the doctor's attention was María's marital status. We can conclude that María did not receive a comprehensive counseling session. The consultation did not resolve the need of the user given that the method was unavailable. The doctor wrote the prescription and gave instructions to buy it at a pharmacy—an out-of-pocket expense for María. We want to draw attention to the fact that, in the absence of emergency contraceptives, the doctor did not propose alternatives such as using oral hormonal contraceptives or an IUD as an emergency method. By not providing counseling services, the medical personnel lost the opportunity to comprehensively address the sexual and reproductive healthcare needs of this adolescent. Finally, the ethical principles of confidentiality and privacy were violated, given that on several occasions communication took place in front of other individuals in the waiting room.

14.4.1.2 Case 2

Sandra, a 21-year-old indigenous woman, went to a health center comprised of two primary care units. The staff at the center included two medical doctors, two nurses, and two auxiliary health workers. Sandra arrived on a Friday at 10:23 AM; there was only one other person in the waiting room. Four minutes after she arrived, the health worker conducted her intake in a friendly manner and told her that when the next patient was finished, she would be seen. After 17 min she was seen, and the same health worker met with her because the two doctors who normally would have seen her were not there. The health worker apologized for their absence, citing that it was the day that the doctors reported to and delivered documentation to the administration 4 h away as the reason for their absence. The health worker also mentioned that this happens two to three times per month, and their absence is due to reporting or training. The health worker asked Sandra about the reason for her visit to the health center, given that she did not recognize her as a member of the community in the facility's catchment area. Sandra mentioned that she was not originally from the surrounding area, but was embarrassed to go to her local health center because she believed that the private information about her consult might be spread in her community. She explained that she preferred a facility where she was unknown and that she had a cousin in the area.

The provider assured her there was no problem in providing her services. Sandra told her that she was thinking about initiating sexual activity but she did not want to become pregnant. The health worker proceeded to begin a contraceptive method demonstration using a prepared demonstration kit where all methods could be seen, except condoms and emergency contraceptives, and she proceeded to explain all of them. The methods that were not physically included in the kit were explained using printed pamphlets. During this explanation, she also covered the components of a comprehensive consultation, explained that this was a service where privacy was guaranteed.

Sandra perceived that the health worker, who spoke *tsotsil* as her native language, was truly interested in her needs. In addition to explaining each of the contraceptive methods, she also discussed STIs and human immunodeficiency virus (HIV) in depth, citing condoms as the preferred method for protection against these diseases. The session lasted approximately 35 min. Communication was respectful and appropriate, and Sandra felt comfortable expressing any doubts. She commented to the health worker that she was interested in using condoms. The health worker told her this was a good choice. However, although the health center had them available, the nurse in charge of resources had taken the keys to the cabinet where the contraceptives were. She apologized for the situation and asked Sandra to come back Monday to pick up the condoms.

Analysis

Sandra had no problem physically accessing the facility, nor did she have any barriers to receiving care. The 17 min of wait time was reasonable. The health worker was curious as to why Sandra did not seek care at the facility within her catchment area, but this did not lead to any barrier at accessing care. Counseling was provided in a timely manner (35 min) and in a private setting. The delivery had some weaknesses, such as an incomplete demonstration kit; however, this was resolved by showing print images of the missing methods. The explanation provided by the health worker was comprehensive, clear, and delivered in the patient's native language. The provider addressed all of Sandra's questions and doubts. However, the care delivered was inconclusive given that the user's selected method was unavailable at that moment. Unavailability was not due to any supply issues; rather it was an organizational problem—the keys to the drawer where condoms were stored were with the nurse, who was not present.

14.4.1.3 Case 3

Cristina, a 21-year-old woman, went to a health center comprised of three primary care units. The staff at the center included three medical doctors, two nurses, and one auxiliary health worker. Cristina arrived on a Monday at 10:10 in the morning; there were three other individuals in the small waiting room. The entire health center was quite small for a three-unit facility with high demand for care. Five minutes after she arrived, the health worker asked her to wait a few minutes and told a few other women in the waiting room that the doctor would not arrive for several hours and asked them to come back later. The young health worker of about 20 years of age then addressed Cristina and said "sorry they are Oportunidades patients and were coming for their follow up appointment." Immediately after, the health worker asked about the reason for her visit. Cristina said shyly that she had sexual intercourse the previous day and did not want to become pregnant. The health worker invited her into the consultation room. Once in the room, the health worker congratulated her on seeking care, hinting that it was uncommon for young women to come alone to ask for contraceptives. The health worker then opened a demonstration kit and explained all methods, with the exception of injectable hormonal methods. The entire consultation was conducted in her native language of *tsotsil*. The appointment was brief and respectful. Cristina felt comfortable expressing her doubts, and they were immediately resolved. The health worker commented that she did not have much experience providing contraceptive counseling, but knew that emergency contraceptive pills existed for cases like this one. However, she had not been left the keys to the room where they were stored. She recommended Cristina return in the afternoon or go to another health center. Cristina describes her experience as follows:

> I actually felt bad because I could tell the health worker was a little nervous, like a little embarrassed, as she tried to explain that the doctors were not there because the roads were in bad shape and its complicated to get there on time…I really liked her explanation of the methods. She was very nice, and spoke to me the whole time in tsotsil, but when it was time for her to give me that emergency pill she got very embarrassed again because she didn't have keys…but I liked her explanation a lot, you would tell she liked her job.

Analysis

Cristina's access to health services did not have any restrictions or obstacles to receiving care. However, it is worth noting that on a Monday there were no medical staff present, even though appointments had been scheduled with pregnant women. The health worker's explanation emphasized geographic and logistical difficulties in accessing the community given that it was rainy season and the roads were unpaved with difficult terrain. It is also worth noting that despite the medical staff's absence, the health worker provided counseling services in an adequate manner and the user was satisfied. The counseling process overall met the recommendations and guidelines for such a service, with the exception of discussing hormonal injectable methods. Similar to Case 2, no method of contraception was given to the user at the time of consultation because the storage area was locked, an organizational barrier preventing access to the necessary supplies that would complete care in a satisfactory manner.

14.4.1.4 Case 4

Flora, a 21-year-old woman, visited a health center in an indigenous community in the Chiapas Highlands as a simulated user; the day before she had engaged in unprotected intercourse with her boyfriend and did not want to become pregnant. She arrived on a Tuesday at 12:40 PM to the health facility. There were two women in the waiting room and another outside the facility waiting for a presentation as part of the *Oportunidades* program. Flora describes the situation when a man conducted her intake interview:

> Well, the truth is I had no idea what that man's job was. I didn't know if he was a doctor, but when I entered the health center, he began to ask me what I needed. I told him I'd like an explanation on how to avoid pregnancy. He looked at me strange, from my feet to my head, he paused and then immediately turned and yelled into the office 'Who can provide this girl with some information about contraceptive methods?'

A nurse immediately came out and greeted Flora warmly, inviting her to come into her office. She closed the door and before beginning the session, the nurse asked her if she understood Spanish, explaining that the person who helped translate was busy at the moment. Flora said that she did speak a little bit of Spanish and the nurse proceeded to explain each contraceptive method. She did not have a demonstration kit, but she showed Flora drawings that she made using a paper and pencil. The counseling session lasted approximately 30 minutes and all contraceptive methods, as well as STIs, were covered. Flora's perception is that the nurse showed a lot of empathy toward her and the situation she was experiencing. She remembers the nurse telling her:

> Now that you have learned about the methods available, right now the one that meets your need is the emergency pill. There are two pills that are going to make sure the egg does not implant and develop in your uterus, and that will prevent pregnancy.

At the end of the consult, the nurse gave her the contraceptive pills along with instructions on how to take them. However, she did not mention adverse effects, the limited protection it provided, or the possibility of continued protection using another method.

Analysis

Flora's access to counseling services was practically immediate; there was a very short wait time. Nonetheless, confidentiality was breeched at the very beginning when the male interviewer asked in a loud voice and publicly in the waiting room if someone could provide contraceptive counseling to *the girl.* When the nurse began the session, she demonstrated empathy and interest in providing information in the best way possible; however, there was no demonstration kit available. Nonetheless, the nurse fully explained contraceptive methods and STIs using drawings she made herself. Unlike other cases, Flora did obtain her preferred method and the instructions for how to use it. A weakness that this case has is the lack of information provided regarding possible side effects and the importance of continued protection.

14.4.1.5 Case 5

Yolanda, a 21-year-old woman, arrived at a health center in the largest municipality in the Chiapas Highlands at 1 PM, the time of day when patient volume slows. At the entrance there was a sign stating that all users must present their public insurance policy. Upon entering she saw an empty waiting room, and in one of the patient rooms, she noticed a group of three individuals laughing together as they watched a computer screen.

> I went and they saw me, and kept on laughing. One of them got up and said 'It's my turn, I'll handle it.' She was a nurse; I saw it on the credential she was wearing. She asked me in a serious tone, 'What do you need, my dear?' I told her that I was interested in learning more about how to prevent pregnancy because I was considering beginning sexual activity. She looked at me for a while and said, 'Mmmhmm ok, come in, let's talk.' When we went to the consult room she asked me, 'Where are you coming from.' I told her from which community. She stared at me again and said 'It's weird that you would come from so far away for this service.'

They went into the consult room. After closing the door, the nurse asked, "you speak Spanish, right? All of you go to school and speak Spanish, don't pretend you don't." Yolanda answered affirmatively. The nurse then explained each method using a demonstration kit. When the 40-minute session was over, the nurse asked, "Which of these methods are you interested in using?" Yolanda replied that the female condom interested her. The nurse was surprised and told her that method was not appropriate for her culture, and she recommended telling her boyfriend to use a male condom. Yolanda insisted that she wished to use the female condom. The nurse told her that was not possible, due to cultural expectations, and gave her three male condoms and told her, "look, I am going to give you these so you can tell your boyfriend to use them."

Analysis

There were no obstacles to access services despite the sign at the entrance of the facility indicating the need to have the public insurance policy document. This may represent difficulty in service utilization for some users. Yolanda recognized that the explanation was comprehensive and detailed, covering each method and ensuring privacy. However, her decision was not respected, despite the chosen method not having any medical contraindications. This situation breeched the fundamental principal of patient autonomy. The nurse's reasoning for denying Yolanda the female condom was that, in her perspective, the method was not appropriate for her indigenous culture. Yolanda did not receive the method of her choice, labeling this as "unmet need for contraceptive."

14.4.1.6 Case 6

Gloria, a 21-year-old woman, arrived at the health center with an interest in learning about contraceptive methods. She arrived at the waiting room at 8 AM and observed that a pregnant woman was also waiting. Half an hour later, a nurse invited Gloria into the consultation room. Inside there was a doctor, who asked her in a friendly manner about the motivation behind her visit. Gloria explained that she wanted CPF information because she did not want to become pregnant. The doctor snapped his fingers and said, "I am going to introduce you to our star contraceptive counselor." He stood up and said, "follow me." They walked to the hallway, knocked on a door, and walked into the room. There was a woman with her back turned to the door as she organized paperwork. She turned around and courteously introduced herself. She was the health center psychologist. The doctor relayed Gloria's need for care and said, "I'm leaving you in good hands, much better than my own." The psychologist had a full demonstration kit that she used during the consult. The session was smooth, organized, and also provided an environment that was calm, friendly, comfortable, and trusting. The psychologist congratulated Gloria on seeking contraceptive counseling.

"You speak Spanish, right," she asked. "A little," Gloria responded. The psychologist replied, "no, no no, we need you to be able to completely understand this, wait here." She left the room and in less than a minute returned with a female health worker who spoke *tsotsil*. The session lasted 45 min, the explanation was very detailed and covered the methods comprehensively as well as STIs. Once the session concluded, the psychologist asked Gloria which method she would like to choose. Gloria chose the female condom. "Good choice," the psychologist said, "It's a good method for protecting against STIs, just like the male condom. The only problem is that right now we don't have any because we have not ordered them given that almost no one in this region had asked for it." She apologized for not having the chosen method and invited her to come back in a few months to see if they had them in supply. Gloria chose an alternative method.

Analysis

Access to the health service was without any barriers. The wait time of 30 min was reasonable. We wish to emphasize the willingness of the staff to adapt the service as necessary to the needs and conditions of the user: the leadership shown by the doctor to find the "star counselor," as well as the psychologist's recruitment of the health worker to support with translation so that the patient could understand the discussion. Gloria thought that the psychologist must have received specialized training based on how professionally she presented the methods and the detail and trust needed to facilitate the conversation with the user. Despite the evident hard work on behalf of the staff, the result was not as wished given that once a decision about a method was made, the response was that the female condom was not available. This is yet another instance of unmet need due to administrative obstacles.

14.4.1.7 Case 7

Rosa, a 21-year-old woman, sought care at one of the municipal health centers of the Chiapas Highlands. A young nurse asked her the reason for her consultation. Rosa replied that she would like information about contraceptive methods. The nurse asked Rosa if she had her health insurance identification, but Rosa told her she did not. The nurse said that was not a problem and that she would be seen after another woman who was also waiting. Approximately half an hour later, a health worker invited Rosa into the consultation room. There she was seen by a doctor who asked her if she would prefer the information be provided in Spanish or *tsotsil*. Rosa preferred *tsotsil*, and the health worker began acting as the interpreter. Rosa explains:

> …they were very nice. I really liked how they explained each of the methods. I think they were trained because their presentation was interesting and entertaining. Before I knew it, 45 min had gone by, and they congratulated me for coming in.

The doctor used a demonstration kit to explain each of the methods, and mentioned which would be useful for Rosa's situation. "As you've seen there are a lot of methods, but right now I think you need the emergency contraceptives," said the doctor, after she learned during the conversation that Rosa had had sex with her partner the day before and did not wish to become pregnant. Rosa agreed with her; however, the pill was not available at the pharmacy, given that it was infrequently requested. The doctor apologized and suggested Rosa go to another public health center.

Analysis

This case presented no barriers to access services. The wait time was reasonable. Rosa was treated in a kind and respectful manner. Counseling was provided in an adequate space, with care given to privacy and autonomy, and in the preferred language of *tsotsil*. The person responsible for providing counseling had the necessary material and gave a comprehensive and understandable explanation of each contraceptive method. The doctor indicated that the emergency pill was aligned with the user's need, however, it was unavailable. The user left the facility with an unmet need. The reason the emergency pill was unavailable was due to little demand, and thus was not being stocked.

14.4.1.8 Case 8

Marcos, a 22-year-old young man, went to a community hospital that offered primary care services. The unit is located in the municipal head, very close to the city of San Cristóbal de Las Casas. Marcos was a simulated user who wished to learn about methods to avoid pregnancies and STIs. He arrived at the hospital on a Sunday, as he understood that the facility had 7-day 24-hour services, and he preferred to seek care on a day where there were less walk-in consultations. As expected, there were very few people in the waiting room. A doctor approximately 50 years old was smoking at the entrance. When he saw Marcos walk in, he put out his cigarette and gave him a courteous welcome.

> Upon my arrival I was greeted in a friendly manner. I immediately went into the counseling session because there was no one waiting. I told the doctor why I was there, and he wasn't surprised or rude, no negative attitude. It was the opposite, he was very friendly and told me it was great that I was seeking information and taking care of myself because there are risks to contracting diseases or unwanted pregnancies.

The doctor appeared to be familiar with young people looking for CFP services, and he even mentioned to Marcos that he was happy to see an increase in demand for sexual and reproductive care and contraceptives.

> [The doctor] told me that I was not the first person to come seeking information, that young people were often interested in learning how to prevent pregnancy and STIs, and that he was extremely happy that young people in this municipality take care of themselves.

After the warm greeting, the doctor opened a complete demonstration kit. The session began with the doctor speaking *tsotsil*, despite the fact that it was not his mother tongue. This effort surprised Marcos. After approximately 10 min, the doctor told Marcos that there were some words he did not know how to translate from Spanish to *tsotsil*, and asked if there would be a problem if he spoke to him in Spanish to make sure he understood.

> After inviting me into the consult room he asked me which language I preferred for the consult, Spanish or tsotsil. I answered that it would be much better in tsotsil. He answered that would be fine, that he would explain in tsotsil but that since I spoke Spanish it would be better for both of us if he explained in Spanish, because he did not speak tsotsil very well, but he would try. And he did try, but after 10 min he began to explain everything in Spanish. It was honestly better because he was trying so hard with tsotsil but I couldn't understand anything. But I appreciated his effort and his continuing in Spanish.

In Marcos' opinion, the doctor was an expert in the topic and had a good attitude. This built trust and allowed Marcos' to share his doubts.

> He asked me about my origin and what my name was, but that didn't really matter, it was just to be able to address me by my name and have strong communication. I told him 'I'm Marcos and I come from Nachji.' He said with a smile, 'very well Marcos, I congratulate you for decided to become informed and take care of yourself. Not only will you avoid your girlfriend becoming pregnant, you also will avoid contracting STIs.' After, he asked me which I would like for him to explain first: STIs or CFP. I asked for him to first explain STIs and how to avoid them. He began, first mentioning syphilis, then gonorrhea, and ending with AIDS. For each of these he had printed material from a catalog. He mentioned that the most complex of them all is AIDS. He asked me if I had any questions and when I said no, he started explaining the CFP methods. He brought out another catalogue and first explained barrier methods. First the male condom and how to use it. After he explained how to use it and showed me, he asked me to show him and handed me the plastic penis so that I could put it on. The explanation included how to open the package, he told me to open it with my fingers tips, never with my teeth or sharp objects like scissors. He asked me if I had used one before and when I said yes, he told me, 'you know how to do this well.'

The counseling session lasted an hour and 15 min. At the end of the session, the doctor gave Marcos three condoms.

Analysis

The quality of care is notable in this case. From the first moment of contact, it is clear that the service provider has a proactive attitude, pushing himself to adapt the services to the needs of the user. We want to highlight that the doctor managed to speak for close to 10 min in *tsotsil*, despite error and not being fluent. This effort illustrates his interest in adapting practices to meet the needs and cultural context in which he provides services. The provider is able to gain the trust of the young user given his cheery attitude, empathy, and interest in providing the counseling service in the most appropriate manner. Finally, the excellent work realized during the care process culminates with the demand satisfied, as exemplified by the three condoms given to Marcos.

14.4.1.9 Case 9

Fernando visited a community hospital in the Highlands. He arrived on a Tuesday morning, with 13 other people already present in the waiting room. There were no obstacles to checking in: he approached the reception area where there was a young male nurse about 20 years old. He told the nurse that he was interested in information related to pregnancy and STI prevention. The receptionist told him to take a seat and wait. After 3 min passed while Fernando was waiting, the nurse spoke out loud and across the room to a nurse at the other end of the office, "Hey! Do you know where there are condoms?!" Several people turned to look at the nurses when he said this. The other nurse's response was, "the boss probably has them!" while walking into a consultation room. Seconds later the same nurse walked out of the consultation room and up to Fernando, saying, "we only have these because not enough have arrived." Fernando took the two condoms that he was being handed and said he was interested in having a conversation with the doctor about other methods and how to prevent STIs. The response he received was that the doctor was busy and the social worker had not yet arrived. As the nurse walked away, he said to Fernando, "anyways you already know how to use them, you look educated."

Analysis

This case presented a different pattern than previous cases; while the user did receive the method requested, he was not given counseling. In addition to being denied the ability to see a provider, there were also violations to his right to privacy and confidentiality. The communication out loud between nurses seems to be making an example of the user, like a form of public admonishment or disapproval of seeking out CFP. Furthermore, the nurses, based on their own prejudices, assumed the user knew how to use the method because he "looked educated."

14.5 Service Providers' Practices and Perceptions

We conducted 5 semistructured interviews and 3 discussion workshops with 36 service providers from the 12 municipalities with the highest indigenous populations in the Chiapas Highlands (Aldama, Chalchihuitán, Chamula, Chanal, Chenalhó, Larrainzar, Mitontic, Pantelhó, Las Rosas, San Cristóbal, Tenejapa, Santiago el Pinar). In this section we describe our findings related to their self-described perceptions and practices about CFP in the indigenous context in which they work.

14.5.1 Foundation and Goals of CFP Programs

When asked about the foundation and objectives of CFP, providers indicated that the efforts of the programs where they work in indigenous contexts are *a medium* that allows them to reach certain results, as opposed to a solution in and of itself. We specifically asked the question: "Why would health professionals provide CFP services?" The answers discussed results to such an intervention, but it was never identified as a human right and a goal in and of itself.

Contraceptive care is considered both a medical and public health intervention, with clinical and epidemiological foundations, designed to obtain positive outcomes for certain health indicators. For example, the providers we interviewed identified that, first and foremost, *the objective of CFP is to reduce maternal and infant mortality* (interviewee, October 2013). This has been the highest priority in the health policy landscape in the region for over a decade. The argument used is both simple and categorical: *if more women use CFP there will be fewer pregnancies and fewer abortions, longer birth spacing, a decrease in women older than 35 with 3 or more pregnancies, and at the end of the day, that implies less obstetric and neonatal risk* (workshop participant, November 2013). There were no doubts about this, as workshop participants indicated that contraception is *one of the pillars for reducing maternal death* (interviewee, October 2013).

Some of the providers indicated that the CFP program has the objective of contributing to social development, decreasing poverty, and improving the economic conditions of families and the indigenous population. This translates to the program being more than in the realm of health and positions it as both a social and an economic development strategy.

> ...the objective of the CFP program is to improve the quality of life for the family, improve their development, find work, educate themselves. (workshop participant, November 2013)

Other providers, predominantly those with over 15–20 years of experience, considered that the CFP program had the goal of addressing *the problem of demographic explosion*, as one of the workshop participants, an experienced doctor currently in an administration role, described it. The argument is that the population of the country and the state of Chiapas *is too large* and that this overpopulation represents *a social and economic problem* that endangers *the country's own viability*. As such, providers indicated that beyond a public health problem, it was a security issue. They believed the government established the CFP program and policies to control *the demographic explosion.*

> ...the program was implemented due to the demographic explosion that Mexico experienced in the seventies. (workshop participant, November 2013)

> ...the government developed a strategy. If we had continued with the growth rate at the time we would have an enormous population. Having a child is costly, for women too, they are not only providers of children, they are also providers of resources. (workshop participant, November 2013)

There were providers who believed that some societies in Mexico and Chiapas, particularly indigenous ones, have an unequal distribution of power between men and women. Men have superiority over women, and this leads to violent practices toward and subordination of women. The CFP program also has the objective of *contributing to the empowerment of women* (workshop participant, November 2013), beginning with control over their body and reproduction. Furthermore, this can allow a woman to have more control over her life plans and not depend on the decisions and willingness of a man (partner, husband, brother). The CFP program is thus a tool in the larger struggle to decrease patriarchal power and build more equitable gender relationships.

> ... to give the woman the chance to develop another role besides motherhood; as a professional or in another realm to be able to succeed. (workshop participant, November 2013)

These were the primary arguments used to explain the objectives and foundation, technical, legal, and ideological, for the CFP program. This program is *a medium* to reach diverse objectives and outcomes. Not a single participant mentioned that CFP was a human right. No one referenced the Mexican Constitution, where Article 4 states this as a basic right. It wasn't until we specifically posed a question about Article 4 of the Constitution that one participant mentioned that individuals have *the right* to CFP. However, during the three workshop discussions and individual interviews with providers, the notion that the CFP program (particularly within the context of indigenous and socially marginalized communities) is a medium to reach greater goals (improve health, decrease maternal and neonatal death, decrease population size, combat poverty, contribute to economic development, and empower women) was paramount; CFP as a *human right* was not. This finding is relevant because the comprehension of the foundation and objectives of a program determines the way in which aligned actions are implemented.

14.5.2 CFP Among the Indigenous Population

Nobody questioned that the CFP program should be considered a high priority for the health system and service providers' daily workload. However, it was mentioned that during the first decade of the twentieth century, the program was constantly abandoned at the federal and state level alike and, as a consequence, at the health centers. Although there was not a specific explanation given as to the reasons for the perceived abandonment, some participants considered that it may have been due to shifting political priorities, as the federal government in power ideologically opposed CFP.

It is worth noting that among service providers, the primary barrier identified to the use of contraceptive methods is culture. Participants indicated that part of the cultural norms and context includes arranged marriages at an early age, no courtship, no premarital sex (or sex pre-partnership when marriage is not in the legally recognized manner), and that fathers consider their daughters to be material goods to be exchanged for money (as one participant put it: *fathers sell their daughters)*. There was also a mention of the social pressure in communication for young couples to have children—and many—and that children are considered resources in families' reproduction and production because they support both domestic and agricultural work. Overall, these arguments were used to explain why CFP coverage is generally low in indigenous communities. These representations were strongly engrained in the providers' discourse. In addition, not having empirical evidence to support their hypotheses, which were clearly stereotypes, their attitudes also negatively affected their willingness to offer counseling and orientation services.

It was only when we asked participants about the supply side of CFP services that they noted several deficiencies. First, they made critical observations about the availability of CFP and counseling services. They mentioned that there is a reduced availability of contraceptives at health centers and there is usually a shortage of one or many of them. This generates a significant inconvenience for real users who, upon returning for the method of their choosing, often have to switch to another method based on what is available, oftentimes resulting in abandonment of the method. Moreover, the supply of goods is based on current demand, instead of the supply needed to have full coverage among the population; the health centers do not have the adequate physical space to provide counseling in a manner that meets privacy and confidentiality and promotes trust; staff do not always have the proposer training and competencies to provide counseling to the indigenous population; there are insufficient demonstration kits with models of the contraceptives; there is a lack of support materials to provide further information; and there are not enough interpreters or trained staff that can deliver a complete counseling session in users' native language (Fig. 14.7).

14.5.3 Contraceptive Counseling Services Provided to the Indigenous Population

Although, in general, providers consider that CFP services are contradictory to the indigenous worldview, they also recognize that the characteristics on the supply side do not facilitate the practice of counseling. They recognize organizational barriers and issues of availability, for example, the insufficient supply of methods, the limited schedule during which an adequate counseling session can be delivered (*we have to provide the consult in 15 or 20 min' people there are a lot of people waiting, how can we do that?* workshop participant, November 2013), and the lack of trained personnel who can provide information in the local language. The aforementioned barriers, from the providers' perspective, impede in the counseling process being carried out appropriately.

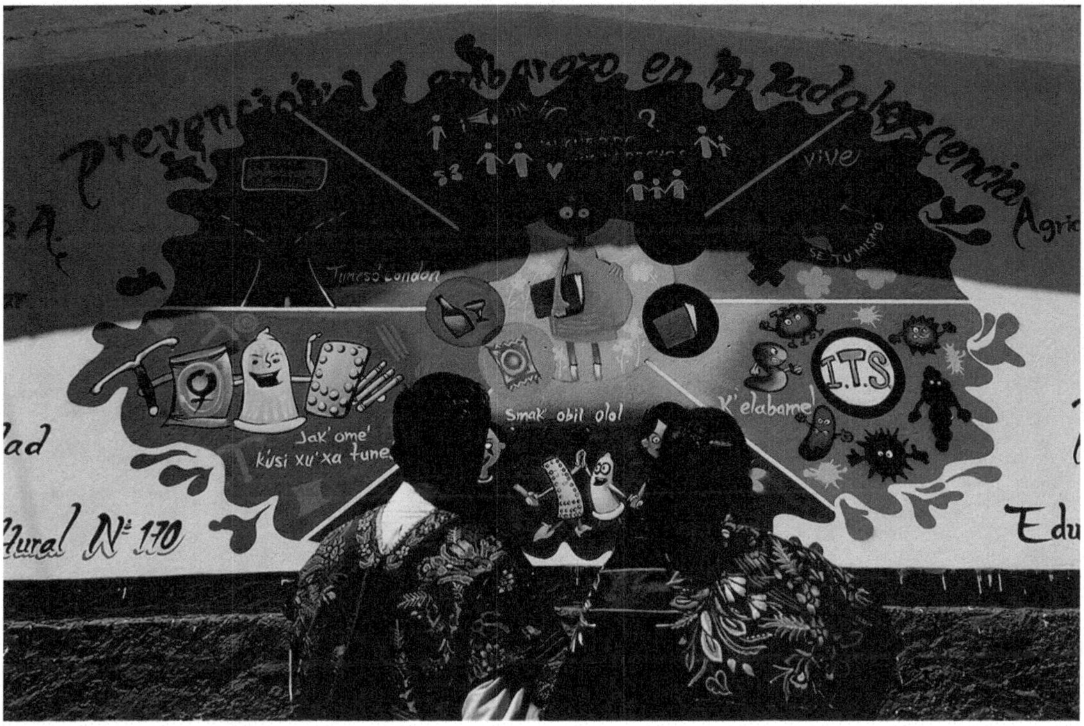

Fig. 14.7 Indigenous adolescents in front of a school mural promoting information on contraceptives in the *Tsotsil* language. Photo by Juan Carlos Martínez

However, providers' also spoke to *the art of persuasion* that they enacted so that the indigenous population would use a CFP method. This was reiterated on several occasions. Providers used the concept of *persuading* the indigenous patient to use CFP.

> You have no idea how difficult it is to convince women, but above all their husbands, to use CFP. There are some times where they just don't understand. (workshop participant, November 2013)

> But, tell me, how do I persuade a woman who is in her ninth or tenth pregnancy, who down the road will come in on a trauma call half dead, if she arrives at all instead of dying at home. (workshop participant, November 2013)

> As health professionals, we have the training needed and it is our responsibility to convince [indigenous] men and women that they use CFP. It's complicated due to language barriers and cultural norms, but, well, it's our job: the art of persuasion. There is no other way. (workshop participant, November 2013)

This finding is in contrast to the previous finding of providers not recognizing the decision about how many children to have and when to have them is a human right and that this right should be carried out with respect for human dignity (as the General Health Law states in Article 67), including respecting individuals' autonomy, expectations, values, and decisions. At the same time, providers recognized the external factors pushing CFP, and its central role in reducing maternal morbidity and mortality, and to a lesser degree related to women's empowerment and education and contributing to the decrease in poverty and increase in development. These may be some of the reasons that providers see their role as *persuading* indigenous populations about the need and convenience of CFP (Fig. 14.8).

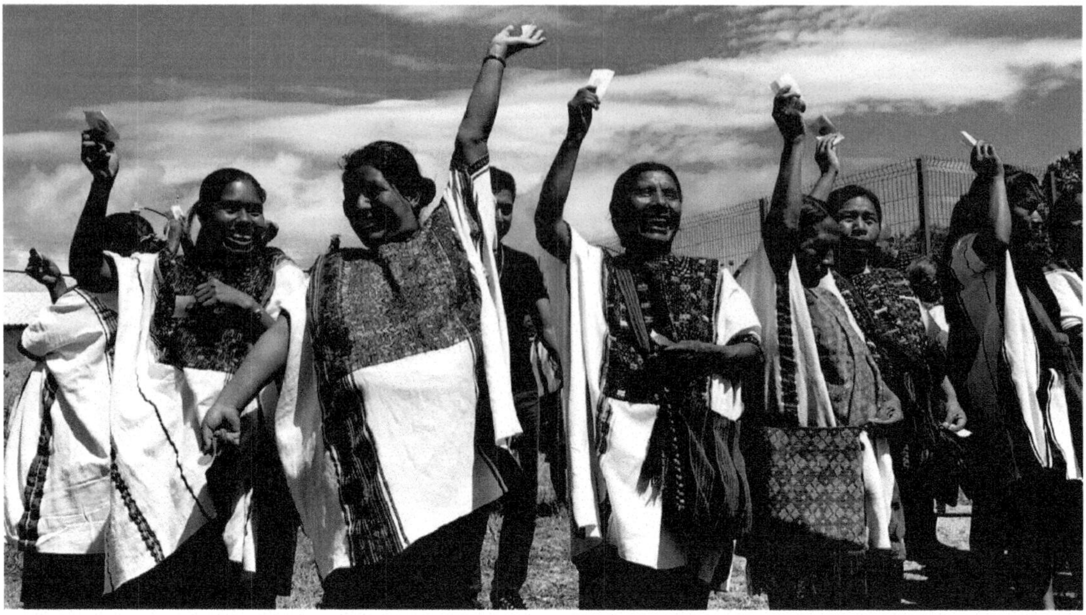

Fig. 14.8 Traditional midwives in the ending of training workshop of family planning and pregnancy monitoring. Photo by Juan Carlos Martínez

Conclusions

It was interesting to observe how providers did not identify CFP services as a basic human right, but did see it as a medium to reach other outcomes, particularly to reduce maternal mortality or morbidity, improve economic and social development, and increase women's empowerment. It is also worth noting that providers emphasized *the need to persuade* the population to use CFP, an idea that seems inextricably linked to CFP being viewed as a medium to reach public health goals and not as a value in and of itself. Moreover, there is a profound subtext about indigenous individuals as passive objects of intervention and not as active subjects with their rights.

We want to highlight the consensus among providers with regard to the insufficient availability of CFP methods in health centers. The experience of the simulated users showed evidence of this situation; in various cases users were not given their method of choice or steered toward another method, both of which are considered as unmet contraceptive need. The simulated user technique also provided evidence of the insufficient availability of demonstration kits. The providers' testimony also emphasized the lack of tools to support counseling. The cases where demonstration kits were available showed that they were of great use in explaining the different methods and contributing toward the comprehension and satisfaction of simulated users, again showing their utility. As such, it should be guaranteed that all health facilities have demonstration kits that are complete and in good condition (Fig. 14.9).

The providers and simulated users' testimonials recognized that an important organizational barrier to contraceptive counseling is the lack of adequate physical space where privacy is guaranteed and trust can be built. Further, the limited service delivery hours and high demand for care do not always allow there to be sufficient time to provide counseling with the level of care that is needed. Because of this, we suggest strategies to provide this service during the hours with the least demand for care or alternatively that the service be provided by non-physician staff (nurses, health workers, social workers).

The simulated user technique allowed us to uncover discriminatory practices used by providers during contraceptive counseling for the population seeking services. Specific instances included the

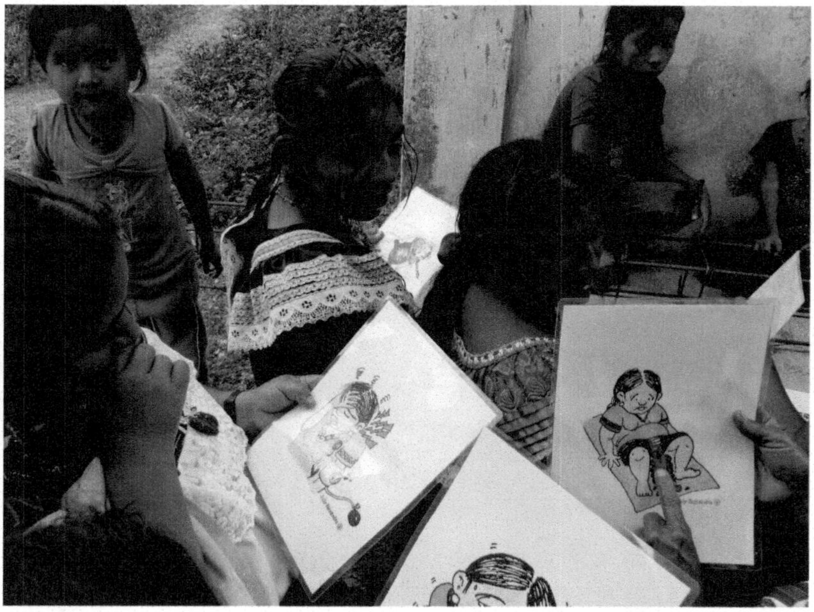

Fig. 14.9 Traditional midwives in a training session. Photo by Marisol Vega

user was not from the immediate vicinity; the user did not have their public health insurance paperwork; the user appeared to be well-educated; and based on gender, age, and marital status. In fact, all women, young adults, and single women faced major barriers to access counseling services and were the most likely to be denied their preferred method. Some of the women were denied CFP because the providers considered that they would be "outsiders," culturally speaking, or because they might encounter challenges with their partners as a result. However, it is worth noting that providers shouldn't be the ones determining whether a contraceptive method is culturally appropriate or not or whether the users' marital status matters. Their responsibility is to provide technical information based on guidelines on best practice and scientific evidence, so that users can make an informed choice about which methods they wish to utilize. It is also important to emphasize the finding that young users encountered greater difficulty seeking care: longer wait times, insufficient privacy, and lack of provision of the desired method.

Counseling was not always provided in the local language. It was frequently given in Spanish or with the assistance of a health worker acting as an interpreter. The use of health workers for interpreting purposes presents the possibility that the information provided by the health professional may not be translated exactly as intended. This is an important element in making services appropriate: training staff (both health workers and nurses) who speak the local language to deliver counseling and protect the dignity of users (Fig. 14.10).

A weakness observed in the health centers was the limited care given to respecting patients' privacy at the time of counseling: open doors, announcing the reason for the visit in the waiting room, and giving instructions in front of third parties. These are factors that affect quality of care. Moreover, the following weaknesses diverge from the counseling process:

- Asking or alluding to a user's marital status to determine whether or not to provide the counseling session
- Lack of availability of a complete demonstration kit
- Lack of anatomical models (male and female reproductive organs) to use in counseling sessions
- Lack of educational materials to facilitate counseling sessions

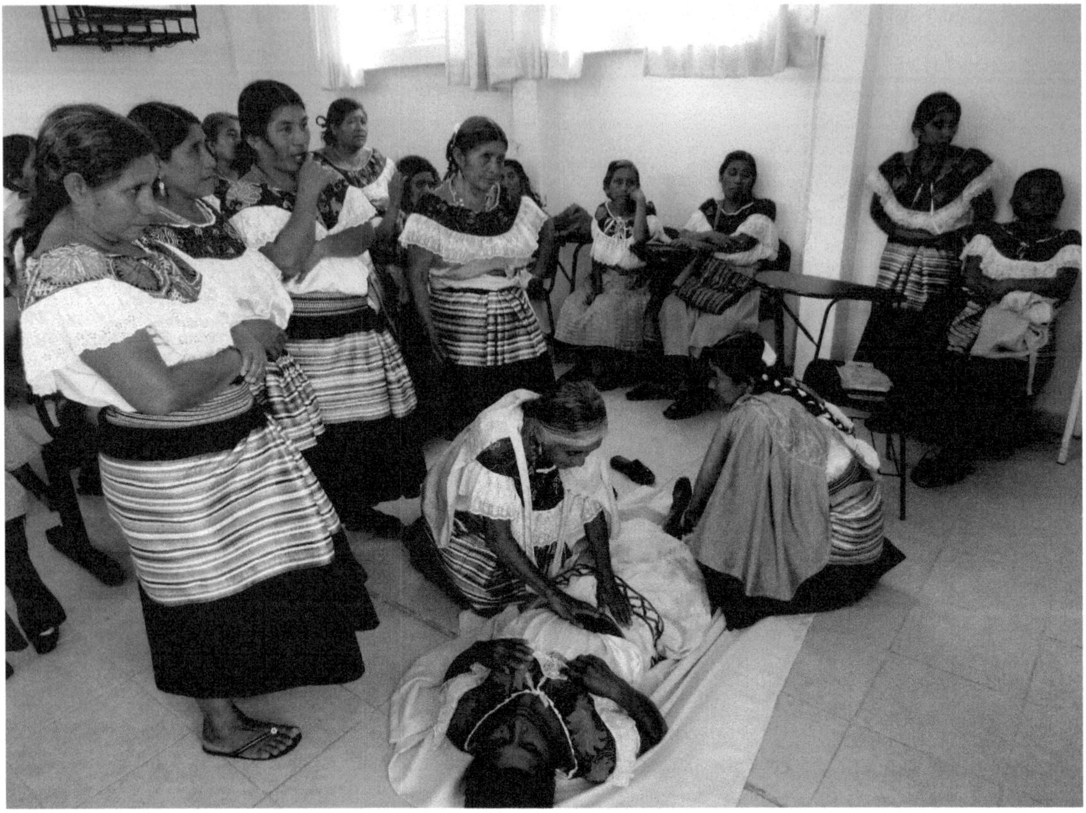

Fig. 14.10 A class of traditional midwives in a training session. Photo by Marisol Vega

- Incomplete counseling that does not cover all components included in the guideline: how to use method, how the method functions, contraindications and warnings, safety, side effects, follow-up, and evaluation needed
- Lack of comprehensive sexual and reproductive healthcare for users (particularly adolescents) that may be beyond the reason for their visit

We were able to identify very positive cases, when it comes to the interpersonal quality of care. In these cases, the provider teams had a positive and, in some cases, even an enthusiastic attitude in general toward contraceptive counseling and answered all of the users' questions. They also went to great effort to provide the information in the users' native language and to ensure they understood. It is notable what providers did to adapt the services to the needs and conditions of the users. However, we also identified certain practices that may serve as a window of opportunity for improving services:

- The objective of counseling is not to *persuade* the use of CFP. It is the users' right to have the information needed, ask questions, and subsequently to decide whether or not to use CFP.
- The provider must be sure to provide counseling in a place where privacy is guaranteed.
- The provider should abstain from expressing his or her own opinions or values about the users' sexuality.
- Providers should avoid public embarrassment or admonishment of users seeking contraceptive counseling.

Specific processes could be improved to ensure the right to CFP services and, simultaneously, have a positive effect on the external outcomes of reducing maternal and infant mortality in the Chiapas Highlands. It is possible to successfully face the challenges through the implementation of improvement processes that involve the population itself, providers, and administrators. For example, our findings suggest important challenges in the development of competencies among health professionals who are currently responsible for providing reproductive health services in public health facilities. The analysis of their job performance in terms of CFP requires deep reflection and transformation in how doctors, nurses, auxiliary staff, and community health workers are trained. Since 2011 the Secretariat of Taxes and Public Credits authorized the code used to hire professional midwives as health professionals in public health facilities, who, according to the International Labour Organization's International Standard Classification of Occupations, can provide contraceptive counseling (OIT 2008). The State of the World's Midwifery report indicates that midwives are authorized to offer at minimum one type of contraceptive in 71 of 73 of the countries evaluated, with the exception of China and Iraq. Professional midwives can complete 87% of the 46 essential intervention in reproductive, neonatal, and maternal health, including contraceptive counseling and provision of methods (OMS 2014). The progressive inclusion of professional midwives in public health facilities could improve the technical and interpersonal quality of CFP in indigenous regions, as well as increase utilization and substantially reduce the unmet meet in rural and indigenous contexts.

References

Banco Interamericano de Desarrollo. (2013). *México SM2015: Censo y encuesta de línea base por hogares, Informe final*. Iniciativa Salud Mesoamérica 2015.

Campbell, O., & Graham, W. (2006). Strategies for reducing maternal mortality: Getting on with what words. The lancet maternal survival series. *Lancet, 368*(9543), 1284–1299.

Castro, R. (2000). *La vida en la adversidad: el significado de la salud y la reproducción en la pobreza*. Mexico: CRIM-UNAM.

CONEVAL. (2014). *Pobreza en México*. México: Consejo Nacional de Evaluación de la Política de Desarrollo Social.

Declaración de Moisés Gandhi. 1997. Por una Salud en Manos del Pueblo. Región Autónoma Tzotz-Choj, Chiapas. Retrieved January 7, 2017, from http://www.cedoz.org/site/content.php?doc=500&cat=83.

Donabedian, A. (1988). *Los espacios de la salud: aspectos fundamentales de la organización de la atención médica*. Mexico: Fondo de Cultura Económica.

Frenk, J. (1994). *La salud de la población: hacia una nueva salud pública. La salud de la población: hacia una nueva salud pública*. Mexico: Fondo de Cultura Económica.

Freyermuth, G. (2003). *Las mujeres de humo. Morir en Chenalhó. Género, etnia y generación, factores constitutivos del riesgo durante la maternidad*. Mexico: CIESAS, Porrúa.

Ibáñez, M., Heredia-Pi, I., Meneses, S., Pelcastre, B., & González Block, M. A. (2015). Labour and delivery services use: Indigenous women's preference and the health sector response in the Chiapas Highlands of Mexico. *International Journal for Equity in Health, 14*(156), 1–10.

INEGI. (2014). *Encuesta Nacional de Dinámica Demográfica 2014. Instituto Nacional Estadística y Geografía. Principales resultados*. Retrieved May 12, 2016, from http://www.inegi.org.mx/est/contenidos/proyectos/encuestas/hogares/especiales/enadid/enadid2014/doc/resultados_enadid14.pdf.

INEGI. (2015). *Encuesta Intercensal 2015*. México: Instituto Nacional de Geografía y Estadística.

ISECH. (2014). *Guía de consejería anticonceptiva con pertinencia cultural*. Chiapas: Instituto de Salud del Estado de Chiapas/Salud Mesoamérica.

Kirsch, J., & Arana, M. (1999). Informed consent for family planning for poor women in Chiapas, Mexico. *Lancet, 354*, 419–420.

Ley General de Salud. 2016. Retrieved July 28, 2016, from http://www.diputados.gob.mx/LeyesBiblio/pdf/142.pdf.

Loewenberg, S. (2010). The plight of Mexico's indigenous women. *Lancet, 375*, 1680–1682.

Meneses, S. (2004). *Semiótica de la otredad. La diferencia como diagnosis. Etnografía de los encuentros médicos interétnicos en Los Altos de Chiapas*. Tesis para obtener el grado de maestro en antropología social. San Cristóbal de Las Casas, Chiapas: Centro de Investigaciones y Estudios Superiores en Antropología Social, Sureste.

Nazar, A., Halperin, D., & Salvatierra, B. (1996). Efectos de las prácticas anticonceptivas sobre la fecundidad en la región fronteriza de Chiapas, México. *Salud Pública México, 38*, 13–19.
Nazar, A., Salvatierra, B., Morales, M., Rodríguez, M. (2011). *Estudio cualitativo de barreras de demanda y oferta con enfoque a nivel local y comunitario y cambio de comportamiento en municipios prioritarios de Chiapas, México*. Banco Interamericano de Desarrollo (unpublished).
OIT. (2008). *Clasificación Internacional de Ocupaciones. Organización Internacional del trabajo*. Retrieved June 4, 2016, from http://www.ilo.org/public/english/bureau/stat/isco/isco08/index.htm.
OMS. (2014). *Informe Mundial del Estado de las Parteras en el Mundo, 2014*, Conferencia Internacional de Matronas, Organización Mundial de la Salud. Retrieved February 20, 2016, from https://www.unfpa.org/sites/default/files/pub-pdf/SoWMy2014_complete-Spanish.pdf.
OPS. (2012). *Plan de acción para acelerar la reducción de la mortalidad materna y la morbilidad materna grave: estrategia de monitoreo y evaluación* (p. 1593). Montevideo: Publicación Científica.
ONU. (2015). Objetivos del desarrollo sostenible. Nueva York: Organización de las Naciones Unidas. Retrieved January 7. 2017, from http://www.un.org/sustainabledevelopment/es/.
Palma, C., & Suárez, M. (1994). Planificación familiar. Diferencias regionales en la práctica anticonceptiva. *Demos, 7*, 39–40.
PHR. (1999). *Health care held hostage: Human rights violations and violations of medical neutrality in Chiapas, Mexico*. Boston: Physicians for Human Rights.
PNUD. (2010). *Objetivos de desarrollo del milenio*. Programa de las Naciones Unidas para el Desarrollo. Retrieved July 28, 2016, from http://www.undp.org/spanish/mdg/goal5.shtml.
SSA. (2008). *Programa de acción específico 2007–2012: Planificación Familiar y Anticoncepción, México*. Retrieved January 7, 2017, from http://www.spps.gob.mx/planificacion-familiar-y-anticoncepcion.
SSA. (2014). Programa de acción específico Planificación Familiar y Anticoncepción 2013–2018. Mexico: Secretaría de Salud. Retrieved January 7, 2017, from http://cnegsr.salud.gob.mx/contenidos/descargas/PlanFam/PlanificacionFamiliaryAnticoncepcion.pdf.
Sesia, P. (2009). El potencial del programa Oportunidades para promover una maternidad segura y abatir la muerte materna en México: una propuesta de política pública para regiones indígenas de alto rezago social. In G. Freyermuth & P. Sesia (Eds.), *La muerte materna. Acciones y estrategias hacia una maternidad segura*. Mexico: Comité Promotor por una Maternidad sin Riesgos en México/CIESAS.

15 Problems with Epidemiological Surveillance and Under-Reporting of Maternal Deaths in Yucatan, Mexico: An Analysis of Six Studies

Elsa María Rodríguez-Angulo, Jolly Josefina Hoil-Santos, and Ricardo Ojeda-Rodríguez

15.1 Maternal Death and Under-Reporting

Researchers in the fields of biomedicine, public health, and the social sciences have always been interested in knowing the actual magnitude of the problem of maternal deaths in various regions or countries. However, classifying the causes of death as a result of pregnancy remains an important problem for decision-making authorities and for those personnel in charge of maternal death epidemiological surveillance.

Maternal and perinatal mortality is an indicator, or proxy, of a country's development. Because of this, maternal morbidity statistics have had an impact on the health information systems—health analysts, public health authorities, and international agencies carefully evaluate it to determine the overall quality of the national health services. For example, in New Zealand, the reporting rate for serious maternal and perinatal events that reach official surveillance networks is low—fewer than 9% of local serious adverse events (SAEs) are captured and reported. This has been attributed to a low level of local review of those events eligible for analysis (Farquhar et al. 2015), with the consequence that the quality of perinatal medical care cannot be adequately monitored.

Despite the progress that has been made in some countries in the registration services of maternal mortality, a true epidemiological surveillance system of maternal deaths that guarantees reliability in terms of the actual magnitude of the problem has not been implemented. In the United Kingdom (UK), attempts to improve the registration of maternal deaths for the past 60 years have been made through the review of several data sources that allow for information triangulation. The UK recognizes that it is insufficient to base the registration of the causes of maternal death solely on the review of the death certificates, as the woman's pregnancy is not a reportable event (WHO 2004).

For many years, the reporting of cases of maternal death has been based on the identification of cases through the retrospective review of death certificates, where the major cause(s) of death are stated, together with information on the woman's condition (if she was pregnant or in the puerperium

E. M. Rodríguez-Angulo, M.D., Ph.D., M.P.H. (✉)
J. J. Hoil-Santos, M.D., M.A.Sc.
R. Ojeda-Rodríguez, B.A.
University of Yucatan, Mérida, Mexico
e-mail: rangulo@correo.uady.mx

D. A. Schwartz (ed.), *Maternal Death and Pregnancy-Related Morbidity Among Indigenous Women of Mexico and Central America*, Global Maternal and Child Health: Medical, Anthropological, and Public Health Perspectives, https://doi.org/10.1007/978-3-319-71538-4_15

at the time of death). However, in some jurisdictions, there are mistakes as to the correct completion of the certificates that deviate from the actual cause(s) of death, resulting in under-reporting or under-notification of the cases of maternal death. In those instances where there are doubts about the causes of death of a pregnant woman, relatives of the deceased woman can be interviewed (termed the verbal autopsy) in order to ascertain information regarding the pregnancy and the onset of the signs and symptoms of the complication(s), up to the moment when care was sought at a hospital or death intervened (Curtis et al. 2015). Moreover, there are important social determinants that can influence the mechanisms and causes of maternal death (Lewis 2003, 2008).

A maternal death is the result of complications that arise during pregnancy, labor and delivery, or the puerperium. The causes are specified in the International Classification of Diseases, Tenth Revision (ICD-10), and the major etiologies include the hypertensive diseases of pregnancy (preeclampsia and eclampsia), postpartum hemorrhage, sepsis, and abortions (PAHO 1995; Schwartz 2015a, 2015b, 2015c). Accidental or incidental causes are not taken into account when counting the number of occurrences, but deaths derived from iatrogenic conditions, misdiagnoses, or incorrect treatments are.

One of the main problems regarding maternal mortality surveillance is that the reference documents used to report maternal deaths and their cause(s) differ between countries. Most of them utilize the ICD-10 and, based on the cause(s) reported in the death certificates, codify the major cause to be considered in the statistical calculation. In 2012, the International Classification of Diseases for Maternal Mortality (ICD-MM) was published by the World Health Organization (2016); suicide was reclassified as a direct cause of maternal death instead of an indirect one. In spite of this reclassification, the registration of pregnancy-related suicides has not been taken into account in the calculation of the maternal mortality ratio (MMR) except in some countries (i.e., United Kingdom) where it was incorporated into the statistics several years ago.

There are many publications regarding the under-reporting or under-notification of maternal deaths in the literature (Farquhar et al. 2015; McCaw-Binns et al. 2015; Simoes and Almeida 2011; Karimiam-Teherani et al. 2002; Turner et al. 2002), but such reports addressing the situation in Latin-American countries are scarce. Even though advanced information technologies have been implemented in some Latin-American countries as part of their surveillance and reporting systems, they have not yet achieved optimal quality standards to capture the total number of mother deaths. In Yucatan in the year 2002, studies were launched to analyze the under-reporting of cases of maternal death, which allowed to demonstrate their existence (Rodríguez et al. 2005, 2007, 2009; Rodríguez 2010). This paper presents the results of the analysis of the problems regarding epidemiological surveillance and the under-reporting of maternal mortality cases in the state of Yucatan.

15.2 Methodology to Analyze Under-Reporting of Maternal Deaths

The state of Yucatan is located in the southeastern region of Mexico. It has 2,097,175 inhabitants (INEGI 2015), out of which 51% are women, and out of them, 27.6% are between 15 and 49 years of age and live distributed in 106 municipalities (INEGI 2016). Between the years 2002 and 2011, six studies were carried out to analyze the under-reporting of cases of maternal death in different communities of Yucatan. Four of the studies examined the period between 1997 and 2001; another compared this period in addition to mother deaths occurring between 2002 and 2010, and one more comprised the first period and extended up to the year 2008. All of them were cross-sectional retrospective studies.

Utilizing diagnostic entities from the ICD-10 as a basis, maternal deaths were classified into two categories: (1) direct obstetric deaths and (2) indirect obstetric deaths. Direct obstetric death results from obstetric complications that occur during pregnancy, delivery, or puerperium, from interventions, omissions, incorrect treatment, or a chain of events resulting from any of the aforementioned circumstances.

Indirect obstetric deaths result from a previously existing disease or one that developed during pregnancy, which was not due to direct obstetric causes but was aggravated by the physiologic effects of pregnancy. These two categories were considered in analyzing the classification of maternal death. Other categories include late maternal death and pregnancy-related death. The former is the death of a woman from direct or indirect obstetric causes, more than 42 days but less than 1 year after the termination of pregnancy. The latter is the death of a woman during pregnancy or puerperium, regardless of the cause (ICD-10).

Following the methodology described by Laurenti (1988) based on a list of diagnoses associated with maternal death, death certificates and medical/necropsy records were reviewed, and interviews with the relatives of the deceased women (whose deaths were due to an obstetric complication with an unspecific diagnosis or those whose records showed no cause associated to pregnancy, delivery, or puerperium but the pregnant state was recorded) were carried out. The cases of death of women whose ages ranged between 9 and 50 years of age were selected. The Registry Office provided 57% of the death certificates and the Ministry of Health, 100%. Identification information of the deceased women, addresses, and death diagnoses were obtained from the case registry system at the State Ministry of Health. With this information, the domiciles of the deceased women, who resided in the different municipalities of the state of Yucatan, were located. When evidence of pregnancy or puerperium at the time of death was recorded in the death certificate or when the main cause of death corresponded to an obstetric complication, according to causes O00–O95 as codified in the ICD-10, the case was considered as probable maternal death. Once these cases were selected, the information on the obstetric history of the deceased woman, her condition of being pregnant or in puerperium at the time of death, and the circumstances and clinical characteristics involved in her death were compiled. Information was collected by means of semi-structured interviews carried out with the deceased women's relatives (mothers, mothers-in-law, sisters) who were well acquainted with the circumstances of the death and the events occurred during the journey for care of the obstetric complication (verbal autopsy). Before interviewing the relatives, their informed consent was obtained, including the request to record the interviews. When the procedure triggered the relative's tears and sadness, psychological support to achieve resilience was available. When the relative spoke in the Mayan language, a translator was necessary, and the interview was transcribed in Spanish.

When the diagnosis was non-specific, the relatives were asked if the women had been pregnant within 1 year before dying. Thus, it was possible to relate the cause of death to the pregnancy. Information obtained from certificates, records, necropsies, and relatives was cross-checked, processed, and analyzed through descriptive statistical testing. To estimate the under-reporting of maternal mortality, the number of deaths found was compared to the deaths officially reported by the National Institute of Statistics, Geography, and Informatics (*Instituto Nacional de Estadística, Geografía e Informática*) (INEGI 2016) during the period studied. The following variables related to the cases of maternal deaths were analyzed: age at the time of death, place of residence, place of death, main cause of death, and classification of obstetric death. Finally, the percentage of under-reporting corresponding to each study was estimated.

15.3 Studies on the Under-Reporting of Maternal Deaths

15.3.1 First Study of Under-Reporting

During the period between 1997 and 2001, a 19% under-reporting of maternal deaths was found in the state of Yucatan, i.e., there were only 98 deaths reported in the official records, while in reality there had actually been 121. Women had died in 51 municipalities in the state, and not in 37, as it had been reported (Fig. 15.1). Under-reporting was higher in very marginalized areas, where the magnitude of

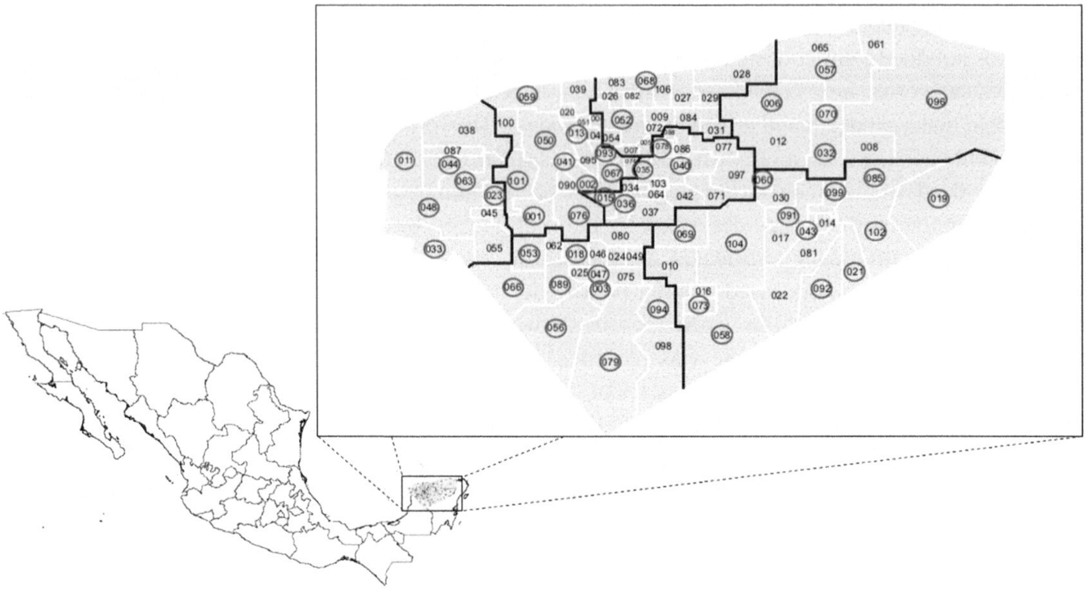

Fig. 15.1 Municipalities with maternal mortality in the state of Yucatan

underestimation of maternal deaths ranged between 50% and 100%. The main causes of under-reporting were mistakes regarding the interpretation of the clinical diagnosis, omission when codifying, and by not taking into account the pregnant condition of the woman recorded in the death certificate. The main regions with under-reporting were Merida, the state capital, 26 eastern municipalities, as well as Tizimin and Chemax.

15.3.2 Second Study of Under-Reporting

In the period between 1997 and 2001, there were 26 cases of maternal death in Merida. Five of these were late maternal deaths, which should not be included in the calculation of the MMR. Out of the 21 (81%) taken into account for the calculation, 16 were officially reported, and five corresponded to cases of under-reporting. The MMR was 0.2 per 1000 children born alive (BA). Furthermore, four (15%) were pregnancy-related deaths, and one (4%) was a case of late maternal death. The mean age of the decedents was 28 years, in a range between 19 and 38. Out of the 21 maternal deaths, 20 (95%) took place in a hospital and one (5%) at home. Seventeen (81%) of the maternal deaths occurred during puerperium and four (19%) during pregnancy. The main causes of maternal death in the cases of under-reporting were septic shock, puerperal fever, choriocarcinoma (a malignant tumor of the placental trophoblast), multiple organ failure, and pulmonary thromboembolism. Nineteen (90.5%) women died from direct obstetric causes based upon criteria according to the IDC-10. Regarding the pregnancy-related deaths, two (50.0%) were suicides (asphyxia by hanging) in women who were 20 and 24 years old. Official data had reported 16 maternal deaths in Merida during the period studied, and we identified five additional cases. The years with under-reporting of maternal deaths were 1997, 1998, and 2000, with 14%, 50%, and 75%, respectively. Twenty-four percent, or almost one quarter, of maternal deaths went under-reporting during the 5 years analyzed in the Merida municipality.

15.3.3 Third Study of Under-Reporting

In our investigation of maternal death under-reporting occurring in nine communities of eastern Yucatan during the same period of study, 757 death certificates and 1316 death certificates were reviewed. Of all the certificates, 543 (41.3%) corresponded to women, and among these, 99 (18.2%) were between 9 and 50 years of age. Twenty-one cases (21.2%) of maternal deaths were identified, six (28.6%) of which had not been reported. The years with highest under-reporting were 1998 and 1999, with 40% and 50% of deaths missed, respectively. The highest MMR was 14 deaths per 1000 children BA in the year 2000. The percentage of under-reporting made the total MMR increase to 3.1 more women dead per every 1000 children BA. Most of the maternal deaths corresponded to women between 20 and 29 years of age (47.6%), followed by women between 35 and 44 years of age (33.3%). The most frequent cause of death was hemorrhage, occurring in five (23.8%) cases.

15.3.4 Fourth Study of Under-Reporting

In another under-reporting study which we conducted in 15 municipalities in the eastern region of the state, a comparison between the deaths occurring during two periods (1997–2001 and 2002–210) was carried out. Thirty-two maternal deaths took place in each period, in 7 and 14 municipalities, respectively. During the first period, no under-reporting was found, but during the second period, one case, corresponding to a maternal death in the Valladolid municipality, was found. The MMR of the two time periods studied were compared, and the highest were recorded in the smallest municipalities, like Uayma (12 per 1000 children BA), Quintana Roo (37 per 1000 children BA), and Sucila (11 per 1000 children BA). When studying the trend in the two municipalities with the highest number of maternal deaths (Valladolid and Chemax), with 14 and 9 deaths, respectively, a decrease in the number of maternal deaths was observed. However, regarding the Valladolid municipality, there was a trend toward increased deaths starting in the year 2010. When comparing the number of deaths between four groups of maternal deaths (1997–2001 vs. 2002–2006 and 1997–2001 vs. 2007–2010), significant differences were found between both comparisons ($p = 0.049$ and $p = 0.0002$, respectively) (Table 15.1).

The leading cause of maternal death in the 1997–2001 period was obstetric hemorrhage and, in the 2002–2010 period, eclampsia. Deaths due to puerperal sepsis were reported only in the first period. Regarding the locations where the deaths occurred, it was observed that the highest number took place during transfer between the women's community and the hospital where they were treated ($p = 0.035$) (Table 15.2).

15.3.5 Fifth Study of Under-Reporting

The study was conducted in the Tizimin municipality, where death certificates from 1997 to 2008 were reviewed, and 31 were selected as probable maternal deaths. After carrying out the interviews (verbal autopsies) with the relatives, 19 cases of maternal death were confirmed, out of which two

Table 15.1 Comparison of maternal mortality according to time periods

Periods	Number of deaths	X^2	p
1997–2001 vs. 2002–2006	32 vs. 21	3.85	0.049
1997–2001 vs. 2007–2010	32 vs. 12	13.74	0.0002

Table 15.2 Location of demise for the maternal death cases in the municipalities of eastern Yucatan

	1997–2001		2002–2010		X^2	
Location of demise	Cases	Percentage	Cases	Percentage		*p*
Hospital with ICU*	13	40.6	5	22.5	1.88	0.17
Hospital without ICU	7	21.9	2	9.1	0.75	0.385
Transfer	2	6.3	7	31.8	4.43	0.035
Home	5	15.6	6	27.6	0.49	0.483

*Intensive care unit

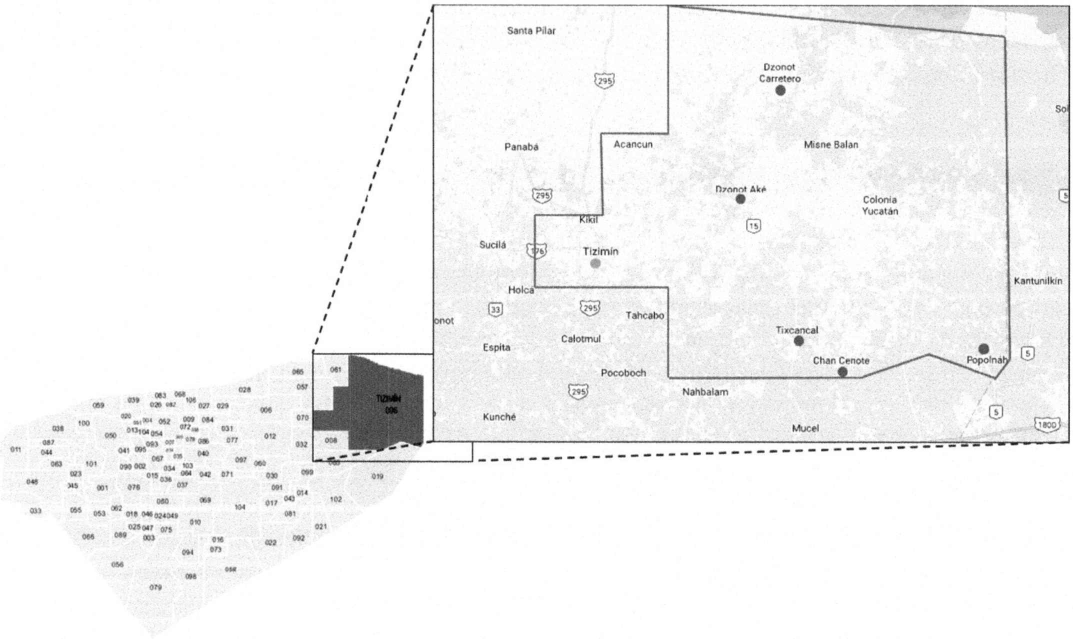

Fig. 15.2 Communities of the Tizimin municipality with maternal death under-reporting

(one from 1997 and one from 1998) had not been recognized or reported. During the 12 years analyzed, a 10.5% under-reporting was found. Two decedents who we classified as late maternal deaths and two pregnancy-related deaths were also identified. The annual MMR had a decreasing trend starting in 2002, which was the year with the highest number of deaths, with 5.4 maternal deaths per 1000 children BA. The main causes of death were hemorrhage in nine (47.4%) cases and hypertensive disorders in six (31.6%). In four (21%) cases of deaths, evidence of pregnancy, delivery, or puerperium at the time of death was recorded, and they were classified as "other causes" since the basic cause of death was not codified by the ICD-10. Out of the total maternal deaths, 15 (78.9%) were classified as direct obstetric maternal deaths and four (21%) as indirect obstetric maternal deaths. The deceased women were from five far-distant communities away from the municipal seat, where emergency services to treat obstetrical complications were not available (Fig. 15.2). Among the 19 confirmed maternal deaths, 12 (63.2%) took place in social assistance institutions, 5 (26.3%) at the deceased women's home, and 2 (10.5%) in private clinics. Underlying diseases (HIV/condylomatosis, cirrhosis, arterial hypertension, and diverticular disease) were found in four (21.1%) of the deceased women. Most deaths took place during puerperium (84.2%), two (10.5%) occurred during pregnancy, one (5.3%) took place during delivery, and six (31.6%) infants died together with their mother.

Table 15.3 Main results of the studies of under-reporting of maternal deaths in the state of Yucatan, Mexico

Region studied	Number of communities	Period	Under-reporting (%)	Maternal death diagnoses	Causes of under-reporting
State of Yucatan	51	1997–2001	19%	–	Misinterpretation of the clinical diagnosis and omission when codifying
Merida	1	1997–2001	24%	Septic shock, puerperal fever, choriocarcinoma, organic failure, pulmonary thromboembolism	
Eastern region	9	1997–2001	28.6%	Acute renal impairment, anemia, wasting syndrome, liver cancer, fulminant liver failure	Basic cause undefined and omission when codifying
Eastern region	15	2002–2010	3%	Suicide	Omission of evidence of pregnancy when codifying
Tizimin	1	1997–2008	10.5%	Hypovolemic shock, hypertensive crisis	Omission of evidence of pregnancy and puerperium when codifying
Chemax	1	1997–2001	22%	Arteriovenous malformations, left hemisphere frontoparietal aneurysm	Incorrect completion of the certificates due to a misreporting of the sequence of events that led to death

15.3.6 Sixth Study of Under-Reporting

This study was carried out in Chemax, a Mayan community considered to be highly marginalized and very deeply rooted in its indigenous cultural traditions, where the population speaks the Mayan language. Nine maternal deaths were found there for the 1997–2001 quinquennium, of which two (22%) had not been officially recognized or reported. The total number of maternal deaths in this community corresponded to 9.2% of the deaths reported in the whole state of Yucatan during that period, and the decedents were distributed equally between the two age groups of 20–24 and 35–39 years. Seven (77.7%) deaths were classified as direct obstetric deaths, and two (22.2%) were indirect. Eight (88.8%) deaths took place during puerperium and one (11.1%) during pregnancy. Four (44.4%) deaths occurred in a tertiary care hospital, and two (22.2%) occurred in a secondary care hospital. Two (22.2%) maternal deaths occurred during transfer, and one (11.1%) while at home. The estimated time between the onset of the complication, the search for medical care, and the actual care was prolonged in the cases of eclampsia (5 h). In the two cases of under-reporting, the time was 4 h for arteriovenous malformations and unknown for the case of left hemisphere aneurysm. Under-reporting was due to the incorrect completion of the death certificates, since the report of the sequence of events that led to death was incorrect, and as a result, the main cause of death was missed.

Table 15.3 summarizes the percentages of maternal death under-reporting, the municipalities where the six studies were carried out, the diagnoses recorded in the death certificates, and the main causes of under-reporting.

15.4 Discussion and Conclusions

The under-reporting of maternal death in the state of Yucatan remains a problem that requires attention, as is evidenced in the six studies discussed in this chapter. Although under-reporting was mainly observed in the 1997–2001 period, which was followed by a trend toward a decrease in the cases of death, it cannot be asserted with certainty yet that the notification surveillance system is working under optimal conditions. The last study included results up to the year 2010, and from that time on, no new studies have been undertaken to discover whether under-reporting of maternal deaths is still occurring.

The magnitude of under-reporting identified in the six studies conducted in Yucatan varied according to the size of the locality. For example, in urban areas like Merida, the rate of under-reporting was lower (24%) in comparison with smaller communities where the phenomenon was occurring in between 50% and 100% of cases. Under-reporting in Latin America and the Caribbean was 10.1% in 2011 (PAHO-WHO 2013). However, there are significant variations between countries, such as the case of Argentina, which has declared an under-reporting level of 9.5% for maternal deaths (CEDES 2004), lower than the one found in our study. Brazil declared a 30% under-reporting (Simoes and Almeida 2011), whereas Bolivia and Haiti reached under-reporting levels of up to 50% (CEPAL 2010), similar to the rates that we found in rural Yucatan.

Even though Latin-American countries have made an effort to improve the maternal death registration system, there is still much work to be done in order for the number of deaths reported to coincide with reality. In other words, there are still lags in the information systems that prevent optimal results regarding the cases of maternal death. International organisms like the UN Maternal Mortality Estimation Interagency Group (MMEIG) and the Institute for Health Metrics and Evaluation (IHME) have created complex calculation models of the MMR based on estimations; however, they have to be taken with caution since they are built on assumptions (Family Care International 2012). Making the estimates of the MMR is difficult when death registers are few because the value per 100,000 children BA cannot be used since the results would include decimals that would hinder interpretation. This was the case of our studies, where we used the constant per 100,000 BA to derive integers. This has made it difficult to contrast our results with other countries' MMR, but it allowed us to identify the areas at higher risk of maternal death in the state (Rodríguez and Ordóñez 2006). Deaths caused by maternal hemorrhage prevailed in the first 5 years studied, in accordance with what has been reported by other authors as the characteristic cause of maternal death in marginalized communities (Islam and Yoshida 2009). However, in the following decade, the hypertensive diseases of pregnancy—preeclampsia-eclampsia—were the major etiology. These conditions can be detected during prenatal consultations through a series of alarm signs, and adequate treatment can be of potential in preventing preeclampsia from progressing (SEGOB 2016). A community intervention designed to improve awareness of the signs of alarm was tested in a Mayan locality. The intervention involved an interdisciplinary team with specialists in medical and social anthropology, public health, psychology, education, and nursing, as well as the participation of health aids from the community who served as Mayan translators. The experience was successful because there was significant progress in the recognition of the signs and symptoms of preeclampsia-eclampsia and hemorrhage by the Mayan women who participated (Rodríguez et al. 2012a). Although cases of puerperal sepsis were the second leading cause of death during the first years studied, there could have been an under-reporting of cases of death by infection, resulting from the increase of such invasive bacteria such as group A Streptococcus (GAS) to the antibiotic resistance, to the rise of cesarean sections, and to the prevalence of obesity among women, as has been reported in the United Kingdom and the Netherlands, which have experienced an increase in maternal deaths due to these causes (Acosta and Knight 2013). In Yucatan, maternal mortality committees have been created in hospitals to address serious cases of obstetrical complications. The Committee analyse the situation in cases of death and determine the medical procedures that had been attempted to treat the complication. When the information on the circumstances surrounding the death is not clear, the deceased women's relatives are interviewed (verbal autopsy) in jurisdictional areas where health information from certain number of municipalities is centralized. After the case has been analyzed at a hospital level, the State Interinstitutional Committee, made up by representatives from the health sector, meet, and the case is presented and analyzed again, and strategies to prevent further deaths are discussed and agreed upon. However, even though this is a well-intended attempt to prevent maternal deaths from occurring, we do not know if there has been a systematic follow-up of the proposed strategies to see if they are implemented. Moreover, it is essential to have permanent surveillance systems of the sociocultural, political, and structural causes involved in the process of providing care for pregnant women with serious complications, since these aspects can result in formidable barriers that delay response to obstetrical emergencies and can ultimately lead to death (Rodríguez et al. 2012b; Rodríguez et al. 2014). Delays in providing care for an obstetrical complication have also been reported due to the difficulty for the pregnant women and her relatives to reach a hospital given the long distances they must travel to reach a hospital with an ICU, indispensable to address emergencies (Rodríguez et al. 2009). This difficulty, representing the second delay of the three delays model of maternal mortality, accounted for some of the cases of maternal death during the study on under-reporting conducted in the eastern municipalities of Yucatan.

After the occurrence of a maternal death in Yucatan, the sequence that the information must follow can delay the updating of the data on the number of cases. This in turn can impact the results when trying to determine the number of deaths occurring at any given moment. When a maternal death takes place, whether it occurs in the home, at the hospital, or elsewhere in the locality, it has to be notified to the next level of information (Sanitary Jurisdiction) within 24 h so it can be reported to the state-level agency (Yucatan State Health Services). The state-level agency reports it to the Health Ministry in Mexico City (central level), where the information from the death certificate, the verbal autopsy, and the rulings of the hospital and interinstitutional mortality committees is analyzed. In other words, at the central level, the case is analyzed once again, and it is finally ruled as a maternal death or not. Then, those cases which are definitely certified as maternal deaths are officially reported to international instances.

The perception of the procedures that are undertaken to reduce maternal deaths has created a puzzling environment among the personnel at the hospitals and the health units regarding the notification process. This is due to attention being focused on the statistics and on fulfilling numerous requests for immediate information on the individual cases, but the personnel do not perceive the changes or improvements proposed by the committees to prevent maternal mortality (oral communication).

There are studies that document that hospital information systems are not monitored for the quality of the data. In other words, the death diagnoses from the certificates are captured digitally, but the quality of the report to confirm that the correct diagnosis was captured is not analyzed (Kihuba et al. 2014).

The major causes of under-reporting which we identified in this study using several search methods and including verbal autopsies, such as the mistakes in the diagnoses stated in the death certificates, have also been reported in Los Altos de Chiapas, Mexico. In this region, 8.4% of maternal deaths were not reported in the year 2001 (Freyermuth-Enciso and Cárdenas-Elizalde 2009).

The delay in submitting forensic reports of maternal deaths has been identified as a cause of under-reporting in other countries, along with the misclassification of the diagnostic reports (McCaw-Binns et al. 2015). The second phenomenon was also identified in our studies. Hence, the importance of training personnel on the correct causes of death and how to report them on the certificates, so they are able to recognize both the diagnoses and the coding details of maternal deaths.

The risk associated with the age of the pregnant woman has always been considered an important factor for maternal mortality. However, there are limitations in asserting that maternal mortality increases in adolescent pregnancies. This can be seen from the results of a study in 144 countries, which showed lower mortality rates in this age group, compared with women older than 30 years (Nove et al. 2014). Greater attention to the study of this risk factor will have to be implemented in the future, as the number of adolescent pregnancies is increasing worldwide. Even though the impact of this condition on human development during adolescence is well known, in Yucatan the magnitude of the risk associated to this age group remains unknown.

It will be particularly important to delve into the under-reporting of violence-related maternal deaths (a component of obstetric violence), since the studies carried out in the eastern region of the state have reported that pregnant women were physically abused by their husbands leading to miscarriages (Rodríguez et al. 2012c). In municipalities such as Chicxulub Puerto and Tahdziú, depression-related violence and low-weight newborns have been found (Oliva et al. 2016). This evidence should alert us to intensify surveillance for cases of pregnant women with emotional disorders such as untreated depression, which can culminate in suicide. Codifying these causes as direct obstetric deaths will allow us to capture those under-reported deaths resulting from maternal suicide. This will have a significant impact in the future when calculating the MMR, and they will be considered when implementing mortality prevention strategies (Knight et al. 2016).

Organizing a highly functional and effective maternal death surveillance system in Yucatan will be a challenge for the health system in the coming years. The effective training of individuals responsible for coding of obstetrical diagnoses will be a challenge to achieve.

It will also be necessary to train health personnel, consisting mostly of registered medical practitioners and those who are fulfilling their social service in different communities throughout the state, as they are the health professionals that recognize and certify the cause(s) of death of women, be it at home, during transfer, or at the hospital.

References

Acosta, C. D., & Knight, M. (2013). Sepsis and maternal mortality. *Current Opinions in Obstetric & Gynecology, 25*, 109–116. https://doi.org/10.1097/GCO.0b013e32835e082

CEDES Centro de Estudios de Estado y Sociedad. (2004). *Mortalidad materna en Argentina. Diagnóstico para la reorientación de políticas y programas de salud.* Área Salud, Economía y Sociedad. Retrieved October 4, 2016, from http://www.fasgo.org.ar/archivos/ComSexRep/CEDES.pdf.

CEPAL Comisión Económica para América Latina. (2010). *Reporte de avance en el ODM5 en América Latina y el Caribe. Mejorar la salud materna.* Retrieved September 20, 2016, from http://www.cepal.org/MDG/noticias/paginas/2/40012/ODM_5.pdf.

Curtis, S. L., Mswia, M. G., & Weaver, E. H. (2015). Measuring maternal mortality: Three case studies using verbal autopsy with different platforms. *PLoS One, 10*(8), e0135062. http://journals.plos.org/plosone/article?id=10.1371/journal.pone.0135062

FCI Family Care International. (2012). *Estimaciones de la mortalidad materna en América Latina y el Caribe: Un breve panorama.* Retrieved September 8, 2016, from http://www.familycareintl.org/UserFiles/File/GTR_SP.pdf.

Farquhar, C., Armstrong, S., Kimm, B., Mason, V., & Sadler, L. (2015). Under-reporting of maternal and perinatal adverse events in New Zealand. *British Medical Journal Open, 5*(7), e007970. https://doi.org/10.1136/bmjopen-2015-007970

Freyermuth-Enciso, G., & Cárdenas-Elizalde, R. (2009). Evaluación del subregistro de la mortalidad materna en Los Altos de Chiapas, mediante las estrategias RAMOS y RAMOS modificada. *Salud Publica de Mexico, 51*(6), 450–457.

INEGI Instituto Nacional de Estadística Geografía e Informática México. (2016). *Estratificador INEGI.* Retrieved October 11, 2016, from http://www.inegi.org.mx/est/contenidos/proyectos/estratificador/.

INEGI Instituto Nacional de Estadística Geografía e Informática México. (2015). Información por entidad. Número de habitantes. Retrieved October 12, 2016, from http://www.cuentame.inegi.org.mx/monografias/informacion/yuc/poblacion/default.aspx?tema=me&e=31.

Islam, M., & Yoshida, S. (2009). Women are still deprived of access to lifesaving essentials and emergency obstetric care. *International Journal of Gynaecology and Obstetrics, 106*(2), 120–124.

Karimian-Teherani, D., Haidinger, G., Waldhoer, T., Beck, A., & Vutuc, C. (2002). Under-reporting of direct and indirect obstetrical deaths in Austria. 1980-98. *Acta Obstetricia et Gynecologica Scandinavica, 81*(4), 323–327.

Kihuba, E., Gahara, D., Mwinga, S., Kospei, R., Mogoa, W., Nyamai, R., et al. (2014). Assessing the ability of health information systems in hospitals to support evidence-informed decisions in Kenya. *Global Health Action, 7*, 24859. https://doi.org/10.3402/gha.V7.24859. eCollection 2014.

Knight, M., Manisha, N., Brocklehurst, P., Kenyon, S., Neilson, J., Shakespeare, J., et al. (2016). Examining the impact of introducing ICD-MM on observed trends in maternal mortality rates in the UK 2003-13. *BioMed Central Pregnancy and Childbirth, 16*, 178–185. https://doi.org/10.1186/s12884-016-0959-z

Laurenti, R. (1988). Marcos referenciais para estudos e investigacoes em mortalidade materna. *Revista de Saúde Pública, 22*(6), 507–512.

Lewis, G. (2003). Beyond the numbers: Reviewing maternal deaths and complications to make pregnancy safer. *British Medical Bulletin, 67*, 27–37.

Lewis, G. (2008). Reviewing maternal deaths to make pregnancy safe. *Best Practice & Research. Clinical Obstetrics & Gynaecology, 22*, 447–463. https://doi.org/10.1016/j.bpobgyn.2007.10.007

McCaw-Binns, A. M., Mullings, J. A., & Holder, Y. (2015). Vital registration and under-reporting of maternal mortality in Jamaica. *International Journal of Gynaecology and Obstetrics, 128*, 62–67. https://doi.org/10.1016/j.ijgo.2014.07.023

Nove, A., Mathews, Z., Neal, S., & Camacho, A. V. (2014). Maternal mortality in adolescent compared with women of other ages: Evidence from 144 countries. *Lancet Global Health, 2*(3), e155–e164. https://doi.org/10.1016/S2214-109X(13)70179-7

Oliva, P., Santana, A., Andueza, G., Hoil, J., Ojeda, R., García, G., et al. (2016). Risk factors associated with domestic violence and homicidal violence of women: The case of Yucatan, Mexico. *Psychology, 7*, 62–73. https://doi.org/10.4236/psych.2016.71008

PAHO (Panamerican Health Organization). (1995). *Clasificación estadística internacional de enfermedades y problemas relacionados con la salud, 10ª revisión*. Retrieved August 9, 2016, from http://www.sssalud.gov.ar/hospitales/archivos/cie_10_revi.pdf.

PAHO-WHO Panamerican Health Organization-World Health Organization. (2013). *Indicadores Básicos 2013. Indicadores demográficos*. Retrieved September 12, 2016, from http://www.paho.org/per/images/stories/D y E/1B2013.pdf.

Rodríguez, E. (2010). Epidemiología sociocultural de las defunciones maternas en Yucatán, México. In G. Rosado (Ed.), *Voces entretejidas* (pp. 275–292). México: Instituto para la Equidad de Género en Yucatán. Gobierno del Estado de Yucatán.

Rodríguez, E., Andueza, G., Montero, L., & Hoil, J. (2005). Subregistro de muertes maternas en Mérida, Yuc. México (1997-2001). *Ginecologia y Obstetricia de Mexico, 73*(7), 347–354.

Rodríguez, E., Andueza, G., Montero, L., & Hoil, J. (2009). Subregistro de muertes maternas en comunidades mayas del oriente de Yucatán, México. *Revista Biomedica, 20*(2), 90–98.

Rodríguez, E., Andueza, G., Rosado, L., Ortiz, E., & Hernández, B. (2012a). Effect of a community-based intervention to improve the knowledge on the warning signs of maternal complications among Mayan women from Yucatan randomized controlled trial. *Revista de Investigación Clínica, 64*(2), 154–163.

Rodríguez, E., Aguilar, P., Montero, L., Hoil, J., & Andueza, G. (2012b). Demoras en la atención de complicaciones maternas asociadas a fallecimientos en municipios del sur de Yucatán, Mexico. *Revista Biomedica, 23*(1), 23–32.

Rodríguez, E., Andueza, G., & Montero, L. (2012c). Un abordaje cualitativo de las defunciones maternas en Tizimín, Yucatán, México. *Alteridades, 22*(43), 145–158.

Rodríguez, E., Montero, L., Andueza, G., & Manrique, W. (2007). Características médico-sociales de las muertes maternas en una comunidad maya de Yucatán, Méx. *Ginecologia y Obstetricia de Mexico, 75*(2), 79–85.

Rodríguez, E., & Ordóñez, M. (2006). Mortalidad materna y marginalidad. *Revista Biomedica, 17*(4), 237–242.

Rodríguez, E., Palma, M., & Zapata, R. (2014). Causas de demora en la atención de pacientes con complicaciones obstétricas ¿qué es necesario atender? *Ginecología y Obstetricia de México, 82*, 647–658.

Schwartz, D. A. (2015a). Unsafe abortion: A persistent cause of maternal death and reproductive morbidity in resource-poor nations. In D. A. Schwartz (Ed.), *Maternal mortality: Risk factors, anthropological perspectives, prevalence in developing countries and preventive strategies for pregnancy-related death* (pp. 425–439). New York: Nova Science Publishers.

Schwartz, D. A. (2015b). The pathology of maternal death - the importance of accurate autopsy diagnosis for epidemiologic surveillance and prevention of maternal mortality in developing countries. In D. A. Schwartz (Ed.), *Maternal mortality: Risk factors, anthropological perspectives, prevalence in developing countries and preventive strategies for pregnancy-related death* (pp. 215–253). New York: Nova Science Publishers.

Schwartz, D. A. (2015c). Interface of epidemiology, anthropology and health care in maternal death prevention in resource-poor nations. In D. A. Schwartz (Ed.), *Maternal mortality: Risk factors, anthropological perspectives, prevalence in developing countries and preventive strategies for pregnancy-related death* (pp. ix–xiv). New York: Nova Science Publishers.

SEGOB Secretaría de Gobernación México. (2016). *Norma Oficial Mexicana NOM-007-SSA2–2016, Para la atención de la mujer durante el embarazo, parto y puerperio y de la persona recién nacida*. Retrieved May 24, 2016, from https://drive.google.com/file/d/0B_Wsl17nCOpWNGtjd1dYSTZXYzQ/view.

Simoes, P. P., & Almeida, R. M. (2011). Geographic accessibility to obstetric care and maternal mortality in a large metropolitan area of Brazil. *International Journal of Gynaecology and Obstetrics, 12*, 25–29. https://doi.org/10.1016/j.ijgo.2010.07.031

Turner, L. A., Cyr, M., Kinch, R. A., Liston, M., Kramer, R. S., Fair, M., et al. (2002). Under-reporting of maternal mortality in Canada: A question of definition. *Chronic Disease in Canada, 23*(1), 22–30.

WHO. (2016). *Application of ICD-10 to deaths during pregnancy, childbirth and the puerperium; ICD-MM*. Retrieved September 12, 2016, from http://apps.who.int/Iris/bitstream/10665/70929/1/9789241548458_eng.pdf?ua=1.

WHO World Health Organization. (2004). *Beyond the numbers: reviewing maternal deaths and complications to make pregnancy safer*. Retrieved October 4, 2016, from http://apps.who.int/iris/bitstream/10665/42984/1/9241591838.pdf.

Contemporary Issues in the Training, Practice, and Implementation of Midwifery for Indigenous Women in Mexico

16

Jennifer Foster and Cristina Alonso

16.1 Introduction

In October 2013, Irma Lopez gave birth in a garden outside of a large hospital in the state of Oaxaca (Fig. 16.1). She had traveled from her village, as she had been strongly encouraged by health authorities to give birth properly in the hospital and avoid the dangers of an unsafe birth at home, attended by an untrained midwife. As her baby plopped on the grass, someone took a photograph and uploaded it to Facebook. The picture went viral, and within days the Mexican maternal health system was also in shock. Days later, a similar incident occurred in the state of Puebla, and sometime later, a woman in the state of Chiapas bled to death after a cesarean section (Grupo de Informacíón en Reproduccíón Elegida (GIRE) 2015). Days later, a similar incident occurred in the state of Puebla, and sometime later, a woman in the state of Chiapas bled to death after a cesarean section (GIRE 2015). These incidents had happened before, but what was new was the capacity of social networks to expose the realities of a health system that cannot adequately serve all of the women it aspires to serve.

These three tragic and preventable events opened a door to a raw examination on the part of nongovernmental organizations (NGOs) of a maternal health system that attends close to three million pregnancies a year (INEGI 2015) and is conceptualized within a dominant moral discourse that all women should deliver in facilities that provide at least basic obstetric care for reasons of safety in case of complications (UNFPA 2014a, b). The issue of distance and infrastructure is well understood as problematic within the health system, but given the variable topography of the country, it remains a challenge for women, in particular indigenous women, who live in areas distant from health centers where births are attended. Moreover, cultural preferences as a factor in deciding to seek care in a facility have not been valued.

J. Foster, Ph.D., C.N.M., M.P.H., F.A.C.N.M., N.A.A.N. (✉)
Nell Hodgson Woodruff School of Nursing,
Emory University, Atlanta, GA, USA
e-mail: Jennifer.foster@emory.edu

C. Alonso, M.P.H., C.P.M.
Project Director, Luna Maya Birth Center, Past President,
Mexican Midwifery Association, Mexico City, Mexico

D. A. Schwartz (ed.), *Maternal Death and Pregnancy-Related Morbidity Among Indigenous Women of Mexico and Central America*, Global Maternal and Child Health: Medical, Anthropological, and Public Health Perspectives, https://doi.org/10.1007/978-3-319-71538-4_16

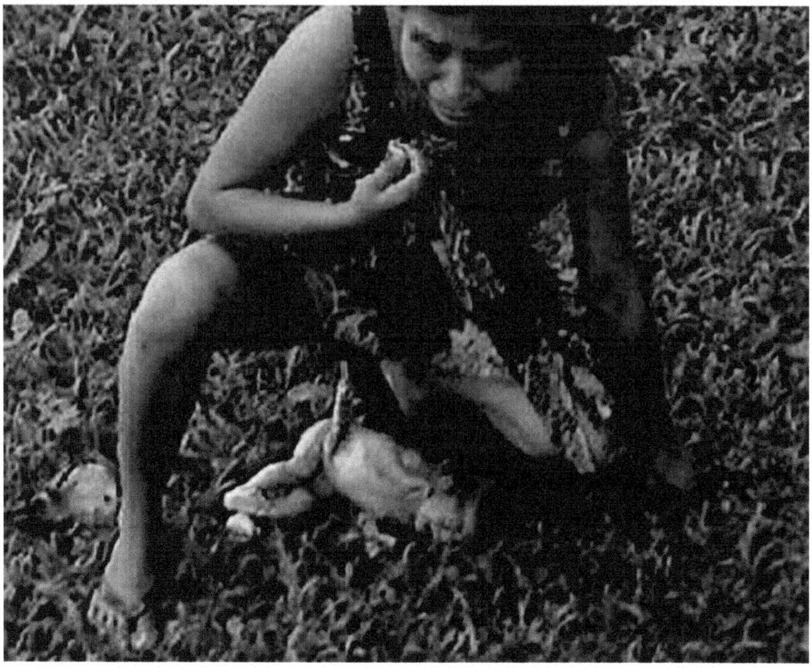

Fig. 16.1 Irma Lopez Aurelio giving birth by herself on a patch of grass across the hospital where she was refused care in Oaxaca. An indigenous Mazatec woman, she did not speak Spanish and was turned away from a rural health center by nurses who could not communicate with her (Photograph courtesy of Eloy Pacheco López, Oaxaca, Mexico)

On one hand, Mexico has constitutional protection for indigenous rights and culture, yet on the other hand, the current maternity health system is primarily based on biomedical values that prioritize intervention on the body, as well as institutional system efficiencies. These priorities are widely divergent from the historical knowledge system of the indigenous peoples in Mexico and Central America. The biomedical system is based on a cosmology of the material body with discrete borders, a space where the skin encases the whole, which is only one aspect of what the body signifies. Since pre-Hispanic contact, the midwife has served as spiritual servant of the Divine (Marcos 2006). This tradition continues, especially in rural Mexico. Mesoamerican indigenous women have a long tradition of home birth attended by community midwives (*parteras*), where birth is not only a physical but also a spiritual and family event.

Midwifery care in Mexico is currently not understood to be a profession, nor is there acceptance of the midwifery model of care as a desirable norm for most women. The midwifery model of care, as outlined by the International Confederation of Midwives, recognizes pregnancy and childbearing as usually physiological processes, which require care that is holistic and continuous, respects ethnic and cultural diversity, and takes place in partnership with women (International Confederation of Midwives 2014).

There are multiple obstacles that preclude midwifery care as an option within maternal health services in Mexico. While there has been a commitment to integrated medicine in the public sector, such as the Intercultural Hospital in San Cristobal de Las Casas, and recently "humanized birth" areas in maternity hospitals in Tula, Hidalgo, and Tlaxcala, there are different and conflicting opinions and visions how to achieve "integrated medicine," which includes midwifery care. The controversy about midwifery continues, even though on a global level, there is an increasingly common understanding that well-trained and supported midwives contribute to reducing maternal and newborn mortality and morbidity, as well as providing satisfying care (Renfrew et al. 2014).

Midwifery has been identified by international experts, including the United Nations Fund for Population Assistance (UNFPA), as the crucial link for decreasing maternal mortality and morbidity (UNFPA 2014a). In 2008, the UNFPA and ICM published a report, *Investing in Midwives and Others with Midwifery Skills*, that stated: "Quality midwifery care, provided close to where women live, can increase families' capacity to self-care during pregnancy, as well as before, during and after childbirth; it can also increase access to Emergency Obstetric Care (EmOC) care by educating and empowering women and their communities. Despite repeated evidence that midwifery care at the community level is inadequate and lacks competent providers with the requisite collaborative support, country plans often fail to address the need." (International Confederation of Midwives 2008).

When midwives are integrated within the health-care system, women's pregnancy outcomes improve (UNFPA 2014b). This chapter examines the current state of maternal health and professional and traditional midwifery in Mexico and its effect on health outcomes for women and its interface with publicly funded care. We initially review the state of maternal health in Mexico. Next, we explore the cultural worldview of Mesoamerican birth ways, which remains an important influence among the various indigenous groups in contemporary Mexico.

Using the state of Puebla as an exemplar, we show how that worldview is beginning to be acknowledged within one state but still exists on the margins of acceptability for obstetric providers. The results for women like Irma Lopez, who traveled to the tertiary hospital, was turned away, and then delivered outside of the hospital on the grass, invoke claims of "obstetric violence" by human rights activists (D'Gregorio 2010).

We argue that professional midwifery is the bridge between the two worlds of contemporary Western biomedical obstetric care with its evidence base in addressing the physical complications of pregnancy and childbearing *and* the more spiritual and holistically driven orientation of indigenous traditional midwifery. We articulate a vision for the way a midwifery model of care could be implemented in Mexico. It is our hope Mexico will choose to build this bridge in a large and systematic way. We believe it is necessary for the reduction of maternal and newborn mortality among the indigenous women who bear this disproportionate burden.

16.2 Current Status of Maternal Health in Mexico

The current care available to pregnant women in various parts of the public sector in Mexico is inadequate, both from a quantitative perspective in terms of mortality, morbidity, and cesarean section rates and in the quality of care. Mexico sustains an inacceptable maternal mortality ratio (MMR) for its economy nationally (38.9 per 100,000 live births), and did not achieve the Millennium Development Goal (MDG) set by the United Nations in this category (Observatorio de Mortalidad Materna en México, 2014). While Mexico has shown concerted effort and significant progress in decreasing maternal mortality nationally, there remain significant pockets of disparity in which indigenous families are overrepresented. Sixty percent of the indigenous populations are located within the lowest income quintile in Mexico. Maternal mortality is 3 times higher among indigenous populations, and infant mortality is 1.7 times higher, in comparison to other populations in the country (Duarte-Gomez et al. 2015).

Nevertheless, a strong and growing movement from within and outside of the government in support of the professionalization of midwifery and its integration into the health sector recognizes the need to create trained and qualified midwives and provide health care that is centered on women's values and choices, particularly given the widespread and varied cultural diversity that constitutes Mexico. The Ministry of Health recognizes the need to integrate multicultural solutions to a multicultural nation. In 2013, the Ministry of Health published the *Program for Specific Action: Maternal and Peri Natal Health 2013–2018* (Secretaría de Salud 2013). The strategy recommended the hiring of nonmedical providers, such as professionally trained midwives, obstetric nurses, and perinatal nurses for prenatal and birth care. In order to achieve this, the hiring code that recognizes obstetric nurses (*enfermeras obstetricas*) was reinstated in 2008 and in 2011, and a hiring code was also adopted that recognizes professional midwives. In 2016, the Norm 007 that regulates the care of women during pregnancy, birth, and postpartum was reviewed; it recognized obstetric nurses and professional midwives as qualified providers, as well as their need to provide training to traditional midwives.

This was an important step. In a country with a population of approximately 121 million persons, however, a total of 23 professionally educated midwives have been hired by the Mexican National Health System to provide care and train traditional midwives at the time of this writing. This contrasts with the 15,000 medical doctors graduating each year (Nigenda & Munoz 2015), many of whom attend the births in rural, publicly funded health centers without specialized training in obstetrics and gynecology.

Since the 1950s with the closing of midwifery schools in Mexico, women were encouraged to attend institutions for prenatal care and birth. With the introduction of the Seguro Popular in 2004, universal access to health care was supposed to phase out what officials felt were "antiquated" and dangerous home births with traditional midwives in indigenous villages. The concept was that women should attend a local health center for prenatal care and a secondary level hospital for birth. This strategy coincided with a shift in maternal health policy toward Emergency Management of Obstetric Emergencies (EMoC), the programmatic objectives of which focused on the premise that any birth could become an emergency at any given moment. Therefore, given that birth emergencies are unpredictable, it would be better that women give birth in institutions with blood banks, surgery suites, resuscitative equipment, and access to obstetricians and anesthesiologists.

The fundamentals of EMoC (as it was implemented in Mexico) include some assumptions that are not aligned with the midwifery model of care nor with the historic cultural practices of indigenous women. The midwifery model assumes that most women are essentially healthy, most pregnancies and births are physiological, and most women require a well-trained, well-supported midwife who is competent to attend a spontaneous vaginal birth as well as to identify and refer complications to a physician who can manage complications in a timely way. The midwives in indigenous communities cannot realistically practice within the midwifery model of care. Although most women birthed at home with midwives, the traditional midwives were often untrained, due to lack of educational opportunities in general for women and specifically a lack of access to quality midwifery education. They were also far from hospitals that could manage obstetric complications. Nevertheless, the Ministry of Health recognized that traditional midwives were often the only people available to attend women in childbirth in many areas, and they have organized trainings through the public system.

The Ministry of Health has registered 9000 traditional midwives in Mexico. Although some have received 3-day trainings (see below for more on training), none have received any formal midwifery education. In fact, many neither read nor write. It would make sense, therefore, that all women be referred to secondary levels of care, where they would be better attended by skilled personnel. This universal policy did not take into account the fact that hospitals in Mexico are by and large culturally completely foreign to indigenous women.

As a result, birth in Mexico has become a singularly medicalized event, conducted by medical professionals who consistently interpret all birth from a high-risk perspective. According to the INSP "National caesarean percentage increased in the last 10 years at an annual rate of 1%. It was considerably higher in social security institutions and the private sector. Caesareans percentages in 1999 were slightly above 35%" (Puentes-Rosas et al. 2004). The national cesarean section rate currently exceeds 45% (INEGI, 2015), and by 2013 mass media were already reporting rising cesarean rates and unacceptably low breastfeeding rates (Mendez 2017).

Results of studies conducted in public hospitals by the National Institute of Public Health in Mexico (INSP) show that the increased incidence of cesarean section deliveries is associated with nonclinical factors such as size of the hospital and the presence of a birth attendant. They recommend a model of support for women which includes information and counseling, and the presence of a birth attendant during labor can contribute to reducing the risk of unnecessary cesareans in populations such as that studied (Campero et al. 2007).

16.3 Indigenous Cosmology of Birth

Apart from select academics who study indigenous Mexican lifeways, the contemporary general public in Mexico had little public exposure to the spiritual underpinnings of indigenous culture until the First Indigenous Women's Summit of the Americas, a United Nations Meeting, which was held in December of 2002. Approximately 400 indigenous women leaders were in attendance from most countries in the world. Indigenous spirituality cuts across all discussions and was an element of every issue voiced (Marcos 2010).

The concept of the body is understood very differently by practitioners of contemporary biomedicine and traditional Mesoamerican indigenous healers. The worldview of Mesoamerican healers, which includes midwives, does not view the interior and exterior of the body separated by the barrier of the skin. Rather, the body is permeable and open to forces in the cosmos. The body can receive or dispel entities from the exterior. The soul in the *Nahuatl* language is *tonalli*, an aggregate of multiple, psychic entities that reside within the body. The principal location for the *tonalli* is the head; the *tonalli* travels at night during dreams, becoming independent of the body and interacting with the supernatural world. Soul loss is thus a common response to an unexpected event. When the event is negative, the result is *susto* or fright.

The liver is another location for the animated entities of the soul. The concept that there could be emanations from the liver that are harmful is the basis for the notion of "bad airs." The heart is also a dwelling place for the soul. The heart is the seat of memory, knowledge, reason, and intelligence. When the psychic entity, the *teyolia*, leaves the heart, death ensues.

Another core concept that serves as the basis for meaning and action in the Mesoamerican world is the concept of gender duality. Every element of the world is either masculine or feminine. The earth and the sky, the day and the night, sadness and happiness each complements the other; one cannot exist without the other. "God is a pair, a double, both mother and father, female and male," speaks a *Nahua* woman (Marcos 2006 p. 12). These gender categories are not fixed, binary, and hierarchical; rather, they reflect an open, shifting state, with variable valences of masculine and feminine, in religion and everyday life. Scholars of Mesoamerica have found this duality concept prevalent across the whole region (Marcos 2006). The modifier of these dualities is another core concept, which is equilibrium or balance. Balance is understood as a fundamental, primordial characteristic of the universe, and there is a collective understanding that humans have a moral code to participate in achieving it and then sustaining it. Attainment of this cosmic balance requires embodiment of interrelatedness with the world, as well as interconnection with all life.

Historically, midwives were "the great priestesses" of the indigenous world, encouraging women on their "first battlefield, the birth ceremony" (Marcos 2006). They used herbs and rituals and chants that gave the woman's body cosmic significance and encouraged her to align her body with all the forces that give life. Midwives empowered the women they attended, and still today indigenous women feel deeply connected to them. The indigenous women's movement openly confirms the prevalence of orally transmitted traditions over time, and their cosmic vision is very aligned with the global calls for dignity, respect, and justice.

It is of no surprise, then, that indigenous women are afraid of leaving their families, communities, and respected midwives, to travel to the hospital for birth, where they are treated, too often, as objects. Anecdotal reports, personal stories, and local gossip about women who went to the hospital in labor with a normal and healthy pregnancy and emerged with an unexpected and unwanted vertical cesarean scar, in shock, and with a baby unable to breastfeed are being shared among women who are increasingly disappointed by the care. The typical length of stay for a vaginal delivery is 8 hours or 24 hours for a cesarean delivery.

The dominant message indigenous women and midwives hear is the recommendations from the medical community—the message that homebirth is dangerous and midwives are unprepared. Traditional midwifery training calls for all primigravid women to be transferred to the hospital. Anecdotal evidence and testimony gathered by the Mexican Midwifery Association report that midwives in some areas are punished for attending births (AMP 2017).

In the contemporary global human rights discourse, the lack of options and repression of birth choices among indigenous women is spoken about as a violation of both basic human and reproductive rights, where women are forced to birth or undergo surgery in places or for reasons that they would not consent to, if they had another choice. Current discourse and literature disclose that women are often caught between too much care too soon and too little care too late (Miller et al. 2016). Indigenous women in Mexico are often trapped between too little care by family members or traditional midwives who have not been trained for several years or formally educated as midwives. When obstetrical complications occur, midwives may refer too late for medical intervention to be effective, and women may be attended in an overstressed hospital where staff are exhausted, beds are full, and the conditions for physiological birth are completely lacking. Thus, they often receive either too *much* care (a cesarean section without a proper medical indication) or too *little* care (they birth alone on a bed or in the hallway).

16.4 The Relation of the State to Traditional Midwifery in Puebla: An Exemplar

States within Mexico vary to the degree they have chosen to actively pursue training of traditional midwives. In Mexico, midwifery training is coordinated at a statewide level, a jurisdictional level, and at the primary care level. The Secretariat of Public Health (SSP) in the state of Puebla serves as one example which has elected to be active in training traditional midwives at the statewide level.

The population of Puebla state is approximately six million persons, of which approximately 18% are of indigenous origin. Indigenous persons are identified as speakers of *Náhuatl* (72.5%), or *Totonaca* (17.2%), or those who self-identify as indigenous (personal communication, Duarte, October 13, 2016). In 2015, there were 52,959 births in Puebla state, and 3332, or approximately 16%, were attended by indigenous midwives (Fig. 16.2).

The SSP defines the traditional midwife (termed *partera*) as a community person who is strictly linked with health, especially with respect to pregnancy, birth, and postpartum, and who obtained her knowledge from family and direct experience. They classify the traditional midwives, as active, and within active or inactive, midwives may be trained or untrained.

An active traditional midwife is a person recognized by her community as a midwife, whether or not she is trained, and who is linked with health services, incorporating practices of modern medicine with traditional medicine. For purposes of health programming, she is considered active when she has attended at least one birth in the last year, or she fulfills any activity related to reproductive health, such as care of pregnant women, postpartum, or newborns, or family planning.

A second category, termed trained midwives, are those women who have attended at least one course of training per year by the Ministry of Health, which allows her to practice standardized prenatal, birth, postpartum, and newborn care, focused on the detection of obstetric risk factors and timely transfer, along with general health promotion in accordance with established protocols. It is important to mention that the Ministry is not training *new* traditional midwives.

In 2014, there was an initiative to train 100% of traditional midwives in the state of Puebla in the integrated care of mother and newborn, before, during, and after birth. A total of 562 midwives received this training, covering 57.3% of active midwives. The training course took 3 days (8 hours per day).

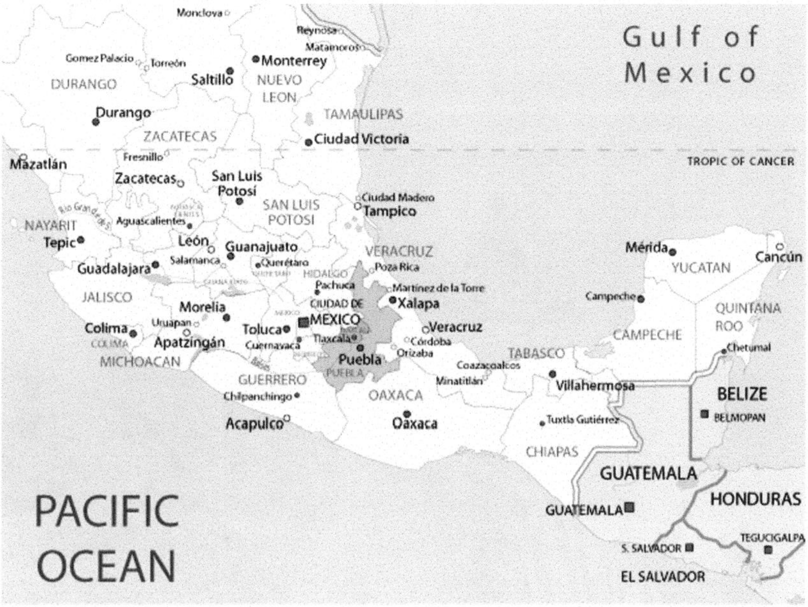

Fig. 16.2 Location of Puebla state in Mexico (Source: Maps of world. com http://jedu.tk/map-puebla-mexico/)

The training for midwives is conducted by the health center personnel linked to the midwife's geographic area, if possible, or by the regional jurisdiction, or the state department of reproductive health. The reason that health center personnel may not be available to do the training is because there are some centers or posts that do not have the necessary personnel, especially in the more rural regions of Puebla state. During 2015, some midwives did not attend any births, a result of few incentives and the predominant message that all births are supposed to happen in hospitals.

The most skilled and participatory active midwives are selected by trainers to become *accredited* (vs. simply trained). The process of accreditation verifies the midwife's knowledge, skills, and weakness by using *the Manual de la Partera Tradicional* (Secretaria de Salud 1992). Accreditation is voluntary. The Ministry identifies which midwives are most likely to succeed in the process of accreditation and invites them to pursue this level. Of the 946 midwives in the state, 563, or 57%, are accredited from the year 2014. Accreditation must be repeated every 2 years. There is a competency practice evaluation, performed on a one-to-one basis between the instructor nurse from the Puebla state SSP and the midwife student. The nurse trainer conducts these competency tests, usually 10 per day, in a central location near where the midwives live. The Ministry has records of which midwives are actively in practice, which are trained, and which provide documentation to the health centers.

The nurse trainer has described the necessary acculturation process for these midwives, who travel from afar to even come to be evaluated. They prefer to prepare their own meals and to stay in very simple lodging, such as cabins or cottages (Personal communication, Lic. Rosaura Cervantes Contreras, nurse trainer, Puebla SSP, February 16, 2016).

In addition to the training of traditional midwives, the public health system in Puebla includes 15 structures, or annexes, which are sites where traditional medicine practice takes place, adjoining the secondary level hospitals that offer allopathic medicine. These annexes host the practice of a total of 382 practitioners, including naturopathic physicians, bone setters, *curanderos* (shamans), and midwives that offer services there. A birthing room, a *temazcal* (steam room), herbal pharmacy, and a maternity waiting home are available. The birthing room was designed by the traditional medicine program at the Federal Secretariat of Health, and it has physical supports for women to give birth vertically or squatting (Fig. 16.3).

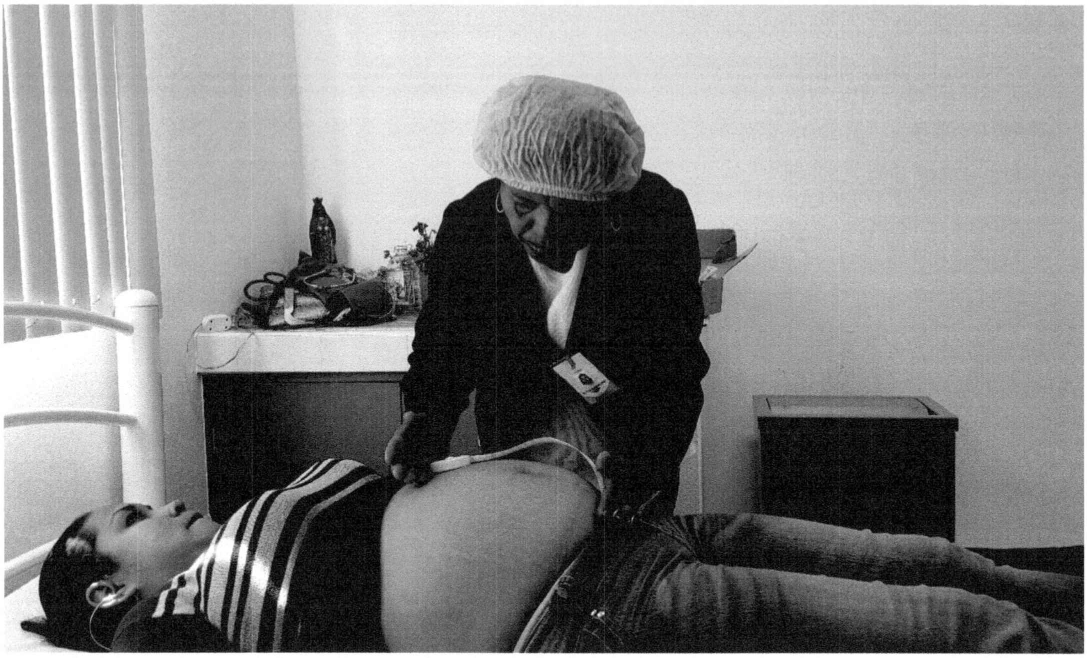

Fig. 16.3 Midwife from Puebla conducts prenatal visit in the integrated medicine annex, 2016 (Photograph by Jennifer Foster)

The maternity waiting home is a place that hosts pregnant women from rural areas to arrive before labor in order to avoid travel during labor in case of complications. Additionally, the role of "godmother," a traditional community role, is promoted by the program, "An Equal Start in Life," and about 25% of pregnant women in the state have them. The godmother is to serve as an advocate and emotional support to the pregnant woman.

A visit to the birth room in one of the traditional medicine annexes in a secondary hospital in Puebla state in February 2016 indicated these were vastly underutilized. Only two births had occurred in the birthing room in 9 months, although several women had begun labor there and transferred to the main hospital before delivery. To be permitted to give birth in the birth room in the traditional medicine annex with a midwife, every woman was required to see the obstetrician at least five times throughout their pregnancy. The reasons for the underutilization of the birth room are unknown but reflect the complex, multilayered, present reality of Mexico's traditional midwives in modern times. The next section explores the diversity of traditional midwifery practice in Mexico overall.

16.5 Traditional Midwifery Practice in Modern Times

Traditional midwifery practice is enormously diverse, and there is a large variation in the way midwives are inducted and trained, as well as variation in how they practice. Cultural norms vary among indigenous groups, and some traditional midwives have received training in the Mexican Institute for Social Security (IMSS) or the public health sector. These trainings are heavily oriented to medical procedures, such as using intravenous equipment and injecting oxytocin as a routine intervention. Some midwives have been practicing for over 40 years; some young midwives are trained by their mothers, grandmothers, or apprenticeship. Some are trained via nongovernmental organizations

(NGOs) through workshops. Midwives may work in extremely rural communities, where health services are nonexistent due to distance, superstition, or violence. There are midwives working in communities that are better connected to cities or health systems and receive government or NGO training. Other traditional midwives live in cities and have verbal collaborative agreements with obstetricians, are activists and have an active relationship with the health sector, may have created networks for humanizing childbirth with the support of medical personnel and local NGOs, and understand their role as midwives to be in the defense of human rights and sexual and reproductive health care.

There are some traditional midwives who are organized as local or statewide associations and have learned to work with other organizations, where they advocate for recognition and protection of their profession. Other midwives work in isolation, with no formal relationships to organizations or the established health sector, and are simply recognized by their community as the midwife.

Within all of this diversity, all self-identify as traditional midwives *(parteras)*, but not all believe they need to be or are recognized by the public health system. In workshops carried out by the Mexican Midwifery Association in four states with traditional midwives during 2016, some of the midwives expressed the belief that their gift was given by God and can only be inherited by lineage, and others also believe that training and continued education will help them be better midwives, contributing to the strengthening of midwifery and ensuring it does not disappear. Traditional midwifery is contextually defined: the existing inequities of Mexico clearly shape its practice.

There is a huge chasm between isolated and illiterate traditional midwives of the mountains of Guerrero and the dynamic midwives of Morelos who have Facebook and web pages and communicate via "WhatsApp," traveling the world giving "Rebozo" workshops. Location and class determine their opportunities and realities.

Since the inception of universal health care in Mexico (Seguro Popular), traditional midwives on average attend very few births, approximately one delivery each month. Women have been frightened away from homebirth, between claims that their lives are at risk and threats that they will lose social programs and preference for access to medicalized care. In many sites, traditional midwives are limited to the role of pregnancy massage and postpartum care.

It is rare that births are compensated, particularly in rural areas. Payment can be 200 pesos ($12 US) per birth. Due to this meager income, midwives attend to general family health and provide massage and fetal positioning for pregnant women, charging about 30 pesos a visit ($2 US). Midwives feel compelled to provide care even when families are unable to pay, and since the work is regarded as a Divine gift, generating income from their services is not culturally obligatory.

Traditional midwives face constant institutional abuse and violence, criminalization, and threats and are often denied birth certificates. When midwives request birth certificates, they are often bounced around between different government offices and the hospital, or a payment is requested, even though birth certificates are free and a constitutional right for all babies born in Mexico.

In some jurisdictions, midwives must be accompanied by the mother and her newborn to be a witness to the birth. This contradicts cultural norms that women must remain at home for the first 42 days after birth. In some situations, women are thoroughly checked to "make sure" they were actually pregnant. This may include "manual revision of the uterus," where the provider manually cleanses the internal walls of the uterus to check for lochia and placental remains, a procedure long ago abandoned by Western obstetrics and currently deemed dangerous by the World Health Organization (WHO 1999).

Midwives have been told that they will go to jail if they continue to provide planned homebirths but at the same time are told they will be criminalized if they refuse to care for a woman who shows up in labor with no prenatal care. Midwives are instructed to fill out the "Registry of Activities among Certified Traditional Midwives" with detailed information about each pregnant woman which they must submit each month to the government. These documents enable the local health center to keep track of who is pregnant and ensure that she goes to her local hospital for birth. If births do occur at

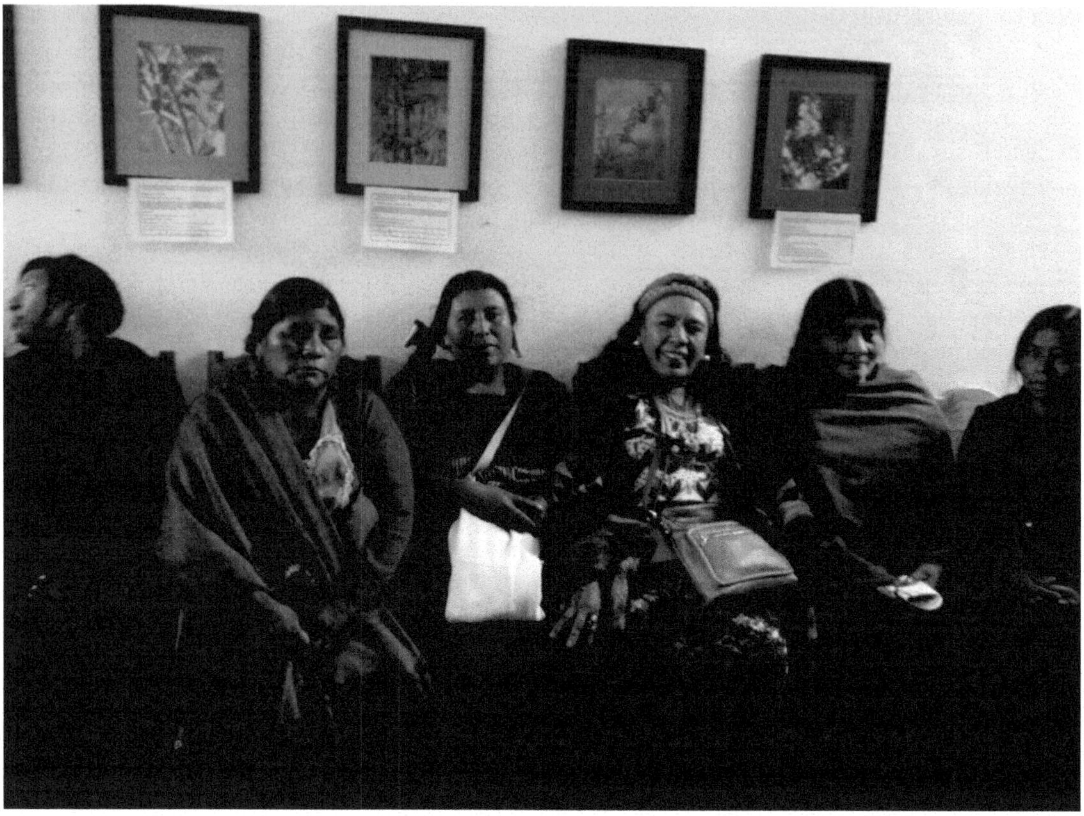

Fig. 16.4 Traditional midwives in Mexico (Photograph from the Mexican Midwifery Association) (AMP 2017)

home, midwives are often told to let the health center know as soon as the woman is in labor and check in regularly to make sure the birth does not "get complicated from taking too long." In their training sessions that discuss high-risk pregnancy and referral, first-time mothers, women under 18 and over 35, and single mothers are all generically categorized as too high risk to be attended by midwives.

When midwives attend a birth and transport a woman to the hospital because of complications, they report being scolded and mistreated by hospital staff and blamed for causing the complication. Women who arrive with the midwives become frightened when hospital personnel announce the medical staff will not be held accountable if the woman or the baby dies. Despite cultural and linguistic protection of indigenous groups that guarantees that women may be accompanied by a translator or traditional midwife during medical procedures, the experience of most of the traditional midwives is that they are not allowed into hospital to explain the situation or to advocate for their patient (Fig. 16.4).

16.6 The Mexican Midwifery Association

The Mexican Midwifery Association (Asociación Mexicana de Partería, or AMP) developed from a working group that included expert organizations and individuals in maternal health and midwifery. These groups were the Center for Adolescents of San Miguel de Allende (CASA), CIESAS (Center for Research and Education in Social Anthropology), CIMIGEN (a private hospital that employs obstetric nurses for birth in Mexico City), the Committee for Safe Motherhood, the National School for Nursing and Obstetrics (ENEO), Luna Maya Birth Center, the Midwives Alliance of North

America (MANA), Mujeres Aliadas, Nueves Lunas, Parto Libre as well as independent midwives, including some traditional midwives. Within this shifting political and social climate, the newly formed Mexican Midwifery Association seeks to position itself as the expert entity on national midwifery. The AMP's mission and vision reflect the multicultural reality of Mexican midwifery and Mexican birth, acknowledging that there is no simple or unilateral solution to solving maternal health problems in Mexico. However, having received support through the MacArthur and Kellogg Foundations to establish itself in 2012, the AMP seeks to increase membership to represent the diversity of midwives practicing in Mexico. AMP is also working to unify criteria as to the future of midwifery in Mexico, ensure basic standards for preservice education and continuing education, and act as representative for the midwifery model of care at public health and policy discussions and decisions.

Currently, there is no standardized regulation of the practice of midwifery across Mexico, and only obstetric and perinatal nurses, as well as graduates of the two recognized midwifery schools, can be hired within the health system. Traditional midwives are increasingly coerced to stop attending births. However, other than directing all women to secondary-level institutions for birth, which are often far from the homes of many indigenous women, the health system does not provide a feasible primary care alternative for many indigenous women, much less one that is culturally acceptable and available in their communities.

The mission of the AMP is to strengthen the profession of midwifery in Mexico as a model for sexual and reproductive health that promotes women's autonomy and rights, is sensitive to their needs, and trusts the wisdom of their bodies.

The AMP vision is to represent midwifery in Mexico, promote education and training of new midwives, and impact legislation and public policy. The AMP strives to create an independent organism that certifies and regulates the practice of midwifery. The position of the AMP was strengthened when, in June 2016, the AMP became an associate member of the International Confederation of Midwives, advancing its status as an organization within and outside of Mexico.

16.7 What Traditional Midwives Tell the Mexican Midwifery Association

During 2016, the AMP carried out six group discussions in four states with 10–30 traditional midwives in each group, with attendees coming from the states of Morelos, Guerrero, Chiapas and Michoacán, to gather information on their current status and needs. In general, the traditional midwives feel that they are being used by the government in official events, invited and paraded around, given gifts and told they are essential to primary health care, but then told not to continue their work as midwives. In every group, midwives expressed anger and exhaustion over being used as cultural icons in the political discourse but ignored or threatened in daily life. In some states, the government resources allocated for midwifery training programs are not spent, disappear, or are reassigned to other programs. The example, described previously about Puebla state, is an exception.

When midwifery schools open, traditional midwives are often told they will have special privileges to attend educational programs or will be hired as teachers. However, in practice, lack of formal education makes it impossible for traditional midwives to register as students and to be hired as midwives. De facto, midwifery education programs do not have traditional midwives as teachers and mentors.

Despite their exclusion from formal education, many of the traditional midwives recognize their work as important. Women like their care because they experience more kindness from them and the midwives "don't cut them." Traditional midwives express that training and unity among midwives will strengthen all of them collectively. Traditional midwives are also concerned about the lack of training on the part of some traditional midwives, recognizing a concern with patient safety and the potential of some to soil the reputation of all midwives. Traditional midwives feel their communities trust them and are willing to continue their education to avoid maternal mortality and improve maternal health.

Traditional midwives also believe in teaching the younger generations, who express that generally they are not interested in becoming midwives for all the reasons described above. Not infrequently, however, traditional midwives have daughters and granddaughters as assistants. Some of these continue to become midwives themselves, and some who have the opportunity go to midwifery or nursing school. However, traditional midwives are concerned that their wisdom will disappear, as fewer and fewer women are becoming midwives.

Through the conversations, the AMP identified the following needs of traditional midwives: (1) a certificate or license that recognizes midwives as legitimate birth attendants such that society will trust them and acknowledge their skills and their kindness; (2) the establishment of a functional system to enable unrestricted distribution of birth certificates for those in active practice; and (3) the creation of support networks for their personal wellbeing, stress management, and resilience.

Even statewide organizations have identified the need for creating national unity and strengthening of the profession and are particularly concerned about the situation of birth certificates at a national level. Traditional midwives are lacking national leadership and a unified voice. The AMP is working with midwifery groups to develop leadership capacity at a local level. Traditional midwives are very concerned that the health sector is actively seeking to push them out of providing health care and frightening women into institutional birth. Women are increasingly more afraid of birth as a concept, and they may request a cesarean delivery, to "avoid suffering."

16.8 A Vision for Midwifery in Mexico

The level of exclusion and discrimination that traditional midwives have endured in Mexico is unconscionable. Despite this, midwives persist in their work and continue to struggle, even where health services are unavailable, ensuring women have access to culturally appropriate midwifery. Traditional midwives suffer the triple burden of being indigenous, women, and midwives.

The AMP has therefore insisted on supporting and protecting the well-being of traditional midwifery beyond cultural heritage and as primary health providers. The AMP seeks to:

1. Contribute to better positioning and strengthening the identity of midwives within the health sector.
2. Improve traditional midwives' knowledge how to claim their human rights.
3. Improve interpersonal relationships within their local community networks.
4. Improve communication between midwives and midwifery supporters across the country.
5. Create a support network among traditional midwives across states.

Mexico is at a transition in maternal health. Funding provided by the MacArthur foundation in recent years with a concrete initiative to support the integration of professional midwifery into the health system has opened the possibility for change. The concern, however, is that professionalization of midwifery will exclude traditional midwifery and will once again exclude indigenous women through another shift in health-care policy. The Mexican Midwifery Associations' insistence that "a midwife is a midwife" provides a vision to build a future where basic competencies are universal and adapted to the cultural milieu and birth location. The Mexican health sector has an opportunity to spearhead an inclusive health-care system that honors its roots and tradition while integrating scientific best practices. An inclusive maternal health system would include educational opportunities for young indigenous women who want to become midwives, trained within their own communities by both professionally trained midwives and traditional midwives, to bridge an increasing age gap between aging traditional midwives and young birthing women.

A healthy inclusive system would include maternity-led units or birth centers that would service regions or areas so that women could be transferred for advanced care and attended to by professionally trained midwives. A midwife-led continuity model provides care from the same midwife or team of midwives during the pregnancy, birth, and the early parenting period (Sandall et al. 2016). Similarly, traditional midwives and indigenous women leaders should be consulted in the creation of maternal hospitals and birth centers to ensure cultural relevance in terms of physical space, and traditional midwives could be integrated into the public-sector hospitals as doulas, in partnership with professional midwives or physicians. It is neither feasible nor sustainable for all women to birth in secondary care hospitals, both from the perspective of the women trying to get there and from the perspective of the institution, which does not have the capacity to provide quality care for the larger volume of women currently giving birth at home.

A vision for the future would include multi-tiered levels of care where the heart of midwifery—kind, compassionate care—could shape the physical space for most births and convey respect to every woman's beliefs about her body and her capacity to give birth. In a country torn apart by drug violence and corruption, birth can provide a peaceful beginning where citizens are honored for their wisdom while co-participating in a healthful care milieu with compassionate service provision.

References

Asociación Mexicana de Partería, or Mexican Midwifery Association (AMP). (2017). *Asociación Mexicana de Partería*. Retrieved March 15, 2017, from www.asociacionmexicanadeparteria.org.

Campero, L., Hernandez, B., Leyva, A., Estrada, R., Osborne, J., & Morales, S. (2007). Trends in caesarean sections associated with non-clinical factors in a birthing educational center in Mexico City. *Salud Pública de México, 49*(2), 118–125.

D'Gregorio, R. P. (2010). Obstetrical violence: A new legal term introduced in Venezuela. *International Journal of Gynecology & Obstetrics, 111*, 201–202.

Duarte-Gomez, M. B., Nuñez-Urquiza, R. M., Restrepo-Restrepo, J. A., & Richardson-Lopez-Collada, V. L. (2015). Determinantes sociales de la mortalidad infantil en municipios de bajo índice de desarrollo humano en México. *Boletin Medico Hospital Infantil México, 72*(3), 181–189.

Grupo de Información en Reproducción Elegida (GIRE). (2015). *Omisión e Indiferencia: Derechos reproductivos en Mexico*. Retrieved February 10, 2017, from http://informe.gire.org.mx/.

Instituto Nacional de Estadística y Geografía (INEGI). (2015). *Encuesta Nacional de la Dinámica Demográfica, Boletín de Prensa Num 271/15*, Retrieved, March 19, 2017, from http://www.inegi.org.mx/saladeprensa/boletines/2015/especiales/especiales2015_07_1.pdf.

International Confederation of Midwives (ICM). (2008). *Investing in midwives and others with midwifery skills to save the lives of mothers and newborns and improve their health*. Retrieved February 10, 2017, from https://www.unfpa.org/sites/default/files/pub-pdf/midwives_eng.pdf.

International Confederation of Midwives. (2014). *Philosophy and model of midwifery care*. Core document. Retrieved March 15, 2017, from http://www.internationalmidwives.org/assets/uploads/documents/CoreDocuments/CD2005_001%20V2014%20ENG%20Philosophy%20and%20model%20of%20midwifery%20care.pdf.

Marcos, S. (2006). *Taken from the lips: Gender and eros in Mesoamerican religions*. Boston: Brill Press.

Marcos, S. (2010). Indigenous spirituality, gender, and the politics of justice: Voices from the first summit of indigenous women of the Americas. In S. Marcos (Ed.), *Women and indigenous religions* (pp. 45–68). Santa Barbara, CA: Praeger.

Mendez, C. (2017). Half of Mexicans are born by Cesarean. *El Universal*. Retrieved from http://www.eluniversal.com.mx/articulo/periodismo-de-datos/2017/01/22/nacen-por-cesarea-la-mitad-de-los-mexicanos.

Miller, S., Abalos, E., Chamillard, M., Ciapponi, A., Colaci, D., Comandé, D., et al. (2016). Beyond too little, too late and too much, too soon: A pathway towards evidence-based, respectful maternity care worldwide. *Lancet, 388*(10056), 2176–2192.

Nigenda, G., & Munos, J. A. (2015). Projections of specialist physicians in Mexico: A key element in planning human resources for health. *Human Resources for Health, 13*, 79. https://doi.org/10.1186/s12960-015-0061-z.proceso

Observatorio de Mortalidad Materna en México. (2014). *Indicadores de mortalidad materna*. Retrieved March 28, 2017, from http://www.omm.org.mx/images/stories/Documentos%20grandes/INDICADORES_2014_Web.pdf.

Puentes-Rosas, E., Gómez-Dantes, O., & Garrido-Latorre, F. (2004). Las cesáreas en México: Tendencias, niveles y factores asociados. *Salud Pública de México, 46*(1), 16–22.

Renfrew, M. J., McFadden, A., Bastos, M. H., Campbell, J., Channon, A. A., Cheung, N. F., et al. (2014). Midwifery and quality care: Findings from a new evidence-informed framework for maternal and newborn care. *Lancet, 384*(9948), 1129–1145.

Sandall, J., Soltani, H., Gates, S., Shennan, A., & Devane, D. (2016). Midwife-led continuity models versus other models of care for childbearing women. *Cochrane Database of Systematic Reviews, 2016*(4), CD004667.

Secretaria de Salud, Gobierno de México. (1992). *Manual de la partera tradicional*. Mexico City: Secretaria de Salud.

Secretaria de Salud, Gobierno del Estado de México. (2013). *Programa de Acción Específico: Salud Materna y Perinatal, 2013–2018*. Retrieved March 19, 2017, from http://cnegsr.salud.gob.mx/contenidos/descargas/SMP/SaludMaternayPerinatal_2013_2018.pdf.

United Nations Fund for Population Assistance (UNFPA). (2014a) Setting standards for emergency obstetric care. Retrieved March 14, 2017, from http://www.unfpa.org/resources/setting-standards-emergency-obstetric-and-newborn-care.

United Nations Fund for Population Assistance (UNFPA) (2014b) The state of the world's midwifery: A universal pathway. A woman's right to health. UNFPA. New York, NY. Retrieved September 1, 2016, from http://www.unfpa.org/publications.

World Health Organization, Department of Reproductive Health and Research. (1999). *Care in normal birth, a practical guide*. Geneva: World Health Organization.

17 Registration of Vital Events by the Civil Registry Office in an Indigenous Context: Implications for the Registration of Maternal Deaths

María Graciela Freyermuth Enciso

17.1 Introduction

Over the past 30 years, the region of Los Altos de Chiapas, in Mexico, has undergone a profound transformation. Throughout its history, it has been an isolated area with limited communication, not only with the rest of the country (due to its poor road infrastructure) but also with the state government, public health services, and even between the different communities that comprise the region (Fig. 17.1).

Several elements have changed this region in recent decades, including the emergence of Zapatismo, the decentralization of federal resources through Ramo 33,[1] and the implementation of targeted social development programs that have changed the way the government interacts with the local indigenous population.[2]

Los Altos de Chiapas is a *sui generis* region in which more than 80% of the inhabitants speak an indigenous language (ILS), which means that it has the highest percentage of indigenous inhabitants

[1] "Ramo 33." Federal Contributions for Federal Entities and Municipalities; is a budget mechanism designed to transfer resources to states and municipalities that enable them to strengthen their capacity to respond and meet government demands in the areas of education, health, basic infrastructure, financial strength, and public safety, as well as to implement food, welfare, and educational infrastructure programs. The distribution of these resources is regulated by the Fiscal Coordination.

[2] Chiapas received a large amount of resources following the emergence of the Zapatista movement. In 1998, the budget assigned to Chiapas through the Ramo 33 Contribution Fund for Health Services (FASSA) was $654,961.35, and total health expenditure amounted to $2,060,823.71 (De la Torre 2006). In 2012, Chiapas received through FASSA $2,909,862,005 (SHCP 2014) and through the People's Insurance (Seguro Popular) $3,533,300,000 (SP 2012), making a total of $6,443,162,005; that is to say, between 1998 and 2012, the federal budget assigned to Chiapas increased 3126 times. This does not take into account the additional resources that the states received through Ramo 12 of the Ministry of Health. In 2011, the resources allocated to the program Oportunidades amounted to 59,908 million pesos, which decreased to 32,053 in 2015. In 1998, the year in which this program started operating in Chiapas, the state received 3% of the national budget allocated to the program. In 2015 it received 7%, slightly less than that received by the Federal District, whose population is much higher (Presidencia de la República 2015 C 173). In 2015, 696,339 families in Chiapas (68% of the total) were affiliated to the program Prospera (Presidencia de la República 2015, 177–178 C). These figures placed Chiapas as the state with the highest percentage of families affiliated to Prosepera in the country.

M. G. F. Enciso, M.D., Ph.D.
CIESAS-Southeast,
San Cristóbal de Las Casas, Chiapas, Mexico

D. A. Schwartz (ed.), *Maternal Death and Pregnancy-Related Morbidity Among Indigenous Women of Mexico and Central America*, Global Maternal and Child Health: Medical, Anthropological, and Public Health Perspectives, https://doi.org/10.1007/978-3-319-71538-4_17

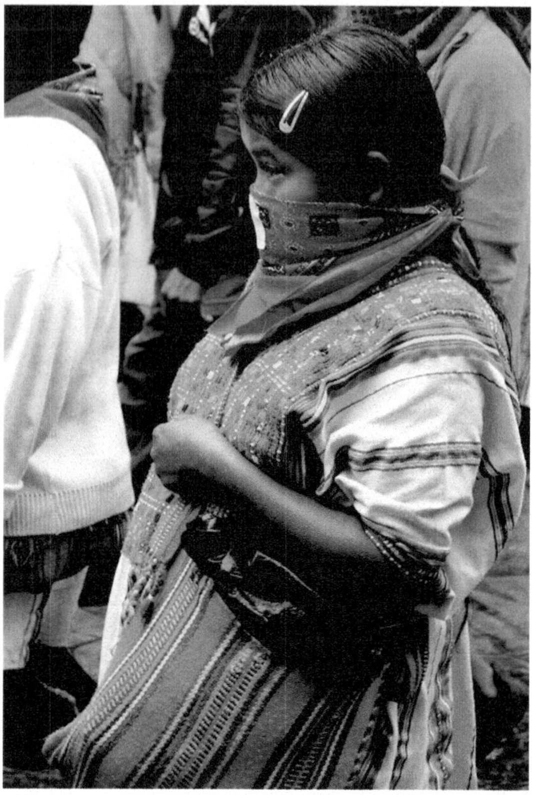

Fig. 17.1 Pregnant Zapatista girl. Photo courtesy of Juan Carlos Martínez Pérez

in Mexico (INEGI 2016). Most of the residents of this region belong to the Tzeltal and Tzotzil ethnic groups[3]; these indigenous languages predominate in 13 of its 16 municipal districts (Fig. 17.2).

Although illiteracy has declined by 20% in the last 20 years, 44.3% of the women are still illiterate. In municipal districts with a mestizo population, illiteracy is 20% for women and 11% for men. In both types of municipal districts, there are two illiterate women for every illiterate man (INEGI 1990, 2010).

Twenty-five years ago, the only type of health problems identified in the region were sanitary, and health services were limited to vaccination and malaria programs. Only rarely did local nursing homes and clinics (IMSS-Oportunidades) offer the services of a medical intern; most of the time there were only local health promoters. It is important to note that this region did not benefit from the medical-health programs implemented in 1928 after the creation of the Plan to Coordinate the Health Services of the Republic (Bustamante 1984), nor from those implemented in 1936 through the Cooperative Rural Medical Services created by President Lazaro Cardenas (Álvarez et al. 1984); both initiatives targeted rural areas of economic importance, excluding the most vulnerable regions and sectors of the country.

The Zapatista uprising brought about major changes in the regional landscape. Before 1994, the federal and state governments were almost totally absent in indigenous communities, but the guerrilla outbreak triggered an intense activity of international nongovernmental organizations (NGOs) and

[3]The main indigenous languages spoken in Chiapas are *Tzeltal* and *Tzotzil*. Of the total the population in Chiapas over three years of age (which according to the intercensal survey of 2015 was estimated at 4,863,092), 28%, or 1,361,249 persons, were indigenous language speakers. Of these, 29.9% did not speak Spanish and spoke only one indigenous language. Of the speakers of an indigenous language, 39.48% spoke *Tseltal* and 34.78% spoke *Tzotzil*.

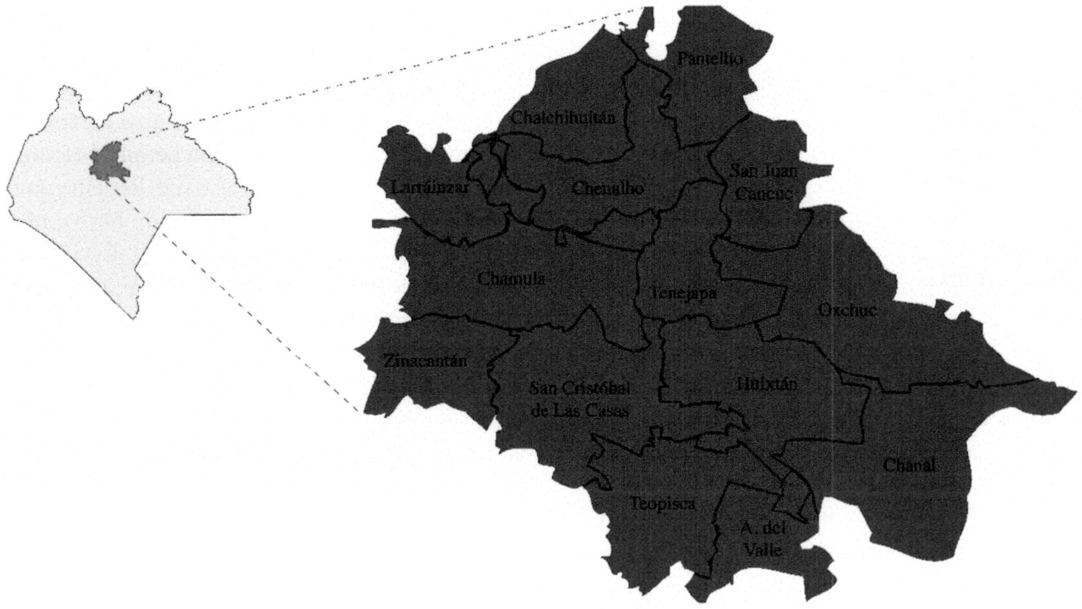

Fig. 17.2 Map of Chiapas, Altos de Chiapas Municipalities, 2010. Reproduced according to data from INEGI

agencies, making Chiapas an important element of the international image of Mexico. Following the Zapatista uprising, a substantial amount of resources from federal and international agencies began flowing into the state of Chiapas, while military needs led to the construction of highways and roads that linked previously inaccessible communities and regions.

As both a response and a strategy against the Zapatistas, the federal government implemented a number of programs through which cash transfers were made to poor households. Previously, these programs transferred resources to organizations, and it was through them that the living conditions of the population were supposed to have improved. However, this corporatist strategy allowed the resources to be exploited for political purposes and for maintaining the status quo. The changes introduced in response to the Zapatista uprising included the policies implemented by the National Development Plan of 1995–2000 that were designed to combat poverty, such as the Education, Health and Food Programs (PROGRESA) as well the Program for Expansion of Coverage (PAC). The latter program was aimed at fulfilling the agreements of the Declaration of Alma-Ata (OMS UNFPA 1978): Health for all by the year 2000.

This context of regional transformation has framed the study of the relationship between indigenous peoples, particularly in the region of Los Altos de Chiapas, and the federal government over the past 25 years. These relationships are a result of the establishment of an administrative entity: the Civil Registry Office (CRO). The purpose of this research is to analyze the registry of deaths, specifically maternal deaths.

17.2 Background

Focusing on the region of Los Altos de Chiapas allows us to document the processes of change related to the registration of female deaths in complex sociocultural systems. It also allows us to analyze the relationship between the national government and the population in terms of the concrete actions carried out by institutions to implement government policies, such as the administrative procedures and practices that are established over time (Foucault in Castro 2011); in this case, the processes underlying the registration of life events in an indigenous population.

Administrative records are essential for citizens to exercise their rights, and are also a primary source of statistics that permit the monitoring of vital events in the life of common people (Álvarez 1960). The Civil Registry (CR), which depends of the General Directorate of Civil Registry and whose director is appointed directly by the state executive, is in charge of documenting births, recognitions of children, adoptions, marriages, divorces, deaths (Periodico Oficial del Estado de Chiapas 2011) and judgments related to guardianships, absences, death and disability assumptions or limitations for administering property. These vital events are recorded in books that are kept by the Civil Registry Offices, which issues certified copies of the death records of each of these vital events. The death record, for example, contains the basic information about the context and causes of the death of a person.

The death records are of public interest as well as an indispensable tool for the design of health policies. Maternal deaths (MM) are those that occur to women during pregnancy, childbirth, or within the 42 days following the end of pregnancy for reasons directly related to it or to previous illnesses aggravated by it. Monitoring maternal deaths has been a priority during the last 25 years in the member countries of the United Nations to measure the progress of public policies; in this context, the role played by an administrative body such as the Civil Registry cannot be overestimated.

The death records issued by the CR are based on medical certificates of death issued by health authorities or by authorized persons. Death certificates are used to build databases that include information such as (1) the sociodemographic characteristics of the deceased: date of birth, sex, age, education, occupation, marital status, nationality, geographical location of habitual residence, and affiliation; (2) characteristics related to death: date of registration and occurrence, geographical location of occurrence and registration, address of occurrence, health care, necropsy conditions, causes of death, pregnancy status, and person who certified the death; and (3) a special section for accidental or violent deaths: homicide, suicide, or legal or war operations (Y35, Y36, and Y89, according to the International Classification of Diseases, ICD-10). This latter section also has information related to the presumption of accident, occurrence of death during work, and the place where it occurred and on family violence (INEGI 2014). The definitions and criteria for these variables are based on the work of Mexican health institutions and the World Health Organization/Pan American Health Organization (WHO/PAHO).

Death records are used to estimate the maternal mortality ratio (MMR), which is the indicator used to evaluate the success of each country in reducing MM. The MMR is estimated by dividing maternal deaths over live births occurred during a given period and multiplying the result by 100,000. For example, in 2014 there were 872 maternal deaths in Mexico, according to official figures, while the number of live births recorded during the same year was 2,239,268; this gives an MMR of 38.9 for every 100,000 live births.

There is another indicator that can also be estimated using the number of maternal deaths: the maternal mortality rate (MMRate), which is a measure of the frequency of maternal deaths during a specific period. It is calculated by dividing the number of maternal deaths by the number of women in the same age group who died during a given period. For example, if 872 MM were recorded in 2014 and the number of women of reproductive age (from 15 to 49 years) was 33,076,163, the MMRate for that year is 2.6 per 100,000 women of reproductive age. As is evident, the documentation administered by the CT is critical to estimate both indicators.

It is important to note that it is increasingly common for women to die from maternal causes greater than 42 days after delivery. In 2014, these deaths constituted 16% (140) of all maternal deaths, a significant increase compared to 2009, in which the proportion was only 5% (60).

There are two characteristics of the MMR which make it a particularly interesting and significant statistic. The first is that it identifies inequalities between women in different environments, being a pregnancy statistic that shows the largest differences between countries. For example, in 2013 (and prior to the onset of the Ebola virus epidemic) the women of Sierra Leone (with an MMR of 1100 deaths per 100,000 live births) were 275 times more likely to die during pregnancy compared with women in Spain or Italy, whose MMR was 4. In the Americas, the gaps between countries are smaller in magnitude but no less profound; it is enough to compare the MMR of Haiti (380) and that of Canada (11), which is 34 times smaller. Although it might be unexpected, Chile (14) and Uruguay (22) each have a smaller MMR than the United States (28). Thus, this indicator reveals the inequalities between women living in different countries, regions, states, and municipal districts. Secondly, pregnancy is a relatively short process (between 37 and 42 weeks at term gestation), which allows the evaluation of policies aimed at improving the health system in the short term. These two characteristics explain why the MMR is an ideal indicator to evaluate public health policies.

Since the early 1980s, and despite the lack of figures about global maternal deaths, there was a perception, from a medical point of view, that women were dying unjustifiably during pregnancy, childbirth, postpartum, and from abortion. A meeting held in Nairobi in February 1987 by the World Bank, World Health Organization (WHO), and United Nations Fund for Population Activities (UNFPA) led to the creation of the Safe Motherhood Initiative: A Call to Action, whose main purpose was to reduce maternal deaths by one-half by the year 2000. This initiative claimed that the MM indicator had not been duly considered as a way to measure quality of care and quality of life (Starrs 1987, p. 6).

The first fruits of this initiative were seen in 1994 and 1995, at the IV International Conference on Population and Development in Cairo, Egypt (Naciones Unidas 1994), and in the Fourth World Conference on Women in Beijing (Naciones Unidas 1995). Three of the goals set out in Cairo and Beijing coincided with the concerns of the Call to Action of 1987: to reduce the maternal morbidity and mortality levels of 1990 by one-half by the year 2000, and reduce them again by one-half by 2015; furthermore, the disparities between countries, geographic regions, and ethnic groups regarding maternal death should also be reduced. Another objective of these conferences was to improve the quality and scope of basic information on birth and death rates disaggregated by gender and ethnicity.

In September 2000, the member countries of the United Nations signed the Millennium Declaration on Development and Poverty (Naciones Unidas 2000)—Millennium Development Goals (MDGs), in which it was agreed to reduce maternal deaths by 75% between 1990 and 2015 (MDG 5: Improve maternal health), an objective that had already been established in the Cairo and Beijing conferences on women. The Millennium Declaration identified the proportion of births attended by skilled personnel as another indicator that could help achieve the proposed goals (Naciones Unidas 2000). The signing of this declaration prompted the Mexican government to issue a report every five years to monitor the compliance with these objectives, even though the declaration was not mandatory. Until 2012, these reports constituted an important incentive to improve maternal health and, above all, the health information systems that generate the figures needed to estimate the indicator of maternal mortality (Presidencia de la República 2005).

In this context, the objective of this work is to report the changes and persistent elements in the documentation of vital facts by the Civil Registry Office. In particular, this chapter discusses the registration of female deaths from obstetric causes from the 1990s to the year 2015 in an indigenous enclave: the *Tzotzil-Tzeltal* region of Los Altos de Chiapas, referred in this work as Los Altos de Chiapas (Fig. 17.3).

During the nineteenth century there was a dispute in Mexico over the control of statistics of vital events between the Church and the State. During the twentieth century, in the indigenous region of

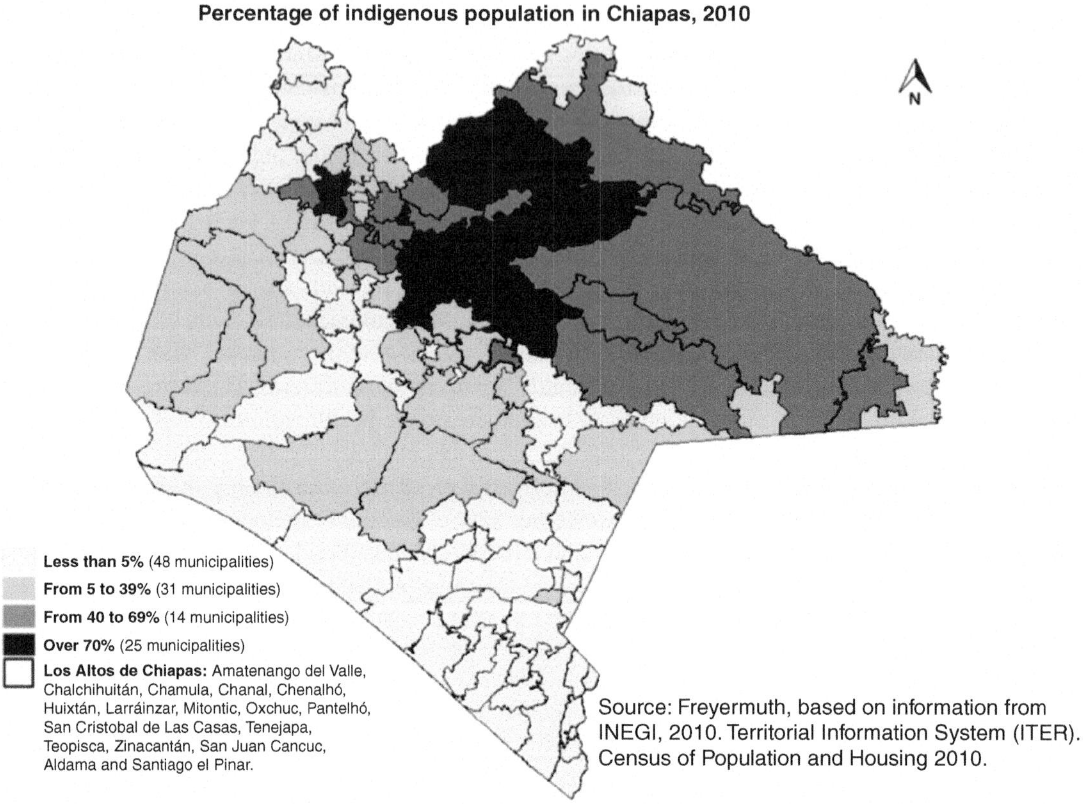

Fig. 17.3 Map of Chiapas, demonstrating the percentage of indigenous population in the region. Reproduced according to data from INEGI

Los Altos de Chiapas, this dispute was between traditional and national authorities. The index of MM reflects some of the changes that have occurred in the last 25 years in the relationship between the State and the indigenous peoples of Mexico, regarding both their status as citizens and as part of the nation.

The records generated by the CRO are of utmost importance, since they are the primary source of information on deaths in our country. The procedures and protocols that are used to build these records are critical to the quality of the information they provide. In the so-called "information age," civil registry records have become a fundamental reference for the planning of population, health, and migration policies, as well as for electoral registers and population control measures; they are also a valuable tool for assessing compliance with national and international commitments. The CRO is a good example of the medicalization of society, understood as the political role of medicine and the extension of medical knowledge to the administrative field (Castro 2011, p. 272).

Two administrative entities are involved in the registration of mortality: the Secretariat of Health (SSA), responsible for establishing and conducting national health policy under the terms of applicable laws and in accordance with the provisions of the Federal Executive,[4] and the Civil Registry[5] (CR), responsible for registering, authorizing, and publishing events related to the civil status of

[4]This is its main function; its powers may be consulted in the Ley General de Salud, Nueva Ley, published in the Diario Oficial de la Federación on February 7, 1984. Last reform published DOF 28-06-2005.

[5]Article 348, Chapter V, Title fourteenth "Donation, transplantation and loss of life" of the Ley General de Salud.

individual persons. It is the Civil Registry which authorizes the burial of corpses, subject to the presentation of the medical certificate of death. This is a document that must be issued by the attending physician, a physician with professional license or authorized personnel, according to the current standards on Health Information (Diario Oficial de la Federación [DOF] 2012).

17.3 Information Sources

The temporal boundaries of this study begins some years before the Zapatista uprising. During this period the movement received a great deal of media attention and at the same time the social assistance program Solidaridad-Progresa-Oportunidades-Prospera was implemented. This work belongs to a series of studies on maternal mortality that have involved in-depth archival research in the CROs, direct observation of their operation, and interviews with officials of the institutions involved. The first study focused on the registration of maternal mortality in the region of Los Altos de Chiapas from 1990 to 1993. Subsequently, a second work was focused on the underreporting of maternal mortality in Chenalhó from 1995 to 1996 (Freyermuth and Garza 1996). A more recent study, sponsored by the Sectoral Funds CONACYT (Consejo Nacional de Ciencia y Tecnología), investigated the underreporting of maternal mortality in the indigenous region of Los Altos de Chiapas from 2003 to 2006, and proposed an alternative indicator to identify it (Freyermuth et al. 2007). Finally, in 2015 our research efforts focused on the study of the health information systems in the region of Los Altos de Chiapas. Our visits to the CRO in 1989, 1995, 1996, and 2003 lasted from three days to three weeks depending on the volume of information available in each office. The archival work of 1995–1996 was complemented with interviews with officials working in the CROs. From 2014 to 2015, a study was conducted to determine the dynamics of the registration of birth certificates in the civil offices of the indigenous municipalities of Los Altos de Chiapas; this study included interviews with officials that were similar to those conducted in 1995–1996.

This chapter is structured as follows: the first section provides a background of the CR in Chiapas, and of the beginnings of the documentation of vital events in the region. The second section presents the results of more than two decades of follow-up of the activities of these institutions, focusing on the registration of maternal deaths. The last section presents the conclusions of this study.

17.4 The Establishment of the Civil Registry in Los Altos de Chiapas

In the seventeenth century, Catholic churches were built in the main towns of Los Altos de Chiapas; each of them had a sacristan, a prosecutor, and priests in charge of organizing the celebrations of religious festivals and administering the sacraments accepted by the indigenous population. The population paid for the upkeep of the priests and for the sacraments and the corresponding taxes. With the advent of national independence, the priests continued to document births and raise taxes. The increasing workload on the Indians and a series of disagreements led to the start of the Caste War (Rus 1995),[6] which saw the priests permanently abandon the churches of the region until the late twentieth century (Guiteras 1996). These events created particular problems for the registration of sacramental events in this region, resulting in irregular reporting—the population associated the registration of vital events with plundering and exploitation.

In the second half of the twentieth century, the indigenous municipalities of Los Altos de Chiapas were governed by two bodies: the indigenous council (cabildo indígena) and the municipal presidency

[6]The so-called Caste War took place from 1867 to 1870 between Chamulas and state authorities.

(presidencia municipal). The political-religious authorities included the "mayordomo," "mayor," governing mayor (regidor alcalde), and governor. The municipal authorities included an indigenous "president" and a "síndico" (both speaking Spanish) and, well into the twentieth century, a "*ladino*" secretary appointed by the authorities of San Cristobal de Las Casas. These authorities were in charge of the Civil Registry until 1991 (Guiteras 2002).

17.4.1 The Operation of the Civil Registry in the Early 1990s

The events recorded by the Civil Registry are births, registration of children, adoptions, marriages, divorces, deaths, and judgments declaring absence, presumption of death, guardianship, and loss or limitation of the legal capacity to administer property. However, the civil registry records that have been most used in Los Altos de Chiapas in recent decades are, in order of importance, those of births, deaths, marriages, divorces, registration of children, and fetal deaths.

Before 1991, the Civil Registry Office (CRO) was operated by the municipal presidency. Depending on the municipality, the powers of the Civil Registry were part of the duties of the municipal president[7] or the municipal secretary.[8] The municipal president frequently appointed a secretary whose functions and responsibilities included those of the presidency and the CRO. The municipal presidency financed the CR, whose activities were considered of secondary importance; the president signed death records in his spare time, and delays were thus very frequent.[9]

The requirements for the registration of birth and death were lax, as it was the municipal president who guaranteed that villagers belonged to a particular place of origin. In the 1980s, the presence of the parents was not necessary to register a birth, or a marriage certificate to attest to the paternity or maternity; the municipal president signed the record and he himself attested the validity of the document, even in the absence of the newborn or the parents.[10]

To serve as an official or assistant in the CRO, the only requirement was to have typing skills and notions of spelling. It was also required to have basic education[11]; some officers had completed only primary school, but had typing skills. Another aspect that characterized this period was the flexibility of opening hours of the CRO, which were the same as for the municipal presidency.

In 1991, the CROs were separated from the municipal presidencies, and the hiring of the staff was carried out by the Directorate General of Civil Registration (DGRC). The change of affiliation of the CROs involved the professionalization of their staff. This led to a continuous increase in the requirements for working as a civil registry official during the 1990s.

17.4.2 Registration of Deaths in Los Altos de Chiapas During the 1990s

The possibility of being enrolled in the public-school system became an incentive to obtain a birth certificate. Furthermore, the death certificate had no practical use for the indigenous population of Los Altos de Chiapas. However, its relevance was essential in the case of an inheritance. Marital status is

[7]Officials of the CR, Municipality of Huixtán, Chiapas, 1994, October 26; Municipality of Larráinzar, Chiapas 1994, October 4.

[8]Official of the CR, Chenalhó 1996, May 18.

[9]Official of the CR, Municipality of Chenalhó and Chiapas 1996, May 18.

[10]Official of the CR, Municipality of Zinacantán, Chiapas, 1994, March 30.

[11]Official of the CR, Municipality of Zinacantán, Chiapas 1994, March 30, Official of the CR, Municipality of Chenalhó, Chiapas 1996, May 18.

Table 17.1 Causes of death among people aged 15–49 years in Zinacantan, Chiapas, México in 1980

Cause	Occurrences
Inflammation	1
Vomit	1
Cough	1
Psychiatric	1
Inflammation of the whole body	1
Acute colitis	1
Giving birth	1
Respiratory insufficiency	1
Total	8

Source: Based on archival work in Civil Registry Offices, 1995

very important when dealing with heritable property, as it establishes rights and obligations with respect to third parties—children, parents, or spouses. However, in a population in which all acts of life are regulated by uses and customs beyond the National State, the registration of the civil status of persons is meaningless. Mexican indigenous peoples felt a deep distrust of the National State, which was perceived more as an agent of dispossession than a guarantor of rights. This is the reason they were not interested in the legal definition of marital status or identity, or in the registration of deaths. The registration of marital status in this region reflects the troubled relationship and misunderstandings between the indigenous population and the National State.

The small regional influence of health services during the 1980s reflected how the State conceived the indigenous population, whose production was mainly subsistence-oriented.[12] The SSA had no presence in Chiapas before the 1940s, and even then only through control programs of tropical diseases such as river blindness (onchocerciasis, an insect-borne parasitic disease caused by a roundworm, *Onchocerca volvulus*), yellow fever, pinta (a tropical skin disease caused by *Treponema pallidum carateum*), malaria, and smallpox.

In the late 1980s, the region had only two hospitals, both of them with limited resources. In addition, the capital of each municipal district had a precarious medical service, where it was possible to obtain a medical certificate of death which, as noted above, had been mandatory since 1986. This very limited presence of medical services can be deduced from the causes of death recorded in the CRO (see Table 17.1) of the municipality of Zinacantan in 1980, which list only the symptoms and conditions under which the death occurred.

The analysis of greater than one thousand death records in the municipalities of Chamula and Huixtán showed that, between the years 1989 and 1991, the percentage of certification was 1–4% in Chamula and 4–10% in Huixtán (Freyermuth and Fernández 1997). Consistent with these data, and during the same period, the percentage of women who lived in the indigenous region and who had received medical attention before dying from maternal causes was less than 17%. This percentage was lower (8%) when considering overall deaths, and very different from the percentage of women who died in predominantly *mestizo* municipalities (65%) (Tables 17.2 and 17.3).

[12]Before the 1917 Constitution, public health was the responsibility of local entities and municipalities. There was no public system of health services, and medical care was provided through other public services or charity. The 1917 Constitution transformed this system, and the foundations of the current National Health System were established in the first half of the twentieth century. The rural population was not provided with medical care until 1928; however, the provision of public health services in Chiapas came later, mainly because the rural economy in this state was based on subsistence agriculture, and the public programs implemented in 1928 and 1936 focused on farmers of economic importance, excluding regions such as Los Altos de Chiapas (Freyermuth, 1993).

Table 17.2 Evolution of maternal mortality deaths according to the medical care provided in Los Altos de Chiapas[a] México, 1988–2013

Year of death	Had medical care (%)	No medical care (%)	Total
1989–1995[a]	16.8	83.2	100
2002–2007	44	56	100
2008–2013	83.3	16.7	100

Sources: Based on vital statistics of INEGI 1989–1996, and Database of Maternal Deaths DGIS/SS, 2002–2013
[a]Amatenango del Valle, Chalchihuitán, Chamula, Chanal, Chenalhó, Huixtán, Pantelhó, Tenejapa, San Juan Cancuc, Zinacantán, Aldama, Santiago el Pinar

Table 17.3 Evolution of the percentage of overall deaths of women and men of reproductive age according to medical care provided before their death

	Women		Men	
Year	Had medical care (%)	No medical care (%)	Had medical care (%)	No medical care (%)
1990	8.1	91.9	7.9	92.1
1995	26.3	73.7	20.9	79.1
2000	39.0	61.0	34.0	66.0
2005	42.9	57.1	33.8	66.2
2010	41.6	58.4	28.2	71.8
2014	43.9	64.6	35.4	64.6

Indigenous municipalities of Los Altos de Chiapas[a] México, 1990–2014. Sources: based on databases of overall deaths (INEGI/SALUD, 1990, 1995, 2000, 2005, 2010 and 2014)
[a]Amatenango del Valle, Chalchihuitán, Chamula, Chanal, Chenalhó, Huixtán, Larráinzar, Mitontic, Oxchuc, Pantelhó, Tenejapa, San Juan Cancuc, Zinacantán, Aldama y Santiago el Pinar

At that time, the civil registry could issue death records without a medical certificate of death. The officials argued that they could not leave people without them,[13] and they often had the permission of the municipal president, who signed all records issued by the civil registry.[14] The population of Los Altos lacked health services, as seen in Table 17.4, which shows that until 1990 there was no presence of social security institutions in that region.

Despite the ease with which death records could be obtained, a significant part of the population was buried without them. The officials interviewed during the years 1994–1996 noted the existence of people who died without their families giving notice of their death. After 1992, it was a requirement to present a notice of death issued by the authorities or a medical certificate of death issued by the health services, but this made the process of obtaining a death certificate more difficult, especially in remote locations that lacked health services and where funerals were held inside houses. Approximately 92% of the men and women of reproductive age who died in 1990 did not receive medical attention before dying, and the few medical certificates in which health personnel attested to the death of the person were usually contained information provided by a declarant who was often not a close relative of the deceased, but someone commissioned to give notice of the death (Freyermuth, personal workbook, based on fieldwork 1992–1996).

The Civil Registry official of Chamula acknowledged that stating eliminar the cause of death was witchcraft, and did not reveal the true cause of death. The fact that in earlier times people would go to traditional healers to seek treatment for health and other problems was one of the biggest challenges of the civil registry.[15] Documents from the end of the 1980s state that in the municipalities of San Juan

[13]Official of the CR, Municipality of Altamirano, Chiapas, 1994.
[14]Official of the CR, Municipality of Mitontic, Chiapas 1996.
[15]Official of the CR, Municipality of Chamula, Chiapas 1994, March 3.

Table 17.4 Evolution of the deaths of women and men of reproductive age, according to their affiliation to the health system in indigenous and *mestizo*[a] municipalities of Los Altos de Chiapas[b], 1981–2013

	Indigenous municipalities				*Mestizo* municipalities			
	Women		Men		Women		Men	
Period of death	None and unspecified	Affilitation to the health system	None and unspecified	Affilitation to the health system	None and unspecified	Affilitation to the health system	None and unspecified	Affilitation to the health system
1981–1985	100	0	100	0	100	0	100	0
1986–1990	99.9	0.1	99.6	0.4	100	0	100	0
1991–1995	98	2	97.2	2.8	86.4	13.6	86.5	13.5
1996–2000	96.4	3.6	96.2	3.8	81.4	18.6	89.1	10.9
2001–2005	97.2	2.8	97.5	2.5	83.7	16.3	91.1	8.9
2006–2010	85.3	14.7	92.2	7.8	71.1	28.9	86	14
2011–2013	71.4	28.6	82.6	17.4	46.9	53.1	91.3	8.7

Sources: Dirección General de Información en Salud (DGIS). Database of overall deaths, 1979–2013 [online]: National Health Information System (SINAIS). [Mexico]: Secretariat of Health [query: April 15, 2015]

[a]Teopisca and San Cristobal de Las Casas

[b]Amatenango del Valle, Chalchihuitán, Chamula, Chanal, Chenalhó, Huixtán, Pantelhó, Tenejapa, San Juan Cancuc, Zinacantán, Aldama, Santiago el Pinar

Chamula and Huixtán, the municipal judge decided how to "choose" the causes of death reported by respondents, since they could not be registered as "cortar vela,"[16] "aire" (*ic'*),[17] "sueño,"[18] "potzlom,"[19] or "*me'vinik.*"[20] In the absence of the judge, the person in charge of preparing the certificate in the municipal presidency made these reinterpretations.

Another challenge was the small number of types of blank certificates (12) provided to the health center. The Civil Registry official of Larráinzar[21] said they had to work around this problem so that people could have a death record (it was registered without a medical certificate). Besides the precarious relationship between the population and the health services, frequent absenteeism of staff in health units, even in the municipal capitals, determined that it was the municipal judges or officials

[16]Casting evil ("mal echado"), envy or cutting the candle ("cortar vela") are actions that require the use of witchcraft and are used in response to conflicts between individuals or families.

[17]Air, or *ic'*, is one of the most common ailments among pregnant women, but it is dangerous only during this stage of pregnancy. Air can cause abdominal pain, back pain, and malposition of the child. In some cases, air can lead to death, causing a condition characterized by severe abdominal pain and accompanied by the perception of visual phosphenes. The air may be encapsulated by water, and when this happens the discomfort disappears when the water breaks (rupture of the amniotic membranes).

[18]During sleep, people are more vulnerable and can acquire different types of diseases. An unpleasant experience in a dream can cause a disease, especially if the dream repeats itself.

[19]This disease is acquired through sexual dreams or bad dreams.

[20]For the *Tzotzil* people, "*me'vinic*" or "alteration" is something inherent to human beings, a sign of life that is present in children, women, men, Indians, and *mestizos*; it is located in the mouth of the stomach and can be recognized by its beat (pulsation of the abdominal aorta). The modification of this beat is what causes illness or death, and is known as "*me'vinic.*" When a person is sick, the alteration rises, and if the person is weak, it can cause death.

[21]Official of the CR, Municipality of Larráinzar, Chiapas, 1994, October 4.

Table 17.5 Evolution of the registration of deaths of women of reproductive age, according to death records and medical certificates of death, Chenalhó, Chiapas, México 1988–1993[a]

Year	Number of death records	Medical certificates of death
1988	68	1
1989	126	2
1990	126	1
1991	100	41
1992	83	83
1993	56	55

Based on archival work
[a]Freyermuth and Garza, Maternal Death in Los Altos de Chiapas, unpublished results, 1995

who established the causes of death. In 1988 there were a total of 43 doctors for the 15 municipalities in the region of Los Altos, and the number of death records that had a corresponding medical certificate of death was very low (less than 2% between 1988 and 1990). In the case of Chenalhó, the number of medical certificates of death increased since 1991, as can be seen in Table 17.5. After 1991, civil registry officials began an information campaign so that people knew their obligations in cases of death. They also said that issuing death records demanded of them to be available 24 h, 365 days a year, and that some of them alternated with an assistant.

The causes of death recorded did not always correspond with reality because, as already mentioned, it was those relatives and friends who had attended the funeral who were generally entrusted to notify the authorities as declarants and witnesses.[22] It is not surprising that almost all causes of death stated on the death records were in the category of signs, symptoms, and ill-defined morbid states. The most common diagnoses recorded on death records between 1989 and 1991 were: fever, swelling, nonspecific signs and symptoms related to the gastrointestinal tract, nonspecific signs and symptoms related to the respiratory system, old age, violent or accidental death, alcohol poisoning, and tuberculosis (Freyermuth and Fernández 1997).

In Larráinzar, when a person died in an isolated place, an official document of death ("oficio de defunción") was completed and filed by the municipal agent; this document served as a medical certificate of death. The municipal agent of each community notified the officialdom of the death, and the death record was prepared from 24 to 48 h afterwards.[23] The only requirement was to notify the municipal agent that a person had died, after which he authorized the burial.[24] In Chamula, it was the municipal judge who attested to all natural or violent deaths.

A study on the causes of death recorded in the Civil Registry of Chenalhó (Freyermuth and Garza 1996) identified 117 records of deaths of women between 10 and 49 years of age between 1988 and 1993; 11 of these death records mentioned diagnoses compatible with maternal death. After investigating 38 cases suspected of having been wrongly recorded, it was found that nine more cases were directly related to maternity (Freyermuth 2003).

Thus, 88% of all maternal deaths in the period were underreported in the CR, a percentage that rose to 96% when compared with the cases that had medical certificates. An important aspect is that only 10% of the deceased women had sought medical care at the regional hospital of San Cristobal de Las Casas.

[22]Official of the CR, Municipality of Chamula, 1992, October 8 and 1994, March 3, Official of the CR, Municipality of Chalchihuitán, 1996, May 14.

[23]Official of the CR, Municipality of Chalchihuitán, Chiapas, 1996, May 14.

[24]Official of the CR, Municipality of Zinacantán, Chiapas 1994, March 30.

Table 17.6 Underreporting of maternal deaths found during fieldwork and in the study of death records and medical certificates of death, Chenalhó, Chiapas México 1988–1993

Year	Death record A	Medical certificate B	Total identified A and B	Total with fieldwork	Live births
1988	1	1	1	2	1008
1989	0	0	0	4	1018
1990	1	1	1	1	1381
1991	1	1	1	4	1299
1992	3	1	4	4	1389
1993	3	1	4	5	1431
Totals	9	5	11	20	7526
MMR	119.58	66.43	146.16	265.8	
Underreporting	55%	75%	45%		

Based on fieldwork and archival work, 1988–1993

Table 17.6 shows that in the early 1990s the reporting of maternal deaths was still very sporadic, even years after the compulsory certification of deaths had been established.

In the mid-1990s, the presence of the health system in this region was still very marginal, even in those situations with a high risk of death. By then, Mexico had already committed to attain the goals of the Cairo conference of halving the number of maternal deaths that had occurred in 1990 by the year 2000. However, in this region where there were not even the necessary conditions to certify the cause of death, the State was in no position to provide appropriate care in cases of obstetric emergencies. The system of administration of justice was also absent, since according to Civil Registry officials, in the 1990s the role of the public prosecutor in indigenous areas was exercised by municipal judges; this meant that the investigation of serious crimes was often done according to the local traditions and customs.

17.4.3 The Operation of the Civil Registry Offices in the Early Twenty-First Century and the Registration of Deaths in Los Altos de Chiapas[25]

By 2003, the secretarial staff of the CROs in the region were mostly indigenous, while judges were both indigenous and *mestizo*. An interesting case was that of the Civil Registry Office of Chalchihuitán, which in 1993 operated only erratically and death registration was virtually nonexistent, with an average of two cases per year. By the first half of 2000, it was maintained by indigenous staff, who received a recognition from the General Directorate for good performance. Throughout the region of Los Altos de Chiapas, there was a significant improvement in the management and conservation of records and certificates, as well as in the order of the books kept by civil registry offices.

According to official data, in 2000 the majority (68%) of adult women in the villages of Los Altos de Chiapas with less than 2000 inhabitants were still dying in their homes (65.5%) without proper medical care and beyond the reach of the health services or of a doctor who could certify their death (Table 17.4). This situation was very different from that of other regions. Nationally, only 33.6% of women were dying at home, while 78% received medical care, and only 1.8% lived in towns with less than 2000 inhabitants.[26] By the year 2000, access to health services in the

[25] Reproductive Age Mortality Survey (RAMOS), Measure evaluation.

[26] Sources: Dirección General de Información en Salud (DGIS). Database of overall deaths, 2001 [online]: National Health Information System (SINAIS). [Mexico]: Secretariat of Health [query: April 10, 2003].

nonindigenous municipalities of Los Altos had changed somewhat. At the moment of death, 13.6% of the nonindigenous women in those municipalities were affiliated in some way to social security, compared to only 2% for indigenous women (Table 17.4). There was an increase in the percentage of women who received medical care before death. The number of women who received medical care before dying from general causes increased four times, even though only 2% had social security. Of the women who died from maternal causes between 2002 and 2007, 44% received medical care before death; this means that access to health services for women with maternal complications increased twofold in a decade.

When death occurred, the family could follow-up in two ways to give official notice, depending on the importance of the town. If there were civil authorities or community representatives in the town, the family notified them of the death and they prepared an official document that stated the circumstances in which it had occurred. With this kind of certificate, a person entrusted by the family traveled to the Civil Registry Office to testify before the authorities.

But if the death occurred on holidays, Saturdays or Sundays, the burial was carried out before notifying the authorities, as had been done in the 1990s. These two methods carried important implications for the documentation of deaths, since the process of certification was performed by people who did not know the development of the illness that led to the death of the women, and therefore could not provide additional information beyond that found in the official document prepared by the local authorities when a doctor tried to perform a thorough anamnesis.[27]

Information was excluded that could be considered problematic. For example, a case of maternal death involving a stillbirth required two documentation procedures, and thus sometimes the people chose to report a common disease as cause of death to avoid the additional bureaucratic procedure.

In 2003, we analyzed 245 cases of deaths of women aged 10–49 years that occurred in Los Altos de Chiapas in 2001, in order to identify underreporting of maternal deaths. To do this, we conducted an exhaustive review of the archives of the Civil Registry Office and compared them with databases of medical certificates of death. As in the research project of 1995, we also conducted verbal autopsies with the families of the dead women.[28]

One of the findings in this study was that in 85% of the cases in which the declarant did not have a medical certificate of death when he arrived at the CR, the employees of this office sent him to an establishment of the Institute of Health of the State of Chiapas (ISECH) so that the doctor in charge would issue the medical certificate. In 25% of these cases, however, no doctor was found. When this occurred, an official of the Civil Registry, the municipal judge, a health promoter, or any member of the local health committee was forced to issue a kind of death proof. Of the medical certificates issued in the region of Los Altos, the most reliable, as expected, were those prepared by doctors working in health units. These accounted for only 7.6% of the total number of deaths recorded in 2001, according to data from INEGI.

It is important to note that there were cases in which the neighbors reported that the relatives of the deceased woman had negligently let her die or even murdered her. When a family member became aware that he was under such suspicion, he asked the judge to come to the home to certify the cause of death, and the deceased was not buried until the authorities recognized the context and the causes of the death.

[27]A doctor in the health clinic of Chamula told us about the difficulties to confirm a diagnosis.

[28]Research project: "Maternal Mortality in Indigenous Regions."

17.4.4 Dissimilarities that Hinder Communication Between the Informant and the Doctor Issuing the Medical Certificate of Death

According to INEGI (INEGI, Dirección General de Información en Salud [DGIS], Database of overall deaths, 2001), 53.6% of the deceased women analyzed in this study had no schooling, 21% had incomplete primary education, and only 8% had higher education. Data from the CR showed that 29% of the declarants were illiterate. Illiteracy in this region was high; the average among men was 24%, but it was higher than 30% in five municipalities. The illiteracy rates for women were twice those of men. In 14 of the 17 municipalities, virtually all inhabitants were indigenous language speakers (ILS), and Spanish was only marginally used. This created communication problems with the *mestizo* population, most of whom did not know the indigenous languages; in particular, it made it difficult for declarants to communicate with the doctor issuing the medical certificate. These communication problems were aggravated by the different world views of the certifying agent and the declarant, ignorance about the traditional nosology used by the inhabitants of Los Altos, and that a significant number of people died without medical attention (Table 17.3). Among the causes of death reported by relatives were witchcraft, envy, evil cast, the death of animal companions (*wayjelel*), and that the deceased had their "time cut" ("cortado la hora"). We have already documented these causes in the 1990s (Freyermuth 2003).

Doctors generally prepared the medical certificate of death in the medical units; they almost never traveled to or visited the community. Many times, the burial had already occurred, making it difficult to establish a clear diagnosis, and so the doctors were forced to take as authentic the document or certificate presented by the declarant. When a death certificate was issued without a medical certificate of death, the Health Institute of the State of Chiapas (ISECH) sent community health coordinators to look for the family of the deceased in order to conduct a verbal autopsy.

17.4.5 Maternal Death, a Problematic Death

In the first five years of the twenty-first century, maternal mortality began to be recognized as a priority by the health authorities of the state of Chiapas. Since then, health personnel have been pressured to bring it down, often without providing the material support required by the relevant institutions to achieve this goal (Meneses 2007). Maternal deaths have since then been a stigma for health jurisdictions where such deaths are more frequent.

We were interested in identifying underreported maternal deaths for 2001 with the method used in 1995, called the RAMOS method (Reproductive Age Mortality Survey).[29] This method delimits the study to deaths of women of reproductive age, or other defined age range, in order to identify the causes of each death and ways to prevent them (WHO 1987). To accomplish this, we searched in the CR and in the municipal offices of Los Altos de Chiapas for all deaths of women aged 15–49 years that occurred in 2001; since we found no deaths of women under 15 years of age, we excluded that age group from the discussion of the results. According to the results of our work in the field and in the archives of municipal offices, 226 women aged 15–49 years died in 2001. Table 17.7 shows the

[29] Maternal Mortality in 2000. Estimates developed by WHO, UNICEF, and UNFPA. https://books.google.com.mx/books?hl=es&lr=&id=2valPKR-7v4C&oi=fnd&pg=PT4&dq=Reproductive+Age+Mortality+Survey+(RAMOS)&ots=xicEo-PeXS&sig=vurcvK2fCRuc-_dtWRp6dNQCLGs&redir_esc=y#v=onepage&q=Reproductive%20Age%20Mortality%20Survey%20(RAMOS)&f=false. Accessed 27 June, 2016.

Table 17.7 Underreporting of maternal deaths for women of reproductive age (15–49 years), Los Altos de Chiapas, 2001

Total of deaths of women of reproductive age Altos occurring in Chiapas in 2001[a]	226
Verbal autopsies	190
MM based on research results	30
MM recorded by municipal offices[a]	9
MM incorrectly recorded/municipal offices	20
MM recorded by INEGI	11
MM incorrectly recorded by INEGI[b]	20
Underreporting of MM by municipal offices	70%
Underreporting of MM by INEGI	63%

Source: Maternal mortality and underreporting in the indigenous region of Los Altos de Chiapas, 2005
[a]Fieldwork in 17 Civil Registry Offices
[b]The number of cases incorrectly recorded in INEGI coincides with those of Civil Registry Offices

Table 17.8 Underreporting of maternal deaths for women of reproductive age (15–49) against the variable of receiving medical care before death

	Had medical care	No medical care	Unspecified	Total
Cases officially identified	1	7	3	11
Underreported cases	5	14	0	19
Total cases	6	21	3	30
Percentage of underreported cases	83%	67%		

Municipalities of Los Altos de Chiapas, 200. Source: Field work

underreporting of maternal deaths in the region of Los Altos; the municipal offices reported nine cases; INEGI reported 11; our field work allowed us to identify 30. Therefore, the underreporting of maternal deaths in 2001 was 63% for INEGI and 70% for the municipal offices. These data are important to validate the reliability of different sources of information; a previous study of maternal deaths in Chenalhó between 1988 and 1993 found greater underreporting of MM in the data from INEGI, which was based on medical certificates, but our study now found that the underreporting was a little higher in the data from municipal offices.

When analyzing the relationship between the underreporting of maternal deaths with the receipt of medical care prior to death, we found that in the 30 cases identified as maternal deaths, there were differences depending on whether or not the women had received medical care before death as shown in Table 17.8. Based on the information provided by medical certificates of death, the underreporting of maternal deaths was 83% for women who received medical care and 67% for women who did not receive medical care. From these results it is inferred that medical care before death did not ensure a proper diagnosis of the cause of death.

Despite this, there was an improvement (still not satisfactory) in the certification of maternal deaths. The underreporting of MM decreased by 20% in almost ten years; certification increased over the previous decade and, despite the scarce availability of health services, providing attention to women with obstetric emergencies was prioritized.

17.4.6 The Operation of the Civil Registry Offices in 2015

By 2015, there were several differences between different offices of the CRO. Larger municipalities such as Chamula and Oxchuc, with populations of 76,000 and 43,350 inhabitants, respectively (INEGI 2010), have two CROs with a larger staff. Some of the CROs have become part of the Interactive Module of the State Government (MIGO), which includes Banchiapas, Chiapas Solidario, and the Secretariat of Finance and the Administrative Office. Nine of the sixteen CROs included in our fieldwork were located in these modules, which have newer infrastructure. When they first set up the office in these modules, the civil registry official of Chenalhó[30] said that they even had internet connectivity, but conditions have deteriorated since then with the change of governments. The worst conditions were those of the civil registry office of Santiago el Pinar, located in an office next to the municipal presidency; it had one desk and a file cabinet but not even a typewriter; the official in charge had to go to office of the Court of Peace and Conciliation to use a typewriter to be able to issue the death records. Due to the lack of resources, the civil registry office was often closed.[31] It is important to note that this office was previously located in the MIGO module, but it was ransacked and the stolen equipment was not replaced.

In Chamula, the CRO is located next to the municipal presidency, and even though it is not very well organized, there is more staff and equipment; they have several typewriters and five computers, as well as typists and stenographers. An official[32]of this CRO said that they no longer keep books, unlike the rest of the CRO, because all data are stored in the computers.

Usually, the CROs are open from 9:00 to 15:00; however, some have established culturally appropriate opening times; in Chalchihuitán, for example, the official said[33] that the CRO opens at 6:00 and closes at 3:00; the CRO of Zinacantán[34] opens on Saturdays and Sundays and closes on Mondays and Tuesdays; the office of Chamula opens on Saturdays, which is market day and is convenient for people who come from other towns; in Chenalhó, the civil registry official[35] goes to different neighborhoods in the evenings to issue birth records when there are more than five children who require the service.

Most civil officials have only worked in the indigenous region of Los Altos de Chiapas, except for the official of Chamula, one of the few who does not speak an indigenous language (ILS); he has 26 years of experience and has worked in 20 different civil registry offices in two different regions: La Frailesca and Los Altos. A distinctive feature of the CROs in 2015 is that almost all officials speak an indigenous language, and they consider that this is a quality that makes them ideal for the office. Still, it is not a requirement for the job, even though more than 80% of the population are speakers of indigenous languages (INEGI 2010).

As in the previous decade, the position of civil registry official is a position of confidence, and the designated person can occupy it for long periods until he decides to resign or is discharged for not doing his work properly. They have to deliver monthly reports about each of their main administrative activities, so that their work is constantly evaluated. The officials train an auxiliary, whose willingness to learn is essential to keep the job.

17.4.7 The Registration of Deaths in 2015

The conditions under which the civil registry offices operate have undergone significant changes over the last 25 years. However, the main factor influencing the underreporting of maternal deaths, as stated by civil registry officials, is that Zapatista villages have their own registration systems.[36]

[30] Official of Chenalhó 2015, June 18.

[31] Official of Santiago el Pinar 2015, July 16.

[32] Official of Chamula 2015, June 15.

[33] Official of Chalchihuitán 2015, July 23.

[34] Official of Zinacantán 2015, July 15.

[35] Official of Chenalhó 2015, June 18.

[36] Aldama 2015, June 24; Altamirano 2015, July 7.

Table 17.9 Evolution of the percentage of certificates of deaths of women of reproductive age issued by nonmedical staff, Los Altos de Chiapas, México 1990–2014

Municipality	1990	2000	2013
Aldama	ND	77.8	71.4
Amatenango Del Valle	5.0	3.6	76.4
Chalchihuitán	92.0	25.0	76.5
Chamula	93.3	20.6	3.4
Chanal	45.3	0.0	45.8
Chenalhó	95.3	12.2	5.3
Huixtán	94.1	63.3	77.0
Larráinzar	64.9	5.0	19.1
Mitontic	50.0	11.8	27.5
Oxchuc	1.7	0.0	46.2
Pantelho	69.9	2.0	23.5
San Juan Cancuc	98.2	91.6	88.7
Tenejapa	89.2	35.0	81.0
Zinacantán	91.9	78.3	90.4
Santigo el Pinar	ND	ND	ND
Total	77.4	30.7	45.7

Source: Dirección General de Información en Salud (DGIS). Database of overall deaths, 1979–2013

Another important problem is the persistent lack of blank certificates in some health units, which are sometimes provided by the municipal capitals; the officials themselves have to request the Secretariat of Health for new supplies. The civil registry officials of San Juan Chamula, Mitontic[37] claimed that medical certificates of death had been issued for virtually all death records. This was due to the presence of health centers in the municipal capitals, and that requests of these death records were sent to these health centers,[38] Zinacantán and Chalchihuitán, the officials said that although most people die outside of the health system, there was coordination between the Secretariat of Health and municipal officials to provide the medical certificate and issue the death record. This was performed by the municipal agent, the secretary, the municipal judge, as well as staff of the Health System. Table 17.9 illustrates the evolution of the percentage of certificates issued by nonmedical staff; it can be seen that Chamula, Mitontic, and Larrainzar are the municipalities with the lowest percentage of medical certificates issued by such staff.

The data obtained from DGIS are interesting. According to the Intercensal Survey of 2015, 86% of the indigenous population of Chiapas declared an affiliation (in some way) to the health system, and 76.3% said they used the Popular Insurance (Seguro Popular), although the only tertiary hospital in Los Altos de Chiapas is located in the city of San Cristobal, identified as a *mestizo* town. By 2014, 65% of the women in this region received no medical care before death (Table 17.3); however, this percentage is four times lower when the death is due to maternal causes (83.3%). This indicates that pregnant women, women in labor or in the postpartum period have better access to health services (Table 17.2).

According to officials of Chamula, Mitontic, and Larráinzar, the declarant should ideally be a close relative, but in reality it can be anyone. The declarant and the witnesses are generally men, but the

[37]CR official Chamula and Mitontic, 2015, June 15.

[38]CR official of Chamula, Larráinzar, 2015. July 8.

officials noted that it is common for women to go to the CRO either as companions or as declarants. The predominance of men is attributed to the need for traveling to the CRO from outside the town.[39]

The population is aware that they should inform the authorities about any death within 24 h to avoid committing an irregularity. However, the official of Zinacantán said the death certificate can be issued with a notice of death.[40] The municipal agent issues a death notice specifying the circumstances of the death, and this document is sufficient to avoid having to go through the bureaucratic procedure of an extemporaneous registration.

The CROs of Chamula, Mitontic, and Larráinzar reported that the Justice of the Peace is responsible for mediating between the Public Prosecutor's Office (Ministerio Público; MP) and the population in cases of violent deaths. In other municipalities, the officials indicated that the MP does all the paperwork. Even though a higher percentage of women received medical care before dying, 14.3% of the 77 women who died from maternal causes in Chiapas in 2014 died in their homes, and 26% were indigenous (Freyermuth et al. 2016).

Although the Civil Registry officials said that no cases remain unregistered, in 2014 the Global Pediatrics Alliance documented two unreported cases of maternal mortality, neither of which had been certified or reported to the CR. When the General Directorate of Health Information (ISECH) was notified about these cases, they carried out an investigation and concluded that only one of the cases could be classified as a maternal death.

The compliance that is demanded by the assistance program Prospera (formerly Oportunidades) has created incentives to register deaths and births in the civil registry offices, but has also led to some deaths not being recorded, or to being evasive or even dishonest about the causes of death. According to the Intercensal Survey of 2015,[41] 75% of the indigenous population in Chiapas receives money from some social program; this percentage is higher than the national average, which is 60% for the indigenous population.

This is very important, because transfers from social programs have come to represent a significant proportion of the income of many families in Los Altos, thus becoming one of the main incentives for compliance with the registration of civil acts and, apparently, also for the concealment of certain causes of death, such as those related to maternity.

Conclusions

The Civil Registry was consolidated in the second half of the twentieth century, involving the participation of a large number of actors who determine the way in which it operates. During that period, the State Health System established the guidelines for issuing death records and appropriated the authority to issue a preliminary document, the medical certificate of death; it also started comparing its information with that generated by INEGI. The scarcity of health services in the most dispersed and remote towns has limited the registration of vital events by the CR or the SSA, which means that the activities of these institutions are limited by their presence, especially in populations living beyond the reach of the benefits provided by health protection or social security institutions.

The factors that prevent, in the short term, the documentation of vital events are of a structural nature and are related to the historical context. In the nineteenth century and the first half of the twentieth century, the secularization of the registration of vital events occurred in the broader context of the independence from Spain and of the struggle for power between the State and the Church. In the late twentieth century, the Civil Register offices were part of the structure of municipal

[39] Official of the CR, Municipalities of Aldama and Chalchihuitán 2015, April 1.

[40] Official of the CR, Municipality of Zinacantán, 2015, Feb 13.

[41] Our own estimates based on the Intercensal Survey of 2015.

governments, with all that this implied. This period was marked by processes of decentralization and greater presence of the State in local affairs, which led to the normalization of these offices and to conflicts between the State and local authorities.

Armed conflicts and natural disasters in Central America during the 1980s resulted in migrants coming to Mexico, which in turn caused internal migrations throughout the country, sometimes with the United States as the final destination. This led to the involvement of other government institutions in the definition of the activities of the CR, explaining why, in the late twentieth and early twenty-first century, the Interior Secretariat (Secretaría de Gobernación) has coordinated the definition of such activities. Thus, in the twenty-first century the CR could become what Cosme Varela envisaged after the Independence: an institution responsible not only for documenting vital events but also for public and finance administration and for the political control of the country's inhabitants.

In 2016, there are three government institutions with data bases related to the Civil Registry: (1) the Secretariat of Health, (2) the INEGI, and (3) the National Database of the Civil Registry of RENAPO. This illustrates the poor efficiency in which the government databases are generated. Although each database is used in a different way, it would be more efficient to have an integrated database.

The results of the analysis of the records of maternal deaths of 2001 showed that contact with the health services did not ensure a proper diagnosis of the cause of death. This paradox suggests that health workers could be intentionally concealing maternal deaths, as the reduction of the MMR is considered a priority under the Millennium Development Goals (MDGs). In this context, it could be said that the goverment's actions to reduce maternal deaths had a negative impact on the registration of MM and on the objective to improve the quality of medical care. The failure to register maternal deaths is a bad practice of middle managers aimed at artificially improving statistics or avoiding sanctions for poor management, as maternal death is preventable with the medical resources available in the country. However, the issuance of medical certificates improved over a period of eight years, as shown by the similarity of underreported cases between the information provided by civil registry offices and the databases based on medical certificates of the SSA; this contrasted with the number of underreported cases identified in the 1990s when the use of medical certificates was not so frequent.

This study also recognized how an entity such as the Civil Registry can reflect the relationship of the people with the state and local governments, as well as with the national government; in the case of the region of Los Altos de Chiapas, we saw that, up to the 1990s, the inhabitants of Los Altos had no need to be part of the Mexican nation. When a population regulates all acts by local uses and customs beyond the laws of the National State, the registration of the civil status of persons is meaningless. It was not until after the outbreak of the neo-Zapatista uprising that the federal and state governments undertook initiatives focused on this population and began to provide it with benefits in the form of social programs and public infrastructure.

Our analysis of the documentation of maternal deaths which occurred over a relatively short period of time allows us to appreciate the difficulties that must be overcome to implement even this apparently simple public service. This is true not only in view of the obvious underreporting of maternal deaths that has prevailed for two decades, but also of the faulty registration of the various causes of death. Of course, is also partly the result of the limited presence of health services in this region.

Monitoring federal government programs in this region over nearly three decades has allowed us to recognize their forms of intervention and the influence exercised by the exigencies of the government and the registration of vital events on the practices and representations of the people.

A key role has been played by the social development programs and funds that, since 1998, have been channeled to municipal governments.

Despite the leadership of the Secretariat of Health in the standardization and systematization of demographic information, the discontinuous presence of state health services in this region has created conditions for other local actors to have a great influence on the registration of vital events, including violent deaths, such as Justices of the Peace, municipal presidents and agents, and other local authorities. Due to the importance of population control, civil registry officials have been involved in midwifery and in the creation of a register of midwives outside the public health system.

An important lesson made clear by this study is that public policy initiatives must necessarily be long-term projects, with strategies that transcend the interests of single-term governments, and that involve direct benefits for the population.

References

Álvarez, J. (1960). Historia de la salubridad y de la asistencia en México. (History of health and medical care in Mexico). In J. Álvarez (Ed.), *Tomo I: Historia de la salubridad desde 1910 hasta 1960*. México: SSA.

Álvarez, J., Bustamante, M., López, P. A., & Fernández, F. (1984). Servicios Médicos Coopertativos en la Historia de la Salubridad y Asistencia en México. (Cooperative medical services in the history of health and medical care in Mexico). In H. Hernández (Ed.), *La atención médica rural en México, 1930–1980, Colección Salud y Seguridad Social. Serie Manuales de Estudio*. México: Instituto Mexicano del Seguro Social.

Bustamante, M. (1984). La Coordinación de los Servicios Sanitarios federales y locales como factor de progreso en México. En H. Hernández, (comp.). (Coordination of federal and local health services as a factor of progress in Mexico). In H. Hernández (Ed.), *La atención médica rural en México, 1930–1980, Colección Salud y Seguridad Social, Serie Manuales Básicos de Estudio*. México: Instituto Mexicano del Seguro Social.

Castro, E. (2011). *Diccionario Foucault: temas, conceptos y autores*. (Foucault dictionary: Themes, concepts and authors). Buenos Aires: Siglo XXI Editores.

De la Torre, C. (2006). *El proceso de descentralización y los presupuestos del sector salud en el estado de Chiapas: un análisis del Fondo de Aportaciones para los Servicios de Salud y su impacto en la muerte materna, (Tesis de licenciatura)*, [The process of decentralization and health sector budgets in the state of Chiapas: an analysis of the Contribution Fund for Health Services and its impact on maternal death (Thesis)]. Universidad de Autónoma de Chiapas, México.

Diario Oficial de la Federación (DOF). (2012). *Norma Oficial Mexicana NOM-035-SSA3-2012, en materia de información en salud* (Official Mexican Standard NOM-035-SSA3-2012, In health information), segunda sección. Edición matutina, Editor. Retrieved November 12, 2015 from http://dof.gob.mx/nota_detalle.php?codigo=5280848&fecha=30/11/2012.

Freyermuth, M. G. (1993). *Médicos Indígenas, Médicos Alopatas. Un encuentro difícil en los Altos de Chiapas* (Indigenous physicians, allopathic physicians. A difficult encounter in the Chiapas Highlands). Chiapas: Co-edition of the Goverment of the state of Chiapas and CIESAS-Sureste, Chiapas.

Freyermuth, M. G. & Garza, A. (1996). Muerte Materna en Chenalhó. Informe final presentado al Programa de Salud Reproductiva (Maternal Death in Chenalhó. Final report submitted to the Reproductive Health Program of El Colegio de México) de El Colegio de México, San Cristóbal de Las Casas.

Freyermuth, M., & Fernández, M. (1997). Factores culturales en el registro de la muerte de mujeres en dos municipios de los Altos de Chiapas (Cultural factors in the register of women death in two municipalities in the Altos de Chiapas). In E. Tuñón & U. J. El Colegio de la Frontera Sur (Eds.), *Género y salud en el sureste de México* (pp. 34–54). México: El colegio de la Frontera Sur, Universidad Juárez, Autómona de Tabasco.

Freyermuth, M. G. (2003). Mujeres de humo. *Morir en Chenalhó durante la maternidad* (Women of smoke. Dying in Chenalhó during maternity). CIESAS, Porrua, México.

Freyermuth, M. G. & Cardenas, R. Sesia, P. (2007). *Tercer informe ténico. Mortalidad materna en regiones indígenas: una propuesta metodológica para identificar a municipios de alto riesgo en salud matern.* (Third technical report. Maternal mortality in indigenous regions: A methodological proposal for identifying high-risk municipalities in maternal health) *a.* Cd.: (01-08-2005 a 01-02-2006).

Freyermuth, G., Luna, M. & Muños, J (2016). *Indicadores* 2014. *Mortalidad Materna en México.* (Indicators 2014. Maternal mortality in Mexico). México: Observatorio de Mortalidad Materna.

Guiteras C. (1996) *Los peligros del Alma. Visión del mundo de un tzotzil* (Perils of the soul: The world view of a Tzotzil Indian). 1ª edición 1962, Fondo de Cultura Económica, México.

Guiteras, C. (2002). Diario de San Pablo Chalchihuitán. (Field Journal of San Pablo Chalchihuitán) Pensamiento Contemporáneo, Biblioteca Popular de Chiapas, Consejo Estatal para la Cultura y las Artes de Chiapas, 1ª edición 1946, Tuxtla Gutiérrez, Chiapas.

INEGI. (1990). *Sistema de integración territorial (ITER). Censo de población y vivienda 1990.* Instituto Nacional de Estadística y Geografía. (Territorial integration system, population and housing census 1990). México: INEGI. Retrieved January 20, 2016 from http://www3.inegi.org.mx/sistemas/iter/default.aspx?ev=5.

INEGI. (2010). *Censo de población y vivienda 2010.* Instituto Nacional de Estadística y Geografía. (Population and housing census 2010). México: INEGI. Retrieved July 22, 2016 from http://www3.inegi.org.mx/sistemas/iter/entidad_indicador.aspx?ev=5.

INEGI. (2014). *Estadísticas de Mortalidad.* Instituto Nacional de Estadística y Geografía. (Mortality statistics) México: INEGI. Retrieved June 27, 2016 from http://www.inegi.org.mx/est/contenidos/proyectos/registros/vitales/mortalidad/presentacion.aspx.

INEGI. (2016). *México en cifras. Información nacional, por entidad federativa y municipios.* Instituto Nacional de Estadística y Geografía. (Mexico in figures. National information by state and municipalities). México: INEGI. Retrieved April 27, 2016 from http://www3.inegi.org.mx/sistemas/mexicocifras/default.aspx?e=12.

Meneses, S. (2007). *¿Acceso universal a la atención obstétrica? El seguro Popular de Salud Frente al reto de Mortalidad Materna en Los Altos de Chiapas* (Universal access to obstetric care? The popular health insurance against the challenge of maternal mortality in Los Altos de Chiapas). In D. Diaz (Ed.), *Muerte materna y seguro popular.* México: FUNDAR, Centro de Análisis e Investigación A.C..

Naciones Unidas. (1994). *Informe de la Conferencia Internacional sobre la Población y el Desarrollo. El Cairo, 5 a 13 de septiembre de 1994* (Report of the international conference on population and development. Cairo, September 5ft to 13th, 1994). A/CONF.171/13/Rev.1., Nueva York.

Naciones Unidas (UN). (1995). Conferencia Mundial sobre la Mujer: La mujer indígena se hace cargo de su destino 4 de septiembre de 1995 (Beijing, China [Internet]. Nueva York: Naciones Unidas; 1995 [consultado el 1 de septiembre 2016]. Recuperado de: http://www.cinu.org.mx/biblioteca/documentos/dh/ConfBeijing1995.htm.

Naciones Unidas. (2000). *A/RES/55/2. Resolución aprobada por la Asamblea General* (Resolution adopted by the general assembly). Retrieved March 10, 2015 from http://www.un.org/spanish/milenio/ares552.pdf.

OMS & UNFPA. (1978). Conferencia Internacional sobre Atención Primaria de Salud. *Alma-Ata, URSS, 6–12 de septiembre de 1978 (*International Conference on Primary Health Care. Alma-Ata, USSR, September 6th–12th, 1978). Organización Mundial de la Salud, Ginebra.

Periodico Oficial del Estado de Chiapas. (2011, December 28). Última reforma publicada en el reglamento del registro civil para el estado de Chiapas. (Last reform published in the regulation of civil registration for the state of Chiapas). *Reglamento publicado en la segunda sección del Periódico Oficial del Estado de Chiapas*, México.

Presidencia de la República. (2005). *Los Objetivos de Desarrollo del Milenio en México: Informe de Avances 2005* (The millennium development goals in Mexico: Progress report 2005). Presidencia de la República, Naciones Unidas, México.

Presidencia de la República. (2015) *Tercer Informe de Gobierno 2014–2015, Enrique Peña Nieto* (Third governmental report 2014–2015, Enrique Peña Nieto). Presidencia de la República, Naciones Unidas, México. Retrieved March 29, 2016 from http://www.presidencia.gob.mx/tercerinforme/.

Rus, J. (1995). ¿Guerra de castas según quién?: indios y ladinos en los sucesos de 1869. (Caste War according to whom?: Indians and ladinos in the events of 1869). In J. Viqueira, & M. H. Ruz, *Chiapas: los rumbos de otra historia* (pp. 145–174). UNAM, CIESAS, CEMCA-UDG, México. Available via DIALOG. Retrieved July 30, 2016 from https://books.google.com.mx/books?isbn=9683648363.

SHCP. (2014). Secretaría de Hacienda y Crédito Público. *Aportaciones federales de los fondos que comprenden el ramo 33 por trimestre.* (Federal contributions of funds bouquet comprising branch 33 per quarter). SHCP, México. Retrieved April 10, 2016 from http://www.hacienda.gob.mx/ApartadosHaciendaParaTodos/aportaciones/33/aportaciones.html.

Starrs, A. (1987). *Preventing the tragedy of maternal deaths: a report. International Safe Montherhood Conference. (No. DERAJ-401).* DC; Nairobi, Kenia: PAHO, UNFPA, World Bank Group, Washington.

World Health Organization. (1987). Studying maternal mortality in developing countries: Rates and causes: A guidebook. WHO/FHE/87.7.

18 Misconceived Mortality: Solitary Birth and Maternal Mortality Among the *Rarámuri* of Northern Mexico

Janneli F. Miller

18.1 Introduction

The general assumption in international health circles is that solitary birth is dangerous. The World Health Organization (WHO), the United Nations (UN), The International Confederation of Midwives (ICM), and the International Federation of Gynecologists and Obstetricians (FIGO) all assert that the proven way to reduce infant and maternal mortality is to ensure that all women give birth with a skilled assistant. In addition, they suggest that pregnant women receive at least four antenatal visits during pregnancy and have access to contraception counseling. These efforts have been stated clearly in the UN's Millennium Development Goals (MDGs). Goal 4 addresses the reduction of child mortality and Goal 5 targets the improvement of maternal health.

While there has been some moderate success in many regions of the world, the MDG 2015 report stated that "Improving maternal health is part of the unfinished agenda for the post-2015 period" (Way 2016:43). Notably, the women who are still not receiving skilled assistance at birth tend to live in rural indigenous regions of the world. "Data on maternal care revealed that around 2000, the proportion of births attended by health professionals was 38 percentage points lower among indigenous women than non-indigenous women in Mexico" (MDG 2015:11).

The rural indigenous *Rarámuri* women of Northern Mexico present an interesting case as regards the idea that maternal mortality will decrease by making sure all births have a skilled attendant present, since they have a long-standing tradition of solitary birth. In this chapter I suggest that providing culturally appropriate reproductive health care is as important—if not more important—than ensuring a skilled attendant is present at birth. If reproductive health care services are not provided to women in culturally congruent ways, then the very services designed to reduce maternal mortality may actually impede these efforts. After presenting *Rarámuri* birth practices and information on maternal mortality among this indigenous group, I conclude by discussing the trajectory by which efforts designed to improve maternal mortality actually end up being deleterious to women and their families, as outlined in Fig. 18.1.

J. F. Miller, Ph.D.
Independent Scholar, Dolores, CO, USA

D. A. Schwartz (ed.), *Maternal Death and Pregnancy-Related Morbidity Among Indigenous Women of Mexico and Central America*, Global Maternal and Child Health: Medical, Anthropological, and Public Health Perspectives, https://doi.org/10.1007/978-3-319-71538-4_18

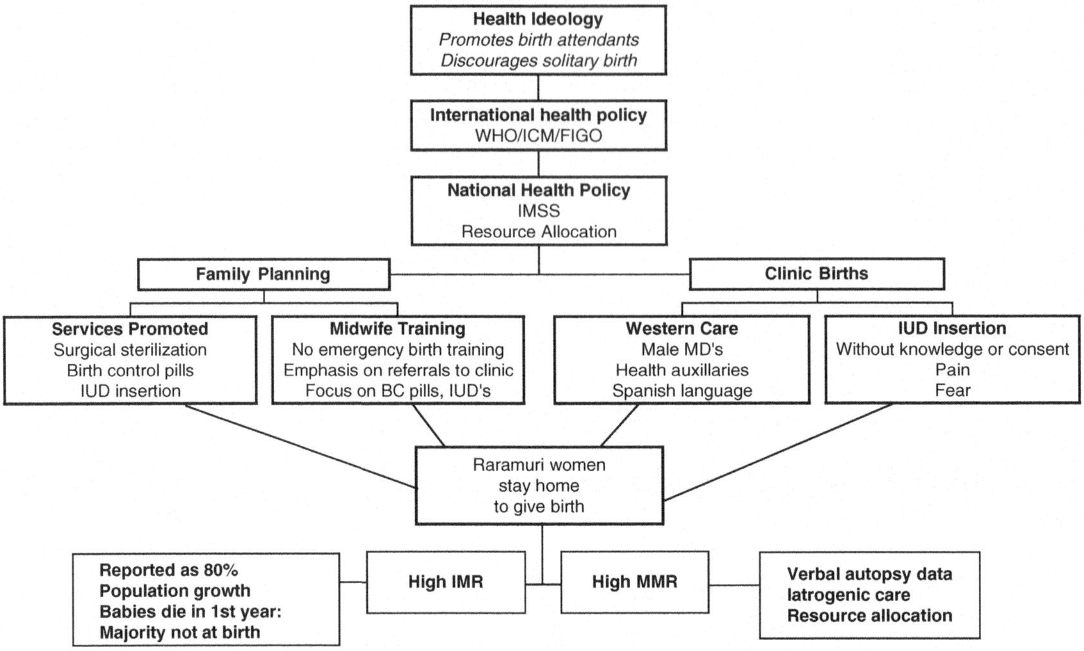

Fig. 18.1 Global health ideology dictates policy and impacts local practices (Miller 2010). Published with kind permission of © Janneli F. Miller 2017. All Rights Reserved

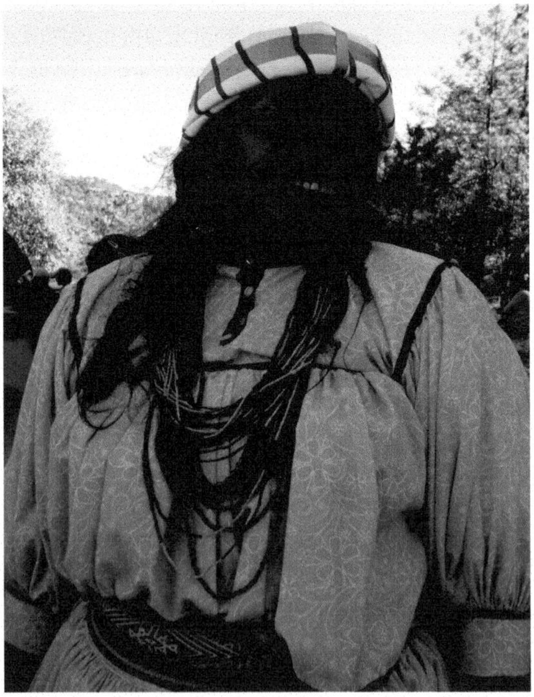

Fig. 18.2 This *Rarámuri* woman has five children, all born at home. Published with kind permission of © Janneli F. Miller 2017. All Rights Reserved

This *Rarámuri* example affirms and complements the work of Mounia El Kotni (El Kotni, this book, Chap. 6) among indigenous women, since in Chihuahua as in Chiapas, structural violence is indeed a root cause of maternal and infant mortality among indigenous women. Much of what is presented in El Kotni's chapter as regards international and national health policy in Mexico pertains to Chihuahua, thus will not be repeated here. Yet among the *Rarámuri* we see how not only structural violence, but also "euphemized violence" (Ginsburg and Rapp 1995) is at work, since the idea that solitary birth is dangerous is never called into question. Instead, rural indigenous women are blamed for not utilizing available services, while efforts to provide skilled attendants, contraceptive care, and train midwives are normalized and augmented, often exacerbating the very conditions they intend to prevent.

18.2 Methods

This chapter is based upon ethnographic research carried out in Mexico from 1998 to 2015, in two settings. I lived in a *Rarámuri* village in the *municipio* of Guachochi, in the Sierra Madres of Chihuahua, from 1999 to 2001, returning annually through 2010 and again in 2015. In 1998/9 I conducted research among *Rarámuri* living in the urban *asentimientos* or *barrios* of Chihuahua City, in order to determine if solitary birth practice was impacted by increased access to medical care, as is often suggested.

I used typical anthropological methods including extensive participant observation in both the Sierra Madre and Chihuahua City, observing hospital births and visits, clinic births and health interactions, as well as participating in the daily life of the village, including ceremonies, foot races, food preparation, planting and harvesting of crops, and all other aspects of *Tarahumara* life. I conducted both semi-structured and open-ended interviews with *Rarámuri* women, men, and children; *Rarámuri owirúame* (healers) and village governors; *mestizo* health care professionals including doctors, nurses, hospital directors, and health auxiliaries; social workers, educators, politicians, priests, Mexican anthropologists, and *mestizo* citizens. I elicited reproductive narratives from over fifty *Rarámuri* women in both settings. I also interviewed and conducted life histories with thirteen *mestizo* midwives

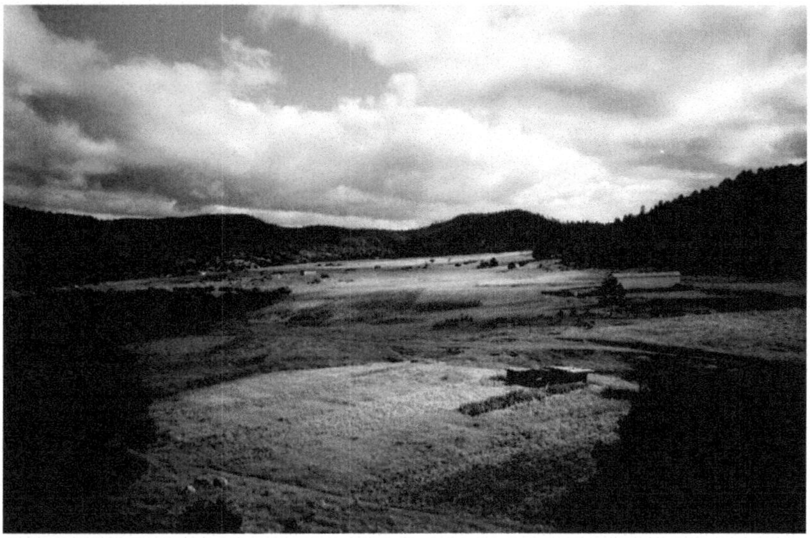

Fig. 18.3 View of the village where author lived for 2 years. Corn and bean fields in foreground by traditional house. A seventeenth century Franciscan church is on the right. Published with kind permission of © Janneli F. Miller 2017. All Rights Reserved

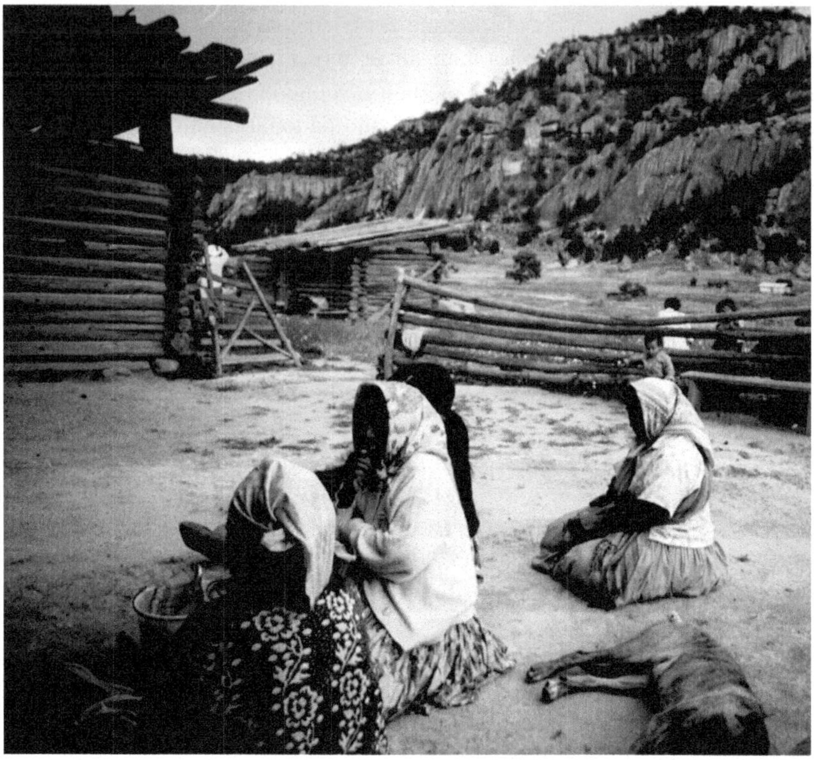

Fig. 18.4 *Rarámuri* women chat and gossip during a *tesguinada* while their children play. Published with kind permission of © Janneli F. Miller 2017. All Rights Reserved

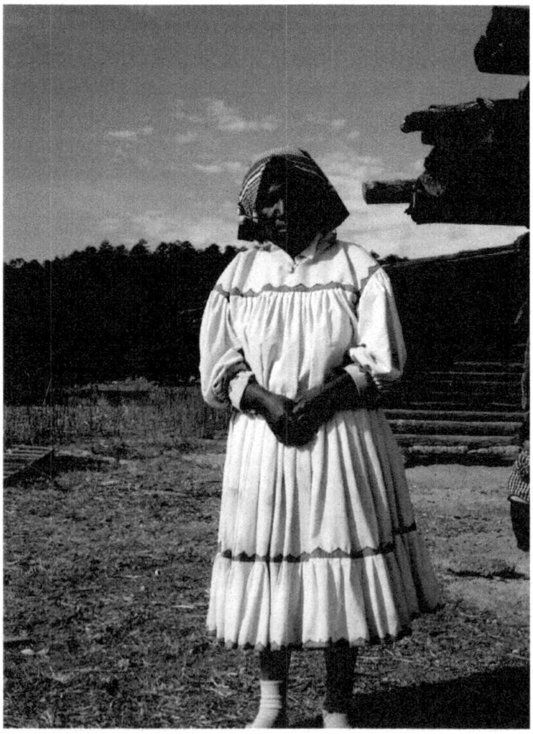

Fig. 18.5 A *Rarámuri* woman from rural Chihuahua. Published with kind permission of © Janneli F. Miller 2017. All Rights Reserved

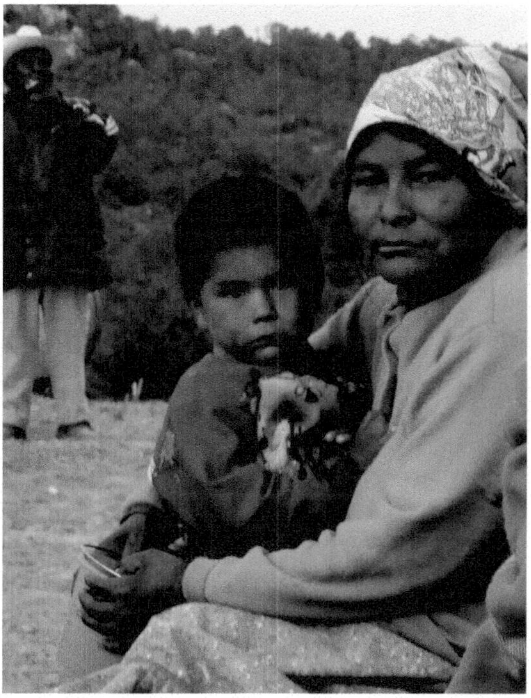

Fig. 18.6 A *Rarámuri* grandmother holds her grandson. Published with kind permission of © Janneli F. Miller 2017. All Rights Reserved

living in Guachochi, and attended thirteen of their monthly training sessions (1999–2000) provided by the Mexican Social Security agency (IMSS). My research in the Sierra was sponsored by a Fulbright Garcia-Robles dissertation grant, as well as Spicer-Comins, Riecker, and summer research grants from the University of Arizona).

18.3 *"Se Alivian Solas, Como Las Chivas"*

Rarámuri women have a long-standing tradition of giving birth alone, outside. Most people with any knowledge of the *Rarámuri* know they give birth alone, and may repeat verbatim the pejorative phrase above which translates as "they give birth alone, like goats" (Miller 2003). Interestingly, the same phrase has also been used to title a recent publication (Chopel 2014). The practice and knowledge of solitary birth among the *Tarahumara* has been publicly documented since Norwegian explorer Carl Lumholz trekked through Mexico in the late 1800s (Lumholz 1902:271). Scholars working in the Sierra Madre have noted the practice (Bennett and Zingg 1935:234) and usually the more generalized the account the more dramatic the description becomes, with women not only compared to goats, but the childbearing experience described as "primitive, often tragic" (Cassell 1969:110), or as taking place "without any other help than that of a branch" (Espino Loya 1987:13). Generally, portrayals of the solitary birthing customs of the *Rarámuri* align with the international health ideologies, suggesting that the practice is dangerous and women birthing alone outside are in need of "rescue" (Miller 2003:307).

My research focused on normative cultural values that explain how and why giving birth alone is not perceived to be dangerous or risky by *Rarámuri* women. While most of that discussion is beyond the realm of this chapter, several key points are cogent to the discussion of mortality. The Rarámuri do not have a word in their language (*Tarahumara*, a member of the *Uto-Aztecan* language family) for

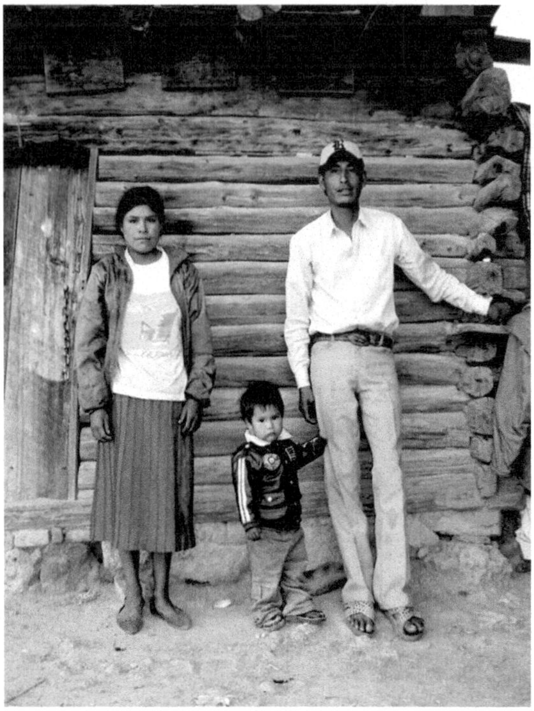

Fig. 18.7 A young *Rarámuri* family in front of their home. The child is a year and a half old, and was born in the clinic when his mother was 15 and her husband 17. Note the adoption of *mestizo* clothing. She received an intrauterine device (IUD) when her son was born, and when she asked about it was told that it couldn't be taken out. Published with kind permission of © Janneli F. Miller 2017. All Rights Reserved

someone who is a "midwife" or "helper" at birth. Giving birth is perceived to be a normal function of a woman's body, and the risks associated with it are not any more or less than risks associated with the vagaries of living a subsistence lifestyle in a remote canyon region.

Rarámuri value modesty and do not draw attention to themselves, especially when pregnant. After a woman notifies the local *owirúame* (healer) of her pregnancy, she pretty much carries on with her daily duties. There are no food restrictions nor taboos associated with pregnancy, other than refraining from heavy lifting and living a moral life—speaking well and working well and participating in ceremonies. A pregnant woman does not talk about her own pregnancy, and minimizes her exposure to danger by staying home where she is surrounded by trusted people. Women, men, and children know about pregnancy and birth, and women learn about birth from female kin as children.

I documented place of birth among women in the Sierra, and of 179 births to forty-one women, eighty percent of births took place at home, six percent at hospitals, six percent at clinics, and eight percent in the *"monte"* (outside). At the time of my research, women were moving away from the *monte* and into their homes to deliver, because it was not as safe due to increasing presence of loggers, *narcos* (drug growers and traffickers), and tourists. In Chihuahua City, where reproductive services were available, sixty-five percent of women gave birth at home, and fifteen percent in hospitals and clinics. The higher number of women giving birth in hospitals and clinics was explained by the fact that many of the women lived in the urban settlements, where they were often watched by social workers who would take them to the clinic if they complained of labor pains. Indeed, many women living in the *asentimientos* explained that they had to hide out to give birth at home, where they felt safer alone than surrounded by strangers.

In the Sierra, 53% of women giving birth at home were attended by their husbands, similar to the forty-nine percent who were attended at home by their husbands in the city. Twenty percent of women delivering at home in the Sierra gave birth alone, while 25% did so in the city. Other attendants at home birth in the Sierra included mothers (11%), husband and mother (9%), husband and mother-in-law (6%), and grandmother (1%). In Chihuahua City, mothers and grandmothers were each present at 13% of the home deliveries. Reasons and patterns for these numbers are further explained in another publication (Miller 2009), but it is apparent from the above numbers that women choose to deliver at home in both the urban and *serrano* setting, and that if they are not alone, their husbands are their preferred attendants, followed by female relatives.

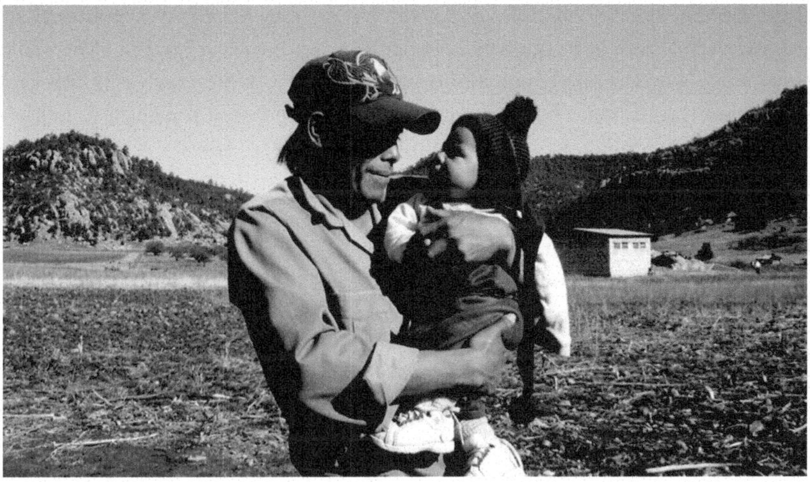

Fig. 18.8 A *Rarámuri* father and his third child, born at the clinic. Men are involved in child care as much as women. Published with kind permission of © Janneli F. Miller 2017. All Rights Reserved

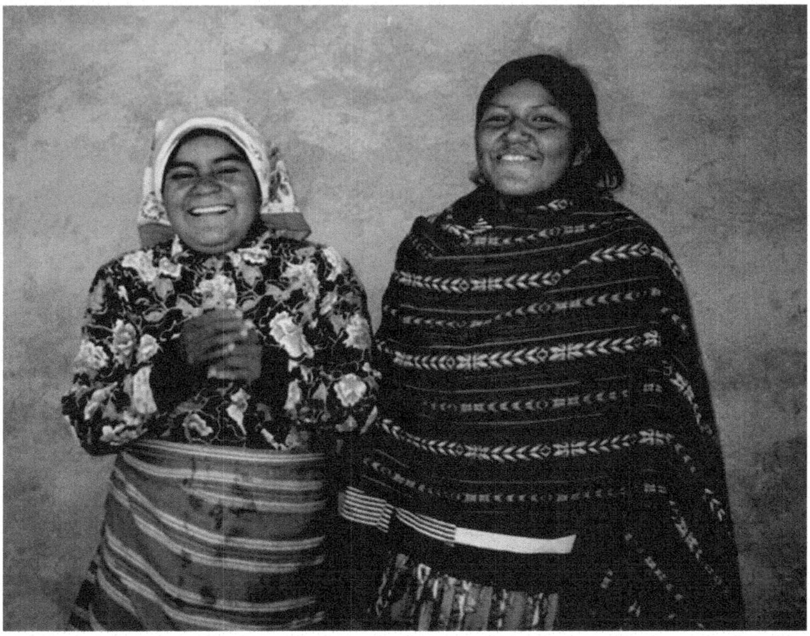

Fig. 18.9 Two young *Rarámuri* women sharing a joke. Lola, on the left, is pregnant with her first child. Alma on the right gave birth to her first child at her mother's house at age 15. Published with kind permission of © Janneli F. Miller 2017. All Rights Reserved

18.4 Maternal Mortality in the Sierra

18.4.1 Maria's Story

Maria had three children and was expecting her fourth in the summer of 2001. She lived in La Laja with her husband Santiago, but they also farmed fields given to her by her parents, in the *ranchería* of Ricubichi. It was about a three-hour walk between these two places, and the family had homes in each, since they spent equal amounts of time in both *ranchos*. La Laja was adjacent to the highway, and thus closer to the clinic than Ricubichi, which was approximately four hours walk away from the nearest road. Maria visited the clinic during her pregnancy several times, at first because her husband wanted her to, and subsequently because the auxiliaries (clinic health workers with no medical licensure) were worried about her blood pressure (BP), which was running high. Because of this worry, they convinced her and her husband that she should wait for labor to begin in the clinic's *albergue,* a small building adjacent to the clinic with two rooms, a kitchenette, and bathroom facilities. Convalescing *Rarámuri* stay here when they are still too weak to return to their *ranchos*, but well enough not to be hospitalized. Maria and her husband Santiago agreed, and stayed in town for two weeks in early July when Maria was due. But as the days passed and she did not go into labor, Maria and her husband became anxious. They had left their three children with Maria's parents, and nobody was tending their fields. It was a rainy summer, meaning the cornfields needed frequent weeding so that the weeds would not choke out the nascent corn. Santiago left several times for a day or two during this period to tend the *rancho* in La Laja, but nobody was taking care of their crops in Ricubichi. They also missed their children and grew tired of staying in town, where they had nothing to do but wait. Maria had her BP checked several times during this two-week period, and it was normal each time. Finally, one morning at dawn, she and her husband left the *albergue* without telling the auxiliaries. The auxiliaries were upset that she returned to her *rancho,* but then again, they understood that Maria and her husband were more comfortable in the *rancho* than in town, and besides, her BP was normal and Maria had no other risk factors other than the usual ones of being *Rarámuri* and a multipara. What could they do?

Maria and Santiago stopped in at La Laja to check on their animals and corn, and then proceeded on to Ricubichi, where their children were. They were happy to be home, and even more so to receive invitations to drink *batari* (fermented corn drink) at the home of one of Santiago's brothers. Unfortunately, during the *tesguinada* (drinking party) tragedy struck in the form of a lightning bolt, which landed in the center of the patio, killing one man and knocking over several others. Maria was close to the lightning bolt strike, receiving a burn on the right side of her body. During this season afternoon storms are a daily occurrence, and lightning bolts are common. People scurry about their afternoon chores with an anxious look toward the sky. When it rains heavily people huddle inside their houses or under rock overhangs, and children are scolded to come in so they will not be hit by lightning. This particular lightning strike was unusual, in that it killed one man and injured several others. There was much talk about witchcraft, because powerful *sukurúame* (sorcerers) are said to be able to control lightning. In this case, the man who died was thought to be having sexual relations with a woman in another nearby *rancho*. Apparently, his jealous wife had gone to a *sukurúame,* who had contrived to kill the man by sending the lightning bolt.

There was a somber death *fiesta* for the man killed by lightning, with people wary of lightning or afraid of *sukurúame*. In quiet conversations, villagers wondered why *Onorúame* (god) had sent such powerful storms. The storms increased in intensity, flooding fields and causing streams to run dangerously fast. *Rarámuri* who had waited anxiously through a dry spring, wondering if their corn would sprout, now watched it turn yellow under the grey skies and torrents of rain. People were tense.

One day, about a week after the ill-fated *tesguinada*, a *Rarámuri* man came to my house asking me to help a woman in labor. Maria had gone into labor in Ricubichi that morning, but by late afternoon she was "very sick" and the baby had still not arrived. (Most labors only last from 6 to 8 h). The villagers knew that I had something to do with the clinics, or medicines, and wanted me to come to a nearby *rancho* to wait for Maria, who was being brought up the trail in a wheelbarrow. Maria's relatives thought we could get her to the clinic faster if I was at the trailhead with my truck. I agreed and set off with a graduate student, Estela, who was visiting me to learn more about the *Rarámuri* in preparation for her fieldwork. An excerpt from my field notes continues the story:

6 pm. Everyone said it would take 2 h to get from Ricubichi to Basigochito, and I was notified at 5 pm, so we were thinking that sometime soon they would come. I worried about my ability to help, wondering what I could really do here on the trail if labor was protracted. And would I know what was wrong and how to help? I was thinking of the woman in labor, who was now being wheeled up the trail in the rain, because she could not walk.

8 pm. It got real cold. Colder and colder and colder. We put on one layer of coats, then another, then another. Then we got in the truck to stay warm, then we shut the doors of the truck. It was amazing how fast it got cold, too cold for July. Heavy fog rolled in down canyon where the trail toward Ricubichi was, and where we kept looking for any sign of people coming. Nothing, nobody. Now and then Estela or I said something about the cold, but mostly we just waited in anxious silence. It was growing dark.

8:15 pm. It was cold and grey, damp with fog roiling in over the canyon, thick and grey and ominous looking. We shivered. I talked with Estela and decided that the best we could do when the woman arrived was to get her vital signs, listen to the heart tones and perhaps check her dilation—I'd then decide from there. I got my BP cuff, a glove, and the doptone (fetal heart monitor) ready so I could check vitals fast—because of the cold and the oncoming dark. All of a sudden a younger man comes out of the fog telling us that they will be here soon. "How are they carrying the woman I ask?" "*En lomo, como muerto, casi es muerto, yo no se*". (On their backs like dead are carried, she is almost dead, I don't know). This really concerned me and put me in a whole other mind set. It is way more serious than I thought, out of my control. "Can the woman talk?" I am trying to find out if she is conscious. "*No, no habla*," (no, no she doesn't speak) and she's choking, *basquiando*, kind of spitting up, vomiting. We wait together silently another 15 or 20 min or so and then he says, "There they are."

Out of the darkness, materializing out of the fog, Santiago appears. I don't even recognize him because of the tortured expression on his face, and upon seeing me he says, "*Ya se pasó.*" (She already passed.) I am not sure what he means, thinking they already passed by us in the dark, so I say "*Donde*?" (where), and he motions over to a group of people who are walking: three women and five men. They have tied blankets on a pole and Maria is in the blankets. "*Ya se pasó.*" They say it again, "Just now, just a few minutes ago." They bring her up to where I am standing, Estela is in the truck, and I finally understand that it means Maria just died, just barely before they arrived, and Antonio tells me two times how she choked, how she was vomiting, and then she choked, and then she passed, and this just happened.

I ask if I can check her, and they stand around, "*ayena, ayena*," (yes, yes) looking at each other, and I reach in to find her arm, a wrist, unwrapping the blanket tentatively, not sure what I should or should not do. But if she is dead, she is dead, and I find her arm. It is warm. I feel her wrist; no pulse, but her body is warm. I am disturbed by the contrast between the cold night and the warm body. What to do?

I stand up and everyone looks at me. Someone says again, "it just happened." I have this terrible thought: what if the baby is still alive? I ask if I can listen to the baby's heartbeat to see if the baby is still alive, and they all give me permission, all her relatives, nodding their heads and standing solemnly around the blanket and the pole, looking at me, and watching my every move.

Maria's head is covered, and Santiago, the father, *desesperado* (desperate) just wringing his hands literally and so grief stricken he can barely comprehend the situation. The others are calmer, silent, wary. I get the doptone, turn it on, and search for the heart tones, with everyone continuing to watch me intently. But no familiar rhythm comes, the doptone is silent, and part of me is glad, because, what would I do if the baby was alive? I don't think I have the guts to cut the baby out.

It was so sad and intense, but I don't get any heart tones. So tragic to feel her warm belly, and think of the hearts that just stopped beating. I cover Maria's belly back up, and I tell the relatives that the baby has also died.

This seems to be a relief to them, her aunts and brothers and sisters and husband. "*Ayena*," they say. Her brother continues, "Yes, we know, that is probably why she died. She was hit by lighting and the lightning probably killed the baby and that's why she died, that's why the baby wouldn't come. A week ago when the man was killed by lightning, she too was right by him, so we think that the lightning also did her some damage."

The words spill out into the cold bleak night.

Maria was buried the next day, without ceremony. A handful of family members gathered to perform the rituals associated with death. Women bathed Maria at sunrise, peeking and then wincing at the bruised and burned skin on her right leg, abdomen, and neck. Her hands were joined together and a small wooden cross placed in them. The men built a simple coffin, and when they had placed Maria's body inside it, the small group stood quietly around while one of the *sontasi* (soldiers) gave a *nawésari* (public speech), admonishing Maria to stay away from her relatives and leave her husband and children in peace. After this brief ceremony or *velación*, the body was taken to the graveyard, where other male relatives had already dug the grave. Only men are allowed to participate in burials, and in this case, Maria's husband was so distraught he did not attend, instead returning to La Laja with his children as soon as the *nawesari* was completed.

18.4.2 After Maria's Death

Maria's death was attributed to the lightning bolt. Her husband wandered around grief stricken for a few days in a state of shock. When you looked into his eyes it was as if he did not hear or see you. He weeded his fields and attended *tesguinadas,* but clearly he was in an altered state. The children returned to Ricubichi to stay with Maria's mother. There was some conjecture about how close Maria had been to the man who died, and whether or not the lightning bolt had really killed her. At the *velación,* some of the women moved Maria's clothing to see if her body had really been burned. There was a purple bruise on the right side of her neck and shoulder, and a dark patch on her leg. General consensus was that the lightning bolt had killed the baby, which is why it would not come out, and this was why Maria died.

Notably, Maria's death was not recorded in any clinic records. The auxiliaries at the clinic had heard about Maria's death, and I queried them as to whether or not they thought she had died from eclampsia. This was my best assessment, since it appeared she had mini-seizures before her death. The auxiliaries really did not know, since Maria's BP had been normal in the last weeks of her pregnancy, during her stay at the clinic, and they had not made a diagnosis. Eclampsia is associated with abnormally high blood pressure at the end of pregnancy, which causes seizures that often kill both mother and child if left untreated. Normal treatment is bed rest and medication. Maria had not received this treatment regimen, since her BP had been normal for those two weeks she was at the clinic, and nobody knows what her BP was once she left for Ricubichi. One auxiliary voiced the opinion that she would not have died if she would have only stayed at the clinic where they could have monitored her. Yet clearly, staying at the *albergue* was not tenable for their lifestyle, since daily responsibilities required both Maria and Santiago's presence at home. I mentioned the *tesguinada* and the lightning bolt, and what Maria's relatives had said and thought about the death. Upon hearing this, another of the auxiliaries, a *mestiza*, looked at me and stated gravely, "Well, yes, then I believe the lightning killed her. Who knows, it could be true".

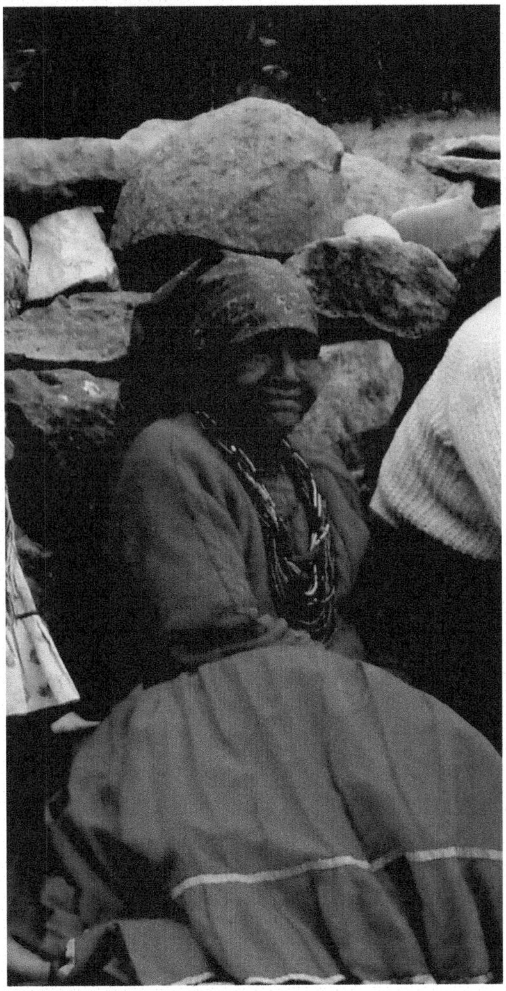

Fig. 18.10 This *Rarámuri* woman gave birth to her children alone in the *monte*. Published with kind permission of © Janneli F. Miller 2017. All Rights Reserved

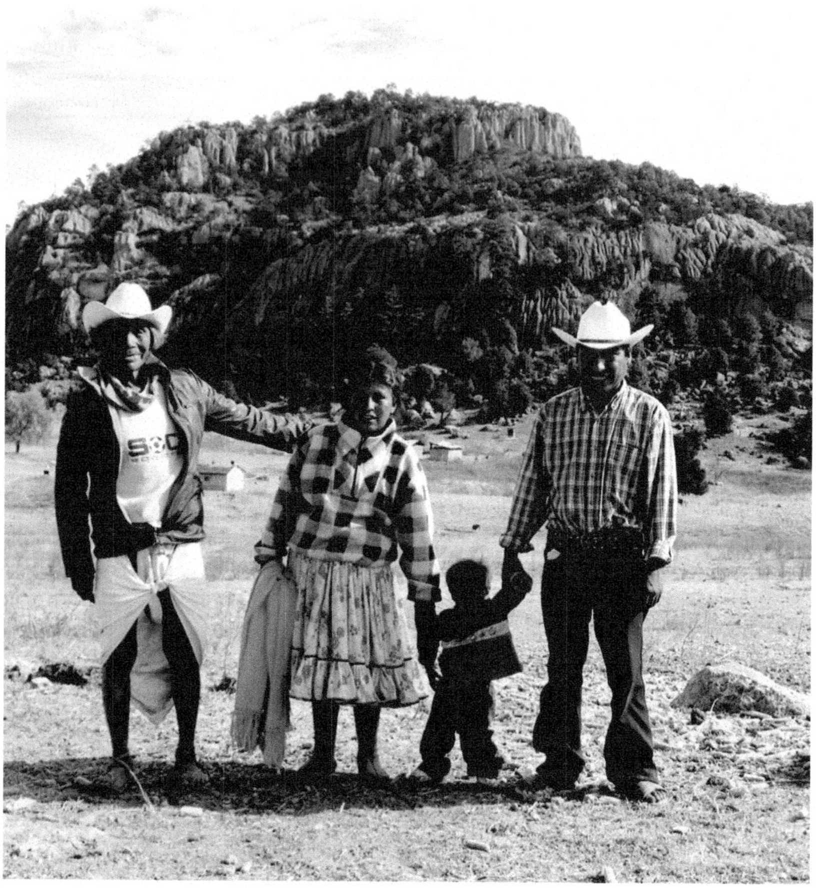

Fig. 18.11 A *Tarahumara sipaame* (shaman) on the left stands with his granddaughter and her family. She gave birth to this child in the clinic and an IUD was inserted, causing her much distress, emotionally and physically. Published with kind permission of © Janneli F. Miller 2017. All Rights Reserved

18.5 The Rarámuri Do Not Fear Birth

Rarámuri women I spoke with did not fear birth. They regarded it as a natural body process, fraught with the same kind of risk and uncertainty that any other physical condition might be. Pregnancy is not considered to be an illness, and although people recognize that babies die, and less frequently, women themselves; death during pregnancy or birth is not particularly feared. Rarámuri do not speak of death directly. Instead they say that a person's life "went out," or "stopped." The verb *suwimea* means to go out or stop, and is used in reference to one's life, as well as to other things, like money or clothing (Brambila 1976:543). Another word, *mukumea*, is also used, but when *Rarámuri* in Basigochi translated either word they used the Spanish *acabar*, which means to stop. The sense is that one's souls go out of the body, and when they go out, the life in the body stops. Souls come and go from one's body in life, usually when sick or drunk (Merrill 1988:88), but when they go out and cannot be coerced to return (usually by an *owirúame*), then the person dies. Death, of course, comes from illness, but can also come from shock or fright, as well as witchcraft; thus the idea that one can be killed by a lightning bolt incorporates not only the physical danger of electrocution, but also the social danger of being so frightened that one's souls cannot be retrieved. This idea of fright or shock chasing and scaring the souls out of the body is similar to the Mexican notion of *susto*, but *Rarámuri* do not use this term.

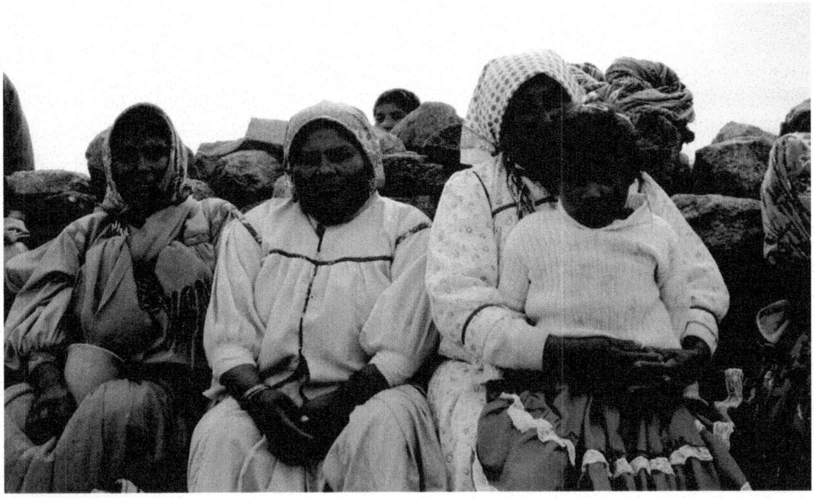

Fig. 18.12 Four generations of Rarámuri women—the mothers all gave birth at home, with their husbands. Published with kind permission of © Janneli F. Miller 2017. All Rights Reserved

Rarámuri do not usually fear death itself. Instead, because it is something they come into contact with frequently in life, they understand it as an inevitable part of life and sometimes it is even desired (Merrill 1988:160). They experience sadness and grief from the loss of a loved one, but their expression of these emotions is different than western practice, in that they believe it is not healthy to remain sad for long periods of time. They try not to dwell on the strong negative feelings they have, so as not to draw sickness to themselves, or make the dead person feel bad. Death *fiestas* warrant drinking, joking, dancing, and demonstration of happiness just as any other occasion would. The dead are said to be lonely and want to return to the living. For this reason it is the responsibility of the living to make sure the dead do not return. This is accomplished by death *fiestas,* which are held three times for a man and four for a woman. During these *fiestas* people talk to the dead, an altar is made with the dead person's possessions, and food and *tesguino* are offered. Usually the home where the dead person lived is abandoned or destroyed, so the dead person will not return. The *fiestas* have the purpose of reassuring the dead that their relatives are happy, and also that the dead should leave them alone. Sadness may cause a dead person to return, since the dead will want to return to comfort their loved ones. Thus, *Rarámuri* valiantly attempt to overcome their grief and enjoy life.

Pregnant *Rarámuri* women do not see themselves as any more vulnerable to death than when they are not pregnant. Instead, pregnant women's fears focus on witchcraft and *sukurúame*. This is an important reason why a woman must demonstrate the ideal behaviors of thinking well and behaving well. By doing so, she will not draw attention to herself, or her condition, since it is aberrant behavior that may attract the attention of a potential sorcerer. She further protects herself by engaging an *owirúame* (doctor/shaman) to watch over her pregnancy in his dreams. The *owirúame* will be able to determine if a *sukurúame* intends the pregnant woman harm, and will be able to inform the woman of any precautionary measures she needs to take, or whether or not a curing ceremony is necessary.

However, these measures do not protect her from the dangers inherent through contact with outsiders, including *mestizo* health care providers, or other clinic patients, all of whom are unknown and carry a very real threat of exposing her to danger. Fear of witchcraft is one reason women fear clinics and hospitals, and indeed, any kind of western medical care includes this threat, since it involves contact with *mestizos*. Women with more knowledge and exposure to *mestizos* have less fear of the clinics and hospitals, although they too make sure to protect themselves by accessing *owirúame* and participating in curing ceremonies.

Thus, in general, pregnancy and birth are not necessarily feared by the *Rarámuri*—instead, contact with outsiders is what is considered dangerous during these times. Staying home to deliver a baby at home (or in the woods) alone or with a trusted family member, such as her husband, a child, or a

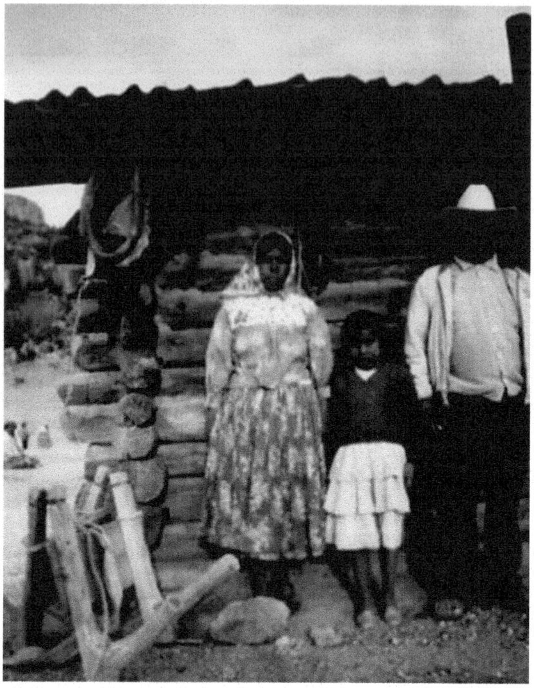

Fig. 18.13 *Tarahumara* family with their only daughter. Lupe was not able to have any more children after having her first in the clinic—she may have been surgically sterilized without her knowledge or consent. Published with kind permission of © Janneli F. Miller 2017. All Rights Reserved

mother or mother-in-law, is perceived to carry less risk than venturing out to the *mestizo* world where things cannot be controlled and people cannot be trusted. Giving birth in a clinic or hospital carries the risk of the unknown, and places the woman entirely outside of her cultural norms.

Maternal mortality is defined as the death of a woman while pregnant or within 42 days of terminations of pregnancy, irrespective of the duration and site of the pregnancy, from any cause related to or aggravated by the pregnancy or its management but not from accidental or incidental causes (Ghosh 2001:429; Schwartz 2015a).

As with infant mortality, there are many acknowledged factors contributing to maternal mortality, including access to health care facilities and quality of health care services received, socioeconomic conditions influencing the nutritional and health status of women, use of family planning services, fertility rate, and health-seeking behaviors including cultural and political factors (Ghosh 2001; Janes 2001; Royston and Armstrong 1989; Schwartz 2015b). Unassisted births have been identified as one of the primary causes of maternal mortality (AbouZahr and Wardlaw 2001:563; Family Care International 2002). Causes of maternal mortality may be categorized as either direct, indirect, or coincidental. Direct causes are those that occur only during pregnancy, indirect causes refer to underlying diseases complicated by pregnancy, such as diabetes or tuberculosis, and coincidental causes of deaths have nothing to do with the pregnancy, such as car accidents. Sociocultural influences leading women to hesitate seeking medical care are listed as indirect causes, while postpartum hemorrhage is a direct cause. The number one cause of maternal mortality globally is hemorrhage, followed by infection and eclampsia (Schwartz 2015a,b).

All indirect causes are listed together and account for twenty percent of maternal deaths worldwide (Ghosh 2001:430; Langer et al. 1994; Family Care International 2002). In Mexico, the medical causes of maternal mortality are the same as elsewhere (Lozano et al. 1994). Pregnant women die from hemorrhage, seizures, and infection, no matter where they live or what their ethnic heritage may be. Notably, the indirect causes of status of women and quality of services have been singled out, in addition to direct causes, as the three essential factors contributing to high levels of maternal mortality and morbidity in Mexico (Langer et al. 1994). Medical causes of maternal mortality, which account for fifty percent of maternal deaths, are thought to be preventable, since hemorrhage can be medically or surgically stopped, infection is treated with antibiotics, and the hypertensive diseases of pregnancy (preeclampsia and eclampsia), if discovered prenatally, can usually be avoided or treated with medications and/or cesarean section. Given these circumstances, the key to lower maternal mortality is thought to be increased access to medical services.

Indirect causes account for one-quarter of maternal deaths (Ghosh 2001) and include conditions influencing a woman's ability to access services—which, in addition to transportation or economic access, must include cultural predilections such as Rarámuri modesty, fear of sorcery, and subsequent aversion to contact with outsiders.

Although Mexico's maternal mortality ratio (MMR) decreased from 90 to 38 maternal deaths per 100,000 live births between the years 1990 and 2015, the ratio remains high in those rural areas where most indigenous women reside. A woman living in a community with less than 2500 residents has double the risk or dying during childbirth than does a woman residing in an urban area (Lozano et al. 1994). Women who live in marginalized households without electricity or running water, who have less education, and who are indigenous are all at higher risk of dying in childbirth. There is also a geographical distribution, in which northern Mexican states report lower rates of maternal mortality than do southern states (Lozano et al. 1994). While this is true using aggregate data, it has led to a situation in which, according to Dr. Pérez, director of the IMSS hospital in Guachochi, attention in Mexico is focused on improving conditions in the south, while the northern regions, such as the Sierra Tarahumara, are ignored.

Health care administrators in Guachochi (Dra. Judith Zazueta, Director of Reproductive Health for the Secretary of Health Services, Dr. Pérez, the Director of the IMSS hospital, and Dr. Roque of the National Indigenous Institute) have insisted that Guachochi has the highest maternal mortality of any *municipio* in the country of Mexico because the *Rarámuri* give birth alone. The *municipio* of Guachochi has the largest indigenous population in the state of Chihuahua, with seventy percent of the residents over five speaking an indigenous ethnic language. This statistic is calculated based upon the assumption that most people speaking an indigenous language in Guachochi are *Tarahumara*. The high maternal mortality rates in Guachochi are explained by the fact that indigenous women do not use clinic facilities during pregnancy or labor. I was told this by all of the administrators above, in addition to Dra. Veronica Villegas, the subdirector of reproductive health for the state of Chihuahua.

However, I complied verbal autopsy data for the five *Rarámuri* women who died at birth in *municipio* Guachochi in 1999, and found that out of these five, only two of them fit the stereotype of women not utilizing services (Table 18.1). The other three did indeed receive prenatal care, and three of them died in the hospital, not at home, including one maternal death from an indirect cause (tuberculosis) and another from a cause that is not considered "preventable" (embolism). It should be noted that all *Rarámuri* women are classified as having such pregnancy risk factors as alcoholism and nutritional deficiency since they drink *batari* at ceremonies even when pregnant (although they usually only take a few sips), and their diets are found to be lacking in protein and iron.

Table 18.1 Verbal autopsy data for women dying at birth in Guachochi in 1999. Source: Secretary of Health, Department of Reproductive Health, Guachochi, Chihuahua

Age	Ethnicity	Pregnancy	Prenatal care	Nutrition	Risk factors	Site of death	Cause
25	Rarámuri	Second	None	Deficient	Alcoholism	Home	Postpartum hemorrhage
28	Rarámuri	Fourth	3 visits	Deficient	Alcoholism	Hospital	Eclampsia
28	Rarámuri	Third	2 visits	Deficient	Alcoholism	Hospital	Embolism
34	Rarámuri	Seventh	None	Deficient	Alcoholism	Home	Postpartum hemorrhage
35	Rarámuri	Seventh	None	Deficient	Alcoholism	Hospital	Tuberculosis

Maternal mortality data for Guachochi is clinic and hospital based, with information collected from government and private health care facilities. As mentioned earlier and as seen in the vignette, *Rarámuri* women may hesitate to access these facilities. State and national population and health statistics including actual rates of fertility, pregnancy, live birth, as well as infant and maternal mortality among the *Rarámuri* are estimates, may or may not be accurate, and should not be generalized.

It is not surprising that health care administrators blame the practice of unassisted birth among the *Rarámuri* for the elevated maternal mortality rates in Guachochi. Medical causes of maternal mortality are thought to be preventable, and "the single most important way to reduce maternal deaths is to ensure that a skilled health professional is present at every birth" (Family Care International 2002). "There is a clear clinical justification for the presence of a skilled attendant at delivery, as this may reduce both the incidence of complications and case fatality" (AbouZahr and Wardlaw 2001). Unassisted births have even been touted as "process indicators," which can be used to measure maternal mortality (AbouZahr and Wardlaw 2001:563). It is noted in the MDG 2015 report that "A key strategy for reducing maternal morbidity and mortality is ensuring that every birth occurs with the assistance of skilled health personnel, meaning a medical doctor, nurse or midwife. Progress in raising the proportion of births delivered with skilled attendance has been modest over the course of the MDG time frame, reflecting lack of universal access to care. Globally, the proportion of deliveries attended by skilled health personnel increased from 59% around 1990 to 71% around 2014. Yet this leaves more than one in four babies and their mothers without access to crucial medical care during childbirth" (Way 2015: 39). Clearly, unassisted births bear the brunt of the blame for maternal mortality worldwide. But what about the indirect causes? Where is the accounting for the resistance to access culturally inappropriate reproductive services provided?

18.6 Victim Blaming Is Counterproductive

To conclude, I now trace the trajectories of global health ideology as applied to on-the-ground services provided to indigenous *Rarámuri* women, as displayed in Fig. 18.1. As discussed, global health ideology and policy implementation stigmatize the practice of solitary birth. Women who give birth alone are encouraged, and sometimes coerced, to deliver their children in the presence of a "skilled" attendant. The *Rarámuri* have a long-standing and culturally congruent tradition of giving birth alone or accompanied by husbands and female kin, none of whom meet the definition of "skilled" attendant, defined as "an accredited health professional—such as midwife, doctor or nurse—who has been educated and trained to proficiency in the skills needed to manage normal (uncomplicated) pregnancies, childbirth and the immediate postnatal period, and in the identification, management and referral of complications in women and newborns" (WHO/ICM/FIGO 2004).

In the name of "improving" maternal health and "decreasing" maternal mortality, *Rarámuri* women are encouraged to give birth in clinics and hospitals attended by (mostly) male doctors, and/or (*mestizo*) nurses, or auxiliary health care workers with no "accredited" medical training. Women who do deliver in clinics and hospitals are subjected to experiences that contradict normative cultural behavioral standards, similar to experiences of women from other indigenous ethnic groups such as the Maya in Mexico and Central America, which increases their fear and discomfort. In the course of my time among the *Rarámuri* I heard a 50-year-old woman tell me that the delivery of her seventh child in the hospital (after seven births at home, including one stillborn) was the "most shameful" thing that had ever happened to her. Another 20-year-old woman told me in 2010 that she delivered her second child alone at home, after a cesarean section delivery in the hospital, because she was too afraid to go back to the hospital. Another woman in her early twenties said she went to the clinics for the checkups, "But the doctors did not do anything—nothing" (Miller 2003:314). I observed another pregnant woman run away from social workers who visited the village to conduct prenatal visits. These women's fears are real, but disregarded, hence the lack of any efforts to provide culturally appropriate reproductive health services results in women's hesitance to utilize services provided. Since women are blamed for not using services, resources are not allocated proportionately, and what care there is continues to be inadequate, haphazard, and inappropriate.

Local *mestiza parteras* (traditional birth attendants or TBAs) often serve as the first line of resort for *Tarahumara* women, who would rather go to them instead of a clinic when in need. However, these *parteras* are not provided with training in emergency birth protocols, but instead are taught to get everyone on birth control and refer all women to clinics or hospitals. Seven of thirteen training sessions for the IMSS *parteras* (2000–2001) consisted of educational sessions on birth control pills and IUDs. Not a single session covered such important topics as how to control hemorrhage at birth, how to identify preeclampsia and what to do about it, or neonatal resuscitation. Instead, in order to comply with international mandates about birth control, the focus was on "family planning," and *parteras* and auxiliary health workers were taught how to insert IUD's, which often happened at clinic births.

In 1999, sixteen of eighteen *Rarámuri* women delivering in the local clinic had an IUD inserted, and one was referred for surgical sterilization (tubal ligation). In 2000, 17 *Rarámuri* delivered in the clinic, 12 received IUD's, and 3 were taken to the hospital for tubal ligations. One woman who had a cesarean delivery because of a fetal demise at 40 weeks was surgically sterilized without her knowledge or consent—an act of obstetric violence. She asked me if I had any pills to help her to have babies, since she knew there were pills women took to not have babies… IUD's cause pain, increased menstrual bleeding (which leads to anemia), and fear since the women do not know what has been put inside of them. Consequently, it is not surprising that for many *Rarámuri* women, their fear of the clinics and hospitals, or what may happen as a result of going there, is greater than the fear of death.

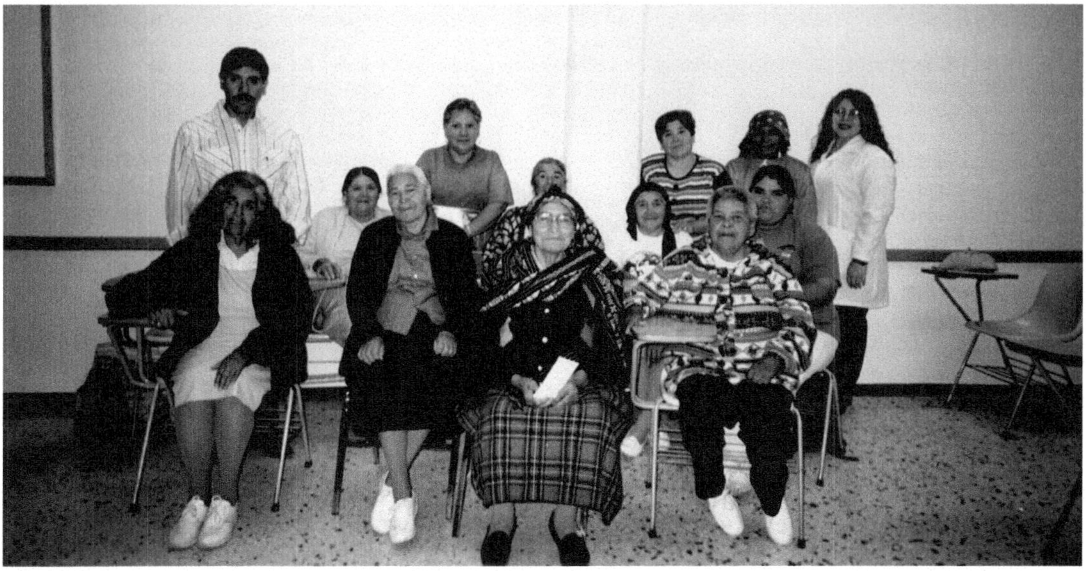

Fig. 18.14 A meeting of IMSS sponsored *mestiza* midwives in Guachochi. The social worker and doctor leading the training are pictured standing at either end of the back row. All of these *parteras* have stories of *Rarámuri* women knocking on their doors asking for help in labor. Published with kind permission of © Janneli F. Miller 2017. All Rights Reserved

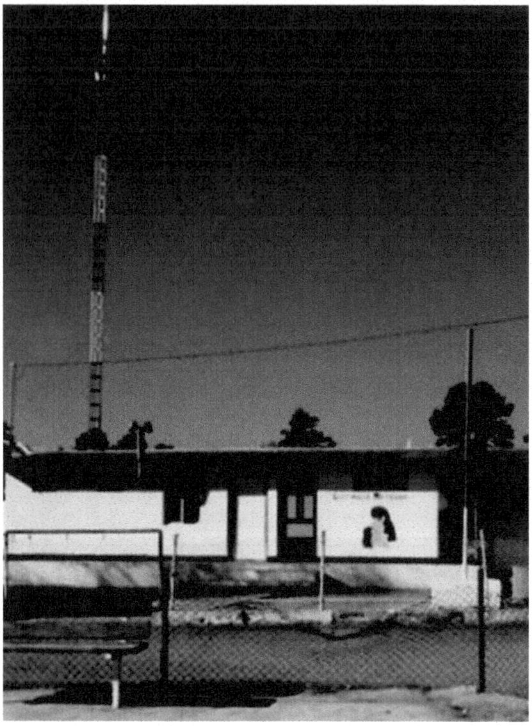

Fig. 18.15 The IMSS health clinic in 2000, where I observed clinic births (and where Maria and Santiago stayed.) It was being rebuilt in 2005. Published with kind permission of © Janneli F. Miller 2017. All Rights Reserved

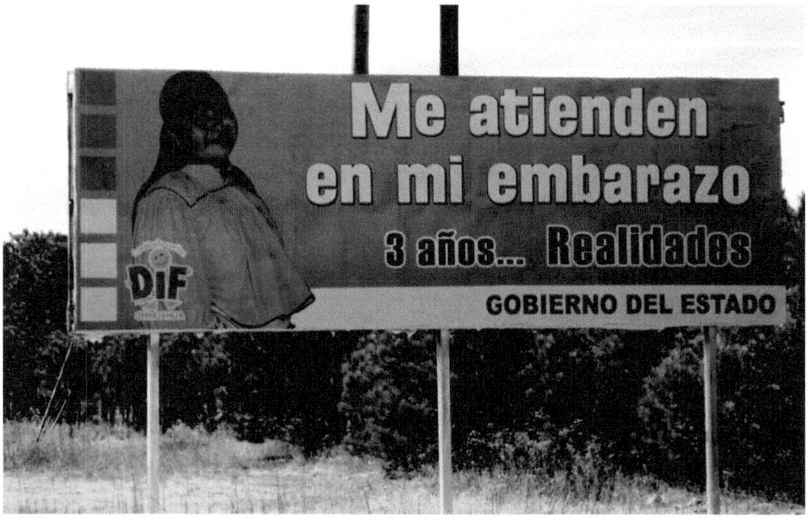

Fig. 18.16 Sign demonstrating that *Rarámuri* women give birth in the clinics and hospitals ("They attend me during my pregnancy") on the main highway linking Chihuahua City with the Sierra Tarahumara (note that the sign is written in Spanish, not in the indigenous *Tarahumara* language). Published with kind permission of © Janneli F. Miller 2017. All Rights Reserved

Reproductive health services provided to indigenous *Rarámuri* women are based on Western concepts of risk, ignore the *Rarámuri* cultural world and belief system, and stigmatize the traditional practice of giving birth at home alone or attended by kin. This, in turn, ensures that many women choose to stay home rather than go to clinics, or may only go as a last resort. It is easier to blame the (rural uneducated indigenous) women for not taking advantage of services provided, since this thinking matches the accepted ideology that birthing alone is dangerous and to be discouraged.

If reproductive health services were provided with proper respect and acknowledgement of traditional cultural beliefs, perhaps they would be better utilized. What to do? Here is a simple list of interventions that could be easily implemented among the *Rarámuri*:

Provide culturally and gender appropriate caregivers (female physicians).
Promote *Rarámuri* (*Tarahumara*) language training for all health care practitioners.
Discourage racism on all fronts.
Define risk categories according to local population health status and practices.
Train midwives in emergency birth care and neonatal resuscitation.
Educate all practitioners about indigenous *Rarámuri* health practices.
Base resource allocation on need instead of politics or ideology.
Eradicate victim blaming and stigmatization of solitary birth.
Permit *Rarámuri* women to choose for themselves where and with whom they want to give birth, and provide culturally appropriate support systems to facilitate their decisions.

Maternal mortality can indeed be decreased by providing better access to reproductive health care, as has been demonstrated by the drop in maternal deaths worldwide as reported in the MDG 2015. Skilled attendants doubtlessly help improve maternal child health outcomes in certain situations. But when there is a cultural tradition of giving birth alone or with trusted kin, as among the *Rarámuri*, the continued stigmatization of solitary and kin-assisted birth, combined with efforts to eliminate it completely, actually contribute to the very conditions international, national, and local health care policy and providers hope to prevent. In order to decrease maternal mortality among the *Rarámuri* and other indigenous peoples, we must acknowledge, respect, and incorporate cultural beliefs and practices, and the women who carry on these traditions, even if they run counter to Western health ideology.

References

AbouZahr, C., & Wardlaw, T. (2001). Maternal mortality at the end of a decade: signs of progress? *Bulletin of the World Health Organization, 79*(6), 561–573.
Bennett, W. C., & Zingg, R. M. (1935). *The Tarahumara*. Chicago: University of Chicago Press.
Brambila, D. (1976). *Diccionario Rarámuri-Castellano (Tarahumar)*. México, DF: Obra Nacional de la Buena Prensa.
Chopel, A. M. (2014). Reproductive health in indigenous Chihuahua: giving birth "alone like the goat". *Ethnicity & Health, 19*(3), 279–296.
Espino Loya, S. (1987) *Kuira*. Chihuahua City, ENAH: Dirección General de Desarrollo Social, Dept. de Educación, Coordinación de Fomenta a la Expresión Cultural.
Family Care International. (2002). Safe motherhood fact sheet. Retrieved from www.safemotherood.org.
Ghosh, M. K. (2001). Maternal mortality: A global perspective. *The Journal of Reproductive Medicine, 46*(5), 427–433.
Ginsburg, F. D., & Rapp, R. (1995). *Conceiving the new world order: The global politics of reproduction*. Berkeley & Los Angeles: University of California Press.
Janes, C. R. (2001). *Free markets and dead mothers: economic transition and the collapse of health care in Mongolia*. Paper presented at the Annual Meetings of the Society for Applied Anthropology, Merida, Mexico.
Langer, A., Hernández, B., & Lozano, R. (1994). La morbimortalidad materna en México: niveles y causas. In M. Elu, A. Langer, & A. (Eds.), *Maternidad sin riesgos en México* (pp. 23–29). IMSS: México, DF.
Lozano, R., Hernández, B., & Langer, A. (1994). Factores sociales y económicos de la mortalidad materna en México. In M. Elu & A. Langer (Eds.), *Maternidad sin Riesgos en México* (pp. 43–51). México DF: IMSS.
Merrill, W. (1988). *Rarámuri souls: Knowledge and social process in Northern Mexico*. Washington DC: Smithsonian Institution Press.
Miller, J. (2003). *Birthing practices of the Rarámuri of Northern Mexico*. PhD. Dissertation. Tucson, AZ: University of Arizona. Retrieved from http://hdl.handle.net/10150/289917.
Miller, J. (2009). Husband-assisted birth among the *Rarámuri* of Northern Mexico. In M. Inhorn, T. Tjørnhøj-Thomsen, H. Goldberg, & M. la Cour Mosegaard (Eds.), *Reconceiving the second sex: Men, masculinity, and reproduction* (pp. 327–348). New York & Oxford: Berghan Books.

Miller, J. (2010). Solitary, husband, and kin-assisted birth among the *Rarámuri* of Northern Mexico: Considerations for normal birth. Paper presented at the 5th International Normal Labour and Birth Research Conference Vancouver: University of British Columbia.

Royston, E., & Armstrong, S. (Eds.). (1989). *Preventing maternal deaths*. Geneva: World Health Organization.

Schwartz, D. A. (2015a). The pathology of maternal death—the importance of accurate autopsy diagnosis for epidemiologic surveillance and prevention of maternal mortality in developing countries. In D. A. Schwartz (Ed.), *Maternal mortality: Risk factors, anthropological perspectives, prevalence in developing countries and preventive strategies for pregnancy-related death* (pp. ix–xiv). New York: Nova Science Publishers, Inc..

Schwartz, D. A. (2015b). Interface of epidemiology, anthropology and health care in maternal death prevention in resource-poor nations. In D. A. Schwartz (Ed.), *Maternal mortality: Risk factors, anthropological perspectives, prevalence in developing countries and preventive strategies for pregnancy-related death* (pp. ix–xiv). New York: Nova Science Publishers, Inc..

Way, C. (Ed.). (2016). *The Millennium Goals Report 2015*. Geneva: United Nations.

WHO, ICM & FIGO. (2004). *Making pregnancy safer: the critical role of the skilled attendant*. Geneva: World health Organization. Retrieved from http://www.who.int/maternal_child_adolescent/documents/9241591692/en/.

19 Lessons from Chiapas: Caring for Indigenous Women Through a Femifocal Model of Care

Cristina Alonso, Alison Danch, Jenna Murray de López, and Janell Tryon

19.1 Introduction

Although Mexico is now considered a high middle income country, there remain significant disparities in health, wealth, and social issues across the 32 federal entities. Situated in the south east on the border of Guatemala, Chiapas is one such region that presents challenges to Mexico's image as a global economic power (Fig. 19.1). On the one hand, Chiapas is extraordinarily rich in natural resources and is the most geographically and culturally diverse state in Mexico. On the other, is among the top five most marginalized states, with the highest recorded unemployment levels and lowest educational attainment by gender (completing secondary school) of all thirty-two federal states (OECD 2015). Access to health services is particularly poor and is associated with wider political economic and social issues. Chiapas has the second highest maternal mortality ratio (MMR) at 68.1 per every 100,000 live births, and the highest infant mortality rate (IMR) at 17.9 per every 1000 children under 5 years in the country as a whole (INEGI 2015).

Approximately twenty-seven percent of the total population of Chiapas self-identify as indigenous Mexicans (INEGI 2010). Indigenous populations are most concentrated in the rural highlands, though internal conflict and economic disparities have led to widespread displacement and transmigration over recent decades. Changes in migration patterns and the impact of national and global recession have resulted in the rural-urban poverty divide being less apparent. The Organization for Economic Co-operation and Development (OECD) reported in 2015 that the urban population is no longer significantly better-off in having access to health services than rural populations. This observation is also

C. Alonso, M.P.H., C.P.M. (✉)
Luna Maya Birth Center, Mexico City, Mexico

A. Danch, M.S.W., M.P.H.
Indiana Institute on Disability and Community, Indiana University, Bloomington, IN, USA

J. M. de López, Ph.D.
University of Manchester, Manchester, UK
e-mail: jenna.murray@manchester.ac.uk

J. Tryon, M.P.H.
San Francisco Department of Public Health, San Francisco, CA, USA

D. A. Schwartz (ed.), *Maternal Death and Pregnancy-Related Morbidity Among Indigenous Women of Mexico and Central America*, Global Maternal and Child Health: Medical, Anthropological, and Public Health Perspectives, https://doi.org/10.1007/978-3-319-71538-4_19

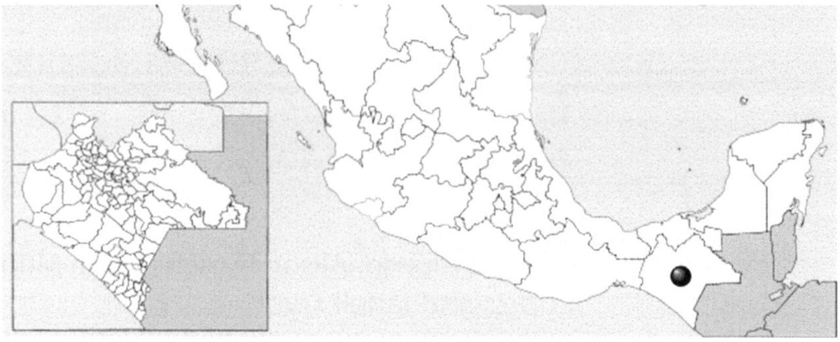

Fig. 19.1 Map of Chiapas. Adapted from Wikimedia Commons, https://commons.wikimedia.org/wiki/Chiapas

reflected in a narrowing in the division between the occurrence of rural and urban maternal mortality and morbidity in both indigenous and mestizo populations.

As with all critical global health debate the aim of this chapter is to look beyond the "abstract and bureaucratic considerations of public policy" (Biehl and Petryna 2013: 3) to recognize how lives are actually lived and cared for. By highlighting the various ways in which indigenous women in the colonial city of San Cristóbal de Las Casas manage maternal health and birth care, in this chapter we intend to provide a counter-narrative to the dominant approach which conflates medicalized maternal health with low mortality ratios, regardless of the quality of interventions and the cultural preferences of diverse populations. While the majority of the female urban indigenous population will access public services when they need to give birth, others seek out alternative models of care more closely related to traditional model of care. This occurs on a timeline, as indigenous women may migrate to the city and never find safety and relevance in medical maternal health models, or they may have always lived in a neighborhood where all women birth at home with traditional midwives. In other cases, some women have crossed the cultural boundary to the medicalized model and now desire a return to homebirth due to personal preferences related to family, respect, and privacy. In such cases, they may no longer find a traditional midwife and are confronted with having to choose a "postmodern midwife," crossing a second boundary to being cared for by a mestizo or foreign midwife (Davis-Floyd 2001, 2005).

In the following pages we will describe how the type of maternity and birth care indigenous women will access in the city is dependent upon age, social networks, fluency in Spanish, and their economic and housing situation. Together with other anthropological studies of the southern region, our research and experience shows that indigenous and nonindigenous women throughout Mexico continue to seek the services of midwives and out-of-hospital care, regardless of the improvements in access to public services (Sesia 1996; Murray de López 2015; Flores and Espejel 2015; Smith-Oka 2013). This observation alone raises important questions about the division between the type of public services available to indigenous and low-income women, and their needs and desires around the lifecycle process of motherhood. This chapter is divided into three sections, discussing reproductive rights, choice, and policy, midwifery in San Cristobal, and focusing on Luna Maya as a femifocal Birth Center. Drawing from research and the experience of the authors, the chapter draws on narratives and interview transcripts to provide case examples.

Established on August 25, 2004, the Luna Maya Birth Center has provided over a decade of services to women and their families in San Cristóbal de Las Casas in Chiapas, Mexico and, more recently, in Mexico City. In addition to expanding beyond traditional midwifery services, Luna Maya broadened the very meaning of midwifery: "We see birth as the beginning of a whole bunch of processes about becoming aware of your body, of your system, of your relationship to your health" (Alonso 2014). From its inception, Alonso understood that the state of maternal services in Chiapas necessitated a woman-focused, humanized intervention to employ the broadest meaning of women's health.

Since the medical model of pregnancy and birth took hold in Mexico, women have been offered an increasingly narrow set of maternal health services, which are highly medicalized and often obstetrically violent. Responding to this environment of limited care options, Luna Maya has not only stressed the importance of holistic care, which addresses the psychosocial needs of its clients, but has also provided alternative healing as an alternative to the allopathic framework of popular medical models of maternal care. Moreover, Luna Maya has created a model that understands that the individual is linked to and informed by her environment, which includes her family and community.

19.2 Reproductive Rights, Choice, and Opportunities

San Cristóbal de Las Casas is the third largest in Chiapas with a population of 158,102 and with 62,208 inhabitants identifying as being indigenous Mexicans in the most recent census (INEGI 2010). As mentioned in this chapter's introduction, internal conflict and broader economic precarities conflict has led to a forced displacement of whole indigenous communities and mass migration of families and individuals from rural to urban areas, of which women, children, and older people have been particularly affected (FrayBa 2012). This has led to a significant increase in population (both transient and permanent) in cities close to the highlands, subsequently resulting in heightened pressure on public services. Within the municipal boundaries there are a total of eleven public hospitals and seven (registered) private maternity clinic/hospitals—one of which includes a charitable hospital which also targets low-income families. Of the eleven public institutions two are part of the conditional cash transfer (CCT) program IMSS-PROSPERA (previously known as IMSS-Oportunidades) and another three are open to the basic assistance program Seguro Popular. Most significant for the transient indigenous population is the Seguro Popular Hospital de las Culturas, built specifically in 2010 to serve the incoming rural and mainly *Tsotsil-* and *Tseltal*-speaking indigenous population (Secretaria de Salud 2013). Upon its launch, the Hospital de Las Culturas was celebrated for being "the first hospital in the country to include traditional medicine, taking into account the traditions and customs of indigenous peoples" (Periodico La Jornada 2011). In the Traditional Medicine Section of the hospital there are four traditional midwives working as doulas who can attend to pregnant or postpartum women. However, the Hospital de las Culturas does not attend births, and women who attend the Traditional Midwifery Section of the hospital are then referred to the city Maternity Hospital where doulas or traditional midwives are not permitted entry (Fig. 19.2).

As previously mentioned there are two main assistance programs running throughout Mexico that provide for those individuals and families without any health insurance and living below globally defined poverty levels. Seguro Popular (also known as the People's Health Insurance) was created in 2003 and is intended to cover all families that are otherwise uninsured. Seguro Popular is a voluntary family health insurance program funded by the federal government with resources allocated and delivered at a state level. Seguro Popular is means-tested with a sliding fee-scale for services, and with all fees waived for families in the lowest two income deciles (Homedes and Ugalde 2009). Services

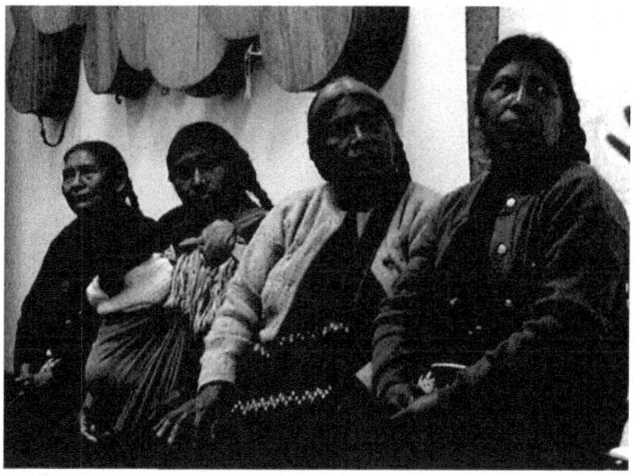

Fig. 19.2 Indigenous midwives from Tenejapa participate in midwifery training sessions conducted by the Luna Maya Birth Center

provided via Seguro Popular are delivered through existing state and federal institutions, and can also be contracted out to private services. Seguro Popular is currently providing services to approximately 61.7% of the population of Chiapas, while 21.5% of the state population remain beyond its reach (ENSANUT 2012) (Fig. 19.3).

The second main assistance program is the aforementioned IMSS-PROSPERA. This is a CCT program that originally targeted impoverished rural areas and, in more recent years, has been extended to impoverished urban areas. Its overall aim is to improve education, health, nutrition, and living conditions for population groups in extreme poverty, as well as to break the "intergenerational cycle" of poverty. The maternal health element focusses on the provision of prenatal services to help the proper development of the pregnancy, to protect the mother's health, and to identify high-risk pregnancies. In combination with other national health policies there is also an emphasis on offering contraception choice and family planning advice to all women as part of the regular *platicas* (educational program) and in prenatal appointments (Fig. 19.4).

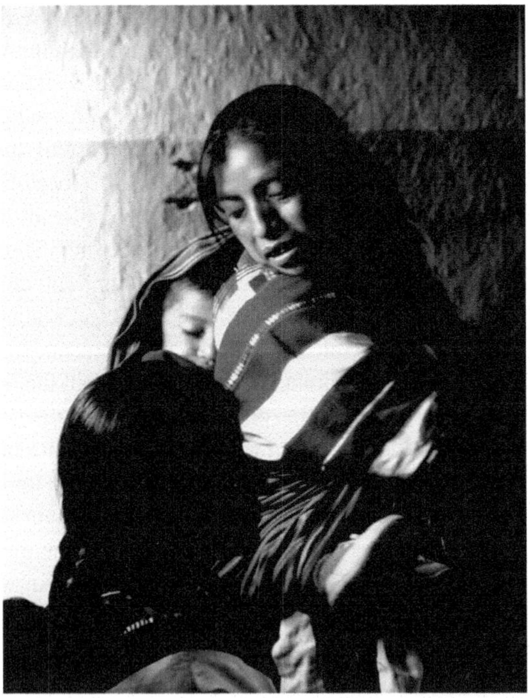

Fig. 19.3 An indigenous pregnant woman attends Luna Maya for prenatal care with her small child on her back

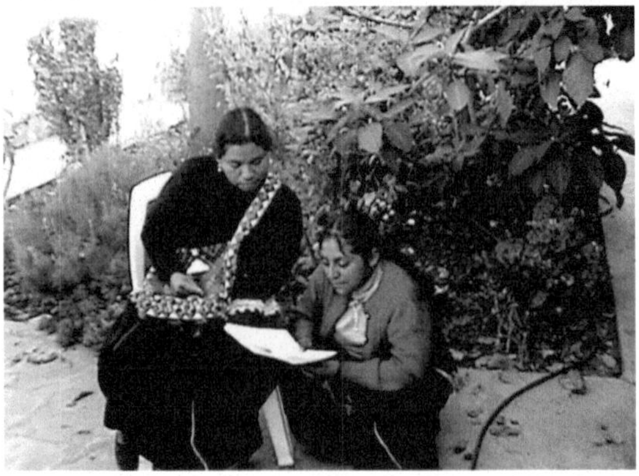

Fig. 19.4 Health promoters participate in Emergency Obstetric training in Luna Maya to create a network that supports infrastructure and support to women and rural areas

As a consequence of its high MMR, Chiapas is a principal federal target for the PROSPERA program. Recent government figures suggest that approximately 32.8% of the urban population and 80.7% of the rural population are in receipt of assistance from PROSPERA (ENSANUT 2012). While the program has had some relative success with lowering the MMR among the rural population of Chiapas, the MMR between urban (mestiza and indigenous) beneficiaries and non-beneficiaries is reported to be less than ten percent (Freyermuth and Sesia 2009). Furthermore, while over one-half of the state population receives aid *Seguro Popular* or *PROSPERA*, the overall maternal mortality rate in public institutions is improving at just one percent per year (Freyermuth and Sesia, 2009). This questionable impact on urban and rural MMR is steeped in the misconception, despite much evidence to the contrary, that maternal mortality is a quandary to be solved by medicine alone. The reduction of maternal mortality to a distinctly medical—rather than social—problem, "means that the only outcome can be life or death" (Berry 2010). The management of pregnancy and birth, in global and local policy, thus becomes framed by a medical rhetoric of saving lives at any cost—mother death for the medical practitioner is synonymous with failure. This in turn leads to an overemphasis in localized contexts on access to emergency obstetric services and a model of prenatal care that is hypersensitive to diagnosing and managing risk. Pregnant women, as principal benefit recipients and potential agents of social change, become defined within a medical framework as difficult subjects with risky bodies—particularly in terms of their reproductive and sexual behavior. This is further complicated by social prejudices based upon ethnicity, class, and gender. Each category further adds to the health professionals' calculation of perceived risk.

In everyday practice "risk" is a tricky concept to pin down, as it becomes not one measurable thing but a multilayered relationship of things dependent upon the actors involved. The competing cultural metaphors of risk at play in the medical environment culminate in an oversimplified idea that women in need of CCTs equate to a potential danger to themselves and wider society. When these "risky bodies" enter into a high-pressured, under-resourced public hospital, they are, in turn, subjected to a particular type of treatment. One way to understand how poor women embody biosocial ideas about risk is to examine the interactions between them and health professionals in the medical environment. When we bring attention to the marked ethnic and class differences between patients and health professionals, we begin to see the ways in which women are framed by competing notions of risk.

During a period of ethnographic fieldwork carried out in 2011–2012, Murray deLópez interviewed Ricardo, a recently qualified doctor, about his experience of attending recipients of Seguro Popular and PROSPERA at various maternity hospitals throughout the state. Below he describes the type of contact doctors have with women during what is referred to in the medical lexicon as "*control prenatal*" (prenatal care) or more loosely by many women as "*el control*":

> … in hospital the first appointments … they will give the diagnosis [of pregnancy] or they will give the first appointments. So when they next come to the hospital they are seen in a group for the *platicas*. In my experience the '*control prenatal*' actually happens in the ultimate appointments. They do an ultrasound if the equipment is there, very quickly just to check that everything is okay, to measure how low the baby is, to check the position of the product. And well, when we carry out this evaluation of the product we do a quick evaluation of the patient. Then we will advise [her] when her dates are, the possible due dates … we tell the woman to be conscious of these dates and understand what the alarm signals are …

Ricardo's description highlights the emphasis on "detection of risk" in the approach to *control prenatal*. The phrase itself is an intriguing one as it suggests something, in this case a body or a process, in need of control or management. This terminology is part of a wider medical lexicon that in itself shapes ideas about women's bodies as precarious, at risk of harm, or of harming. The type of interaction that takes place in the prenatal care appointment firmly positions the pregnant woman as passive, yet at the same time responsible, for recognizing the warning signs that mean she is "at risk" of giving birth.

Increased access to institutions in urban areas via Seguro Popular and PROSPERA has contributed in practical terms to a national statistic of 94% recorded live births now taking place in hospital clinics (ENSANUT 2012). In comparison, in Chiapas it is estimated that a more conservative 60.5% of live births take place in a hospital or clinic, despite the large coverage of PROSPERA (Lazcano-Ponce et al. 2013). It would be wrong to assume that women who are not included in the 54.9% are simply failing to access hospital care, or indeed that they all require access to a welfare program. The paucity of data available for women across the social strata who have out-of-hospital births in urban areas of Chiapas makes it difficult to indicate the level of choice involved in doing so. The small amount of research that does exist raises important questions about the actions that women in Chiapas take when presented with the restrictions of the public health care system, or when they feel for whatever reason that the pregnancy, birth, and postpartum stages of the lifecycle process should be cared for in other ways.

19.3 Midwifery in San Cristobal

There is a popular assumption in Mexico that where possible women, and particularly mestiza women, prefer to give birth in a clinical environment in the presence of an obstetrician. The hiring of a midwife (to attend birth at least) in the dominant social imagination is associated with something that ignorant, uneducated, and poor women do—those who have not yet learnt what it means to be a modern citizen of Mexico. Smith-Oka argues across Mexico "a tussle exists between tradition and past, represented by the *parteras* (traditional birth attendants), and modernity and the future, represented by clinicians" (Smith-Oka 2013: 83). In the urban environment, this oversimplified dichotomy of traditional and modern is more readily challenged. As the focus of this chapter demonstrates, the reason why Luna Maya continues to thrive arises from the needs of women across the local social spectrum who, for a variety of reasons, seek out-of-hospital maternal health care and the intercultural knowledge base and practices of midwifery.

Murray de López (2015) has observed three different types of midwife practicing in the urban context of San Cristóbal: The first is the traditional midwife or traditional birth attendant as described in policy initiatives and whom many people associate with the practice of midwifery in Mexico. This image of the traditional midwife is that of an indigenous woman, attending poor women in a rural context, and is reinforced by media representations and development policy alike. Despite this stereotype, there are various traditional midwives practicing in the cities of Chiapas, attending only other indigenous women. The second and most common type of midwife is found in low-income urban barrios, and represents the empirical midwife. The third type of midwife is found in the urban context and is the professional or autonomous midwife, the only practitioner to be working across class and ethnic boundaries, as shall be discussed further below.

The term empirical midwife is sometimes used to denote women who learned midwifery, either through attending women in childbirth or through apprenticeship to another experienced midwife (Mills and Davis-Floyd 2009). Murray de López has extended this definition in her work to distinguish mestiza traditional midwives who employ a combination of traditional and lay-allopathic techniques. This distinction is necessary in areas where homebirth and midwife-supervised aftercare remains popular among the low-income mestiza population. Local ethnic divisions between mestiza and indigenous populations mean that an indigenous traditional midwife is unlikely to attend the birth of a low-income mestiza woman. Under Mexican law the title of *partera tradicional* (traditional midwife) is protected as an indigenous custom and traditional practice. This means that the numerous mestiza women practicing as empirical midwives remain without recognition or regulation by the state, and their contribution to maternal health is effectively "disappeared" from debate. The empirical midwife, who is generally hired via mestiza families or close social networks, as well as the women hiring an empirical midwife are more likely to be combining her services with those available in the public and private health system. The empirical midwife plays a significant and under-researched role in an integrated model of maternal and women's health care beyond pregnancy and birth. For low-income mestiza families, she is particularly significant in the postpartum healing period and the spiritual wellness of the mother-infant unit (Fig. 19.5).

Each year there are fewer and fewer empirical midwives regularly practicing and attending births in the barrios of cities like San Cristóbal. There are multiple factors that contribute to the trend of decreasing out-of-hospital births attended by an empirical midwife. These include women's improved access to public health care as previously mentioned, the success of CCT programs and Seguro Popular, and general changes in the perceptions of risk associated with childbirth. In addition, women are told directly that they will lose access to Seguro Popular/IMSS-PROSPERA and social benefit programs if they give birth outside of government institutions. Although this is not stated anywhere in policy, it has become an "oral" policy, and has been perpetuated long enough for many physicians to believe this is actually the case. The overall aim of IMSS-PROSPERA is to "reflect the priority that births should be attended by qualified personnel in an institution as an effective strategy for reducing risks in maternal and infant health" (IMSS 2015). As a woman is also unlikely to find an IMSS-PROSPERA-affiliated midwife in an urban context, giving birth in an institution is the only likely way that a woman can access the paperwork needed to apply for welfare for her child (Fig. 19.6).

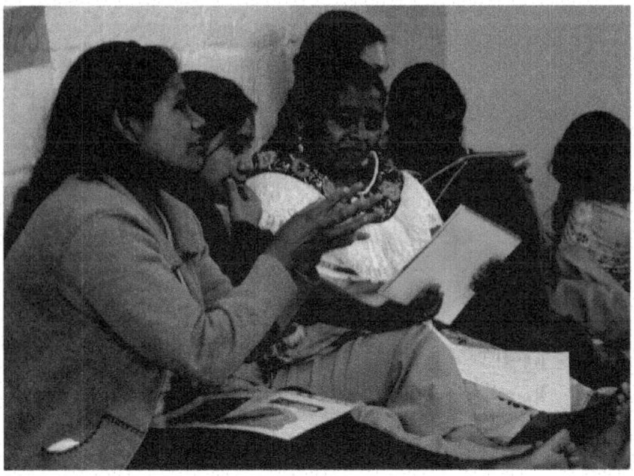

Fig. 19.5 Indigenous women and midwives participate in women's circles at Luna Maya to learn about their bodies

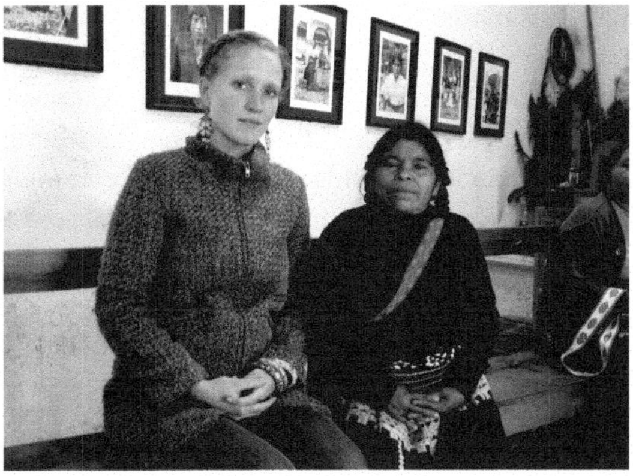

Fig. 19.6 A midwife apprentice at Luna Maya exchanges with a traditional midwife

In 2001 Robbie Davis-Floyd described the postmodern midwife in Mexico, which she describes as building an emerging identity of a professional midwife (Davis-Floyd 2001).

Although it is impossible to say when the postmodern movement of midwifery emerged in Mexico, there are key events that mark its integration into the maternal health conversation at a national level. By 2014, literature describing the midwifery movement in Mexico had described a new term, the "autonomous midwife" (Laako 2016). According to Laako, the autonomous midwife "emphasizes the political and autonomous aspects of this type of midwife. The concept of autonomy is fundamental in the collective action of these midwives as their profession lacks autonomy in Mexico. However, the concept of autonomy also emphasizes the anti-systemic character of these midwives: their critique of the biomedical system with its pathological perspective of birth and the defense of a rights-based approach to birth" (Laako 2016: 171).

Luna Maya was founded three years after the death of Doña Graciela, a renowned traditional midwife who, according to San Cristobal folklore, attended most births from the 1980's to the millennium. Luna Maya was founded on a rights-based approach, as witnessed by its vision and mission statements establishing humanized birth and respectful care as human rights. Women who had birthed with Doña Graciela then shifted their care to Luna Maya without even realizing they had become activists of an emerging political movement—they just wanted peaceful births within their own home with a trustworthy midwife.

The establishment of Luna Maya occurred concurrently with a national movement that spoke of peaceful birth, respect for tradition and culture, women's empowerment, and continuity of care as essential aspects of millennial midwifery. This practice weaves traditional ceremony and technique with modern tools such as Facebook, conferences, WhatsApp conversations, and websites.

19.4 Luna Maya Vision and Mission: Empowering Women, Empower Communities at a Femifocal Birth Center

Luna Maya was founded in 2004 to provide humanized health services including respectful maternity care under the vision "to achieve safe motherhood through the empowerment of women" (Alonso cited in Banet Lucas and Tryon 2014). Established as a birth center and midwifery training program, Luna Maya has become a model in Latin America for out-of-hospital birth and integrative care. Highly informed by its international and regional context, Luna Maya's founding vision outlined the ways in which it would adopt an evidence-based midwifery model of care in an effort to alleviate the burden of maternal morbidity and mortality, deficiency of birth-related and postpartum care services, and obstetric violence on the local level. Luna Maya's model of care offers a continuum of women's and maternal health services in a community setting, of which it is an integral part. Luna Maya set in motion a particularly innovative conceptual lens for the midwifery model of care (Table 19.1, Fig. 19.7).

Matrifocal, a term used to describe matrilineal communities and mother-centered political and cultural structures, necessarily hinges on the figure of the woman. The use of this term has extended beyond these initial fields and forums, becoming one that is used to describe types of ideologies relating to and guiding health care service and delivery. While this represents a positive development in terms of the incorporation of a women-specific discourse, there is still the need for further development of the related concepts and phrases used to represent these philosophies. The most notable shortcoming is that the term does not represent all women; namely, it excludes all those who fall outside of the parameters of motherhood, no matter what the reason. Many health care services, globally, are focused

Table 19.1 The goals and mission of the Luna Maya birth center

Vision: To achieve safe motherhood through the empowerment of women.
Mission: Luna Maya works to ensure that all women of Chiapas have access to a safe and humanized birth and birth experience. They believe that the women of Chiapas have the right to make informed decisions about their bodies and access and the right to the necessary means to ensure their health and wellbeing. The believe that safe motherhood is a human right that contributes to the empowerment of women, the improvement of the quality of life, and the strengthening of families.
Goal: To contribute to the reduction of maternal mortality in Chiapas, Mexico.
Objective: To improve access to safe motherhood through the empowerment of women utilizing the Professional Midwifery Model of Care and access to the emergency obstetrical care, as needed, in Chiapas Mexico.
Expected Results: 1. An autonomous and sustainable birth center, run by professional midwives 2. Better knowledge and awareness about sexual and reproductive rights, including humanized birth, as it is defined by the World Health Organization 3. A training program for local, Mexican, and international midwives 4. A network of service providers, governmental institutions, and women's organizations that aims to increase access to humanized birth through collaboration and referral

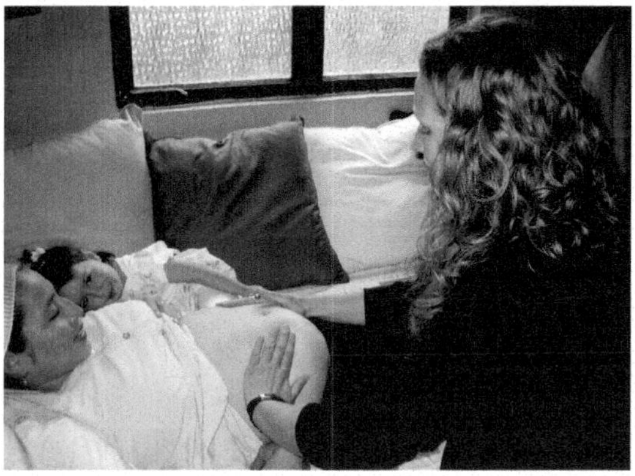

Fig. 19.7 A pregnant woman receives prenatal care from a midwifery student, supervised by a midwife

specifically towards mothers, thereby excluding women who are not mothers. While the matrifocal movement has covered important ground by creating a politically palatable way to move the discursive focus towards women from a legacy of male-centricity, there is still the need to broaden the focus to explicitly include all women. Therefore, in order to acknowledge motherhood as one option among many that are presented to women, we suggest the use of the term *femifocal*, thereby encompassing all those who identify as women, regardless of their relationship to having children (Fig. 19.8).

To date in the literature, the term femifocal has been used sparsely. When used, however, it has been ascribed to certain types of women-led kinship structures and household patterns that move beyond the strict relationship of a mother to her child (Alber et al. 2013). Specifically, femifocal describes the transition in kin roles that occurred as men began to adopt more migratory work patterns, thereby leaving the home in the full care of a female. This specific shift to femifocality happened through shared experiences and hardships most regularly between sisters. Alber et al. (2013) suggest that "social practices and changing household patterns reconfigure kin, gender, and generational patterns" (p. 49). In a similar vein, through invoking the term femifocal in regard to conceptualizations of health care services and delivery, we are recognizing that there are a multiplicity of experiences for women that must be acknowledged and embraced (Lucas and Tryon 2014) (Fig. 19.9).

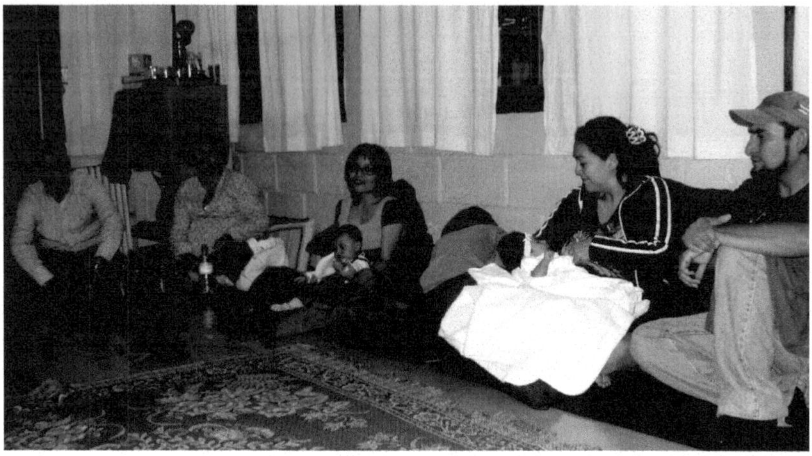

Fig. 19.8 Building community: couples share their birth experience in Childbirth Preparation class

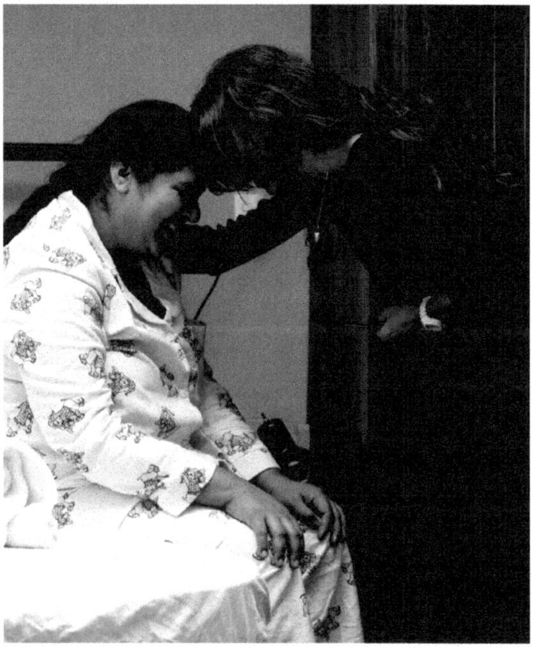

Fig. 19.9 A midwife and new mother share an intimate moment to rejoice in a beautiful, empowering birth

Femifocal can be understood as a mindset, which can then inform policy and behavior. When we discuss femifocal care, we are specifically referring to how this mindset or lens is applied in terms of policy and best-practices development in the fields of medical and health care services and provision methods. Femifocal recognizes that a woman is at the center of her own social, political, and cultural ecology. This includes women and girls who are mothers, have been mothers, those who have never been mothers, those who hope to become mothers, those who intend to never become mothers, and all girls and women who define their own category of relating to their experience as women. Femifocal care is humanized. It views a woman as containing many spheres of experience and existence, rather than solely as a biological machine that needs medical attention (Fig. 19.10).

Similarly, femifocal care understands that humans are nested within larger contexts that can be positive and negative, often comprising loved ones, family, friends, community, culture, political structures, built environment, and natural geography. Femifocal care works with a woman within these multiplicitous contexts. Femifocal care works with a woman across and throughout her life

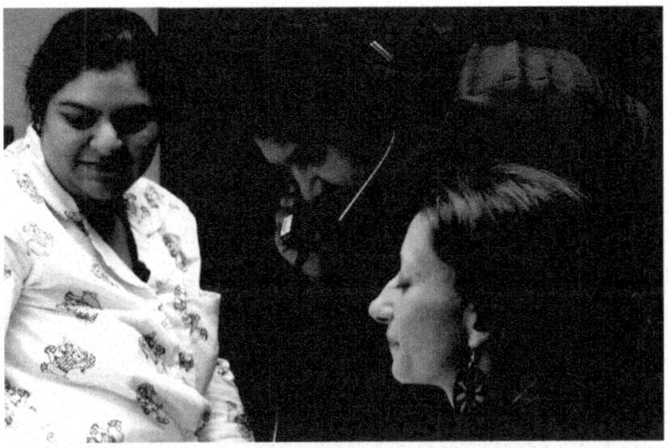

Fig. 19.10 A grandmother listens to her grandbaby's heartbeat at the mother's bedside as the midwife carries out the well-baby check

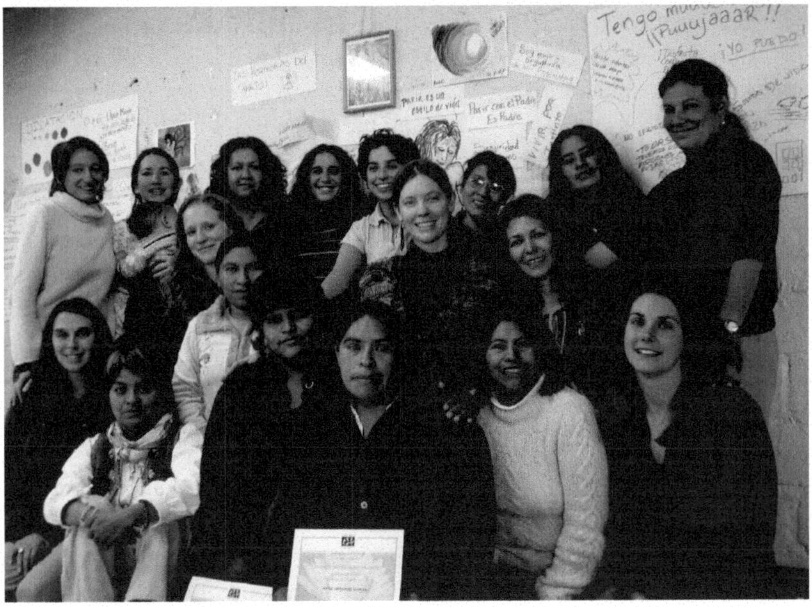

Fig. 19.11 A new group of doulas and birth activists graduate from a one-year training program at Luna Maya

course, realizing that she is accumulating experiences and history as she grows and develops. The ability to understand the woman in many of her changes throughout her life course is enabled by the fact that ideally she is seen by the same provider the whole time, thereby infusing the traditional patient/provider dynamic with more relational and temporally consistent elements. All femifocal care is rooted in a woman's desire to participate (with her informed consent) in the treatment and care, as well as on her elucidation of what her unique health goals are. Femifocal care is women-centered, and individually driven (Fig. 19.11).

19.5 Tenejapa and the Highlands of Chiapas

The Altos of Chiapas is one of eight socioeconomic regions in which the state is divided. With 18 municipalities, 15 have majority indigenous population. A third of the state indigenous population is concentrated in this region, with almost 75% of its population above 5 years and a monolingual rate (indigenous language) above 32.6% compared to the state average. Most of the population can be considered rural and almost 70% is dispersed among ranches and other places of difficult access and communication, lacking basic services. Although one of the smallest regions of the state, after the Sierra region, it has a higher population density than both the national and state averages.

Almost all indigenous municipalities are classified as having a very high degree of marginalization, leading this region to be the most marginalized in Chiapas. One-half of the total population of 30,640 are below 15 years of age, and 99.5% of the population is Tzeltal. Over 33% of women are illiterate, three times more than their masculine counterparts. In the year 2000, 4500 women were of reproductive age with an average of 4.6 children, above the national average for indigenous populations (3.9) (INEGI 2010).

19.5.1 Traditional Midwifery in Tenejapa

According to the Ministry of Health there were 13 midwives in Tenejapa in the year 2000. A baseline survey carried out by Luna Maya in 2003 identified 25 in the 20 communities. However, through a six-year relationship with Tenejapa and with midwives, Luna Maya was able to work with over 50 in 6 years. Midwives attend between 2 and 6 births a month. Although traditional midwives can have a relationship with health institutions, they are generally selected by women, mothers-in-law, or husbands in the community. In Tenejapa, Luna Maya found that many midwives preferred not be registered with health authorities, in order to avoid having to travel for long meetings and for fear of arrest or punishment in the case of maternal deaths. Most of the midwives that Luna Maya worked with were above 40 years of age, monolingual (Tzeltal), and illiterate.

19.5.2 Midwifery Training

During the period from 2005 to 2010 Luna Maya worked alongside 55 traditional midwives in the indigenous area of Tenejapa. This program aimed to empower traditional midwives as community leaders as well as to educate them on basic lifesaving skills and safe birth practices. Adult learning techniques were utilized, focused on self-exploration, mind-body therapeutic techniques, and circles of knowledge. When our work began in 2005, maternal mortality had remained stable, with mother deaths occurring seven or eight times per year, and representing almost one maternal death every month. The midwives were disorganized, divided among themselves, working alone, and were disregarded. Instead of "teaching" them about risk management in labor, the group has focused on a model which was called "circles of knowledge." Through this it was anticipated that traditional midwives already have an immense amount of knowledge and wisdom about birth and women's health. The facilitators, indigenous women themselves, listened to their beliefs and discussed with them additional knowledge from other models, such as biomedical beliefs. In this way, the midwives' knowledge was expanded and their resources were increased. A principal component to the training was leadership and organization as a group. Luna Maya worked via the belief that traditional midwives are primary community leaders and women's health advocates.

This program had several accomplishments: the midwives named themselves as a formal association (Metik U, Association of Traditional midwives of Tenejapa) and presented themselves to the local authorities. The Association negotiated direct transport with the taxi company and the local government to ensure that all women with obstetric emergencies were transported to the San Cristobal hospital with the local authorities covering 50% of transport costs. The midwives secured funding to participate in several national conferences and meetings regarding maternal health and midwifery. The midwives also created a network where Luna Maya served as a recipient site in nonemergency transport sites, enabling traditional midwives to work alongside professional midwives in collaborative care.

19.5.3 Reaching Out to the Barrios: El Molina, Peña Maria, Hogar Comunitario

Through building relationships with individuals, Luna Maya became known within several outlying neighborhoods of San Cristobal. These neighborhoods are created by migrant indigenous groups who move to San Cristobal fleeing religious or political conflict, or simply in search of better financial opportunities. What is characteristic of these neighborhoods is they often lack a traditional midwife. Two neighborhoods in particular stand out in their relationship with Luna Maya: Ranchería Peña María and El Molino. Both are impoverished and homes are precarious, made of plywood, plastic sheeting, and lack indoor plumbing. Most homes have dug-out latrines and connect to a neighborhood electric grid. Women marry young, often before 18 years of age, and have an average of three or four children. Men work in the service industry or construction and, on some occasions, migrate to the United States.

Luna Maya began working with El Molino when one woman who was at a birth that had lasted two nights, decided to call one of the midwives to ask for assistance. The traditional midwife attending the birth was asleep and could not provide more support or diagnosis. The baby was in an asynclitic position, meaning the head was sideways, and posterior, meaning the baby's back was lying towards the mothers' back. Using the *reboso* (Mexican shawl) to help better position the baby, the midwife helped the mother have a gentle, natural birth and avoid transport to the local hospital. From this moment, women from El Molino would chose to birth with Luna Maya midwives, or call Luna Maya when births were not going well to ask for assistance. Women who birth in El Molino attend late in their pregnancy and are mostly concerned with the baby's position. They do not attend childbirth education classes and inherently believe that birth is a natural event that should occur at home with other women. They are afraid of the local hospital and believe that all women who birth there are given cesarean sections and are mistreated.

The first birth attended by Luna Maya in Ranchería Peña María was a breech delivery. It was the woman's second pregnancy, and she had been told by the hospital that she would have to be delivered by cesarean section. She began asking for support for a vaginal breech birth and eventually found Luna Maya, who offered to attend the birth. The birth went very well, and since that time the women from Ranchería Peña Maria have selected Luna Maya for maternal, pediatric, and family health care. The community has no traditional midwives or healers and is desperately poor—on average, families subsist on one plate of beans a day. Alcoholism is rampant among males and therefore violence against women is at a high rate.

For six years Luna Maya worked with the Hogar Comunitario, Yatzil Antszetik (Community Home). The Hogar Comunitario was founded in 1994 to provide a safe house for single mothers. Although levels of sexual violence are extremely high, when indigenous women and girls become pregnant, if they are not married they are forced to flee their communities. Abortion is not legal or available in Chiapas. Prior to 2016, therapeutic abortion was not legal in cases of rape without a judge's order, which was complex process which women often chose not to carry out. The Hogar Comunitario therefore offered a safe space for pregnant women to live during the final stages of their pregnancy and after. Before Luna Maya was established, all births were referred to the hospital where women were further victimized, including obstetric violence and unnecessary cesarean sections. Luna Maya worked with the Hogar Comunitario from 2005 to 2010 to attend births in the safe house, and to apprentice the nurses who worked in the Hogar to learn midwifery skills. Water birth was included, as well as placental encapsulation. The Hogar nurses eventually developed the necessary skills to provide the care themselves, and Luna Maya remained at a consulting role for the staff.

Luna Maya has provided a safe space to poor and victimized women to recover their power and strength. Through respectful care, informed consent, and careful relationships based on mutual trust and communication, Luna Maya provides a unique space for women whose lives are difficult, violent, and very sad, to find the joy in their own power and connect deeply with their newborns. The work Luna Maya has done with each woman from the Hogar and marginal neighborhoods embodies the essence of midwifery. It is one of the aspects that Luna Maya is most proud of—being able to bring the midwives model of care to any economic or social reality and find connection with women.

According to an indigenous woman who has had two children and received well-woman care from Luna Maya:

> "Luna Maya midwives have more experience than traditional midwives. The midwives are very impatient in my community. I felt very safe when my babies were born, I wasn't afraid, I felt very satisfied and felt that I had the birth I wanted. The midwives are kind, they are very loving. Doctors have never been an option for me to have my baby." (Ana Elizabeth, interview, 2016)

Luna Maya therefore provides a service where women from all socioeconomic and cultural backgrounds can access evidenced-based care that involves antihemorrhagic medications, diagnostic tests, resuscitation equipment, and respect for and honoring of cultural traditions and choice, such as when and how to cut the cord, the importance of massage and fetal positioning, and the choice of who is present at the birth. The following story illustrates an example of how the Luna Maya model of care extends into even the most disenfranchised women.

19.5.4 Sara's Birth Story

Sara lived alone in one of San Cristobal's poorest barrios, having been sent by her family to the city to work, and she was about to become a single mother. Sara had been sent to Luna Maya by Guadalupe, another woman who works at the market and had participated in a doula training at Luna Maya. She often referred market women to birth peacefully at Luna Maya and avoid the hospital, where it is common knowledge that young, single, indigenous women are mistreated.

Following the onset of labor, the process was taking its toll on her body, with no family support and little physical will left to begin this new phase of her life, and she was pleading the midwives for help. Just as she thought she could take no more, there was a powerful contraction and the head emerged. The midwife took Sara's hand and placed it under the water and between her legs to let her know there wasn't far to go. She rested for a few moments before the next wave of pain came along. Feeling the baby's head had given her hope that the birth would soon be over, but at the same time filled her with dread at the realization she was about to become a mother.

The next contraction began with more force than the others, bringing her back down to earth as the urge to push took over her body. The baby was born at 8.15 PM rising from the warm water of the bath and being placed on her mother's chest without making a sound. The baby lay limp and motionless while her mother stared into space, glad that the immense physical pain had subsided. The midwife quickly checked and found a faint heart beat establishing that the tiny baby was alive. With umbilical cord still attached and the placenta yet to be delivered the midwife started resuscitation. Sara looked on without saying a word as the midwife worked to bring life into her child. The midwife told her to speak to the baby by her name, that she would respond to her voice. Sara replied that she couldn't think of a name and didn't know what to say. The apprentice midwife said forcefully "how about Daniella?" and so Daniella she became without any disagreement from Sara. Half an hour later with the placenta delivered and Daniella out of danger both mother and daughter lay in bed together and contemplated what lay ahead. As they slept until the following afternoon, the midwives decided not to disturb them, only to bring her more food, as they wanted to prolong Sara's return home to an empty house.

Conclusion

Well-intended improvements in the ability of indigenous women to have access to medicalized care have decreased maternal mortality rates. However, a global trend is beginning to be observed where indigenous women are opting to return to traditional maternity care and midwives, seeking kindness, human contact, and a rights-based approach (Molina et al. 2016). This trend appears to indicate that, despite increased technology, some indigenous women still perceive birth as a normal and healthy experience, and as a result, may prioritize familiar relationships and connections over medical safety within a hospital or other medical institution. Within this landscape, birth centers like Luna Maya provide a viable, medically safe, and equitable alternative where both evidence-based care and culturally appropriate kindness are woven together in order to bridge gaps between technology and ritual.

References

Alber, E., Coe, C., & Thelen, T. (2013). *The anthropology of sibling relations. Shared parentage, experience, and exchange*. New York: Palgrave Macmillan. Retrieved from http://www.palgraveconnect.com/pc/doifinder/10.1057/9781137331236.

Alonso, C. (June 6, 2014). Personal Communication.

Banet Lucas, A. & Tryon, J. (2014). The Luna Maya model of care: A femifocal family care birth center. *Manual for replication*. Luna Maya Birth Center and Midwifery Training Institute. San Cristobal de las Casas, Chiapas, Mexico. August 2014.

Berry, N. (2010). *Unsafe motherhood: Mayan maternal mortality and subjectivity in post-war Guatemala*. New York: Berghahn Books.

Biehl, J. G., & Petryna, A. (2013). Critical global health. In J. G. Biehl & A. Petryna (Eds.), *When people come first: Critical studies in global health* (pp. 1–22). Princeton: Princeton University Press.

Davis-Floyd, R. (2001). La partera profesional: Articulating identity and cultural space for a new kind of midwife in Mexico. *Medical Anthropology, 20*(2–3), 185–243. https://doi.org/10.1080/01459740.2001.9966194

Davis-Floyd, R. (2005). Daughter of time: The postmodern midwife. *MIDIRS Midwifery Digest, 15*(1), 32–39.

ENSANUT (Encuesta Nacional de Salud y Nutricion). (2012). Retreived March 3, 2013, from http://ensanut.insp.mx/informes/ENSANUT2012ResultadosNacionales.pdf.

FrayBa. (2012). *Entre la política sistémica y las alternativas de vida. Informe sobre la situación de los derechos humanos en Chiapas durante los gobiernos federal y estatal 2006–2012*. Centro de Derechos Humanos Fray Bartolomé de Las Casas. Retrieved from http://www.frayba.org.mx/archivo/informes/130212_informe_frayba_prov.pdf.

Flores Hernandez, A., & Espejel Rodriguez, A. (2015). Una cadena de acompanamiento: La experiencia entre la red de parteras y promotoras communitarias y la semujer del estado de Guerrero, Mexico. In G. Sanchez Ramirez (Ed.), *Imagin Instantanea de la Parteria* (pp. 111–132). Mexico: EcoSur.

Freyermuth, G., & Sesia, P. (2009). *Maternal death. Actions and strategies towards safe motherhood*. México: Comité Promotor por una Maternidad sin Riesgos en México.

Homedes, N., & Ugalde, A. (2009). Twenty-five years of convoluted health reforms in Mexico. *PLoS Medicine, 6*(8), e1000124.

INEGI (Instituto Nacional de Estadística y Geografía). (2010). Censo de Población y Vivienda 2010. Retrieved from http://www.inegi.org.mx/default.aspx.

INEGI (Instituto Nacional de Estadística y Geografía). (2015). México en cifras. Retreived from http://www3.inegi.org.mx/sistemas/mexicocifras/default.aspx?e=7.

IMSS. (2015). *Informe al Ejecutivo Federal y al Congreso de la Unión 2014–2015*. Mexico. Retrieved from http://www.imss.gob.mx/conoce-al-imss/informe-2014-2015.

Laako, H. (2016). Los derechos humanos en los movimientos sociales: el caso de las parteras autónomas en México. *Revista Mexicana de Ciencias Políticas y Sociales, 61*(227), 167–194.

Lazcano-Ponce, E., Schiavon, R., Uribe-Zúñiga, P., Walker, D., Suárez-López, L., Luna-Gordillo, R., & Ulloa-Aguirre, A. (2013). Cobertura de atención del parto en México: Su interpretación en el contexto de la mortalidad materna. *salud pública de méxico, 55*, S214–S224. Retrieved from http://www.scielo.org.mx/pdf/spm/v55s2/v55s2a19.pdf.

Lucas, A. B., & Tryon, J. (2014). The Luna Maya model of care: A femifocal family care birth center. *Tuftscope Interdisciplinary Journal of Health, Ethics, and Policy, 14*(1), 22–27. Retrieved from http://tuftscope.squarespace.com/#/fall-2014/.

Mills, L., & Davis-Floyd, R. (2009). The CASA Hospital and Professional Midwifery School: An education and practice model that works. In R. Davis-Floyd, L. Barclay, B. Daviss, & J. Tritten (Eds.), *Birth models that work*. London: University of California Press.

Molina, R. L., Patel, S. J., Scott, J., Schantz-Dunn, J., & Nour, N. M. (2016). Striving for respectful maternity care everywhere. *Maternal and Child Health Journal, 20*(9), 1769–1773.

Murray de López, J. (2015). Conflict and reproductive health in urban Chiapas: Disappearing the *partera empírica*. Anthropology Matters, 16(1). Retrieved from http://www.anthropologymatters.com/index.php/anth_matters/article/view/339/584.

OECD. (2015). Measuring wellbeing in Mexican states: Executive summary [Online]. Retreived November 3, 2015, from http://www.oecd.org/gov/regionalpolicy/Mexican-States-Highlights-English.pdf.

Periodico La Jornada. (2011). *Hospital de Las Culturas acerca la atención a la población de los Altos*. Retrieved September 12, 2011, from http://www.jornada.unam.mx/2011/09/12/sociedad/045n2soc.

Secretaría de Salud. (2013). *Dirección General de Información en Salud: CLUES*. Retrieved from http://plataforma.salud.gob.mx:8091/.

Sesia, P. M. (1996). "Women come here on their own when they need to": Prenatal care, authoritative knowledge, and maternal health in Oaxaca. *Medical Anthropology Quarterly, 10*(2), 121–140. Retrieved from http://www.jstor.org/stable/649324.

Smith-Oka, V. (2013). *Shaping the motherhood of indigenous Mexico*. Nashville: Vanderbilt University Press.

Maternal Mortality of Indigenous Women in Mexico: An Analysis from the Perspective of Human Rights

20

María Graciela Freyermuth Enciso
and Hilda E. Argüello Avendaño

20.1 Introduction

Maternal mortality (MM) is defined as "[...] the death of a woman while pregnant or within 42 days of termination of pregnancy, irrespective of the duration and site of the pregnancy, from any cause related to or aggravated by the pregnancy or its management but not from accidental or incidental causes" (OMS 2012, p. 9). One of the most important and widely used indicators of maternal mortality is the Maternal Mortality Ratio, or MMR. It is calculated by dividing the number of deaths from complications during pregnancy, childbirth, or postnatal period in 1 year by the number of live births (LB) in the same period and multiplying the result by 100,000 (Cárdenas 2009, p. 35). Maternal deaths are classified into two distinct groups: "direct obstetric deaths are those resulting from obstetric complications of the pregnant state (i.e., pregnancy, labor, and the puerperium), from interventions, omissions, or incorrect treatment, or from a chain of events resulting from any of the above. Indirect obstetric deaths are those resulting from a previously existing disease or a disease that developed during pregnancy and which was not due to direct obstetric causes but which was aggravated by the physiological effects of pregnancy" (OMS 2012, p. 9). Late maternal deaths are those from "direct or indirect obstetric causes, more than 42 days, but less than 1 year after termination of pregnancy" (Ibid.).

The MMR is a powerful indicator of health inequalities. Since maternity is a relatively short process (10 months and 12 days for pregnancy, childbirth, and postpartum), it allows us to identify the short-term effect of the measures aiming to reduce it; it can thus be used to evaluate public policies and identify the various structural, institutional, and personal factors that influence the risk of death of women during maternity. Moreover, this indicator is sensitive to the inequalities between women living in different parts of the world, different regions, different countries of the same region, and even

M. G. F. Enciso, M.D., Ph.D. (✉)
Center for Research and Higher Studies in Social Anthropology-South East Unit, Chiapas, Mexico

H. E. Argüello Avendaño, Ph.D.
Department of Anthropology, Philosophy and Social Work, Rovira i Virgili University, Tarragona, Spain

Maternal Mortality Observatory in Mexico, Chiapas, Mexico

D. A. Schwartz (ed.), *Maternal Death and Pregnancy-Related Morbidity Among Indigenous Women of Mexico and Central America*, Global Maternal and Child Health: Medical, Anthropological, and Public Health Perspectives, https://doi.org/10.1007/978-3-319-71538-4_20

different localities within the same country. In Mexico, the MMR indicates important differences in pregnancy-related health between states; according to official figures for 2014, the highest MMR was recorded in Durango (71 maternal deaths per 100,000 LB), and the lowest in Morelos (9 maternal deaths per 100,000 LB) (Freyermuth et al. 2016a, b).

There are significant poverty-related inequalities in the probability of survival of Mexican women during their maternity. The MMR in municipalities with more than 40% of people living in extreme poverty is 98, compared with an MMR of 35 for municipalities with less than 20% of people living in extreme poverty. The MMR for women living in indigenous municipalities is 94, while the MMR for women living in municipalities with less than 40% of indigenous language speakers is less than one-half of that, or 44. Therefore, it can be safely stated that in Mexico indigenous women are twice more likely to die from maternal causes than women who live in nonindigenous municipalities. The risk of death varies also with the age group; the MMR for women under 15 years of age is 81, and for women over 45 years of age is 91; thus, the risk of death for women in these age groups is three and nearly four times higher than the MMR (25) for women aged 20–24 years.

In this chapter, we are interested in analyzing maternal deaths among indigenous women from the perspective of human rights. We conducted a quantitative analysis of the differences in MM between women living in indigenous municipalities (40% or more of ILS) and women living in nonindigenous municipalities (less than 40% of ILS) in the states of Oaxaca and Chiapas. This analysis allowed us to identify several protective and/or risk factors (such as schooling, place of occurrence). We also made a qualitative analysis of maternal death among Mexican indigenous women based on the three delays model and on an assessment of the elements that characterize the right to public health care (availability, accessibility, acceptability, and quality). This analysis tries not only to clarify the inequalities that emerge from official statistics but also to show, through narratives of death, the ways in which these inequalities are constructed and limit the survival of Mexican indigenous women.

20.2 International Framework

The Universal Declaration of Human Rights, adopted by the United Nations General Assembly on December 10, 1948, enshrined the right to health. The International Covenant on Economic, Social and Cultural Rights (ICESCR) and its Optional Protocol, adopted in 1966, "are the international instruments of the Universal System of Protection of Human Rights that govern the protection of economic, social, and cultural rights"[1] (Comisión Nacional de Derechos Humanos (CNDH) 2012, p. 5). All states should recognize the right of everyone to the enjoyment of the highest attainable standard of physical and mental health (Naciones Unidas-Derechos Humanos 1966). These principles were ratified at the World Population Conference, held in Bucharest in 1974, where it was established that family planning is a basic right of all couples and individuals (Ferrer and Martínez 2006, p. 2). The Mexican State ratified the ICESCR on May 23, 1981 (CNDH 2012, p. 5).

The Alma Ata Conference (September 1978) again recognized health as a fundamental human right (Organización Mundial de la Salud (OMS) 1978, p. 2). Inequality in the health status of the world population was considered politically, socially, and economically unacceptable (Ibíd.). The Convention on the Elimination of All Forms of Discrimination Against Women (CEDAW) was signed by the Mexican government in 1979 and published in the Official Journal of the Federation (DOF in Spanish) on January 9, 1981 (DOF 1981). This Convention is mandatory and

[1] "Economic, social, and cultural rights are considered material equality rights by means of which people can satisfy their basic needs and attain the highest possible level of dignity." (CNDH, 2012, p. 6).

includes two important articles: Article 3, which seeks to ensure the full development and advancement of women, and Article 12, related to health:

> "States Parties shall ensure to women appropriate services in connection with pregnancy, confinement and the post-natal period, granting free services where necessary, as well as adequate nutrition during pregnancy and nurturing lactation."

In 1987, the Initiative for Safe Motherhood recognized maternal death as a public health problem and called to reduce the number of MM cases and morbidity by half by the year 2000 (Maine 1992, p. 5; Freyermuth 2010, p. 9). In 1989, the World Summit for Children established the reduction of MM as a goal that should be monitored.

The Programme of Action of the International Conference on Population and Development, held in Cairo in 1994, and the Declaration and Platform for Action, held in Beijing in 1995, reaffirmed the commitments of States Parties regarding the reduction of MM and the provision of universal access to reproductive health care. The Millennium Declaration of 2000 (resolution 55/2 of the UN General Assembly) also discussed maternal health from the perspective of human rights. Objective 5 of the Declaration focused on improving maternal health by reducing maternal deaths by 75% by 2015, compared to 1990 figures; this objective was reaffirmed in the Final Document of the World Summit 2005 (resolution 60/1 of the General Assembly).

On August 11, 2000, the United Nations published the General Comment 14 on The Right to the Highest Attainable Standard of Health. This Comment states the need to implement "measures to improve child and maternal health, sexual and reproductive health services, including access to family planning, pre- and post-natal care, emergency obstetric services and access to information, as well as to resources necessary to act on that information." (Organización de las Naciones Unidas 2000, p. 5).

For its part, the Inter-American Commission on Human Rights (CIDH in Spanish) considers MM as a violation of human rights, and has established the following obligations for States Parties: to respect and guarantee human rights without discrimination, particularly the right to personal integrity, in order to help overcome inequalities in access to maternal health services, particularly for those who have been historically marginalized, so that they can enjoy effective access to these services (Comisión Interamericana de Derechos Humanos 2010, p. 1).

20.3 Framework in Mexico

In 1990, under the presidency of Carlos Salinas de Gortari (1988–1994), it was proposed to include the recognition of the cultural rights of indigenous peoples in the second article of the Constitution. This was approved, and 2 years later was published in the DOF on January 28, 1992 (Page 2002, p. 43):

> "The Mexican nation has a multicultural composition originally based on its indigenous peoples. The law shall protect and promote the development of their languages, cultures, habits, customs, resources and specific forms of social organization, and ensure effective access to the jurisdiction of the State. In the trials and agrarian proceedings in which they are party, their legal practices and customs shall be taken into account in the terms established by law." (Ibid.)

On August 14, 2001, several amendments made to the second article of the Constitution were published in the DOF (2001); these amendments tried to improve the conditions of indigenous people by ensuring their access to health services and expanding social services (subsection B, paragraphs II and IV) IV) (Argüello-Avendaño, 2018):

> B. In order to promote equal opportunities for indigenous people and to eliminate discriminatory practices, the Federation, the Federal District, the States and the local councils shall establish the necessary institutions and policies to guarantee indigenous people's rights and comprehensive development of indigenous communities. Such institutions and policies shall be designed and operated together with them. (Ibid.)
> In order to overcome the scarcities and backwardness affecting indigenous peoples and communities, authorities are obliged to:

III. Enforce an effective access to health services by increasing the coverage of the national health services, while making good use of traditional medicine and also to improve the indigenous people's nutrition through food programs focusing especially on children. (Ibid.)
IV. Improve the living conditions of indigenous communities and the spaces used for social activities and recreation through policies that enable the access to public and private financing for housing construction and home improvements, as well as policies that extend the coverage of basic social services (Ibid.).

Maternal mortality, one of the most persistent gaps in Mexican women's health, must be analyzed in this context.

Mexico joined the Initiative for Safe Motherhood in the year 1993 (Freyermuth 2000, p.19). This led to the formation of the National Committee for Risk-Free Motherhood (CPMSR in Spanish)—now called Safe Motherhood—with the aim of contributing to the decline of MM at the national level. The Committee has been an important component in the recognition of maternal death as a serious public health problem in the country.

The year 2002 saw the publication of the specific action program Even Start in Life ("Arranque Parejo en la Vida" in Spanish, or PAE APV), with normative character for the whole country, whose purpose was to "achieve universal coverage and equal conditions of quality care for women during pregnancy, childbirth, and the postpartum period, as well as for children before birth and up to two years of age" (Secretaría de Salud (SSA) 2002, p. 13). The implementation of this program prioritized the regions with the highest incidence of maternal deaths. The PAE APV for the period 2007–2012 was the main instrument of public policy to achieve the fourth and fifth MDGs, respectively: reducing child mortality and reducing MM (SSA 2007, p. 12).

A public policy was promoted during the presidential term of 2006–2012 that sought to ensure access to health services: the Agreement of the Technical Council of the Mexican Institute of Social Security (IMSS in Spanish) for the care of women without medical coverage referred for obstetrical complications from the IMSS-Opportunities program (now Prospera); however, this policy had no budget allocated to pay for these services. IMSS-Prospera makes cross payments to the regular IMSS system.

In 2008, at the first technical meeting between civil society organizations, academic researchers and officials of the State Health Services (SESA) and the Secretary of Health (SSA in Spanish), the CPMSR promoted universal access to obstetric care, which led to the creation of the "Healthy Pregnancy Program" (Sesia 2015), which consisted in affiliating all pregnant women and their families to the Popular Health Insurance (SPS). As a result of this, by 2015 the SPS attended 65% of the indigenous language-speaking population in Chiapas (Instituto Nacional de Estadística y Geografía 2015).

In 2009, the Secretary of Health launched a comprehensive strategy to accelerate the reduction of maternal mortality in Mexico, which included the signing, on May 28, 2009, of the General Convention of Interagency Collaboration for Obstetric Emergency Care (CAEO in Spanish) (ratified in 2015) to ensure universal attention. This Convention states that all women with obstetric complications must be treated in any hospital of the Mexican Social Security Institute (IMSS in Spanish), the Institute for Social Security and Services for State Workers (ISSSTE in Spanish) or of the Secretariat of Health (SSA in Spanish), regardless of their affiliation status. This requires crossed payments between institutions, but no special budget was allocated for the implementation of the Convention. In 2013, IMSS-Prospera was incorporated into the Convention. Currently, obstetric emergency care is guaranteed by a decree which adds various provisions to the General Law of Health, the Social Security Law, and the Law of ISSSTE (Diario Oficial de la Federación (DOF) 2015).

Furthermore, the Agreement for Strengthening Public Health Action in the States (AFASPE in Spanish), signed in 2008, allows the transfer of financial resources from the federal government to the states of the republic to pay for specific action programs. The initial intent of these transfers, in the case of PAE APV, was to reduce gaps in MMR among the states.

Also, there was a recent update (4 April 2016) to the Mexican Official Standard NOM-007-2016-SSA2 for the care of women during pregnancy, childbirth, and postpartum, and of newborns, which sets guidelines for providing timely obstetric emergency care.

The Special Program for Indigenous Peoples 2014–2018 (2014), which is mandatory for the National Commission for the Development of Indigenous Peoples (CDI in Spanish), as well as other agencies of the Federal Public Administration (DOF 2014, p. 1),

> "seeks to guarantee the indigenous population access to health services, particularly to health centers and clinics in all indigenous communities, and to promote the creation of spaces and the availability of supplies for childbirth care in indigenous communities" (Ibid.: 28).

This legal framework is intended to ensure the survival of women with obstetric complications; therefore, all these instruments ensure justiciability (the possibility of recurring to a legal process or legal enforceability) in cases of maternal deaths that could have been avoided.

20.4 Methods

The quantitative analysis was based on data obtained from databases of mortality of the General Directorate of Health Information (DGIS in Spanish) of the SSA: the Epidemiological and Statistical Subsystem of deaths (SEED in Spanish), particularly the sub-base of maternal mortality and the Birth Information Subsystem (SINAC in Spanish). Data from the intercensus survey were also used in this study.

The population was divided according to the prevalence of indigenous language speakers or ILS using the categories found in the databases of mortality of DGIS: municipalities with greater than 40% of ILS are considered indigenous municipalities, while those with less than 40% ILS or with 5000 indigenous people or more are considered municipalities with indigenous presence; there are also municipalities with scattered indigenous population or minority languages, and municipalities with no indigenous population. Regarding MMR, the analysis was performed comparing two populations: the indigenous population and the remainder of the population.

The variables used for the description included the National Population Council (CONAPO in Spanish) marginality index of the United Nations Development Programme (UNDP). Analyzing this index according to the grouping based on ILS allowed us to have a clearer idea of the relationship between maternal deaths and the level of development of each type of municipality. Other variables included living in a town with less than 15,000 inhabitants and with less than 2500 inhabitants; this allowed us to analyze maternal deaths as a function of the dispersion of the population. The last variable was place of death, which was used to assess the access to health services of different types of population.

The case studies were based on the documentation generated by DGIS in 2012 and 2015 regarding cases of deaths of women occurring in 2010 and 2014.

20.5 Maternal Mortality Is a Sensitive Indicator for Identifying Inequality in Terms of Human Rights—The Case of Chiapas and Oaxaca

In a previous study, Freyermuth and Luna (2014) showed that the highest rates of maternal deaths from preventable causes for the period 2002–2006 were those of Guerrero (83.7%), Chiapas (77.2%), and Oaxaca (75.9%). For the period 2007–2011, the rate of maternal deaths in these three states decreased to 76.4%, 70%, and 70.1%, respectively. Chiapas and Oaxaca[2] are the states with the highest densities of indigenous population.

[2]In Chiapas and Oaxaca, many people face adverse contexts associated with poverty. In 2014, 76.2% of the population of Chiapas lived in poverty, and 31.8% in extreme poverty, while 78.7% of the population had an income below the limit of welfare. In the same year, 66.8% of the population of Oaxaca lived in poverty, 28.3% in extreme poverty and 68.8% of the population had an income below the welfare limit. (CONEVAL estimations based on the MCS-ENIGH 2010, 2012 and 2014).

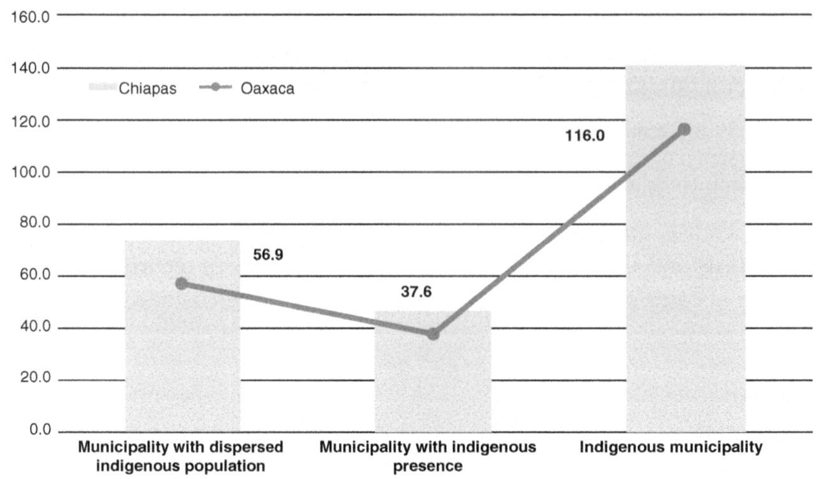

Fig. 20.1 MMR for Chiapas and Oaxaca according to the presence of indigenous populations, 2010–2014. Source: Freyermuth, G., 2017, General Directorate of Health Information (DGIS). Database of maternal deaths 2002–2014 (online) and database of child births—SINAC 2012: National Health Information System (SINAIS). (Mexico): Secretariat of Health. (Date of query: August 10, 2016). Note: The analysis considered all maternal deaths in Chiapas and Oaxaca

In 1990, the estimated MMR for Mexico in its entirety was 89, for Oaxaca 175, the highest in the country, and for Chiapas 121 (28th place). Twenty-five years later, the MMR for Chiapas was 68 (31st place) and for Oaxaca 47 (24th place), while the national MMR was 39. According to these data, Mexico seems to be on track to meet the new Sustainable Development Goals (SDG) by 2030. However, analysis of the MMR from 2010 to 2014 using the official data available shows a gap associated with the indigenous population. In this period, the national MMR for indigenous women was 94, twice that of the rest of the population, which is 47. This trend is similar in Oaxaca and Chiapas, as shown in the following chart (Fig. 20.1).

Education allows women and their families to develop capabilities to make informed decisions, improves their working conditions, and enhances horizontal and vertical support networks. However, in the case of women living in municipalities inhabited by indigenous languages speakers (MILS), the protective effects of education are weaker than in municipalities of nonindigenous language speakers (MnoILS in Spanish). In MnoILS, the MMR for women with high school, undergraduate, or graduate education was 57 times lower as compared with unschooled women. In contrast, the MMR of women with high school education or higher who died in MILS was only five times lower when compared with unschooled women living in the same type of communities. The same trend can be recognized in Chiapas; the MMR is six times lower among women with professional-level studies as compared with unschooled women. In Oaxaca, the risk of death for unschooled women is only three times higher when compared with educated women. This shows that the Mexican indigenous population is still very far from reaching the SDG (Fig. 20.2).

It is evident that factors such as education, which could increase the survival rate of a person, have an important effect only when structural conditions allow it. The degree of marginalization is an example of this: the lower it is, the lower is the MMR, as shown in Fig. 20.3.

A factor that merits further analysis is the location in which childbirths occur. Nationwide, the MMR of women who live in MnoILS and who have social security or SPS is very similar: the MMR of women affiliated with IMSS is 30, compared with 38 for those affiliated with SESA and 44 for those affiliated with ISSSTE. The lowest MMR (18) corresponds to IMSS-Prospera, which is even

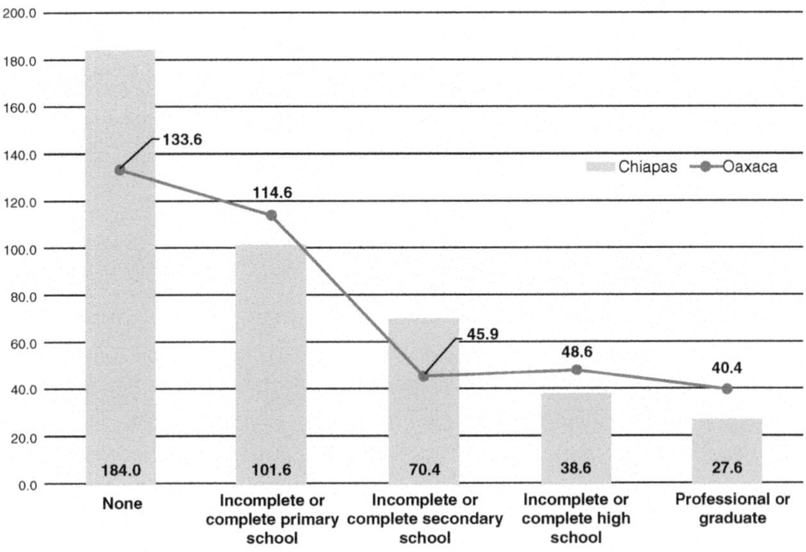

Fig. 20.2 MMR for Chiapas and Oaxaca in relation to the education of women, 2010–2014. Source: Freyermuth, G., 2017, General Directorate of Health Information (DGIS). Database of maternal deaths 2002–2014 (online) and database of childbirths—SINAC 2012: National Health Information System (SINAIS). (Mexico): Secretariat of Health. (Date of query: August 10, 2016). Note: The analysis considered all maternal deaths in Chiapas and Oaxaca

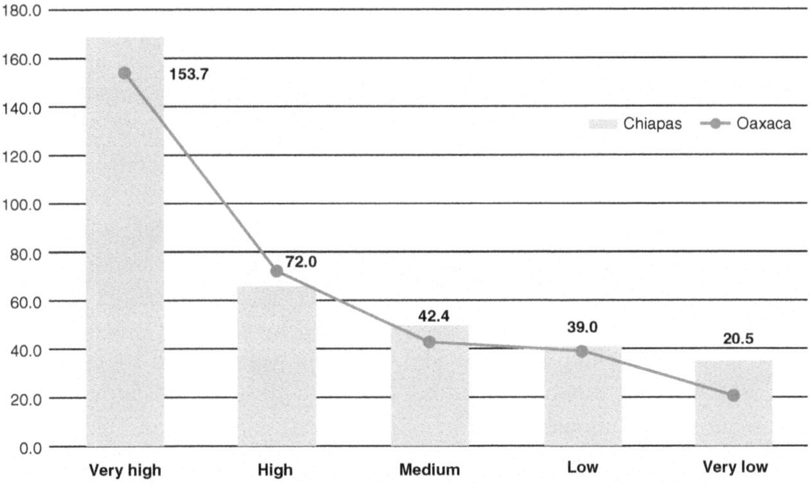

Fig. 20.3 The MMR for Chiapas and Oaxaca according to the degree of marginalization, 2010–2014. Source: Freyermuth, G., 2017, General Directorate of Health Information (DGIS). Database of maternal deaths 2002–2014 (online) and database of childbirths—SINAC 2012: National Health Information System (SINAIS). (Mexico): Secretariat of Health. (Date of query: August 10, 2016). Note: The analysis considers all maternal deaths in Chiapas and Oaxaca

lower than the MMR of Petroleos Mexicanos (PEMEX in Spanish), Secretariat of the Navy (SEMAR in Spanish) and the Secretariat of National Defense (SEDENA in Spanish), which is 21. However, this trend is not the same for women who live in MILS, for whom the MMR of those affiliated to social security institutions (IMSS, ISSSTE, SEDENA, Pemex and SEMAR) is on average much higher (107) than the MMR of those affiliated to SESA (63) or IMSS-Prospera (24) (Table 20.1). This could be the result of the spatial distribution of medical units, since access is better in institutions open to all

Table 20.1 Factors associated with maternal mortality in different municipalities in Mexico according to their percentage of indigenous language speakers, 2010–2014

Characteristics		MMR	
		Other municipalities	Municipalities with more than 40% of ILS
Education level of the mother	None	116	263
	Incomplete primary school	90	158
	Completed primary school	60	88
	Incomplete secondary school	46	62
	Completed secondary school (9 years of school)	36	55
	Completed high school (academic or technical)	2	41
	Professional or graduate	2	53
Affiliation of the mother	None	37	83
	IMSS	37	44
	ISSSTE	55	75
	PEMEX, SEDENA or SEMAR	35	69
	SP	46	88
	Other	39	327
	IMSS-Oportunidades	176	314
Place of delivery care	Secretariat of Health	38	63
	IMSS-Oportunidades	18	24
	IMSS	30	128
	ISSSTE	44	39
	PEMEX, SEDENA or SEMAR	21	81
	Other public unit	30	82
	Private medical unit	25	32
	Public space	221	385
	Home	187	353
	Another place	67	116

Source: Freyermuth, 2016, based on information from the DGIS 2010–2014

population groups or those working with the SPS, whereas women with social security may have access problems. Alternatively, it may also be that women with severe obstetrical complications are referred to social security institutions.

The case of IMSS-Prospera is interesting. Although it has the lowest MMR among public institutions, its target population has an MMR of 174 in MnoILS and 314 in MILS in cases where the women did not die in medical units of that institution, which suggests that its beneficiaries are having difficulty accessing medical care during obstetric emergencies. Living in a municipality with a high percentage of ILS, combined with other factors, is detrimental to the survival of women during an obstetric emergency, and is often associated with death during the transfer to a more specialized medical unit.

In this context, the "Three Delays" model may be useful for a qualitative analysis of the medical attention received by women with obstetric complications. A study published in 1994 became a precedent for future analysis and implementation of public policies focused on reducing maternal death: "Too Far To Walk: Maternal Mortality In Context" by Sereen Thaddeus and Deborah Maine (Thaddeus and Maine 1994). Their analysis focused on the factors (social, cultural, and medical) that come into play in the interval between the onset of an obstetric complication and its outcome, and proposed a conceptual framework called the "Three Phases of Delay": (1) delay in deciding to seek care on the part of the individual, the family, or both, which is related to acceptability, availability, and cultural accessibility; (2) delay in reaching an adequate health care facility, which is closely linked to economic and geographic accessibility; and (3) delay in receiving adequate care at the facility, which is related to the quality of medical care (Thaddeus and Maine 1994, p. 1092; Organización de las Naciones Unidas 2000, p. 3–4). It is important to note that although any of these delays can determine the death of a person, often the death of women in comprehensive hospitals is caused by a complicated path that can result from the first and second delays. As will be seen in the narratives of personal experiences, the characteristic elements of the right to health may be involved in any of the three delays as underlying causes of death.

20.6 The First Delay

In the first delay, the women die without having sought medical attention. This delay is influenced by socioeconomic and/or cultural factors (such as recognizing an emergency or the severity or etiology of a disease; the status of women, economic solvency, education, accessibility in terms of distance, transportation, roads, costs, the perceived quality of care given its reputation or previous experience, the effectiveness of treatment, the attitude of the health personnel, privacy, access of visiting or accompanying relatives, medical procedures, and waiting time).

From a human rights perspective, it is necessary that the holder can claim these rights. Poor and indigenous women typically face numerous difficulties in this respect because they themselves do not think they are entitled to these rights. The first delay shows the need for human rights organizations not to confine their recommendations to public institutions and instead to emphasize the importance of private dynamics that hinder or disempower women as subjects of rights; as Susana Chiarotti points out (2006), it is in the private sphere where the subordination of women is constructed and where most limits to the exercise of their rights exist.

The acceptability of health services and health workers among the indigenous population is often compromised due to unsatisfactory or unsuccessful previous experiences. Dissatisfaction with health services does not necessarily depend on an unsuccessful outcome from a medical point of view; even when people have their health restored, their experiences with medical services may discourage their use in a new event of illness. In Mexico, almost no measures have been taken to ensure the availability of translators/cultural mediators in health units located in towns, municipalities or entities with high density of indigenous population. The indigenous population is faced with a medical culture that not only is conducted in Spanish, but whose particular language, routines, and operation are almost completely alien to them (Freyermuth and Argüello-Avendaño 2011). Indigenous women often face more obstacles than their male counterparts do because most of them have less contact with urban centers and are more likely to be monolingual and illiterate: "The invisibility of the indigenous population to public institutions naturalizes the skills that people must possess to make use of public services" (Ibid. p. 205). The limited opening hours of medical units in health centers or clinics (they usually only operate in the morning), long waiting times, and lack of basic materials or complementary diagnostic resources (in indigenous communities, there is very limited access to laboratory studies, for example) also discourage the use of public health services (Argüello-Avendaño 2018).

20.6.1 The First Delay Applied to the Analysis of a Case of Maternal Death from Hemorrhage—Magdalena Was as if Unconscious (*Tseltal from Chiapas*)

Magdalena was 28 years old, married, and had four children; she had not finished primary school, spoke *Tseltal* and Spanish, and was affiliated with the "seguro popular" (SP in Spanish). Her previous deliveries had occurred without mishap. She lived in a municipality where 95% of people live in poverty, 65% in extreme poverty and 95% of the population has an income below the welfare line. Only 11.7% of inhabitants from this municipality have no access to health services, according to CONEVAL (2014). She was in her ninth month of pregnancy, and from the first trimester she had been treated at the clinic of the municipality; she attended more than five prenatal consultations and had undergone basic laboratory tests.[3] Magdalena's husband narrates her misfortune:

> My wife started with labor pain yesterday at six o'clock in the morning. Around 11 we went to call the midwife, who went to see my wife; the strongest pains began at four in the afternoon and by 6 pm my son was born; he cried and breathed at birth, but my wife was unconscious, and the placenta did not come out. Since my house is very far from town and is a long climb up, we did not want to take her out; so, at 7, we went to look for the owner of the pharmacy. When she arrived, she injected my wife with a drug to force the placenta to come out, but it didn't, and so my brother went to look for a doctor at the health center; he arrived at the health center of Tenejapa at 8 and asked the nurse to come to my house to see my wife because she was seriously ill. But when the nurse arrived, my wife had already died; the nurse was kind enough to cut the cord for my son and to attend him.

When an obstetric emergency occurs, structural limitations, such as lack of geographic access or available transportation 24 h/365 days a year, determine that people seek attention within the range of their possibilities; in this case a midwife, a pharmacist, and a nurse.

In the case of Magdalena, the delays in seeking care can be explained by the lack of availability and lack of physical accessibility to medical services, but it shows the cultural acceptability of preferring local health agents.

In the case of indigenous women, who have traditionally given birth in their homes, the policy of attending deliveries within a hospital discourages them from seeking assistance at the primary care level. Thus, it can be said that the acceptability criteria is essential to reduce this delay:

> "All health facilities, goods and services must be respectful of medical ethics and culturally appropriate, i.e. respectful of the culture of individuals, minorities, peoples and communities, sensitive to gender and life-cycle requirements, as well as being designed to respect confidentiality and improve the health status of those concerned." (Organización de las Naciones Unidas 2000).

20.7 The Second Delay

In the second delay, seeking care is delayed by the difficulty of reaching an adequate health facility. The accessibility of medical units depends on distance and travel conditions (travel time, unforeseen events occurring during travel such as weather, conditions of roads, etc.); availability of public transport and cost (if it exceeds planned costs or the ability to afford it). According to the Committee on Economic, Social and Cultural Rights (CESCR), availability is understood as a sufficient number of facilities, goods and public health services and centers, as well as the existence of health programs with sufficient material and human resources. In physical terms, accessibility implies that goods and services must be within safe physical reach for all sections of the population, especially for vulnerable or marginalized groups, such as ethnic minorities.

[3] The basic laboratory studies to which all pregnant women should have access include: blood count, blood sugar, blood type, urinalysis, and rapid HIV test.

20.7.1 The Second Delay Applied to the Analysis of a Case of Maternal Death from Abortion: Ana Maria—The Pills Came Wrapped in Paper (*Chatina from Oaxaca*)

Ana Maria was 37 years old; she lived in free union, was illiterate, spoke only *Chatino*, and had six children. She died at home 4 months into her seventh pregnancy (17 weeks gestation). She had no prenatal care and she was not affiliated to the Popular Insurance (Seguro Popular or SP) or to IMSS-Prospera.

Ana Maria lived in a municipality where 92.4% of the population live in poverty (with an income below the welfare line) and 64.5% in extreme poverty. According to CONEVAL (2014), only 15.9% of the population of this municipality has no access to public health care; Ana Maria belonged to this small part of the population.

On January 10, 2010, Ana Maria went to a nearby town "to buy pills"; her husband does not know exactly what it was that they sold to her; they came wrapped in paper without a prescription. She ingested the pills at 7 o'clock that night; he doesn't know how many. The next day, Ana Maria began to feel bad, and at 7 o'clock in the morning, she started feeling pain in her belly. She "took out the child," and then started bleeding. The husband, seeing her worse, went to the municipality to ask for an ambulance at around four in the afternoon. The ambulance arrived an hour later, but Ana Maria had already died.

This case shows a paradigmatic story of women who cannot continue with a pregnancy for reasons of extreme poverty and who live in a place where abortion is not a legal option. The decriminalization of abortion for people living in extreme poverty would increase the probability of survival for women like Ana Maria, who left behind six orphaned children. In Mexico, there are precedents for the decriminalization of abortion for economic reasons. In Mexico City, women can opt for this procedure, and it is thus possible to say that women in the rest of the states suffer an unfair disadvantage.[4] This means that the Mexican State has failed to comply with the obligation: "…to adopt appropriate legislative, administrative, budgetary, judicial, promotional and other measures towards the full realization of the right to health." (Organización de las Naciones Unidas 2000, p. 9). This cause of death is found mainly among poor and uneducated women. Between 2010 and 2014, six women, all without education and living in MILS, died at home from abortion without having sought medical care; some of these abortions were sought, other were spontaneous. Taken together, these six women had had 33 pregnancies among them, and each left behind an average of four orphaned children.

20.8 The Third Delay

The third delay occurs from not receiving adequate and appropriate treatment. The quality of the service may be related to the number of patients admitted in critical condition or to the lack of health personnel in medical units, or to the lack of skill of the existing personal; it may also be related to material deficiencies (nonavailability of blood, drugs, or other necessary equipment), or to improper handling of the existing equipment (incorrect diagnosis or disease management). According to the CESCR, health facilities, goods and services not only should be acceptable from a cultural point of view but they should also be adequate from a scientific and medical point of view, and provide good quality service. This requires, among other things, the presence of skilled medical personnel, scientifically approved drugs and hospital equipment in good condition, clean and potable water, and adequate sanitation.

[4] Inequalities produced by legislation that undermines human rights (unfair disadvantage) (Art. 23 of the General Law). When local laws do not provide the same guarantees to all people.

20.8.1 The Third Delay Applied to the Analysis of a Case of Maternal Death from Severe Preeclampsia: Sandra—Seeking Care by Her Own Means (*Mixe from Oaxaca*)

Sandra was 37 years old; she had five children, lived in free union, had finished primary school, and spoke only *Mixe*. She lived in a town in which there was only a nursing home attended by a traveling medical team; she was affiliated with the popular insurance (SP) and Prospera 4 months into her sixth and final pregnancy, and was provided care by a male nurse working in the nursing home. Sandra lived in a municipality where 90.9% of people live in poverty (with an income below the welfare line) and 61.9% in extreme poverty. According to CONEVAL (2014), 38.8% of the population of this municipality lack access to health care.

Sandra attended four prenatal consultations. In three of them, her blood pressure was found to be rather low, 90/60 mm Hg; she was a small woman, less than 1.50 m in height. During the fourth prenatal consultation, on January 19, 2010, her blood pressure was 100/70 mm Hg. She had no access to basic laboratory studies throughout her prenatal care.

On February 7, she started suffering from headache, leg edema, vomiting, dizziness, retroocular pain, a perception of lights (*phosphenes*), and ringing in the ears (*tinnitus*). She traveled, by her own means, to the nearest Basic Community Hospital located in a neighboring town; there they measured her blood pressure and sent her back to her home. She continued with the same symptoms in the following days, and on February 15th she traveled again by her own means to the Basic Hospital, where she was seen at 9:50 pm by the emergency service. By then, she had also conjunctival jaundice. After several clinical studies, it was determined that she had severe preeclampsia; she was administered antihypertensive medications and sent to a third-level hospital in the state capital.

In the early morning of the next day, February 16th, Sandra had a normal delivery but with abundant meconium. Her baby was in poor condition; a pediatrician was called to care for the newborn but he did not come. In the afternoon, Sandra worsened, developed cardiac shock symptoms with very low blood pressure and kidney damage; she was transferred to intensive care. She died later that night.

This case shows that even when the indigenous population seeks help from public health services, they do not receive quality care, which constitutes a violation of their right to access health care. Sandra had prenatal care, but had to overcome the structural deficits of her community with her own money; she had no institutional support to access third-level medical care and was rejected the first time she tried. This story also shows that the blood pressure of many women is outside the "norm." What in Sandra was a hypertensive crisis was not perceived as such by health personnel because her blood pressure was within "normal" parameters.

Between 2010 and 2014 there were a total of 5222 maternal deaths; 1069 of these women died from hypertensive disorders related to pregnancy. Thus, hypertensive disease of pregnancy was the cause of death in 21% of all maternal deaths, including late ones. Of these, 187 deaths occurred in MILS and 879 in the rest of the municipalities; eclampsia was the most common cause of death in these women, accounting for 59% and 52% of maternal deaths, respectively. The second leading cause was severe gestational hypertension or preeclampsia (pregnancy-induced) with proteinuria, accounting for 36% and 42% of deaths, respectively (Table 20.2).

Hypertension during pregnancy is one of the costliest causes of maternal death, not only for the monetary-related costs of treating it on an acute basis but also because it may require long stays in the Intensive Care Unit (ICU).

Virtually all women who die from hypertension do so in a medical unit; only a few die in their homes. Of those living in MILS, only three died in their homes, and only one of the 879 who lived in

Table 20.2 Number and percentage of maternal deaths in Mexico by type of hypertensive diseases of pregnancy in municipalities categorized according to the percentage of indigenous language speakers, 2010–2014

		Rest of the population		More than 40% of indigenous population	
Hypertensive disease of pregnancy	Code CIE-10	No def	%	No def	%
Eclampsia	O15	459	52.2	110	58.8
Gestational hypertension (pregnancy-induced) with proteinuria	O14.1	370	42	68	36.4
Preexisting hypertension complicating pregnancy, childbirth, and postpartum	O10	18	2	2	1.1
Preexisting hypertensive disorders with proteinuria	O11	13	1.5	2	1.1
Gestational hypertension (pregnancy-induced) without proteinuria	O13	15	1.7	3	1.6
Unspecified maternal hypertension	O16	4	0.5	2	1.1
Total		879	100	187	100

Source: Freyermuth, 2017, based on information from the DGIS 2010–2014

Table 20.3 Number of hospitals in Mexico according to the level of medical care provided and to municipalities with indigenous population

	Level of medical care				
Municipalities by indigenous population	High	Low	Basic	Medium	Overall total
Scattered indigenous population	43	4	11	147	205
Indigenous presence	117	8	1	98	224
Indigenous municipality	0	0	2	31	33
No indigenous population	0	1	0	0	1
Overall total	160	13	14	276	463

Source: Freyermuth and Gomez with information from the General Cooperation Agreement signed by the Secretariat of Health, the Mexican Social Security Institute and the Institute for Social Security and Services for State Workers for the Management of Obstetric Emergencies, Annex 1 updated in September 2015

MnoILS did so. Thus, survival depends on two issues: first, early diagnosis, and second, good quality of care. Pregnancy-related hypertensive disease often presents with bleeding. The availability of safely matched blood, blood products (platelets), and ICU transfusion banks are critical for the survival and good handling of women with obstetric complications, as most of them die due to the limited availability of these resources.

Estimates based on the intercensus survey 2015 show that 73.35% of indigenous women are affiliated with the Seguro Popular (SP), and only 13.35% do not have any health protection. In the states of Chiapas and Oaxaca, 79.34 and 76.26% of indigenous women are affiliated with the SP, and only 14.03% and 12.26% lack affiliation to a public health service, respectively. Notwithstanding this, these women remain twice as likely to die from maternal causes compared to other Mexican women.

The basic risk factor for having maternal death among these women resides in the accessibility and availability of hospital care resources; for example, throughout Mexico, no third-level hospital can be found in municipalities defined as indigenous (Table 20.3).

These data demonstrate that being affiliated with the SPS or IMSS-Prospera is almost the same as not being affiliated with any of them; that is, there is no difference between the quality of care received.

Conclusions

Although Mexico had pledged to reduce its MM to 22 per 100,000 live births (LB) by 2015, this goal has been abandoned. According to the new Sustainable Development Goals, MM should reach 70 deaths per 100,000 LB by 2030. However, Mexico is a diverse country with large disparities between its different groups of citizens, even though access to health protection has increased among the indigenous population as indicated by the National Health Survey (ENSANUT in Spanish) of 2006 and 2012. Among the indigenous population, affiliation with the popular insurance programs rose from 14 to 61.9% (Leyva-Flores et al. 2013, p. 125), but this has not guaranteed, as we have shown, improved access to health services or a positive trend in reducing the risk of dying from maternal causes in MILS. Although hospital care of indigenous women during their delivery rose from 63.8% in 2006 to 76.4% in 2012, the use of outpatient health services was lower among the indigenous population as compared with the nonindigenous population in the same period (Ibid.: 127). This poses major challenges not only for public policy but also for the public health and the human rights framework.

We can conclude that the cases presented here show that the living conditions of indigenous women are so precarious that the decrease in the percentage of women who lack access to health services does not ensure that they receive adequate medical attention. Most of them must still pay to travel outside their communities pay to travel outside their communities to third-level care units or buy medicines and other necessities that are not provided by medical units. They also face rejection by hospitals, lack of cooperation and coordination between the first and second level of care, lack of access to family planning methods, and to the possibility of exercising their sexual and reproductive rights without risking their lives.

Even though 16 years ago it was decided that the MILS should be targeted through multisectoral actions to improve their health and welfare, available indicators show they still lack the necessary conditions for exercising their human rights.

References

Argüello-Avendaño, H. (2018). *Maternal mortality at the beginning of the 21st century in Los Altos of Chiapas, Mexico: Structural violence and care seeking, Doctoral Thesis in final review*. Tarragona: Universitat Rovira i Virgili.

Cárdenas, R. (2009). *Selected indicators for the evaluation of health conditions*. Mexico: Comité Promotor por una Maternidad Sin Riesgos, Asesoría Capacitación y Asistencia en Salud A.C..

Chiarotti, S. (2006). Women and human rights: Convergences and tensions between two social movements. In A. E. Yamin (Ed.), *Economic, social and cultural rights in Latin America. From the invention to the tool* (pp. 85–102). Mexico: Plaza y Valdés.

Comisión Interamericana de los Derechos Humanos (CIDH). (2010). Acceso a servicios de salud materna desde una perspectiva de derechos humanos, OEA/Ser.L/V/II. Doc.69. Retrieved March 30, 2017, from http://cidh.org/women/SaludMaterna10Sp/SaludMaterna2010.pdf.

Comisión Nacional de Derechos Humanos (CNDH). (2012). *International covenant on economic, social and cultural rights, and its optional protocol*. México: CNDH.

Consejo Nacional de Evaluación de la Política de Desarrollo Social (CONEVAL). (2014). *Anexo Estadístico de pobreza en México 2014*. México: CONEVAL. Retrieved March 31, 2017, from http://www.coneval.org.mx/Medicion/MP/Paginas/AE_pobreza_2014.aspx

Diario Oficial de la Federación (DOF). (1981). Decree approving the International Covenant on Civil and Political Rights, opened for signature in New York City, USA, on December 19, 1966, with the interpretative declarations to articles 9, paragraph 5, and article 18, and reservations to article 13 and subsection B) of article 25, to be made by the Executive of the Union upon accession. Retrieved January 9, 1981, from http://dof.gob.mx/nota_detalle.php?codigo=4603452&fecha=09/01/1981.

Diario Oficial de la Federación (DOF). (2001). Decree approving the article by which a second and third paragraphs are added to article 1, article 2 is reformed, the first paragraph of Article 4 is repealed; And a sixth paragraph is added to article 18, and a last paragraph to the third fraction of article 115 of the Political Constitution of the United

Mexican States. Retrieved from March 30, 2017, from http://www.dof.gob.mx/nota_detalle.php?codigo=762221&fecha=14/08/2001.

Diario Oficial de la Federación (DOF). (2014). Special Program of the Indigenous People 2014–2018. Retrieved March 30, 2017, from http://www.dof.gob.mx/nota_detalle.php?codigo=5343116&fecha=30/04/2014.

Diario Oficial de la Federación (DOF). (2015). Decree to add various provisions of the General Health Law, the Social Security Law and the Law of the Institute of Social Security and Social Services of State Workers. Retrieved July 20, 2016, from http://www.dof.gob.mx/nota_detalle.php?codigo=5415150&fecha=12/11/2015.

Ferrer, M., Martínez, J. (2006). Population, development and human rights: A proposal for its adoption in Latin America and the Caribbean. Santiago de Chile: CELADE- División de Población de la CEPAL, Naciones Unidas. Retrieved March 30, 2015, from http://www.cepal.org/sites/default/files/events/files/ferrer-martinez.pdf.

Freyermuth, G. (2000). *To die in Chenalho. Gender, ethnicity and generation. Risk factors during maternity,* PhD thesis in Social Anthropology, Mexico, Universidad Nacional Autonoma de Mexico.

Freyermuth, G. (2010). Unequal in life, unequal to die. Maternal mortality in Chiapas: an analysis from inequality. Mexico: United Nations Development Program in Mexico, Report on Human Development in Chiapas, Working Paper 2010/1. Retrieved August 26, 2016, from http://docplayer.es/17067177-Desiguales-en-la-vida-desiguales-para-morir-la-mortalidad-materna-en-chiapas-un-analisis-desde-la-inequidad.html.

Freyermuth, G., & Argüello-Avendaño, H. (2011). The premature death of women in Los Altos of Chiapas. An analysis from violence. *Pueblos y Fronteras Digital, 6*(10), 181–216.

Freyermuth, G., & Luna, M. (2014). Maternal death and avoidable deaths in excess. Methodological proposal to evaluate public health policy. *Realidad, Datos y Espacio Revista Internacional de Estadística y Geografía, 5*(3), 44–61. Retrieved March 17, 2014, from http://www.inegi.org.mx/RDE/rde_13/rde_13_art4.html.

Freyermuth, G., Argüello Avendaño, H. E., Mera, A. Z. (2014). *Monitoring of sexual and reproductive health care in indigenous adolescents.* Friendly Services of the State Health Institute of Chiapas and Paired Services of Asesoría, Capacitación y Asistencia en Salud, A.C., in the Tsotsil-Tseltal Zone of Los Altos of Chiapas. Mexico: CIESAS-INMUJERES. Retrieved May 14, 2016, from http://cedoc.inmujeres.gob.mx/cendoc/documentos_download/101242.pdf.

Freyermuth, G., Luna, M., & Muños, J. (2016a). *Indicadores 2014. Mortalidad materna en México.* México: Observatorio de Mortalidad Materna.

Freyermuth, G., Luna, M., & Muñoz, J. (2016b). 2014 Indicators. In *Maternal mortality in Mexico.* Mexico: Observatory of Maternal Mortality.

Freyermuth, G. (Ed.) (2017). The Right To Health Protection For Indigenous Women in Mexico. National Analysis And Cases From A Human Rights Perspective. México: Centro de Investigaciones y Estudios Superiores en Antropología Social, Comisión Nacional de los Derechos Humanos.

Instituto Nacional de Estadística y Geografía (INEGI). (2015). *Intercensal survey.* Aguascalientes: INEGI. Retrieved March 31, 2017, from http://www.beta.inegi.org.mx/proyectos/enchogares/especiales/intercensal/

Leyva-Flores, R., Infante-Xibille, C., Pablo-Gutiérrez, J., & Quintino-Pérez, F. (2013). Persistent inequity in health and access to services for the indigenous peoples of Mexico, 2006–2012. *Public Health of Mexico, 55*(2), S123–S128.

Maine, D. (1992). *Safe motherhood programs: Options and issues.* Nueva York: Center for Population and Family Health, Columbia University. Retrieved August 5, 2015, from http://www.amddprogram.org/v1/resources/SMProgOptionsandissuesSP.pdf

Naciones Unidas-Derechos Humanos. (1966). *International covenant on economic, social and cultural rights.* New York: UN. Retrieved March 10, 2017, from http://www.ohchr.org/SP/ProfessionalInterest/Pages/CESCR.aspx

Organización de las Naciones Unidas. (2000). Economic, Social and Cultural Rights Committee. Observation 14 The right to the enjoyment of the highest attainable standard of health (Article 12). Substantive issues addressed in the implementation of the International Covenant on Economic, Social and Cultural Rights. New York: UN. Retrieved May 11, 2016, from http://conf-ts1.unog.ch/1_SPA/Tradutek/Derechos_hum_Base/CESCR/00_1_obs_grales_Cte_Dchos Ec Soc Cult.html#GEN14.

Organización Mundial de la Salud (OMS). (1978). *Alma-Ata 1978 primary health care.* Geneva: WHO. Retrieved April 18, 2016, from http://apps.who.int/iris/bitstream/10665/39244/1/9243541358.pdf

Organización Mundial de la Salud (OMS). (2012). *WHO guide for the application of CIE-10 to deaths during pregnancy, childbirth and puerperium: CIE-MM.* Geneva: WHO.

Page, J. (2002). *Health policy aimed at the indigenous peoples of Mexico and Chiapas 1875–1995.* Mexico: Multidisciplinary Research Program on Mesoamerica and the Southeast, National Autonomous University of Mexico, Institute of Indigenous Studies, Autonomous University of Chiapas.

Secretaría de Salud (SSA). (2002). *Action Programme: "start even in life".* Mexico: SSA. Retrieved August 18, 2016, from http://www.salud.gob.mx/unidades/cdi/documentos/DOCSAL7106.pdf

Secretaría de Salud (SSA). (2007). *Specific action program 2002–2012, start even in life.* Mexico: SSA. Retrieved August 18, 2016, from https://www.google.com.mx/url?sa=t&rct=j&q=&esrc=s&source=web&cd=1&ved

=0ahUKEwi6j6_9x4DTAhUM6CYKHZTvDSoQFggiMAA&url=http%3A%2F%2Fsalud.edomexico.gob.mx%2Fhtml%2Fdescarga.php%3Farchivo%3DMedica%2FARRANQUE%2520PAREJO%2520EN%2520LA%2520VIDA.%2520PROGRAMA%2520%25202007-2012.PDF&usg=AFQjCNFiw3_OvUZARFlxMdti07Gb3kce0w&sig2=dJculDm2AYZysHVa_jNiRw&cad=rja

Sesia, P. (2015). Technical meetings for the promotion of maternal health in Chiapas, Guerrero, Oaxaca and Veracruz. In G. Freyermuth (Ed.), *25 years of good practices to reduce maternal mortality in Mexico. Experiences of civil society organizations and the academy* (pp. 37–43). Mexico: Center for Research and Higher Studies in Social Anthropology, Observatory of Maternal Mortality in Mexico, Promoting Committee for Safe Maternity in Mexico.

Thaddeus, S., & Maine, D. (1994). Too far to walk: Maternal mortality in context. *Social Science & Medicine, 38*(8), 1091–1110.

Part III

Honduras

21 The Consequences of Social Inequality: Maternal Morbidity and Mortality in Honduran *Miskito* Communities

Shahna Arps

21.1 Introduction

Indigenous people in Latin America experience higher rates of morbidity and mortality than their national nonindigenous counterparts (Gracey and King 2009; Montenegro and Stephens 2006; Valeggia and Snodgrass 2015). For indigenous women in particular, a combination of poverty, political oppression, limited access to education and quality biomedical health care, and stressful environments increase their risks for poor health outcomes (Castro et al. 2015; Locklear et al. 2013; PAHO 2004). Although the World Health Organization's Safe Motherhood Initiative and more recently, the United Nations' Millennium Development Goals have focused international attention on improving maternal health, women in marginalized populations continue to suffer disproportionately from maternal mortality and morbidity (WHO 2005). We know that women who reside in remote, indigenous communities are vulnerable, but more detailed ethnographic accounts of how globally recognized risk factors manifest at the local level are needed. Local, national, and international forces converge and influence maternal health in varied, and yet often unexamined ways (Janes and Chuluundorj 2004; Miller et al. 2003; PMMN 1992; Wall 1998). To help fill this gap, I describe the specific challenges that women contend with during pregnancy and childbirth in indigenous *Miskito* communities along the northeastern coast of Honduras. Comprehensive information about the sociocultural and economic conditions that influence maternal health and health-seeking behaviors is necessary for designing effective public health policy and improving reproductive outcomes (Chapman 2003; Berry 2006).

The key threats to maternal health in *Miskito* communities are inadequate health services, poverty, gender inequality, young maternal age, sorcery, and witchcraft. To situate these risk factors within the specific local context, I begin by describing the *Miskito* ethnic group and the demographic and health trends in the region where I conducted fieldwork. A summary of the methods of data collection and analysis I used follows, and then the results section examines how each of the key problems identified

S. Arps, Ph.D.
Department of Sociology and Anthropology,
University of Toledo, Toledo, OH, USA
e-mail: shahna.arps@utoledo.edu

D. A. Schwartz (ed.), *Maternal Death and Pregnancy-Related Morbidity Among Indigenous Women of Mexico and Central America*, Global Maternal and Child Health: Medical, Anthropological, and Public Health Perspectives, https://doi.org/10.1007/978-3-319-71538-4_21

influence women's health and well-being. The chapter concludes with an explanation of how the findings can benefit public health initiatives in *Miskito* villages and recommends avenues for intervention that are designed to address the particular circumstances of women in these communities.

21.2 Methods

21.2.1 Setting and Ethnographic Background

The *Miskito* (also written *Miskitu*) are an Amerindian group who live on the Mosquito Coast of eastern Honduras and Nicaragua. Hundreds of thousands of people maintain their *Miskito* ethnic identity today, with the majority living in Nicaragua and about one-third residing in Honduras (Herlihy 2012). In Honduras' 2013 census, 80,007 people were identified as *Miskito*. The *Miskito* comprise 11.2% of the total indigenous population in Honduras and are the second largest indigenous group in the country (INE 2013). Over 90% of *Miskito* people reported living in Gracias a Dios, a department with low population density and limited infrastructure (INE 2013). The research discussed in this chapter was conducted in Gracias a Dios and focused specifically on rural villages located on a spit of land between the Caribbean Sea and the Ibans lagoon in the Rio Plátano Biosphere Reserve. The reserve is a large protected area established in 1980 (Herlihy 1997). Culturally diverse people inhabit the reserve, including the *Miskito*, *Pech*, *Garifuna*, and nonindigenous Hondurans; and its rainforest, coastal lowland, and lagoon habitats support abundant and varied plant and animal species. Approximately 5300 people were living in the villages where data collection occurred (Fig. 21.1).

Unlike the historical experience of many indigenous peoples in Latin America, the *Miskito* actually grew in population size and geographic territory after European contact (Dodds 1994; Hale 1994; Herlihy 1997; Offen 1999). Their physical and cultural survival has been linked to the ways they interacted socially, economically, and politically with outside groups (Helms 1969, 1983; Herlihy 2012). Their relations with African, European, as well as other indigenous peoples have been characterized by frequent intermarriage, economic trade, and cultural exchange since the colonial era (Helms 1971, 1977). According to Herlihy (2002), *Miskito* people base their ethnic identity less on common ancestry or physical appearance and more on their shared culture and language. The *Miskitu* language is part of the *Misumalpan* language stock that also includes the *Sumu* of Honduras and Nicaragua, and *Matagalpa-Cacaopera* of El Salvador (Mason 1973). The term *Misumalpan* is formed by use of the names of the

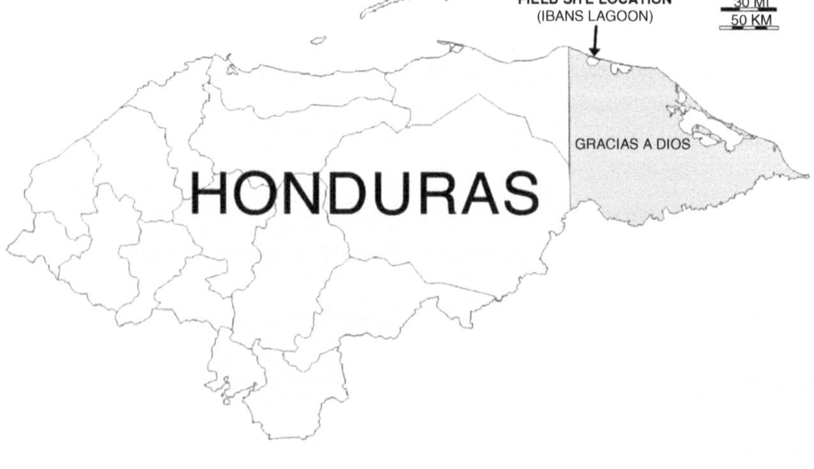

Fig. 21.1 Map showing the fieldwork location along the Ibans Lagoon, Gracias a Dios, Honduras

linguistic family's subgroups—*Mi*skito, *Sumu*, and Matag*alpan*. It is spoken by approximately 150,000 persons, and is the most widely used of the *Misumalpan* family of languages which include a number of dialects (Lewis et al. 2016). *Miskitu* is a dynamic language that uses many nouns borrowed from other languages, particularly English (Heath 1913; Helms 1971), Creole, and more recently, Spanish.

Early trade with Europeans involved the exchange of natural resources found in the region (dyewoods, animal skins and meat, sarsaparilla, rubber, indigo, and cacao) for foreign goods (clothes, machetes, rum, tools, muskets, gunpowder, cooking pots) (Helms 1971). The *Miskito* used the guns they acquired through trade to raid other indigenous and Spanish settlements (often in alliance with the British) and gain control over coastal areas (Dennis and Olien 1984; Dodds 1994; Helms 1983). During the colonial era, men began leaving their communities for prolonged periods of time to participate in militia activities or to work for international companies in extractive industries (Helms 1971). Matrifocal social practices developed in response to their frequent absence (Helms 1971; Herlihy 2007). Herlihy (2007: 133) describes *Miskito* women as the society's "conservative cultural core" as they continued to pass their language, culture, and identity on to their children. Male absence in villages is still common today, as most men spend two or more weeks of the month away from their homes while they work wage labor jobs at sea. Matrilocality is the cultural ideal, and women typically live with their spouses and children in houses clustered around their mothers' and sisters' homes (Fig. 21.2). Women also inherit land and other material goods from their parents.

While coastal *Miskito* villages are not far from La Ceiba (the fourth largest city in Honduras) in actual distance, the lack of roads in the department makes reaching them slow and difficult. Community members travel primarily by canoe, foot, motorcycle, or airplane and have little access to electricity, improved water sources, and sanitation. Supplies generally arrive by boat; therefore, the availability of goods depends on weather conditions and other forces outside local people's control. Despite the remote location of villages, coastal peoples have participated in the global economy as wage laborers and consumers of Western goods for over 250 years (Helms 1971; McSweeney 2004; Nietschmann 1973). Today, men primarily work as wage laborers on lobster, shrimp, and other fishing boats. Approximately 90% of boys and men in the Río Plátano Biosphere Reserve have worked in the lobster industry in particular (Herlihy 2012). Deepwater diving for lobster using scuba equipment is dangerous work, and men frequently suffer health problems associated with decompression sickness (e.g., pain, paralysis, and death). However, they earn substantial amounts of cash for their involvement in these export industries, and contribute over US three million dollars a year to the coastal economy (Herlihy 2006).

Many families also plant bananas, manioc, beans, rice, and maize on inland agricultural fields for their own consumption and for sale. Less commonly, people are employed as teachers, nurses, doc-

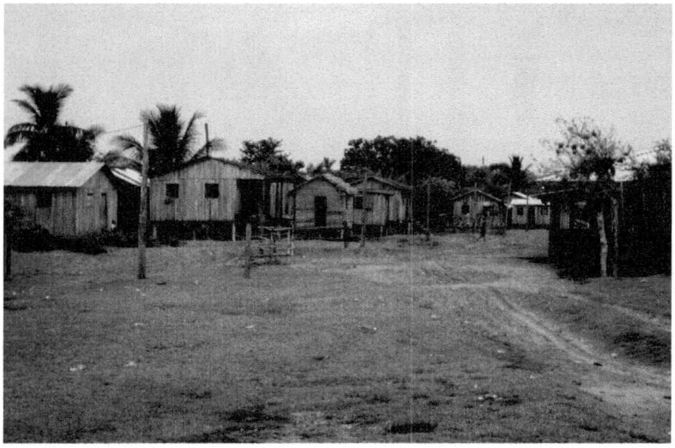

Fig. 21.2 A coastal Miskito village

tors, pastors, or work for governmental agencies or nongovernmental organizations. Some families also receive remittances from city-dwelling kin. Small local stores and traveling vendors sell clothes, tools, gasoline, and food items in *Miskito* communities (Fig. 21.3).

Labor is divided on the basis of gender, with women's responsibilities including mostly domestic tasks. Women manage large households and perform chores such as cooking, cleaning, laundry, and childcare. While men's economic prospects have grown with market integration, women have fewer wage labor opportunities. They often supplement household income by selling baked goods, cooking and cleaning for other families, and running boarding houses. Although some women generate income, they usually depend on money their spouses earn to pay for food, clothes, costs associated with children's education, and other necessities. Men decide how much money they will give their wives to use for household needs and how much they will keep to spend for themselves. Because men are the primary wage earners in the family, large economic expenditures, such as hospital visits or educational programs for children, require their approval.

Children attend primary school (kindergarten through sixth grade) in their communities. Primary education is free, but families must pay for uniforms and school supplies. Opportunities for post-primary education are increasing locally, but most villages currently share facilities. Some parents send older children to schools in other Honduran towns or cities for further education. However, relatively few children have the chance to attend secondary schools or college given the high costs of transportation, school fees, and room and board (Fig. 21.4).

People have access to multiple health care centers in the communities along the Ibans lagoon. Centers are staffed by (or share on a rotating basis) a doctor and multiple nurses. Patients pay a con-

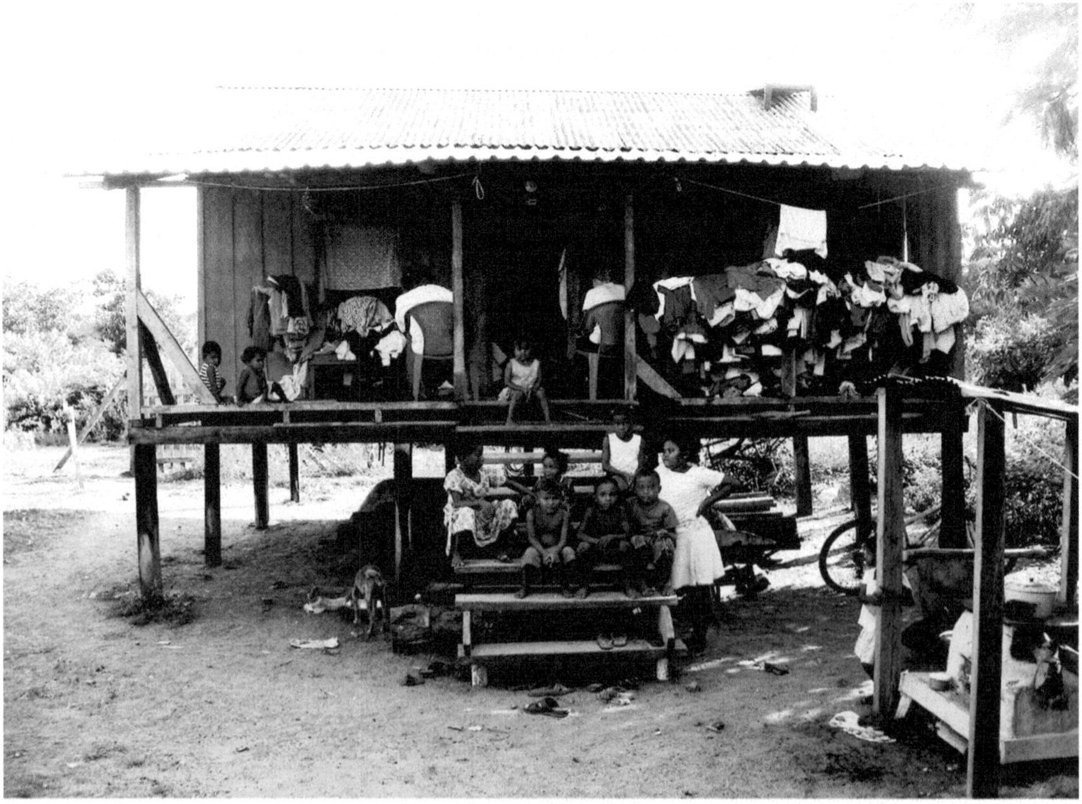

Fig. 21.3 Women may earn income from selling items like secondhand clothing from their homes

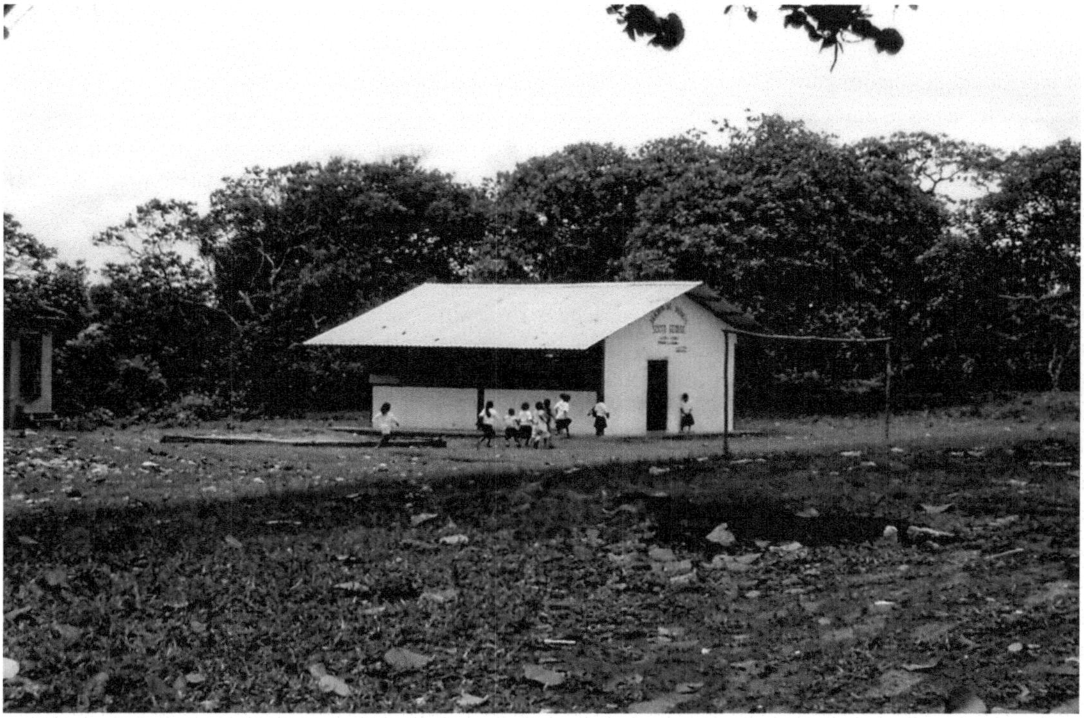

Fig. 21.4 *Miskito* children rushing into the school to start their lessons

sultation fee for services (5–10 Lempiras depending on their time of arrival; US $0.30–0.60). Despite an adequate number of health centers in the area, diagnostic and treatment services remain limited, because they lack laboratory testing facilities and their pharmacies are poorly stocked. People must travel outside of their communities for more comprehensive biomedical care. A health clinic in the village of Palacios, about a one- to two-hour trip in a motorized canoe, performs some minor surgeries. A wider range of services is available at the private hospital in Ahuas and the public hospital in Puerto Lempira. Traveling to these facilities requires an all-day trip by motorized canoe, pick-up truck, and motorcycle or chartering a faster, but expensive airplane. Most community members cannot afford to seek care at either hospital due to the cost of transportation and treatment. The delay associated with traveling to the hospitals is especially problematic in emergency situations.

Given the remoteness of the region, collection and analysis of demographic information have been limited. In 1990, a national maternal mortality survey estimated a maternal mortality ratio (MMR) of 878 maternal deaths per 100,000 live births in Gracias a Dios (Danel 1998). In comparison, the national MMR for Honduras was 182 maternal deaths per 100,000 live births. Despite being substantially lower than the MMR in Gracias a Dios, the national ratio was still one of the highest MMRs in Latin America at the time (Castellanos et al. 1990; Danel 1998). Based on these troubling findings, the Honduran Ministry of Health implemented plans to improve maternal health outcomes and received assistance from international donors to build maternal health clinics, increase access to emergency obstetric care, and train local midwives (Danel and Rivera 2003; Danel 1998). By 1997, the national MMR decreased by 40% to 108 maternal deaths per 100,000 live births (Meléndez et al. 1999; Shiffman et al. 2004). The rate of maternal deaths has continued to improve, albeit more slowly. In 2013, Honduras estimated a national MMR of 88 maternal deaths per 100,000 live births based on census results (INE 2013). While these improvements are promising, disaggregated data suggest that MMRs vary considerably across different regions of the country (Danel 1998). Although maternal health interventions have proven successful at the national level, risks for maternal mortality persist in communities that continue to lack adequate health care resources. The department of Gracias a Dios is one region where public health interventions have been insufficient to date. A relatively small population size and inadequate reporting of deaths also prevents reliable estimation of maternal mortality rates for the area. For instance, in the 2013 national census, four cases of maternal mortality were reported among the 44 total deaths of women who were age 12–49 years in Gracias a Dios (INE 2013).

Although health statistics for the department are scarce, current development indicators suggest that women who live in Gracias a Dios continue to experience high risk for pregnancy- and childbirth-related deaths. Widespread poverty, limited access to health care, and high rates of infectious and noninfectious disease are major threats to health and survival (UNDP 2003). The department's 2002 per capita income was less than US 2056 dollars, and approximately $265 below the national average at the time (UNDP 2003). Families with low earnings have difficulties meeting household needs for food, clothes, and other resources, which are generally more expensive in the department due to the added cost of importing the goods to remote communities. The government also restricts extractive marine industries on a monthly basis each year. Many wage labor jobs on the coast are unavailable during the annual government-imposed moratorium on lobster fishing, which has lasted up to 5 months in the past. Since the local economy relies so extensively on cash from lobster diving, even households that pursue other livelihood strategies experience hardship during the moratorium. Declining lobster populations and competition among divers for limited harvests have also reduced incomes.

Lack of improved water sources and sanitation combined with the presence of tropical disease vectors leads to high prevalence of infectious diseases (e.g., malaria, dengue, and diarrhea) (UNDP 2003). Parasitic infections and poor quality diets cause nutritional deficiencies that further compromise health status. These conditions are particularly relevant to maternal health outcomes because women's health status influences their risks of experiencing and withstanding complications during pregnancy and childbirth (Koblinsky 1995; Schwartz 2013).

Despite the growing economic costs of raising children, large families continue to be the cultural ideal in *Miskito* communities. Children provide long-term economic, social, and psychological benefits for their parents, and are therefore highly valued (Herlihy 2002). National census data and smaller scale demographic studies indicate high fertility rates in the region (Arps 2009; Dodds 1998; INE 2001, 2013). During their lifetimes, women in *Miskito* communities experience, on average, about eight live births (Arps 2009; Dodds 1998). Each of these reproductive events provides an additional opportunity for complications to occur during pregnancy and/or childbirth (McCarthy and Maine 1992). Women are at higher risk of maternal morbidity and mortality not only because of the large number of pregnancies they experience, but also because they do not have adequate access to emergency obstetric care if a complication does occur. Doctors and nurses at the local health centers rarely attend births, and few women travel to hospitals or other facilities to give birth. Most home-births are managed by a local midwife, family member, or nurse with a private practice. In Honduran *Miskito* communities, women must therefore contend with a myriad of challenges during their reproductive years, including economic insecurity, limited transportation infrastructure, compromised health status, and high fertility (Fig. 21.5).

21.2.2 Data Collection and Analysis

To examine maternal morbidity and mortality among *Miskito* women, I use an anthropological perspective, integrating findings from previous ethnographic work and national and regional health statistics with my firsthand research in *Miskito* communities. I draw heavily on data collected during

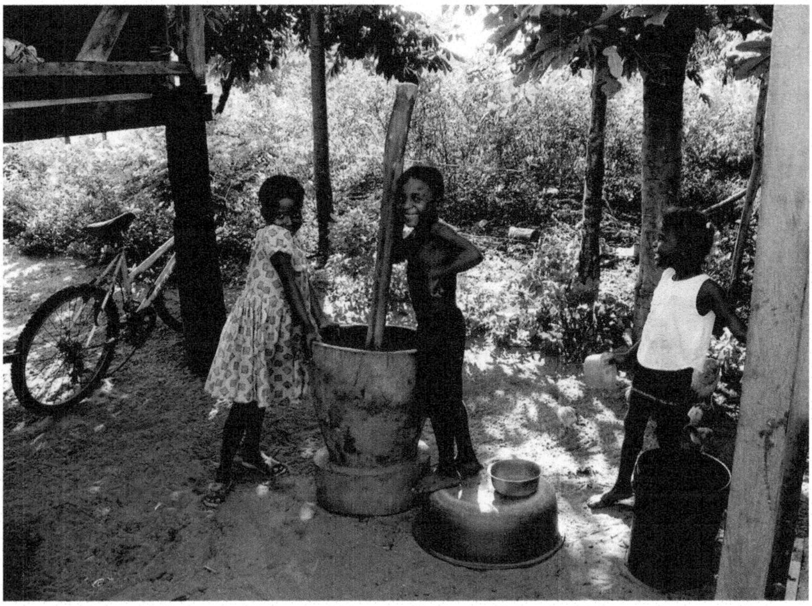

Fig. 21.5 Children help pound rice to remove the husks

fieldwork in 2004–2005 and 2009 in Honduran *Miskito* villages. These data come from a larger project that focused on a wide range of topics including fertility, nutritional status, illness/disease, and maternal morbidity and mortality. I used multiple methods, including group discussions, maternal death histories, individual interviews, health assessments, informal conversations, and participant observation to examine reproduction and health across the life course.

Data collection began with four community discussions held in local schools and churches. While I attempted to limit group size to ten discussion participants, many additional women attended the meetings and were not turned away. Discussion group sizes varied from 10 to 25 attendees. Participants included women aged 16–82 years who resided in the village where the discussion took place. Local research assistants and I conducted the group discussions in Spanish and Miskitu. Participants responded to open-ended questions about pregnancy, childbirth, and maternal morbidity and mortality. I asked each group to describe their perceptions about risks to women's health and the causes of maternal deaths in their community. We recorded responses on site and I later translated comments into English. Transcripts were analyzed by categorizing participants' comments into codes and then identifying major themes in women's perceptions about the underlying causes of maternal death.

I also conducted a maternal mortality survey in the communities along the Ibans lagoon. Local research assistants and I began by asking women age 15 and older ($n = 927$) if any of their female relatives had died due to causes related to pregnancy or childbirth using a verbal autopsy format. If women reported a maternal death, we collected further information about the circumstances of the death. Structured interviews included questions about age at death, date of death, where and when the death occurred, cause(s) of death, prenatal care received, birth attendant(s), birth outcome, and previous number of live births. We cross-checked the original reports by interviewing other family members and birth attendants. While memory lapses, diagnosis errors, and disagreements among relatives can cause limitations in these kinds of surveys, this method provides a general picture of the causes of maternal mortality (Shahidullah 1995). Because most women give birth at home with traditional birth attendants in *Miskito* villages, I also interviewed five local midwives to learn about their perspectives on maternal mortality. The interviews were semi-structured and focused on their training, experiences, and perceptions of maternal health. I transcribed women's responses during on-site interviews and later translated responses into English and coded them for analysis.

In addition to the group discussions, maternal death survey, and interviews with midwives, local research assistants and I conducted individual interviews with 218 women. Interviews focused on childhood and family life, household organization and economics, social support, reproduction, and general health. Two interviews were conducted with each of the participants, who were selected from various age and parity groups. They ranged in age from 17 to 73 years, with 1–14 live births. This systematic sampling ensured that women with diverse experiences who were representative of the broader communities were included. During reproductive histories, participants reported their age at menarche, marriage history, pregnancies, and live births (including birth attendants, birthplace, outcome, birthdates, complications experienced, postpartum activities, and recovery time). They discussed ideal family size and composition, contraceptive use, birth spacing, and perceptions of risks related to reproduction. Statistics related to reproductive morbidity, decision-making autonomy, and socioeconomic status were calculated based on data collected during these interviews.

Women also participated in basic health assessments that included screening for anemia ($n = 314$) (anemia is a pathological condition in which there is a deficiency of hemoglobin or red blood cells in the blood). Local research assistants and I measured hemoglobin concentration using a portable Hemocue B-Hemoglobin Photometer. The photometer required one drop of blood from a finger prick to measure hemoglobin concentration in grams per deciliter. Anemia is defined based upon the laboratory finding of a hemoglobin concentration below 12.0 g/dL in nonpregnant women and less than 11.0 g/dL in pregnant women, following World Health Organization recommendations. The cutoff for anemia is lower among pregnant women to control for hemodilution due to an increase in blood volume during gestation. I considered anemia status to be an important indicator of pregnant and nonpregnant women's health, with crucial links to reproductive outcomes. Previous research suggests that anemia contributes substantially to maternal morbidity and mortality risk (Chi et al. 1981; Llewellyn-Jones 1965). Anemia may decrease women's abilities to withstand excessive blood loss related to childbirth and increase their risk of infection and fatigue (Alauddin 1986; Brock 1999; Kandoi et al. 1991) (Fig. 21.6).

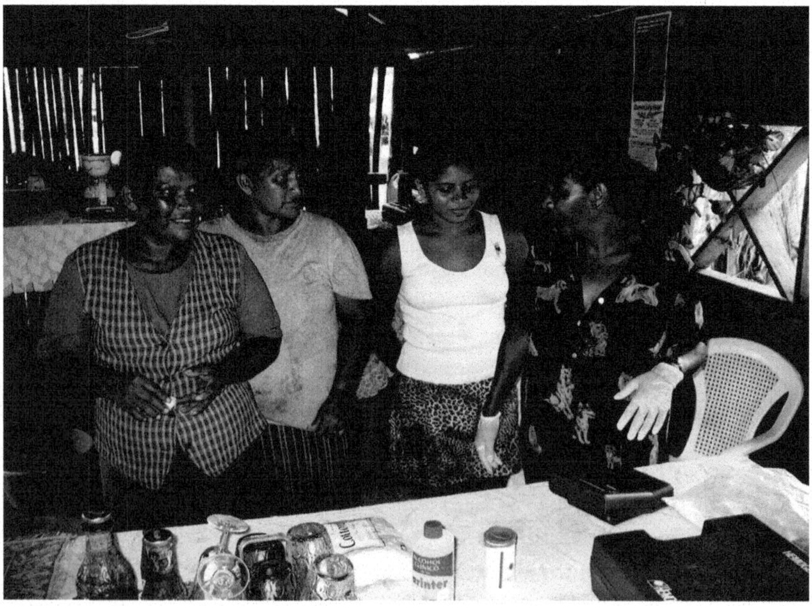

Fig. 21.6 *Miskito* women gather for a demonstration of how the screening for anemia is conducted

Individual interviews and group discussions were supplemented by observations and informal conversations during the 13 months of ethnographic research. Participant observation sites included health centers, churches, group or community events (e.g., soccer games, school productions, parties), and unstructured visits to private homes. Daily interaction helped to establish familiarity and close relationships between the researcher and community members, which made collection of detailed and accurate data possible. Informal conversations with participants' spouses, pastors, herbalists, nurses, and doctors were also conducted throughout the fieldwork period. The Institutional Review Board of The Ohio State University reviewed all data collection methods and research procedures for the original study, and East Carolina University's Institutional Review Board approved the protocol for the subsequent project. Procedures for conducting research with human subjects were followed closely. All participants provided informed consent prior to data collection. Pseudonyms are used for women whose histories are described in the chapter.

Multiple, complimentary methods were used to investigate the complex issues of maternal morbidity and mortality in *Miskito* communities. The findings from group discussions, individual interviews, health assessments, and participant observation create a comprehensive picture of the risks women face during pregnancy and childbirth, as well as local perceptions about those risks. In the following section, I begin by summarizing maternal morbidity and mortality data collected during individual interviews and the maternal death survey, and then discuss the key risk factors for poor maternal health outcomes.

21.3 Maternal Morbidity and Mortality in *Miskito* Communities

21.3.1 Maternal Morbidity

During individual interviews, women frequently reported experiencing complications during reproductive events. Table 21.1 shows the frequency of women who reported morbidity during their most recent reproductive event as well as during any previous reproductive event. Nearly 62% ($n = 135$) of women reported health problems related to their most recent reproductive event and over 85% ($n = 186$) experienced reproductive morbidity in the past. The most often reported problems during pregnancy were severe pregnancy sickness, abnormal swelling, and abdominal pain. Prolonged labor, retained placenta, and severe bleeding were the complications most commonly reported during childbirth. Abdominal pain, fever/infection, and severe bleeding were the most frequent types of morbidity experienced during the postpartum period.

Table 21.1 Women's reports of reproductive morbidity during individual interviews ($n = 218$)

Reported morbidity during:	n	%
Most recent pregnancy	78	35.8
Most recent childbirth	93	42.7
Most recent postpartum period	74	33.9
Most recent pregnancy, birth, or postpartum period	135	61.9
Any previous pregnancy	124	56.9
Any previous childbirth	156	71.6
Any previous postpartum period	136	62.4
Any previous pregnancy, childbirth, or postpartum period	186	85.3

21.3.2 Maternal Deaths

During the maternal mortality survey, women reported 60 maternal deaths that occurred between 1952 and 2009. Of these deaths, 46.7% ($n = 28$) took place after 1997, the year that marked the 40% decrease in the national MMR. Despite the small population sizes of the communities included in the study, from the year 2000 through 2009, 20 mothers died. The majority of women died in the postpartum period ($n = 40$, 66.7%) following a live birth ($n = 32$, 53.3%). More than 26% of the women ($n = 16$) had never experienced a prior live birth. Sixteen (26.7%) of the women who died were under the age of 20 (see Table 21.2). Only two women were age 40 or older (3.3%). The most commonly reported causes of death were severe bleeding (46.7%, $n = 28$), prolonged/obstructed labor (23.3%, $n = 14$), infection (13.3%, $n = 8$), and hypertensive disorders of pregnancy (6.7%, $n = 4$). While relatives reported these as the direct causes of death, in 13 cases (21.7% of deaths) witchcraft or sorcery was thought to be the ultimate cause of mortality (see Table 21.3). In 30.0% ($n = 18$) of the maternal deaths, no skilled practitioner ever attended the woman even after she experienced complications. Midwives and/or private nurses attended 40.0% ($n = 24$) of the women and doctors provided medical attention to 30.0% ($n = 18$). Ten of the women died while en route to a health clinic/hospital (16.7%). Of the 35 live births (which included three sets of twins), 17 of the children were currently alive. Maternal grandparents, aunts, or cousins were caregivers to 15 of the 17 living children and a father and paternal grandmother raised the other two children.

Based on data from the maternal death survey, group discussions, and interviews, five key issues emerged as critical for understanding maternal morbidity and mortality in *Miskito* communities: inadequate access to health services, poverty, gender inequality, young maternal age, and local perceptions

Table 21.2 Reports of maternal deaths, by age cohort and cause of death ($n = 60$)

Reported cause of death	Age ≤ 19	Age 20–24	Age 25–29	Age 30–34	Age 35–39	Age 40–44	Total
Hemorrhage	9	5	5	3	5	1	28 (46.7%)
Obstructed labor	4	4	2	2	1	1	14 (23.3%)
Sepsis/infection	1	2	2	3	0	0	8 (13.3%)
Hypertensive disorders	2	1	1	0	0	0	4 (6.7%)
Other	0	1	3	1	1	0	6 (10.0%)
Total	16 (26.7%)	13 (21.7%)	13 (21.7%)	9 (15%)	7 (11.7%)	2 (3.3%)	60

Table 21.3 Results from the maternal death survey: timing, birth attendant, outcome, and sorcery reports ($n = 60$)

Circumstances of maternal death	Age ≤ 19 ($n = 16$)	Age > 19 ($n = 44$)	Total ($n = 60$)
Primigravida	9 (56.3%)	7 (15.9%)	16 (26.7%)
Death during pregnancy	2 (12.5%)	7 (15.9%)	9 (15.0%)
Death during childbirth	4 (25.0%)	7 (15.9%)	11 (18.3%)
Death postpartum	10 (62.5%)	30 (68.2%)	40 (66.7%)
Attended by doctor	3 (18.8%)	15 (34.1%)	18 (30.0%)
Attended by midwife or nurse	9 (56.3%)	15 (34.1%)	24 (40.0%)
Attended by relative(s)	4 (25.0%)	14 (31.8%)	18 (30.0%)
Died en route to hospital/heath center	6 (37.5%)	4 (9.1%)	10 (16.7%)
Live birth	9 (56.3%)	23 (52.3%)	32 (53.3%)
Child currently alive	5 (31.3%)	10 (22.7%)	15 (25.0%)
Sorcery reported as cause of death	5 (31.3%)	8 (18.2%)	13 (21.7%)

of sorcery/witchcraft as a cause of life-threatening complications. I explain the relevance of each of these factors to maternal health in the next sections of the chapter.

21.3.3 Inadequate Access to Quality Health Care Resources

The majority of women identified in the maternal death survey died of causes that are considered preventable and/or treatable given adequate health services (WHO 2005). However, the low number of births attended by doctors and the high number of women who died en route to a health care facility suggest that opportunities for obstetric care in these communities are insufficient. While these figures are partially related to a general lack of local health care resources, women also avoided using services that were available due to their perceived low quality. Pregnant and birthing women often chose not to seek care from doctors and nurses at the health centers. In the maternal death histories (verbal autopsies), family members reported that women who were attended by doctors did not receive care from them until after complications arose and problems were considered too severe for a relative or midwife to handle.

During group discussions, individual interviews, and informal conversations, women reported a low reliance on local health care centers because they often lacked diagnostic tests, medicines, and other supplies. They were discouraged by long wait times to see a doctor and spending money on consultations only to receive a prescription that the health center could not fill. They could not always find or afford to buy the drugs or vitamins they needed at local private pharmacies (which also have limited amounts and types of medicine) either. Women were also critical of health centers' limited hours of operation and the perceived unwillingness of doctors and nurses to help during urgent situations outside of those hours. Experiences of being disregarded and disrespected also contributed to negative opinions about local health services. Women recounted incidents of exorbitant compensation demands by health center employees and outright refusals to help during emergencies. One woman commented, "some nurses and doctors have a real love for people, but most don't. It's about money. 'I won't get out of bed to come help unless you give me 2,000 Lempiras', the doctor says. It's only a business to them".

Emelina's case study illustrates how the lack of health care resources endangers women's health. Emelina, a 32-year-old mother of four, died soon after giving birth to her fifth child. When labor first began, one of her relatives went to the local health center and asked for a doctor or nurse to come attend the birth at her home. They refused to help. Her mother located a midwife who was willing to support her delivery. She had a healthy baby boy, but the midwife soon realized that Emelina was not expelling her placenta. She began to hemorrhage. While the midwife tried desperately to remove the placenta, Emelina's sisters sent a relative to try to convince a nurse or doctor to assist, once again. By the time a nurse arrived, Emelina was unconscious. Although the nurse was eventually able to remove the placenta, Emelina had experienced significant blood loss and died within hours of delivering her son.

Like Emelina, most women prefer to give birth in the comfort of their own homes with supportive family members and friends inside (and in the case of male relatives, just outside) of the house. They often described giving birth in a hospital as potentially stressful, due to the unfamiliar and intimidating environment. Women reported that birthing mothers may be surrounded by doctors and nurses who treat them poorly, not just because they are strangers, but also based on their ethnicity or socioeconomic status. As a result, women usually rely on local midwives or nurses with private practices (rather than nurses who work at health centers) to attend their births. Among the 218 living women interviewed, midwives and/or nurses attended 64.3% ($n = 805$) of their births ($n = 1251$). Nurses and midwives have undergone varying levels of biomedical training. Most of their knowledge and techniques for ensuring successful childbirths come from actual experience attending women in their communities. Since midwives and their clients live in the same villages, they share social connections, as well as cultural beliefs, norms, and customs.

Despite the frequent and important health care services midwives and private nurses provide, they rarely receive acknowledgment or support from the ministry of health for the work they do in these resource-deprived villages. While midwives have cultural authority in their communities, their autonomy is increasingly limited within the larger health care system. Public health officials have encouraged them to refer women to biomedical practitioners if problems arise during childbirth, rather than attempt to treat complications themselves. Three of the five midwives interviewed expressed dissatisfaction about the lack of instructional seminars and other support offered by governmental agencies in recent years. Ideally, health centers provide midwives with gloves, gauze, iodine, and alcohol as needed. However, they often must locate and purchase their own supplies because health centers are not stocked with sufficient resources.

Rather than feeling like they work in partnership with government agencies, midwives reported growing fears about being punished if women in their care die during pregnancy and childbirth. Health center personnel report maternal deaths to the Ministry of Public Health, which then sends representatives to investigate deaths. Ostensibly, "case reviews with TBAs [traditional birth attendants] are intended to occur in an atmosphere meant to encourage learning and not to place blame" (Danel 1998: 9). However, three midwives described tense relationships with government officials. A midwife who had been attending births for almost 20 years explained, "we have been told not to touch a woman who is having complications. We must get her to a doctor. But where should we take her and how? Some midwives still insist on handling everything themselves, but if someone reports you, you could be sent to jail." Although no one actually knew of anyone who had been imprisoned, some midwives and private nurses reported being told that if women died under their care, they would be prohibited from attending births or providing any other health care services in the future. These warnings further limited local health care options for pregnant women, because some midwives refused to attend women at high risk of experiencing complications (for instance, women under age 15) due to concerns that these threats may be carried out in the future.

Women in *Miskito* communities have limited access to health care, not only during childbirth, but also throughout their lives. Injuries caused by accidents and violence often go untreated and have long-term effects on physical and mental health. Women also suffer from infectious and noninfectious diseases prior to and during pregnancy. Among women screened for anemia, 56.9% of pregnant women (n = 58) and 39.1% of nonpregnant women (n = 256) were anemic (see Table 21.4). In the maternal death histories, hepatitis, tuberculosis, hemorrhagic fever, and anemia were reported as contributing to maternal mortality in six cases. However, many women never receive an exact biomedical diagnosis of these diseases due to the lack of local laboratory testing facilities. As a 33-year-old mother of eight described the situation, "the doctor just has to guess what is wrong by looking at you." Even when the specific cause of illness is identified, resources for preventing and treating these diseases are rarely available at local health centers.

Table 21.4 Prevalence of anemia, pregnant women and nonpregnant women, by age cohort (n = 314)

	Pregnant women		Nonpregnant women		All women	
Age cohort (year)	n	Anemia prevalence[a]	n	Anemia prevalence[a]	n	Anemia prevalence[a]
15–19	18	9 (60.0%)	15	13 (72.2%)	33	22 (66.7%)
20–24	15	18 (43.9%)	41	8 (53.3%)	56	26 (46.4%)
25–29	12	18 (42.9%)	42	5 (41.7%)	54	23 (42.6%)
30–34	7	10 (24.4%)	41	3 (42.9%)	48	13 (27.1%)
35–39	6	11 (34.4%)	32	4 (66.7%)	38	15 (39.5%)
40+	0	34 (40%)	85	34 (40%)	85	34 (40.0%)
Total	58	100 (39.1%)	256	33 (56.9%)	314	133 (42.4%)

[a]Anemia was classified as Hb < 11 g/dL in pregnant women and as Hb < 12 g/dL in nonpregnant women

21.3.4 Poverty

While many people were critical of the care available locally, they generally described the treatment provided by the hospitals in Ahuas and Puerto Lempira as more varied and comprehensive. Yet, their access to these hospitals is limited due to the distance and cost of transportation to and from the facilities. In emergency cases, these barriers are particularly critical as arranging transportation and collecting money, as well as the long-distance trip itself, delay treatment. Even if a doctor, nurse, or midwife recommends that a woman should give birth at a hospital prior to the onset of labor, most families cannot afford the costs of travel and health care. During the annual moratorium on lobster harvesting, when economic insecurity is highest, families have a particularly difficult time finding enough money and transportation services to travel. Like household finances, community resources are especially limited during the moratorium. Local providers discontinue collective transportation services (*colectivos*) by truck, motorcycle, and canoe because few people have the funds to travel. In the absence of these more affordable *colectivos*, families have to charter a small airplane (which typically costs more than US $275) or a canoe with an outboard motor to send a woman to the hospital. In addition to transportation costs, families also have to raise money to pay for food, lodging, and treatment for the woman and any relatives who plan to travel with her. Because of these financial and logistical difficulties, seeking care at a hospital is often a family's last resort for health care. The ten cases in which women died either waiting for transportation to a hospital (by canoe or airplane) or en route not only point to the lack of local emergency obstetric care, but also reflect how delays are further prolonged by poverty. Relatives of deceased women who were attended by a doctor (n = 18) often reported that medical interventions failed because they were administered too late.

Yolanda's story demonstrates the ongoing need for affordable emergency obstetric care. Eighteen-year-old Yolanda was in the eighth month of her pregnancy with twins when she started to experience labor pains. A nurse with a private practice attended her. Delivery was not progressing, and she began to bleed. The private nurse administered synthetic oxytocin, to move delivery along, but the severity of bleeding increased. As her condition worsened, her family decided to send her to the hospital in Ahuas for care. This proved challenging due to their economic circumstances, and her sister reported that it took too long for them to collect sufficient funds to charter a plane to the hospital and arrange for transport. Yolanda and her undelivered twins died at the village airstrip, while waiting for the plane to arrive.

During interviews and group discussions, participants reported that poverty was the primary cause of maternal mortality. Multiple women used the same phrase to describe the dire situation: "if a woman doesn't have money, she just has to die." Women "just have to die" not only because they are too poor to seek health care at a hospital, but also because they cannot afford the costs associated with purchasing uncontaminated drinking water or nutritious food to support a well-balanced diet. Nutritional deficiencies that result from poor quality diets may compromise immune function and increase women's risk for infection (Koblinsky 1995; Schwartz 2013). Healthy food choices are limited at local stores and prices are high, but most families do not have other options, since few households produce their own food. During interviews, women often linked poor health to inadequate diets. They explained anemia, in particular, as the result of eating too little meat (*upan*). Although animal protein is considered a much loved and integral part of the *Miskito* diet, meat is more expensive than other foods (such as rice and beans), so consumption is lower than people would prefer. Although anemia screenings did not assess the underlying causes of low hemoglobin concentrations, the high rates of anemia are worrisome given its association with higher risks for infection, fatigue, and death associated with excessive blood loss during childbirth (Alauddin 1986; Kandoi et al. 1991; Brock 1999) (Fig. 21.7).

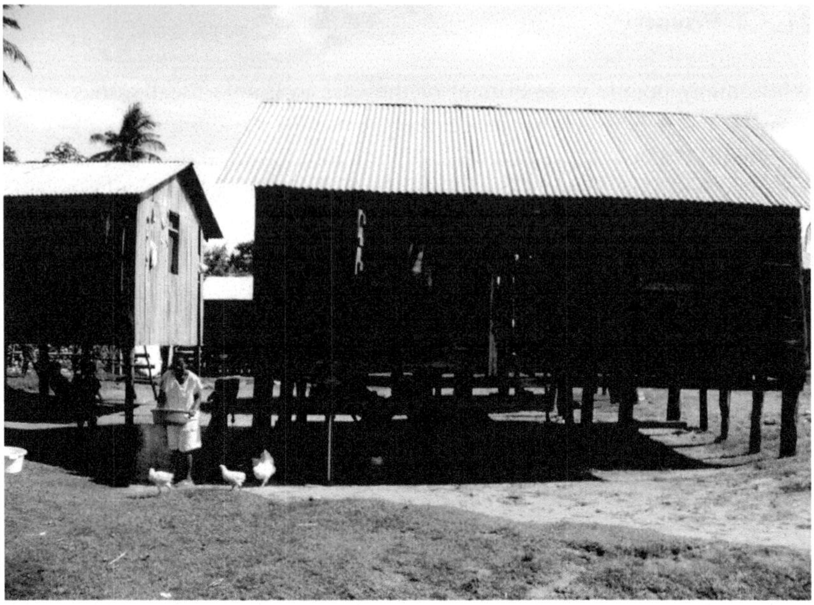

Fig. 21.7 A woman feeds her chickens, which are important sources of meat and eggs

21.3.5 Gender Inequality

Women were particularly susceptible to poverty because they lack employment opportunities due to their gender. Of women interviewed ($n = 218$), 53.3% earned some income, but their work tended to be low paid and temporary. They could not support their families on the money they earned doing laundry, selling baked goods, or cleaning, so they relied on men for economic support. Women used various strategies to convince men to share their earnings (see also Herlihy 2006), but their success varied. As the primary breadwinners, men retained control over major financial decisions in the household. When men chose to spend the greater part of the money they earned on alcohol, luxury items for themselves, or other women, this created stressful conflicts between spouses. During interviews and informal conversations, women reported that these fights became violent at times, particularly when drugs and alcohol were involved (Fig. 21.8).

Gender violence also emerged as an important factor in the maternal death survey. Relatives reported neglect and/or physical abuse by the woman's husband as contributing to three cases of maternal death. In several more cases, respondents mentioned that spouses delayed women from receiving medical attention by withholding permission or financial resources necessary for receiving care. Because childbirth is common and most women do not die giving birth, husbands generally underestimated women's risk of death. They assumed their wives would survive; therefore, there was no reason to spend large amounts of money for travel and treatment at a hospital. Ledetenia and Juliana's deaths provide examples of how women's limited autonomy with regard to decision-making about health care and large monetary expenditures can end tragically.

When Ledetenia, age 26 years, delivered her second child, she was in a canoe, with only her spouse accompanying her. The baby was stillborn and her uterus came out of her body when she gave birth. However, her husband did not take her to receive medical attention for the prolapsed uterus. Even after she developed a high fever, he refused to allow her to seek health care. She shared her health concerns with her brother and sister-in-law. Worried about her deteriorating health, they implored her husband to take her to the hospital, but he declined, claiming he could not afford the costs of travel and treat-

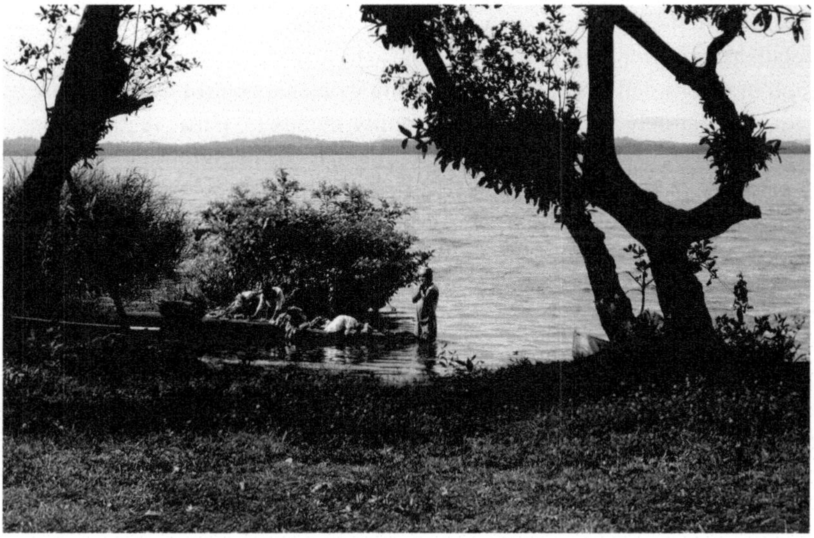

Fig. 21.8 Women washing clothes in the lagoon, a typical domestic chore and a way for some to earn income in coastal villages

ment. Never having received any medical attention, she died 3 weeks after childbirth. Her family blames Ledetenia's death on her husband, who they believe had been physically abusive throughout their relationship.

Juliana, age 34 years, suffered from severely swollen veins in legs during her seventh pregnancy. The doctor at the local health center advised her to travel to the hospital in Ahuas to deliver the baby. However, her husband reportedly told Juliana (and her family) that she was just as capable of giving birth at home this time as she had been in the past. He felt that a trip to the hospital was expensive and unnecessary. Juliana was able to deliver a healthy baby girl after 13 h of labor. However, she was bleeding from her mouth, nose, and vagina. Two local midwives and a nurse attempted to save her life, but she died approximately 20 min after childbirth. Her husband was away from home at the time, working on a lobster boat.

During individual interviews and group discussions, women often criticized their husbands' behavior. Men were frequently referred to as "irresponsible," because wives believed they acted selfishly and in ways that compromised their family's well-being. Women often pointed to how men would refuse to share money to meet household needs, and instead spend critical resources on frivolous goods for themselves (such as clothing, radios, and rum). The costs of alcohol abuse, economically and socially, were particularly distressing for families. In my informal conversations with participants' spouses and other male relatives, men acknowledged that their decisions and actions sometimes contributed to hardships and health consequences for women. Both men and women described that husband's "jealousy" affected women's access to health care and family planning. Some husbands forbade women from seeking medical attention from male doctors (including prenatal care), because of worries that the men would become too intimate with their wife. They also prevented their wives from using contraceptives, assuming that if women could avoid pregnancy then they would be able to have and hide relationships with other men.

Herlihy (2006) describes how multiple factors such as national policies, church doctrines, and men's involvement in export industries are linked to male dominance in *Miskito* communities. Yet, during interviews and group discussions, participants stressed that current economic conditions perpetuated gender inequality rather than focusing on the cultural or religious basis of male-dominant ideologies. They believed that if women had better access to income-generating opportunities, they could make their own decisions about health care services. They would also have more power in their relationships with men, and could choose to leave abusive husbands. Compared to husbands, discussion of other relatives' roles in restricting women's control over reproductive and health care discussions was largely absent. Women's family members, particularly their mothers and other maternal relatives, have substantial influence on their lives, including how and when they bear children and seek medical attention. Nevertheless, when women described the underlying causes of maternal mortality in their communities, they specifically blamed husbands, rather than these other relatives, for making choices that threatened maternal health.

21.3.6 Witchcraft and Sorcery

The underlying causes of maternal morbidity and mortality discussed so far correspond with biomedical ideas of risk. Yet, *Miskito* explanations of maternal death also recognize supernatural forces and techniques as important causes of complications during pregnancy and childbirth. In 21.7% of the maternal deaths reported in the survey, at least one family member cited witchcraft or sorcery as the ultimate cause of death. Two of the local midwives also believed that witchcraft and sorcery were the principal causes of maternal mortality in their communities. The most common types of sorcery reported were referred to as "*poison*," "*trick*," or "*trick poison*." Although the techniques and motives for using these supernatural methods varied, women perceived them as responsible for producing biological complications like severe bleeding, convulsions, and prolonged/obstructed labor. A woman's enemy (or an enemy of her kin) could cause health problems by poisoning her food with physical and supernatural substances and/or by reciting a curse and burying an object or spell along a path she would cross or come into contact with in some way. Sorcerers gathered substances from dead animals, wrote the victim's name on a piece of paper, or recited incantations, spells and "secrets" to induce illness and death. People described complications caused by witchcraft and sorcery as medical emergencies that required immediate care from traditional *Miskito* healers. Women and their relatives consulted with herbal specialists in *Miskito* medicine for remedies if they suspected sorcery or witchcraft; and they perceived biomedicine as ineffective for healing these conditions. Since people also believed that complications during pregnancy and childbirth can occur naturally, determining whether supernatural forces were at work could be difficult. Family members and traditional healers analyzed women's physical symptoms and social situations carefully to diagnose the cause of the complication or illness. They explained that if time was wasted on biomedical care (which cannot address the root cause of the complication in the cases of witchcraft and sorcery), women may not receive the appropriate cure (*sika*) in time to save their lives.

Family members also suspected witchcraft and sorcery after the fact, especially if complications did not appear to be severe and/or death was particularly unexpected. During the maternal death survey and community discussions, people reported that envy, resentment, and revenge were the typical reasons supernatural methods were employed to cause illness. Women who had tense social relations with another person in the community or who broke social norms were particularly at risk of these attempts on their lives (e.g., women who were disliked by their spouse's family, women who had a relationship with a married man or refused a man's attention). Women who were materially better off than their neighbors (referred to as "living well") could also become targets of sorcery. Even poor women were victims, because their pregnancy could evoke feelings of jealousy among childless women. In some cases, women became pawns in supernatural blood feuds, killed to avenge some wrong-doing committed by her kin. Olivia and Miriam's stories show how their families perceived sorcery, motivated by jealousy and vengeance, as the cause of their deaths.

Olivia, age 18 years, was in the eighth month of her first pregnancy when she suddenly began to experience a severe headache and stomach pains. Her symptoms escalated to include vomiting, dizziness, and eventually, convulsions. Her mother, sister, and a midwife attended her, but her family could not afford to send her to a hospital. She died just as they were preparing to take her to the local health center. Her relatives (and others in the community) attributed her death to *Trick poison*, carried out by her former lover, Carlos. They reported that Carlos had been furious that Olivia was living with another man and jealous that she was expecting a child with him. Two years after Olivia's death, Miriam, Carlos' 15-year-old sister, began to experience complications in the 9th month of her first pregnancy. She was bleeding severely and her relatives were unable to help her. They decided to take her to the health clinic in Palacios, but she died in the canoe during the trip. Her family believed that she was killed by *Trick poison* in retribution for Olivia's death. By murdering Olivia, Carlos had started a family feud. Rather than retaliating directly against him, someone in Olivia's family used sorcery to kill his sister. Miriam became a casualty in this feud, not because of anything she had personally done, but simply because she was Carlos' sister.

Local beliefs about the causes of complications during pregnancy and childbirth influenced how women and their families attempted to prevent and treat these issues. If people believed that witchcraft or sorcery caused an illness, biomedical care and resources (or the lack thereof) were irrelevant. More doctors, nurses, and health facilities would not decrease the incidence or improve the outcomes of these complications. Beliefs about supernatural causes lend more support to perceptions that local health centers were ineffectual, not only because they lacked biomedical resources, but also because the resources they offered were useless against sorcery and witchcraft. For instance, one midwife stated, "pregnant women can't get a blood test to check for anemia or *poison* at the health center." Women who sought prenatal care from a local health center received no protection against sorcery. In fact, just being present at the health center on prenatal care days brought public attention to their vulnerable condition. Some women avoided prenatal care because they believed that as community members learned of their pregnancy, potential enemies might see their chance to inflict harm due to feelings of envy or hostility.

Sorcery and witchcraft are only part of a whole range of supernatural and natural factors perceived to cause illness and death. Women and midwives often described the risks that women face during pregnancy and childbirth as numerous, varied, and unpredictable. Given these cultural understandings, women pursue a health care strategy that allows them to maintain diverse treatment options. Families measure the cost of seeking obstetric care at hospitals beyond economic terms, because by choosing this route they become limited to solely biomedical therapies. Conversely, in women's home communities they can draw simultaneously on different types of treatment. For example, three of the midwives interviewed reported using both biomedical knowledge and *Miskito* herbal medicine to treat complications that arose during childbirth. Women also described receiving concurrent care from a *Miskito* healer who administered *sika* for *poison* or *trick* and a biomedically trained private nurse. The traditional healer addressed the ultimate cause of the complication, while the nurse focused on the immediate factors that endangered survival (i.e., the severe bleeding, obstructed labor). Beliefs about the causes of complications in this pluralistic ethnomedical system may therefore prevent women from seeking obstetric care at hospitals, because they prefer what Chapman (2003: 364) calls the simultaneous "layering of protection and treatment from different sources." In their own community, women can depend on a variety of healers that they know personally and trust to address the diverse causes of complications that occur during pregnancy and childbirth.

The perceived need for varied types of health care will likely remain important in the long-term because community members reported that sorcery and witchcraft activities have become more prevalent in recent years. While individual feelings of envy, frustration, and hatred have always been social problems, people believe that socioeconomic changes have fueled more of these negative emotions. Community members specifically reported that increasing inequality has promoted social discord. Some individuals have benefited from opportunities provided by market integration. People with relatively high paid jobs in education, health care, or with governmental agencies or nongovernmental organizations have built more expensive homes and acquired material goods (i.e., televisions, cell phones, stereos, freezers). For others, these goods are visible, yet unattainable, and they struggle to afford basic necessities. During interviews and informal conversations, people reported that traditional values and practices of reciprocity were breaking down. Poorer community members accused their wealthier relatives and neighbors of hording resources and failing to follow traditional norms of sharing that ensured mutual security (and more equality) in the past. Suyapa's story illustrates how local perceptions about socioeconomic differentiation relate to sorcery and maternal death.

Suyapa, age 28 years, began to bleed during the sixth month of her fourth pregnancy. Her relatives were concerned about the blood loss early in pregnancy, so they made arrangements for an airplane to take her to the hospital in Ahuas. As they were waiting for the plane to arrive, the hemorrhaging became severe and her mother was unable to stop the bleeding. Suyapa died at the airstrip. Suyapa had been in good health prior to this time. The rapidness and severity of bleeding caused her family to suspect *poison* as the cause of her death. Her sister believed the trip to Ahuas would have been in vain. Even if she would have survived long enough to receive medical care, no doctor would have been able to save her life. Her family reported that people in the community probably resented Suyapa's economic prosperity. Jealous of her nice house, abundant material goods and food provisions, someone who was less fortunate had used sorcery to cause her sudden death.

Beyond the increasing disparities in wealth among households, a general sense of declining social conditions pervades the communities. Market integration has brought increasing dependence on cash and greater emphasis on consumption, as well as greater interaction with other societies. Self-sufficiency has declined and outside forces have substantial influence over local conditions. The local economy depends not only on a continuing international demand for lobster, but also on national policies that restrict extractive practices to certain times of the year. Community members rely more on imported food and other goods and have less control over resource use and availability. The movement of people and goods through the region has also brought new social and health problems, from HIV/AIDS to cocaine. Drug trafficking (and attempts to stop it) affects peoples' daily lives, and violence, imprisonment of community members, and murders have been consequences (see also Gaynor 2014). In 2012, two pregnant women were shot and killed when the Honduran police and US DEA agents mistook their canoe traveling on the Patuca River for a drug-trafficking vessel (AP 2012). Two others died during the encounter and four more were injured.

One midwife described current problems, "In the past women didn't die as often as they do now. These are bad times and people are thinking and doing bad things. People become jealous of others more often. Drugs, new sicknesses, and other evil things have come [into the community], especially in the past ten years," These perceptions about current conditions have intensified fears and accusations of witchcraft and sorcery in *Miskito* communities. These widespread concerns about supernaturally inflicted harm are likely to affect how pregnant women and their families make health care decisions for the foreseeable future.

21.3.7 Maternal Age

Data from the maternal death survey, individual interviews, and health assessments indicate that young women are particularly vulnerable to maternal mortality and morbidity. Although adolescent fertility rates were relatively low compared to older age cohorts (see Table 21.5), in 16 of the 60 maternal deaths reported (26.7%), women were under age 20. Based on death histories

Table 21.5 Comparative data for maternal deaths ($n = 60$) and fertility, by age cohorts

Age cohort (year)	Maternal deaths *n*	Maternal deaths: Percentage of deaths reported (%)	Age-specific fertility rates[a]	Proportion of total births[b] (%)
15–19	16	26.7	1.28	14.1
20–24	13	21.7	1.78	33.0
25–29	13	21.7	1.78	23.9
30–34	9	15.0	1.43	13.7
35–39	7	11.7	0.99	9.5
40–44	2	3.3	0.34	14.1

[a]Arps (2009)

[b]For women in the Department of Gracias a Dios (INE 2001)

Table 21.6 Socioeconomic variables and participation in decision-making by age cohort ($n = 218$)

Age cohort (year)	*n*	Lives in her own home (%)	Earns some income (%)	Participates in decision-making about: Health care (%)	Travel (%)	Household finances (%)
15–19	7	0.0	28.6	42.9	57.1	57.1
20–24	32	62.5	40.6	83.3	66.7	80.0
25–29	36	72.2	36.1	72.7	84.8	84.8
30–34	35	88.6	57.1	78.8	84.8	90.9
35–39	34	88.2	64.7	81.8	81.8	97.0
40–44	23	95.7	65.2	78.3	95.7	91.3
45–49	23	100.0	73.9	90.5	90.5	100.0
50+	28	100.0	50.0	85.2	81.5	96.3
Total	218	82.6	53.2	79.7	82.1	89.9

(see Table 21.3), adolescents died while en route to a hospital/health center more often than older women, and only 18.8% were attended by a doctor. Witchcraft was cited as the ultimate cause of death in 31.3% of adolescent maternal deaths, compared to only 18.2% of the women age 20 and older.

Among women who had given birth in the last 2 years, 41.7% of adolescents reported experiencing morbidity during their most recent pregnancy and 50.0% during their most recent childbirth. Adolescents' rates of morbidity were more than 10% higher than for women in their 20s. Anemia was also most commonly identified in adolescents, among both pregnant women and nonpregnant women (prevalence was 72.2% and 60.0%, respectively, see Table 21.4). Lower rates of participation in health care, travel, and household financial decision-making were found in adolescents compared to other age cohorts (see Table 21.6). Similarly, adolescents reported the lowest rates of home ownership and income generation of all age cohorts.

Physiological immaturity may partially explain their vulnerability, but social and economic factors likely interact with biology in complex ways to increase risks for adolescents. In *Miskito* communities, adolescents are caught in the ambiguous social space between child and adult. Young women who reside in their parents' houses (even if they have their own children and spouses) are not fully recognized as adult women. Given their low social and economic status, young women have little control over the management of household resources. Their limited abilities to influence decisions about health care and financial expenditures may lead to delayed or inadequate access to obstetric care. In other words, a young woman who is still growing and developing is not only more likely to experience a complication like obstructed labor, but also less likely to receive emergency treatment for the condition due to her social position (Fig. 21.9).

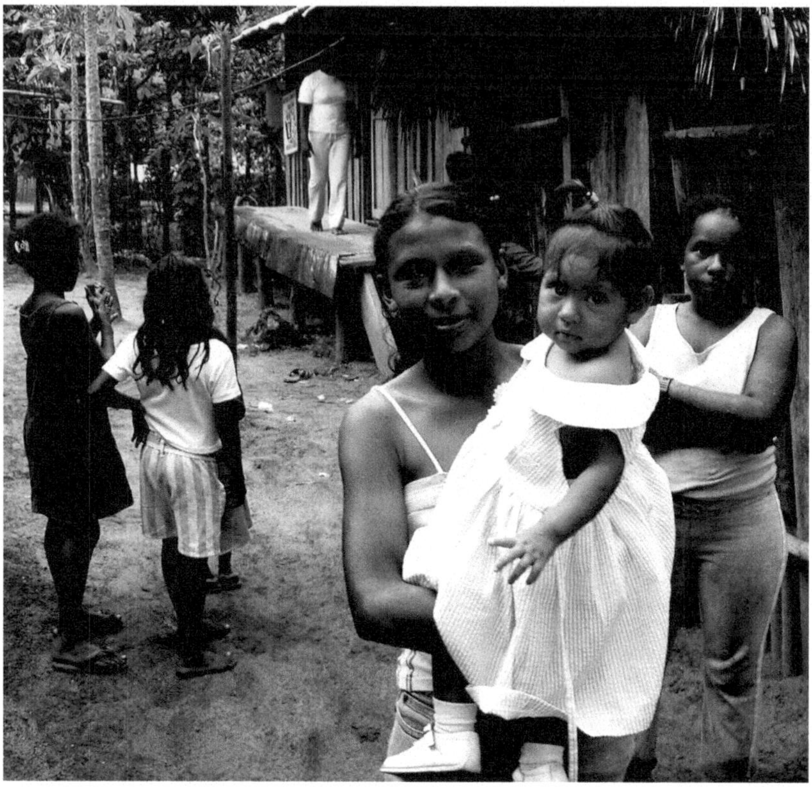

Fig. 21.9 Young women and girls socialize before a child's first birthday party

Maria's death history provides an example of how a young woman from a poor family was unable to access the type of care necessary to save her life. Maria was 18 years old when she died. Her mother and health center staff reported that during prenatal visits the doctor had encouraged her (on at least three different occasions) to give birth to her second child at a hospital. She had almost died during her first childbirth due to prolonged labor. The doctor said that her body was "too small" and that she needed a cesarean section to deliver this baby. Her family, who earned a meager living through agricultural activities, said they were simply too poor to send her to the hospital. Despite the advanced warning that Maria should go to the hospital, her mother stated that they were unable to come up with enough money for transportation and treatment. Instead, they decided to pay a local private nurse to attend her birth. She delivered her baby and placenta after about 3 h with the nurse. However, she immediately began to bleed and the nurse could not stop the hemorrhaging. She sent Maria by canoe to the health clinic in Palacios, but by that time, her blood loss was so severe that the staff there could not save her life. Maria's mother raises her two orphaned children now, which she described as a large financial burden. A local nurse said that the cost of raising the grandchildren could have been avoided if Maria's family would have made the smaller financial commitment to take her to the hospital as the doctor recommended. "It's like their [young women] lives aren't worth anything," she also commented.

The finding that witchcraft was a commonly reported cause of adolescent maternal death also suggests that emic ideas of social vulnerability exist for this group. Local conceptions of age-related maternal mortality risk parallel the J-shaped curve recognized by biomedical perspectives. People believe that adolescents, especially those under age 16, face some heightened risks during pregnancy and childbirth. However, they considered older women to be at greater risk of maternal mortality than young women. In particular, women emphasized that chances of complications and susceptibility to death increase after age 30. Yet, older women can buffer themselves against these risks more effectively than younger women, because they have more autonomy over reproductive and health care decisions. While older women have higher status in *Miskito* societies, as the nurse's statement above implies, adolescents do not command the same level of concern, support, or financial commitment from their families.

21.3.8 Varied and Contested Causes of Maternal Death

From data collected during group discussions, the maternal death survey, and interviews with mothers and midwives, a number of causes emerged as important for understanding maternal morbidity and mortality. Inadequate health care resources, poverty, gender inequality, young maternal age, and sorcery increase risks of negative health outcomes. Although these risks are recognized as important among community members, people often disagreed about which underlying cause was most common or critical. Whereas younger married women were more likely to identify gender inequality, and specifically men's control of household finances, as most important, older women focused on declining social and economic conditions that produced poverty, sorcery, and witchcraft. Men similarly tended to cite large-scale forces as paramount, emphasizing the inevitable constraints caused by poverty, and downplaying their personal decision-making roles and actions. In some cases, men condemned the choices that women themselves made. One participant's uncle specifically focused on women's health care decisions, "Many women don't go to the health center for prenatal care or take prenatal vitamins like they're supposed to. They don't take care of themselves," he said. Even the local midwives emphasized different factors. Three midwives downplayed the importance of supernatural forces, instead citing limited health care resources as the primary obstacle to better outcomes, while the other two midwives reported that sorcery and witchcraft were to blame for most complications. Nurses and doctors at the health center identified the lack of local emergency obstetric care as problematic, but also bemoaned women's preferences for home births, and often described difficulties they faced trying to convince at-risk women to seek care at a hospital.

Not only did community members disagree about the key cause of maternal morbidity and mortality, they sometimes subscribed to different explanations for specific cases of maternal death. Despite similar reports about the physiological complications leading up to death, controversies about which person or which forces were ultimately to blame were frequent. Following a fatal tragedy, family members, neighbors, health center employees, and midwives begin to sort through and critically examine the events that surrounded the woman's death and evaluate the actions of those involved before, during, and after the crisis. People raise and debate charges of sorcery, neglect, and medical wrongdoings. When Justina, a young primigravida, died during the fieldwork period, I observed how perceptions of her death shifted over time and varied among community members. Justina, who was 16 years old, gave birth to a large (she weighed approximately 9 pounds), healthy baby girl with the help of her grandmother and a private nurse. Just after delivering the baby, she began to bleed severely, her blood pressure dropped, and her body began to shake. According to her grandmother, she began to say strange things about dying that indicated she was the victim of sorcery. Her grandmother immediately started administering traditional herbal therapy to address what she suspected was an advanced case of *poison*. The treatment, as well as the nurse's care, failed to save her life. Her grandmother and other family members accused her in-laws of sorcery as soon as she died, just 2 h after the delivery. It was well known in the community that Justina's mother and father-in-law disapproved of her relationship with their son. Her mother-in-law's hatred was no secret, and many people had witnessed her insult Justina publicly. She reportedly told Justina that she hoped she would die during childbirth. This statement later served as proof of her guilt to Justina's family, as well as others in the community.

However, as details of Justina's death filtered throughout the village, some people doubted that sorcery was the cause of her death. In particular, individuals with biomedical knowledge and training argued that the private nurse who had attended Justina, rather than her mother-in-law, was to blame. They accused the nurse of administering too much synthetic oxytocin during the delivery. Although Justina's grandmother said that she delivered the placenta and buried it immediately, no one else observed this. According to this theory, Justina's grandmother was protecting the private nurse. They thought that she convinced others to stay quiet about what happened. The nurse emphasized sorcery as the ultimate cause of Justina's death to preserve her reputation as a health care provider in the community, which was essential to maintaining her private health care practice.

This case study shows how different explanations of maternal death can emerge and become contested by members of the community. It also draws attention to what different actors stand to gain or lose depending on community perceptions about the cause of death. If sorcery is the accepted cause of death, then those accused of using *poison* are solely to blame, and they may face social consequences and supernatural retribution. The diagnosis of sorcery absolves anyone who tried to help the victim, including relatives, midwives, nurses, and doctors who have limited (or no) abilities to counter the effects of supernatural forces. Individuals who are accused of sorcery, on the other hand, may try to shift attention to natural, rather than personalistic, causes of complications. Community members expect that midwives, nurses, and doctors can address natural causes, and family members are responsible for getting women appropriate care in a timely manner. If relatives neglect their duties by failing to take birthing women to a hospital or nurses mismanage complications (by giving too much pitocin, for example), they become culpable for the death, which can decrease their standing in the community and jeopardize their health care business. Different actors may therefore attempt to manipulate public perceptions in order to protect their social positions and their livelihoods. This, in turn, makes examining, explaining, and preventing maternal death more complicated.

21.4 Discussion

The causes of maternal morbidity and mortality in *Miskito* communities may seem familiar to public health experts, physicians, and epidemiologists. Global health and development campaigns like the Safe Motherhood Initiative and the Millennium Development Goals (MDGs) have emphasized poverty and gender inequality as underlying causes of maternal mortality. Yet, solving these problems remains difficult given the diverse and powerful forces that create and maintain inequality. Ultimately, there are no magic bullet solutions that will prevent all maternal deaths around the world. Instead, effective interventions should be based on detailed studies that identify specific factors that prevent safe motherhood and the mechanisms through which they work. Public health policies can then be designed to reflect the specific circumstances and needs of vulnerable populations. This analysis draws attention to how global problems of social and economic insecurity play out in a specific local context. Here, an ethnographic, anthropological perspective is useful for understanding how large-scale forces, historical and present, have implications for women's lives.

In *Miskito* communities, interventions to address inadequate health services, widespread poverty, and gender inequality would benefit from understanding why mothers are poor and lack access to adequate obstetric care. Communities have integrated into the global economy, but wage labor opportunities are seasonal and only available to men for the most part. As the primary breadwinners, husbands dominate financial decisions, including whether women can travel to a hospital for health care. Seeking care at a hospital is rarely an option, because household resources are limited (especially during the moratorium on lobster harvesting) and husbands often downplay their wives' needs for obstetric care. Women also prefer to maintain access to traditional healers in their own community in case they experience complications caused by sorcery or witchcraft. Local biomedical resources are limited, and health center personnel are disinclined to attend births. Women therefore give birth at home with relatives, or with local midwives and/or private nurses. Midwives and private nurses receive little training and support from the ministry of health, and some have recently received threats from government officials due to their involvement in cases of maternal death. Some midwives have decided to avoid attending births of high-risk mothers, further decreasing women's options for support during childbirth.

Emic perceptions of risk that emphasize sorcery and witchcraft as causes of maternal death are also relevant to understanding and addressing maternal health risks. The communities in this study are remote, but modernizing. People's lives are increasingly influenced by outside forces that determine the (seasonal) demand for labor, types of jobs available, and goods offered for consumption. *Miskito* people have little influence over the national and international policies that dictate their access to and use of natural resources. For instance, conservation organizations and multilateral institutions have pressured the Honduran government to address the environmental and human costs of lobster diving (i.e., declining lobster populations and widespread illness and death experienced by divers). In 2009, Honduras agreed to ban scuba diving for lobster by 2011. Since then, two extensions have occurred to provide more time to transition to new fishing practices and jobs for local people (Jorge 2013). Whether (or when) commercial diving for lobster, on which the majority of *Miskito* households depend, will be banned remains unknown. The economic and social effects a ban will produce are equally uncertain (see also Herlihy 2012). Many families have already experienced financial declines due to poorer and shorter lobster harvests in recent years (Fig. 21.10).

As individuals have fared differently under capitalism, disparities in wealth have become more pronounced and social tensions have grown. Changing conditions have fueled conflicts and heightened fears of witchcraft and sorcery in communities. Women, who already suffer disproportionately from social and economic insecurity, are also perceived to be especially vulnerable to supernatural attacks. Personalistic disease etiologies have a long history of importance in *Miskito* society (Dennis 2004); however, community members believe that incidences of *poison* and *trick* have actually increased in response to negative social conditions. Under current circumstances, people have devel-

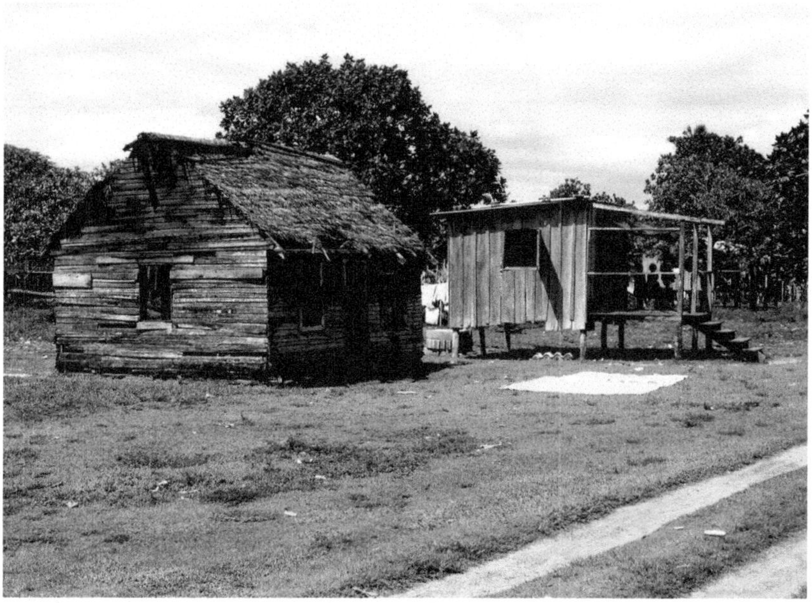

Fig. 21.10 Children playing on the porch of a small home, while recently harvested rice dries on a tarp in the sun

oped motives to "do bad things" to others. Thus, inequality, uncertainty, and poverty cause not only material deprivation, but they also create dangerous social environments. Only traditional medicine can cure witchcraft and sorcery. Biomedicine, a symbol of the modernization processes that have generated these negative changes, has nothing to offer.

Given these findings, a number of important interventions, targeted at entire communities, not just pregnant women, are necessary to improve health outcomes. Improving quality of life by increasing access to nutritious food, clean water, and health care services is crucial for addressing multiple types of insecurities. National and international donors are willing to support these types of projects, and have already been involved in financing water systems, health clinics, and supplemental food programs for school children in some villages in Gracias a Dios. Successful community projects should serve as models for extending resources in other *Miskito* villages in the region. Given local perceptions about increasing social tensions, development programs need to avoid introducing new problems into communities or contributing to inequality that is already present. For example, focusing jobs or leadership positions on affluent community members could lead to further social stratification. Project managers should expect that community members will respond to new forms of inequality with leveling mechanisms such as sorcery. To avoid exacerbating wealth disparities and social conflicts, governmental and nongovernmental agencies need to pay close attention to local power structure, select their employees from different economic backgrounds, and spread benefits as widely as possible (Fig. 21.11).

Community members voiced concerns about the lack of medicines and diagnostic equipment at local health centers, as well as insensitive and disrespectful treatment by health center staff. While health center employees would benefit from training that focuses on helping them support local women effectively in the context of limited resources, the health ministry must commit to stocking health centers with the basic supplies they need to function. Greater governmental assistance (with supplies and

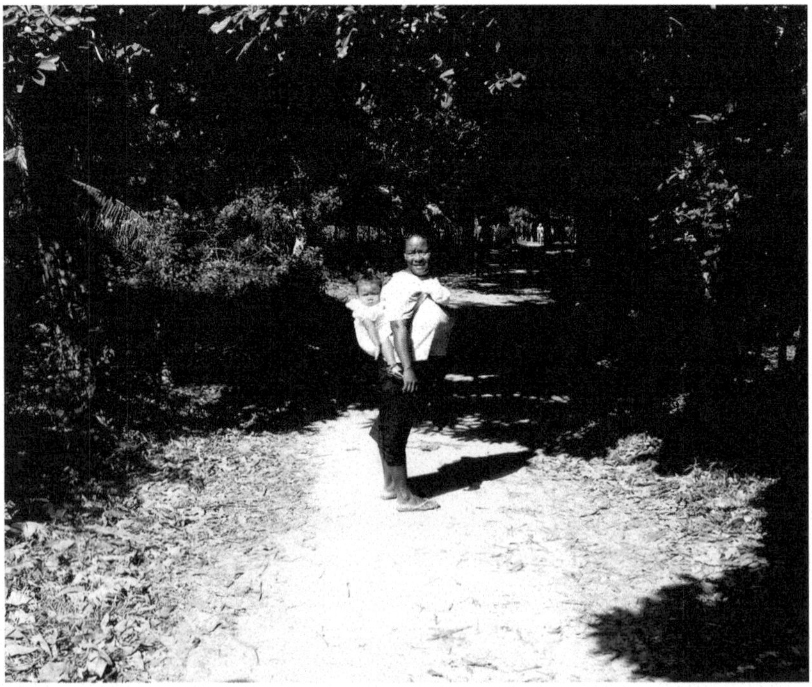

Fig. 21.11 A grandmother carries her granddaughter on her back as she walks along a village path

training) to local midwives is also important, as is building communication, trust, and respect among the different types of healers in *Miskito* communities. Ultimately, health center staff, midwives, private nurses, and traditional healers need to work together to identify at-risk pregnant women and help them obtain appropriate care. Midwives have significant cultural authority, so they should not be overlooked as potential health care partners by biomedical practitioners or government agencies.

Given the obstacles of seeking care outside of coastal communities, the policy of having midwives or doctors at the health center refer women to regional hospitals without providing any logistical support is inadequate. Women and their families need inexpensive transportation services that can be accessed quickly, as soon as a medical need arises. Creating social networks to facilitate trips to hospitals and organizing collective transportation systems could drastically improve women's access to care. Mobilizing these resources is especially important during periods of economic downturn (e.g., the annual moratorium on lobster extraction and fishing activities). Improving access to emergency obstetric care is often cited as key to decreasing maternal mortality in developing countries (Paxton et al. 2005; Razzak and Kellermann 2002), and the recommendations discussed here could be accomplished with small financial commitments.

Promoting earlier access to emergency obstetric care by improving referral and transportation systems may increase the use of biomedical care in many health emergencies. However, treatment can be delayed (or entirely avoided) for a variety of reasons (Berry 2006; Thaddeus and Maine 1994). In *Miskito* communities, disease etiologies, beliefs about healing, and women's perceptions of security and comfort influence health care decision-making. Women may prefer to remain at home during childbirth, not solely to avoid the distance and cost involved with traveling to a hospital, but also to maintain diverse treatment options that are available in their community. In their strategies for managing pregnancy and childbirth, women tried to minimize both natural and supernatural risks to their health. These findings suggest a need, once again, for more coordination between biomedical and traditional healers. Women often viewed biomedicine and traditional medicine as complementary; *Miskito sika* addresses the root cause of the illness, and then biomedicine works to counter the physical cause of a complication (e.g., obstructed labor or severe bleeding). To respect women's desires for varied types of health care and improve health outcomes, biomedical facilities (e.g., local health centers and hospitals) should not prohibit *Miskito* healers from simultaneously monitoring and treating patients.

Decisions about diagnosis and treatment have social, economic, and spiritual dimensions for women and their relatives. As such, pregnant women rarely make choices about health care by themselves. In fact, women's input is particularly limited when they are young and when they rely on spouses or other relatives for financial support. *Miskito* communities are female-centered and male-dominated. Therefore, both maternal relatives and husbands have authority over women. Cultural and economic factors can restrict their options for both preventative and emergency health care. Young women, in particular, face numerous challenges in indigenous *Miskito* communities—they have few economic opportunities, are excluded from decision-making, and wield little control over income or property. Being young and female puts them at the bottom of the socioeconomic ladder, which in turn compromises their health and well-being. Since women often lack the resources or rights to seek obstetric care, interventions to improve maternal health should also target men, families, and entire communities (see also Roth and Mbizvo 2001). To address inequities created by gendered differences in wealth, development efforts should focus on expanding women's economic opportunities. Increasing their access to income-generating activities may improve women's abilities to afford health care and influence household financial decisions (Fig. 21.12).

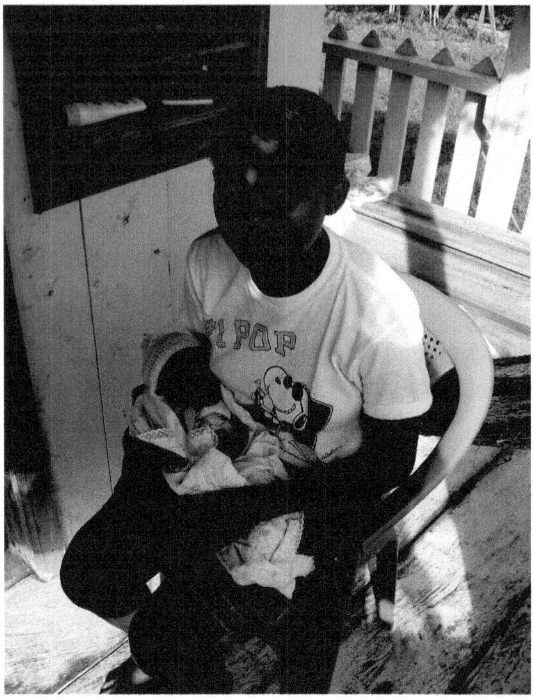

Fig. 21.12 A young *Miskito* mother holds her newborn son

Conclusions

Improving maternal health outcomes in *Miskito* communities requires confronting numerous factors that contribute to poor living conditions, limited emergency obstetric care, and inequalities related to gender, age, and socioeconomic status. While complicated challenges exist, clear avenues for interventions have emerged from this detailed ethnographic study of maternal morbidity and mortality. Despite being one of the poorest countries in the western hemisphere, Honduras has an impressive record of reducing maternal mortality in the past. Political commitments and donor support proved sufficient for improving safe motherhood at the national level. Now, further efforts are necessary to improve maternal health outcomes in geographically and socially marginalized communities like those described here. In *Miskito* communities, public health interventions must be attentive to the larger social, economic, and gendered context in which pregnancy and childbirth occur. Attempts to prevent maternal deaths need to focus on the local and large-scale forces that endanger women's health, while also respecting cultural perceptions about illness and healing.

References

Alauddin, M. (1986). Maternal mortality in Bangladesh: The Tangail district. *Studies in Family Planning, 17*, 13–21.

Arps, S. (2009). *Explaining fertility patterns among women in an Amerindian population: Childbearing goals and perceptions of risk*. Paper presented at the Human Biology Association Annual Meeting, Chicago, IL, April 1–2, 2009.

Associated Press (AP). (2012, May 16). DEA admits to role in deadly Honduras helicopter shooting. *CBS News*. Retrieved September 15, 2016, from http://www.cbsnews.com/news/dea-admits-to-role-in-deadly-honduras-helicopter-shooting/

Berry, N. S. (2006). Kaqchikel midwives, home births, and emergency obstetric referrals in Guatemala: Contextualizing the choice to stay at home. *Social Science & Medicine, 62*(8), 1958–1969.

Brock, J. H. (1999). Iron and the immune system. In J. J. Bullen & E. Griffiths (Eds.), *Iron and infection* (pp. 289–325). New York: John Wiley and Sons.

Castellanos, M., David, V., & Ochoa, J. C. (1990). *Mortalidad de mujeres en edad reproductiva y mortalidad materna*. Tegucigalpa, Honduras: Ministerio de Salud Pública.

Castro, A., Savage, V., & Kaufman, H. (2015). Assessing equitable care for indigenous and afrodescendant women in Latin America. *Revista Panamericana de Salud Pública, 38*(2), 96–109.

Chapman, R. R. (2003). Endangering safe motherhood in Mozambique: Prenatal care as pregnancy risk. *Social Science & Medicine, 57*(2), 355–374.

Chi, I., Agoestina, T., & Harbin, J. (1981). Maternal mortality at twelve teaching hospitals in Indonesia—An epidemiologic analysis. *International Journal of Gynecology & Obstetrics, 19*(4), 259–266.

Danel, I. (1998). *Maternal mortality reduction, Honduras, 1990–1997: A case study*. Washington, DC: World Bank.

Danel, I., & Rivera, A. (2003). Honduras, 1990–1997. In M. A. Koblinsky (Ed.), *Reducing maternal mortality: Learning from Bolivia, China, Egypt, Honduras, Indonesia, Jamaica, and Zimbabwe* (pp. 51–62). Washington, DC: World Bank Publications.

Dennis, P. (2004). *The Miskitu people of Awastara*. Austin: University of Texas Press.

Dennis, P., & Olien, M. (1984). Kingship among the Miskito. *American Ethnologist, 11*, 718–737.

Dodds, D. (1994). *The ecological and social sustainability of Miskito subsistence in the Río Plátano biosphere reserve, Honduras: The cultural ecology of Swidden horticulturalists in a protected area*. Doctoral dissertation, University of California, Los Angeles. University Microfilms International, Ann Arbor.

Dodds, D. (1998). *Informe preliminar sobre demografía de tres pueblos indígenas en la Reserva Biósfera del Río Plátano*. Working paper 98-1, Population Institute for Research and Training, Indiana University, Bloomington.

Gaynor, T. (2014, June 23). *Honduran indigenous groups caught in crosshairs of global drug trade*. *Al Jazeera America*. Retrieved September 15, 2016, from http://america.aljazeera.com/articles/2014/6/23/honduran-indigenousgroups-drugwar.html

Gracey, M., & King, M. (2009). Indigenous health part 1: Determinants and disease patterns. *The Lancet, 374*(9683), 65–75.

Hale, C. (1994). *Resistance and contradiction: Miskitu Indians and the Nicaraguan State, 1894–1987*. Stanford: Stanford University Press.

Heath, G. R. (1913). Notes on Miskuto grammar and on other Indian languages of Eastern Nicaragua. *American Anthropologist, 15*(1), 48–62.

Helms, M. W. (1969). The purchase society: Adaptation to economic frontiers. *Anthropological Quarterly, 42*(4), 325–342.

Helms, M. W. (1971). *Asang: Adaptations to culture contact in a Miskito community*. Gainesville: University of Florida Press.

Helms, M. W. (1977). Negro or Indian? The changing identity of a frontier population. In A. Pescatello (Ed.), *Old roots in new lands: Historical and anthropological perspectives on black experiences in The Americas* (pp. 157–172). Westport, CT: Greenwood Press.

Helms, M. W. (1983). Miskito slaving and culture contact: Ethnicity and opportunity in an expanding population. *Journal of Anthropological Research, 39*, 179–197.

Herlihy, P. H. (1997). Indigenous peoples and biosphere reserve conservation in the Mosquitia rain forest corridor, Honduras. In S. Stevens (Ed.), *Conservation through cultural survival* (pp. 99–129). Washington: Island Press.

Herlihy, L. H. (2002). *The mermaid and the lobster diver: Gender and ethnic identities among the Río Plátano Miskito peoples*. Doctoral dissertation, University of Kansas, Lawrence.

Herlihy, L. H. (2006). Sexual magic and money: Miskitu women's strategies in northern Honduras. *Ethnology, 45*(2), 143–159.

Herlihy, L. H. (2007). Matrifocality and women's power on the Miskito Coast. *Ethnology, 46*(2), 133–149.

Herlihy, L. H. (2012). *The mermaid and the lobster diver: Gender, sexuality, and money on the Miskito Coast*. Albuquerque, NM: UNM Press.

Instituto Nacional de Estadisticas (INE). (2001). *Censo de Población y Vivienda 2001*. Tegucigalpa, Honduras: INE.

Instituto Nacional de Estadisticas (INE). (2013). *XVII Censo de Población y VI Vivienda*. Tegucigalpa, Honduras: INE.

Janes, C. R., & Chuluundorj, O. (2004). Free markets and dead mothers: The social ecology of maternal mortality in post-socialist Mongolia. *Medical Anthropology Quarterly, 18*(2), 230–257.

Jorge, M. (2013, April 23). Time for Honduras to end scuba diving for lobster. *National Geographic Voices*. Retrieved September 15, 2016 from http://voices.nationalgeographic.com/2013/04/23/time-for-honduras-to-end-scuba-diving-for-lobster/

Kandoi, A., Bhatia, B. D., Pandey, L. K., Pandey, S., Sen, P. C., & Satya, K. (1991). Cellular immunity status in anaemia in pregnancy. *Indian Journal of Medical Research, 94*, 11–14.

Koblinsky, M. A. (1995). Beyond maternal mortality–magnitude, interrelationship, and consequences of women's health, pregnancy-related complications and nutritional status on pregnancy outcomes. *International Journal of Gynaecology and Obstetrics, 48*, S21–S32.

Lewis, M. P., Simons, G., & Fennig, C. D. (2016). *Ethnologue: Languages of the world* (19th ed.). Dallas, TX: SIL International. Retrieved from http://www.ethnologue.com

Llewellyn-Jones, D. (1965). Severe anaemia in pregnancy (as seen in Kuala-Lumpur, Malaysia). *Australian and New Zealand Journal of Obstetrics and Gynaecology, 5*(4), 191–197.

Locklear, T. D., Perez, A., Caceres, A., & Mahady, G. B. (2013). Women's health in Central America: The complexity of issues and the need to focus on indigenous healthcare. *Current Women's Health Reviews, 9*(1), 30–40.
Mason, J. A. (1973). The native languages of Middle America. In C. L. Hay, R. Linton, S. Lothrop, H. Shapiro, & G. Valiant (Eds.), *The Maya and their neighbors* (pp. 52–87). New York: Cooper Square Publishers.
McCarthy, J., & Maine, D. (1992). A framework for analyzing the determinants of maternal mortality. *Studies in Family Planning, 23*(1), 23–33.
McSweeney, K. (2004). The dugout canoe trade in Central America's Mosquitia: Approaching rural livelihoods through systems of exchange. *Annals of the Association of American Geographers, 94*(3), 638–661.
Meléndez, J., Ochoa Vasquez, J. C., & Villanueva, Y. (1999). *Investigación sobre mortalidad materna y de mujeres en edad reproductiva en Honduras: Informe final correspondiente al año 1997.* Tegucigalpa, Honduras: Ministerio de Salud.
Miller, S., Sloan, N. L., Winikoff, B., Langer, A., & Fikree, F. F. (2003). Where is the "E" in MCH? The need for an evidence-based approach in safe motherhood. *Journal of Midwifery & Women's Health, 48*(1), 10–18.
Montenegro, R. A., & Stephens, C. (2006). Indigenous health in Latin America and the Caribbean. *The Lancet, 367*(9525), 1859–1869.
Nietschmann, B. (1973). *Between land and water: the subsistence ecology of the Miskito Indians, Eastern Nicaragua.* New York, NY: Seminar Press.
Offen, K. (1999). *The Miskitu Kingdom. Landscape and the emergence of a Miskitu ethnic identity, Northeastern Nicaragua and Honduras, 1600–1800.* Ph.D. dissertation, Department of Geography, University of Texas.
PAHO. (2004). Maternal and child mortality among the indigenous peoples of the Americas. *Bulletin of Indigenous Health, 1*, 1–3.
Paxton, A., Maine, D., Freedman, L., Fry, D., & Lobis, S. (2005). The evidence for emergency obstetric care. *International Journal of Gynaecology and Obstetrics, 88*(2), 181–193.
Prevention of Maternal Mortality Network (PMMN). (1992). Barriers to treatment of obstetric emergencies in rural communities of West Africa. *Studies in Family Planning, 23*(5), 279–291.
Razzak, J. A., & Kellermann, A. L. (2002). Emergency medical care in developing countries: Is it worthwhile? *Bulletin of the World Health Organization, 80*(11), 900–905.
Roth, D. M., & Mbizvo, M. T. (2001). Promoting safe motherhood in the community: The case for strategies that include men. *African Journal of Reproductive Health, 5*(2), 10–21.
Schwartz, D. A. (2013). Challenges in improvement of perinatal health in developing nations—Role of perinatal pathology. *Archives of Pathology & Laboratory Medicine, 137*(6), 742–746.
Shahidullah, M. (1995). A comparison of sisterhood information on causes of maternal death with the registration causes of maternal death in Matlab, Bangladesh. *International Journal of Epidemiology, 24*(5), 937–942.
Shiffman, J., Stanton, C., & Salazar, A. P. (2004). The emergence of political priority for safe motherhood in Honduras. *Health Policy and Planning, 19*(6), 380–390.
Thaddeus, S., & Maine, D. (1994). Too far to walk: Maternal mortality in context. *Social Science & Medicine, 38*(8), 1091–1110.
United Nations Development Programme (UNDP). (2003). Desarrollo humano y capital social en Gracias a Dios: La necesidad de una perspectiva multicultural. In UNDP (Ed.), *Informe sobre desarrollo humano: Honduras* (pp. 101–133). Tegucigalpa, Honduras: PNUD.
Valeggia, C. R., & Snodgrass, J. J. (2015). Health of indigenous peoples. *Annual Review of Anthropology, 44*, 117–135.
Wall, L. L. (1998). Dead mothers and injured wives: The social context of maternal morbidity and mortality among the Hausa of northern Nigeria. *Studies in Family Planning, 29*(4), 341–359.
WHO. (2005). The World Health Organization Annual Report for 2005. *Make every mother and child count.* Geneva: World Health Organization.

Part IV

Belize

Managing Maternal Mortality: On-the-Ground Practices of Traditional Birth Attendants in Southern Belize

22

Aminata Maraesa

22.1 Introduction

The rain-drenched Toledo district of southern Belize is often called "the forgotten district" (Dickinson 2008).[1] Bordering Guatemala to the south and west with the Stann Creek and Cayo districts to the north (Fig. 22.1), this 1669-square mile district has only one town: Punta Gorda, population just under 5500. The early inhabitants of this district were the pre-Columbian Maya, and the district contains numerous archaeological sites including Lubaantun, Nim Li Punit, and the earliest settled city, Uxbenka, with evidence of habitation dating to the Early Classic Period (250–500 CE). Currently the Toledo district contains the largest numbers of indigenous *Kekchi-* (also spelled *Q'eqchi'*) and *Mopan*-speaking Maya who migrated to the area from neighboring Guatemala in the late 1800s. It also includes a substantial population of *Garifuna* people, who are the mixed-race descendants of West African, Central African, Arawak, and Island Carib people and speak a unique offshoot of the Island Carib language. This ethnically diverse and linguistically complex region is the poorest and least developed with some of the most remote and difficult to access villages in the country. It is also the area marked by the highest rates of fertility and intentional home births. Interestingly, its infant and maternal mortality statistics are on par with the rest of the country. Nonetheless, the Belizean Ministry of Health [MOH] has made a concerted effort to move all births into the hospital located in the town center or, in the interim, to ensure that all births in Toledo take place with a medically trained birth attendant.

In 1952 the World Health Organization [WHO] advocated for midwifery skills-training for individuals identified as "traditional birth attendants" [TBAs]. This was the official label given to "the untrained or partially trained indigenous midwife" (WHO 1952 cited in Oakley and Houd 1990: 175), who was to be targeted for standardized midwifery training programs undertaken by ministries of

[1] Toledo has the highest rainfall countrywide at 800 mm. during the month of July, more than twice the national average and nearly four times Belize's central and northern regions.

A. Maraesa, Ph.D.
Departments of Anthropologys, NYU-School of Professional Studies and Fordham University, New York, NY, USA
e-mail: amikole@sheabutter.net

D. A. Schwartz (ed.), *Maternal Death and Pregnancy-Related Morbidity Among Indigenous Women of Mexico and Central America*, Global Maternal and Child Health: Medical, Anthropological, and Public Health Perspectives, https://doi.org/10.1007/978-3-319-71538-4_22

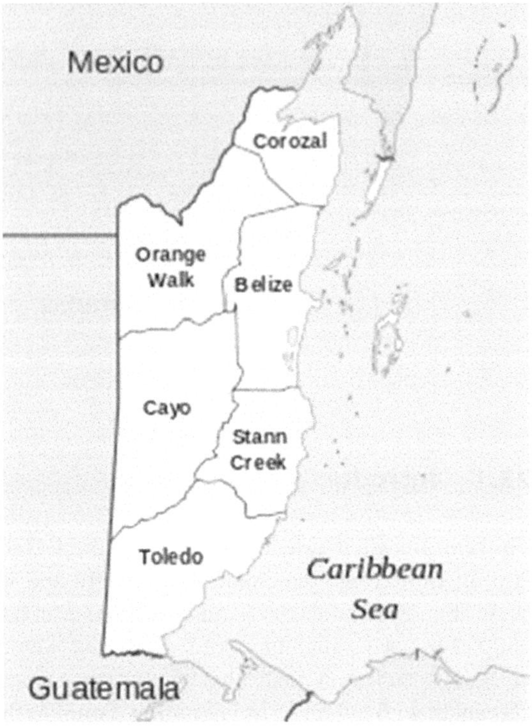

Fig. 22.1 Location of Toledo in Belize

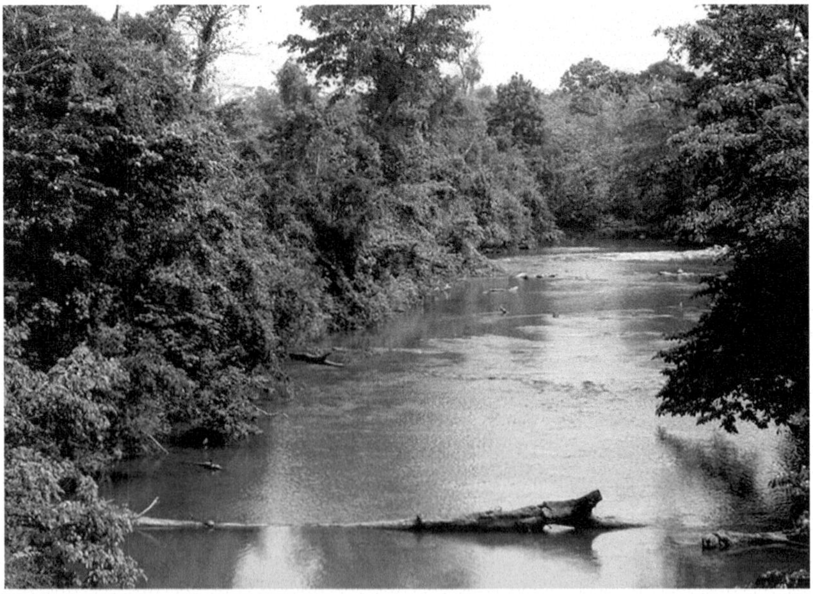

Fig. 22.2 A river in the Toledo district. Published with kind permission of © Aminata Maraesa 2017. All Rights Reserved

health and NGOs worldwide. It was argued that so-called traditional behaviors were an impediment to the modernization process and that maternal and child health outcomes in poor and developing nations could be ameliorated through a training and certification process that emphasized biomedical risk assessment and medical referral (Figs. 22.2, 22.3, and 22.4).

Since 1957, the Belizean Medical Department (now the MOH) has actively trained TBAs throughout the country to improve childbirth outcomes and reduce maternal fatalities. A proposal made to the United Nations Children's Fund [UNICEF] in the late 1990s opened the local world of women's

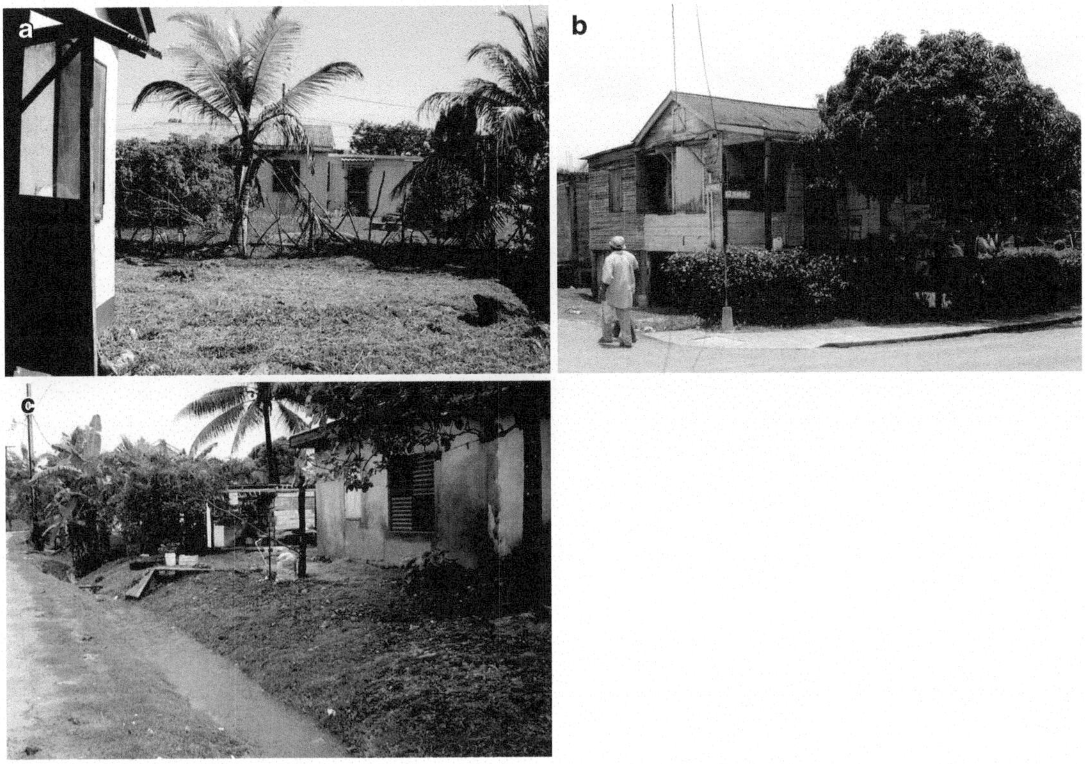

Fig. 22.3 (**a**)–(**c**) Typical urban housing in the town of Punta Gorda. Published with kind permission of © Aminata Maraesa 2017. All Rights Reserved

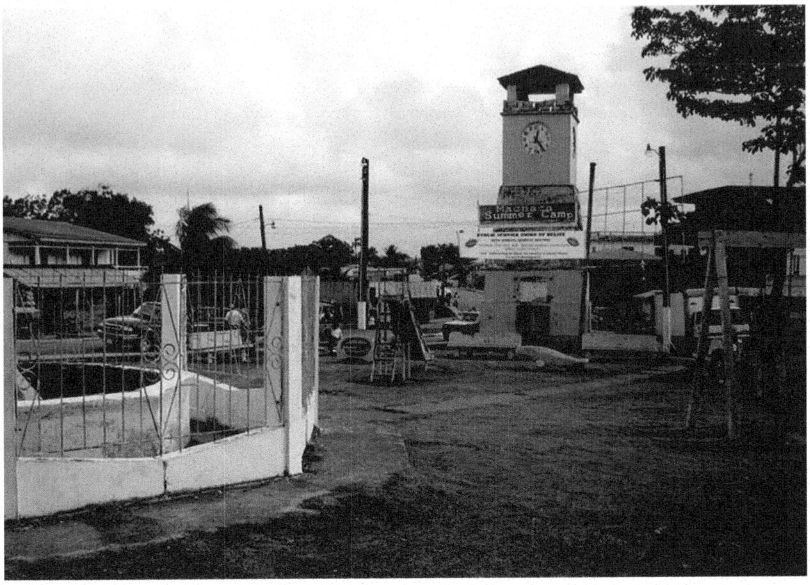

Fig. 22.4 Central Park in Punta Gorda town. Published with kind permission of © Aminata Maraesa 2017. All Rights Reserved

reproductive health care in the Toledo district to the involvement of a global player. In 2000, Giving Ideas for Tomorrow [GIFT], a United States-based nongovernmental organization [NGO] active around areas of health, food, and nutrition began the training of 22 TBAs from the rural areas of Toledo, of which only a handful remain practicing (Figs. 22.5, 22.6, and 22.7).

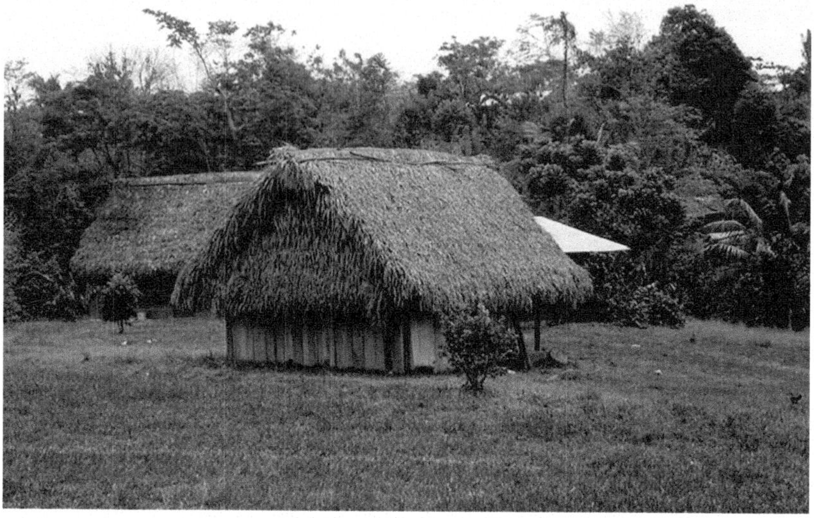

Fig. 22.5 Typical rural housing in a Mopan village in Toledo. Published with kind permission of © Aminata Maraesa 2017. All Rights Reserved

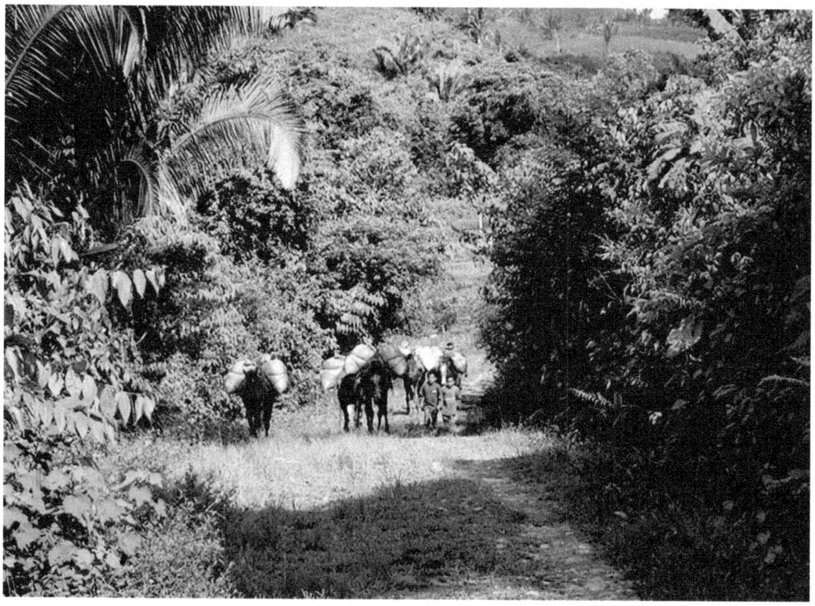

Fig. 22.6 Life in the country—leading horses saddled with beans for the Guatemalan marketplace. Published with kind permission of © Aminata Maraesa 2017. All Rights Reserved

In 2006 I conducted anthropological fieldwork among the TBAs in Toledo, with official follow-up research in 2007–2008. I have maintained informal relationships with these birth attendants up to the present day. This chapter describes the on-the-ground practices of two TBAs trained by GIFT in 2000 and 2001.[2] Both attendants are typical in their "fearless" cultural attitudes and understandings of childbirth and reproductive processes; yet, they stand distinct for their gendered behaviors and practices. This confidence and conduct may, in fact, play a role in their successes as birth attendants. Nonetheless, the "failure" or underutilization of one TBA may

[2]Both TBAs remain active at the time of this writing (2017).

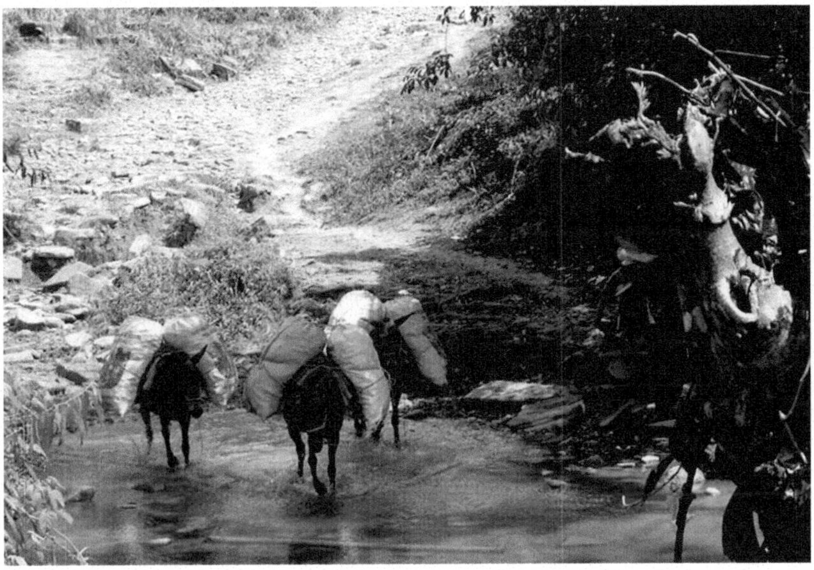

Fig. 22.7 Horses headed for the Guatemala market, loaded with beans and crossing the river separating Belize from Guatemala. Published with kind permission of © Aminata Maraesa 2017. All Rights Reserved

have more to do with his adoption of biomedical protocols and statistical risk analyses rather than the other's reliance on her experiential repertoire when asserting her ability to skillfully attend even the "riskiest" of births.

22.2 Sergio

When my child born, he already born when I gone there. I just helped my wife. I mi 'fraid for her.[3] *And I didn't know I should catch the baby. (Sergio reflecting on the birth of his first son)*

Sergio lives in Santa Madre, a *Kekchi* Maya village of about 350 inhabitants located roughly 25 miles (close to 1 hour vehicular travel time) from the Punta Gorda hospital. Sergio, age 36, has been both the local health post caretaker and the "community nurses aide" [CNA] since 1990. Since the Santa Madre rural health post has neither nurse nor doctor on permanent staff, Sergio holds regular office hours to distribute low-level medication and provide rudimentary medical services. After completing his TBA training in 2001, Sergio added weekly prenatal clinic checkups to the services he offers at the health facility. After meeting Sergio through a MOH-sponsored event, I went to the village of Santa Madre to conduct a recorded interview during which Sergio candidly discussed his personal and professional experiences with childbirth.

Sergio's first child was born when he was 21 years old; his wife was 15. Before engaging in work with the MOH, Sergio, like many rural-dwelling Maya, was a farmer, and he was working in his cornfield when someone informed him that his wife was in labor. Sergio rushed home to find his mother, who lived within a short walking distance from Sergio's home, tending to his wife. However, among the Maya in Toledo, attending to one's wife during childbirth is considered one of the duties a husband should perform. As such, older village women who attend the deliveries of their daughters or daughters-in-law explained to me that they should only have to show the husbands what to do at the first birth clarifying, "I done teach he once, I no wah teach he again." For Sergio, his wife had already

[3] "Mi" creates the past tense of the verb it precedes.

delivered their baby by the time he arrived home. As his newborn son laid on the ground with an intact umbilical cord, Sergio's mother explained to him that he must wait for the delivery of the placenta before touching the baby and cutting the cord. Sergio remembers,

> I wait 'til the placenta born before I went and attend to the baby. And then the baby's crying there. I didn't worry about that much, I 'fraid for my wife. Then my mother is beside me telling me that there's another thing is going to come out. But I don't know 'cause it's my first child. I only there beside my wife, trying to comforting her and trying to give her help. But not with the baby, not helping her pick up the baby. Just trying to hold my wife right here. And my mother mi do the same thing, 'cause that's their culture.

Indeed, all of the Maya men and women I spoke with during my fieldwork period told me that a newborn baby is left on the ground untouched until the placenta is delivered. Only then can the umbilical cord be cut and the baby tended to and breast fed. There is ample evidence supporting the health benefits to the newborn of leaving the cord intact until it stops pulsating (whether or not the placenta has detached) (Ceriani Cernadas et al. 2006); however, the reason cited by an overwhelming number of lay individuals in Toledo is the fear that the umbilical cord will slip back inside the womb if cut loose from the baby before expulsion of the placenta (see Cosminsky 1982a: 243 for similar beliefs among the *Quiché* Maya in Guatemala; Paul 1978 for a similar belief among the *Zutuhil* Maya in Guatemala; and Pinto 2006: 227 for a similar belief in Uttar Pradesh, India). This custom is respected and also believed by many of the hospital-based nurse midwives of *Garifuna* descent who explained to me that they clamp the cord after it stops pulsing, but cut it before the placenta detaches, in order to attend to the baby. Even though this is done before the placenta is delivered, one nurse explained how she leaves a clamp attached to the end of the portion of the umbilical cord that is still inside the woman so that "it can't go nowhere with that clamp right there."

By the time Sergio's second son was born, he had been trained by the MOH to serve as his village's CNA. Included in this training was basic information about prenatal care such as prenatal dietary recommendations and signs of perinatal risk, but little information about the stages of pregnancy or childbirth. Sergio recalls,

> I didn't learn nothing about midwife. They only just tell us advise the mother to seek help during pregnancy, advise them to eat foods that's rich with vitamins and iron, advise them to rest, you know. 'Cause it's danger they say during pregnancy. It's danger sometimes in the middle of pregnancy there's heavy bleeding or maybe water bags break. As soon as you see those people, refer them. But they don't give us detail how it cause and how to prevent it, how to help. We only watch the nurse examine the patient, giving antenatal care to the patient. But we didn't do it and we don't watch the delivery.

Even though Sergio received minimal information about pregnancy and childbirth and had not been given any information or training on attending a delivery, Sergio felt confident after having received Ministry-issued nurse's aide training to help his wife during her second birth. Sergio explained, "I was not trained as a TBA, but I have the idea already because I was a community health worker on that time. Since I already know about health, I do the delivery." Even though his "health" training did not include any midwifery skills other than how to recognize and refer high-risk pregnancies, his exposure to biomedical practices and a new command of risk assessment helped Sergio to overcome the fear he recalled feeling— "I 'fraid for my wife"—during the birth of his first child to go on to attend the deliveries of both his second and third children without additional or trained assistance.

After the births of his own children, Sergio was trained as a TBA. This training made him critically assess and reconsider how his wife delivered their first baby:

> When I first got a child I don't know. Like there is nobody could help them if anything arrive. Like for example placenta or like breeches. But when I get in this training, then I know the danger. And we no use a table or one clean place where we could do the delivery. It's totally on the ground, totally on the ground, without anybody catch the baby. The baby just lying down, crying on the dirt. I don't know that before. I mi think it's normal. But after I get my training, it's absolutely not. Because the baby is in a warm place, and when the baby born, it need to be covered, you know?

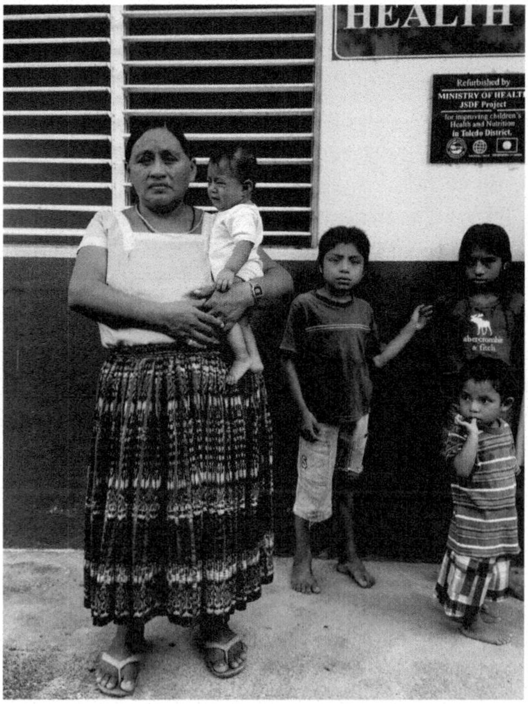

Fig. 22.8 *Kekchi* woman and her child in traditional dress. Published with kind permission of © Aminata Maraesa 2017. All Rights Reserved

Sergio never thought about the "danger" due to complications arising from a retained placenta or fetal malpresentation (an abnormal position of the fetus within the uterus) until after his TBA training. This training made him question what he would have done without any "help" available to him had these scenarios presented. Sergio's training also taught him to speak using a biomedical language of statistically based and normalized risk that he reinforces with his reference to the hypothetical "if anything arrive" and the abnormality of his behavior towards the newborn: "I mi think it's normal. But after I get my training, it's absolutely not" (Fig. 22.8).

Sergio's TBA training also made him shift his attention to the newborn, who he now believed needed a "clean" place for the delivery and to be kept warm after the birth. Before gaining exposure to biomedical procedures, Sergio concentrated on his wife: "And then the baby's crying there. I didn't worry about that much, I 'fraid for my wife." Now, as a trained TBA, Sergio thinks about the baby—especially since many of these births take place under conditions similar to the birth of his first child. According to Sergio,

> In some of the village where I went and do my delivery, some they just stoop down. They having one string there to make them hold themself there and the baby drop on the ground.[4] Nobody pick it up. Even if the mother will be there for one hour or for two hours, the baby will be still there. They no touch the baby 'til they bathe the baby, clean the baby, wash the baby then they put the baby in one cloth and then they put it on the mother for suck. That is their tradition.

Thus, Sergio has been trained to recognize and redirect risky birth behaviors. However, he does not assert absolute authority as a trained birth attendant. Nurse midwives working in the hospital insist on a lithotomy position (in which the woman lies on her back with her hips and knees flexed and her thighs apart), which enables the nurses to actively observe and conduct literal hands-on manipulation

[4]The "string" Sergio refers to is actually a thick rope that is suspended from the rafters of thatch roof houses. Women hold the string for support while they kneel on the ground. The rope can also be looped; women put their torsos through the loop and support themselves with the rope under their armpits.

of the birth process. Contrastingly, Sergio allows the birthing woman to squat or "stoop" so that the newborn is birthed vertically between the mother's legs. He also does not cut the umbilical cord until after the birth of the placenta. Although he places a cloth or plastic sheet (usually made from a flattened plastic shopping bag) on the ground to protect the newborn from the dirt floor of the house and covers the baby with a cloth to keep it warm, for the most part, Sergio permits the birth to progress without interfering or asserting authoritative control.[5]

Sergio's attention to the newborn may not necessarily disrupt the birthing process. However, this was the second time in the interview that he referred to "their" culture or "their" tradition to ideologically distance himself from birthing practices within his own culture that he has been trained to identify as "risky" or outright dangerous. And there are some interventions Sergio deems necessary to monitor the delivery process, which further distance him from his own culture's practices. As opposed to simply being next to the laboring woman and "comforting" her, Sergio tells them "not to relax, or not to lay down. They want a fast birth, so I advise them to walk around." Furthermore, he implements his training by conducting vaginal examinations and telling them,

> When the pain come, they no have to strain themselves 'cause it's not time yet and they push too soon. We exam them. We measure the opening to see if it's opening. You know if it is crowning [the baby's head emerging], it will be soon and they can push.

Nurse midwives claimed in frustration that Maya women begin to push too soon in the labor process and before the cervix is fully dilated. This can cause the cervix to swell or tear, resulting in hemorrhage. Ten centimeters dilation marks the beginning of the pushing stage, before which time women should allow the contractions to hasten dilation without actively bearing down. During his TBA training, Sergio learned to measure cervical dilation through internal vaginal examination: by inserting two fingers into the vaginal canal to feel the diameter of the cervical opening. However, he has encountered resistance to vaginal examinations from both pregnant women and their husbands. According to Sergio, opposition arises in part because he is a man, but it is also due to the fact that there is a general shame surrounding women's genitals. To overcome both of these culturally influenced hesitations Sergio explains, "I talk with them before I do the exam. I talk to them as a human being that this delivery is just going to stay with me and that's it." In this manner he tries to alleviate the woman's shame by telling her that he will not discuss what he has done or seen with others; he respects her shame. Indeed, he feels his own: "Well, most of the times I feel a little shame for me. But I say, 'I'm in a job, and I was trained to do this.' I encourage myself that I could do this, and I do it." Despite his efforts, there are still times when the pregnant woman or her husband refuses to let him perform a vaginal examination. When this occurs Sergio believes he is unable to determine when the baby will be born and feels like he "just go there to be around and just watch." To overcome this uncertainty, Sergio might give the husband a sterile glove and explain how to check for the baby's head—which is different than measuring dilation; nonetheless, feeling the head can indicate cervical effacement and the nearness of the pushing stage. Sergio also shows the husband how to clamp and cut the cord—just as Sergio's mother showed him at the birth of his first child.

According to the former director of GIFT's training program, Sergio was a "star" in class. He understood basic midwifery concepts and accepted the biomedical understandings of the risks related to pregnancy and childbirth. Sergio was clear throughout our interview that he refers all primaparas (women pregnant for the first time) and grand multiparas (women having their fifth or greater pregnancy) to the hospital for delivery. Moreover, he strongly advises women to seek trained assistance during childbirth, because "it dangerous to deliver without help." By initiating his own prenatal clinic

[5]At other births, women might spread a banana leaf on the ground onto which the baby can fall.

hours at the health post and allying himself with the MOH in various ways as the CNA, caretaker, and TBA—in addition to proactively holding regular clinic hours and distribution of medication—Sergio is the epitome of the public health ideals pronounced by the WHO. On the one hand, his training is a success. On the other hand, he remains underutilized for the majority of the births that take place in his village even though he actively provides prenatal care and has been called upon in cases of potential postnatal emergency when the placenta was slow to detach.

Interestingly, Sergio denied what could be considered an "obvious" reason for his underutilization—the fact that he is a male birth attendant in a society regulated by shame and covert female sexuality. A closer analysis of the history of GIFT's TBA training program suggests that Sergio's position as the village TBA is more complicated. GIFT began its programming by first identifying which villages in Toledo lacked a trained birth attendant. Then they requested a village-level meeting to nominate a candidate for the group TBA training sessions that were to be led by a representative from GIFT. The first round of trainees was comprised exclusively of women, and the MOH had minimal involvement in the community vote or training processes. In contrast, the trainees for the second round were chosen in large part by the local public health officials who believed it made more sense to train people already serving within the Ministry's public health system and known to the community as local-level health workers: CNAs or caretakers—three of which were men. Although Sergio admitted, "It's not a nice job. You see, I'm a man, and I'm comfortable to work with a man. But if I go to a woman, it's different. Sometimes I'm nervous, and sometimes I don't want to be there." Sergio underscored his willingness to do his job by saying, "I say [to myself], 'I'm in a job, and I was trained to do this.' I encourage myself that I could do this, and I do it." Moreover, he has the backing of the Ministry of Health. Thus, Sergio is well integrated into the MOH's public health campaigns, locally dominated by female nurses and outreach workers. This association with a maternalist public health department (Macpherson 2003) may serve to soften his manhood, making him an appealing man-midwife.

As such, Sergio's "maleness" is mitigated by the various activities with which he is involved (notably the care he provides at the village health post and his position as a pastor for the local Baptist church), and the activities in which he does not partake (most importantly, the drinking of alcoholic beverages—a common past-time for men in the Toledo district). At the time of our interview, Sergio had only attended a small handful of deliveries. However, he had been called on six occasions to help expel a retained placenta. Using abdominal massage techniques he learned during his TBA training, Sergio was able to assist all six women by manually expelling the placenta, thereby avoiding possible postpartum hemorrhage and infection. These feats furthered his reputation in the community as a reliable caregiver. Moreover, his willingness to teach husbands how to check the vagina for the baby's head and how to cut the umbilical cord likens him in many ways to the older mothers and mothers-in-law who have the task of teaching the young men how to assist at subsequent births.

However, Sergio repeatedly brought up the differences between his biomedical training as both the CNA and TBA and Maya cultural practices that, according to Sergio, affect his ability to practice in his village in the manner according to which he was trained—or even to be called upon at all. Sergio is also very vocal about what he believes should be changed about the laissez-faire cultural traditions regarding the treatment of the newborn baby:

> It [care for the neonate] needs to be changed, because when I was being trained they say there's a chance of the baby could catch asthma or bronchitis if the baby was keep in a cold place, because where the baby come out [the womb] it's not cold; it's hot. So as soon as the baby born you need to wrap that baby in a clean cloth or warm cloth. But nowadays a lot of bronchitis, a lot of asthma due to that [being left uncovered after birth]. Or it could cause infection or skin infection. This is what is very difficult to change the people. *Maybe that's why they're not using me a lot, because we do totally different* (*emphasis mine*).

In accordance to the humoral configuration of health and illness that is prevalent in both Garifuna and Maya cultures, Sergio places emphasis on keeping the newborn warm to avoid "catching" sickness.[6] He rationalizes that the baby must be kept warm because it has just emerged from the womb—a warm place. While this should not conflict with lay understandings of health and illness, Sergio's focus on the baby's well-being may conflict with cultural priorities. Attending to the child before it is severed from the umbilical cord may be misunderstood as care performed at the expense of the mother who is still laboring. Prior to his training, Sergio was preoccupied with the comfort and safety of his wife—not the fetus or the newborn, as he expressed fear on behalf of his wife. When Sergio diverts attention from the laboring woman to the newborn, this may result in resistance to his TBA practice.

Furthermore, Sergio concedes that his own children are healthy after having been delivered onto the floor and left unattended until the placenta was birthed. "Maybe it's people saying, 'My kids are fine. What is he talking about?' That's another thing, they're fine. So there's a chance that it [infant sickness] could happen *but when they don't see it happen they say it's no chance*" (*emphasis mine*). Statistics and probabilities—integral to the creation of risk discourse—are quite distant and foreign to the embodied understanding of birth. I argue that pregnant women in Toledo (and their husbands) understand risk and reason their realities "dramatically, not quantitatively" (Dowie 1980: 108). Despite what is framed as dangerous birthing practices, maternal and infant mortality is relatively low in Belize when compared to neighboring Latin American countries.[7] Notwithstanding exacerbated poverty conditions in Toledo, the average infant mortality rate during my fieldwork period [2006–2008] for the Toledo district (23/1000) was only slightly more than the national average for the same time period (18/1000) (knoema.com, accessed Sept. 1, 2016).[8] Given these statistics and his characterization of what he refers to as particularly Maya cultural practices, Sergio asserts that until people concretely experience the theoretically deleterious effects of these traditions, they will continue.

I also suggest that when Sergio distinguishes between the purported health of children who, by his observations, suffer from asthma and bronchitis more than the children of his imagined past, he is romanticizing a golden era when midwifery practices that appear alive and well among the *Q'eqchi'* Maya people of Guatemala may have been similarly ubiquitous in southern Belize.[9] For many Belizean *Kekchi*, Guatemala is the homeland for traditional spiritual practices (Tedlock 1992: 462–3), where midwives dominate the realm of childbirth in the Maya communities (Cosminsky 1972, 1982a, b; Glei et al. 2003; Greenberg 1982; Hinojosa 1998; Lang and Elkin 1997). However, within the collective memory of the women currently of childbearing age living in the rural areas of southern Belize, village midwives are a thing of the past (Woolfrey 2002). And a distinction must be made between nostalgia of timeless cultural traditions (Fabian 1983) and the contemporary reality of these

[6]A humoral medical system is based on the belief that sickness is caused by hot/cold imbalances that refer to actual temperature as well as qualities labeled "hot" or "cold" that are independent of thermal energy.

[7]Statistics around the time of my research period cited maternal mortality in Belize at 140/100,000 live births, while in Mexico it was 83/100,000 and in Guatemala it was 240/100,000 live births (WHO 2000). Infant mortality in Belize was 15/1000 live births, while in neighboring Mexico it was 22/1000 and in Guatemala it was 32/1000 (UNICEF 2005). Of note, the most recent statistics show lowered mortality rates for all three countries, with Belize's health indicators remaining better than its neighbors (knoema.com, accessed Sept. 1, 2016).

[8]It should be noted that infant mortality rates are calculated per 1000 births. In a country that experienced approximately 7000 births in 2007, every seven children who die under the age of 1 year raises the rate by one. In the Toledo district, where approximately 600 births took place in 2007, every one death raises the infant mortality rate by two. As such, only two or three actual deaths account for the statistical difference between Toledo and the rest of the country.

[9]Kekchi can also be spelled *K'ekchi'* or *Q'eqchi'* to transcribe the two epiglottal stops in pronunciation with the latter spelling asserting an ethnic identity that spans national borders to include *Q'eqchi'* speakers in Belize, Guatemala, and El Salvador. I have chosen to use the standard Belize Creole spelling of *Kekchi* as this is the one most commonly transcribed by Belizeans in both official and popular texts; however, I use *Q'eqchi'* here to refer to the group living in Guatemala as this is the agreed upon pan-*Q'eqchi'* spelling.

women who have neither the midwives of a previous era nor ready access to modern medical facilities. Sergio has been trained to be a "traditional" birth attendant for a group of people with no recent history of this tradition. As a man, his association with the maternalist MOH, older mothers, and Christian morality gain him entry to the female domain of pregnancy and childbirth. However, his repudiation of his own culture's practices and his iteration of the "danger" that he has been trained to acknowledge alienates him in many ways from the majority of women who approach their pregnancies with the intention of giving birth at home without trained assistance, without complication, and without fear.

22.3 Lucia

"Todas las mujeres vienen conmigo. Todas" [All the women come with me. All of them]. (Lucia's proud declaration regarding her TBA practice)

Lucia is a 40-year-old *Kekchi* Maya woman born and raised in Guatemala. Since 1987 she has lived with her Belizean-born husband in the mountainous village of San Lazaro (population approximately 390) located minutes by foot from the Guatemalan border and nearly 4 hours by public transportation from Punta Gorda hospital.[10] Aside from the school bus and a cattle rancher's converted pick-up, there is little vehicular activity on the road leading to town. However, there is much travel by foot to and from neighboring Esperanza village as well as daily treks back and forth between the Guatemalan border town for small shopping needs and larger unregulated commercial transactions (Fig. 22.9).

In 2000, Lucia was chosen by her village community to participate in GIFT's TBA training program. Her previous birth experiences were limited to the unassisted deliveries of her six children and the assistance she provided at the births of all four of her grandchildren. She is a person of high stand-

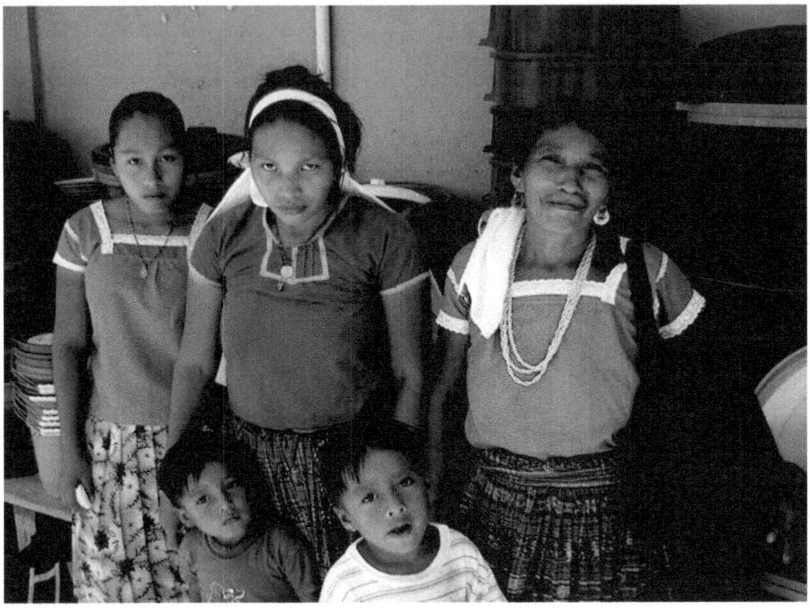

Fig. 22.9 A *Kekchi* TBA with her four children. Published with kind permission of © Aminata Maraesa 2017. All Rights Reserved

[10]By 2016 a significant portion of the roadway connecting San Lazaro to Punta Gorda town was paved, reducing the vehicular transportation time from 4 to 2 hours..

ing in her community, and her charismatic and outgoing personality is somewhat anomalous among the more reserved rural-dwelling *Kekchi* women.

As a relatively young village founded in 1984 by Guatemalan *Q'eqchi'* and a few "Spanish" who were seeking virgin farmland and "bigger yards," San Lazaro has no history of midwives or so-called "traditional" birth attendants. Rural health nurses from the MOH conduct prenatal examinations on their rounds of the mobile clinic on a six-week interval schedule. And, prior to Lucia's presence as a TBA, pregnant women seeking additional maternity services traveled to Guatemala for care where both government midwives and doctors are available at relatively little cost (Fig. 22.10).

Like Lucia, many women living in San Lazaro are Guatemalan by birth and may or may not have legalized their status as either Belizean residents or citizens. As such, immigration concerns by and large dictate where a woman gives birth. Undocumented women prefer to deliver their babies in Guatemala where their legal status ensures treatment and legitimizes their child's nationality. A child born in Belize is an automatic Belizean citizen, but the undocumented women I spoke to were hesitant about registering their children with the authorities out of fear that they would be deported. Even though the Guatemalan healthcare facilities were markedly closer, Belizean women in San Lazaro did not want to deliver their babies into a foreign bureaucratic system. They preferred to give birth in Belize even if they had crossed the border for prenatal care. However, giving birth in San Lazaro village, located some distance from the town hospital, meant that the birth would be conducted, like Lucia's children and grandchildren, without trained supervision. Only since Lucia's participation in GIFT's program have pregnant women in San Lazaro had a trained birth attendant living in the village to assist during labor and delivery.

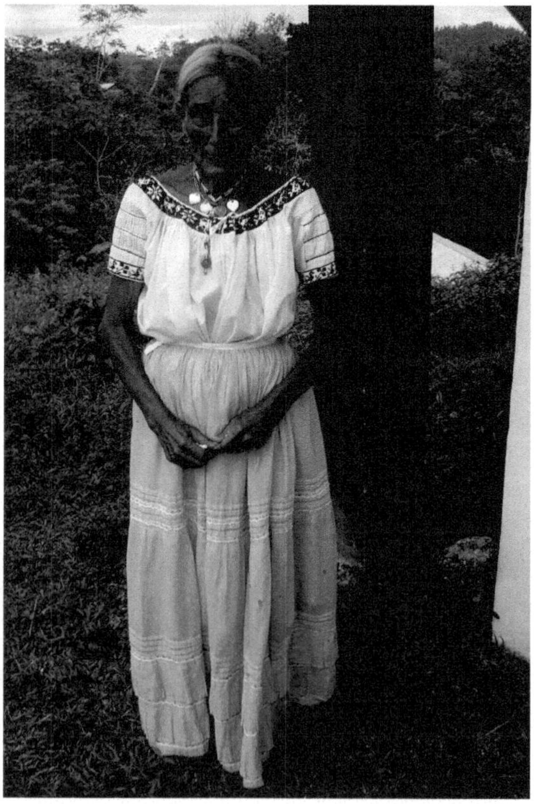

Fig. 22.10 A *Mopan* woman in traditional dress. Published with kind permission of © Aminata Maraesa 2017. All Rights Reserved

I first made contact with Lucia while staying with another GIFT-trained TBA living in neighboring Esperanza village from whence we made our way together on the three-mile journey over the unpaved mountainous road to arrive in San Lazaro a little over 2 hours later. Lucia's home is located on a hill and separated from the village center by a small river that often swells in the rainy season. In this river we found her—knee deep and washing clothes. The note I had sent on the school bus to inform her of my visit had gone undelivered. After an awkward moment of surprise for both of us, Lucia invited me into her home where we had a lively discussion (in Spanish) about her practice.

Lucia is the most active of all of the TBAs trained by the NGO and in 2006 claimed to have delivered over 70 babies since her training in 2000. Lucia proudly asserted that all of the pregnant women in San Lazaro, regardless of immigration status (and even some in neighboring Guatemala), delivered their babies with her. Like Sergio, she regularly provides prenatal care for the pregnant women in her village, but she does not service women at the rural health post or assist during the mobile clinics, prompting a hospital-based nurse midwife to slander Lucia's disengagement with the MOH as "self-interest" at the expense of the community. While Lucia makes regular door-to-door house calls to the pregnant women in her village, she is the only TBA in the entire Toledo district to do so independently of MOH supervision.

Since Lucia cannot read, write, or speak English, she is precluded from holding one of the paid "volunteer" public health positions such as CNA or health post caretaker. Although the TBAs were advised during their training sessions to work closely with the village CNA as well as to assist at the mobile clinic visits, Lucia does not have a working relationship with the CNA and is often "haciendo otras cosas" [doing other things] when the mobile clinic comes to the village. Nonetheless, Lucia has made herself known in her community as "la partera de la comunidad" [the village midwife] and keeps careful record of her prenatal visits in the small green Midwives' Book issued to her during her TBA training.

Lucia has never had a maternal death. One infant died an hour after birth; however, Lucia claims no responsibility for this death. According to Lucia, the delivery went without complication, so the newborn's death was unforeseeable and unexpected. Lucia stated, "Sólo Dios sabe" [Only God knows]—a common explanation for adverse experiences that precludes acknowledgment of statistical risk factors—why the baby died. Lucia also boldly declares that she has never transferred a woman to the hospital. Yet, this assertion, of which Lucia is quite proud, is what makes her so unpopular with the MOH. Both international and local maternal and child health protocols emphasize that high-risk pregnancies, including women having their first or their fifth or greater pregnancy, should deliver under hospital supervision. Lucia, however, laughs at the thought of "high-risk" pregnancies, instead declaring, "Yo no tengo miedo de eso. Voy para chequear las mujeres todos los meses. Están bien así" [I am not afraid of that (official definitions of and protocols for high risk). I go to check the women every month. They are good like that].

Although Lucia's fearlessness has hampered her relationship with local MOH personnel and created a wall of mistrust and animosity between them, Lucia continues to work quite successfully as a TBA independent of the MOH. Indeed, the ambivalent status of TBAs within the Belizean medical system—recognized as a care provider, yet the only community worker within the system of public health that does not receive a stipend—lends itself to Lucia's independent approach to servicing her community.

This independence, however, also lends itself to financial insecurity. In a more formalized interview Lucia lamented, "Cuando hay mujeres embarazadas, allí, sí me pagan. Pero cuando no hay, no hay pago. No hay pisto" [When there are pregnant women, when women get pregnant, then they pay me. But when there are none, there is no pay. There is no money].[11] Since Lucia is not paid by the

[11] *Pisto* is the name of a Spanish dish of tomatoes, onions, eggplant, zucchini, and sweet peppers similar to French ratatouille. In Guatemala *pisto* is slang for money. Lucia's use of the expression "no hay pisto" alludes to the hand-to-mouth nature of the subsistence economy in which she lives such that if there is no money, there will be no food.

MOH, she must survive on the few dollars she receives for prenatal care and the larger (but still meager) sum of money she earns when she attends a delivery. Even though she is married, Lucia never made mention of her husband or his ability to provide for the family. By declaring that if there are no pregnant women to pay for her midwifery services she will not have money (*pisto*) and may go hungry, Lucia is indexing herself as the primary breadwinner (literally and metaphorically) and claiming the responsibilities of the male head of household. Moreover, she is asserting her independence from the MOH by stating the official healthcare system does not pay her salary. Hence, she owes them nothing in return and does not feel beholden to their regulations. The freedom Lucia affirms within her personal life as the economic head of her household is likewise expressed in her independent midwifery practice.

Although she lived 4 hours by vehicular transportation each direction from town, I would often see Lucia on market days making small purchases, catching up on the latest news and gossip with her friends from other villages, and sipping from a glass bottle of Coca-Cola under the awnings of the semi-enclosed shops of Main Street. On these occasions we would chat about the people we knew in common, I would tell her about any news I may have heard at the hospital, and she would tell me about her most recent deliveries. The latest one was exceptionally interesting: during her prenatal visits, Lucia had dismissed the preeclamptic condition of a pregnant woman, Medina, and, indeed, successfully attended her birth without complication. "Además" [Furthermore], she smiled, "habían gemelos" [it was twins]. Was she aware of this prior to the delivery I questioned in amazement? "Claro que sí, pero no quiería hacerse miedo que no pudiera nacer bien" [Of course, but I did not want to make her afraid so that she would not give birth well].

Lucia was nonchalant in her discussion of Medina's delivery. Indeed, she was quite proud of herself. Yet, when I told a nurse midwife about the birth, she was livid. This nurse actually knew the mother's case quite well: "I see the gal two times on the mobile. I see her [on the street] in town. I tell her, 'You should have the baby da hospital. Your foot swell up, your blood low [low hemoglobin level or anemia], this is your first baby.' And then she had twins! Lucia like take risk. She no *see* the danger" (*emphasis mine*). It is true that Lucia's experiential repertoire does not include any of the dangers that are purportedly associated with definitions of high risk and grounds her perinatal decisions in this experiential knowledge base—one that is increasingly supporting her open renunciation of the "risks" maintained by the medical community and the nurse midwife who ended her admonition by saying, "Even if she do the delivery, she should have called the ambulance to back her up should in case anything happen." However, nothing did happen, and Lucia will add this potentially complicated birth to her list of successful actual deliveries that she has *seen* and conducted despite the hypothetical outcomes formulated in medical risk discourse. For Lucia, and the pregnant women in her community, the statistical risks expressed by the MOH will stay distant while homebirths successfully conducted without complication—or fear of complication—remain near.

Conclusion

At the international level, TBA training programs have been implemented in efforts to lower maternal and child death. Many of these training programs have been analyzed for their effectiveness and cultural relevancy, and the practicing TBAs assessed for their ability (and willingness) to engage with biomedical protocol. This chapter has added to these analyses by looking at the on-the-ground practices of two TBAs to look at how they interacted with and performed according to relationships of power, categories of knowledge, and gender constructs as they navigated international and local understandings of maternal risk in their TBA practices. Although both differed in the means and manner of services they provided to the pregnant women in their villages, I argue that their high level of activity is related to their ability to agentively position themselves within the local hierarchy of the MOH, draw on their personal and collective "ethno-obstetric" (McClain 1975) experiences, and negotiate local gender conventions. TBAs like Sergio and Lucia substantiate their practices through reasoning informed by both their biomedical training and life histories—reasoning that sometimes is at odds with an abstract risk discourse. And both merged standardized biomedical procedures and technology with local meaning and understandings of pregnancy and maternal risk to provide culturally relevant perinatal care to the rural-dwelling women in the Toledo district.

Throughout this chapter, relationships of power are present in the stories of birth attendants who negotiate their standing within a hierarchy of knowledge systems. Gender, as a performative role, is one such relationship of power that is agentively harnessed by Sergio and Lucia in order to effectively serve their communities. In 1978, Paul described how midwives among the *Zutuchil*-speaking Maya of southwestern Guatemala act in opposition to the patriarchal gender code: to do her job, she must be aggressive and overcome the intense shame that surrounds the female sexual organs. Paul rhetorically asks, "For what young man will court a girl who is to become a midwife?" (1978: 132). Nearly 30 years after Paul's research, female midwives in the Toledo district likewise encounter difficulties from men—and women—who do not approve of publicly unescorted women. Of the TBAs trained by GIFT, nearly all the women explained that they could not leave their homes in the middle of the night to attend a birth if their husband did not accompany them. There was even one TBA whose husband stopped her from finishing the training course because he refused to let her leave the house for extended periods of time. Other women, however, enjoy their mobility and, like Lucia, even appropriate the male role in the household by earning the money to feed the family through their TBA practices.

Discussions about female sexuality and reproductive practices—including female gender impropriety—were usually accompanied by references to shame. As such, male birth attendants, like Sergio, had to overcome gendered obstacles to effectively assist women during pregnancy and childbirth. In my analysis, I suggest that Sergio negotiated his position as a TBA by proving himself faithful to the community through health-related and religious service, by deviating from allegations of generic male laziness—often accompanied by accusations of drinking, and by aligning himself with a maternalist health care system and the older women in the community whose job is to teach the young husbands how to assist women through childbirth. Although he maintained certain cultural traditions—including some that were at odds with MOH recommendations, he distanced himself from certain birthing practices that he identified as "risky" according to the TBA training he received. Sergio was very active in providing prenatal care, but he remained underutilized as a birth attendant.

In my discussions with pregnant women, TBAs, and even Ministry personnel, fear emerged as a locally defined risk factor that often entered into the decision-making process of where and with whom to give birth. Nurse midwives often warned pregnant women of the purported risks involved in birthing at home. These risks are certainly grounded in the realities specific to the Toledo district such as access to transportation and distance to the nearest medical facility, but they are also constructed using internationally standardized statistical data concerning parity and blood pressure. Yet nurse midwives also routinely asked women if they were feeling "worried" about the delivery or "nervous" about their pregnancies or approaching births. Likewise, Lucia assessed the pregnant woman's level of fear as a determining factor in whether or not a birth could be managed outside of a hospital setting. Hence, Lucia expressed the need to assuage maternal fear, choosing to withhold information concerning a twinned pregnancy rather than explain the risks she has been trained to recognize. In her practice, Lucia appropriated her own biomedical authority in addition to local understandings of healing to avoid scaring the pregnant woman while increasing her own confidence as a fearless birth attendant.

Indeed, expressions of fear—or, more commonly, lack thereof—are used by TBAs to justify their behaviors, which at times are perceived as risky by the rural health nurse midwives who are to supervise their practices. While Sergio would not attend the deliveries of women who are classified according to medical standards as high-risk, he and Lucia emphasized that they are not afraid of certain conditions or procedures the MOH considers to be high risk. Lucia outright asserted, "Yo no tengo miedo de eso" [I am not afraid of that (official definitions of and protocols for high risk)]. Likewise, Sergio explained that even though some nurses will try to scare a TBA away from so-called risky procedures such as external version, he declared, "I no 'fraid for that." All expressed their own personal confidence in overriding the statistical signs of risk.

Despite Sergio's overall fearlessness, he does not agree with many of the birthing practices that take place in the homes of villagers that, since his training, he now identifies as risky. Sergio points out, "Maybe that's why they're not using me a lot because we do totally different." Ironically, it may be that Sergio's presence in the village serves to reinforce the contemporary cultural traditions that he finds so problematic. According to many of the recently trained TBAs who, like Sergio, are rarely called upon to deliver babies, villagers feel a level of security to continue their traditions knowing that trained assistance is nearby. Hence, TBA training may actually increase resistance to medical protocols and risk compliance when Lucia attends a birth or Sergio asserts his presence within the village. Women are not afraid to birth at home, because if there is a problem, at least there is someone to call.

References

Ceriani Cernadas, J., Carroli, G., Pellegrini, L., Otaño, L., Ferreira, M., Ricci, C., et al. (2006). The effect of timing of cord clamping on neonatal venous hematocrit values and clinical outcome at term: A randomized, controlled trial. *Pediatrics, 117*(4), e179–e786.

Cosminsky, S. (1972). *Decision making and medical care in a Guatemalan Indian community*. Ph.D. dissertation, Brandeis University, Waltham.

Cosminsky, S. (1982a). Knowledge and body concepts of Guatemalan midwives. In K. Artschwager (Ed.), *Anthropology of human birth* (pp. 233–252). Philadelphia: Davis Company.

Cosminsky, S. (1982b). Childbirth and change: A Guatemalan study. In C. MacCormack (Ed.), *Ethnography of fertility and birth* (pp. 205–229). New York: Academic.

Dickinson, O. (2008). The forgotten district. LVP.

Dowie, J. (1980). Bounds and biases. In C. Wooldridge, N. Draper, & T. Hunter (Eds.), *Risk and rationality* (pp. 99–156). Milton Keynes: The Open University.

Fabian, J. (1983). *Time and the other*. New York: Columbia University Press.

Glei, D., Goldman, N., & Rodríguez, G. (2003). Utilization of care during pregnancy in rural Guatemala: Does obstetrical need matter? *Social Science and Medicine, 57*(12), 2447–2463.

Greenberg, L. (1982). Midwife training programs in highland Guatemala. *Social Science and Medicine, 16*(18), 1599–1609.

Hinojosa, S. (1998). *Spiritual embodiment in a highland Maya community*. Ph.D. dissertation, Tulane University, New Orleans.

Knoema. (2016). *World data atlas*. Retrieved September 1, 2016, from knoema.com

Lang, J., & Elkin, E. (1997). A study of the beliefs and birthing practices of traditional midwives in rural Guatemala. *Journal of Nurse-Midwifery, 42*(1), 25–31.

Macpherson, A. (2003). Colonial matriarchs: Garveyism, maternalism, and Belize's black cross nurses, 1920–1952. *Gender and History, 15*(3), 507–527.

Oakley, A., & Houd, S. (1990). *Helpers in childbirth: Midwifery today*. New York: Hemisphere Publishing Corporation.

Paul, L. (1978). Careers of midwives in a Mayan community. In J. Hoch-Smith & A. Spring (Eds.), *Women in ritual and symbolic roles* (pp. 129–149). New York: Plenum Press.

Pinto, S. (2006). Divisions of labour: Rethinking the "midwife" in rural Uttar Pradesh. In J. Chawla (Ed.), *Birth and Birthgivers: The power behind the shame* (pp. 203–238). New Delhi: Shakti Books.

Tedlock, B. (1992). The role of dreams and visionary narratives in Mayan cultural survival. *Ethos, 20*(4), 453–476.

United Nations Children's Fund [UNICEF]. (2005). *Info by country*. Retrieved October 21, 2007, from http://www.unicef.org/infobycountry/latinamerica.html

WHO. (2000). *Core health indicators*. Geneva: World Health Organization.

Woolfrey, J. (2002). *Safe motherhood: A matter of life and death for women in Belize (An exploratory study on pregnancy related death, illness and disability in Belize: Its causes, and how to address them)*. Washington, DC: Pan American Health Organization.

Curse or Cure? The Phenomenon of *Obeah* Pregnancy Among Belizean Maya

23

Aminata Maraesa

23.1 Introduction

In the Maya villages of southern Belize, it is whispered that there are hills down which unwanted newborns are thrown. If found, the babies are dead and usually have been gnawed at by stray dogs—thankfully unrecognizable for the women who refuse their recognition. Rumors of these babies, and their actual discovery, circulate along with allegations of "*obeah*"—a supernatural force that is thought to cause a pregnancy-like state but without a human fetus; the *obeah* fetus is animal. Very often it is lamented that a woman who has been *obeahed* with a pregnancy will die unless she seeks counteractive spiritual assistance to rid her of the condition. However, it is also quietly discussed that *obeah* is responsible for unwanted pregnancies that result in [human] fetal or even newborn demise. This chapter looks closely at how women's reproductive behaviors that transgress ideal gender norms and sexual propriety may, at times, rely upon a discourse of supernatural power to deflect involvement with socially inadmissible reproductive activity. However, this form of avoiding social sanction may, nonetheless, result in maternal, fetal, or infant death.

23.2 The Place

Belize is a geographically small, English-speaking, multi-ethnic, postcolonial nation located in Central America, adjacent to Guatemala (Fig. 23.1), with an ideological commitment to providing universal healthcare to its population of just under 400,000. Similar to the rest of the country, the southernmost Toledo district comprises a heterogeneous population; however, the region differs significantly in terms of its ecological specificity, economic status, and particular ethnic composition—all of which play a role in women's reproductive health and behaviors (Fig. 23.2).

A. Maraesa, Ph.D.
Departments of Anthropology, NYU-School of Professional Studies
and Fordham University, New York, NY, USA
e-mail: amikole@sheabutter.net

D. A. Schwartz (ed.), *Maternal Death and Pregnancy-Related Morbidity Among Indigenous Women of Mexico and Central America*, Global Maternal and Child Health: Medical, Anthropological, and Public Health Perspectives, https://doi.org/10.1007/978-3-319-71538-4_23

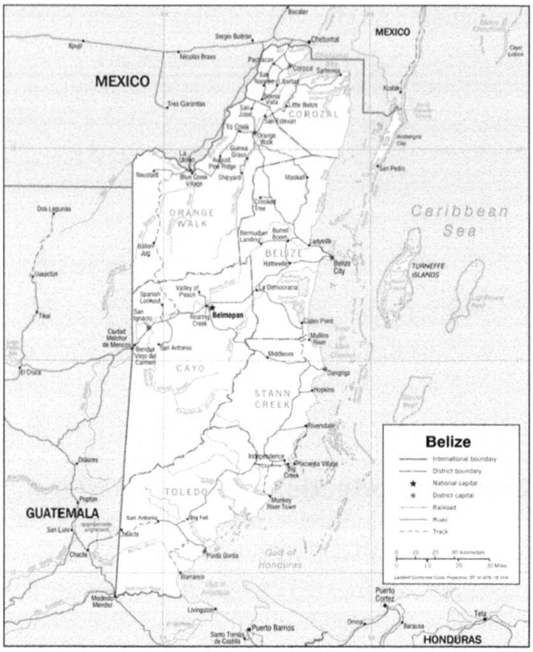

Fig. 23.1 Map of Belize and the Toledo District (Courtesy of Wikimedia Common Atlas of the World. Available from: https://commons.wikimedia.org/wiki/Atlas_of_Belize#/media/File:Belize_pol_03.jpg)

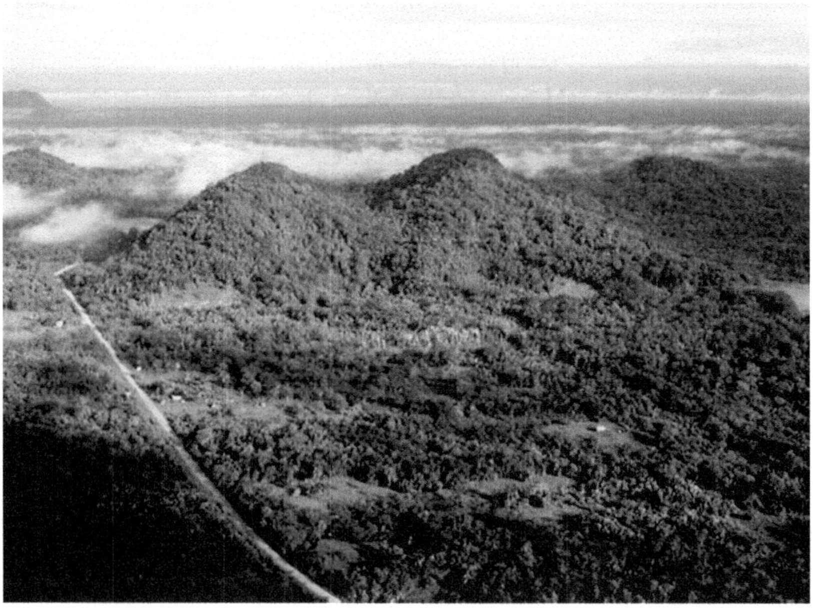

Fig. 23.2 Aerial view of the coastal lowland area of Toledo, approaching Punta Gorda by air. Published with kind permission of © Aminata Maraesa 2017. All Rights Reserved

The district's only urban center, the town of Punta Gorda, was initially settled in 1802 by the *Garifuna* people, an ethnic group boasting of a proud *Arawak* and never-enslaved African heritage who freely entered the shores of the now-named Toledo district by boat from Honduras (Avila and Avila 2008). They comprise the majority of the urban population where *Garifuna* cultural practices and language are prevalent. The *Garifuna* language is spoken by approximately 14,000 persons in Belize. It is an *Arawakan* language containing vocabulary from *Arawakan* and *Carib*, and to a lesser degree French and English. While the majority of *Garifuna* people are officially Catholic, they

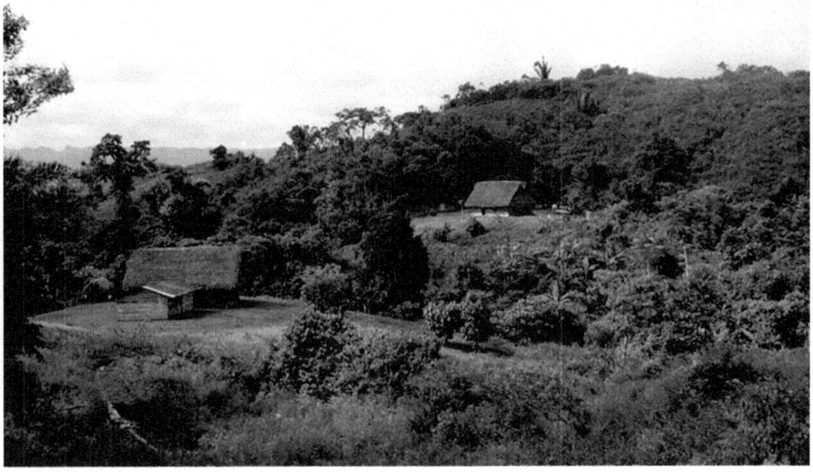

Fig. 23.3 Housing in Jalacte, a small community of *Kekchi* Maya farmers in the Toledo district of southern Belize, west of San Antonio village. Published with kind permission of © Aminata Maraesa 2017. All Rights Reserved

practice a type of syncretic Catholicism in which they incorporate traditional beliefs and rituals, and use a shaman (termed a *buyei*) to direct *Garifuna* religious practices. Comprising the majority of the district's rural areas are two linguistically distinct Maya groups, *Mopan* and *Kekchi*, both of which date their overland migration from Guatemala into what was then British Honduras in the late 1880s (Rambo 1962). The region is also populated by small percentages of Creoles (English speakers of African descent), Mestizos (Spanish-speakers of Guatemalan and Mexican origin), East Indians, Chinese, Mennonites of European descent (both Amish and proselytizing), other ethnic groups, and retirees from the United States of America (Figs. 23.3 and 23.4).

As a whole, Belize has a hot and humid climate, prone to heavy rains and hurricanes. Toledo, however, has the highest annual rainfall and is the most rural and underdeveloped region of the country; here, quotidian life is profoundly impacted by the environment. Imported supplies—like medical equipment—tend to degrade under these adverse conditions, rivers flood onto roads and bridges causing difficulties in both basic and emergency transportation, and infectious and parasitical diseases are easily spread. Far from taming the forces of nature, local ingenuity has developed a mode of existence accepting of life's precarious condition. Adversity, misfortune, and death are understood as factual and unavoidable circumstances, and Belizeans of all ethnic groups hold strong religious beliefs in a Christian God and the spirit world to which their fates are beholden—including their reproductive destinies. "Only God knows" is an oft-heard refrain when discussing the future or when specifically questioning how many children one "plans" to have.

Poverty is not the only determining factor in rapid population growth; however, multiple characteristics of poverty contribute to high fertility (Aassve et al. 2005; Birdsall and Griffin 1988; Central Statistics Office 2001b; Cameron 1997). Correspondingly, Toledo has the highest fertility in Belize with a total fertility rate of 5.6 among women aged 15–44, while the national average is markedly less at 3.65 (Central Statistical Office 2001a).[1] Indeed, Toledo is characterized as the poorest region of Belize, having 79% of the inhabitants classified as poor (defined as unable to meet basic food and

[1] The most recent national statistics available from 2011 to 2015 indicate the average total fertility rate to be 2.6 (World Bank 2014). District-specific statistics are not readily available.

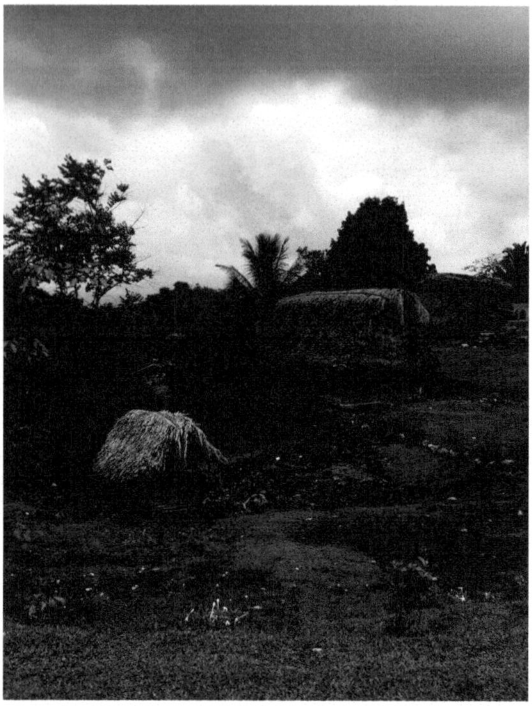

Fig. 23.4 Another view of rural housing in Jalacte, the last village on the border with Guatemala. Published with kind permission of © Aminata Maraesa 2017. All Rights Reserved

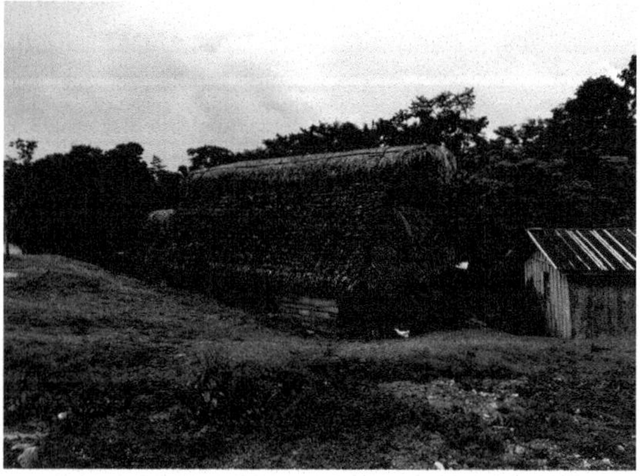

Fig. 23.5 Typical housing of the Belizean Maya in the area of Toledo. Published with kind permission of © Aminata Maraesa 2017. All Rights Reserved

nonfood costs) and 56.1% classified as indigent (defined as unable to meet basic food costs) (Central Statistics Office 2004; UNICEF 2005).[2] Unemployment rates in Toledo are likewise the highest in the country (Central Statistics Office 2004). Women's reproductive behaviors, including access to and use of healthcare services, susceptibility to unwanted and/or unplanned pregnancies, and their beliefs about fertility are undoubtedly influenced by environmental factors and poverty. I argue that they are also heavily conditioned by cultural norms and practices that include gendered constructs of propriety and a belief in spiritual practices that may, at times, be agentively—or unwittingly—harnessed to obscure reproductive misfortune (Fig. 23.5).

[2]The national averages are strikingly lower at 33.5% poor and only 10.8% indigent.

23.3 Beliefs About *Obeah* Pregnancy

In 2006, I conducted anthropological research that was focused on women's reproductive health and decision-making processes. I worked closely with nurse midwives from the Ministry of Health [MOH], traditional birth attendants [TBAs], and pregnant women to understand how cultural beliefs and practices influence reproductive health, mortality rates, and the implementation of development initiatives. A few months into my research I was introduced to the term "*obeah* pregnancy" by Petrona, a *Mopan* Maya woman who had been trained as a TBA to provide midwifery services for her rural community and with whom I had begun to work closely (see Maraesa 2012). Petrona, in her 40s, was unmarried and without children. Despite her lack of personal experience with childbirth, she was deemed an ideal candidate for TBA training since her lack of marital constraints would allow her freedom of movement to attend to the pregnant women in her village. One day as we chatted about childbirth, she digressed to describe this harrowing phenomenon: "For nine months, a lady belly get bigger and bigger. But there is no baby. Her belly get big because the man go to the bush doctor for *obeah* the lady. Maybe he get vexed because she no want to have sex with him, so the man mek the bush doctor *obeah* she. Then blood come out from between her legs and she dead."

Heretofore I had understood "bush doctors" to be healing practitioners who utilized plant-based medicine and prayer to treat various ailments of diverse origin, including maladies of pregnancy, but never had I heard that a bush doctor could *cause* a pregnancy—and a fatal one at that! This was also the first time I heard the word "*obeah*" used by a Maya to describe a type of supernatural magical practice commonly referred to by people of African descent. Indeed, *obeah* is a term widely employed throughout the English-speaking African diasporic communities of the Caribbean and the southern United States (Chambers 2009; Paton and Forde 2012) and appears only to surface among indigenous populations in Belize where they have been in close contact with diasporic Africans for hundreds of years (McClusky 2001).

Although historically and conventionally, *obeah* (and its practitioners) has been associated with counter-hegemonic activities like slave rebellions while concomitantly typified as a superstitious cultural practice that is inferior to scientific European rationality (Earle 2005; Bell 1893; Richardson 1997), a number of *obeah*-practicing Maya bush doctors have been incorporated into the world of rational biomedical care as "certified nurse's aides" [CNA] by the MOH's public health outreach campaigns (Belize Ministry of Health 1987: 21). Primary healthcare is based on community participation (World Health Organization 1978), and the integration of individuals like bush doctors, who are already positioned as community-based healthcare providers, is a local adaptation to this international objective. Arguably, the local attraction to bush doctors-cum-MOH service providers is their ability to span both worlds.

Included in a bush doctor's healing repertoire are certain skills that fall under the domain of midwifery—most notably, *hile'ek*, a form of uterine massage that is accompanied by prayer to ascertain and remedy fetal malpresentation.[3] *Hile'ek* may be conducted throughout the pregnancy, but a bush doctor may also be called during labor to perform *hile'ek* if the laboring woman experiences pain or if the labor is not progressing normally. At times, the bush doctor may determine that the laboring woman is experiencing difficulties because she has been "*obeahed*," and the bush doctor will perform additional spiritual healing practices to counter the negative spell, thus enabling a successful delivery (Fig. 23.6).

[3] *Hile'ek* is in the Kekchi language, but Mopan Maya also refer to uterine massage as *hile'ek*. In the Belizean Creole it is called '*nointing*.

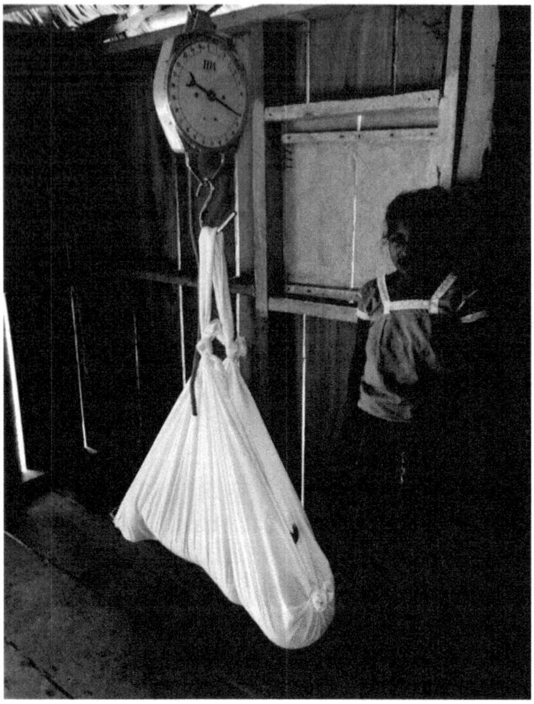

Fig. 23.6 A baby inside a *lepob* suspended from a scale at a well-child mobile clinic visit. Published with kind permission of © Aminata Maraesa 2017. All Rights Reserved

23.4 Encounters with *Obeah* Pregnancy

On the day Petrona opened my anthropological world to *obeah*, we made plans to talk again later that week. This second conversation, however, was postponed by her hospitalization. Unbeknownst to me—or to anyone, Petrona had been 9 months pregnant. She went into labor that very evening but suffered from placenta previa (note: an abnormal implantation of the placenta where it extends across the opening of the cervix in the lower uterus). When the low-lying placenta detached, she began to hemorrhage, causing massive bleeding and fetal demise. When her brother found Petrona the next morning, he rushed her to the hospital where she underwent an emergency cesarean section (Fig. 23.7).

Four weeks later I saw Petrona when she was in town to have her stitches removed, and we met at a café while she waited for her village bus. We made awkward small talk until I finally asked about her pregnancy-related hospitalization, whereupon she denied all knowledge of the pregnancy because she had continued to menstruate and adamantly claimed (without my asking) never to have had sex—ever. Petrona then exclaimed, "It was *obeah*!" Henceforth we walked in uncomfortable silence toward the bus until she made a stop at a public latrine. A few minutes after entering the bathroom, Petrona called for me: raising her skirt, she nervously asked what I saw. Fresh blood was seeping from the bandages around her abdomen. I quickly called for a taxi to take her back to the hospital where she was resutured and readmitted until her body was fully recovered from the cesarean delivery.

For the remainder of my fieldwork tenure, Petrona and I maintained a professional relationship; yet, the topic of her reproductive experience remained an unspoken albatross. Indeed, Petrona undeniably had an emergency surgery to remove a dead human-shaped fetus from her womb, yet she continued to proclaim (and believe?) that her pregnancy was the result of *obeah*—not out-of-wedlock sexual intercourse. However, once my ears were open to this phenomenon I encountered other stories of women who had survived an *obeah* pregnancy but were not innocent to sex, nor were their births of human form. Treena, a Creole woman, 17 years old at the time, was having sex with a 34-year-old

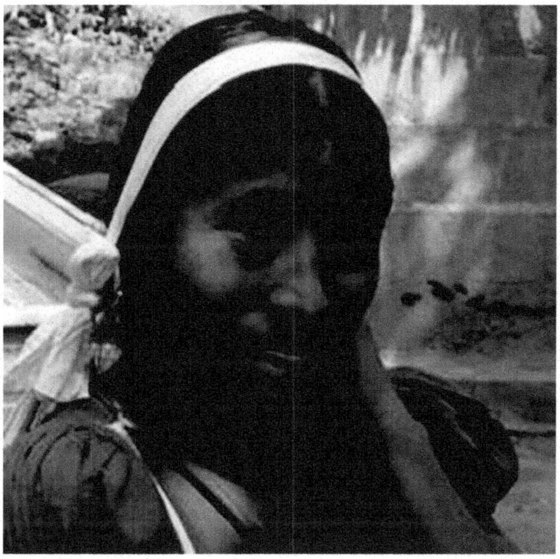

Fig. 23.7 Felicia, a *Kekchi* Maya women carrying her baby in a *lepob* suspended from her forehead. Published with kind permission of © Aminata Maraesa 2017. All Rights Reserved

married man. His wife threatened Treena by saying that if she got pregnant, "it [the pregnancy] will give you a lot of trouble because you messed with my husband knowing he was married!" The wife then went to a bush doctor who *obeahed* the teenage girl to become pregnant with a stingray. According to Treena, the obstetrical ultrasound even confirmed that a stingray was inside her womb, and the nursing staff said they could not help with situation. When she began to experience intense abdominal pain, Treena sought the help of a bush doctor who gave her bush medicine and recited prayers to counter the initial *obeah* of the angered wife's bush doctor. This brought on the labor, and Treena gave birth to the stingray. According to the bush doctor who recounted this story, if Treena had not sought spiritual help, she would have stayed pregnant with the stingray past 9 months and eventually would have died.

Then there was the story told to me by one of the MOH's top nurse midwives who denied the phenomenon of *obeah* pregnancy—"except for one case, which was my grandmother. Her belly mi swell, swell and you could even see a wiggling under her skin. When she was dying she said to us that something di come out from inside of her. Then a rat come out of her and fluid pour out. Then she take her last breath and she dead. They say that dah *obeah,* but I no know. Maybe."[4] Nurse Ical explained how an *obeah* pregnancy could be a case of fibroid tumors that distend the abdomen as they grow (note: benign tumors of smooth muscle origin that develop in the uterus, also termed leiomyomas). Often by the time a woman seeks medical assistance to check the "pregnancy," the fibroid is too large to treat without a total hysterectomy, an operation that usually cannot be performed due to a combination of distance to the medical facility, cultural miscommunication, and finances. Untreated fibroids may result in complications, including obstetrical hemorrhage, that affect the health of the "pregnant" woman. This then would "confirm" the power of the *obeah*. According to Nurse Ical, fibroid tumors account for some of the "*obeah* deaths" of women in southern Belize. His grandmother's "rat" could also have been a hydatidiform mole, or molar pregnancy, a chromosomally abnormal pregnancy that grows in place of the placenta that can be removed through dilation and curettage.[5] However, in

[4]Regarding her research in the Toledo district among the *Mopan* Maya population, McClusky asserts that "Maya frequently use 'maybe' even if they are certain. In fact, it sometimes signals great certainty, but an uncomfortable topic. Maya also use it to express what someone else thinks" (2001: 278).

[5]In the United States and Europe, hydatidiform moles occur in approximately 1 pregnancy out of 1000. Symptoms of this condition include rapid growth in the size of the uterus with no fetal heart tone (American Cancer Society 2016).

southern Belize, where women often do not seek prenatal care until the second or third trimester, a molar pregnancy usually self-terminates in a spontaneous first trimester abortion. The passing of unidentifiable tissue without acknowledging the possibility of a "true" pregnancy may also validate the compelling power of *obeah*.

23.5 Community of Silence

In southern Belize, belief in the supernatural thus joins biomedical explanation to become part of the profoundly mundane "ways of knowing the world" (Khan 2004: 103). And as I made further inquiries into the different forms that *obeah* pregnancies could manifest, I was told they included a range of animals from small rodents like Nurse Ical's rat to aquatic animals such as Treena's stingray. So varied were the manifestations that the only consistency was a non-human form (see Sobo 1993 for a similar belief system in Jamaica). So what of human-like *obeah* pregnancies like Petrona's? Could women allege *obeah* to cover up their reproductive improprieties? Or could others assert *obeah* to cover improprietous actions toward women that occurred under their watch?

In the summer of 2011, I returned to southern Belize to find out more about *obeah* pregnancy. A woman who self-identified as *Kekchifuna* [ethnically mixed *Kekchi* Maya and *Garifuna*] told me the story of her neighbor, Leila, a 14-year-old *Kekchi* Maya girl who lived in the section of town known as Indianville. First populated by rural dwelling *Kekchi* and *Mopan* Maya families who were to temporarily relocate to town so their children could attend high school, many of these residents stayed on to create a pocket of rurality within the urban *Garifuna* landscape. It was here that Leila resided in her two-room home with her parents, her newly married sister, and the sister's husband. A few months after sharing sleeping quarters with her brother-in-law, Leila's stomach began to grow. Her parents told the neighbors that they believed her daughter had been *obeahed* with a "pregnancy" due to jealousies regarding the family's business. Their store was gaining in prosperity once the new husband had moved in to work full-time. The neighbors, however, were suspicious about the concurrence and questioned whether Leila's growing belly was the result of *obeah* or incest.

Although I left Belize before this situation was resolved, I stayed in communication with Leila's neighbor who told me a few months later that Leila's "big belly" was gone, but there was no new baby at the house. What happened to Leila cannot be known for sure, as no official investigation was ever made, and the parents continued to seek help only from bush doctors. Proclaiming an *obeah* causation for their daughter's distended abdomen, Leila never engaged prenatal care services or went to a hospital for treatment. Her family and neighbors preferred to turn a blind eye and tacitly agree with the presence of *obeah* in the girl's womb rather than call attention to other social problems like allegations of incest or a teen pregnancy.[6]

[6]It is widely acknowledged that incest is a social problem that often goes unreported or unpunished (Di Capua 2006). So widespread is this recognized social problem that it was even the subject of an instructional comic book entitled *D(B) addy* published in 2003 by a local nongovernmental organization. The first of the five stories included in the book is entitled "Family Affair" which begins with the story of a young girl raped by her step-father who proclaims, "I am the king of all I survey!" After the forced sexual intercourse, he reasserts his patriarchal authority with the rhetorical question, "Who your daddy now?" (Youth Empowerment Services 2003: 2–4). Indeed, there was a cultural understanding prevalent among the many men that I spoke to in the Toledo district that they had a patriarchal right to marital (including common-law) property, which explains and may even justify—or allow them to "turn a blind eye" to—father/daughter incest. And boisterous allegations of sexual encounters between these relations were often made by women in the community when discussing clandestine out-of-wedlock pregnancies, some of which were terminated through illegal abortion or the pregnant woman's death.

Throughout my fieldwork in 2006, I worked closely with the rural health nurses who provided prenatal care at a village health post. Arriving to the clinic one morning I found Ana, a 15-year-old *Mopan* Maya girl, in active labor. Ana had showed up to the clinic that morning complaining of a stomachache. When she was told she was pregnant, Ana denied any knowledge of it and incredulously asked how she could be pregnant if she never had sex. Upon birthing a baby girl, Ana left the clinic—and her baby—never to return. Her daughter was subsequently adopted.

Filomena, the TBA living in Ana's village, was actively engaged with her community's reproductive needs by providing rudimentary prenatal care for the pregnant women in her village and attending home births, the most recent of which was for Ana's mother. Throughout her twelfth pregnancy, Ana's mother had received in-home prenatal services from Filomena—at the same time that Ana was living in the house and hiding her own pregnancy. While I reasoned that Filomena should have recognized Ana's pregnancy, offered prenatal care, and spoken to her about attending the prenatal clinic, Filomena's response to my inquiry emphasized the cultural logic of a community of silence: "Yeah, I mi know she pregnant. I see she belly. But she no ask me nothing. So I no say nothing."

Like the *obeah*-practicing bush doctors who are also members of the public health team, the position of TBAs vis-à-vis socially problematic reproductive states, rumored infanticide, and *obeah* pregnancy is emblematic of the pervasiveness of cultural knowledge and practices that defy healthcare initiatives, yet that "make sense" at the local level and that of the individual. Indeed, the discretion with which Filomena answered my impudent inquiry impressed upon me the extent to which the tangible realities of everyday life in southern Belize are shaped by the invisible cultural walls that uphold the social world. These walls are extra thick when it comes to the public discussion of women's reproduction. As such, Filomena could not introduce any discussion of prenatal care until Ana disclosed her pregnancy. Because Ana chose to conceal her pregnancy, the presence of a TBA in the village did nothing to influence the outcome of her pregnancy—except maybe to prompt her to seek more anonymous care outside of her village when she went into labor.

Ana was familiar with Filomena and the midwifery services she provided—Filomena had previously delivered Ana's mother's baby. However, Ana looked for childbirth assistance outside of her community. By going to the rural health center located 10 miles from her village to birth her baby, Ana ensured that she could return to her community with no evidence of ever having been pregnant. Although her "secret" was a façade (if Filomena knew it can be assumed that others in her community were aware of her pregnancy—especially her own mother), Ana was able to effectively guard her private affairs by disposing of the baby outside of the community.

While Ana's baby was safely delivered into the world, other babies are not. Four years after I witnessed Ana's birth, I talked to Antonia, a *Kekchi* TBA living in a village 35 miles from Punta Gorda town, about clandestine births in her village and possible allegations of *obeah*. Was it coincidence, or was it pervasive practice, that only a week ago she saw a newborn baby hanging from the mouth of a stray dog as it walked through the village streets? Harrowingly similar to Tsing's "monster stories" (1990) about "bad mothers" in the United States who leave their newborns floating in toilets or bathtubs, Antonia's neighbor appears to have left her baby in the yard where it was picked up by the dog. However, unlike Tsing's mothers who were prosecuted for perinatal endangerment, Antonia's neighbor was never investigated. Even after village officials traced a trail of blood to the neighbor's back door, the explanation she offered: "That not a baby" suggests that what was later determined to be a premature stillbirth could have been the real "monster" in the eyes of the mother who was rumored to be having an affair with a married man.

Conclusion

While Petrona's training as a TBA should have alerted her to (1) her pregnancy and (2) the symptoms of placenta previa that include vaginal bleeding for which she should have sought out medical attention, she could have been trying to convince herself that she was spontaneously aborting. Maybe she was even taking an abortifacient when she went into labor and perceived that she was completing the induced abortion. Or maybe Petrona was trying to give birth clandestinely with the intention of absolving her shame through one final act of denial: leaving the baby in the bush for dead. In a culture where adulterous jealousies, gendered sexual impropriety, or incestuous relations spawn fetuses construed as rats or stingrays, masking the products of an unwanted pregnancy under the guise of *obeah* may be a way for women—and the larger social world—to conceal reproductive practices that, despite their ubiquity, carry a greater stigma and shame if openly acknowledged.

Throughout this chapter I have argued that *obeah*, dominantly portrayed as a counter-hegemonic force, can be agentively commanded by women to uphold normative representations of female sexuality and reproduction while engaging in illicit or immoral sexual activity—as agent or victim. In southern Belize, where women's reproductive behavior is highly scrutinized, *obeah* discourse may be a way to help conceal reproductive impropriety. Whether one believes in the power of *obeah* or accepts the cultural conditioning that tacitly sanctions problematic sexual encounters, social recognition of *obeah* pregnancy influences women's reproductive decisions—some of which may end in their own death, or that of their babies, when this belief results in clandestine perinatal behaviors.

References

Aassve, A., Engelhardt, H., Francavilla, F., Kedir, A., Kim, J., Mealli, F., et al. (2005). *Poverty and fertility in less developed countries: A comparative analysis*. ISER Working Paper 2005–2013. Colchester: University of Essex. Retrieved from https://www.iser.essex.ac.uk/files/iser_working_papers/2005-13.pdf

American Cancer Society. (2016). *What are the key statistics for gestational trophoblastic disease?* Retrieved September 4, 2016, from http://www.cancer.org/cancer/gestationaltrophoblasticdisease/detailedguide/gestational-trophoblastic-disease-key-statistics

Avila, T., & Avila, J. (2008). *Garifuna world*. Providence, RI: Milenio Associates.

Belize Ministry of Health. (1987). *The Belize national primary health care manual*. Photocopied document obtained from the files at the Punta Gorda Town Hospital.

Bell, H. (1893). *Obeah: Witchcraft in the West Indies*. London: Sampson Low, Marston & Co..

Birdsall, N., & Griffin, C. (1988). Fertility and poverty in developing countries. *Journal of Policy Modeling, 10*(1), 29–55.

Cameron, S. (1997). *From girls to women: Growing up healthy in Belize*. Belize City: Government of Belize.

Central Statistical Office. (2001a). Belize family health survey: Females. Belize.

Central Statistical Office. (2001b). Abstract of statistics for Belize: 2000–2001. Belize.

Central Statistical Office. (2004). *Environmental statistics for Belize: 2004*. Belmopan, Belize: Ministry of National Development.

Chambers, D. (2009). *Murder in Montpelier: Igbo Africans in Virginia*. Jackson: University Press of Mississippi.

Di Capua, A. (2006). *Child sexual abuse in Belize 2002–2005: An analysis of the criminal justice response*. Belize: National Committee for Families and Children.

Earle, W. (2005). In S. Aravamudan (Ed.), *Obi; or, the history of three-fingered Jack*. Peterborough: Broadview Press.

Khan, A. (2004). *Callaloo nation: Metaphors of race and religious identity among south Asians in Trinidad*. Durham, NC: Duke University Press.

Maraesa, A. (2012). Saving face, losing life: Obeah pregnancy and reproductive impropriety in southern Belize. *Culture, Health and Sexuality: An International Journal for Research, Intervention and Care, 14*(Supp 1), S95–108. https://doi.org/10.1080/13691058.2011.626075

McClusky, L. (2001). *"Here, our culture is hard": Stories of domestic violence from a Mayan community in Belize*. Austin: University of Texas Press.

Paton, D., & Forde, M. (Eds.). (2012). *Obeah and other powers: The politics of Caribbean religion and healing*. Durham: Duke University Press.

Rambo, A. (1962). The Kekchi indians of British Honduras: An ethnographic study. *Katunob, 3*(3), 40–48.

Richardson, A. (1997). Romantic voodoo: Obeah and British culture, 1797–1807. In M. Fernández Olmos & L. Paravisini-Gebert (Eds.), *Sacred possessions: Vodou, santería, obeah, and the Caribbean* (pp. 171–194). New Brunswick, NJ: Rutgers University Press.

Sobo, E. (1993). *One blood: The Jamaican body*. New York: SUNY Press.

Tsing, A. L. (1990). Monster stories: Women charged with perinatal endangerment. In F. Ginsburg & A. L. Tsing (Eds.), *Uncertain terms: Negotiating gender in American culture* (pp. 282–299). Boston: Beacon Press.

United Nations Children's Fund. (2005). *The Belizean child: A situation analysis of children and adolescents in Belize, 2004*. Belize: Cubola.

World Bank. (2014). *Fertility rate, total (births per woman)*. Retrieved October 30, 2016, from http://data.worldbank.org/indicator/SP.DYN.TFRT.IN

World Health Organization. (1978). *Declaration of Alma Ata*. Retrieved November 1, 2016, from http://www.euro.who.int/en/publications/policy-documents/declaration-of-alma-ata,-1978

Youth Empowerment Services. (2003). *Torn pages: D(B)addy—5 stories of sexual abuse and exploitation*. Belize City: YES.

Part V

Guatemala

24 Childbirth as a Lens of Medicalization on a Guatemalan Plantation

Sheila Cosminsky

24.1 Introduction: Change and Continuity in Traditional Midwifery and Biomedicine

Based on a study of midwifery and childbirth beliefs and practices in Guatemala, I will discuss some of the continuity and change that have occurred over a period of 40 years. These include midwives' incorporation of biomedical practices, sometimes adding them to their own practices, substituting them, and at other times resisting or even rejecting them (Cosminsky 2016). Most studies have focused on the changes or resistance to such changes in the local ethnomedical system, both voluntary and imposed (Berry 2010; Cosminsky 1994; Hinojosa 2004, 2015; Rogoff 2011). During this period, the biomedical system has also been changing, as a result of which new scientific information and improvements in clinical medical practices and treatment becomes available. However, when biomedical practices are presented in the government midwifery training programs, they are presented as an absolute. Both outdated and newer biomedical practices are presented as the only proper, safest, or best alternative, often not acknowledging or unaware that these have actually changed and progressed. In some cases, midwives are practicing what they had been taught in earlier training programs, only to be now criticized and told to do something else, with the current biomedical personnel unaware that the midwives had already changed due to the pressure from previous medical personnel. In other cases, the newer biomedical practices are similar to the traditional or ethno-obstetric ones that the midwives or mothers actually practice, but the biomedical personnel are unaware of this.

The purpose of this chapter is to analyze the problems of change through a series of examples of beliefs and practices of traditional midwives and mothers that have changed, been modified, or persisted over a 40-year period of research during which time biomedical thoughts and practices have also changed. These observations were conducted on a *finca* (a ranch, plantation or country estate) in Guatemala and in the highland *aldeas* (hamlets) of Chuchexic and El Novillero of Santa Lucia Utatlán. The Guatemalan biomedical practitioners (those that I encountered in the training sessions or health

S. Cosminsky, Ph.D.
Department of Sociology, Anthropology, and Criminal Justice, Rutgers University, Camden, NJ, USA
e-mail: Cosminsk@rutgers.edu

D. A. Schwartz (ed.), *Maternal Death and Pregnancy-Related Morbidity Among Indigenous Women of Mexico and Central America*, Global Maternal and Child Health: Medical, Anthropological, and Public Health Perspectives, https://doi.org/10.1007/978-3-319-71538-4_24

facilities or were told about by either midwives or mothers) either were not aware of the changes that had taken place within the larger biomedical community, and in the case of some practices do not acknowledge that the practice has changed, or they were unaware that midwifery practices had changed. In other cases, they did not acknowledge that the practices carried out by the midwives were the ones that were currently being recommended by the larger biomedical community—e.g., semivertical delivery position, and breastfeeding on demand.

Although biomedicine is constantly changing as new information and evidence becomes available, it is often presented as an absolute and unchanging truth in the training programs. Similarly, although midwives in Guatemala have been shown to change and incorporate aspects of biomedicine while rejecting others, biomedicine often portrays them as static, with midwives stubbornly continuing their practices in the face of "modern" medicine, and sometimes blaming the midwives' old age, illiteracy, or their traditional culture. They blame the midwives for the continuing high rates of maternal and infant morbidity and mortality, without due consideration of the underlying structural factors involved in persistent poverty, discrimination, government corruption, and problems in the public health system (Cosminsky 2012).

24.2 Shifting Policies of the World Health Organization

In addition to changes occurring in biomedical practices, the World Health Organization (WHO) has shifted their policy concerning traditional birth attendants (TBAs) during this time, with pressure placed on member governments, including Guatemala, and nongovernmental organizations (NGOs) to follow its latest policy. In the 1960s and 1970s, WHO promoted a policy of utilizing or incorporating traditional healers, including midwives, to promote primary health care with the goal of Health to All by the Year 2000. These programs included training both community health workers and midwives. The aim of the latter was to "upgrade" their practice to reduce maternal and infant mortality. However, in the 1980s and 1990s, WHO shifted their policy based on their conclusion that maternal mortality had not declined sufficiently, and blamed this lack of success on the traditional midwives. The training programs then emphasized teaching "risk factors," and midwives were to refer mothers who possessed such "risk factors" to the hospital and not attend these deliveries themselves. Such "risk" factors include: first time mothers (primaparas), teenage mothers, women over 35 years of age, those who had undergone previous cesarean section deliveries, signs of preeclampsia, a malpositioned fetus (breech, transverse, etc.), bleeding, and a "long" labor. These exclusionary factors severely limited not only the midwife's clientele but also her livelihood.

WHO policy shifted again around 2000 at the time of the Millennium Development Goals (MDGs) which had been set at the 2000 Millennium Summit in New York. They concluded that maternal mortality rates still had not declined sufficiently with the emphasis on risk factors, and the blame was again placed on the traditional midwives. The emphasis was then placed on "emergency obstetrics," termed EmOC (Emergency Obstetric Care). A pregnant woman, together with the midwife and her family, had to prepare an "emergency" plan. Such a plan included recognizing these risk signs, but also saving money for transportation, arranging for transportation to the hospital in case of an obstetric emergency (which included prolonged labor and complications such as retained placenta and hemorrhaging), and arranging who would take care of her other children if she had any. The emphasis was again placed on midwives, who were instructed to refer mothers to the hospital (Berry 2010). WHO has again shifted policy, since the emphasis on "emergency obstetrics" did not produce the desired results of sufficient decline in maternal mortality. The emphasis now is on delivery by "skilled attendants." According to WHO, a traditional birth attendant cannot be a "skilled attendant"—i.e., one trained in some degree of biomedical obstetrics (WHO 2004).

The current WHO policy is the eventual replacement of *comadronas* or traditional midwives on the assumption that the maternal mortality goals (Target 5.A) of the Millenial Development Goals were not met because of these midwives. The rationale given for the need to replace the midwives' practice is that it is biomedical practice that is lifesaving, and the midwives' practices are harmful or risky, thus increasing the likelihood of morbidity or mortality (Highland Support Project Blog 2016). New training programs are emphasizing the training of young, literate women who act primarily as referral agents for hospital deliveries (Maupin 2008) rather than the older, highly experienced and locally respected midwives, who are assigned the fault for persistently high maternal mortality rates.

Despite WHO's policy, the Guatemalan government has continued to support training programs for both old and new midwives (Berry 2010; Cosminsky 2016), through the Ministry of Health and through many NGOs.

24.3 Methods

This chapter is based on ethnographic fieldwork carried out intermittently over a period of more than 40 years. Between 1968 and 1979, and then in 1996, I interviewed and observed three *K'iche'* Maya midwives and one *Ladina* midwife in the hamlets (*aldeas*) of Novillero and Chuchexic of the town of Santa Lucia Utatlán as part of an investigation of decision-making and health care. In 1970, a team of physicians from the United States carried out surveys and interviews on a coffee and sugar plantation (*finca*) as part of a training course in nutrition sponsored by INCAP (Institute of Nutrition of Central America and Panama) and MIT (Massachusetts Institute of Technology) under the supervision of Dr. Nevin Scrimshaw. I had access to these unpublished studies, which provided important baseline data. I made several visits between 1974 and 2013 to this plantation where a midwife (*comadrona*), Doña Maria, and her daughter, Doña Siriaca, lived. The latter carried on Maria's practice in her later years and after her death. I also interviewed and observed two other midwives who occasionally attended births on the *finca*. Training and review sessions for the midwives carried out by the Ministry of Health in Retalhuleu or neighboring towns were observed. I trace the changes in biomedicine as presented in review classes in health centers, the hospital, and from interviews with the midwives. In addition, most of the mothers on the *finca* were interviewed at various times during the 40-year period, including gathering reproductive histories. I also carried out interviews and observations of other healers including shamans or daykeepers (K'iche': *ajq'ijab*), spiritists, bone-setters and herbalists (Cosminsky 2012, 2016) in both field locations.

I also collected specimens of medicinal plants and herbs. These were identified by Dr. Lorin I. Nevling of the Field Museum of Chicago.

24.4 Setting, Ethnomedical Concepts

Ethnographic fieldwork was carried out in the hamlets of Novillero and Chuchexic of Santa Lucia Utatlán, which are in the Department of Solola and located at about 8000 ft altitude in the western highlands of Guatemala. The population is primarily *K'iche'* Maya. The nearest hospitals are in Solola and Quetzaltenango, each at least 1 h away by road. A Catholic mission-run clinic in Novillero has provided basic health care services since the 1960s, and at least until 2000 it was also providing health promoter and midwifery training programs. A public health clinic is in the Santa Lucia town center. Ninety-seven percent of the births in Santa Lucia Utatlán are still assisted by *comadronas* (Guatemala 2005).

Houses are primarily made of adobe with tile or tin roofs and dirt floors, although some poorer ones have wattle and daub walls with thatched roofs. Until the mid-1990s people had no electricity or running water, and there were very few latrines. Residents have small plots of corn and beans (*milpa*), and many migrated seasonally to coastal plantations. Since the 1980s, when the political violence targeted the area, migration to the United States increased and housing conditions have improved from the remittances sent back from the migrant workers.

The plantation, Finca San Luis, lies in the *boca costa*, in the Department of Retalhuleu, with an altitude ranging from sea level to approximately 1500 ft. The area is 12.5 *caballerias* or 1384 acres. The main crops were sugar and coffee, and some land was devoted to pasture for the dairy cattle that were being raised. The resident population is of mixed Maya and *Ladino* descent. The Maya are mainly third and fourth generation descendants of migrants who came from various parts of the highlands. Status differences exist according to ethnicity in that most of the salaried workers, such as the administrator, office manager and chauffeur are Ladino and live in better housing than the field workers. In 1976 there were 610 people living in 130 houses, whereas in 2010, 310 were living in 45 houses. This decline in population is due to the *finca* owner eliminating almost all full-time workers or *colonos,* and using temporary or day laborers from both on and off the plantation. Workers are given small plots of land to grow their own corn and beans. Housing is poor and overcrowded—most are constructed of wood boards for walls, a corrugated metal roof, and a dirt floor. Latrines are virtually nonexistent. Defecation occurs in the fields, woods, or nearby stream, contributing to poor environmental sanitation and risk for gastrointestinal infections. As *colonos* retired or died, the house would be knocked down and the younger members would move if they previously had not already left the plantation. Another factor affecting the population size is the *finquero* (finca owner) stopped growing coffee in 2003. During the coffee boom in the mid-1800s until around 2000, this land was prized for its coffee and sugar. However, the demand for coffee has recently shifted to higher quality coffee grown at higher altitudes. In addition, the world market price of coffee dropped because of expansion of coffee grown in Southeast Asia. Since women's main source of income was picking coffee, this change has had a significant impact on their access to cash. The women are more dependent on men, yet are still responsible for the health and nutrition of their children.

Most *finca* mothers give birth in the home attended by a local *comadrona.* The nearest hospital to which people will go for births and emergencies is the National Hospital in Retalhuleu.

24.4.1 Hot–Cold Balance

One of the primary conceptual principles of the traditional Maya ethnomedical system is that of the humoral balance of the body, involving the hot–cold principle. The body is made up of substances that have qualities that vary along a hot–cold continuum, and normally should exist in balance. Too much of a quality can cause illness. When a woman is pregnant, she is in a hot condition, resulting from the accumulated blood in her body, and because she doesn't get her period. Thus, a pregnant mother must be careful to avoid hot foods, such as chili peppers.

After the birth, she is in a cold state, because of losing blood and expelling the placenta and the baby. The mother must restore the balance after delivery by eating and drinking substances classified as hot and by taking hot baths. She is regarded as vulnerable to cold states and illnesses, and must keep covered, drink hot teas, etc. Similarly, the baby is in a cold state and susceptible to cold illnesses, and thus must be well covered, usually with a cap and swaddled in several layers of cloth.

Although bodily balance is restored by intake or application of substances opposite of one's body quality, too great a contrast can also cause illness, such as getting caught in the rain while sweating and being overheated from working.

24.4.2 Emotional Balance

A healthy body is an emotionally balanced one, and strong emotions can cause illness. Emotional states are also linked to the humors—anger is considered a hot emotion, and fright is a cold one. A pregnant woman and new mother should avoid strong emotions, such as anger, fright *(susto)*, nerves (*nervios*), and sadness as they can cause a variety of unwanted complications including miscarriage, premature labor, retained placenta, a cold, insufficient breast milk, or an ill baby. Such illnesses have been called "idioms of distress" (Nichter 1981) in the anthropological literature, to express somatically the moral outrage associated with violation of norms, and expressing one's powerlessness. The term "*nervios*" is increasingly being used on the *finca* to express anxiety and high blood pressure (*presion)*. One woman has been repeatedly diagnosed as having high blood pressure and *nervios*, the latter causing the former and related to anxiety, and is being prescribed injections for her nerves. Physicians, pharmacists, and patients are confusingly using high blood pressure and nerves as synonymous.

24.5 Prenatal Care

24.5.1 Prenatal Visits

WHO (2016) has just released new guidelines for prenatal care in which it sets eight prenatal visits as the recommended goal. The previously recommended number was four visits. Although these recommendations may be considered as ideal for maximum positive results, and may be available in developed countries for some groups, they are unrealistic in many less-developed societies. In Guatemala, in more rural and/or indigenous groups, prenatal visits to a biomedical clinic, health center, or hospital usually occur once or twice during the pregnancy. The reason is to obtain a tetanus vaccination and vitamins, as well as to check the position and condition of the fetus. According to 2012 statistics, 85% of pregnant women received a neonatal tetanus vaccine and 93% of women had at least one visit for prenatal care (UNICEF 2015). On the other hand, the traditional midwife usually does visit the mother once a month or more frequently during the last month, to examine the progression of the pregnancy, the position of the fetus, the health of the mother, and to perform traditional massage on the mother. Given accessibility issues of cost and lack of transportation, work, child care, and lack of health care facilities, the current WHO recommendation is highly unrealistic for much of Guatemala. In fact, it leads one to argue for the necessity of utilizing the (wo)manpower provided by the midwife and to increase her training in a more effective and efficient manner.

24.5.2 Massage

Massage is an integral part of every phase of the birth process, from prenatal to postnatal. It also serves several purposes. During the prenatal exam, the midwife massages and palpates the abdominal area and measures the height of the fundus, tracks the growth and development of the fetus, and the position (lie) of the fetus. The biomedical personnel are particularly concerned that the midwife not perform external version, and at least some of them seem to assume that the prenatal massage entails this maneuver. The midwife rubs some oil on her hands and warms them over the fire before massaging the woman. She says that the oil helps her hands go over the body easier, and also soothes the woman. In 2013, Siriaca said that the doctor has told her she should not warm her hands before massaging the woman because then when she washes her hands after the massage in cold

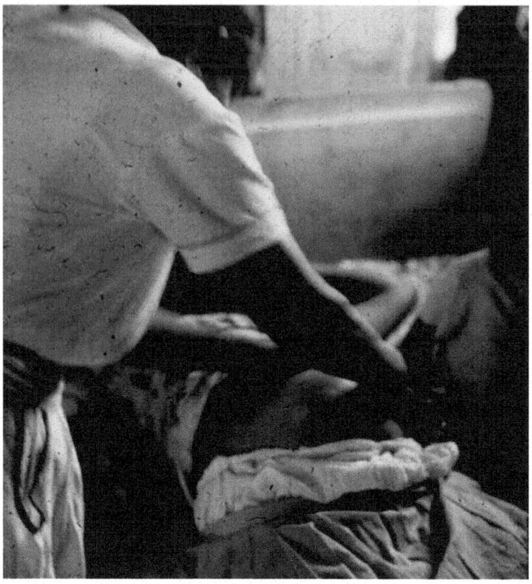

Fig. 24.1 Maria examining and massaging pregnant woman (1974)

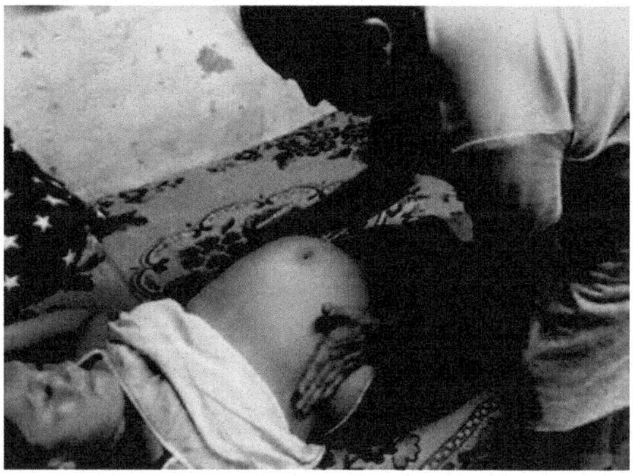

Fig. 24.2 Siriaca examining and massaging pregnant woman (2010)

water, it can cause arthritis in her hands. "The doctor said it is not necessary because the baby has its own heat inside the mother" (Cosminsky 2016: 76). However, by the time Siriaca finishes the massage, her hands are no longer warm. Whereas Siriaca was concerned about the effect of her cold hands on the hotter body of the pregnant woman, the doctor expressed concern about the effect of the contrast on the midwife's hands. Ironically, the doctor is expressing his criticism of the traditional practice in terms of the hot–cold principle that too strong a contrast can cause illness. As with all the practices criticized by the doctors or nurses, they never ask the midwife why they are carrying out a particular practice. These directives by the doctor to the midwife seem at times to be arbitrary and without scientific evidence, but primarily to exert authority (Figs. 24.1 and 24.2).

24.5.3 Preeclampsia

Siriaca said she checks for signs of preeclampsia, such as swelling of the face or hands, and headaches or dizziness, as she has been taught in the training course. She said the birth is considered high-risk (*alto riesgo),* and the woman should go right away to the health center or the hospital. I asked Siriaca what causes preeclampsia, and she said it is because the blood is weak; it has too much water, or the woman doesn't have enough blood and she is pale. Ironically, one of the main signs of preeclampsia is high blood pressure, but since most of the midwives do not have blood pressure cuffs and have not been taught to take blood pressure measurements, they are not taught about this sign which would usually be considered as having strong blood rather than weak blood. Similarly, the midwife should refer the mother to the hospital if there are any signs of eclampsia at delivery, such as convulsions. However, in such cases, the midwives are told to refer the woman to the hospital and are not taught what to do in the meantime as lifesaving measures, especially since it may take well over an hour to get to the hospital (cf. Berry 2010).

Some of the NGOs that have been offering training programs, such as Saving Mothers (Oliveira 2015), have been more willing to teach midwives aspects of biomedicine that the government programs have not, such as teaching midwives how to take blood pressure, listen to the baby's heartbeat, and provide the technology to use such diagnostic instruments as a sphygmomanometer, stethoscope, and fetoscope.

24.6 Labor

The length of labor is highly variable. Attempts have been made, however, to standardize what is considered "normal." The medical advice has been that if strong contractions last and/or no longer progress after 10–12 h, the mother should be sent to the hospital (Verderese and Turnbull 1975). Traditional midwives, however, consider each mother's situation individually, rather than compare it with the statistical average of "normalcy," and don't necessarily consider long labor problematical unless it is accompanied by other complications, such as failure to progress, changes in the baby's breathing, and cord prolapse. However, recently some obstetricians have noted that it has been recognized that today labor progresses at a rate substantially slower than what was historically taught (Caughey 2011; Caughey et al. 2014; Neergaard 2014). This time limit is also a factor in the overuse of Cesarean operations.

Whereas doctors and nurses complain that the midwives don't want to change, ironically, Neergaard points out the difficulty of changing long-term practices among physicians (2014).

24.7 Delivery Position

Various positions are used for birth by Guatemalan woman: kneeling, semi-reclining (leaning against a supporter, usually the husband or mother-in-law, kneeling or sitting behind her with his/her arms around her and, with her arms over his head), squatting, holding on to a rope tied to a rafter, or lying down horizontally on ones back (lithotomy or supine) and holding her legs up by her knees (since there are no stirrups in a local bed). From the first interview I performed with a midwife in 1968 in Santa Lucia Utatlán to the last one on the *finca* in 2013, the message from the medical personnel, whether in a training course or in the hospital, was to have the woman lie down. In Santa Lucia Utatlán, some midwives would tell me they used the horizontal position, because that is what they thought I wanted to hear. The mothers, however, would tell me they delivered kneeling. The most "traditional" midwife told me she had the women delivered kneeling. She said if she lied to me she would be punished by God, because being a midwife was a gift from God and she had to tell the truth. The midwife on the *finca*, Siriaca, said that the doctor told her it was dangerous not to have the mother lie down. And she would be to blame if something happened to the mother and she had used a different position, i.e., that it was dangerous not to use the horizontal position. Despite the fact that many biomedical practitioners have recognized for many years (Gelis 1991; Murphy-Lawless 1998; Thilagavathy 2012) that the supine position can present many problems and promotes interference, the standard practice in Guatemala hospitals is the use of the horizontal position.

24.8 Umbilical Cord and Placenta

24.8.1 Cord Clamping and Cutting

The midwives employ a complex of related practices concerning the umbilical cord and placenta. These involve the cutting of the cord, treatment of the cord, expulsion of the placenta, and disposal of the cord and placenta. Midwives believe that if they cut the cord before the placenta is expelled, the placenta could rise up in the body, which they picture as a tube, and choke the woman. However, in the training courses they have been pressured to cut the cord immediately after the birth, and delay in their cutting is condemned.

One nurse said that the midwife may neglect the baby while waiting for the placenta and delaying cutting the cord. However, she didn't know of any such examples. Both Maria and Siriaca (30 years later) told me that the doctors use clamps when they cut the cord and that prevents the placenta from rising. Since they don't have clamps it is too risky to cut the cord immediately. They do not want to be responsible for endangering the mother and child. However, when I returned in 2000, Siriaca had been given a pair of clamps by the doctor and was using them and cutting the cord immediately after the birth.

Biomedical personnel condemn the local practice of delayed cutting of the cord and assume that what the midwife is doing is wrong and needs to be changed, because the biomedical practice is best. However, several biomedical studies have demonstrated beneficial effects of waiting until the cord stops pulsing before cutting. Grajeda et al. (1997) report the delayed cutting maximizes the amount of oxygen and iron going through the cord to the baby. Ryan McAdams (2014) also argues that delayed cord clamping decreases iron-deficiency anemia and increases iron stores in neonates. Mary Malloy (2013) and Van Rheeman (2011) also promote delayed cord clamping and conclude that there is no benefit and more harm in immediate cord clamping and cutting.

The World Health Organization (WHO 1998) supports delayed clamping and cutting of the cord especially in home deliveries, where there is a tradition of this practice and where there hasn't been active interference in the delivery, as it may help prevent anemia in the infant. As of 2013, the doctors and nurses in Retalhuleu were still telling the midwives to cut the cord immediately. This is another example of a biomedical practice that is changing elsewhere but not in Guatemala. And ironically, it is in the direction of what has always been practiced by traditional midwives, where the opposite practice—the immediate cutting of the cord before the placenta is delivered—is supported and even forced on the midwives.

24.8.2 Treatment of Umbilical Cord

The treatment of the cord is another practice that has changed with respect to biomedical (WHO) recommendations. Maria measured and tied the cord in two places, one an inch way from the cord's attachment to the baby and the other about 6 in. away. She then cut the cord between the two knots, or about four finger widths, with a special string from the pharmacy using scissors which had been soaked in hot water.[1] Maria poured alcohol over the scissors before cutting the cord. She then put merthiolate and alcohol on the umbilicus *(ombligo),* as she had been taught in the training course, after which she cauterized the cord with a candle flame. Next, she put talcum powder and/or licopodia (lycopodium) on the umbilicus after cauterizing the cord, covered it with a white cloth, and tied it. Siriaca treated the cord the same way, except she put a cloth under the cord when she cauterized it so that melted wax would not get on the baby and burn it, which was a concern of the doctor.

[1] I do not know if the water or the scissors had been boiled.

The biomedical personnel have long been against the cauterizing of the cord, even though it leaves it sterile and thus prevents neonatal tetanus (Mata 1995). Siriaca said she continues to cauterize the cord because it leaves it dry and clean, with a smaller umbilicus. Since some women still do not get the tetanus vaccine during the prenatal period, it is a wise precaution. Previously, WHO recommended that the midwives should not put anything on the cord,[2] and to put something on it was considered a harmful practice (Goldman and Glei 2003). WHO has changed this recommendation, and now considers it beneficial to use dusting powders formulated with talc, starch, or zinc oxide to promote healing of the stump (1998).

24.9 Weighing the Baby After Birth

After the baby has been born and the placenta expelled, the baby is swaddled in several layers of cloths to keep it warm. The midwife then weighs the baby with a scale she has been given by the training program. She is supposed to record the baby's weight when she presents her monthly report of births to the health center. However, no account is taken of the weight of the swaddling clothes, and thus the recorded weight of the baby may be greater than the baby's actual weight. This is important and may be misleading in a population in which there is often a high proportion of low birth weight (LBW) babies (Figs. 24.3 and 24.4).

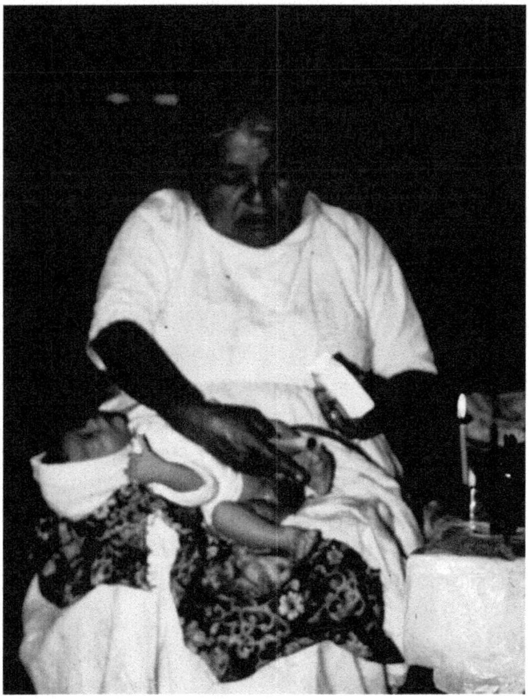

Fig. 24.3 Doña Maria treating umbilical cord with alcohol and talcum powder after cauterizing cord with a candle (1974)

[2]This recommendation was probably based on using substances like cow dung on the umbilicus that were used in some societies in other parts of the world such as India.

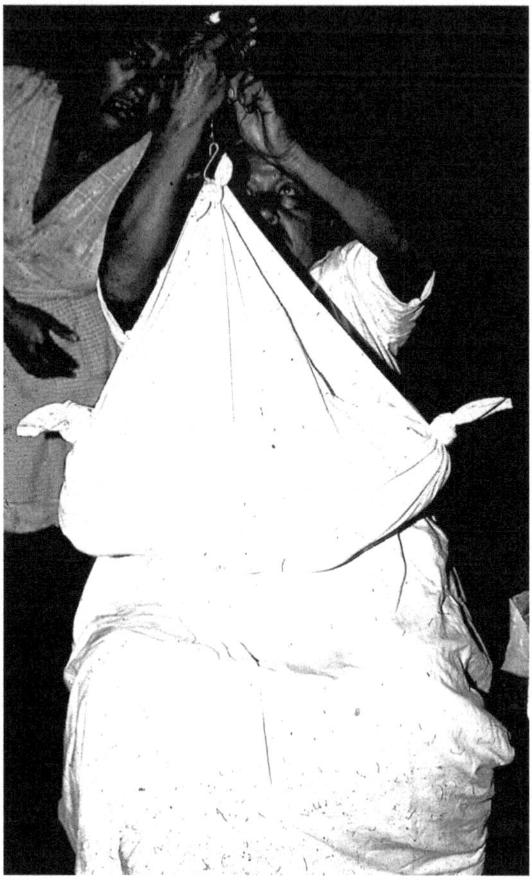

Fig. 24.4 Doña Maria weighing the baby after birth (1974)

24.10 Postpartum Bath

24.10.1 The Sweatbath

In many Maya villages, the sweatbath or *temescal* (Sp), *tuj* (*K'iche'*) is an important element in the postpartum care of the new mother. Another term for the midwife is *ajtuj* or "person or owner of the sweatbath," and as one Luciano midwife said, "the sweatbath is my medicine." Rogoff (2011) reports that they no longer use the sweatbath in San Pedro, and have not for several years. Berry (2010) says that in San Marcos in 2002 and 2003, no one was using the sweatbath, and it had been used primarily "as a postpartum facility," rather than a place to give birth. In Berry's description of an ideal birth in Santa Cruz, the sweatbath was used as an examining room for prenatal and postnatal exams, but not for the birth. In Santa Lucia Utatlán, the sweatbath was still being used for bathing, as well as for postpartum baths in 2000 (Fig. 24.5).

24.10.2 Herbal Bath

On the *finca*, and in some other places on the coast, an herbal bath is used instead of a sweatbath. The midwife usually gives the new mother the bath on the 3rd and the 6–8th postpartum days.

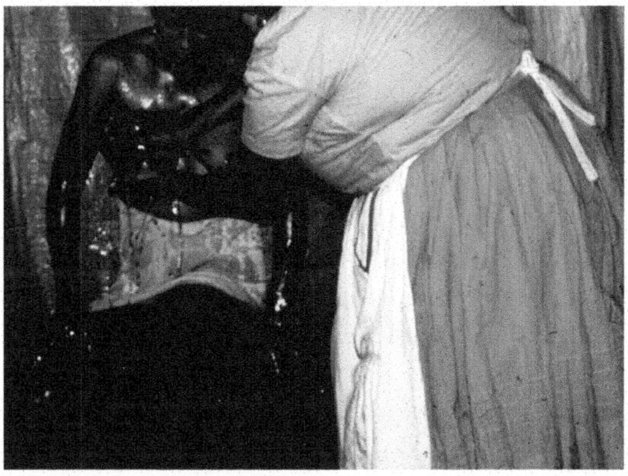

Fig. 24.5 Doña Maria giving postnatal bath and massaging breasts with herbs (1978)

The mother sits on a stool and is undressed except for her half-slip and/or skirt, a covering which is dictated by the value of modesty or "*verguenza*." First the midwife washes the mother's hair with hot water in which onion stalks have been soaked, and then the mother's head is covered with a scarf to keep it warm. The onion stalks are of a hot quality, adding heat to the mother's body since she is vulnerable to a cold state in part due to the loss of blood after the birth. Similarly, the herbs that are used in the bath are of a hot quality to restore the bodily balance and to heat the mother's milk. The midwife then puts a handful of the herbs that have been heated in the bath water on the fire, and puts them on the stool or bench the woman is sitting on and inside her slip in front of the vagina. She then takes a handful of the wet-heated herbs and massages the woman's breasts to heat the milk, beats her shoulders with the leaves' backs, presses the herbs against her knees, and massages her legs, rubbing upward and punching the bottom of the feet. She then places the herbs underneath her feet. The vagina, knees, feet, and head are all regarded as possible points of entry of *aire* (winds or cold), and thus must be heated. Then she pours the remaining bath water over the woman. The herbs used in the bath are *Santa Maria* (*Piper* sp.), *guaruma (Cecropiapletata), cihuapate (Pluchea odorata),* and *siquinai* (*Vernonia* sp.). All of these are considered to be of "hot" quality.

Although Siriaca administers the bath the same way as Maria, recently she has allowed for some changes, some requested by mothers, others demanded by the doctor. Some women wanted the bath but without the herbs because they said got a rash from the herbs. In such cases, Siriaca gives them a plain, hot herbless bath. She says, "For a young woman, even just a plain bath with warm water helps lower the milk." It also cleanses and relaxes the woman. However, Siriaca said that at times, "when there is a woman who has had several children, the milk doesn't come down and then bathing her with the herbs, the milk comes in." In such cases, Siriaca tries to convince the mother to have the herbal bath, exerting her authoritative knowledge. There is also the psychological and social effect of the physical and emotional support of being the center of the midwife's attention.

Another recent change in the postnatal bath has been pushed by the doctor, who has told Siriaca not only not to use herbs but also not to use hot water, only warm water, saying the hot water was too great a contrast to the body. Ironically, this recommendation from the doctor reinforces the hot–cold principle.

The baby is also bathed and the umbilicus checked and redressed. By the last bath, the cord is usually healed. The midwife Maria gave the mother a tea for stomach ache made from cumin, lavender, oregano, three cloves, which are all hot herbs, and some rum (Cosminsky 2016: 156).

24.11 Abdominal Binder

After the bath, the midwife massages the woman and ties a sash or binder around her below the abdomen (Fig. 24.6). The binder is supposed to keep the organs in place and pull the bones together, which are believed to separate when the baby is born. It is also supposed to help prevent fallen or prolapsed uterus. Mothers who are delivered in the hospital and do not use the sash, say they feel "*flojo*" (loose) without it. Some will have the midwife put on the binder when they come home from the hospital. The doctors and nurses at the hospital do not use the binder nor advise it's use.

24.12 Breastfeeding and Bottle-Feeding

Another area in which biomedical advice and practice has changed throughout the years is that of breastfeeding and infant feeding (Fig. 24.7). Maria said the nurses in the training course told her to tell the mothers to breastfeed the baby every 3 h, instead of the usual practice of demand feeding. In addition to being very unrealistic and impractical, it also reflects different attitudes toward child-rearing as well as different work patterns of the rural mother and the medical personnel. The *finca* mother usually carries the baby on her back in a shawl, including when she is in the field or picking coffee, and gives the baby the breast whenever it cries. Maria continued to advise her mothers to breastfeed on demand. Under these circumstances, scheduled feeding is medically and scientifically unsound and can be more harmful than demand feeding. Breast milk production is stimulated by the hormone prolactin, which is produced by the frequency of breastfeeding. Biomedical personnel were pushing a more harmful practice of scheduled feeding instead of the more beneficial and situationally appropriate demand feeding. In a 2013 training session a nurse and a nutritionist were tellling the midwives that they should tell the mothers that they should breastfeed the baby on demand, with either no acknowledgment or knowledge that this is what the women do and have done for years.

Scheduled feeding also was related to bottle-feeding, which was being promoted by the doctors and nurses during the 1970s. Sometimes this began in the hospital if the mother had difficulty nursing or was sick, and the baby was given sugar water in a bottle. Other times the baby was sick, and when the mother took it to the doctor she was told she should stop breastfeeding because the mother's milk was making the baby sick. Blaming the mother's milk or lack of milk may be a reflection of the negative and condescending attitude that many medical personnel have toward the indigenous and *Ladino* rural poor.

Some women on the *finca* said they began bottle-feeding because they didn't have enough milk (insufficient milk syndrome). Early feeding with sugar water will lessen the child's sucking and appetite for breast milk, resulting in a decreased supply of mother's milk. Some mothers, including Siriaca

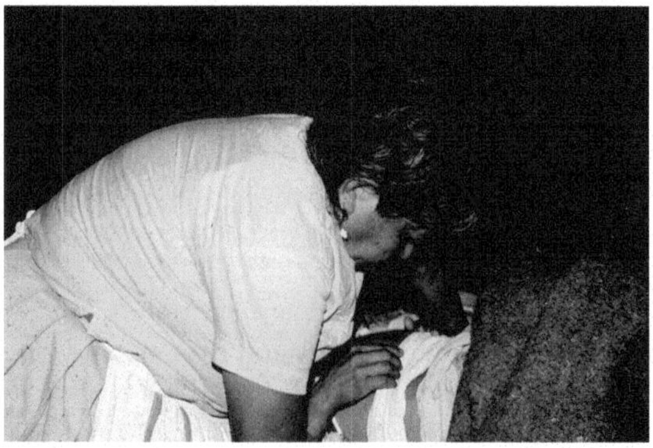

Fig. 24.6 Maria adjusting postpartum abdominal binder (1978)

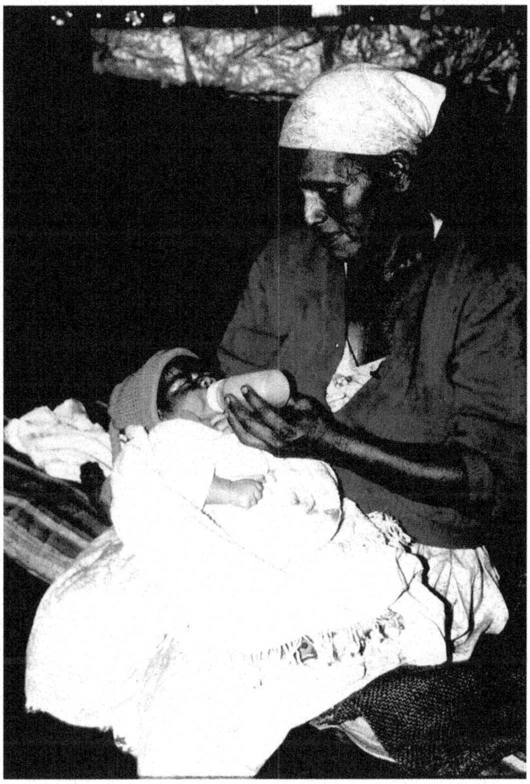

Fig. 24.7 Mother bottle-feeding baby

herself, said they did not have enough milk because of fright, anger, or sadness, relating insufficient milk to strong emotions. Siriaca said that with her last child, the baby got colic from drinking milk after she got angry. In such cases, blame is again placed on the mother, this time because of her excessive emotions which resulted in insufficient milk or "poor quality" or thin or watery milk (Chary et al. 2011). Boiling gives the water a hotter quality, even if drunk at a cool temperature.

The water is boiled partly because of a belief that boiling changes the quality of crude water, which has a cold quality and is therefore dangerous for a new infant, as well as because people have been told that crude water may contain parasites and thus make the infant sick. Unfortunately, contaminated water is a problem, not only in terms of giving sugar water, but also in the preparation of formula or other mixtures used in the bottle. In addition, the bottle and nipple are easily contaminated, and can cause diarrhea and consequent malnutrition. Mothers then use a variety of other substances in the bottle, including commercial formula, powdered milk, coffee, corn starch *(maizena)*, Harina de San Vicente (a mixture of 13 grains that is bought in the store), *atole* (a thin gruel made from corn dough), and Incaparina, a high protein powdered mix. Dilution is another problem in using infant formula and other substances in bottle-feeding, since it makes the substance less nutritious.

24.13 Social Support

Both in Santa Lucia Utatlán and on the *finca,* birth is not only a medical event but is also a social event. It reinforces kinship ties both generationally and by the participation of both sides of the family.

24.13.1 Support During Labor

Having a support person or companion with the mother during her labor and delivery, whether a relative or a doula, has been shown to be a positive element and decrease anxiety and stress. In a home birth, both in Santa Lucia and on the *finca*, the presence of family support during labor and delivery, such as the husband (if he is available), female kin including mother, mother-in-law, sisters and sisters-in-law, and the traditional midwife talk to the woman (birth talk), help her breathe, massage her, and provide physical support as well as psychological support. In contrast, in the hospital, the woman is alone during labor, except when a nurse comes in to check the progression of labor, examine the extent of dilation, and to call for the doctor when she deems the birth is imminent or there is a problem that may necessitate a Cesarean section. Despite the now accepted practice in medicine in the United States and elsewhere of the importance of having a support person for the mother during her labor, delivery, and postpartum, this is not the situation in some of the hospitals in Guatemala.

24.13.2 Kin-Based Aspects of Birth

A new birth reinforces kinship ties and the linkages between the two sides of the family in a number of ways. As mentioned above, during the birth, the husband (if available) helps support his wife along with other female relatives. In contrast, the hospital in Retalhuleu does not allow anyone other than hospital personnel to accompany the birth mother during labor and the birth. Among the *K'iche'* in Santa Lucia Utatlán, these women, plus other female relatives (aunts, nieces, daughters, etc.), also assist in making the food for the feast and ceremony called *elesan xe ch'a*t which marks the end of the 20 day rest period (Cosminsky 1994). While most of the women stay in the kitchen during the meal, the men from both sides of the family drink and eat at the table together. Bowls of food are also sent to people that visited the mother during this period of restricted activity. The celebration of the birth reinforces the ties between members of the family. Birth is not an individual act but a social and kin-based one, compared to the individualistic one practiced in the hospital.

24.14 Sacred and Ritual Aspects of Birth

Birth is regarded as sacred and is accompanied by a number of ritual acts. The midwife's role is thought to be a sacred calling or a divine gift (Sp. *don)*. This is revealed to the midwife in a number of ways. She may have dreams, find strange objects, have been born with a caul, and have suffered from a serious or life-threatening illness. These signs are interpreted by a diviner or day-keeper as signifying she should become a midwife, and if she doesn't, she will not recover but may get worse. The midwife may have certain bodily sensations like twitches that foretell a birth—if the twitch is on the right side, it predicts a boy infant, and if it is on the left side, a girl. When she feels such a sensation, she says someone is going to call her.

Both Maria and Siriaca lit candles and prayed for a successful birth before they went to attend a delivery. Maria said the spirits of specific dead midwives advise her during a birth and help to guide her. Siriaca said she does not believe in those spirits but says God guides her hands during massages and during a birth. Maria told one mother who was having a hard labor that she should pray to the Virgin Santissima to give her strength and resistance. Praying would also distract her from focusing on the pain. After the baby was born, the placenta expelled and the cord cut and cauterized, Maria rubbed the baby with rue oil (*aceite ruda)* making a cross over his head and saying a prayer. She said this was to prevent the illness *mal de siete dias* (illness of 7 days) or neonatal tetanus. She said the illness was caused by infection of the umbilicus, which she had been taught in the training course. Nevertheless, she still sacralized the procedure through using rue oil, the sign of the cross, and prayer. She also made a cross over the baby after swaddling him.

In Santa Lucia Utatlán, a ceremony is held at the end of the mother's period of restriction, usually 20 days after the birth. The midwife gives the mother the last postnatal massage and sweatbath, cleans out the ashes from the sweatbath, lights candles, burns incense, places white roses on the hearth, and prays and gives thanks to God, Mary, Saint Ann, and El Mundo (Earth Spirit) for a safe birth. She crosses herself before and after praying. The midwife then goes into the house and takes off all the bed coverings from the woman's bed, and shakes them out. She crosses herself, prays, and says the name of the baby. She sweeps out all the pine needles and dirt from under the bed that were collected during the 20 days. She burned and buried this together with the ashes from the sweatbath.[3] The sweatbath and this cleansing ritual may symbolize birth, renewal, and purification. Changes in these birth rituals occur primarily due to conversions to Evangelicism. An evangelical midwife will pray to God but not to the saints or to El Mundo. Biomedical personnel either are unaware of or consider the beliefs and rituals about the sacredness of birth outside their sphere of interest or importance or regard them and demean them as superstitions and a problem to be ignored or eliminated.

Conclusions

Medicalization of childbirth in Guatemala has occurred primarily through training courses given to *comadronas* (traditional midwives) by the Ministry of Health and various NGOs. In this chapter, we have focused on training or review sessions or classes given by the Ministry of Health over a 40-year period. During that time, biomedicine has also been changing as new scientific evidence becomes available. However, there is a time lag and accepted practices that have become outdated in modern obstetrics continue to be taught and practiced in Guatemala. In other cases, recent recommended biomedical practices are actually similar to indigenous ones that have previously been criticized by the biomedical personnel. In the process of medicalization of traditional births, midwives may have changed some of their former indigenous practices; ironically, these same traditional practices are now recommended by biomedicine and acknowledged as beneficial, compared with the biomedical ones that now have become outdated.

Practices in biomedicine which have changed, or have been recommended to change, which have been made and resemble indigenous ones include (1) changing the delivery position from supine to semivertical; (2) changing immediate cutting of the umbilical cord to delayed clamping and cutting; (3) acknowledging that normal labor may take longer than the 10–12 h previously assumed, rather than being deemed dangerous with the result of speeding up labor with oxytocin or performing a C-section; and (4) changing from breastfeeding every 3 h to breastfeeding on demand.

During this same time period, many *comadronas*, as represented by Maria and Siriaca, have altered their traditional birth practices because of pressures from biomedicine, changing from having the mother give birth in a vertical or semivertical position to the supine position, from considering individual variation in labor to standardized limits of time for labor, and delayed cord cutting to immediate cutting. These are all practices which, as mentioned above, are now being recommended in biomedicine as new evidence for their benefits have become available.

Furthermore, increasing restrictions are being placed by the Ministry of Health on whom the midwife can attend and whom she should refer to the hospital. The latter include primiparas, teenage mothers, women over 35 years of age, fetal malpresentation, preeclampsia, history of a previous Cesarean delivery, multiple births, and other complications which are considered to be high risk. The midwife can lose her license if she attends home deliveries in such cases and a problem occurs.

[3] For a structural and symbolic analysis a la Mary Douglas of this ritual cf. Cosminsky (1994).

The goal of WHO is to have all births attended by a "skilled attendant," usually in a hospital, and to eventually replace all traditional midwives. Given the current situation in Guatemala where hospitals have been estimated to be able to attend only 20% of the births, the lack and deteriorating conditions of health facilities, the lack of medicines, vaccines, and other medical supplies, and the current poor health situation of many women and infants' especially among the indigenous and rural population, the WHO policy of stopping midwifery training programs and replacing traditional midwives seems very inappropriate and short-sighted. Given such conditions, the traditional midwives are needed more than ever. Hopefully, the Ministry of Health will support the expansion of midwifery training programs, both for traditional midwives and for new younger more educated midwives, and the medical staff in these programs and health care facilities will be less authoritarian, dogmatic and condescending and more willing to listen to and respect both the traditional midwives and the mothers.

References

Berry, N. (2010). *Unsafe motherhood: Mayan maternal mortality and subjectivity in post-war Guatemala*. New York: Berghahn Press.

Caughey, A. B. (2011). Is there an upper time limit for the management of the second stage of labor. *Obstetric Anesthesia Digest, 13*(1), 27–39.

Caughey, A. B., Cahill, A. G., Guise, J.-M., & Rouse, D. J. (2014). ACOG/SMFM Concensus: Safe prevention of the primary cesarean delivery. *American Journal of Obstetrics and Gynecology, 21*(3), 179–193.

Chary, A., Dasgupta, S., Messmer, S., & Rohloff, P. (2011). But one gets tired: Breastfeeding, subjugation, and empowerment in rural Guatemala. In M. Walks & N. McPherson (Eds.), *An anthropology of mothering*. Ontario, Canada: Demeter.

Cosminsky, S. (1994). Childbirth and change: A Guatemalan case study. In C. MacCormack (Ed.), *Ethnography of fertility and birth* (2nd ed., pp. 195–213). Prospect Heights: Waveland Press.

Cosminsky, S. (2012). Birth and Blame: Guatemalan midwives and reproductive risk. In L. Fordyce & A. Maraesa (Eds.), *Risk, reproduction, and narratives of experience* (pp. 81–101). Nashville, TN: Vanderbilt University Press.

Cosminsky, S. (2016). *Midwives and mothers: Medicalization of childbirth on a Guatemalan plantation*. Austin: University of Texas Press.

Gelis, J. (1991). *History of childbirth*. Boston: Northeastern University Press.

Goldman, N., & Glei, D. (2003). Evaluation of midwifery care: Results from a survey in rural Guatemala. *Social Science and Medicine, 56*, 685–700.

Grajeda, R., Escamilla, R., & Dewey, K. (1997). Delayed clamping of the umbilical cord improves hematologic status of Guatemala infants at two months of age. *American Journal of Clinical Nutrition, 65*(2), 425–431.

Hinojosa, S. (2004). Authorizing tradition: Vectors of contention in highland Maya midwifery. *Social Science and Medicine, 59*, 637–651.

Hinojosa, S. Z. (2015). *In this body: Kaqchikel Maya and the grounding of spirit*. Albuquerque, NM: University of New Mexico Press.

Malloy, M. (2013). Optimal cord clamping. *Midwifery Today, 108*, 9–12.

Mata, L. (1995). The Santa Maria Cauque study: Health and survival of Mayan Indians under deprivation, Guatemala. In N. Scrimshaw (Ed.), *Community-based longitudinal nutrition and health studies* (pp. 28–78). Boston: International Foundation for Developing Countries.

Maupin, J. (2008). Remaking the Guatemalan midwife: Health care reform and midwifery training programs in highland Guatemala. *Social Science and Medicine, 28*(8), 1456–1463.

McAdams, R. (2014). Time to implement delayed cord clamping. *Obstetrics and Gynecology, 123*(3), 549–552.

Murphy-Lawless, J. (1998). *Reading birth and death: A history of obstetric thinking*. Bloomington: Indiana University Press.

Neergaard, L. (2014). No rush to C-sections, new guidelines urged. *Philadelphia Inquirer.* February 20, p. A6.

Nichter, M. (1981). Idioms of distress: Alternatives in the expression of psychosocial distress. *Culture, Medicine and Psychiatry, 5*, 379–408.

Oliveira, J. (2015). Escuela de POWHER par alas comadronas (proporcionando, cobertura en salud, la educacion y los recursos de las mujeres). Saving Mothers. Unpublished draft.

Rogoff, B. (2011). *Developing destinies: A Mayan midwife and town*. Oxford: Oxford University Press.

Thilagavathy, G. (2012). Maternal birthing position and outcome of labor. *The Journal of Family Welfare, 58*(1), 68–73.

UNICEF. (2015). *State of the world's children 2015 country statistic tables*. Retrieved from www.unicef.org/infobycountry/guatemala_statistics.html

Van Rheeman, P. (2011). Delayed clamping and improved infant outcomes. *British Medical Journal, 343*(1), d7127.

Verderese, M., & Turnbull, L. (1975). *The traditional birth attendant in maternal and child health and family planning health*. WHO Offset Publication No.18. Geneva: World Health Organization.

World Health Organization [WHO]. (1998). *Care of the umbilical cord: A review of the evidence (WHO/RHT/MSM/98.4)*. Geneva: World Health Organization.

World Health Organization [WHO]. (2004). *Making pregnancy safer: The critical role of the skilled birth attendant, a joint statement of the WHO, ICM, and FIGO*. Geneva: World Health Organization.

World Health Organization [WHO]. (2016). *Pregnant women must be able to access the right care at the right time*. Media Centre. Retrieved November 8, 2016, from http://www.who.int/mediacentre/news/releases/2016/antenatal-care-guidelines/en/

25 Approaching Maternal Health from a Decolonized, Systemic, and Culturally Safe Approach: Case Study of the Mayan-Indigenous Populations of Guatemala

Anne Marie Chomat, Bry Kring, and Luis Paiz Bekker

25.1 Introduction

Persisting, and in some cases widening, ethnic and socioeconomic disparities have been extensively documented throughout the world (CSDH 2008), especially affecting maternal and child health (Hogan et al. 2010; Mumtaz et al. 2014; WHO 2012). Nowhere is this more apparent than among indigenous populations, which consistently face worse health conditions and reduced life opportunity than their nonindigenous counterparts (Montenegro and Stephens 2006; Stephens et al. 2006).

Since 2003, the World Health Organization (WHO) and the Pan American Health Organization (PAHO) have promulgated new initiatives in what has become known as the Renewal of Primary Health Care, Integrated Health Services. In October 2014, the Directing Council of the PAHO approved the "Strategy for universal access to health and universal health coverage" (WHO/PAHO 2014). In these initiatives, the need to incorporate or strengthen integral, integrated, and continuous care, as well as inter-sectorality, is emphasized, seeking equity and compliance with the right to health for the entire population.

The hegemonic model of biomedicine focuses on an individual and curative approach, rarely establishing a dialogue with alternative care models and systems of medicine that possess knowledge and practices that could contribute to more integral solutions to complex obstacles in guaranteeing equal

A. M. Chomat, M.D., Ph.D., M.P.H.
CIET international Guatemala (Community Information and Epidemiological Technologies), Guatemala City, Guatemala

Participatory Research at McGill (PRAM), Department of Family Medicine, McGill University, Montreal, QC, Canada
e-mail: anne.chomat@mail.mcgill.ca

B. Kring, B.A.
Asociación de Comadronas del Área Mam (ACAM), Concepcion Chiquirichapa, Guatemala

L. P. Bekker, M.D., M.T.M. (✉)
CIET international Guatemala (Community Information and Epidemiological Technologies), Guatemala City, Guatemala

D. A. Schwartz (ed.), *Maternal Death and Pregnancy-Related Morbidity Among Indigenous Women of Mexico and Central America*, Global Maternal and Child Health: Medical, Anthropological, and Public Health Perspectives, https://doi.org/10.1007/978-3-319-71538-4_25

access to, and outcomes in, maternal and child health across populations. This is particularly relevant to indigenous populations, groups that face some of the worst maternal and child health outcomes worldwide. Intersecting inequalities place some women in very marginalized positions, while the systemic neglect of the role of traditional culture in health has been described as "the single biggest barrier to advancement of the highest attainable standard of health worldwide," especially among marginalized groups (Napier et al. 2014). Indeed, culture is a way of life shared by a group of people, that encompasses a collection of principles of human existence (values, norms, beliefs, attitudes), and shared understandings and patterns of behavior, that allow those people to survive within, and adapt to, their unique, complex environment and live together in relative harmony and sometimes in ways very distinct from other populations (Kipuri 2009). It is this divergence from the dominant cultural framework that makes local cultures an especially easy target for discrimination and neglect. As a result, local, culturally distinct communities are rarely consulted in decision-making processes relating to the health of their populations, and health facilities are rarely adapted to the sociocultural realities and needs of the populations they serve (CIHR 2007; Napier et al. 2014).

In this chapter, we will explore the nature and significance of factors relating to maternal health among the Mayan-indigenous populations of Guatemala. This should provide a framework to contextualize and improve our understanding of the root causes of maternal health inequity, as well as preventable morbidity and mortality of pregnant women, in such marginalized and socioculturally distinct populations. The Mayan example clearly illustrates why it is of paramount importance to recognize local systems of knowledge and praxis and transcend the biomedical health model as the only way to achieving health and to integrate different ways of knowing, practicing, and healing within the health system.

25.2 Inequity in Life and Maternal and Child Health of Indigenous Populations of Guatemala

25.2.1 Country Overview

With roughly 15 million inhabitants, the Republic of Guatemala is the most populous nation in Central America (INE 2012). Fifty-one percent of the population lives in rural areas (INE 2012). With an estimated 60% of the Guatemalan population belonging to one of 21 cultural-linguistics groups descending from the original Mayans (Montenegro and Stephens 2006; IWGIA 2017),[1] indigenous populations make up an important, though often marginalized, sector of Guatemala's diverse society.

Despite having the biggest economy in Central America, Guatemala has the lowest indices of human development and one of the highest measures of inequality in Latin America, with some of the worst poverty, malnutrition, and maternal-child mortality rates in the region, especially in rural and indigenous areas (World Bank 2016). The country ranks 125 out of 187 in the Human Development Index, a measure of life expectancy, access to education, and standard of living, adjusted for levels of inequality (UNDP 2014). The World Bank's Poverty Assessment in Guatemala (World Bank 2009) reported that the country had reduced its poverty rate from 56 to 51% between 2000 and 2006; however, official figures indicate that poverty rose to 59% in 2014 (World Bank 2016). The situation is particularly difficult for the country's indigenous populations, where 75% live below the poverty line, compared to 36% among their nonindigenous counterparts (World Bank 2016). The govern-

[1]The official figure of 41% (INE 2012) is heavily contested and most experts agree with a prevalence closer to 60% (Montenegro and Stephens 2006; IWGIA 2017).

ment's ability to provide social services to its population is largely hampered by weak tax systems, with Guatemala's tax revenue of 12% of GDP being among the lowest in the region (OECD 2015).

25.2.2 Maternal Health Statistics

With a total fertility rate (TFR) of 3.1 births per woman (3.6 among indigenous versus 2.8 among nonindigenous women) (MSPAS 2015a), the Guatemalan population is growing at double the average rate of other Latin American and Caribbean countries (2.5 vs. 1.1%) (WHO 2014). According to the National Survey of Maternal and Child Health (*Encuesta Nacional de Salud Materno Infantil, ENSMI*) 2014–15, 61% of Guatemalan women of reproductive age and in a relationship use modern methods of contraception, but significant differences remain between utilization in urban (68%) versus rural (55%) areas, and among indigenous (52%) versus nonindigenous (68%) populations (MSPAS 2015a). These disparities reflect not only differences in preferences, but also the lack of access to contraceptives. Indeed, according to ENSMI 2014–15, the unmet need for contraceptives was 14% of women of reproductive age—11% among nonindigenous women and 18% among indigenous women (MSPAS 2015a). However, these rates may be as high as 28 and 51%, respectively (Ishida et al. 2012).

Significant disparities between indigenous and nonindigenous populations also exist in the place of delivery, with only 30% of indigenous women versus 71% of nonindigenous women delivering in health facilities (Avila et al. 2015). In the Western Highlands, a predominantly indigenous region, four out of every five women deliver at home (Avila et al. 2015; Chomat et al. 2014, 2015).

Although the maternal mortality ratio (MMR) in Guatemala decreased from 219 per 100,000 live births in 1989 to 113 per 100,000 live births in 2013, large gaps still exist between wealthier, urban regions and the poorer, rural regions (MSPAS 2015b) (Fig. 25.1). The Western and Northwestern departments, in particular, are those that registered the majority of maternal deaths in 2013, with

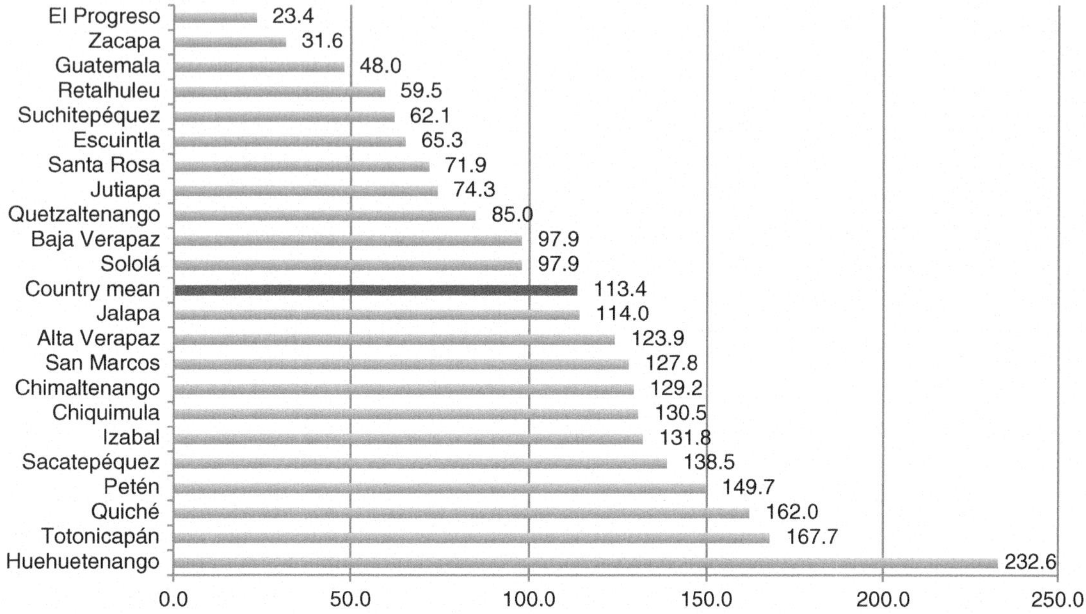

Fig. 25.1 Maternal mortality ratio (MMR) by mother's department of residence, 2013. *Source*: Adapted from MSPAS (2015b)

Huehuetenango alone accounting for 20% of all maternal deaths (MSPAS 2015b). In fact, according to these data, women living in Huehuetenango are ten times more likely to die during childbirth than are women living in the Northeastern department of El Progreso. The Western and Northwestern departments of Guatemala tend to have predominantly rural populations, and to have higher rates of illiteracy, greater poverty, and higher fertility rates than other regions of Guatemala (MSPAS 2015b). They were also particularly affected during the 36-year civil war that ended in 1996 after decimating many indigenous communities in this area.

Maternal mortality also disproportionately affects indigenous women (68% of all maternal deaths in 2013), with an overall maternal mortality ratio of 159 per 100,000 live births, compared to 70 per 100,000 live births among nonindigenous women (MSPAS 2015b). The leading causes of maternal mortality are hemorrhage (41%) and eclampsia/preeclampsia (25%); infection and abortion each accounted for another 6% (MSPAS 2015b).

Finally, women in Guatemala face high rates of gender inequality, prevalent throughout the country and across ethnicities and often characterized by violence and a concentration of resources and decision-making in the hands of men (Chomat 2016; MSPAS 2015a). The femicide rate is the third worst worldwide, and one-half of Guatemalan women have experienced intimate-partner violence at least once in their lifetime, and 25% in the last year (MSPAS 2015a; USAID 2009). The added marginalization of indigenous women and girls contributes to low levels of education, poor health, and rare control over productive or financial resources, all of which generate reluctance or inability to act independently, and with correspondingly low rates of self-esteem, agency, and self-determination (Chomat 2016; USAID 2009). These factors all combine to result in indigenous women exerting little control over their reproductive health and pregnancy care choice.

25.2.3 Looking Beyond Statistics: The Complex Interplay of Social, Political, Cultural Factors

Despite repeated assertions that reducing inequity and reaching indigenous populations is a top government priority, and despite overall reductions in maternal mortality in Guatemala, maternal mortality ratios remain very high in local populations. This is especially true for those living in the poor, marginalized, and predominantly indigenous regions of the country. These statistics clearly indicate that indigenous women in Guatemala face significant obstacles to health care access.

The structures and processes restricting indigenous people's access to health care are complex and intractable (Mumtaz et al. 2014). The notion of structural violence describes how embedded social structures supported by normalizing ideologies systematically oppress and exploit particular groups within societies, resulting in poor health within these populations (Farmer et al. 2006; Galtung 1969). The notion of intersecting inequalities describes how several, interlocking processes—poverty, ethnicity, caste, religion, gender—place some women in very marginalized positions (Kabeer 2010). Finally, the systemic neglect of the role of culture in health has been described as "the single biggest barrier to advancement of the highest attainable standard of health worldwide," especially among marginalized groups (Napier et al. 2014).

In order to understand the complex interplay of the many social, economic, political, and cultural factors which affect the reproductive health of indigenous women, it is important to view their daily lives in context to guide development of interventions which are not only helpful, but also culturally appropriate.

25.3 Historical and Sociopolitical Context

Guatemala is part of what once was a Maya civilization extending from Mexico to regions of Honduras and El Salvador. It is estimated that since at least 15,000 BCE people in these regions have been planting beans, maize, squash, and chili peppers (Grandin et al. 2011). In 1524, the Spanish invaded Guatemala and manipulated preexisting conflicts between Mayan populations to achieve military victory. The Europeans also wiped out a significant portion of the indigenous population through fatal and non-autochthonous infectious diseases (Cook 1998). The indigenous peoples suffered immensely under Spanish rule, when they were profoundly discriminated against and exploited to supply the Crown with cacao, textiles, and export crops and were forced to relocate into *pueblos de indios* (Indian towns) and to reorganize their social, economic, and political lives (Grandin et al. 2011). Mayan cosmology and traditional practices were suppressed in favor of Christianity, the religion of Spanish colonialism.

Following the country's independence in 1821, "liberal" militarized dictatorships began privatizing lands and enacting free-trade policies. Independence, however, did not alter the political order and the social inequality and exclusion of indigenous people. By the 1870s, liberal insurgents under the dictator Justo Rufino Barrios had enacted land and labor reforms to promote coffee cultivation and exportation (Kurtenbach 2008). Many indigenous communities were stripped of their land and forced into labor, the likes of which had been encountered under colonial rule. Moreover, the rural and largely indigenous population began to feel the effects of an expanding world capitalist economy, and was forced to transition from subsistence to export agriculture (Grandin et al. 2011).

Guatemala's October Revolution of 1944 led to an array of social and political reforms including abolition of forced labor, the creation of a national health care system, and agrarian reforms favoring the redistribution of uncultivated lands to peasants (Grandin et al. 2011). However, these reforms posed a significant threat to the United States' economic interests and corporate control, especially those of the United Fruit Company, the most lucrative corporation in Guatemala and a strong political force. In 1954, a Central Intelligence Agency (CIA)-backed coup d'état brought them to an abrupt end (Grandin et al. 2011). Supported by the United States, the newly instated military regime increased a state of inequality and repression, erupting in 1960 in a 36-year civil war. The war began with state violence against "subversive" groups, such as activists, students, and unionists, through "disappearances," torture, and the use of death squads (Kurtenbach 2008). The violence escalated as guerrilla insurgents hid and recruited in the Highlands. Seen as guerrilla supporters, rural indigenous populations were killed in large numbers by the army or forced into Civil Self-Defense Patrols, where they had to kill presumed guerrilla sympathizers (Godoy-Paiz 2005). During the worst period of violence, the army enacted a series of scorched-earth campaigns and destroyed as many villages as possible to overcome resistance through attrition (Godoy-Paiz 2005).

The armed conflict officially ended in 1996 with the signing of the Peace Agreements, after an estimated 200,000 people had been killed or disappeared (83% of which were Mayan)—669 massacres were documented and more than one million people were displaced. According to the United Nations' Commission for Historical Clarification, "the massacres, scorched earth operations, forced disappearances and executions of Mayan authorities, leaders and spiritual guides, were not only an attempt to destroy the social base of the guerrillas, but, above all, to destroy the cultural values that ensured cohesion and collective action in Mayan communities" (CEH 1999). The United Nations established that such acts constituted acts of genocide by the Guatemalan government against the Mayan population (CEH 1999).

To this day, Guatemala's political and social relations have their roots in an economic structure marked by wealth for a minority at the expense of the majority (CEH 1999; Anonymous 2014). The Guatemalan state has played a strong role in protecting this structure, establishing profound exclusion, racial discrimination, and mass injustice, and using political violence to maintain a state of structural violence (CEH 1999; Grandin et al. 2011). Despite the Peace Accords, a state of instability has characterized the past 15 or so years, tied to scars left over from the armed conflict and exacerbated by socioeconomic changes brought about by rapid globalization and open trade agreement (Burrell 2009). Effects have included heightened levels of domestic and social violence, increasing inequality, and large-scale work migration to the United States, all of which continue to weaken the social fabric, especially among indigenous people (Burrell 2009; Foxen 2007).

Such structural and historical elements likely shape safe motherhood outcomes of indigenous populations in several ways. First, following 500 years of colonization and state-sponsored repression and recently targeted by the army during the country's civil war, many Mayans view the state with suspicion and are reluctant to approach any of its institutions, including its health care facilities (Shiffman and Garces del Valle 2006). Second, while a peace accord signed in 1996 included a separate agreement on the identity and rights of indigenous peoples, Mayans continue to be far more impoverished than their nonindigenous counterparts. Discrimination against the Mayan population and their cultural practices remains strong, including within public and health services, perpetuating an overwhelming sense of disunity and abandon (Anckermann et al. 2005; Cabrera et al. 2009). Third, the many years of civil war left a profound mark on indigenous populations in the form of sadness, low self-esteem, uncertainty, and loss of hope and social participation, and many families and communities have been destroyed by a climate of mistrust and fear (Anckermann et al. 2005). Fourth, it is believed that structural violence entered indigenous family dynamics partly as a result of shifting social and gender roles in the wake of twentieth-century capitalism, when the traditionally complementary gendered division of subsistence activities gave way to a new market economy geared towards men, leading to economic dependence and vulnerability of women (Green 1999). Finally, the prevalent use of sexual violence against women and the disappearances of husbands during the armed conflict further increased women's vulnerability as many were stigmatized, blamed for atrocities, and forced to live as single mothers and heads of households with no resources and limited opportunity to make a living—a form of social upheaval that today is perpetuated by the frequent absence of men due to work migration.

25.4 Barriers to Indigenous Women Accessing Formal Health Care Services

25.4.1 Institutional Barriers Within the Formal Health System

There exist several important barriers to indigenous women accessing care within the formal health system. First, the hegemonic biomedical model of health has provided a narrow, fragmented, and individual-level focus on health and illness and delivered standardized packages through vertical programs targeting specific diseases, population groups, or life stages—an approach diametrically opposed to the conceptions and practices of indigenous populations (MMN 2016). Such an approach has isolated maternal health from its holistic sociopolitical and cultural context and the realities of daily life, reducing women to only one facet of their identity, defined by their reproductive health status and disconnected from their wholeness, their complex roles in individual, family, and community spaces, and those social determinants that impact a woman's health by conferring vulnerability or resilience. It follows that the formal health system has mostly overlooked interventions in health promotion and prevention by omitting attention at the family- and collective-level, dimensions that are important to indigenous populations' health and healing processes (MMN 2016). Moreover, levels of health services, ranging from the community to tertiary hospitals, are poorly articulated and formal health services lack a referral and counter-referral system, limiting communication between traditional healers, community-based health staff, and acute care biomedical providers (MMN 2016). In addition, data collected by the official health information system—in itself limited by being exclusively oriented to the reporting of isolated illness—has been largely underutilized with most health priorities not based on rigorous epidemiological analysis (MMN 2016).

Second, financial mechanisms within the formal health sector have generated segmentation and inequities. Indeed, while government health expenditures amount to only 1.1% of the gross national product (GNP), health care spending favors tertiary hospitals, which receive 40% of all funding, and urban areas (Avila et al. 2015). There also have existed significant disparities in the flow of resources by region, with per capita health expenditures ranging from US $212 in the metropolitan region of Guatemala City to US $5 in the northern rural region of Petén—disparities that for the most part correlate with rates of maternal mortality (Avila et al. 2015).

Third, institutionalized gender inequality, racism, and discrimination against women and indigenous populations has translated into discriminatory standards of care and health staff attitudes, the subordination of traditional midwives, or *comadronas*, and other indigenous healers to biomedical healers, the invisibilization of the medical knowledge and resources of traditional healers, and poor articulation between formal and indigenous medical models (MMN 2016). Relations between formal and traditional providers have often been tense due to their different approaches to health, a long history of discrimination and devaluation of indigenous knowledge and practices, and the fact that biomedical providers occupy a privileged, dominating position conferred by their institutional knowledge (van Dijk et al. 2013; Hurtado and Saénz de Tejada 2001)—all reflections of a postcolonial health care system. *Comadrona* training programs are frequently criticized for using teaching methods that are culturally inappropriate for older, frequently illiterate, rural women (Chary et al. 2013; Greenberg 1982; Hurtado and Saénz de Tejada 2001). Most efforts aimed at incorporating *comadronas* into the formal health care system have focused on the dismissal of *comadronas'* knowledge and skills and modification of their practices, rather than on the provision of culturally appropriate, culturally safe, high-quality services.

Last but not least is the suboptimal level and fragmentation of health services that has historically been provided to indigenous communities. The signing of the Peace Accords of 1996 provided a new impulse for the health system, in recognition of the urgent need to extend coverage of basic health services to the 46% of the country's population—primarily indigenous communities—without access to health services (Avila et al. 2015). Faced by many challenges, the Ministry of Health and Social Assistance (*Ministerio de Salud Pública y Asistencia Social*, MSPAS) elected to contract local nongovernmental organizations (NGOs) to expand coverage to underserved communities through the Extension of Coverage Program (*Programa de Extensión de Cobertura*, PEC). With additional funding from the international donor community, this program expanded rapidly to cover most of the rural population of Guatemala (Avila et al. 2015). However, a growing dissatisfaction with what was perceived as a lower level of health services provided to indigenous communities under the PEC and little to no evidence of impact of programs (MMN 2016), together with accusations of high levels of corruption, inefficiency, and a lack of transparency in the award of PEC contracts to NGOs, led to the cancellation of most of the NGO contracts in 2014. This resulted in the suspension of all public health care services to the majority of Guatemala's rural, indigenous population. Consequently, approximately four million people were left without access to any sort of publicly funded health care, including reproductive health services (Avila et al. 2015). Since then, health services have been slowly and gradually assumed by the Ministry of Health, but huge gaps still remain.

25.4.2 Logistical Barriers

Given the longstanding political turmoil that Guatemala has faced, there has been little possibility that health could become a priority sector or that an effective health system could develop, particularly in poor, rural, and indigenous areas. As of the early 1990s, the country had the institutional capacity to provide birthing care to only one-fifth of Guatemalan women (Schieber and Delgado 1993)—statistics that likely remain true to this day.

The distance to health facilities and qualified service providers constitute a major barrier to accessing health services. There exists a severe shortage of health workers in Guatemala, with only 12.5 health workers (physicians, nurses, and midwives) per 10,000 Guatemalans (MSPAS/PAHO 2013), the lowest health worker density in Central America (MSPAS/PAHO 2013).[2] Furthermore, stark regional inequalities in the accessibility to health workers exist. Seventy-one percent of doctors and biomedical staff are concentrated in metropolitan areas with better access to economic resources and public infrastructure (Becerril-Montekio and López-Dávila 2011), with 25.7 health workers per 10,000 population in urban areas compared to only 3.0 in rural areas (MSPAS/PAHO 2013). Finally, many communities are located far from any health centers and health posts. As many as three million Guatemalans, or 20% of the total population, live further than 5 km from a health facility—a significant distance for families without access to motor vehicles or who live in mountainous regions with difficult terrain (Avila et al. 2015). Consequently, remote location, poor public transportation infrastructure, cost of travel, and frequent impassability of roads in inclement weather make distances to the closest public health center or public hospital major obstacles to the indigenous populations who live in remote areas (Chomat et al. 2014) (Fig. 25.2).

Moreover, women often travel great distances to health facilities only to sometimes find them closed at times when they are supposed to be open (Hurtado and Sáenz de Tejada 2001). As an indigenous woman explained (ALIANMISAR 2009),

> We walked 3 h and a half to the health center and when we arrived there was no doctor, and there were no remedies to cure the hemorrhage of my daughter who had just given birth. We fought to take her to the hospital, but she had lost a lot of blood and could not hang on any more, and she died on the way.

25.4.3 Sociocultural Barriers

Interestingly, a study by Glei and Goldman (2000) suggests that disparities in maternal and child health utilization may lie more in demand-side cultural influences than on supply-side variations with respect to access to services. Indeed, they showed that although many indigenous women had equal or better access to health care services relative to their nonindigenous counterparts, their utilization of such services was significantly lower and mainly driven by ethnicity and sociocultural influences, rather than by measures of accessibility (Glei and Goldman 2000). In fact, indigenous women who sought out some form of care were only one-quarter as likely as nonindigenous women to see a formal medical provider during pregnancy, even after controlling for other variables (Glei and Goldman 2000). Hence the overwhelming use of *comadronas* among indigenous women is undoubtedly tied to local cultural norms and preferences and greater trust in traditional practices.

[2]Of note, this health worker density is only about one-half of the 22.8 per 10,000 population ratio that the WHO recommends as the minimum for a functioning health system, and much lower than the estimated 59.4 per 10,000 required to reduce maternal deaths to less than 50 per 100,000 live births (Campbell et al. 2013).

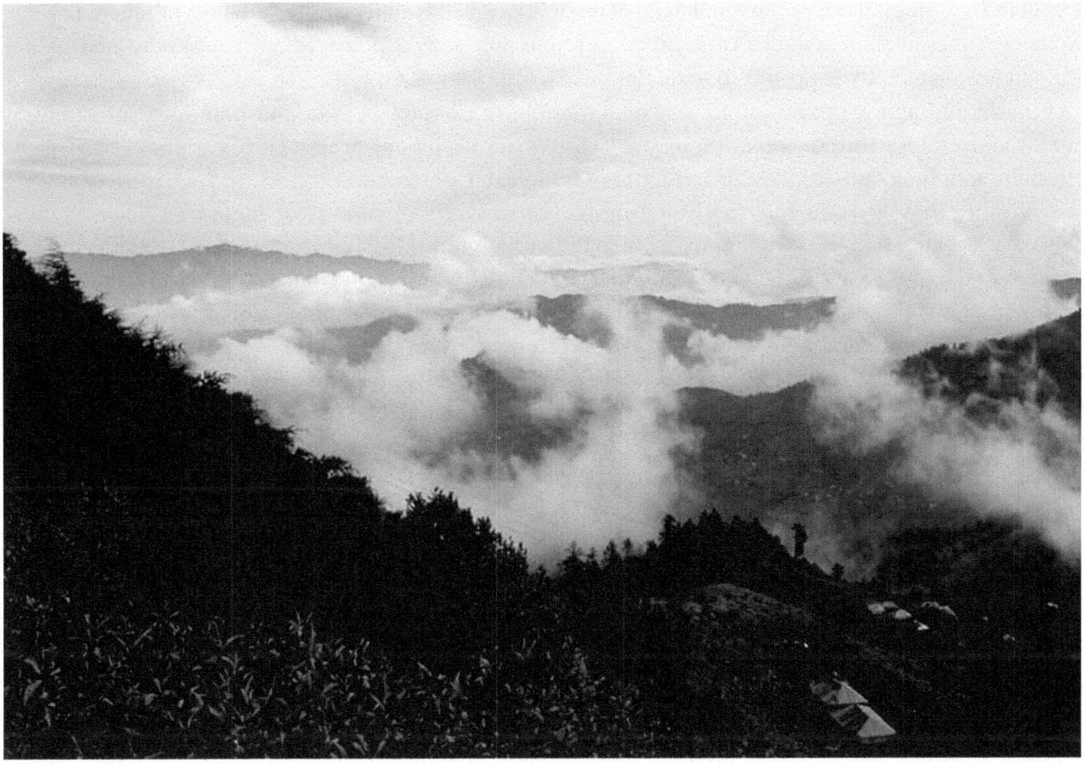

Fig. 25.2 Rugged landscape of the Western Highlands of Guatemala (San Marcos). Photograph by Luis Paiz Bekker

Historical, political, social, and economic exclusion of and discrimination against the Mayan population has made them generally suspicious of institutions associated with the state, including state-run medical institutions (Hurtado and Sáenz de Tejada 2001; Cosminsky 2001a). Many lack confidence in or are suspicious of modern biomedical treatments and often question the quality of care received, referring for instance to medications as "chemicals" and to hospitals as "places where people go to die." In addition, women often feel alienated from the formal health sector due to experiences of poor treatment and discrimination and embarrassment over being examined (Hurtado and Sáenz de Tejada 2001; Rohloff et al. 2011). Few medical personnel speak any Mayan language, and many *comadronas* and indigenous women speak Spanish poorly, if at all, creating significant communication barriers and contributing to many indigenous women feeling uncomfortable in the hospital setting (Berry 2006). These language barriers further exacerbate patients' fears of biomedical practices and limit women from being able to fully participate in decisions relating to their own health (Berry 2006). Most often not allowed to be accompanied during hospital deliveries, many women become silenced and isolated, unable to advocate for their needs and preferences. Gender inequality reinforces women's reluctance or inability to act independently, due to generalized low levels of self-esteem, agency, and self-determination (Chomat 2016; MSPAS 2015a).

Comadronas, respected members of their communities, are potential important mediators as they are conversant with traditional values and practices and also with Western medical techniques (Greenberg 1982). However, they are also often treated poorly, reprimanded and treated in discriminatory or condescending ways by medical personnel, and not allowed to accompany their patients during delivery (Hurtado and Sáenz de Tejada 2001). Most *comadronas* have many stories relating to the discrimination they experience from hospital staff, including racial slurs, being referred to as a "dirty, stupid Indian" or blamed for a woman's difficult delivery. Many *comadronas* are also reluctant to refer women to the hospital because of local perceptions that it is a place where people die and where women are shamed by exposure to male doctors (Cosminsky 2001a).

Finally, indigenous populations of Guatemala have distinct beliefs and practices surrounding health and childbirth that make them wary of Western medical practices (Cosminsky 2001a, b; Hurtado and Saenz de Tejada 2001; Santiso-Galvez and Bertrand 2004; Metz 2001). Most hospitals do not allow a space for traditional indigenous beliefs or practices, including during childbirth. Although taboo for indigenous women and not commonly practiced, women are expected to undress and expose their naked body and genitals, which many experience with shame and embarrassment (Greenberg 1982). Moreover, the vital balance between "hot" and "cold" (based in a humoral theory of disease, as described below) in the perinatal period is usually overlooked, and women are not offered warm beverages or the use of the traditional sauna, termed a *tuj* or *temascal* (Greenberg 1982). As an indigenous woman who had experienced both hospital and home deliveries explained:

> My experience in the hospital was very bad. When the baby was born, they didn't give me anything, not even some *atole*, even though my birth was normal. They didn't let my husband come in. Only the next day they let him in. I was alone. And I didn't have a sweater or nothing to wear. And they use cold water to bathe us, although at home we use hot water that we boil and we put in the *temascal* with fire. There they covered me in soap after I gave birth and it was so cold when they bathed me. Here that is never done. When a woman gives birth she uses the *temascal* to bathe. Water is put over the stones and the vapor rises. When I had my first child my whole body ached, and when I entered the *temascal* I felt so well when I came out. And when one gets out, one drinks a glass of hot *atole*. This is how women always recover. But not in the hospital. And here at home, after giving birth a woman can lie down and she doesn't have to do anything, but in the hospital they force us to get up and walk. The position of giving birth too is different. It was easier giving birth seated than lying down. It is difficult having strength lying down. If I have another baby I would prefer to have it at home.

It is not uncommon to hear rural indigenous women say that they would rather die, and die at home, rather than go to the hospital, even if their *comadrona* recommended them to seek formal care.

25.5 Indigenous Concepts of Health and Illness

Long before health care practice began situating itself within a curative biomedical model, focused on the individual, the biomedicalization of health and illness, and the use of standardized technologies often poorly suited to local realities, other visions of health had flourished in the Americas. Before, during, and after the arrival of Western medicine, indigenous societies of Latin American have held unique systems of knowledge and practice and in many cases developed their own health care models. These incorporate a profound ecological vision and dimensions that transcend those of conventional medicine, such as energetic and spiritual dimensions (MMN 2013).

For indigenous peoples, health is equivalent to the harmonious coexistence of human beings with nature, with themselves, and with others, aimed at integral well-being, in spiritual, individual, and social wholeness and tranquility (Cunningham 2009). The indigenous concept of health typically articulates physical, mental, spiritual, and emotional elements, from both individual and communal points of view, and involves political, economic, social, and cultural aspects. It is shaped by indigenous peoples' historical experiences and worldviews, and is expressed in the rules and norms that are applied in the community and practiced by its members. To promote health and prevent illness, an indigenous community seeks to recuperate and maintain its interior and exterior equilibrium, including the harmony between community members who are sick and the world around them (Cunningham 2009).

25.5.1 The Mayan Cosmovision[3]

The vitality and desire of continuity and permanence of indigenous populations in Guatemala are steadfast, despite the adverse conditions they have, and continue to, endure. Knowledge relating to health and illness has been transmitted from generation to generation and remains prominent in indigenous communities (Villatoro 2001). Within the Mayan cosmovision, similarly to other indigenous populations, a profound relationship exists between the human being, the natural world, and the supernatural world. To the Mayans, the world consists of a unique and indivisible whole, where the harmonious development of life depends on the actions of each and every living being and where a state of equilibrium is achieved through equality, equity, and respect with others, with society, and with the universe as a whole (PIES de Occidente 2009). Hence the "ceremony of presentation," performed some time after the birth of a child, is meant to reveal to mother nature the new being that has come to form part of her. Further, any act or failure to act that breaks the state of equilibrium within the body or with the soul, the social collective, the natural world, or the universe results in illness (Icú Perén 2007; PIES de Occidente 2009). Hence the understanding of health and illness transcends the field of biology to also include economic, social, spiritual, and moral dimensions as etiologies of illness.

25.5.2 The Mayan Medical Model

The indigenous peoples of Guatemala possess a health system that has persisted through history, finding its roots in one of the greatest ancient civilizations of America and evolving and adapting to changing times (Villatoro 2001). The Mayan medical system has its roots in the prehispanic period and is made up of a system of healers with different specialties, operational categorization of illness, and a wide array of therapeutic resources—vegetal, animal, mineral, and spiritual (Villatoro 2001). Over the last 500 years, medical knowledge and practices from Europe, especially Spain, were integrated into the Mayan medical system (i.e., concept of "hot" and "cold," illness of *susto*, or soul loss), and more recently, from popularized modern—or allopathic—medicine, resulting in a complex and comprehensive system of medicine that remains to this day poorly studied or understood.

To the Mayans, the practice of medicine has always held a sacred dimension (Villatoro 2001). Among the deities, guardians and protectors intervening in different processes of health and illness include: *Itzamná*, god of the sun, provides life to all beings on earth and is invoked in times of illness; *Ix Chel*, the moon goddess and wife of *Itzamná*, looks over pregnant women and is invoked for a safe childbirth and to resolve infertility (Fig. 25.3); *Zuhuykak* and *Ixlition* look after the well-being of boys and girls, respectively; and *Temazcalteci*, is the goddess of the steam baths, or *temascal*, often used to recover a state of "heat" lost during pregnancy, childbirth, or postpartum, and to cure other "cold" illnesses (Girón Mena 1979; Villatoro 2001).

Illness is typically classified into two main groups, whether they have supernatural or a natural etiology (Villatoro 2001). Illnesses that have a supernatural influence either involve transgression of social, moral, or spiritual conduct and represent a form of supreme punishment, or are willed by someone due to resentment or envy and enacted by supernatural beings. Therapeutic rituals take on the form of the sacred and use the patient's difficulties as an opportunity to resolve personal, familial,

[3] A cosmovision refers to how a culture perceives, interprets, and explains the world. It is a collection of presumptions and assumptions (i.e., ideas, symbols, myths, religion) that a group sustains, practices, and maintains on the world and how it was, is, and will be (Macleod 2013).

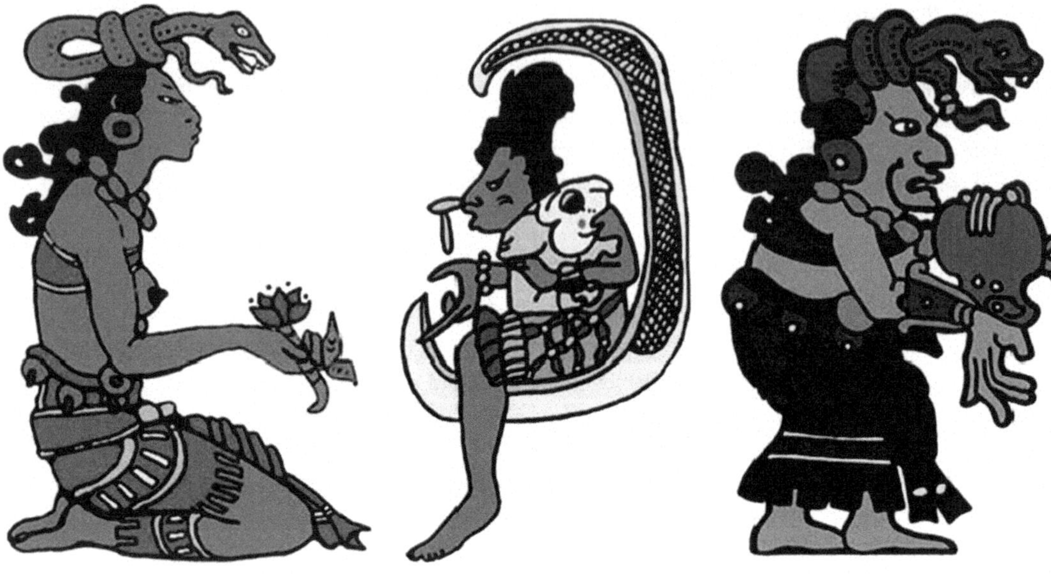

Fig. 25.3 The Maya Goddess *Ixchel* (Adapted from Maya Moon Healing Arts, http://mayamoonhealingarts.com/ixchel-maya-goddess/). "*Ix*" in Maya means goddess, or the feminine sacred, and "*Chel*" means rainbow or light. *Ix Chel* is represented in three different forms. *Ix Chel* the maiden (left) is the ancient Maya goddess of weaving, fertility, and childbirth. She wears a snake on her forehead to signify that she is the goddess of medicine and to symbolize intuitive knowledge and control over earthly forces. She sits in the kneeling position because she is in front of a back-strap loom, weaving. She is responsible for the formation of the baby in the mother's womb, and is considered to be the weaver of humanity. Maya midwives placed her image carved in wood under the birthing bed. *Ix Chel* the mother (middle) is the Maya goddess of fertility, motherhood and the moon. She is considered to be the mother of all the Maya. She sits on a crescent moon representing the cycles and phases of a woman's reproductive life and holds a rabbit in her arm representing fertility. She is no longer depicted with the snake on her head because she is no longer the village healer; in this phase of life she is taking care of her own family. *Ix Chel* the crone (right) is the Maya goddess of medicine and the moon, tending after medicinal plants, healing and the moon phases. Once again, *Ix Chel* wears the snake on her forehead symbolizing medicine, intuitive powers, spiritual knowledge, and control over earthly forces. She has a clay pot full of rainwater and herbs from which she pours blessings upon the world or, if vexed, storms, floods, and hurricanes

or group problems, hence restoring collective unity and harmony and concerting as a social action (Villatoro 2001). On the other hand, "natural" illnesses are based on the concept of equilibrium. States of disequilibrium can be due to (1) disruption of the mechanical balance of the body, (2) disruption in emotional balance, (3) disruption in the body's balance between "hot" and "cold," (4) soul loss (i.e., *susto*), for example, due to a particularly strong or disturbing lived experience, (5) the influence of other beings, natural or supernatural (i.e., evil eye), and (6) the effect of intestinal parasites (Hurtado 1973; Villatoro 2001). Most of these illness categories are recognized not only by Guatemala's indigenous but also its general population, independent of educational level (Villatoro 2001).

Health depends on an effort to keep or restore physical, emotional, social, and spiritual balance, in the realm of the individual, the family, and the community, and in harmony with the cosmos (Icú Perén 2007). Given this systemic worldview, ways of maintaining or restoring health are holistic and include the use of minerals, animals, plants, gesture, prayer, offerings, ceremonies, and other symbolic practices, with the healer being merely an intermediary between the divine and the terrestrial (Icú Perén 2007; PIES de Occidente 2009). The prehispanic Mayans developed extensive knowledge in natural remedies from the plant world. Men and women took on roles as healers under what they perceived to be divine mandate, as spiritual guides, midwives, bonesetters, and traditional healers, among others—professions that are to this day in possession of Mayan ancestral medical lore and whose legitimacy is rooted in the trust placed in them by their communities (Icú Perén 2007; Villatoro 2001).

25.5.3 The Traditional Midwife: The *Comadrona*

Comadronas are vital members of any indigenous community (Fig. 25.4). According to national statistics, traditional midwives, or *comadronas*, attend the deliveries of 29% of the overall population of Guatemala—43% of indigenous and 14% of nonindigenous women (MSPAS 2015a, b). However, in many indigenous communities, the large majority of births (i.e., greater than 80%) are attended by *comadronas* (Chomat et al. 2014).

Traditionally, initiation into their work is determined by their gift or mission, sometimes called "destiny," which is revealed in different ways, in dreams, signs, or through suffering or illnesses (Cosminsky 2001b; Icú Perén 2007; Rogoff 2011a). If this sacred calling is ignored, it is seen as the woman going against the flow of the Mayan cosmovision, and she is not completing what the universal flow is asking of her. Mayan midwives, who at first rejected their vocations, report falling ill and only becoming healthy when they accept their work as a midwife, as quoted by Walsh (2006):

> After having four children I got an illness. A lot of fever, very high fever, and diarrhea and fever at the same time… it was a signal that I had to start. I didn't get better and didn't get better so my mother-in-law used a shaman. [The shaman said] "No don't be ashamed that your daughter in law [is sick]. It is because she has a job and she has not started to do it. It is because of this that she is sick. And when she is going to start to be a midwife, that will go away." And from then the work started and the illness went away. The shaman also told her, "[The work as a *comadrona*] is a gift from God. You cannot go against what God has decided. From here on after now, you can start your work." And it was true. A month later a [pregnant] woman arrived seeking her services.

After discovering their gift or mission, *comadronas* typically acquire additional skills and understanding through their parents, elders, or others in the community, and sometimes through *comadronas* who have passed away or through God (Cosminsky 2001b). This knowledge and understanding are handed down through the generations, are rooted in the Mayan view of the world, the cosmovision, and form part of a living culture (Icú Perén 2007), well explained by one *comadrona* (ALIANMISAR 2009):

> We have listened to what our grandmothers said and from there we learned. And so the recommendations that we give women, on how to care for their pregnancy, what are the foods that they are to eat, what are the herbs that they can have, all of this is part of the knowledge that was transmitted to us and for this reason we pass it on.

Acknowledging spiritual or divine assistance is one way in which *comadronas* are able to maintain authoritative knowledge despite the pressures of medicalization (Cominsky 2001b). Research suggests that *comadronas* who are supernaturally selected and instructed are still preferred to those who have learned their profession from the formal health care system, as a *comadrona's* mystical experiences are proof that she is blessed with supernatural powers to assist women in childbirth (Cosminsky

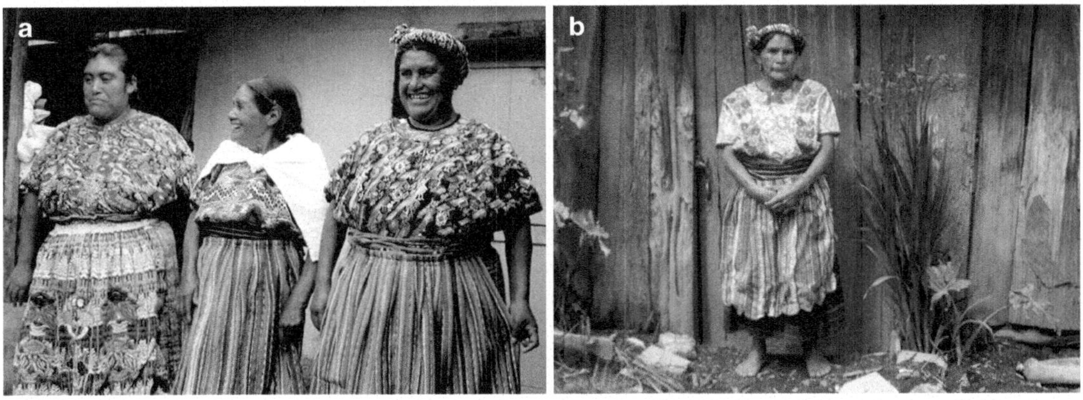

Fig. 25.4 (Top and bottom) *Comadronas* from *Mam* communities of Quetzaltenango. Photos by Anne Marie Chomat

2001b; Paul 1978). Belief in supernatural assistance during childbirth is thought to endow confidence in the face of danger and uncertainty, while giving a deeper layer of meaning to life and its processes. Some *comadronas* have reported feeling twitches in their body and fingers indicating that they will soon be called for a birth (Cominsky 2001b). Others receive such signaling from birds (Cominsky 2001b), or from the sound made by the fire used for cooking (ACAM personal communication 2016). Many *comadronas* will explain that they are guided in their work "by God's hands" or by the spirits of dead midwives, as well as by experience and training (Cominsky 2001b).

The role of the *comadrona* is highly respected in most Guatemalan communities (though not among biomedical personnel), and clear trust exists between *comadronas* and the Mayan population (Cosminsky 2001b). The knowledge and practices of *comadronas* correspond not only to the epidemiological profile of the culture, but also to the same worldview and way of understanding life (Icú Perén 2007). *Comadronas* do more than simply attend births; they provide prenatal and postnatal care, especially through massages and herbal baths; they treat children's illnesses and women's gynecological problems; and they can be both an agent of sociocultural change and of continuity and resistance. *Comadronas* provide comprehensive prenatal, delivery, and postnatal services through psychological comfort, massage, use of the *temascal*, advice on diet, and care for the newborn. For instance, many *comadronas* will counsel pregnant women to avoid such negative experiences as anger or unfulfilled wants such as food cravings, in order to protect the health of the fetus and to keep from miscarrying (Rogoff 2011b). During childbirth, a woman and her *comadrona* not only engage in a biological event, but in a social and cultural one as well, which include various pragmatic and symbolic elements (Greenberg 1982).

Most Mayan women prefer to deliver at home with *comadronas* who, unlike formal health personnel, can attend to their spiritual and psychological needs (Glei and Goldman 2000). As one *comadrona* at the *Asociación de Comadronas del Área Mam* (ACAM) explained,

> The *comadrona* takes her time, listens to her patients, attends with patience, with kind words, pays attention, maybe only psychologically if the woman is ill, and with a simple tea, that's all! During childbirth, what I tell a woman is… we talk to her, we chat, we encourage her, we stroke her head, sometimes her hands, or her shoulders, we tell her, "be patient, the moment will soon be here. Everything, and especially what we are waiting for, is a gift of God. After the pain there will be happiness."

Comadronas form part of the same culture and share the same worldview and language as the Mayan women they tend to, and have an approach based on dialogue and a horizontal approach to care. The social support implicit within many of the *comadronas*' practices, such as the *temascal* bath and massage, as reviewed below, stand in sharp contrast to the impersonal nature of the formal biomedically based health care system, especially as manifested in the hospital (Cosminsky 2001b).

25.6 Practices Around Childbirth

Many Mayans accord cosmic significance to birth. Pregnancy and childbirth are accompanied by rituals of spiritual significance, some of which are particular to the different local worlds and sociocultural contexts within Guatemala. In many areas, pregnant women attach metal safety pins or a piece of red string to their belt or underwear during a lunar eclipse, to protect their growing child from harm, and avoid walking over a rope to keep the umbilical cord from twisting around the baby's neck (PIES de Occidente 2014). Prior to childbirth, the birthing room is often purified with candles, incense, and liquor or holy water sprayed into its four corners, to rid the room of any evil spirits or bad influences that may negatively affect the mother and her child (PIES de Occidente 2014). Sometimes candles are lit during childbirth for protection (Hurtado and Sáenz de Tejada 2001; Cosminsky 2001b). When the umbilical cord is cut, a prayer is often made in gratitude and to help the child find his or her path in life, stating, "Thank you heart of the sky, heart of our mother earth, you who are our grandparents" (PIES de Occidente 2014). In the *Mam* populations of the Western Highlands of Guatemala, the baby is clothed immediately after birth, usually in traditional clothing, and a cloth wrapped around its legs, doubled at the feet and tucked back into a belt to keep the baby from falling into bad habits or a bad lifestyle when he or she is older (personal communication, ACAM, 2016). The placenta is usually brought home with the family and buried deep in the ground, as it is a bad omen if an animal digs it up. All rituals and practices surrounding childbirth are deeply symbolic and linked to the greater Mayan Cosmovision of the universe.

25.6.1 Mother Earth, Maize, and the Cycle of Life

To the Maya, the earth is seen as the Great Mother, or Mother Earth. As one *Mam*-Mayan woman explained to us, "the earth is that which gives, like one's mother, it breastfeeds one, because it brings the harvest and the maize. The earth is like the mother of human beings, because it gives life, and the harvest, and the air. One cannot live without these things." Many Mayans recognize themselves as children of Mother Earth's entrails, dependent on the substances that she offers as a life-giving force (Fig. 25.5).

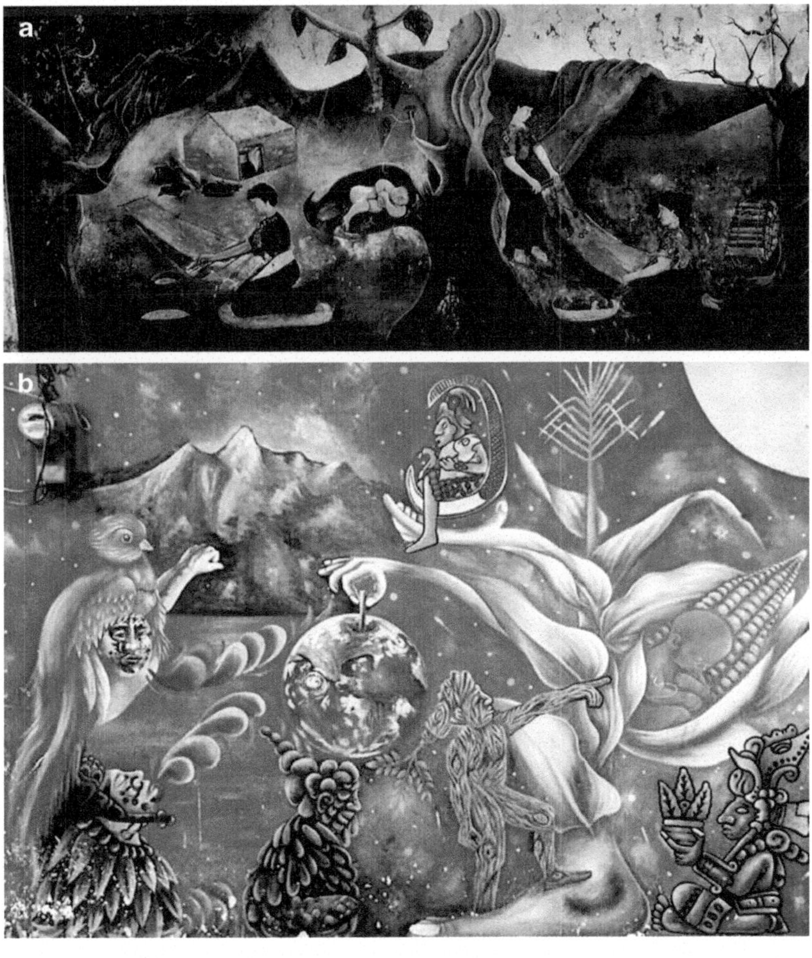

Fig. 25.5 Murals representing different facets of the Mayan Cosmovision. Top: This mural, from Concepcion Chiquirrichapa, depicts women in the feminine landscape of Mother Earth, where trees take on the full symbolism of the woman as reproductive being. Corn kernels and a *temascal* can be seen on the left. Bottom: This mural from Sololá depicts the creation story of man being made of corn, with corn symbolized as the tree of life, and a child being born out of kernel. *Yam Kaax*, the Mayan god of corn, is depicted at the lower right corner. Photos by Bry Kring (top), and Kristen Smith (bottom)

Just as the Mother Earth is sacred and honored, so too are the mother, her pregnancy, and childbearing (Callister and Vega 1998). As a *comadrona* at ACAM explained,

> In Mayan culture, motherhood is an important goal and role to reach as a woman. Being a woman who chooses not to have children is like having a perfectly good, healthy plot of land, with sun and soil and water, but not growing any crops or plants. For Mayan culture, being a mother means growing crops that will use the land that a woman has been given in this life.

In the Mayan world, maize plays a vital role because of the association between the germination of maize and the human life cycle (Fig. 25.5). Maize is seen as the most important symbol of life, vital for the health and balance of every being (Adams and Hawkins 2007; Gómez Bravo 2010). According to the *Popul Vuh* (1954), the sacred narrative of Maya creation, the earliest human beings were created from maize:

> Here then is the beginning of when it was decided to make man, and when what must enter into the flesh of man was sought. And the Forefathers, the Creators and Makers, said: "The time of dawn has come, let man appear, humanity, on the face of the earth." They assembled, came together and held council in the darkness and in the night; then they sought and discussed, and here they reflected and thought. In this way their decisions came clearly to light and they found and discovered what must enter into the flesh of man. And thus they found the food [the yellow ears of corn and the white ears of corn], and this was what went into the flesh of created man, the made man; this was his blood; of this the blood of man was made. And from [ground yellow and white corn] came the strength and the flesh, and with it they created the muscles and the strength of man. Only dough of corn meal went into the flesh of our first fathers.

Closely tied to the Mayan cosmovision, maize constitutes the foundation and staple of the Mayan diet throughout the life cycle (Gómez Bravo 2010). Consuming maize is critical because its essence generates and replenishes the basic fluids of life: blood, sweat, semen, and breast milk (Adams and Hawkins 2007). Maize is also a form of connection to the earth. Feeding a mother or child maize is giving them the essence of Mother Earth.

During pregnancy, *atole de maize* (a warm gruel prepared with corn) is given to the woman to warm her body, nourish her, and provide her with a visceral connection to the very origin of human life: maize. Mayan midwives will often offer a woman warm maize-based beverages during the early stages of labor and following childbirth as maize is thought to restore life force to a body that has just gone through the process of growing a new life, and giving birth. During the postpartum period, such beverages are believed to help facilitate breast milk production and return strength to the mother. And so begins life: through breast milk, the child drinks the essence of maize and grows (Gómez Bravo 2010).

25.6.2 Restoring Hot and Cold Balance

The correct balance between "hot" and "cold" is believed to strongly influence maternal and newborn health. According to the "hot and cold" theory of disease, human beings are made up of a delicate balance between both forces. The "heat" is vitality, energy and bringer of life, while "cold" is linked to death (Villatoro 2001). Since much of the world is categorized in terms of "hot" and "cold," including activities, foods, herbs, medicines, colors, environmental conditions, and other people, health implies a state of harmony between person and environment (Greenberg 1982).

During pregnancy and the postpartum period, women are thought to be especially vulnerable to "cold," and the correct balance of "hot" and "cold" is especially important for the mother and the health of the growing child (Cosminsky 2001b; Greenberg 1982). Hence many *comadronas* proscribe eggs, milk, beans, and avocadoes as they are considered "cold" and thought to produce colic (Greenberg 1982, personal communication[4]). Meat soup, herbal infusions, and corn-based *tamales*,

[4]Where not otherwise indicated, personal communications are from our respective experiences working with indigenous populations in Guatemala, and are from a variety of sources over a significant range of time up to the present.

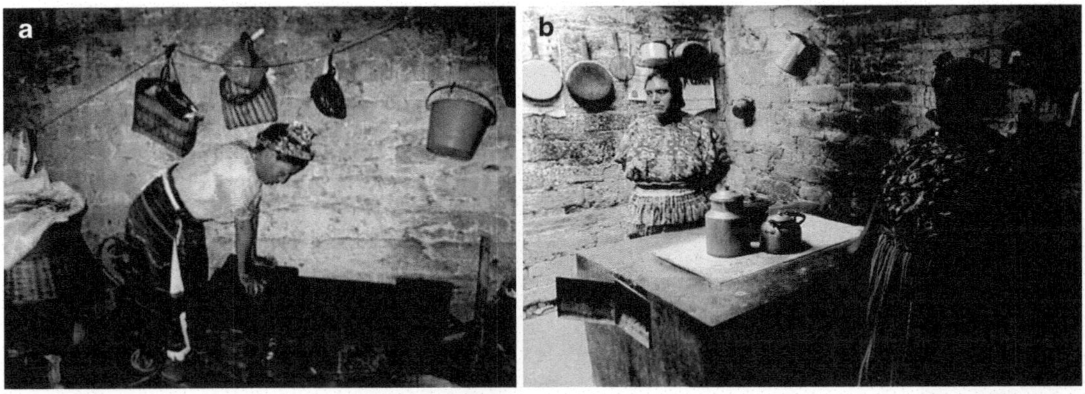

Fig. 25.6 Top: A woman grinds corn on *metate*, or grindstone. Bottom: *Comadronas* preparing *atole* (warm, corn-based gruel) for birthing woman. Photos by Anne Marie Chomat

tortillas, and *atoles* on the other hand are considered "hot" and are recommended to warm a mother's body and make her milk thick and warm (Greenberg 1982, personal communication). Pregnant and breastfeeding women are typically guarded against drinking cold beverages, washing clothes in cold water, or not dressing warmly, as such activities will make a woman's breast milk "cold." Conversely, they are encouraged to use the traditional sauna, or *temascal*, because of its warming properties (personal communication).

During and after labor, Mayan women are typically wrapped in many layers to keep the heat in and the cold air out (Greenberg 1982; personal communication, ACAM 2016). Women typically stay clothed throughout labor in their traditional *huipils* (thick, hand-woven blouse) and *cortes* (wrap-cloth skirt), often simply lifting up or opening their *corte* for childbirth (personal communication, ACAM 2016). Mayan women believe that at the moment of delivery there is an opening of the entire body; if the body is not fully covered, the cold can enter, which would result in illness.

Immediately after birth, the newborn is immediately wrapped in layers. The mother is given a warm beverage, most frequently an *atole* or herbal tea, to restore the "heat" lost during childbirth (Fig. 25.6). The midwife will give warm baths to the mother and her child several times a week in the days following birth, usually in the *temascal*, so as to strengthen and reheat the woman's weakened body, increase breast milk production, and warm the milk (Cosminsky 2001a, b; Greenberg 1982, personal communication). Abdominal massages with hot oils and medicinal herbs are also often carried out in the *temascal* to maintain "heat" during pregnancy and restore the "heat" that is lost during childbirth (Greenberg 1982).

25.6.3 Use of the *temascal*

The *temascal*, or *tuj*, is a traditional sauna used in many indigenous communities of Guatemala and Latin America, although its use has declined in some areas (Fig. 25.7). Spanish priests had tried to stop frequent bathing in the *temascal*, and colonial Guatemalan religious leaders were also suspicious of it because inside the *temascal*, a person was regarded as encountering goddesses connected with healing, midwifery, and the earth (Few 2002). More recently, the government has prohibited its use in certain areas (Rogoff 2011c).

The term *temascal* is derived from the Aztec name of *teme*, "to bathe," and *cali*, "house." The *temascal* is a small mud, adobe, or cement hut, which is heated by lighting a wood-fire underneath a stove of rocks, and pouring warm water over the rocks to create steam. In Guatemala, the *temascal* is

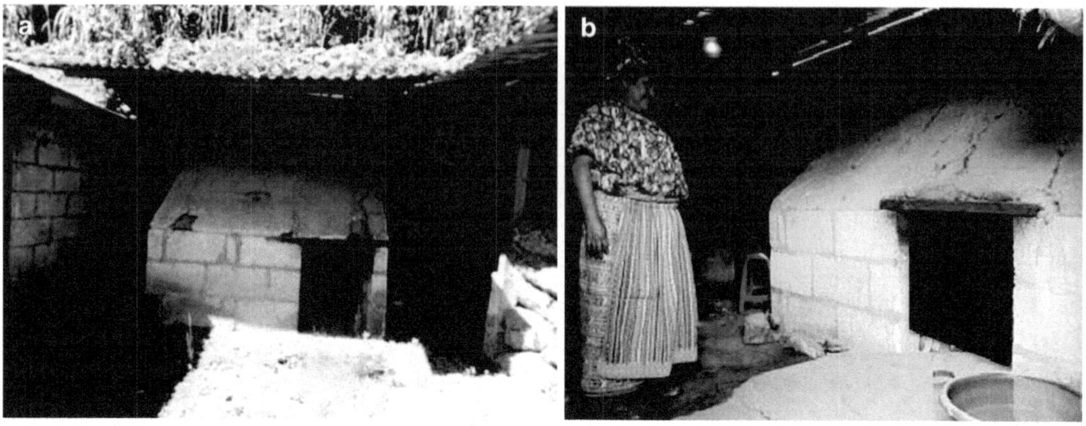

Fig. 25.7 Top: A *temascal* in a home in a *Mam*-Mayan village in the Western Highlands of Guatemala. Bottom: A *comadrona* in front of a traditional sauna, or *temascal*, in her home where she attends births

typically used by all members of a household weekly or biweekly for cleansing (Radoff et al. 2013). Through its "heat" properties, the *temascal* is also used for the prevention of illnesses, for restoring health, and plays an important role throughout the perinatal period. The *temascal* has been referred to as "the domain of the mother goddess who exercises her power over the sick and the pregnant" (Sullivan 1966).

A woman typically uses the *temascal* throughout pregnancy and the postpartum period. The "hot" properties of the *temascal* are thought to help prepare a woman's body for childbirth, which requires a lot of "heat" and energy. Exposing her body to heat throughout pregnancy helps a mother better prepare for the physical demands of the birthing process (MSPAS 2009; PIES de Occidente 2014). The *temascal* is thought to be healing for both mother and newborn following birth. During childbirth, a woman will transition from the "hot" state of pregnancy to a "cold" state, due to blood loss and the detachment of the placenta (Radoff et al. 2013). Ideally, the mother enters the *temascal* a few hours after giving birth to warm the uterus, helping to restore her "hot" and "cold" balance, to cleanse her body and to heal any tears or injuries in the bones, skin, muscles, and internal organs (PIES de Occidente 2014, personal communication). The newborn is also thought to benefit from the heat and ritual of the *temascal*. The *temascal* is thought to help heal and regulate the body temperature of newborns, especially if born prematurely (personal communication, ACAM, 2016). Additionally, the *temascal* allows for intimate skin-to-skin contact between a mother and her newborn. The *temascal* is also thought to bring down milk and make breastfeeding easier (PIES de Occidente 2014).

25.6.4 Childbirth Position

Throughout history, women have given birth in a variety of positions, many of which are "vertical." Only recently, with the medicalization of childbirth and the routine use of anesthesia, has a "horizontal" position—referred to as *lithotomy*, lying flat on back with legs pulled back to either side—been used predominantly, mostly for physician convenience (Oxorn 1986; Villatoro 1994). *Comadronas* have traditionally offered pregnant women a diversity of options, prioritizing the vertical position, and many Mayan women prefer to give birth kneeling compared to lying down because they feel they have more strength and because it is the customary and more modest position (Greenberg 1982; MSPAS 2011). Preference for a vertical birth is one of the reasons behind women's preference not to have a hospital delivery (MSPAS 2011).[5] However, many *comadronas* today use the supine position, a clear example of the impact of medicalization on traditional birth practices (Cosminsky 2001b; personal communication, ACAM, 2016).

25.6.5 Herbal Remedies

Herbal remedies are still widely used among Mayans, and *comadronas* use a variety of hot herbal teas during different stages of pregnancy. All herbal teas are considered "hot" and are used to heat the body. Some teas are used for general ailments such as headaches and nausea, others are used during labor (i.e., to speed childbirth) while still others are used to relieve pain and stimulate milk flow directly following childbirth (Greenberg 1982).

Comadronas have a deep understanding of the earth and the specific uses of various plants. Several herbs are commonly used by *comadronas* in Guatemala during pregnancy, childbirth, or the postpartum period (see Table 25.1). For instance, Lemon verbena (Maria Luisa, *Alosia citadora*) and rue (ruda, *Ruta chalepensis*) are used for strong nerves, stress, and fright (*susto*), although the latter can advance labor and is not to be used during pregnancy (personal communication, ACAM, 2016). Burnet (Pimpinela, *Sanguisorba minor*) can be used to advance labor, dilation up to 8 cm and to augment contractions. Black nightshade (hierba mora, *Solanum nigrum*) can be used as an analgesic, an anti-inflammatory and to reduce hemorrhage. Ixbut (*Euphorbia lancifolia*) can stimulate breast milk production. Finally, orange leaf (hoja de naranja, *Citrus sinensis*) and aniseed (anise, *Pimpinella anisum*) are consumed as teas by mothers to reduce colic of the young infant (personal communication, ACAM, 2016).

25.7 Inclusion of the Mayan Medical System

In most state health systems, the cultures and worldviews of indigenous peoples are ignored, dismissed, or actively opposed. Instead, most states promote *monocultural* health systems[6] based exclusively on Western medicine that do not fully reflect the multiple cultures and ethnicities of their populations, marginalizing indigenous peoples, denying them access to basic health services, and devaluing their traditional health systems (Cunningham 2009).

The formal health system of Guatemala has historically been defined by a hegemonic biomedical approach to health that takes little if any account of the life, knowledge, practices and worldviews of its indigenous population. With the Spanish invasion and colonization of the Americas, biomedical knowledge, considered superior, was implemented with no regard to the medical systems already in

[5]Mayan women's preference for a vertical birth is not unfounded. The choice of labor and birth positions plays a critical role in a mother's comfort level during birth and how quickly and effectively her labor progresses. Research has shown that vertical positions increase both the force of gravity and the diameter of the pelvic outlet, facilitating the baby's descent through the mother's pelvis, and are associated with reduced back pain, reduced pain during pushing, fewer perineal tears and need for episiotomies, and overall easier pushing (Gardosi et al. 1989; Roberts et al. 2005; De Jonge et al. 2004). Furthermore, the risk of fetal distress is reduced by avoiding compromising major blood vessels and interfering with fetal oxygenation (Humphrey et al. 1973). Finally, most women feel that they have more strength and force in a vertical position, and greater control over the birth process.

[6]Monocultural health systems are based on a concept of society being homogeneous, and privileging the dominant national culture over all other cultures, without the systematic participation or consultation of indigenous communities. Health issues that are determined by gender, socioeconomic class, or ethnicity may not be recognized, and training of health practitioners is based on a biotechnological approach that ignores the contributions of indigenous cultures and does not prepare them to work in multiethnic contexts (Cunningham 2009).

Table 25.1 Medicinal plants used during pregnancy, childbirth, or postpartum in indigenous communities of Guatemala

Common name	Scientific name	Origin	Use	Comments	Illustration
Black night-shade (Hierba mora)	*Solanum nigrum*	Eusasia, Naturalized in Americas, Australia, South Africa	Analgesic Anemia Anti-inflammatory Anti-hemorrhage		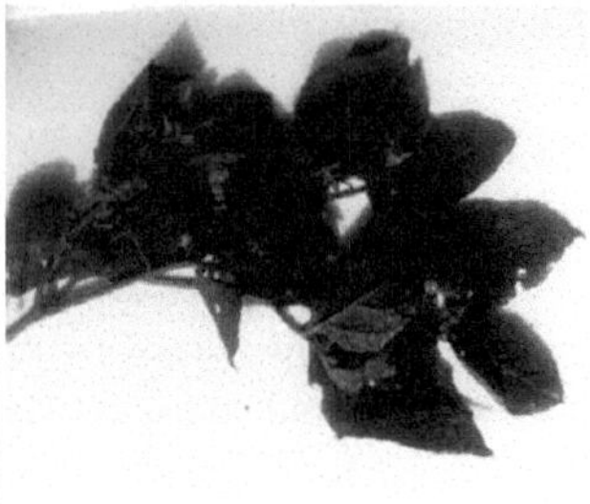
Burnet (Pimpinela)	*Sanguisorba minor*	Africa, Asia, Europe	Can be used during labor for contractions and to advance dilation	Use only until 8 cm of dilation	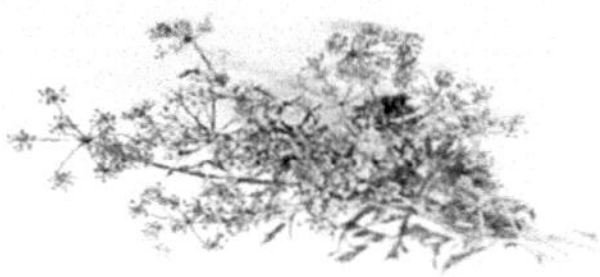
Ixbut (name in *Mam*)	*Euphorbia lancifolia*	Mexico, Central America	Production of breast milk	Can begin to drink a week before baby is born to bring down the milk, or after baby is born	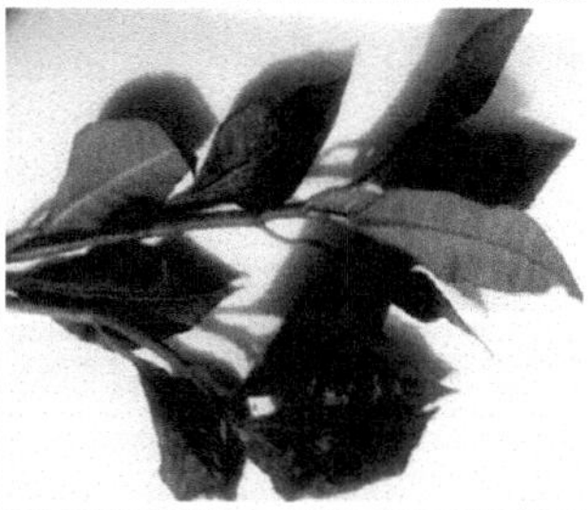
Lemon Verbena (Lemon Beebrush, Maria Luisa)	*Alosia citadora*	South America	Strong nerves, stress, fright (*susto*) After birth, can be combined with sage to relieve body pains		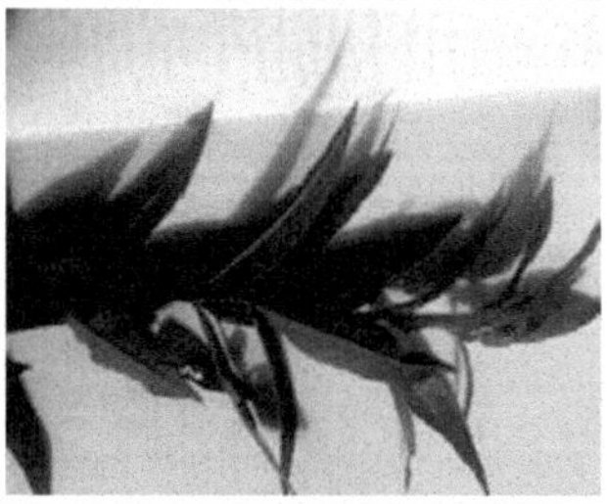
Mugwart (Common wormwood, Artemisia)	*Artemisia vulgaris*	Asia, Africa, Europe, Naturalized in North America	Can be used during labor to advance to full dilation Urinary tract infections		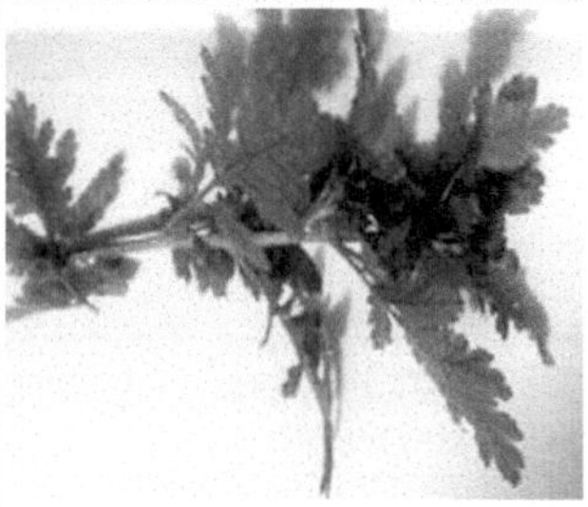

Table 25.1 (continued)

Common name	Scientific name	Origin	Use	Comments	Illustration
Orange leaf (Hoja de Naranja)	*Citrus sinensis*	Asia, Naturalized in majority of the world	Strong nerves, infant colic		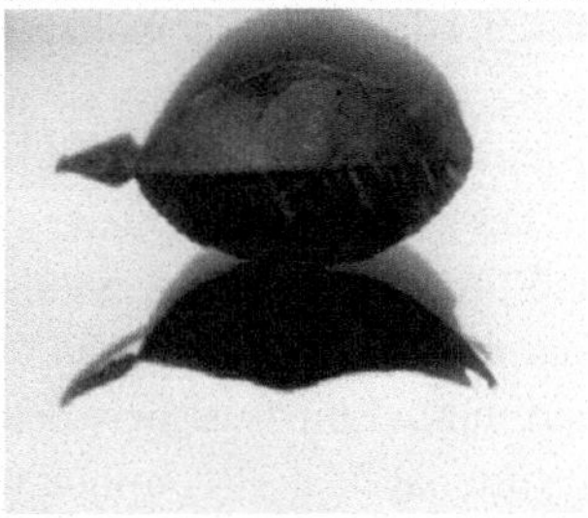
Rue (Fringed rue, Ruda)	*Ruta chalepensis*	Eaurasia, North Africa	Strong nerves, stress, fright (*susto*) Can be used during labor to advance to full dilation	Can be toxic in large quantities Not safe during pregnancy	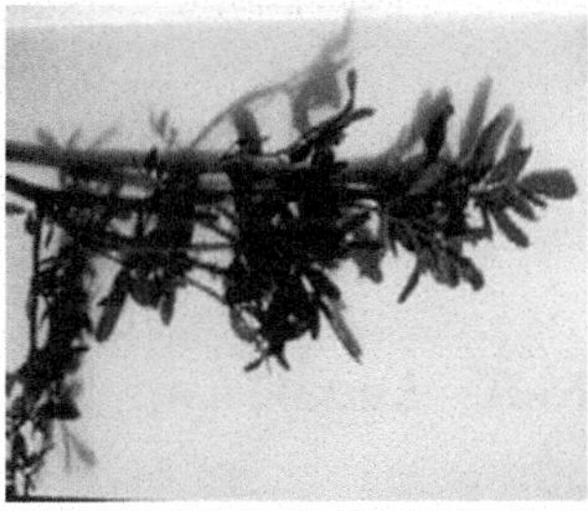
Sage (Salvia Santa)	*Salvia officinalis*	Mediterranean, Naturalized in majority of the world	Menstrual cramps Ovarian cysts After birth, can be combined with lemon verbena to relieve body pains		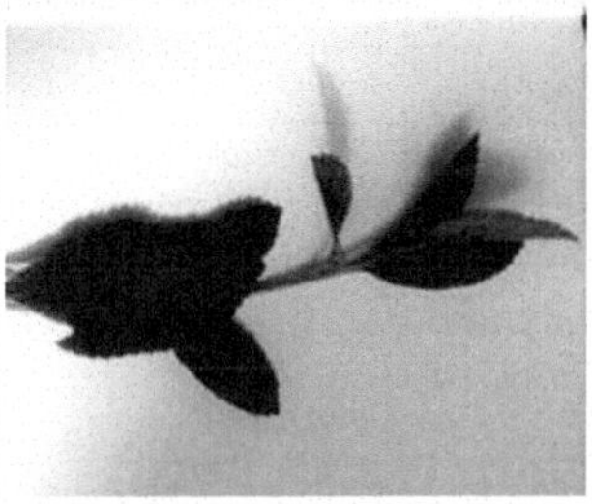
Tarragon (Pericón)	*Tagete lucida*	Mexico, Guatemala	Strong stomach pains		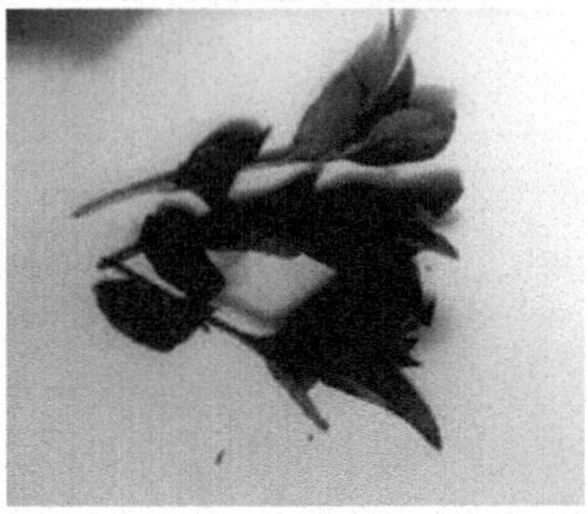
Yarrow (Milenrama)	*Achillea millefolium*	Asia, Europe, North America	Inflammation of uterus Blood coagulant Helps remove inflammation in the uterus after birth or miscarriage	Not safe during pregnancy	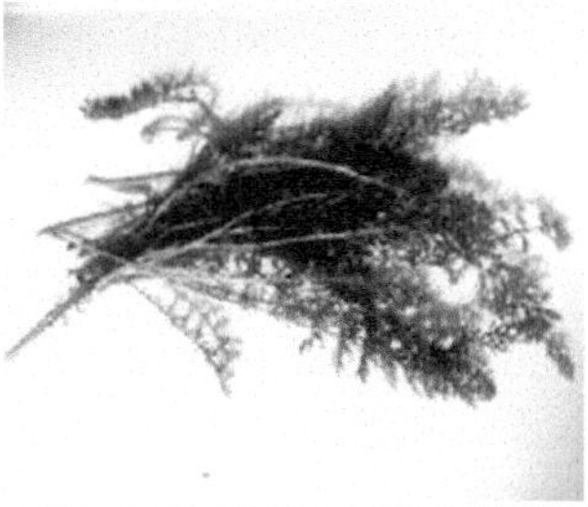

Information: Personal communication, ACAM 2016
Photo credit: Cristina Gomes

place (Cunningham 1997). Under colonial rule, rural health services run by missionaries focused primarily on maternal and child health, while indigenous health care providers were prosecuted, and branded as witches, warlocks, and servants of the devil (Packard 2013). Today, Mayan spirituality, practiced by many *comadronas* who embrace the syncretism of Mayan and Catholic beliefs, continues to be labeled as witchcraft and superstition, and it is not uncommon to hear the rites and methods of traditional healers described as the devil's work (personal communication).

Despite the conceptual richness and the resources of Mayan medicine and the largely unquantified and unrecognized contribution it makes to society in health care, it is considered an inferior system, marginal in importance, and worthy of discrimination and rejection. This has generated a deep chasm and mutual mistrust between the formal (biomedical) and traditional medical systems, especially as traditional healers continue to provide the majority of medical care to the country's indigenous, rural populations. Moreover, it implies that the epidemiological and cultural profile of the Maya population is not represented within the formal health care sector (Icu Perén 2007). This "cultural exclusion" explains to a great extent the difficulties in achieving the fulfillment of the full right to health of indigenous peoples and to equalize health indicators across the Guatemalan population (MMN 2013).

25.8 Legal Framework for Addressing the Health of Indigenous Peoples

The chasm between formal and traditional health systems in Guatemala has been perpetuated by the overall lack of public policies related to intercultural approaches in health that would allow its indigenous populations to exercise their right to health within their own sociocultural contexts. This is despite strong international and national legislations that together establish a framework for addressing the health of indigenous peoples, including the obligation to provide accessible, quality health care and to respect and promote indigenous health systems.

In 1977, the World Health Organization (WHO) formed a working group to emphasize the importance of diverse and ancestral systems of medicine, particularly to resolve illnesses with a sociocultural foundation, and to integrate traditional medical knowledge within national health care programs (WHO 1978). In 1978, the International Health Conference at Alma Ata defined a global strategy to carry forth this integration through the recognition and incorporation of traditional medical practices into community-level programs; the use of traditional healers within the primary health care system; and the training of health professionals and students in the principles of traditional medicine, so as to promote dialogue, communication, and understanding (Alma Ata 1978). Relevant to Latin America, in 1983, the Pan-American Health Organization (PAHO) developed a working group on Health and Traditional Medical Cultures in Latin America and the Caribbean meant to define a fundamental, multi-causal approach to health and illness processes, where culture would play a fundamental role, especially in culturally diverse countries. It stated that the viability and efficacy of health programs could be increased through the promotion of traditional medical cultures but that a dearth of studies limited their recognition and importance for health in the region (PAHO/WHO 1985). Convention 169 of the International Labour Organization on Indigenous and Tribal Peoples (ILO 2003), ratified in Guatemala in 1996, provided that "governments shall ensure that adequate health services are made available to the [indigenous] peoples concerned, or shall provide them with resources to allow them to design and deliver such services under their own responsibility and control, and take into account their traditional preventive care, healing practices and medicines."

More recently, the United Nations Declaration on the Rights of Indigenous Peoples stated that "indigenous peoples have the right to promote, develop and maintain their institutional structures and their distinctive customs, spirituality, traditions, procedures, practices and, in the cases where they exist, juridical systems or customs, in accordance with international human rights standards"

(UN 2007). Finally, the most recent WHO/PAHO initiative, the Strategy for Universal Access to Health and Universal Health Coverage (WHO/PAHO 2014), reaffirms the need for the transformation of health systems and services to combat health inequities and achieve health and well-being for all, based on the right to health:

> Universal access to health and universal health coverage imply that all people and communities have access, without any kind of discrimination, to comprehensive, appropriate and timely, quality health services determined at the national level according to needs… Universal access to health and universal health coverage require determining and implementing policies and actions with a multisectoral approach to address the social determinants of health and promote a society-wide commitment to fostering health and wellbeing. The right to health is the core value of universal health coverage, to be promoted and protected without distinction of age, ethnic group, race, sex, gender, sexual orientation, language, religion, political or other opinions, national or social origin, economic position, birth, or any other status.

25.9 Interculturality: Linking Systems of Knowledge and Practice

Guatemala has passed laws recognizing the rights of indigenous peoples to their cultural identity. These have included: the Law for Healthy Motherhood Decree 32-2010 (articles 2 and 4); the Health Code Acts 18 and 61; the Peace Accords of 1996 clauses pertaining to indigenous and traditional medicine; the Law of Languages (articles 14 and 15); and the Ministerial Agreement 1632-2009 to create the Health Care Unit for Indigenous Peoples and Interculturality in Guatemala. Through this legal framework, the Ministry of Health has made efforts to address the sociocultural factors that affect maternal health service utilization. Hence in 2009, the Guatemalan Ministry of Health in collaboration with the U.S. Agency for International Development (USAID) Health Policy Initiative and the Guatemalan Indigenous Women's Network in Reproductive Health (*Red de Organizaciones de Mujeres Indígenas por la Salud Reproductiva*) put forth recommendations for the establishment of a pluralistic medical model that would incorporate both biomedical and Mayan beliefs and practices in maternal health programs (MSPAS 2009, 2011). Specific recommendations included giving women the choice between *comadrona*-assisted versus physician-assisted deliveries, facilitating the practice of vertical childbearing, and providing women with the option to wear traditional clothes and eat traditional foods, especially those considered vital around the time of childbirth.

However, recommended practices have failed to be integrated into most health care practices nationwide, and programs intended to integrate traditional medicine into the health professional student curriculum have not been implemented, largely blocked by the hegemonic, biomedical model that fails to recognize the added value of the Mayan medical model (PIES de Occidente 2009). Moreover, when it has occurred, the incorporation of elements of Mayan medicine into formal health services has been criticized as superficial, focusing on the isolated insertion of discrete medical practices (i.e., the use of medicinal plants or of the *temascal*, or the presence of *comadronas*), disconnected from their philosophical underpinnings of how indigenous populations relate to life, health and illness, through their relationships with the individual, the family, the collective, and the cosmos (PIES de Occidente 2009). This omission is critical; not understanding that the Mayan medical system is systemic leads to fragmented, disconnected actions echoing Mayan medical practices yet disconnected from a more complex reality. A health system that welcomes and promotes the presence of different cultures present in society, including their respective beliefs, customs, practices, and ways of life (folkways), still falls short if it fails to ensure equality among those cultures or promote mutual learning.

Indeed, intercultural relevance, or interculturality (*interculturalidad*), goes beyond merely recognizing the existence of different cultures. Rather, intercultural approaches seek to develop an equal, horizontal, reciprocal relationship between culturally distinct individuals, populations, departing with historical asymmetries in social, economic, and political power to actively promote the construction of spaces of encounter where listening and mutual enrichment about different ways of life can occur (Cunningham 2009; MMN 2013; Walsh 2005). An intercultural approach is based on dialogue, where both parties are heard and speak, and where each takes what can be taken from the other, or simply respects their uniqueness and individuality. The goal is not to impose or to subjugate, but to harmonize.

Within the realm of health care, an intercultural approach implies articulating within a single health system diverse health models, be they institutional or community-based, starting with a relationship that is respectful rather than subordinating. An encounter or dialogue between actors from different sociocultural frameworks becomes necessary, not only to eliminate discrimination, but also to ensure the right to health of traditionally marginalized groups and achieve greater local relevance and effectiveness of health actions (MMN 2013). Moreover, promoting indigenous systems of medicine enhances the self-esteem of its practitioners, strengthens indigenous identity, and increases populations' confidence in the official health system because their beliefs are respected and their sociocultural illnesses are not only recognized but also addressed (Cunningham 2009). In practice, this implies that both Western and indigenous health systems should be practiced with equal human, technological, and financial resources, with spaces for exchange of knowledge, methodologies, and practices that ensure the ongoing development of both systems. Hence an intercultural approach is not about inserting Mayan medicine into the formal health system. Rather, it has to do with how both systems can work jointly. The challenge lies in creating enabling conditions for such a relationship, which involves changing official, institutionalized conceptual frameworks.

25.10 Looking Ahead

With the health system on the brink of collapse due to its historically weak leadership capacity, the lack of government financing, and the national health crisis that followed dismantling of the PEC, leaving one-quarter of its population without health coverage, promising changes have occurred with the appointment in August 2016 of a new executive team to the leadership of the MSPAS, led by the Health Minister Dra. Lucrecia Hernández Mack. This team has shown clear technical capacity, capacity for strategic planning, and political commitment to reach Guatemala's rural, indigenous population. Under their leadership, the Inclusive Health Model (*Modelo Incluyente de Salud*) will be implemented throughout the country as the official health care model for the first level of care.

For decades, the standard of primary care in rural Guatemala had been a network of Ministry of Health posts and health centers that offer basic primary care services. As discussed earlier, in 1997, the MSPAS had initiated the now defunct PEC, an ambulatory model of primary health care services contracted to NGOs to extend services to underserved areas. In reaction to this, concerned that the PEC would do little to address the needs of the majority rural, indigenous population, a coalition of grassroots organizations called the *Instancia Nacional de Salud* (INS), with the support of *Medicus Mundi Navarra*, began work in 1998 to develop the Inclusive Health Model, designed specifically for the Guatemalan context (INS 2002). This coalition was intent to explicitly address intercultural and gender equality given the systematic exclusion of Mayans, rural peasants, and women from social development programs in Guatemala (Fort et al. 2011).

The Inclusive Health Model, initially piloted in 2002–2007 in the departments of Sololá and Quetzaltenango and later extended to Huehuetenango and Baja Verapaz, has emerged as a long-term strategy to promote a rights-based approach to comprehensive and inclusive care aimed at reducing inequities, in line with the national and international legal framework for addressing the health of women and indigenous populations. Their strategy for the linking of knowledge between formal and Mayan health systems is based on "coordination in parallel." This strategy considers the knowledge, understanding, and strengthening of traditional health models; identification and systematization of sociocultural epidemiological profiles; coordination and horizontal exchange with traditional healers; and the implementation of integrated actions of intercultural relevance at the individual, family, and community levels (MMN 2013). The model has proven to be effective in universalizing attention to all life cycles and in reducing maternal mortality, neonatal and infant mortality, thanks to the real articulation it achieves between individuals, families, communities, indigenous healers, and *comadronas*, among others (Fort et al. 2011; ISIS 2009).

Although institutional change present immense challenges, these positive recent developments represent a very significant step forward in achieving the provision of high-quality, culturally safe care to Guatemala's rural, indigenous population, and a much-needed shift within the MSPAS and the country's health care system. It will be critical that these actions be sustained within a political and programmatic framework.

Conclusions

The colonial thinking behind a hegemonic biomedical model of health care has limited efforts aimed at reducing the high rates of maternal and infant mortality in indigenous populations of Guatemala. There is a strong need within Guatemala's rural, indigenous populations for maternal and child health to be deliberately approached from an inclusive, integral, and multidimensional concept of health and well-being—one that recognizes the existence of diverse perceptions, concepts, knowledge, and practices relevant to health and well-being that form part of people's culture and realms of action not only at the individual but also at the collective level. Of particular importance to the local world of indigenous populations, an individualized, biomedical approach must give way to a bio-psycho-social-environmental approach contiguous across different levels of care, that can be firmly grounded in local needs and address the determinants of health constantly acting and interacting at the individual, family, and community levels and across the life cycle.

While maternal and child health may be a priority, action must take place at diverse levels. Integrated health interventions that include social organization and participation are needed to impact public policies and social determinants of health. A priority is to create the enabling conditions for the appropriate involvement of—and coordination with—indigenous healers, including *comadronas*, who play a fundamental role within their communities in the realm of reproductive health and throughout the reproductive cycle. Further, coordination across systems and healers would facilitate the identification and appropriate referral of high-risk pregnancies. Guaranteeing culturally safe spaces within health care institutions would help women choose the health care setting most suited to her needs during pregnancy and childbirth and access formal services for emergency obstetric care. Finally, transcending the hegemonic model of health and learning from other systems will help generate innovative, decolonized discourses and transfer of knowledge, enabling that all peoples can benefit from the ancestral knowledge of indigenous populations and a health system rooted in an integrated approach to the human being and its relationship with nature and the cosmos.

Acknowledgements The authors would like to thank the many women, midwives, and other individuals and institutions that shared their experiences, personal stories, and ancestral knowledge over the years, and greatly informed the writing of this chapter and the points of view expressed. We extend a special acknowledgment to the women of *Buena Semilla*, to the midwives of the *Asociación de Comadronas del Área Mam* (ACAM) and to the *Instituto de Salud Incluyente*. We would also like to thank Dr. Lucy Manchester and *Health Policy Initiatives* whose invaluable research provided several of the quotes that were used to illustrate women's experiences. Last but not least, we wish to thank our editor, Dr. David Schwartz, for inviting us to contribute to this important book.

References

Adams, W. R., & Hawkins, J. P. (2007). *Health care in Maya Guatemala: Confronting medical pluralism in a developing country*. Norman: University of Oklahoma Press.

Alianza Nacional de Organizaciones de Mujeres Indígenas por la Salud Reproductiva (ALIANMISAR). (2009). La salud reproductiva de la mujer indígena en Guatemala. Análisis situacional y necesidades. ALIANMISAR, Health Policy Initiatives (HPI), United States Agency for International Development (USAID). Power Point presentation to the Ministerio de Salud Publica y Asistencia Social (MSPAS), Guatemala, 17 June 2009.

Alma Ata. (1978). Informe Final de la Conferencia Internacional sobre Atención Primaria de Salud. Alma Ata, URSS, 6–12 September, 1978.

Anckermann, S., Dominguez, M., Soto, N., Kjaerulf, F., Berliner, P., & Mikkelsen, E. N. (2005). Psychosocial support to large numbers of traumatized people in post-conflict societies: An approach to community development in Guatemala. *J Community Appl Soc Psychol, 15*, 136–152.

Anonymous. (2014). *Guatemala: El haz y el envés de la impunidad y el miedo: las estrategias militar-empresarial-gubernamental contra la justicia y la resistencia*. Guatemala. Retrieved February 15, 2017, from http://www.albedrio.org/htm/documentos/GuatemalaImpunidadMiedo.pdf

Avila, C., Bright, R., Gutierrez, J., Hoadley, K., Manuel, C., Romero, N., & Rodriguez, M. P. (2015). *Guatemala health system assessment, August 2015*. Bethesda, MD: Health Finance & Governance Project, Abt Associates. Retrieved February 15, 2017, from https://www.usaid.gov/sites/default/files/documents/1862/Guatemala-HSA%20_ENG-FULL-REPORT-FINAL-APRIL-2016.pdf

Becerril-Montekio, V., & López-Dávila, L. (2011). The health system of Guatemala. *Salud Pública de México, 53*(S2), s197–s208.

Berry, N. (2006). Kaqchikel midwives, home births, and emergency obstetric referrals in Guatemala: Contextualizing the choice to stay at home. *Social Science and Medicine, 62*, 1958–1969.

Burrell, J. (2009). Intergenerational conflict in the postwar era. In W. E. Little & T. J. Smith (Eds.), *Mayas in Postwar Guatemala: Harvest of violence revisited*. Tuscaloosa: University of Alabama Press.

Cabrera LO, Rosales P, Echeverría G, Palma S, López S, Haeussler R, Calan M. Normas con Pertinencia Cultural… hacia la interculturalidad. Ministerio de Salud Publica y Asistencia Social, Departamento de Regulación de los Programas de Atención a las Personas, Guatemala, 2009.

Callister, L., & Vega, R. (1998). Giving birth: Guatemalan women's voices. *Journal of Obstetric, Gynecologic & Neonatal Nursing, 27*(3), 289–295.

Campbell, J., Dussault, G., Buchan, J., Pozo-Martin, F., Guerra Arias, M., Leone, C., et al. (2013). *A universal truth: No health without a workforce. Forum report, Third Global Forum on Human Resources for Health, Recife, Brazil*. Geneva: Global Health Workforce Alliance and World Health Organization. Retrieved February 15, 2017, from http://www.who.int/workforcealliance/knowledge/resources/GHWAa_universal_truth_report.pdf?ua=1

Canadian Institutes of Health Research (CIHR). (2007). *CIHR guidelines for health research involving aboriginal people*. Canadian Institutes of Health Research.

Chary, A., Kraemer Diaz, A., Henderson, B., & Rohloff, P. (2013). The changing role of indigenous lay midwives in Guatemala: New frameworks for analysis. *Midwifery, 29*(8), 852–858.

Chomat, A. M. (2016). Photovoice reveals narratives of hardship and resilience among rural *Mam*-Mayan women in the Western Highlands of Guatemala. In *Maternal stressors impact maternal wellbeing and cortisol and infant growth in rural Guatemala: Insights from qualitative and quantitative approaches*. Doctoral thesis dissertation, McGill University, Montreal.

Chomat, A. M., Solomons, N., Montenegro, G., Crowley, C., & Bermudez, O. (2014). Maternal health and health-seeking behaviors among indigenous Mam mothers from Quetzaltenango, Guatemala. *Revista Panamericana de Salud Publica, 35*(2), 113–120.

Chomat, A. M., Solomons, N. W., Koski, K. G., Wren, H. M., Vossenaar, M., & Scott, M. E. (2015). Quantitative methodologies reveal a diversity of nutrition, infection/illness and psychosocial stressors during pregnancy and lactation in rural *Mam*-Mayan mother-infant dyads from the Western Highlands of Guatemala. *Food Nutr Bull, 36*(4), 415–440.

Commission for Historical Clarification (CEH). (1999). *Guatemala memory of silence*. Report of the Commission for Historical Clarification: Conclusions and Recommendations. Retrieved February 15, 2017, https://hrdag.org/wp-content/uploads/2013/01/CEHreport-english.pdf

Commission on Social Determinants of Health (CSDH). (2008). *Closing the gap in a generation: Health equity through action on the social determinants of health*. Final Report of the Commission on Social Determinants of Health. Geneva: World Health Organization.

Cook, N. D. (1998). *Born to die: Disease and new world conquest, 1492–1650*. New York: Cambridge University Press.

Cosminsky, S. (2001a). Maya midwives of southern Mexico and Guatemala. In B. Huber & A. Sandstrom (Eds.), *Mesoamerican healers*. Austin: University of Texas Press.

Cosminsky, S. (2001b). Midwifery across the generations: A modernizing midwife in Guatemala. *Medical Anthropology, 20*(4), 345–378.
Cunningham, A. (1997). Introduction. In A. Cunningham & B. Andrews (Eds.), *Western medicine as contested knowledge* (pp. 1–23). New York: Manchester University Press.
Cunningham, M. (2009). *Health in state of the world's indigenous peoples*. Department of Economic and Social Affairs, Division for Social Policy and Development, Secretariat of the Permanent Forum on Indigenous Issues. United Nations, New York. Retrieved February 15, 2017, from http://www.un.org/esa/socdev/unpfii/documents/SOWIP/en/SOWIP_web.pdf
De Jonge, A., Teunissen, T. A., & Lagro-Janssen, A. L. (2004). Supine position compared to other positions during the second stage of labor: A meta-analytic review. *Journal of Psychosomatic Obstetrics and Gynaecology, 25*(1), 35–45.
Farmer, P. E., Nizeye, B., Stulac, S., & Keshavjee, S. (2006). Structural violence and clinical medicine. *PLoS Medicine, 3*(10), e449.
Few, M. (2002). *Women who live evil lives: Gender, religion and the politics of power in colonial Guatemala* (pp. 1650–1750). Austin, TX: University of Texas Press.
Fort, M. P., Grembowski, D. E., Verdugo, J. C., Morales, L. C., Arriaga, C. A., Mercer, M. A., & Lim, S. S. (2011). Implementation and progress of an inclusive primary health care model in Guatemala: Coverage, quality, and utilization. *Revista Panamericana de Salud Publica, 30*(3), 217–224.
Foxen, P. (2007). *In search of Providence: Transnational Mayan identities*. Nashville, TN: Vanderbilt University Press.
Galtung, J. (1969). Violence, peace and peace research. *Journal of Peace Research, 6*, 167–191.
Gardosi, J., Sylvester, S., & B-Lynch, C. (1989). Alternative positions in the second stage of labour: A randomized controlled trial. *British Journal of Obstetrics and Gynaecology, 96*, 1290–1296.
Girón Mena, M. A. (1979). Itzamna y la Medicina Maya. *Guatemala Indígena, 14*(3–4), 26–30.
Glei, D. A., & Goldman, N. (2000). Understanding ethnic variation in pregnancy-related care in rural Guatemala. *Ethnicity & Health, 5*(1), 5–22.
Godoy-Paiz, P. (2005). Obstacles to achieving mental health in post-war Guatemala: The intersection of political and structural violence. *The Canadian Student Journal of Anthropology, 18*(1), 34–64.
Gómez Bravo, N. (2010). *Cosmovision y ciencia de la vida del maiz*. Retrieved from http://documentslide.com/documents/cosmovision-y-ciencia-de-la-vida-del-maiz.html
Grandin, G., Levenson, D. T., & Oglesby, E. (2011). *The Guatemala reader: History, culture, politics*. Durham, NC: Duke University Press.
Green, L. (1999). *Fear as a way of life*. New York, NY: Columbia University Press.
Greenberg, L. (1982). Midwife training programs in highland Guatemala. *Social Science & Medicine, 16*, 1599–1609.
Grupo Internacional de Trabajo sobre Asuntos Indígenas (IWGIA). (2017). *Pueblos indígenas en Guatemala*. Retrieved February 15, 2017, from http://www.iwgia.org/regiones/latin-america/guatemala
Hogan, M. C., Foreman, K. J., Naghavi, M., Ahn, S. Y., Wang, M., Makela, S. M., Lopez, A. D., Lozano, R., & Murray, C. J. (2010). Maternal mortality for 181 countries, 1980–2008: A systematic analysis of progress towards Millennium Development Goal 5. *Lancet, 375*(9726), 1609–1623.
Humphrey, M., Hounslow, D., Morgan, S., & Wood, C. (1973). The influence of maternal posture at birth on the fetus. *Journal of Obstetrics & Gynaecology of the British Commonwealth, 80*, 1075–1080.
Hurtado, J. J. (1973). Algunas ideas para un modelo estructural en relación con la enfermedad en el altiplano de Guatemala. *Guatemala Indígena, 8*(1–2), 7–22.
Hurtado, E., & Saénz de Tejada, E. (2001). In B. Huber & A. Sandstrom (Eds.), *Relations between government health workers and traditional midwives in Guatemala. Mesoamerican healers*. Austin, TX: University of Texas Press.
Icú Perén, H. (2007). Revival of Maya medicine and impact for its social and political recognition (in Guatemala): A case study commissioned by the Health Systems Knowledge Network. Guatemala.
Instancia Nacional de Salud (INS). (2002). *Hacia un primer nivel de atención incluyente: bases y lineamientos*. Guatemala: INS. Retrieved March 6, 2017, from https://saludjalapa225.files.wordpress.com/2016/10/hacia-un-primer-nv-de-salud-incluyente.pdf
Instituto de Salud Incluyente (ISIS). (2009). El derecho a la Salud en el Modelo Incluyente de Salud. Documento Técnico. Guatemala: ISIS.
Instituto Nacional de Estadística (INE). (2012). *Caracterización Estadística de Guatemala, 2012*. Retrieved February 15, 2017, from http://www.ine.gob.gt/sistema/uploads/2014/02/26/5eTCcFlHErnaNVeUmm3iabXHaKgXtw0C.pdf
International Labour Organization (ILO). (2003). *ILO convention on indigenous and tribal peoples, 1989 (No. 169): A manual*. Geneva: ILO. Retrieved February 15, 2017, from http://pro169.org/res/materials/en/general_resources/Manual%20on%20ILO%20Convention%20No.%20169.pdf
Ishida, K., Stupp, P., Turcios-Ruiz, R., Williams, D., & Espinoza, E. (2012). Ethnic inequality in Guatemalan women's use of modern reproductive health care. *International Perspectives on Sexual and Reproductive Health, 38*(2), 99–108.

Kabeer, N. (2010). *Can the MDGS provide a pathway to social justice? The challenge of intersecting inequalities*. Institute of Development Studies, MDG Achievement Fund. United Nations Development Programme. Retrieved February 15, 2017, from www.ids.ac.uk/files/dmfile/MDGreportwebstiteu2WC.pdf

Kipuri, N. (2009). Culture. In: *State of the world's indigenous peoples*. Department of Economic and Social Affairs, Division for Social Policy and Development, Secretariat of the Permanent Forum on Indigenous Issues, United Nations. Retrieved February 15, 2017, from http://www.un.org/esa/socdev/unpfii/documents/SOWIP/en/SOWIP_web.pdf

Kurtenbach, S. (2008). *Guatemala's post-war development: The structural failure of low intensity peace*. Germany: Institute for Development and Peace (INEF). Retrieved February 15, 2017, from http://citeseerx.ist.psu.edu/viewdoc/download?doi=10.1.1.465.4544&rep=rep1&type=pdf

Macleod, M. (2013). Mayan calendrics in movement in Guatemala: Mayan spiritual guides or day-keepers understandings of 2012. *Journal of Latin American and Caribbean Anthropology, 18*(3), 447–464.

Medicus Mundi Navarra (MMN). (2013). *Claves para la transformación de los sistemas de salud en América Latina*. Bolivia, Guatemala y Perú: tres experiencias, una sola acción integral e incluyente en atención primaria de salud. Salud Integral Incluyente. Retrieved February 15, 2017, http://www.saludintegralincluyente.com/ftp/saludintegralincluyente/DOCUMENTOS/PDF/Libro/LIBROsaludintegralincluyente.WEB.pdf

Medicus Mundi Navarra (MMN). (2016). Protocolo de Sistematización Avances de La Horizontalización Programática en Cuatro Países Latinoamericanos.

Metz, B. (2001). Politics, population and family planning in Guatemala: Ch'orti' Maya experiences. *Human Organization, 60*(3), 259–271.

Ministerio de Salud Publica y Asistencia Social (MSPAS). (2009). *Normas con Pertinencia Cultural... hacia la interculturalidad*. MSPAS, Departamento de Regulación de los Programas de Atención a las Personas: Guatemala. Retrieved March 6, 2017, from http://www.paho.org/gut/index.php?option=com_docman&view=download&alias=570-2011-normas-con-pertinancia-cultural&category_slug=sfc-salud-reproductiva-materna-y-neonatal-nacional&Itemid=518

Ministerio de Salud Pública y Asistencia Social (MSPAS). (2011). *Manual de adecuación cultural del parto natural/vertical y sus distintas posiciones, en el marco multicultural de Guatemala*. En colaboración con la Alianza Nacional de Organizaciones de Mujeres Indígenas por la Salud Reproductiva (ALIANMISAR), Organización Panamericana de la Salud (PAHO), Population Council: Guatemala. Retrieved February 15, 2017, from http://www.paho.org/gut/index.php?option=com_docman&view=download&alias=569-2011-manual-de-adecuacion-cultural-del-parto-natural-vertical&category_slug=sfc-salud-reproductiva-materna-y-neonatal-nacional&Itemid=518

Ministerio de Salud Pública y Asistencia Social (MSPAS). (2015a). *Encuesta Nacional de Salud Materno Infantil 2014–15 (ENSMI)*. Informe Final: Mujeres. MSPAS/Instituto Nacional de Estadística (INE)/Centros de Control y Prevención de Enfermedades (CDC): Guatemala.

Ministerio de Salud Pública y Asistencia Social (MSPAS). (2015b). *Situación de la mortalidad maternal: Informe de País 2013*. Guatemala. Retrieved January 26 2017, from http://www.osarguatemala.org/Archivos/PDF/201510/255_3.pdf

Ministerio de Salud Pública y Asistencia Social (MSPAS)/Pan American Health Organization (PAHO). (2013). *Segunda Medición de Metas Regionales de Recursos Humanos para la Salud: Informe Final*. Guatemala. Retrieved February 15, 2017, from http://www.observatoriorh.org/sites/default/files/webfiles/fulltext/2013/informe_metas_2013_gua.pdf

Montenegro, R. A., & Stephens, C. (2006). Indigenous health in Latin America and the Caribbean. *Lancet, 367*, 1859–1869.

Mumtaz, Z., Salway, S., Bhatti, A., & McIntyre, L. (2014). Addressing invisibility, inferiority and powerlessness to achieve gains in maternal health for ultra-poor women. *Lancet, 383*, 1095–1097.

Napier, A. D., Ancarno, C., Butler, B., Calabrese, J., Chater, A., Chatterjee, H., et al. (2014). Culture and health. *Lancet, 384*, 1607–1639.

PIES de Occidente. (2014). Encuentro de Comadronas: La comadrona tradicional: Obstáculo o solución a la problemática materno-infantil en regiones de pobreza extrema, exclusión y marginación? Tercera edición. Litografía de Occidente, Guatemala. Retrieved February 15, 2017, from http://asociacionpiesdeoccidente.org/assets/la-comadrona-tradicional-obt%C3%A1culo-o-soluci%C3%B3n-a-la-problematica.pdf

OECD (Organization for Economic Co-operation and Development). (2015). Revenue Statistics in Latin America and the Caribbean.

Oxorn, H. (1986). *Human labor and birth*. University of Ottawa, ON: McGraw-Hill Professional Publishing.

Packard, R. M. (2013). Post-colonial medicine. In R. A. Cooter (Ed.), *Companion encyclopedia of medicine in the twentieth century* (pp. 97–112). New York: Routledge.

Pan American Health Organization (PAHO)/World Health Organization (WHO). (1985). *Informe del Grupo de Trabajo sobre Salud y Culturas Médicas Tradicionales en América Latina y el Caribe* (p. 5). Washington, DC.

Paul, L. (1978). Careers of midwives in a Mayan community. In J. Hoch-Smith & A. Springs (Eds.), *Women in ritual and symbolic roles*. New York, NY: Plenum Press.

PIES de Occidente. (2009). *Conociendo la medicina Maya en Guatemala*. Asociación PIES de Occidente: Guatemala. Retrieved February 15, 2017, from http://asociacionpiesdeoccidente.org/assets/conociendo-la-medicina-maya-en-guatemala.pdf

Radoff, K., Thompson, L. M., Bly, K., & Romero, C. (2013). Practices related to postpartum uterine involution in the Western Highlands of Guatemala. *Midwifery, 29*(3), 225–232.

Recino, A. (Translation Quiche to Spanish), Goetz, D., Morley, S.G. (Translation Spanish to English). (1954). *Popul Vuh. The Book of the People*. Los Angeles: Plantin Press.

Roberts, C. L., Algert, C. S., Cameron, C. A., & Torvaldsen, S. (2005). A meta-analysis of upright positions in the second stage to reduce instrumental deliveries in women with epidural analgesia. *Acta Obstetricia et Gynecologica Scandinavica, 84*(8), 794–798.

Rogoff, B. (2011a). Born to a spiritual calling across generations: Cultural heritage and resistance. In *Developing Destinies: A Mayan Midwife and Town*. Oxford, UK: Oxford University Press.

Rogoff, B. (2011b). Ripples across generations and nations in birth destinies and postnatal care. In *Developing Destinies: A Mayan Midwife and Town*. Oxford, UK: Oxford University Press.

Rogoff, B. (2011c). Ripples across generations and nations in Mayan pregnancy and childbirth. In *Developing Destinies: A Mayan Midwife and Town*. Oxford, UK: Oxford University Press.

Rohloff, P., Díaz, A. K., & Dasgupta, S. (2011). "Beyond development": A critical appraisal of the emergence of small health care nongovernmental organizations in rural Guatemala. *Human Organization, 70*(4), 427–437.

Santiso-Galvez, R., & Bertrand, J. T. (2004). The delayed contraceptive revolution in Guatemala. *Human Organization, 63*(1), 57–67.

Schieber, B., & Delgado, H. (1993). *An intervention to reduce maternal and neonatal mortality*. Guatemala City, Guatemala: Instituto de Nutrición de Centro América y Panamá (INCAP) and Pan American Health Organization (PAHO).

Shiffman, J., & Garces del Valle, A. L. (2006). Political history and disparities in safe motherhood between Guatemala and Honduras. *Population and Development Review, 32*(1), 53–80.

Stephens, C., Porter, J., Nettleton, C., & Willis, R. (2006). Disappearing, displaced and undervalued: A call to action for indigenous health worldwide. *Lancet, 367*, 2019–2028.

Sullivan, T. (1966). Pregnancy, childbirth, and the deification of women who died in childbirth. *Estudios de cultura Nahuatl* (pp. 128–143). Texts from the Florentine Codex, Book IV, Folios.

United Nations Development Programme (UNDP). (2014). *Human development report: Guatemala*. Retrieved February 15, 2017, from http://hdr.undp.org/sites/all/themes/hdr_theme/country-notes/GTM.pdf

United Nations Organization. (2007). *Declaration on the rights of indigenous peoples*. UN Doc. A/61/L.67. Retrieved February 15, 2017, from http://www.un.org/esa/socdev/unpfii

United States Agency for International Development (USAID). (2009). *Gender assessment in Guatemala*. USAID. Retrieved February 15, 2017, from http://pdf.usaid.gov/pdf_docs/Pnado177.pdf

Van Dijk, M., Ruiz, M. J., Letona, D., & García, S. G. (2013). Ensuring intercultural maternal health care for Mayan women in Guatemala: A qualitative assessment. *Culture, Health & Sexuality: An International Journal for Research, Intervention and Care, 15*(S3), S365–S382.

Villatoro, E. (1994). La comadrona a través de la historia en las practicas obstretico pediatricas: una experiencia en el area ixil, quiché. *La Tradicion Popular, 97*, 20.

Villatoro, E. (2001). Promoción de la medicina y terapias indígenas en la atención primaria de salud: el caso de los Mayas en Guatemala. Organización de Promoción, Investigación y Educación de Salud (PIES) de Occidente, Organización Panamericana de la Salud, Organización Mundial de la Salud: Washington, DC.

Walsh, C. (2005). Interculturalidad, conocimientos y decolonialidad. perspectivas y convergencias. *Signo y Pensamiento, 46*, 40–50.

Walsh, L. V. (2006). Beliefs and rituals in traditional birth attendant practice in Guatemala. *Journal of Transcultural Nursing, 17*(2), 148–154.

World Bank. (2009). *Guatemala—Poverty assessment: Good performance at low levels*. Washington DC: World Bank. Retrieved February 15, 2017, from http://documents.worldbank.org/curated/en/803331468254934801/Guatemala-Poverty-assessment-good-performance-at-low-levels

World Bank. (2016). *Guatemala country overview*. Accessed 15 Feb 2017, from http://www.worldbank.org/en/country/guatemala/overview#1.

World Health Organization (WHO). (1978). *Promoción y Desarrollo de la Medicina Tradicional, Serie de Informes Técnicos, 622*. Geneva: WHO.

World Health Organization (WHO). (2014). *World Health Statistics 2014*. Retrieved February 15, 2017, from http://apps.who.int/iris/bitstream/10665/112738/1/9789240692671_eng.pdf?ua=1

World Health Organization (WHO), Pan American Health Organization (PAHO). (2014). *Strategy for universal access to health and universal health coverage*. Retrieved February 15, 2017, from http://www.paho.org/uhexchange/index.php/en/uhexchange-documents/technical-information/26-strategy-for-universal-access-to-health-and-universal-health-coverage/file

World Health Organization (WHO), United Nations Children's Fund (UNICEF), United Nations Population Fund (UNFPA), World Bank (1990–2010). (2012). *Trends in maternal mortality. WHO, UNICEF, UNFPA and the World Bank estimates*. WHO: Geneva. Retrieved February 15, 2017, from http://apps.who.int/iris/bitstream/10665/44874/1/9789241503631_eng.pdf

26 Emergency Obstetrical Planning in Rural Guatemala: A Case Study

Beth Hallowell

26.1 Introduction

This chapter is a story about what happens when care providers try to prevent obstetrical emergencies in rural Guatemala—and why anthropology is crucial to understanding the unexpected challenges they face in doing so. Some of the usual suspects that thwart public health planning efforts in impoverished places have a role to play in this story, like the lack of healthcare facilities, and patients' inability to access the healthcare facilities that do exist. But as I show in the story that follows, the lack of healthcare or the inaccessibility of care is not the whole story. Instead, I use anthropological data to explore how postwar forms of governance that are emerging across the Americas collide with peoples' daily lived experiences to shift what counts as "the right thing to do" in a medical emergency, who is responsible for doing the right thing, and when the right thing should happen. Without anthropology, I argue, we would never be able to see—let alone understand—how and why this happens.

This chapter is divided into five sections. I will first set the scene by describing the ethnographic context for this research: The geographic landscape within which Santiago Atitlán is located, the broader social context that shapes daily life there, and the landscape of maternity care in Sololá, the department where Santiago sits. I will then review some of the anthropological literature to help set the theoretical scene for the argument that follows: Namely, that planning for an obstetrical emergency is a form of governance that seeks to rearrange social, temporal, and moral relationships in rural Guatemala. The reason that it doesn't "just work" is because this model of care is bumping against a whole host of preexisting factors, like social inequality and local notions of responsibility and, especially, of safety and danger. Anthropological methods, I argue, help us to see this conflict from a unique perspective: That of the many different care providers who take responsibility for mothers' well-being in Santiago.

This is not to say that public health or biomedicine has gotten it wrong. Rather, I argue that looking through an ethnographic lens helps any scholar or practitioner to see new things about a particular context, whether that context is familiar or foreign. Doing so can help scholars and practitioners alike

B. Hallowell, Ph.D.
University of Pennsylvania (former affiliation), Philadelphia, PA, USA

D. A. Schwartz (ed.), *Maternal Death and Pregnancy-Related Morbidity Among Indigenous Women of Mexico and Central America*, Global Maternal and Child Health: Medical, Anthropological, and Public Health Perspectives, https://doi.org/10.1007/978-3-319-71538-4_26

develop a more nuanced understanding of the lived realities that shape caregiving and patient-hood. In the conclusion, I offer three takeaways for care providers working in any country who are interested in understanding better how an anthropological perspective can contribute to public health and help improve medical care (Hallowell 2014).

26.2 Why Is It So Hard to Prevent Maternal Mortality?

Most of the time, maternal mortality is preventable (Schwartz 2015; World Health Organization 2015). Yet, this public health problem continues, primarily affecting poor women in rural areas. Considerable work has been done to decrease the maternal mortality rate, in particular by preventing or mitigating obstetrical emergencies with timely healthcare interventions (Mahler 1987; Benagiano and Thomas 2003; Freedman et al. 2007).

While these efforts have had important successes, anthropologists have documented some of the implementation barriers that these interventions have faced, and their iatrogenic effects (Allen 2004; Berry 2010). Throughout, anthropologists have shown that concepts like "safe birth" and "obstetrical emergency" are not universally held, but rather context- and culture-dependent. Specifically, anthropologists have shown that when these concepts are transported from a Euro-American public health planning context to a new social context, like rural Guatemala in the early twenty-first century, they can break down. In this chapter, I demonstrate that as emergency plans to prevent obstetrical emergencies become an increasingly important part of local maternity care in rural Guatemala, we can see new shifts in social and moral relationships take place. This is because of shifts in national and transnational "reproductive governance" in the Americas unfolding today (Morgan and Roberts 2012).

As social theorist Elaine Scarry has shown (2011), contemporary "thinking in an emergency" means that if something is deemed an emergency, it becomes the most urgent and important thing in the world. Contemporary ethics across the Western world hold that systems need to exist to prevent or mitigate emergencies, and constructing these systems occupies an important place in the contemporary role of sovereign states. As a result, preventing emergencies becomes an important cultural norm, shaping social relationships, moral responsibility, and individuals' actions. In the context of a medical emergency, the norm is to stop a medical emergency, or get someone in a medical emergency to the proper authorities (usually a doctor), before anything else can happen. In the USA, examples include Good Samaritan laws that protect people who try to intervene in emergency situations, to encourage everyday citizens to take action if they see someone having a heart attack or witness a car accident. As well, norms of individualism and self-reliance mean that individuals in the USA are also expected to prevent emergencies or help themselves out of an emergency situation. A common parable in the USA tells of a man who knows that a flood is coming. He prays to God to protect him from the rising floodwaters. As he is a praying, someone rows up to his house in a boat and tells him to get in. The man refuses, saying that he is a faithful man and he knows that God will hear his prayers. Then, a rescue team in a second boat rows up to the man's house, and they beg him to get in. Again the man refuses, telling them that God will save him. Finally a third boat comes along, this time as the water is rising above the man's house. Again the man refuses to get in, saying that God will answer his prayers of rescue. When the water subsumes the man's house, he is killed and goes to heaven. The man arrives, angry with God for not saving him from the flood. "I sent you three boats," God explains, "and you refused to save yourself. What more did you want from me?" This parable reflects the US cultural norm that people are expected to save themselves from obvious emergencies. As you read the story about obstetrical emergencies that follows, consider that Good Samaritan laws and imperatives to save oneself from an impending emergency are cultural norms and not moral absolutes. Suspending judgment in this way helps to explain why preventing obstetrical emergencies is harder than it seems, despite decades of public health planning, training, and efforts to make it more straightforward. Suspending judgment in this way also suggests new ways to improve maternity care in Guatemala and elsewhere.

This chapter is intended to help students and practitioners from a variety of health-related disciplines—medicine, nursing, public health, and allied fields—think about rural maternal health in Guatemala in new ways. Even for students who have never or will never travel to rural Guatemala, my hope is that this chapter helps readers learn to be open to the idea that people who don't share one's own cultural norms or background may have assumptions, thoughts, feelings, and constraints that make it difficult to see. This is especially important to consider when working in healthcare or public health because typically, the important work that healthcare providers and public health practitioners do affects people's lives in sometimes intimate ways. Helping people, as I will show in what follows, is not always a straightforward thing to do. In the case of maternal health and obstetrical emergencies in rural Guatemala, international, national, and local-level interventions to save mothers and babies from preventable causes of death is enmeshed in deeply rooted social inequalities that are sometimes difficult to see. Indeed, as I observed in the field, these inequalities shift moral responsibility for poor maternal outcomes onto poor pregnant women and their poorly resourced, frontline caregivers. They also place caregivers in the position of having to fill in the gaps of a broken healthcare system, while also positioning biomedical birth as the primary outcome of moral behavior. Attending to these cultural dynamics can help us understand what may seem like counterproductive health behaviors, as when midwives do not make referrals for high-risk pregnant women.

26.3 Maternity Care in Santiago Atitlán

The maternity-care system in rural Guatemala is a mix of public health centers and private hospitals, staffed by nurses and doctors and occasionally other health professionals such as social workers. In addition, independent midwives practice throughout the region. These women—they are always women—may or may not be affiliated with an institution, and they may or may not have formal midwifery training. These providers work alongside and sometimes in conjunction with a variety of maternal healthcare programs run by the government, nongovernmental organizations (NGOs), and a myriad of international actors from the United Nations to universities. Within this heterogeneous caregiving landscape, many scholars have documented how midwives play a hugely important role in providing prenatal care, referring women to biomedical care providers, delivering babies, following up with women and newborns to provide antenatal care, translating both linguistically (between indigenous languages and Spanish) and culturally between patients and biomedical care providers, and by providing any number of ancillary caregiving services before, during, and after birth, such as housecleaning or care for older children (Cosminsky 1977; Maupin 2008; Berry 2010). Historically, they have also played a role as spiritual or social leaders, able to cut across traditional lines of race and class (Paul and Paul 1975). Because of these important and interlinking roles, they are often the target of government and NGO interventions to change caregiving practices or improve maternal health (Goldman and Glei 2003; Hinojosa 2004; Maupin 2008). Yet, these same actors often blame midwives for the many shortcomings of the system. This is because of their precarious status within the biomedical landscape—they are not typically considered formal providers, and they usually have less formal education than the nurses and doctors they work with—as well as their gender and race (Cosminsky 2012).

As maternal mortality became an increasingly important public health goal at the international level towards the end of the twentieth century, even becoming one of the World Health Organization's Millennium Development Goals (MDGs) in 2000, traditional birth attendants (TBAs) around the world became the targets of public health interventions, most notably through the Safe Motherhood International program. While decreasing maternal mortality is certainly an important public health goal, anthropologists have documented that the programs designed to reach this goal came at a cost. In Guatemala in particular, this cost was the devaluation of indigenous ways of birthing. Because Safe Motherhood emphasized hospital birth over home birth, the program and its implementers downplayed the importance of home birth to forming kinship relations and senses of family and self within indigenous Guatemalan families. Put another way, Safe Motherhood emphasized a western biomedical notion of safety—that is, hospital birth—over local women's family values (Berry 2010). What's more, research has shown that this program put birthing women in harm's way, albeit unintentionally. Because this initiative took the short view of safety, defining safety as a safe hospital birth attended by a formally educated healthcare provider, it ignored other kinds of safety that pregnant women sought: Safety from discrimination, for example, as well as economic safety. Safe Motherhood programs ignored the fact that many indigenous Guatemalan women and their families experienced racism and abuse within hospital settings. These programs also failed to account for the incredible costs associated with hospital care: Paying for the taxi or truck to get to the hospital, lost wages from missed work for accompanying family members, having to find childcare for older children left at home, and of course paying the actual hospital bill were often prohibitive expenses that could be detrimental to low-income and even middle-income rural families (Berry 2006, 2008).

26.4 A Note About Terminology

In this chapter, I use the Spanish term *comadrona* and the English term midwife interchangeably. *Comadrona* is the term most often used in Santiago to mean a woman who provides prenatal and postpartum care, as well as catches babies at pregnant women's homes. Typically, *comadronas* in Guatemala learn midwifery via apprenticeship to an older *comadrona*. They also typically attend trainings like the ones I observed during my fieldwork, and many of them have their own children. Unlike nurse-midwives in the United States, *comadronas* do not typically attend nursing school or receive a formal education in midwifery. Anthropologists have documented in considerable detail how midwifery in Guatemala has changed over time (Cosminsky 2001), while far less has been written about the sociocultural aspects of nursing or doctoring in Guatemala (Hallowell 2014).

26.5 Human Reproduction Through an Anthropological Lens

Anthropological methods have long contributed to our understandings of birth and the body. From Brigitte Jordan's ground-breaking work on birth across different cultures (1978), through Robbie Davis-Floyd's oeuvre documenting the different cultural models of obstetricians, midwives, and pregnant women in the USA (1990, 1994, 2004), medical anthropologists have helped to demonstrate how and why birth is understood in a myriad of socially situated ways. This is to say that medical anthropologists have shown birth to be far from a universal experience that remains constant across time and space. Rather, anthropologists have rigorously documented how peoples' understandings of what birth "is" changes as the result of shifts from colonial to postcolonial nation-states (e.g., Van Hollen 2003), and from wartime to postwar regimes (e.g., Chapman 2010). These scholars have shown that birth has not in fact "always" been viewed as risky business despite this common narrative in US biomedicine.

Rather, the framework of medical risk is only one way to understand pregnancy and birth, and this framework is tied to larger political and economic shifts in the twentieth century (Fordyce and Maraesa 2012)—not the least of which is the rise of the health insurance industry and the medical liability system in the USA (Hallowell 2015). In so doing, these scholars have contributed to our understanding of birth and the pregnant body as something that changes across time and place. Perhaps anthropologists' greatest contributions in this area have been to show that all of these things are deeply influenced by social dynamics like race and racism (Bridges 2011; Gutiérrez 2008; Roberts 2012), economic inequality (Hallowell 2015), and gender and sexuality (Mamo 2007).

In the Guatemalan case specifically, anthropology helps us see that shifts in how powerful actors seek to influence reproduction via local interventions—"reproductive governance"—and turn-of-the-century "emergency thinking"—where states increasingly rely upon emergency planning systems to shore up their own sovereignty—form the cultural framework through which care providers in Santiago learn to place such a premium on planning for obstetrical emergencies (Hallowell 2014). "Reproductive governance" (Morgan and Roberts 2012) is the idea that powerful actors—like nation-states, churches, economic institutions, and NGOs—have a vested interest in how reproduction happens. These actors use the tools at their disposal—such as public policy, incentives, messaging, and even violence—to govern people's bodies. Why do they care? Different actors care for many different reasons. For example, states invest in children's health through national insurance programs and vaccination campaigns to promote healthy families. At the same time, however, these investments are uneven: In the Americas, these investments often differ greatly along racial and economic lines (Gutiérrez 2008; Bridges 2011; Roberts 2012; Hallowell 2015). In this chapter, I argue that anthropological methods show us that one key part of contemporary reproductive governance in Guatemala is something feminist scholars have called "emergency thinking" (Scarry 2011). By emergency thinking, I mean the increasingly narrow focus that planning and action take on when the idea of an emergency is invoked. As I have documented elsewhere, emergency thinking shapes maternity care in a variety of contexts (Hallowell 2015), not just in Guatemala. In this case, emergency thinking is part of a system of reproductive governance that rearranges social and temporal relationships in order to prevent one kind of emergency—maternal death—while ignoring or downplaying the social ripple effects that take place as a result. By treating every woman's pregnancy as a potential emergency, care providers, patients, patients' families, and the health systems of which they are a part learn to see women's bodies and to act in particular ways instead of seeing alternatives.

Why are these contributions important to understanding public health in general, and to understanding the challenges to improving maternal health in rural Guatemala in particular? Because culture shapes how everyone behaves, patients and providers included. Indeed, biomedicine's "culture of no culture" (Taylor 2003) deeply impacts how care providers see themselves as well as how patients see them. Anthropology at its best helps to explain how social systems like biomedicine work empirically, on the ground, in real people's everyday lives. Significantly, it can also show how and why these systems break down: For example, why women in Guatemala who have high-risk pregnancies and the midwives who know they need help still have difficulty going to a hospital (Berry 2010). Put another way, epidemiologists are experts at capturing population-level incidence rates of maternal mortality; public health planners are experts at developing and implementing care models to decrease maternal mortality rates; and obstetricians are experts at the medical interventions necessary to save the lives of pregnant women in medical distress. Anthropologists, for their part, are experts at explaining how and why pregnant women and the people who care for them—like the *comadronas* in Guatemala—sometimes contest public health plans or aspects of medical care, go along with others, or act in ways that seem to the epidemiologist or public health planner or obstetrician to be totally counterintuitive, even dangerous. Why do some women or some *comadronas* seem to put themselves at a high risk for obstetrical emergency, even maternal death, when there are safe hospitals readily available as the result of huge amounts of international funding over many decades? This is the kind of question that anthropologists are good at answering. In the Guatemalan case, the answer has everything to do with how the ideas of minimizing obstetrical risk or averting an obstetrical emergency are at odds with other concerns that people have, other crises that they face, and other values that they hold dear.

26.6 Methodology

To conduct the research for my original pilot study, I spent 2 months in the summer of 2010 in Santiago Atitlán, in central-western Guatemala (Fig. 26.1). Santiago is a medium-sized town, located a few hours by car or bus west of the capital, Guatemala City. A popular tourist destination due to its incredible natural beauty—a crater lake ringed by mountains (Fig. 26.2)—the Lake Atitlán region draws visitors from around the world. It was also the site of some of the Guatemalan civil war's worst atrocities, and markers of that history, including gravestones and memorials, are still apparent throughout the area.

Tzutujil is the most common indigenous language heard in Santiago specifically. It is a Mayan language which is spoken by the *Tzutujil* people in the region south of Lake Atitlán, and is linguistically related to the more widely spoken Mayan languages *Kaqchikel* and *K'iche'*. The *Tzutujil* people are one of 24 ethnic groups in Guatemala. Approximately 100,000 *Tzutujil* people reside in the area around Lake Atitlán. In addition to tourism, agriculture, and fishing, the people of Santiago often migrate seasonally or over a period of years to find work, as is common throughout Guatemala. Others work in education, healthcare, and municipal services. In addition to the Guatemalan residents who call Santiago home, there is a small but highly visible expatriate community, including many people from the United States who have retired or built second homes in the lush forests surrounding the Lake. There is also a steady stream of foreign language students who come to study Spanish, missionaries who come to live semi-permanently, church groups that come to minister for short periods of time, volunteers from around the world including Peace Corps Volunteers, and at least two groups of anthropology students that come from two different universities, one of which I was a part. As well, wealthy Guatemalans from the capital or the coast also occasionally build second homes in the Lake region, adding a relatively new dimension of internal tourism to the highly visible foreign tourism throughout the area (Fig. 26.3).

This research was a pilot study for what would become dissertation research on how social and political factors like health insurance and healthcare markets shape what "counts" as an obstetrical emergency. During this pilot study, I conducted formal interviews, a mix of formal and informal observations, and textual analyses of documents that I collected while in the field. I conducted 12

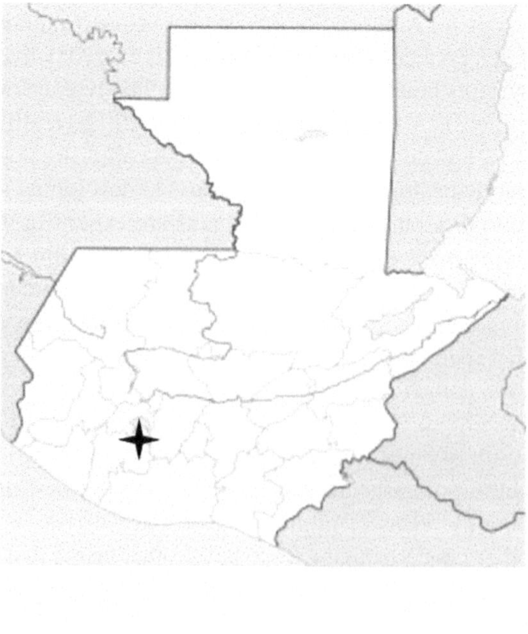

Fig. 26.1 Map of Guatemala showing the location of Santiago Atitlán (star). Modified from Wikipedia Guatemala location map.svg (https://en.wikipedia.org/wiki/Santiago_Atitl%C3%A1n)

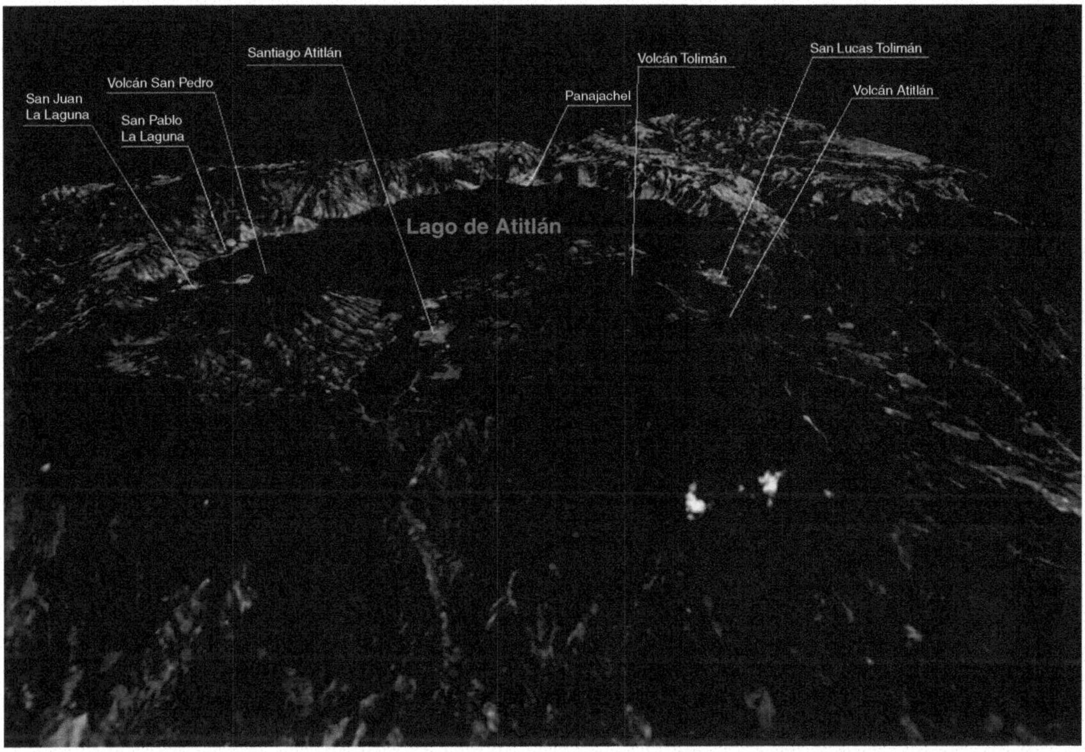

Fig. 26.2 Map of the area of Santiago Atitlán. (By Asybaris0, Topographic data SRTM from NASA and World Imagery) [Public domain], via Wikimedia Commons

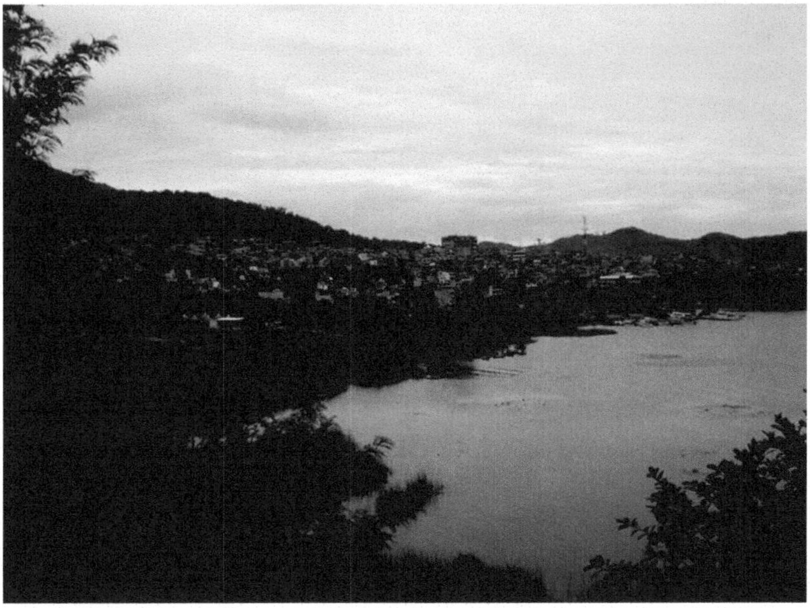

Fig. 26.3 View of Lake Atitlán and Santiago from the private hospital. Photograph by the author, 2010

semi-structured interviews with 10 local care providers, including both midwives and medical staff from the local public health center. These interviewees were selected based on their interest and availability to participate in my study, their role in Santiago's maternity-care system, and their level of Spanish-language fluency. The formal interviews were supplemented with informal conversations during my time "hanging out" at the health center and the hospital (see below). These interviews typically began with a few open-ended questions about the interviewee's work as a care provider, before interviewees typically turned the discussions towards the things that worried them in their daily work—these often involved the pervasive lack of resources for providing good care. I took handwritten notes during all interviews, subsequently coding these notes for key themes after completing my fieldwork (Fig. 26.4).

My observations focused on six health-education trainings that I selected based on their focus, timing, and permission to attend. Three of these trainings took place at the private hospital in Santiago and were conducted by foreign healthcare providers. The other three trainings occurred at health-related NGOs across town. Health center nurses, staff from two local health NGOs, and staff and volunteers from the private hospital led these trainings. Two of these sessions were part of the official state-run training program for *comadronas*; one was also a workshop for *comadronas*, organized by health center staff, but it was not officially part of the state curriculum. These training sessions typically consisted of lectures, didactic games, and report-outs from the *comadronas* about the patients they had attended to in the past month. There was also typically a coffee break and time for social conversations. In addition to observing these trainings, I also observed one planning meeting for the final training I attended, and periodically hung out at both the health center and the private hospital. Hanging out with the night shift doctors at the Centro, foreign volunteers at the private hospital, and with hospital staff helped me understand better how maternity care in Santiago is understood by a number of different kinds of healthcare providers from both Guatemala and elsewhere. I took handwritten notes during formal observations, as well as reflective notes after informally hanging out and at the end of most days in the field. I coded all field notes to identify key themes for analysis, along with the interview notes described above.

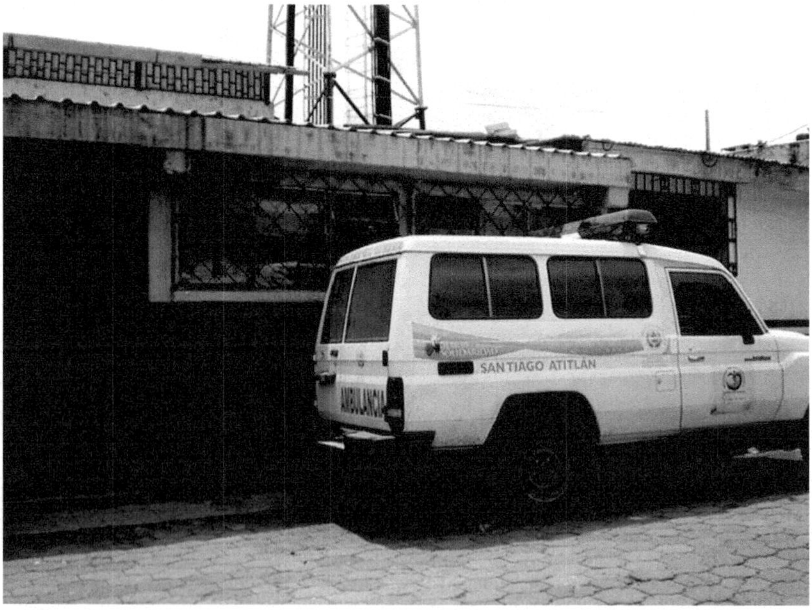

Fig. 26.4 Santiago health center with ambulance. Photograph by the author, 2010

Finally, I also collected documents throughout my time in Santiago related to maternal healthcare. In all cases, either a nurse or a midwife gave these documents to me, to help orient me to their work and models of care. The most important of these documents for this chapter is the Emergency Plan poster. I was also given a copy of the health center's 2010 training curriculum, as well as a copy of the notebook that midwives used to collect official statistics during their daily work. I analyzed these documents within the context of how I saw them used during my observations, as well as how interviewees discussed using these tools during their day-to-day work. The primary limitations of this study were that I only spent one summer in the field, as opposed to years as anthropologists often do (though my background as a former Peace Corps Guatemala volunteer and my affiliation with a university program helped me mitigate this drawback); my lack of *Tzutujil* (I only speak Spanish, so I had to rely on ad hoc translations or follow-up interviews to gather information about what people were saying in *Tzutujil*), and my affiliation with a university program (although this helped me mitigate the drawbacks of a short field stay, it likely shaped who I met and how people on the ground perceived my work).

As I describe in the rest of this chapter, the methods and the qualitative data that they generated were critical in helping me understand how much time and effort—and care—providers put into looking for emergencies during their patients' pregnancies. Rather than taking for granted that planning for emergencies is what "should" happen—as might be the case in a public health context—I suspended judgment, instead noting simply to myself at the time that everyone I talked to took emergency planning very, very seriously. Suspending judgment in this way helped me to see something I would have otherwise missed: That emergency planning systems and management—reflected in and crystallized by the emergency planning poster and the frontline emergency management system of which it is a part—do three things in Santiago. First, this way of thinking and planning generates a moral accountability among care providers and patients for medical outcomes. That is, it makes *comadronas*, nurses, doctors, and mothers morally accountable for medical events that may or may not be within the control of the care provider or the patient. Second, it creates new kinds of collective security, while erasing the need for other kinds of support. Finally, it takes responsibility for moral action out of the present moment and moves it into an imagined future where biomedical care is the only good way to care. In this way, I was able to see that emergency planning—and "emergency thinking" in Scarry's broader terms (2011)—is a "moral regime of reproduction" in the sense of reproductive governance (Morgan and Roberts 2012), just like reproductive rights and rights to life are also moral regimes of reproduction. This insight deepens our understanding of how such moral regimes shape birth in the Americas in the early twenty-first century (Hallowell 2014).

26.7 What Anthropologists See That Others Miss

The Emergency Plan (in Spanish, el Plan de Emergencia) is a public health tool found throughout healthcare spaces in Santiago. It is a colorful, slightly larger-than-legal-sized piece of shiny poster board that visually represents the steps a mother or a care provider in the United States would consider standard prenatal care. There are pictures showing how to go to a prenatal appointment at a health facility, how to care for a baby, and what to do if the mother or her baby looks sick. The poster is didactic: It is meant to be used by midwives and other care providers in educating pregnant women about how to care for themselves and their babies during and immediately after pregnancy.

The audience for the poster is the mother, and the assumed teacher is a *comadrona* working in a rural context. Each one of the boxes shows a different step that the mother should take in order to reach the ultimate goal of the poster and, presumably, the pregnant women the poster is addressing: The safe birth of a healthy baby. Nearly all of the *comadronas* that I interviewed for this study reported making Emergency Plans, following the steps in the Emergency Plan, or both. The plan was passed around at one of the trainings I attended, and was readily visible (or quickly produced upon asking) at midwives' homes and at local clinics (Figs. 26.5 and 26.6).

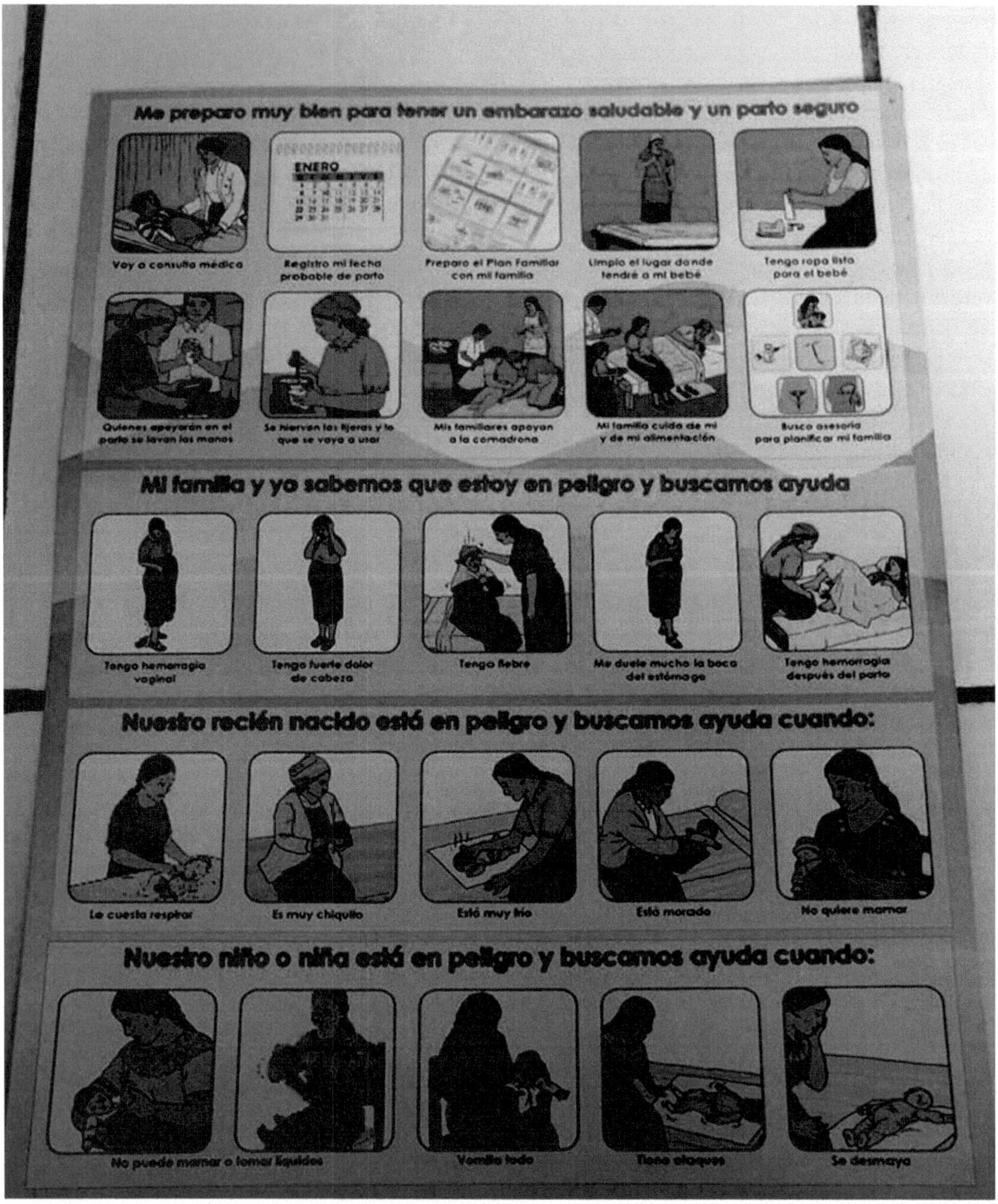

Figs. 26.5 and 26.6 El Plan de Emergencia, posters for mothers illustrating aspects of prenatal care to be used by *comadronas*. Photographs by the author

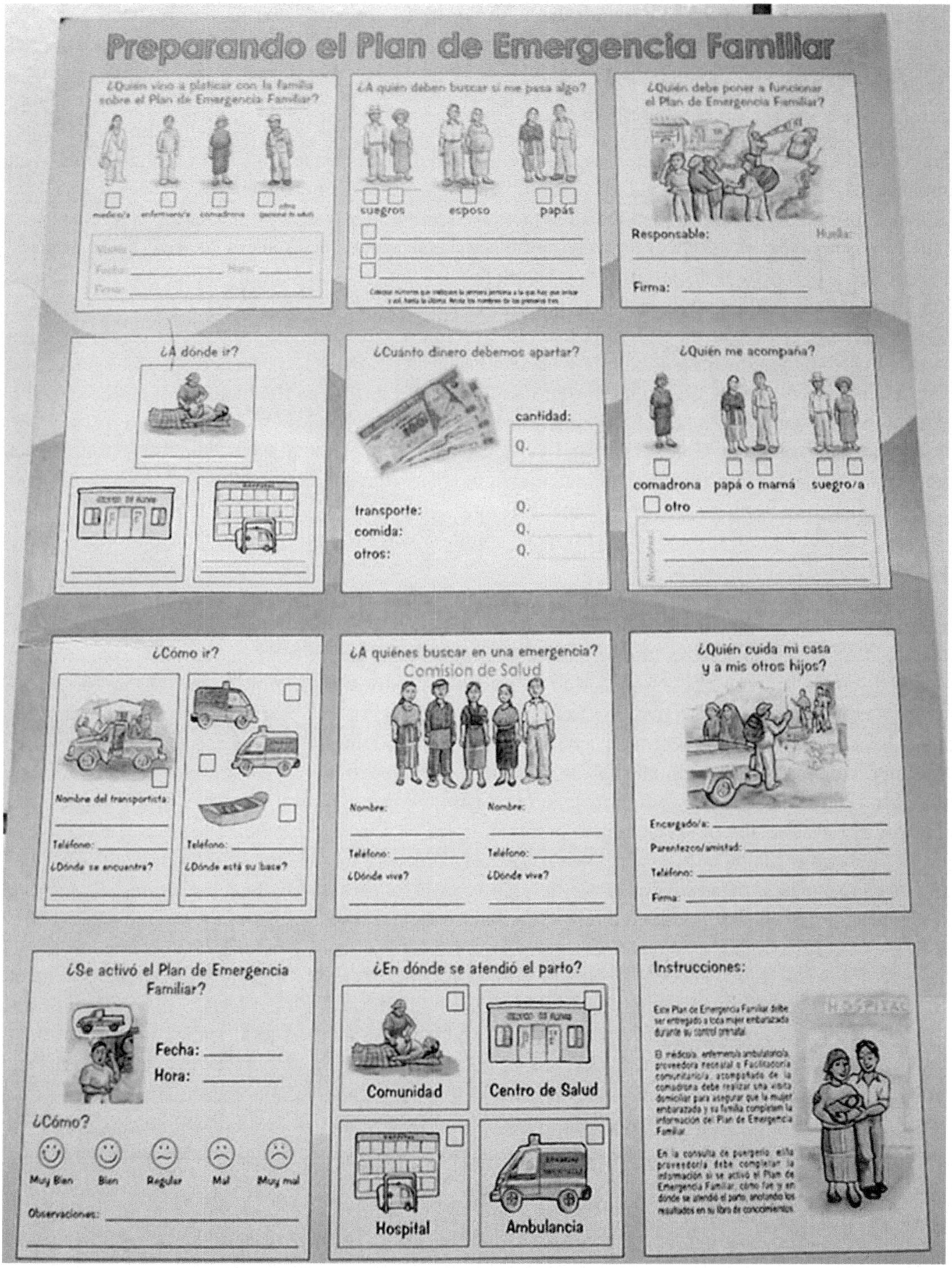

Figs. 26.5 and 26.6 (continued)

To viewers in the United States familiar with western biomedical norms for perinatal care, the poster is deceptively simple. But in the Guatemalan context, the steps described on the poster depicted different—and sometimes competing—models of prenatal care. The idea behind the poster is that a *comadrona* will use it to teach an expectant mother to decide in advance if she will deliver with a midwife at home, in a health center, or at a hospital; to recognize the signs and symptoms of perinatal danger; and to figure out step by step what she will do if she does experience signs or symptoms of an impending obstetrical emergency, like vaginal bleeding or a severe headache.

For example, the poster invites the mother to determine in advance which family members will help her if she experiences one of these symptoms, to keep cash on hand in case there is an emergency and she needs to pay for transportation to a health facility, and to list the family members who can take care of her other children while she is giving birth. There are other pictures on the poster that show a mother how to ensure that she will have a healthy pregnancy, medically speaking. There are pictures showing her how to consult a doctor, how to make sure her *comadrona* practices good hygiene, and even a depiction of how to fill out the poster in advance of a birth. Finally, there are pictures showing when a mother should seek help for a newborn in distress. Yet, because biomedical care is only one system among many in Guatemala, and obstetrical care has not always benefited Guatemalan women—especially poor indigenous Guatemalan women—the value proposition of the poster—that if you look for risks and play by the biomedical rules, you will have a safe and healthy birth—exists alongside and sometimes in tension with more common ways of giving birth, for example, at home with the help of *a comadrona*.

The Emergency Plan poster is the tip of the iceberg when it comes to talk about obstetrical emergencies, risk factors, and planning in Santiago's healthcare scene. Midwives, nurses, and doctors alike all talked at length about the importance of planning, of mothers (and particularly *comadronas*) watching vigilantly for risk factors during pregnancy and after birth, and the terrible possible outcomes—maternal or newborn death—should these practices not be observed. These ideas were also key themes at the trainings I observed and they were addressed throughout the curriculum I was given. Not only were mothers' and infants' lives at stake, but so were people's jobs: Midwives who did not attend trainings, make plans with their patients, or follow through on these plans in the event of an emergency risked losing their licenses to practice.

As the head of the health center, Doctor Tax, explained to me during an interview, the fact that midwives make these plans at all is a sign of huge success for local public health planning. It has been a huge task, he explained, to change midwives' and patients' thinking about the value of going to a doctor—or at least planning to do so. While not everyone is on board—indeed, he explained, some of the older midwives do not necessarily accept the training they receive—they have developed a number of collaborations with local midwives, like Maria, a midwife and a local leader. Like a few of the midwives, she now worked shifts at the local health center in addition to attending patients in their homes, and had become a key local stakeholder over the years. She proudly explained to me during our interview how seriously she and other midwives took this kind of planning, proudly reporting that there had been no cases of maternal mortality in 2010. As she and others explained to me, recognizing risk factors, planning for emergencies, and helping women get to a doctor were among a midwife's most important responsibilities.

The nurses responsible for organizing and running the trainings echoed what I heard throughout my interviews: The most important theme of the trainings is that midwives leave knowing how to look for risk factors and form emergency plans, and the importance of doing so—as well as the risks of not doing so. In this way, midwives bearing posters form the frontlines of emergency planning and response in Santiago today. And because midwives were responsible for this huge task, they could also be held accountable: Not only did they risk losing their licenses and thus their jobs if they failed to perform their duties, one of the private hospital social workers explained to me that midwives could be held legally accountable for maternal deaths, should they fail to refer a patient properly and the mother or baby died as a result.

Yet, following the rules can save a midwife from blame and liability even if her patient dies. As I observed during one of the trainings I attended, Dr. Tax led a review of case where a local woman had recently died shortly after her delivery. The woman's death was investigated as a possible case of maternal mortality, but she was found to have died of a slip and fall injury. As a result, the woman's death was classified as a "muerte subita" (sudden death), and no one was to blame. Dr. Tax went on, however, to point out that because the woman's midwife had properly created an Emergency Plan with the family in advance of the woman's delivery, had she died a "muerte materna" (maternal death), the midwife would not have been found liable for that death. Considered from a US perspective—where specialized first responders working in pairs or teams with ambulances stocked with medical equipment form the frontline of emergency response to obstetrical as well as other kinds of emergencies—the disparity in resources and training alone piqued my interest and concern, even as I sought to honor the stories of what were clearly hardworking, thoughtful care providers laboring diligently under difficult circumstances.

Families also play a key role in responding to emergencies, as several care providers explained to me during our interviews, and as the poster clearly shows. In Guatemala, few medical services are public, there is little in the way of public insurance, and there are no public ambulance systems or 911-type telephonic emergency services. Instead, there are typically private ambulances—usually little more than pick-up trucks whose drivers will come quickly and on short notice. As a result, a woman and her family are responsible—along with the midwife—for getting to a doctor in the event of an emergency. As the poster depicts, this includes keeping enough money on hand during a pregnancy to pay for a possible ambulance transport. Preparing to pay for possible emergency transport is a key step in planning for emergencies. Not keeping this money on hand is an act of bad planning—curious to me, since among Santiago's rural poor having any cash reserves is a huge feat.

In these ways, as I observed and talked with people throughout Santiago, the logic of emergency planning and of the poster itself started to break down. I wondered: How could the burden of first response possibly fall to a group of (typically) working class women with empirical educations (but no formal degrees), little support beyond state-mandated trainings and some basic equipment, and a bunch of posters at their disposal? How is it fair to expect poor families to plan to pay for ambulance transport, and for solo midwives to get them to the doctor, when they have so few resources and support? Is it fair to expect local care providers—midwives, doctors, nurses—alongside patients and their families, to decrease the maternal mortality rate by planning diligently for emergencies, a huge moral responsibility that all of the care providers I spoke with took seriously—especially given this rural, postwar context, where it seemed to me that social and economic factors like racism and poverty were macro drivers of poor public health outcomes?

The data I collected and these questions helped me form my first insight about emergency thinking in Santiago: That in this context, the "right" thing to do is the biomedical thing, like looking for pregnancy-related risks, planning for an emergency, and getting to a doctor if one occurs. These thoroughly biomedical actions are not "wrong" per se, but they are just that: Thoroughly biomedical. Which means that for many people in Santiago, they are different than what they are used to, and carry risks that aren't always obvious, as I discuss below. They are also imbued with different levels of moral responsibility: Midwives are more liable for poor outcomes than others in this system, because they are on the frontlines, even if they are not well resourced in these roles. In anthropological terms, midwives' "good care" (in biomedical terms) is positioned as the most important thing between maternal life and death—which obscures macro threats to maternal life and health, like racism and poverty. As well, care providers learn to think of themselves as moral actors, charged with acting in particular ways—and not others.

The second thing I learned through my fieldwork is that as emergency planning shifts moral responsibility for poor outcomes onto midwives' shoulders, it also seeks to reconfigure other social relationships, like the relationships between birthing women and their neighbors and kin, as well as between citizens and the state. As I observed during my fieldwork, the Emergency Planning poster puts a premium on local, and especially familial, relationships. There are boxes on the planning side of the poster that invite the mother to identify who came to talk with her about making an emergency plan (a doctor, a nurse, a midwife, or "other"), who she will contact if she observes a risk factor or has an emergency (her in-laws, her husband, or her parents), and who is responsible for putting the emergency plan into action if necessary. Still other boxes invite the mother to identify who will transport her to a hospital or health center (local firefighters, a private pick-up truck), who will take care of her other kids while she is incapacitated, who else she could call in an emergency for backup, and which members of the neighborhood health committee she will call on for help as a kind of backup to the backup.

In this way, the poster invites the mother to identify a network of people who will help her in an emergency. It also reflects back the reality of local forms of support that have developed to help people in all kinds of emergency situations (obstetrical or otherwise), such as the common phenomenon in Guatemala of firefighters carrying out emergency transportation, and neighborhood health committees forming to support families with medical crises.

What is so striking about these local networks is not that they are formed in the first place, but that they are necessary in a country which placed such a high premium on primary care for all in the peace accords that settled its civil war in 1996 (MINGUA 1996). Indeed, the providers that I spoke with were adamant that these forms of care were crucial to maternal health in Santiago. And, they were not shy about pointing out the failures of the Guatemalan government to deliver on its many healthcare promises. Elena and Mirsa, two of the health center nurses that I interviewed, explained that the Ministry of Health places the responsibility on them to train midwives, care for pregnant women, and lower maternal mortality rates. The Ministry has failed miserably, however, in giving them the tools to do so. The midwives and the health center were typically responsible for covering the cost of the state-mandated midwifery trainings, for example, and the health center was frequently out of basic supplies like saline. If a pregnant woman came in and needed even these most basic things, she or her family members would have to go out and buy them.

This situation was not new, but it had gotten worse as the result of recent budget cuts, which were incredibly frustrating to the providers I interviewed. As Elena put it, the Ministry of Health puts providers between "la pared y la espada"—between the wall and the sword—by compelling them to keep doing their jobs without the most basic forms of state or institutional support. In this way, emergency planning and thinking in this context relies on local relationships, putting a premium on the roles of family and neighbors. Yet, these plans—and this way of thinking about emergencies—erases the role that the state promised to play in the peace accords, and that arguably any health system should play for the people who need it: The role of an institutional provider, and the ultimate safety net.

The third insight I had as a result of my fieldwork centered on the timing and inevitably of biomedical care in a region that had long placed a premium on other models of perinatal care, like home birth attended by *comadronas* and family members. The logic of emergency thinking and planning shapes what counts as "good care" and specifically, the order or timing of when that care should happen. As I noted above, several of the boxes on the emergency planning poster indicate that a patient can choose a *comadrona* for her care, while offering up nurses and doctors as alternatives. The poster also alludes to the possibility of a home birth in the box that asks the mother to indicate where she will give birth. While one of the options listed is a picture of a *comadrona* examining a woman's pregnant belly, the other options listed are biomedical: An ambulance, a health center, or a hospital.

The providers I spoke with were typically more focused on a biomedical outcome, especially as they talked about emergency planning. They continually stressed, in interview after interview, that looking for risk factors or warning signs and then getting a woman to a doctor in the event one was observed was of the utmost importance. They were also among the first to recognize how poverty shaped what actually happened. As Maria, one of the midwives, explained to me, women of means were likely to be referred to a private hospital, while poor women were more likely to be referred to a public health center or hospital. The high cost of transportation and families' expectations that they would encounter racial and ethnic discrimination in biomedical facilities also shaped who could get care (Berry 2006, 2008).

Moreover, at one of the meetings I attended at the health center, the staff talked in urgent and distressed tones about how some of the midwives had not been making timely referrals, and as a result they had had a few close calls: One such near miss involved a prenatal patient who had had difficulty walking due to circulation problems in her legs, and another involved a postpartum patient who had gone into convulsions following a home birth. Yiomara, a local social worker, later explained to me in an interview that midwives risked their livelihoods and their patients' lives by not making timely referrals to the health center or hospital. It was inconceivable to her that anyone would take such risks: Timing and especially fast action were everything in these cases.

What struck me about this repeated insistence on the importance of timely referrals was how urgent the mothers' and midwives' actions (or inactions) seemed to be to the care providers I spoke with, when there were so many things that prevented midwives from making those referrals, and that prevented patients from following through on them. Why was everyone so focused on making timely referrals, when midwives and families were not following through on them for reasons that were largely out of their control, like a lack of cash? I realized that underneath these conversations was a dynamic wherein talking about emergencies and planning for emergencies shifted everyone's focus towards a biomedical birth as the only logical outcome of moral action in this context. Put another way, in the context of emergency thinking in Santiago, the only way to provide good care was to plan for a future where a woman would be quickly referred to a biomedical facility to give birth in a biomedical context.

Importantly, I noticed, this was not the result of a simple "biomedicine versus traditional medicine" narrative, nor was it the result of unidirectional or hegemonic biomedicalization of a "traditional" context. Indeed, as Mirsa explained, there were lots of reasons to doubt the efficacy of the care providers' efforts: Although there was some evidence that maternal mortality was going down in Santiago, she was concerned that these statistics were not reliable, and that the health center was even witnessing an increase in maternal mortality. Yet, even she stressed the importance of planning in this way. These conversations helped me realize that far from these scholarly narratives of biomedicine vs. traditional medicine and one-way biomedicalization, in fact there were quite subtle dynamics at work in this planning. Through the process of thinking and planning for emergencies, care providers learned to think of timely referrals leading to a biomedical birth as the only good outcome, if everyone in the system did their part.

26.8 Thinking in Anthropology

As I have shown in this chapter, anthropological methods and data reveal that planning for an obstetrical emergency is not as straightforward or a natural as it may seem. It is, like every other set of human actions, a process that is context-dependent. This is to say that the process of designing and implementing emergency plans engenders new kinds of social relationships. It also shifts moral responsibility and moral action. In so doing, this process places the burden of good care and moral action squarely onto the shoulders of mothers and midwives, as well as other local care providers. While new kinds of relationships form to support these shifts, like the neighborhood health committees, these shifts let the state level public health system off the hook for resourcing the midwives, doctors, and nurses that bear the brunt of frontline emergency responses every day. This process also positions timely referrals and biomedical birth as the only good public health outcomes in a region where home birth is a social norm and is in many ways socially valued. This abdication by the state—and the net effect of making already-precariously positioned healthcare providers that much more structurally vulnerable—is especially troublesome given the fact that many of their patients are poor or working class and have historically faced terrible discrimination in medical settings, to say nothing of the decades of brutal civil war that targeted indigenous Guatemalans and hit the central-western part of the country particularly hard. Against this backdrop, care providers in Santiago continue to work diligently and passionately to improve maternal and child health in this region.

Importantly, these findings and this kind of story only become visible through anthropological methods. Although public health studies have long identified some of the challenges associated with improving maternal and child health outcomes in rural Guatemala, without the deep listening and systematic gathering and analysis of qualitative data common to anthropology, stories like Elena, Mirsa, Dr. Tax, Maria, and Yiomara would not come to light—and thus it would be difficult to see how the myriad social pressures that they face link back to structural inequalities and forms of governance. Using the lens of emergency thinking—and considering this squarely in the context of early twenty-first century reproductive governance—helps us connect the dots between local experiences and larger patterns of change across the Americas. Further fieldwork and analysis, either in Guatemala or similar areas, may well reveal that patterns of state abnegation of responsibility for healthcare in the wake postwar (Latin) American promises to provide primary care for all shift moral responsibilities and social relationships in ways that are unexpected or counterintuitive.

Understanding these patterns and shifts, and the reasons that they happen, can help care providers in any context understand what their counterparts are experiencing in other locations. For providers from a US context interested in working or understanding a broader inter-American context, this analysis sheds light on why *comadronas*, health center staff, and other providers feel the pressures that they feel and make the choices they make. In particular, this chapter sheds light on why these providers plan for and react to obstetrical emergencies as they do. As scholars call the efficacy of Safe Motherhood in Guatemala into question (Berry 2010), one way to improve maternal health in this context could be to take these otherwise-invisible social factors into account in future public health interventions.

By shedding light on how and why people do what they do in diverse healthcare and public health contexts, anthropology can make substantive contributions to the study of healthcare and public health. My aim in this chapter is to help students and providers see that public health interventions, well intentioned though they may be, often impact people's lives in unexpected, even iatrogenic ways. I hope that readers will see that without attending to the seemingly mundane details of people's lived experiences, it can be difficult to tease out the full impact of even something as seemingly straightforward and morally compelling as preventing maternal mortality. Because working in healthcare and public health can intimately impact people's bodies, lives, families, and communities, practitioners in these fields face more challenges—and more responsibility—than simply just trying to help.

As the field of global public health continues to grow, the need for anthropological analysis will continue to grow with it, as it is only through the systematic and thoughtful collection of qualitative data—like people's stories and observations of daily life—that we can fully understand the contexts from which our quantitative understanding of the world emerges. Changes in maternal mortality rates belie a complex web of shifting social relationships and moral responsibilities that shape and are shaped by the very systems of planning that public health experts and local frontline providers put into place to improve maternal health outcomes and prevent maternal death. Analyzing these systems helps to shed light on what they are doing besides moving the needle on maternal mortality, where they break down, and why it can be so hard to prevent something that should be easy to prevent, like so many cases of maternal mortality.

References

Allen, D. R. (2004). *Managing motherhood, managing risk: Fertility and danger in West Central Tanzania*. Ann Arbor: University of Michigan Press.

Benagiano, G., & Thomas, B. (2003). Safe motherhood: The FIGO initiative. *International Journal of Gynecology & Obstetrics, 82*(3), 263–274.

Berry, N. (2006). Kaqchikel midwives, home births, and emergency obstetric referrals in Guatemala: Contextualizing the choice to stay at home. *Social Science & Medicine, 62*, 1958–1969.

Berry, N. (2008). Who's judging the quality of care? Indigenous Maya and the problem of "not being attended". *Medical Anthropology, 27*(2), 164–189.

Berry, N. (2010). *Unsafe motherhood: Mayan maternal mortality and subjectivity in post-war Guatemala*. Oxford: Berghahn Books.

Bridges, K. M. (2011). *Reproducing race: An ethnography of pregnancy as a site of racialization*. Berkeley: University of California Press.

Chapman, R. R. (2010). *Family secrets: Risking reproduction in central Mozambique*. Nashville: Vanderbilt University Press.

Cosminsky, S. (1977). Childbirth and midwifery on a Guatemalan finca. *Medical Anthropology, 6*(3), 69–104.

Cosminsky, S. (2001). Midwifery across the generations: A modernizing midwife in Guatemala. *Medical Anthropology, 20*(4), 345–378.

Cosminsky, S. (2012). Birth and blame: Guatemalan midwives and reproductive risk. In L. Fordyce & A. Maraësa (Eds.), *Risk, reproduction, and narratives of experience* (pp. 81–101). Nashville: Vanderbilt University Press. Retrieved August 5, 2013, from http://search.ebscohost.com/login.aspx?direct=true&scope=site&db=nlebk&db=nlabk&AN=467212

Davis-Floyd, R. (1990). The role of obstetrical rituals in the resolution of cultural anomaly. *Social Science & Medicine, 31*(2), 175–189.

Davis-Floyd, R. (1994). The technocratic body: American childbirth as cultural expression. *Social Science & Medicine, 38*(8), 1125–1140.

Davis-Floyd, R. (2004). *Birth as an American rite of passage* (2nd ed.). Berkeley: University of California Press.

Fordyce, L., & Maraësa, A. (2012). *Risk, reproduction, and narratives of experience*. Nashville: Vanderbilt University Press. Retrieved August 5, 2013, from http://search.ebscohost.com/login.aspx?direct=true&scope=site&db=nlebk&db=nlabk&AN=467212

Freedman, L. P., et al. (2007). Practical lessons from global safe motherhood initiatives: Time for a new focus on implementation. *The Lancet, 370*(9595), 1383–1391.

Goldman, N., & Glei, D. A. (2003). Evaluation of midwifery care: Results from a survey in rural Guatemala. *Social Science & Medicine, 56*(4), 685–700.

Gutiérrez, E. R. (2008). *Fertile matters: The politics of Mexican-origin women's reproduction*. Austin: University of Texas Press.

Hallowell, E. (2014). "Between the wall and the sword": Reproductive governance and the technology of emergency in Guatemalan maternity care. *Feminist Formations, 26*(3), 100–121.

Hallowell, E. (2015). *Emergencies that count: Pregnancy and economies of care*. U.S. Dissertation. University of Pennsylvania, Philadelphia, PA.

Hinojosa, S. (2004). Authorizing tradition: Vectors of contention in highland Maya midwifery. *Social Science & Medicine, 59*(3), 16.

Jordan, B. (1978). *Birth in four cultures*. Montreal: Eden Press.

Mahler, H. (1987). The safe motherhood initiative: A call to action. *Lancet, 1*(8534), 668–670.

Mamo, L. (2007). *Queering reproduction: Achieving pregnancy in the age of technoscience*. Durham: Duke University Press Books.

Maupin, J. N. (2008). Remaking the Guatemalan midwife: Health care reform and midwifery training programs in highland Guatemala. *Medical Anthropology, 27*(4), 353–382.

MINGUA. (1996). Agreement on socio-economic aspects and agrarian situation concluded on 6 May 1996 between the presidential peace commission of the government of Guatemala and the Unidad Revolucionaria Nacional Guatemalteca. United States Institute for Peace. Retrieved from http://www.usip.org/publications/peace-agreements-guatemala

Morgan, L. M., & Roberts, E. F. S. (2012). Reproductive governance in Latin America. *Anthropology & Medicine, 19*(2), 241–254.

Paul, L., & Paul, B. D. (1975). The Maya midwife as sacred specialist: A Guatemalan case. *American Ethnologist, 2*(4), 707–726.

Roberts, E. F. S. (2012). *God's laboratory: Assisted reproduction in the Andes*. Berkeley: University of California Press.

Scarry, E. (2011). *Thinking in an emergency*. New York: W.W. Norton & Company.

Schwartz, D. A. (2015). Interface of epidemiology, anthropology and health care in maternal death prevention in resource-poor nations. In D. A. Schwartz (Ed.), *Maternal mortality: Risk factors, anthropological perspectives, prevalence in developing countries and preventive strategies for pregnancy-related death*. New York: Nova Science Publishers.

Taylor, J. S. (2003). Confronting "culture" in medicine's "culture of no culture". *Academic Medicine, 78*(6), 555–559.

Van Hollen, C. C. (2003). *Birth on the threshold: Childbirth and modernity in South India*. Berkeley: University of California Press.

World Health Organization. (2015). *Maternal mortality*. WHO. Retrieved October 1, 2016, from http://www.who.int/mediacentre/factsheets/fs348/en/

Unintended Pregnancy, Induced Abortion, and Unmet Need for Effective Contraception in Twenty-First Century Indigenous Mayan Populations of Guatemala

27

Edgar Kestler and Vinicio Mora

Abbreviations

CPR	Contraceptive prevalence rate
CRP	Center for Reproductive Rights
DMPA	Depomedroxyprogesterone acetate
ENCOVI	Encuesta de Condiciones de Vivienda
FP	Family planning
ICPD	International Conference on Population and Development
ILO	International Labor Organization
INE	Instituto Nacional de Estadistica/National Institute of Statistics
IUD's	Intra-uterus device
LAM	Lactational Amenorrhea Method
LARC's	Long-Acting-Reversible-Contraception
LBMM	Linea Basal de Mortalidad Materna
MDG	Millennium Development Goal
MMR	Maternal mortality ratio
MOH	Ministry of Health
MVA	Manual Vacuum Aspiration
NMCHS	National and Maternal Child Heath Survey
SDG's	Sustainable Development Goals
SDL	Social Development Law/Ley de Desarrollo Social
SEGEPLAN	Secretaría de Planificación y Programación de la Presidencia
TFR	Total fertility rate
UN	United Nations
WHO	World Health Organization

E. Kestler, M.D., M.Sc. (✉) · V. Mora, M.D.
Epidemiologic Research Center in Sexual and Reproductive Health, Guatemala City, Guatemala
e-mail: ekestler@ciesar.org.gt

D. A. Schwartz (ed.), *Maternal Death and Pregnancy-Related Morbidity Among Indigenous Women of Mexico and Central America*, Global Maternal and Child Health: Medical, Anthropological, and Public Health Perspectives, https://doi.org/10.1007/978-3-319-71538-4_27

27.1 Introduction

According to the National Living Condition Survey (INE-ENCOVI 2014), Guatemalan indigenous women (who account for 40–50% of the total population) are disproportionately affected by adverse reproductive and sexual health outcomes, particularly in the districts-departments of Solola (96.8% indigenous), Totonicapan (93.6% indigenous), and Alta Verapaz (93.5% indigenous), where more than 90% of the population is of Mayan ancestry. Indigenous Mayan girls and women tend to live in rural, poor, marginalized areas with very limited access to healthcare and to quality reproductive and sexual health services. Rates of unplanned and unintended pregnancies in adult women over 19 years of age and in adolescents aged 10–18 years are very high in these poor indigenous Mayan populations, and these girls and women face greater risks of abortion-related complications and death than do non-Mayans. These health disparities reflect systemic patterns of institutional-structural inequity and social injustice linked to (a) gender-based discrimination, termed "*machismo,*" (b) ethnic prejudices and biases, and (c) religious, political, and socioeconomic oppression. Despite official policies as well as religious and public discourse that oppose abortion as a moral and legal offense, unsafe induced abortions are widespread and commonly practiced at dangerously high rates on poor, young, and ethnic minority women who bear the brunt of the physical, psychological, and social costs.

In order to fully grasp "on-the-ground situations" and effectively identify possible solutions, the daily routine and experiences of girls and women and their beliefs regarding abortion, together with the circumstances that shape their decisions, must be evaluated within their social-political-cultural context and in light of recent 2015–2016 political, economic, governmental processes, and the new commitments to Sustainable Development Goals (SDGs) signed by Guatemalan government (United Nations 2015). The new government (2016–2020) was believed to have an unprecedented opportunity to establish the solid foundations and the necessary bases to shift the living conditions of Mayan populations onto a path of inclusive and sustainable development; it was and is still hoped that future governments would share this vision and continue to promote, finance, and achieve the SDG's.

It is estimated that about one million unsafe abortions are performed in Central America yearly (WHO 2011). These estimates are most probably very low due to underreporting, poor surveillance, and additional challenges to data collection. Research and accurate statistics are usually hindered by the illegal status of abortion throughout most of Central America as well as incomplete admissions data from urban hospitals, which only account for girls and women who are able and willing to seek hospitalized care for induced abortion complications. Not counted in the statistics are impoverished rural girls, and women who cannot obtain hospital care due to geographic and financial barriers or who do not seek care fearing legal, criminal, or social repercussions.

Across Central America, studies have revealed a myriad of "determinants" of unplanned-unintended pregnancies and unsafe abortions which include poverty, lower education levels, high fertility rates, younger age at first intercourse, early menarche, adolescents "unsafe sex practices," rural areas of residence, "*machismo,*" sexual abuse-violence-rapes of girls and women, and indigenous cultural-language barriers in healthcare facilities (WHO 1992). Many studies have shown that being of Mayan origin is a significant risk factor for unsafe abortion and unplanned-unwanted pregnancy. In Guatemala, the risk of teen pregnancy is eight times greater for girls ages 10–18 years with no education compared to those with higher education, and is two times higher when they relate to girls in the lowest quintile compared with the highest quintile. This suggests that education is critically important, and is even more important than wealth, as a discrete risk factor for teen pregnancy (WHO 1992). Mayan girls and women generally have lower resources and less opportunity than do more affluent middle and upper class girls and women to access effective contraceptives and have safe abortion conducted by trained professionals under sanitary conditions. High-quality reproductive health services are generally located in urban areas. Mayan girls and women living in poor and rural areas have inaccessible geographic and financial access.

Previous publications examining induced abortion among women in Guatemala have reported that between 49 and 63% of Mayan women obtained abortions from unsafe providers; less than 15% were attended by highly trained professionals (as compared to two-thirds of well-off women in urban centers) (Singh et al. 2006). Recent studies show a very high level of fertility/pregnancy in teenagers aged 15–19 years—many have had a live birth or become pregnant for the first time before age 19. One of every 5 girls aged 15–19 years (20%) have had children or have been pregnant; sixteen per cent were "teen-moms" or adolescent mothers, and five per cent were currently pregnant. The percentage of pregnant girls was about 6% among the youngest teens (15 years old) and 41% among the older teens (aged 19 years) (NMCHS 2015).

In addition to reproductive-sexual health/contraception programs and preventative services, adequate postabortion contraception with effective methods like intrauterine devices (IUD's) and implants is imperative to reduce maternal mortality and morbidity associated with unsafe abortion, and to prevent repeat abortions. According to a review of results of ten major postabortion care research projects over a 9-year period in seven Latin American countries, abortion care can be significantly improved with several interventions. Treatment with Manual Vacuum Aspiration (MVA) is safer than the conventional method of sharp curettage, and requires less heavy anesthesia or sedation. In addition, the MVA procedure can be performed in an ambulatory (out-patient) setting, which reduces overall costs and the length of hospital stay. Integration of contraceptive counselling services and the immediate provision of effective contraception with IUD's or subdermal implants before the patient leaves the hospital or clinic are also essential to reduce repeat abortions and decrease maternal mortality and morbidity.

Unsafe abortion refers to a procedure for terminating an unplanned-unintended pregnancy performed either by persons lacking the necessary skills or in an environment that does not conform to minimal medical standards, or both (Schwartz 2015a). Mayan-indigenous girls and women in Guatemala have poorer reproductive health outcomes than do nonindigenous whites and Ladinas, and face considerable barriers in accessing adequate health services. Multiple socio-economic-political and demographic determinants and barriers include such factors as illiteracy, poverty, lack of awareness about access to abortion services, social stigma, and untrained, culturally insensitive or overtly discriminatory health professionals. These factors have continuously resulted in restricted utilization/access of girls and women to safe abortion services. The consequences of unsafe abortion have been alarming, seriously questioning the quality of healthcare delivery system. Global international data indicate that unsafe abortions have existed and continue to exist everywhere; given the nature of these "humanitarian emergencies," the need for safe abortion services has increased for girls and women in "low resource settings" and in all humanitarian crises. Too many girls and women who wish to delay pregnancy have little access to contraceptive services, and too many girls and too many who experience an unplanned-unwanted pregnancy are unlikely to have access to quality abortion care, often leading them to seek an unsafe abortion.

27.2 Context of the Social and Economic Situation in Mayan-Indigenous Populations

Guatemala is one of the poorest countries and one of the most stratified societies in Latin America. It is also one of the countries in the region with the least progress made in population health issues. According to recent estimates (World Bank 2016a) 56% of the families are below the poverty line and 16–20% live in extreme poverty. The poverty levels are most acute for indigenous Mayan groups in which more than three-fourths are below the line of poverty, and greater than one-fourth live in conditions of extreme poverty. As previously stated, the indigenous Mayan populations still account for about one-half of the total Guatemalan population.

According to World Bank reports, indigenous people in Latin America number more than 42 million, and they speak almost 560 languages (World Bank 2016b). The majority (38 million) live in Mexico, Guatemala, Peru, and Bolivia. In recent years, they have acquired more visibility and gained greater participation in political decisions; more than 15 Latin American countries have signed the Convention of Indigenous and Tribal Peoples of the International Labor Organization (ILO) which guarantees a series of protections for these indigenous groups.

There have been significant achievements in most indigenous communities with regard to education, the availability of electricity, access to clean drinking water, and important reduction in poverty in indigenous communities, particularly in Peru and Bolivia. Unfortunately, Guatemala is one of the few countries in the region that has experienced an increase in poverty in recent years (increasing from 51% in 2006 to 59.3% in 2014) despite, paradoxically, one of the best economic performances in Latin America—Guatemala has a growth rate of above 3% from 2012 and reaching close to 4% by 2015. Today, Guatemalan indigenous Mayan communities are the poorest among the poor on the continent, living in worsening conditions and receiving incomes that are worse than non-natives, even with similar levels of education.

Table 27.1 shows the twenty-first century differences and the large gaps existing among the six countries in the Central America Region in terms of population, social conditions, and health. Guatemala has the greatest population in Central America, and also possesses also the greatest rural population (50.2%), followed by Honduras (47.8%) and Nicaragua (42.4%). Panama is the country in Central America with the lowest rural population (24.8%). These data also show that Guatemala is the country in Central America which has the lowest public expenditure on health (2.5%), as compared to Costa Rica, the Central American country with the largest public expenditure on health (7.4%). Life expectancy is lower in Guatemala than in the other five Central American countries (Prado 2013).

Guatemala, one of the largest economies in Central America, is listed among countries with (a) higher levels of ethnic inequality and healthcare disparities in Latin America, (b) high rates of poverty and severe poverty, particularly in rural areas and among indigenous populations, (c) some of the highest rates of chronic and acute malnutrition, and (d) some of the highest maternal mortality ratios (MMRs) and infant-child mortality rates (IMR's and CMRs) in Central America. These discouraging statistics and living conditions are particularly difficult for almost one-half of rural municipalities, where 8 of every 10 people are poor, according to the 2011 Rural Poverty Maps (IFAD 2011).

The large disparities among the Maya and Ladino populations in relation to education, health, poverty, and economics are reflected in the 2014 statistics from INE-ENCOVI on the average number of family members per household. In households living in extreme poverty, the average is 6.9 mem-

Table 27.1 Population, social and health conditions for Central American Region (from Prado 2013)

	Guatemala	Honduras	El Salvador	Nicaragua	Costa Rica	Panamá
Population (millions)	14.8	7.8	6.2	5.9	4.7	3.6
Rural population	50.2%	47.8%	35.2%	42.4%	35.4%	24.8%
GDP per capita	$3178.08	$2225.67	$3701.99	$1243.21	$8675.83	$8590.09
Life expectancy	71.1	73.1	71.9	74.0	79.3	76.1
Adult illiteracy	30.9	20	18.9	32.5	5.1	8.1
Public expenditure on health (% of GDP)	2.5%	4.4%	4.3%	4.9%	7.4%	6.1%
Health expenditure *(per capita)	$196.22	$136.78	$236.78	$103.44	$811.44	$616.39

Fig. 27.1 Family size and poverty level (from INE-ENCOVI 2014)

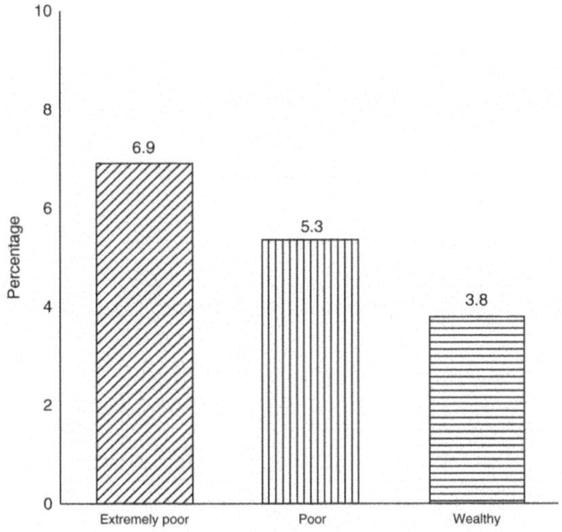

Fig. 27.2 Literacy rates by ethnicity and gender (from INE-ENCOVI 2014)

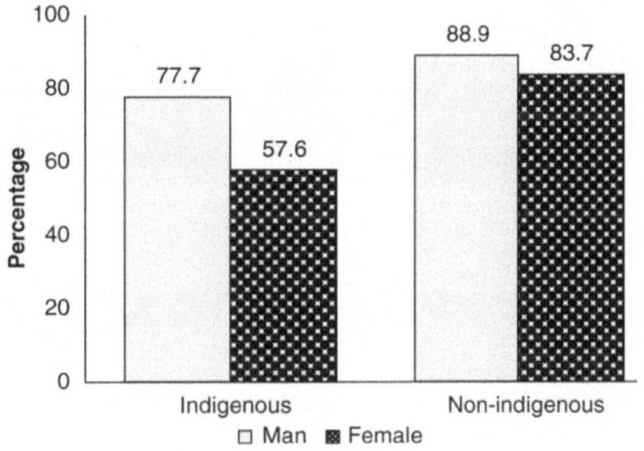

bers per household; it is 5.3 per poor households and 3.8 for nonpoor households (Fig. 27.1). The "extreme poverty households" are predominantly the households of indigenous Mayan, rural and poor population who experience barriers to and have little to no access to the national health system.

Figure 27.2 illustrates the disparities that exist in literacy rates according to gender and ethnic group. Overall, women have lower rates of literacy than do men, and indigenous women have the lowest literacy rates at 57.6%.

27.3 Sexual and Reproductive Rights in Guatemala

Guatemala has had a broad national and international legal framework (from 1948 to 2016) ratified by the Guatemalan government (Table 27.2). There have been multiple legal mandates and instruments aimed at improving the sexual and reproductive rights of Guatemalan girls and women. These include access to effective contraception, induced abortion, and obstetrical and neonatal care to reduce maternal, perinatal, and neonatal mortality. Unfortunately, the mandates of this legal and political framework have not been fulfilled for a multiplicity of reasons (financial, cultural, economic, religious, and political, among others), and the health needs of indigenous Mayan, rural and poor girls and women have not been met.

Table 27.2 Legal national and international framework for sexual and reproductive rights

National	International
Policy Constitution of the Republic of Guatemala	Universal Declaration of Human Rights 1948
Health Code (Decree 90-97, April 29, 1961)	Convention on the Elimination of All Forms of Discrimination Against Women (CEDAW) ONU 1981
Peace Accord, December 29, 1996	The International Conference on Safe Motherhood, Nairobi 1987
Social Development Law (Decree 42-2001)	Children's Rights Convention, 1989
Labour Code (Decree 1441)	World Conference for Children, New York 1990
Protection of Children and Adolescents Law (Decree 27-2003)	International Conference on Population and Development, ICPD (Egypt) 1994
Tax law on the distribution of distilled spirits, beer and other fermented drinks, its regulations, and the dry law (Decree No. 21-2004)	Fourth World Conference on Women, Beijing 1995
Femicide and other forms of violence against women law (Decree 22-2008)	Agreements of Millennium Summit, September 2000
Universal and equal access to family planning services and its integration into the National Reproductive Health Law, Decree 279-2009	UN Special Session on Children, New York 2002
Sexual violence, trafficking and exploitation of people law (Decree 9-2009)	Regional Plan of Neonatal Maternal and Reproductive Health
Enhancing and Advancing Women Law (Decree 7-99)	Convention against Torture and cruel treatment, inhuman or degrading punishment
Safe Motherhood Law (Decree 32-2010) and its regulations (Decree 65-2012)	Children's rights convention
Population Policy and Social Development SEGEPLAN 2001	American Convention on Human Rights ("Pacto de San José, Costa Rica")
Health for Adolescents and Youth Policy (Decree SPM-M-636-2004)	Addendum to the American Convention on Human Rights Protocol on Economic, Social and Cultural Rights ("Protocolo de San Salvador")
K'atun Development Plan "Our Guatemala 2032" (SEGEPLAN 2014)	ILO Convention 169 of Indigenous and Tribal Peoples, 1989
Health Sector Reform in Guatemala (MSPAS 2016)	Inter-American Convention on the Prevention, Punishment and Eradication of Violence against Women ("Convención de Belem do Pará"), 1994
	Millennium Development Goals 2015
	Sustainable Development Goals 2030

Twenty years after the United Nations had established the basic rights of individuals (United Nations 1948), the UN reconfirmed the right of individuals and adult couples "to decide freely and responsibly on the number of their children" (United Nations 1968). The concept of family planning as a human right also was reaffirmed at the UN World Population Conference in Bucharest in 1974 (Mauldin et al. 1974). The World Plan of Action adopted at the Mexico City conference (Isaacs and Cook 1984) affirmed that governments should, as a matter of urgency, make universally available contraception information, reproductive and sexual health education, and should also provide effective means to assist individuals and couples who wish to or do not wish to have children. Particular attention should be given to those marginalized segments of the population that are most vulnerable, and those most difficult to reach. However, the Guatemalan State has failed to respond to this international community call for action and fulfill its obligations (CRP 2003). Why can't the Guatemalan State ensure that all its citizens, especially indigenous Mayan girls and women from rural areas, enjoy their basic human rights, obtain quality and comprehensive reproductive and sexual health services, have free access to effective contraception (IUD's and subdermal implants), and be able to obtain reliable, scientific information on planning family for women and men?

In Guatemala, abortion is against the law except to save a woman's life; however, this law is not enforced. Numerous instruments of international human rights and humanitarian law support improved access to safe abortion. The 179 country signatories of the 1994 Programme of Action of the International Conference on Population and Development (ICPD 1994) committed to addressing the consequences of unsafe abortion and supported women's right to effective contraception and to sexual and reproductive health services. The Sustainable Development Goals (SDG's 2030) ask for a growing awareness of the negative impacts of lack of contraception and of unsafe abortions on the health and lives of girls and women… and declare that access to effective contraception and to safe abortion are fundamental to women's rights and to maternal health goals.

27.4 Unmet Need for Contraception

Unmet need refers to the percentage of women not using contraception who (a) do not wish to get pregnant (or should not get pregnant); (b) want to cease further childbearing (unmet need for "limiting"); or (c) want to postpone the next birth at least 2 more years (unmet need for "spacing"). In general, as access to effective contraceptives increases, the percentage of women with unmet need decreases. However, this relationship is not "linear," since women with little education, lack of knowledge of and little access to contraception may "accept" continued childbearing and get pregnant repeatedly; thus, as they do not express a wish to avoid pregnancy and they are not counted as having unmet need. Unmet need is a politically useful indicator, because it carries no judgment of what contraceptive prevalence rate (CPR) should be in a given country, but rather reflects the voices of many of the women of that country in terms of their stated desires for getting pregnant or for not getting pregnant. The prevalence of modern effective contraceptive methods in use and the percentage of the demands that are met by effective modern methods permit assessing the extent of family planning programs, and whether they are meeting the needs for contraception and family planning services for girls and women.

The total unmet need has reportedly been reduced from 28% in 1995 to 14% according the 2015 estimates (NMCHS 2015). On the other hand, Fig. 27.3 also shows the trends for the

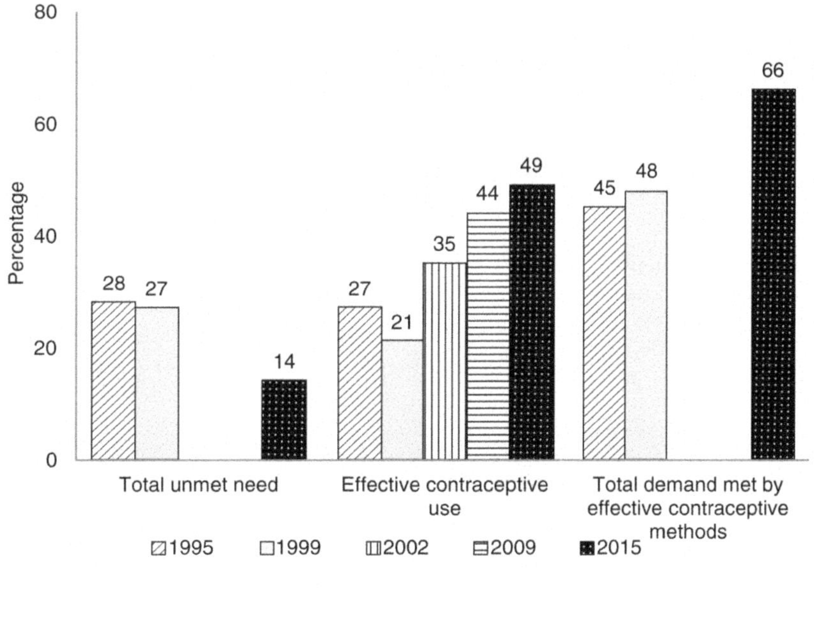

Fig. 27.3 Trends of unmet need for contraceptive methods, prevalence of use of effective contraceptive methods, and total demand met by effective contraceptive methods (from National Maternal and Child Survey 1995–2015)

prevalence of modern contraceptives for the years from 1995 to 2015. An increase from 21% (in 1999) to 49% in 2015 in the use of modern contraceptive is shown. Also, the total demand met by modern contraceptive methods increased from 45 to 66% in the same time period. These figures need to be read with much precaution, however, given that the definition used for modern contraception includes the controversial Lactation Amenorrhea Method (LAM) that must meet three conditions: (1) exclusively breastfeeding; (2) no menstrual period, and (3) no food supplement to the new born for 6 months. It is clear that most indigenous Mayan women start food supplementing their newborns as early as they can. No data are available without the LAM method, and no data are available to compare the difference between the indigenous and nonindigenous population.

27.4.1 Unmet Need for Contraception in Urban and Rural Areas of Central America

Countries in the Central American region have very different levels of unmet need in urban areas as compared to rural areas (Fig. 27.4). For example, unmet need differs by less than 2% between urban and rural areas in Honduras and Nicaragua. By contrast, in Guatemala, there is greater disparity; unmet needs are at least 10 percentage points higher in the rural areas where greater numbers of poor and indigenous women live.

Reports have shown the ethnic disparities for unmet need in married women of reproductive age (15–49 years) in five Latin American countries (Fig. 27.5), and described a higher unmet need among the indigenous populations compared with the nonindigenous population. Data for 2009 demonstrate that the greatest gap occurred in Guatemala—there was almost a 15% difference in unmet need between the indigenous Maya (29.6%) and nonindigenous population (15.1%) (Bertrand et al. 2015).

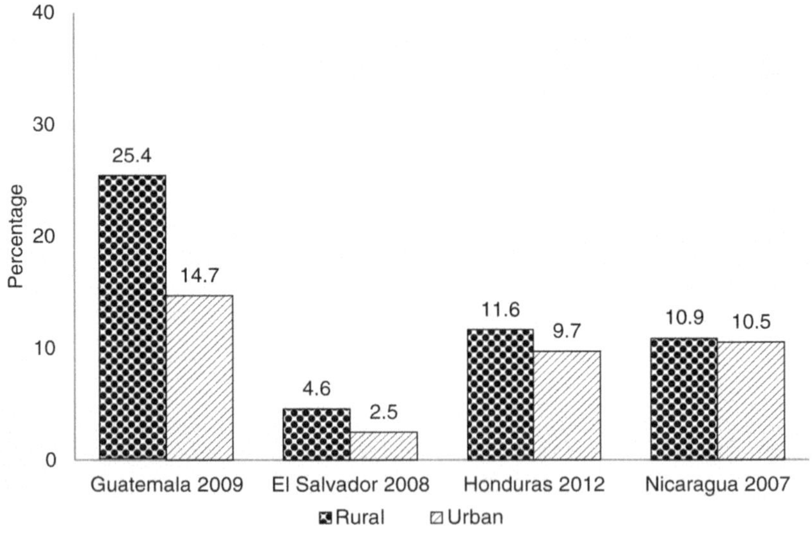

Fig. 27.4 Proportion of unmet need for contraception in four countries of Central America (from National Maternal and Child Survey 2007, 2008, 2009, and 2012)

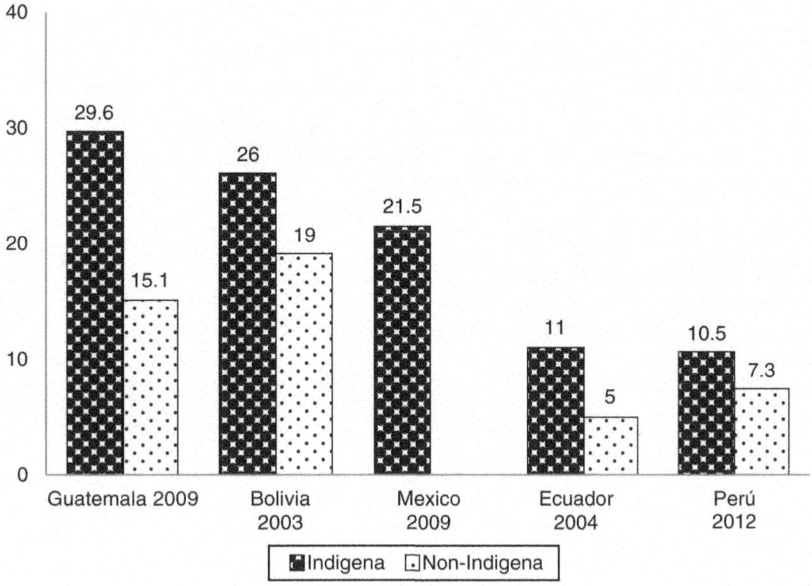

Fig. 27.5 Disparities in unmet need for married women of reproductive age 15–49 years (from Bertrand et al. 2015)

27.5 Total Fertility Rate

Total fertility rates (TFRs) have changed in Central America since 1981 (Fig. 27.6). Fertility rates have dropped in every country in Central America, in most cases by at least 1.5 child per woman (most notably in Costa Rica) over the past four decades (Bertrand et al. 2015). However, Guatemalan fertility rates have remained higher than those of all the other Central American countries.

Despite the disparity with other Central American countries, fertility rates in Guatemala have continued to decline (Fig. 27.7). The decline in total fertility rate from 5.6 children per woman in 1987 to 5 children in 1999, 4.4 children in 2002, 3.6 children in 2009, and to 3.1 children in 2015 (NMCHS 2015) is still considered a "success story." Many factors have contributed to the dramatic decline in fertility in Guatemala as well as in the entire Central American region over the past 40 years. These include increased educational levels, improved economic conditions, decreased infant and child mortality, rapid urbanization, political stability, and changing cultural norms, among others. Unfortunately, in Guatemala, significant ethnic disparities have persisted and are reflected in the observations that the total fertility rate in 2015 was 3.6 children per "indigenous" woman compared to 2.8 children per "nonindigenous" woman.

27.5.1 Fertility Rate in Mayan Populations

The 50% decrease in fertility rates for the indigenous Mayan population over the 28-year period of 1987–2015 was very significant, being as notable as that for nonindigenous women. However, the TFR for indigenous Mayan population has persistently remained higher. The TFR in 1987, which was 6.8 children per indigenous woman in 1987 (compared with 5 children per nonindigenous woman), decreased to 3.6 children per indigenous woman in 2015 (compared to 2.8 children per nonindigenous woman) (Fig. 27.8) (NMCHS 2015).

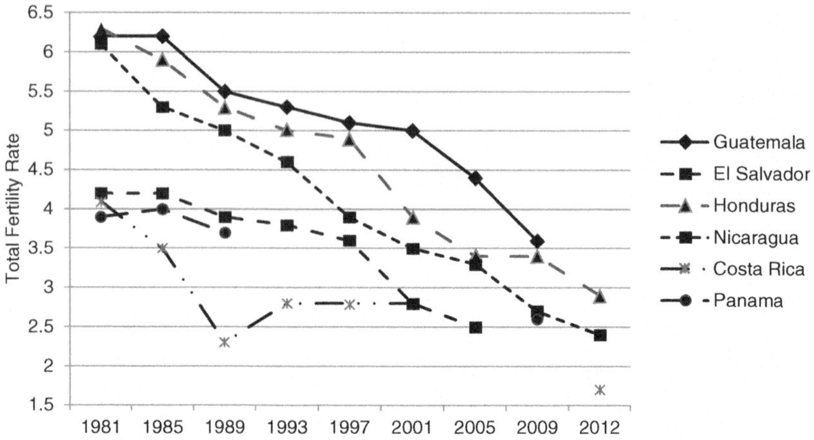

Fig. 27.6 Decreasing trends in total fertility rates in Central America (from Bertrand et al. 2015)

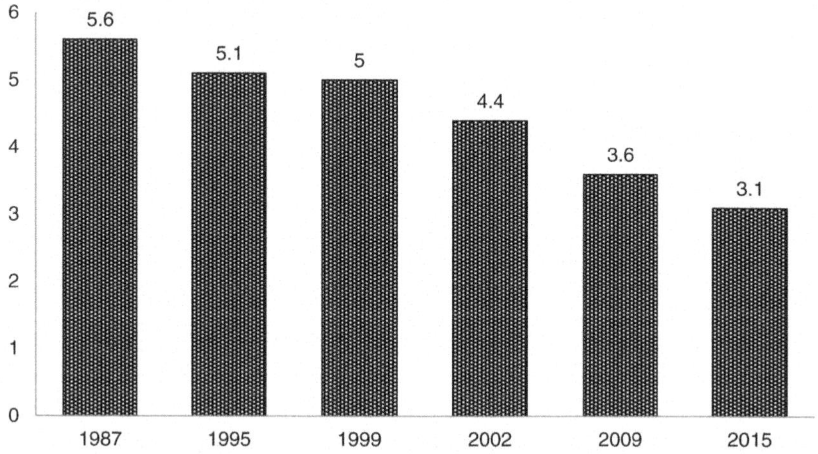

Fig. 27.7 Decreasing trends in Total Fertility Rate (TFR 1987–2015) in Guatemala (from National Maternal and Child Survey 1987–2015)

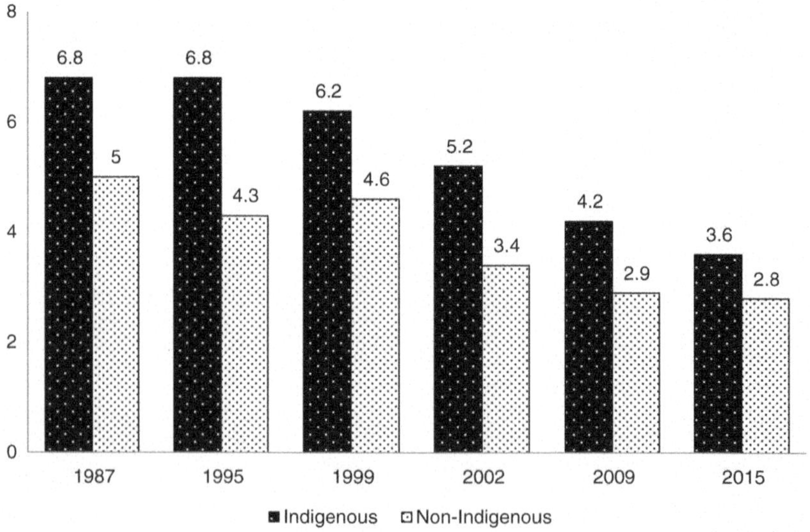

Fig. 27.8 Trends in Total Fertility Rate (TFR) from 1987 to 2015 among indigenous Mayan and nonindigenous women (from National Maternal and Child Survey 1987–2015)

Fig. 27.9 Trends of contraceptive use prevalence rates (modern and traditional methods) (from National Maternal and Child Survey 1977–2012)

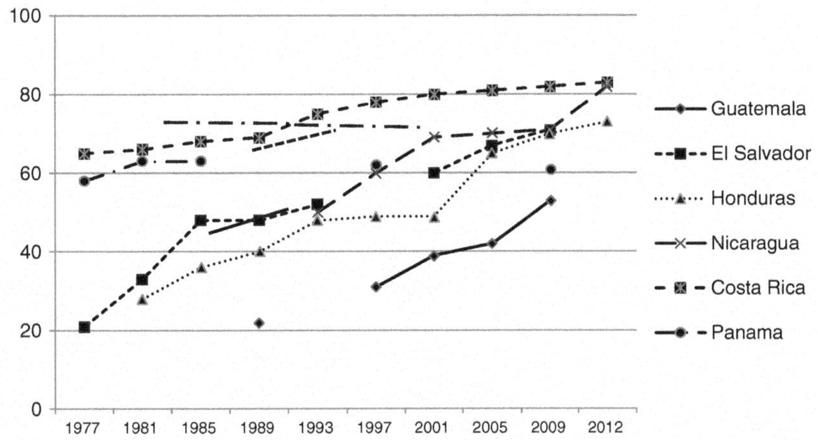

Family planning is defined as a conscious effort "shared-informed decision-making" of a mature adult woman or a couple to limit the size of their family through the spacing or prevention of pregnancy. Contraception is defined as the deliberate prevention of conception or of pregnancy by any or various drugs, techniques, or devices. The term "birth control" has become obsolete and controversial; it is also a bit inaccurate since the goal of family planning and of contraception is to reduce the risks of getting pregnant and hopefully to prevent pregnancy and not to prevent birth.

Family planning evolved from a virtually taboo subject to a widely accepted practice throughout most of the Central American countries. While family planning is still a politically sensitive topic among some religious-evangelical-right-to-life adherents throughout the region, it is widely accepted by the medical community and by the majority of the population in most nations. Over the past 30 years contraceptive prevalence rates (modern and traditional) for married adult women over 18 years of age in selected Central American countries show a steady increase (Fig. 27.9). Data for Guatemala show that in 1989 the contraceptive prevalence was estimated at 22%, and only 20 years later in 2009 the prevalence rates had reportedly increased to 53%. However, these data may be inaccurate and unreliable; they also seem to mix modern, effective methods such as IUD's, subdermal implants, and injections of progestin's with traditional and lesser effective methods including LAM, "withdrawal," "fertility awareness-based methods," rhythm, and abstinence. Nonetheless, they do suggest that Guatemala has one of the lowest contraceptive use prevalence rates in Latin America (Bertrand et al. 2015).

Recent 2015 data from Guatemala (NMCHS 2015) indicate that contraceptive use has increased in association with increases in the number of surviving children, greater education, and increasing wealth. For modern methods[1] contraceptive use was 38% by women with no education compared to 60% for women with higher education. Sixty-one per cent of currently married adult women currently used a contraceptive method; 49% used an effective modern method, and 12% used a traditional method.[2]

In the past 28 years, indigenous Mayan populations in Guatemala have maintained low rates of use of effective contraceptive methods (Fig. 27.10) ranging from 4.5% in 1987 to 11.8% in 2009. Data for the year 2015 show that almost one-third of indigenous women had access to safe and effective contraceptive methods, as compared with greater than one-half of nonindigenous women.

[1]The most effective modern methods are female and male sterilization, implants, and IUD's; progestin injections, pills, patch, rings, and male and female condoms are less effective.

[2]Traditional methods which include "necklace method," Lactating Amenorrhea Method or LAM, rhythm, abstinence, and withdrawal are the least effective.

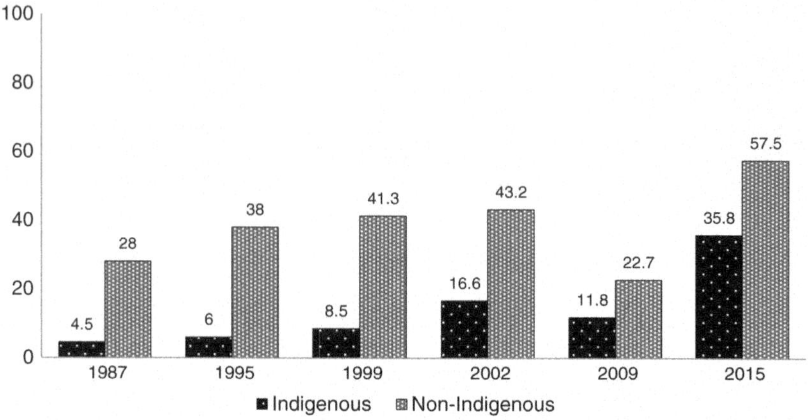

Fig. 27.10 Trends in the use of effective, modern contraceptives by ethnic group (from National Maternal and Child Survey 1987–2015)

Table 27.3 Trends in effective contraceptive use in indigenous and nonindigenous women. Guatemala 1987–2015 (from National Maternal and Child Survey 1987–2015)

		Female sterilization	DMPA	Pill	Condom	Jadelle/ Norplant	IUD	Male sterilization
1987	Indigenous	2.8	0.3	1.0	0	0	0.1	0.3
	Nonindigenous	15.0	0.6	5.7	1.9	0	2.9	1.3
1995	Indigenous	N/A	N/A	N/A	N/A	N/A	N/A	N/A
	Nonindigenous	N/A	N/A	N/A	N/A	N/A	N/A	N/A
1999	Indigenous	4.3	1.9	1.6	0.1	0	0.3	0.3
	Nonindigenous	22.5	4.8	6.6	3.3	0	3.0	1.0
2002	Indigenous	5.9	8.0	1.4	0.4	0	0.7	0.1
	Nonindigenous	22.1	9.5	4.3	3.3	0.1	2.4	1.4
2009	Indigenous	7.2	2.4	0.5	1.6	0	0.1	0
	Nonindigenous	12.3	3.5	2.2	3.9	0	0.6	0.2
2015	Indigenous	12.4	16.5	1.3	2.4	1.7	1.2	0.3
	Nonindigenous	26.8	16.6	4.6	4.9	2.0	1.7	0.9

When we study the trends over the same period of 1987–2009 for the use of effective contraception in both ethnic groups (indigenous and nonindigenous women), the figures are disappointing. In 1987, the use of effective contraceptive methods was greater in the nonindigenous population, but still extremely low: female sterilization (15%); contraceptive pills (5.7%), and IUD's (2.9%). Among the indigenous population, the data were 2.8%, 1%, and 0.1%, respectively (Table 27.3). Twenty-eight years later there are very modest changes for both ethnic groups. Recent data (NMCHS 2015) shows that female sterilization has remained a very attractive option for the nonindigenous group (26.8%), followed by DMPA (depot medroxyprogesterone acetate or Depo-Provera®) (16.5%) and the pill (4.6%). Indigenous Mayan women seem to prefer progestin injections of DMPA (16.5%) followed by female sterilization (12.4%). Table 27.3 shows the breakdown for each of the effective contraceptive methods and their prevalence through time.

27.6 Unintended Pregnancy

Unintended pregnancies are pregnancies that are mistimed, unplanned, or unwanted. An unintended pregnancy results (1) most frequently from "unsafe-unprotected sexual practices" such as engaging in vaginal-penile sexual activity without the use of contraception, or (2) due to incorrect use of a contraception method, but (3) may also arise from failure of the contraception method even when used correctly to prevent pregnancy or reduce the risks of getting pregnant. In Guatemala, as in other countries, women may resort to abortion when they have an unintended pregnancy. Some are unable to care for a child; some already have all the children they want; others do not want the pregnancy because it is the result of forced sex or incest; and some women's lives or health are at risk if they continue with the pregnancy. A number of other factors also contribute to unintended pregnancy and seeking abortion, including insufficient and inaccurate information about contraception, inadequate access to services and supplies, and incorrect and inconsistent contraceptive use.

Measuring or estimating the number of unintended pregnancies in Guatemala is not easy. One previous publication (Singh et al. 2006) "guesstimated" the statistics of unintended pregnancy, and calculated the number of unplanned births by applying the proportion of births that are unplanned, mistimed, or unwanted to the estimated total annual number of live births needed. Combining this number with the number of induced abortions yielded an estimate of the number of unintended pregnancies. The rate of unintended pregnancies per 1000 women in the reproductive age range (15–49 years) and the proportion of pregnancies that were unintended were calculated.

Table 27.4 illustrates that for Guatemala a total of 66 unintended pregnancies occurred per 1000 women, and that more than one-third of all pregnancies were unintended. All but two regions had higher-than-average unintended pregnancy rates (68–77 per 1000). The Northwest region had a noticeably lower-than-average unintended pregnancy rate (46 per 1000), as well the lowest proportion of unintended pregnancy (21%). The Metropolitan region had a somewhat lower-than-average unintended pregnancy rate (59 per 1000), but a higher-than-average percentage of "unintended pregnancies" (37%), presumably reflecting both its higher levels of contraceptive use and its more educated population, which is likely to be more motivated to achieve fertility preferences.

Overall, 205 pregnancies occurred per 1000 women aged 15–49 years. The pregnancy rate varied substantially across regions, being lowest in the Metropolitan region (160 per 1000), and with highest in the Petén and North regions (258 and 264 per 1000, respectively).

Table 27.4 Estimates of number of pregnancies, unintended pregnancy rate, proportion of pregnancy that were unintended, and pregnancy rate according geographical region

Region	Number of pregnancies	Unintended pregnancy rate[a]	Proportion of pregnancy that were unintended	Pregnancy rate[b]
Metropolitan	112,451	59	37	160
North	58,640	77	29	264
Northeast	48,258	70	33	212
Southeast	42,353	68	35	196
Central	57,546	75	38	195
Southwest	141,093	72	32	223
Northwest	76,916	46	21	225
Peten	20,234	77	30	258
Total	**557,492**	**66**	**32**	**205**

[a]Number of unintended pregnancies (unplanned births + abortions) per 1000 women aged 15–49 per year
[b]Number of pregnancies (live births + induced abortions + spontaneous abortions) per 1000 women aged 15–49 per year

27.7 Induced Abortion

The World Health Organization (WHO) defines unsafe surgical abortion as a procedure for terminating a pregnancy carried out either by persons lacking the necessary skills or in an environment that does not conform to minimal medical standards, or both (WHO 1992). Greater than 97% of women of childbearing age in Latin America and the Caribbean live in countries where abortion is restricted, illegal, or banned altogether. Abortion is not permitted for any reason in seven countries in Latin America; three of them are Central American countries (Table 27.5). It is allowed only to save the women's life in two Central American Countries (Guatemala and Panama). Only Panama allows abortion in cases of rape, fetal impairment, or parental authorization.

During the period from 2010 to 2014, an estimated 6.5 million induced abortions were performed each year in Latin America and the Caribbean, compared to 4.4 million during the earlier period of 1990–1994, i.e., an increase of almost two million of induced abortions in the Latina American countries. For these two periods of study, it has been calculated that Central American countries have seen an increase of 500,000 induced abortions annually, and a corresponding increase in the abortion rate (abortions per 1000 women aged 15–44 years) from 27 to 33 (Table 27.6). Central American women are believed to continue to have one-fourth of their pregnancies terminate in abortions (Sedgh et al. 2016).

27.7.1 Quantitative Abortion Data in Guatemala

Induced abortion is highly restricted and allowed only to save a woman's life in Guatemala. However, abortions are commonly performed, and it is estimated that approximately 65,000 abortions are performed each year for Guatemalan women aged 15–49 years; this represents an annual rate of 24 abortions for every 1000 Guatemalan women. As it is the case in all other countries with highly restricted abortion legislation, abortions in Guatemala are quite often carried out clandestinely and in conditions where the risks of injury, infection, and death of girls and women are very high. Indeed, many women and girls die, and many more suffer complications, because a large proportion of abortions are carried

Table 27.5 Legality and illegality of abortion in Central American Region (modified from Center for Reproductive Rights (CRR), *The World's Abortion Laws 2016*, New York CRR, 2016)

Central American Countries according to reasons for which abortion is legally permitted or prohibited	
Reason	Countries
Prohibited altogether, or no explicit legal exception to save the life of a woman	El Salvador, Honduras, and Nicaragua
To save the life of a woman	Guatemala, Panamá[a]
To preserve physical health and to save a woman's life	Costa Rica

[a]Panamá also allows abortion in cases of rape, fetal impairment, and parental authorization

Table 27.6 Regional and Central American estimates of induced abortion, 1990–1994 and 2010–2014

	Number of abortions (millions)		Abortion rate (#per 1000 women aged 15–44 years		% of pregnancies ending in abortion
	1990–1994	2010–2014	1990–1994	2010–2014	2010–2014
Latin America and the Caribbean	4.4	6.5[a]	40	44	32
Central America	0.8	1.3[a]	27	33	24

[a]Difference between 2010–2014 and 1990–1994 is statistically significant

out by unqualified persons and without the proper hygienic and aseptic conditions resulting in such life-threatening complications as postpartum endometritis, puerperal sepsis, genital trauma, intestinal obstruction or perforation, postpartum hemorrhage, and thrombosis (Schwartz 2015a, b).

During the last decades, many studies have reported on the large number of women who have undergone hospitalization for complications from induced abortions, thus confirming that induced abortion is common in Guatemala (Kestler et al. 2006; Grajeda et al. 1995; Figueroa and Schieber 2001). Recent data suggest that increasing numbers of girls and women who have had induced abortion complications have been seeking postabortion care at hospitals and local clinics (Cobb et al. 2001; Haddad and Nour 2009).

The number of induced abortions can be approximated using indirect estimation methodologies previously validated and adapted to the Guatemalan context and published elsewhere (Singh et al. 2006). Using these methodologies, about 65,000 induced abortions are estimated to have occurred in Guatemala yearly (Table 27.7). This number is a mean estimation between 43,000 and 87,000 abortions. These estimates also indicate that, on average, there is probably one woman with abortion-related complications who needs to be hospitalized for every three who have obtained an induced abortion.

In 2003, the "estimated national abortion rate" was 24 induced abortions per 1000 women aged 15–49 years; the low estimate was 16 per 1000 women, and the high estimate was 32 per 1000 women in the reproductive age group (Fig. 27.11). Rates are higher than averages in the Metropolitan and Southwest regions (29 and 30, respectively), followed by the Northeast, Southeast, Central, and Peten regions (21–24 per 1000). The North and Northwest regions have substantially lower rates (8–15 per 1000).

Table 27.7 Complications of induced abortions and estimated number of induced abortions (after Singh et al. 2006)

Region	Number of women 15–49 years treated in hospital for complications of induced abortions	Estimated number of induced abortions
Metropolitan	7021	21,094
North	605	1818
Northeast	1723	5177
Southeast	1692	5084
Central	2330	7001
Southwest	6056	18,195
Northwest	1650	4957
Peten	548	1647
Total	**21,625**	**64,974**

Source: Singh et al. (2006)

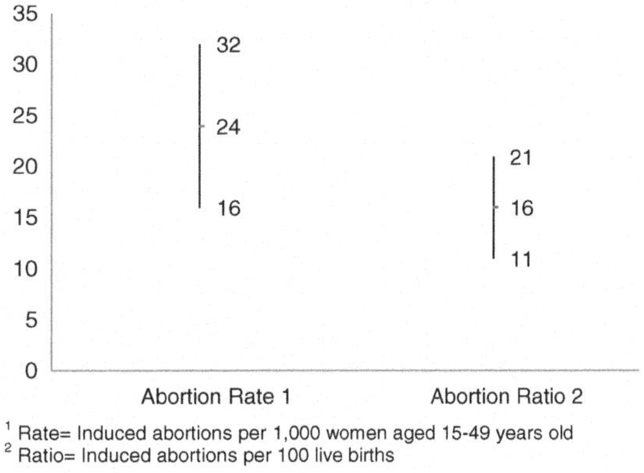

Fig. 27.11 Estimates of the abortion rates and the abortion ratios for women not treated in a hospital setting (from Singh et al. 2006)

The abortion rate is the number of abortions per 1000 women ages 15–49 years; the abortion ratio is the number of abortions per 100 live births. The "national abortion ratio" estimates for Guatemala lie between 11 and 21 abortions per 100 live births, with a yearly average of 16 abortions per 100 live births. This means that in Guatemala as a whole, approximately one pregnancy is voluntarily aborted for every six that results in a live birth.

27.7.2 Qualitative Abortion Data

Although an induced abortion is medically safe when performed in accordance with WHO recommended guidelines (WHO 2012), many women undergo unsafe procedures that put their well-being and lives at risk (Schwartz 2015a). Previous studies on abortion from a population health perspective (Saenz de Tejada et al. 2006) describe some of the postabortion morbidity or "abortion complications" that are not treated in health institutions or clinics. These also described many of the perceptions and opinions of a group of indigenous men, women, and ancestral health providers in Mayan communities. In these traditional Mayan communities, motherhood is highly valued, and the essence of marriage is believed to be for purposes of procreation. Some have reported that the concepts of fertility control and the notions of contraception and family planning may seem foreign to most Mayans, and that the interruption of an unplanned pregnancy may appear inconceivable to many. However, this report also revealed that numerous rural Mayan women who experience a "delay in their menstrual period" will often attempt to bring about their menstruation through the use of Mayan traditional methods.

Many Mayan girls and women with an unplanned-unwanted pregnancy may therefore try to induce an abortion themselves by taking "special community beverages" or other homemade remedies, perform traditional Mayan practices, and/or ingest massive doses of analgesics. If these fail, many go on to seek induced illegal abortions by someone in the community who, too often, may use unsanitary methods. Others may consult a "pharmacist"—typically an inexpensive healer or a trusted Mayan practitioner who is readily accessible, who appears more compassionate regarding their situation, and who more closely shares their Mayan cultural identity.

The following graph (Fig. 27.12) depicts the proportion of women seeking abortion, according to their economic status and different abortion providers. It is clear that poor rural indigenous women are

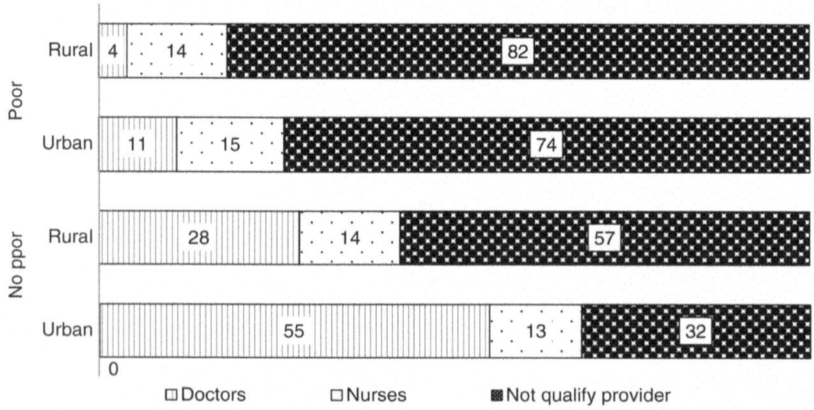

Fig. 27.12 Proportion of induced abortion by different providers (from Singh et al. 2006)

Fig. 27.13 Proportion of poor/nonpoor vs. urban/rural women with complications secondary to induced abortion (from Singh et al. 2006)

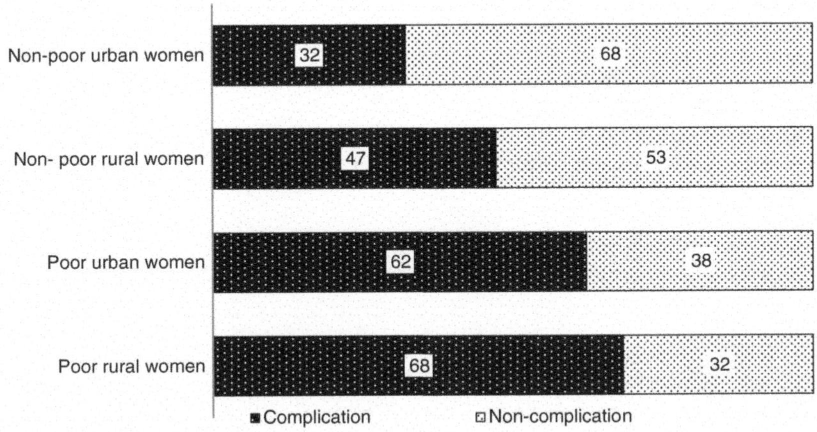

much more likely to use the services of abortion providers who are not qualified (82%). The graph also suggests that urban women with greater economic resources tend to seek the medical services of trained and well-qualified medical doctors and nurses.

The bar graph below (Fig. 27.13) shows that poor women in rural areas experience the majority of complications from having an induced abortion (68%), followed by poor urban women (62%), while 47% of nonpoor rural women and 32% of nonpoor urban women have postabortion complications.

27.8 Maternal Mortality and Induced Abortion

According to the most recent estimates, in Latin America and the Caribbean at least 900 (10%) of all maternal deaths were due to unsafe abortion, and 760,000 women are treated annually for complications from unsafe abortions. Limited access to effective modern contraceptives and restrictive abortion laws are the main causes of a significant number of deaths of girls and women due to unsafe abortions (Kestler et al. 2008)

The definition of maternal mortality has recently been stated to be "the death of any woman dying of any cause whatsoever while pregnant or within 1 year after the termination of the pregnancy, irrespective of the duration of the pregnancy at the time of the termination or the method by which it was terminated". It is not yet universally accepted.

Maternal mortality is a very sensitive issue in Guatemala. Reaching a low maternal mortality ratio (MMR) should be among the main priorities in the public health sector. Guatemala had been committed, as have many countries in the region, to reach the United Nations Millennium Development Goal #5 (United Nations 2000) to reduce maternal mortality by 75% by 2015. Unfortunately, this goal was not reached. Although Guatemala has recorded a slight progress in reducing maternal mortality, the official report for the MDG5 still shows that there were greater than 100 maternal deaths per 100,000 live births (Fig. 27.14).

It is unfortunate that many, and perhaps even most, of these mother deaths are preventable (Schwartz 2015c). These unnecessary maternal deaths indicate and reflect the extent of social injustices, neglect, inequities and biases against poor Mayan women in rural areas. Induced abortion continues to be one of the leading causes of avoidable maternal deaths in Guatemala, and a formidable population health challenge. In the year 2000, induced abortion accounted for 10% of all

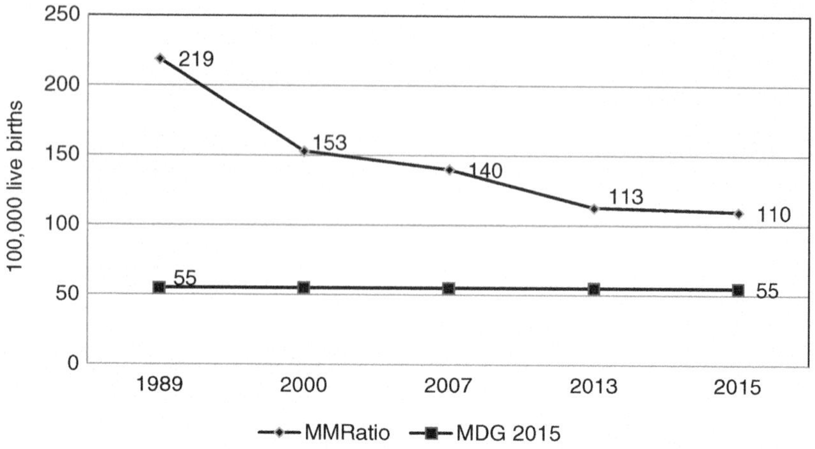

Fig. 27.14 Trends for the Maternal Mortality Ratio (MMR) in Guatemala 1989–2015 (from SEGEPLAN, http://metasdelmilenio.segeplan.gob.gt/odm/?page_id=686)

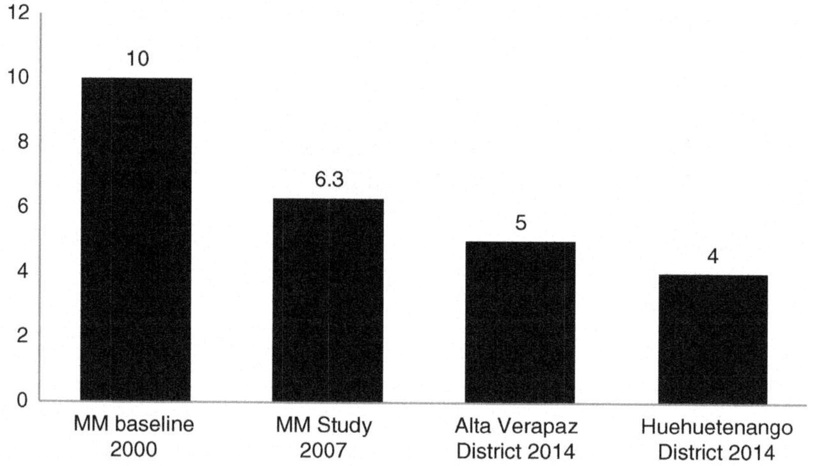

Fig. 27.15 Proportion of women dying as a result of induced abortion from 2000 to 2014 in Guatemala (from MOH-CIESAR 2015, 2016)

national maternal deaths (MOH LBMM 2003), and 7 years later a new national maternal mortality study determined that 6.3% of maternal deaths were still related to induced abortion. More recent reports from two of the main districts/departments in Guatemala (Alta Verapaz and Huehuetenango) which have very large indigenous populations determined that for the 5 years studied, 2000–2014, induced abortions were still responsible for 5% of preventable maternal deaths in Alta Verapaz (MOH-CIESAR 2015) and 4% of preventable maternal deaths in Huehuetenango (MOH-CIESAR 2016) (Fig. 27.15).

It is very sad that abortion continues to be requested, and a surgical abortion is especially dangerous in settings where the procedure is severely restricted legally (Schwartz 2015a). Reducing the risk of unintended pregnancy by offering effective contraceptives decreases the likelihood that young girls and women will need to turn to such procedures as potentially hazardous unsafe abortions. The provision of high-quality postabortion services and of immediate postabortion contraception with IUD's or implants will prevent repeated abortion cases and maternal deaths. There are multiple international examples where the provision of quality postabortion care and of effective contraception has significantly reduced the maternal mortality related to unsafe abortions (Cobb et al. 2001; Haddad and Nour 2009; Azmat et al. 2012).

27.9 Recommendations

Since young adolescents are among the groups at highest risk for unplanned pregnancies and induced abortions, it is critically important that the government provide not only comprehensive sexual education to them but also effective contraceptives, "free LARC's first" to all Guatemalan youth, in compliance with the Social Development Law (SDL 2001). GuateMayan *comadronas*, traditional birth attendants (TBSs), lay midwives and other primary healthcare providers and medical personnel are not likely to be advocates for "post-obstetrical-events contraception" or to provide effective methods of preventing repeat pregnancies, particularly to girls aged 10–19 who have recently been pregnant. Thus, the urgent priority and formidable challenges are to educate, train, and certify new primary care providers who are entirely dedicated to adolescents, and who would routinely provide quality "adolescent medicine services" and routinely offer LARCs after all pregnancies.

Adult men and women who may seem opposed to family planning will need frequent and repeated educational programs to dispel their misconceptions and to embrace strategies that improve their lives and the lives of their children. Culturally sensitive and ethnically competent healthcare providers, hospitals, and clinics are clearly needed to do so. Having at least some familiarity with the language(s) of the ethnic Maya women would be very helpful in providing clear communications regarding the available choices of contraception and their correct usage (see Navarro, S.M. et al. *Contraceptive Counseling and Family Planning Services in the Chiapas Highlands: Challenges and Opportunities for Improving Access for the Indigenous Population*; and Sheedy, C. *Speaking in Tongues: The Importance of Learning Indigenous Languages in Healthcare Amongst Indigenous Populations*, this volume). Posters and public service announcements, both in Spanish and Guatemalan ethnic languages, should broadcast the message that "*Unsafe surgical abortions performed by untrained practitioners kill girls and women*". Unsafe surgical abortions performed by untrained practitioners must be presented to the public as dangerous and deadly procedures which can be avoided by preventing adolescent pregnancies with "free LARCs first," and by offering freely available and effective methods of family planning to adult men and women.

The dissemination of accurate information on the numbers of abortions performed each year, descriptions of their serious and devastating biomedical consequences, and their psychological impact can help reduce the secrecy and the stigma of abortion, helping to counteract the disinformation and by certain groups traditionally opposed to a woman's right to choose her own reproductive alternatives including contraception and abortion. Accurate and reliable records on abortion morbidity and mortality in Guatemala are urgently needed in order to help guide future reproductive health policies. It is necessary that the Ministry of Health, hospital private organizations, and medical societies implement a mandatory system of anonymous registration of postabortion cases handled (including basic demographic and obstetric history of patients) in all health institutions that provide postabortion treatment.

Conclusions

Unsafe abortion has been described as "one of the most neglected sexual and reproductive health problems in the world today" and is a major public health crisis throughout many developing countries and low resource settings. In 2008, 43.8 million abortions were reported to have been performed worldwide; nearly one-half of these abortions were unsafe, and 98% of all unsafe abortions occurred in developing nations (Sedgh et al. 2016). Worldwide, unsafe abortions are believed to result in eight maternal deaths every hour (Schwartz 2015a). Surgical abortion procedures, when performed by trained professionals in appropriate settings, carry very low risks of complications and death. In countries where abortion is criminalized, it must, therefore, occur in clandestine and usually unsafe conditions. Restrictive antiabortion laws have never prevented and will not prevent women from having abortions; indeed, it is reported that the estimated rate of abortions in those countries where abortion is prohibited or only allowed to save the life of the mother is still high—approximately 37 per 1000 women aged 15–44 years. Restrictive abortion laws have always been associated with greater risks of disabilities and deaths for girls and women; these unjust misogynous laws simply make abortion illegal, stigmatized, costlier to society, and inhumanely harmful.

Unsafe abortions, together with the consequent maternal morbidity and mother deaths due to complications of unsafe abortions, continue to afflict the lives of many women, mostly in developing countries like Guatemala. Unsafe abortion is the cause of serious complications, disability, and mortality for millions of women each year (Schwartz 2015a, b). The global numbers of unsafe abortions have risen with the global increase in the number of women of reproductive age. This inhumane trend may, and very likely will, continue unless girls and women have free and easy access to effective contraception and to comprehensive reproductive-sexual services. Unsafe abortions and their medical and psychological consequences are entirely preventable; the disabilities and the deaths from unsafe abortions are avoidable in the twenty-first century. Mayan girls and women of Guatemala need not die from unplanned-mistimed or unwanted pregnancies.

All evidence suggests that a reliance on abortion can be and will be greatly reduced when: (a) girls and women are free to plan their reproductive lives, making their own decisions whether to utilize effective contraception and when and if they desire to become pregnant; (b) access becomes freely available for counselling and reproductive health services to reduce the unmet need for contraception and family planning for both women and men; (c) "free LARC's first" (free Long-Acting-Reversible-Contraceptives like IUD's and contraceptive subdermal implants) are routinely offered and easily provided to adolescent girls between puberty and age 19 years; and (d) an appropriate mix of contraception and sterilization methods are offered to all adult women and men, both married and unmarried.

The 2016 Guatemalan government has recently enacted new policies, programs, and plans to improve women's reproductive health, but it is too early for studies to be implemented and reviewed to assess their impact. Unfortunately, the issue of maternal death and illness resulting from unsafe abortion has not been properly addressed, and the lack of comprehensive and reliable data makes effective action difficult. Because unsafe abortion is a critical factor in causing maternal morbidity and mortality in Guatemala, and because it is financially costly and represents a very significant expenditure for the meagre budgets of Guatemalan hospitals and clinics, reliable and accurate quantitative indicators are needed to assess the extent of the practice, to determine all its negative impact on women's health, and to seek effective means to improve reproductive health services and postabortion care.

Acknowledgment To Roger Duvivier, M.D., F.A.C.O.G., for the review, edition, and constructive comments.

References

Azmat, S. K., Shaikh, B. T., Mustafa, G., Hameed, W., & Bilgrami, M. (2012). Delivering post-abortion care through a community based reproductive health volunteer programme in Pakistan. *Journal of Biosocial Science, 44*(6), 719–731. https://doi.org/10.1017/S0021932012000296

Bertrand, J. T., Ward, V. M., & Santiso-Gálvez, R. (2015). *Family planning in Latin America and the Caribbean: The achievements of 50 years*. Chapel Hill, NC: MEASURE Evaluation. Retrieved January 29, 2017, from https://www.measureevaluation.org/resources/publications/tr-15-101

CRP [Center for Reproductive Rights]. (2003). *La Planificación familiar en Guatemala no se cumple*. New York City, NY: Center for Reproductive Rights. Retieved from http://www.reproductiverights.org

Cobb, L., Putney, P., Rochat, R., Solo, J., Buono, N., Dunlop, J., et al. (2001) *Global evaluation of USAID's Postabortion Care Program*. POPTECH Publication Number 2001-024-007. Washington, DC: The Population Technical Assistance Project. Retrieved January 27, 2017, from http://pdf.usaid.gov/pdf_docs/pnacn773.pdf

Figueroa, W., & Schieber, B. (2001). *Study of the use of financial resources in reproductive health and post abortion care*. New York: Population Council.

Grajeda, R., et al. (1995). *Estudio multicéntrico sobre aborto*. Guatemala City: World Health Organization (WHO).

Haddad, L. B., & Nour, N. M. (2009). Unsafe abortion: Unnecessary maternal mortality. *Reviews in Obstetetrics & Gynecology, 2*(2), 122–126.

ICDP. (1994). *International conference development population*. Cairo, Egypt. Retrieved September, 1994, from http://www.un.org/popin/icpd/conference/offeng/poa.html

IFAD. (2011). *International fund for agricultural development*. Rural Poverty Report. ISBN 978-92-9072-200-7. Retrieved from https://www.ifad.org/documents/10180/c47f2607-3fb9-4736-8e6a-a7ccf3dc7c5b

INE-ENCOVI. (2014). *Encuesta Nacional de Condiciones de Vida*. Guatemala: Instituto Nacional de Estadística. Retrieved January 18, 2017, from http://www.ine.gob.gt/sistema/uploads/2014/01/15/v8ukWQ78M4VJrnYqyN2oCumMy1GiBzaf.pdf

Isaacs, S. L., & Cook, R. J. (1984). Laws and policies affecting fertility: A decade of change. *Population Reports Series E, Law & Policy, 12*(6), E105–E151.

Kestler, E., Valencia, L., Del Valle, V., & Silva, A. (2006). Scaling up post-abortion care in Guatemala: Initial successes at national level. *Reproductive Health Matters, 14*(27), 138–147.

Kestler, E., Silva, A., Del Valle, V., Hernández, E. M., & Barrios, B. (2008). Acceso humanizado a métodos contraceptivo modernos en Hospitales Públicos de Guatemala. *Revista Centroamericana de Obstetricia y Ginecología (REVCOG), 13*(3), 77–84.

Mauldin, W. P., Choucri, N., Notestein, F. W., & Teitelbaum, M. (1974). A report on Bucharest: The world population conference and the population tribune, august 1974. *Studies in Family Planning, 5*(12), 357–395.

MOH LBMM. (2003). *Informe Final: Línea Basal de Mortalidad Materna para el año* 2000. Ministerio de Salud Pública Guatemala. Ciudad de Guatemala: MSPAS.

MOH-CIESAR. (2015). *Tendencia de la mortalidad materna en el departamento de Alta Verapaz 2010–2014*. Ministerio de Salud Pública y Asistencia Social. Guatemala, Alta Verapaz : Centro de Investigación Epidemiológica en Salud Sexual y Reproductiva. ISBN: 978-9929-40-788-6.

MOH-CIESAR. (2016). *Tendencia de la mortalidad materna en el departamento de Huehuetenango 2010–2014*. Ministerio de Salud Pública y Asistencia Social. Guatemala, Huehuetenango: Centro de Investigación Epidemiológica en Salud Sexual y Reproductiva. ISBN: 978-9929-40-789-3.

NMCHS. (2015). National Maternal and Child Health Survey/Encuesta Nacional Materno Infantil Guatemala. Ministerio de Salud Pública y Asistencia Social (MSPAS), Instituto Nacional de Estadística (INE), ICF International.

Prado, A. (2013). *"Propuesta de Intervención" INCAE, 2013*. Central American Health Care Initiative (CAHI). Retrieved from http://ca-hi.org/assets/Una-Propuesta-de-Intervención.pdf

Saénz de Tejada, S., Prada, E., & Ball, G. (2006). *Morbilidad por aborto en Guatemala: Una visión de la comunidad*. Informe Ocasional No. 27. New York: Guttmacher Institute. Retrieved January 20, 2017, from https://www.guttmacher.org/pubs/2006/11/09/or_27.pdf

Schwartz, D. A. (2015a). Unsafe abortion: A persistent cause of maternal death and reproductive morbidity in resource-poor nations. In D. A. Schwartz (Ed.), *Maternal mortality: Risk factors, anthropological perspectives, prevalence in developing countries and preventive strategies for pregnancy-related death* (pp. 425–439). New York: Nova Science Publishers.

Schwartz, D. A. (2015b). The pathology of maternal death—the importance of accurate autopsy diagnosis for epidemiologic surveillance and prevention of maternal mortality in developing countries. In D. A. Schwartz (Ed.), *Maternal mortality: Risk factors, anthropological perspectives, prevalence in developing countries and preventive strategies for pregnancy-related death* (pp. 215–253). New York: Nova Science Publishers.

Schwartz, D. A. (2015c). Interface of epidemiology, anthropology and health care in maternal death prevention in resource-poor nations. In D. A. Schwartz (Ed.), *Maternal mortality: Risk factors, anthropological perspectives, prevalence in developing countries and preventive strategies for pregnancy-related death* (pp. ix–xiv). New York: Nova Science Publishers.

Sedgh, G., Bearak, J., Singh, S., Bankole, A., Popinchalk, A., Ganatra, B., et al. (2016). Abortion incidence between 1990 and 2014: Global, regional and subregional levels and trends. *The Lancet, 388*(10041), 258–267. https://doi.org/10.1016/S0140-6736(16)30380-4

Singh, S., Prada, E., & Kestler, E. (2006). Induced abortion and unintended pregnancy in Guatemala. *International Perspectives on Sexual and Reproductive Health, 32*(3), 136–145. Retrieved January 2, 2017, from https://www.guttmacher.org/journals/ipsrh/2006/09/induced-abortion-and-unintended-pregnancy-guatemala

SDL. (2001). *Social development law*. Ley de Desarrollo Social Decreto número 42-2001. Retrieved from http://www.depadresahijos.org/derechos/ley_desarrollosocial.pdf

United Nations. (1948). *Universal declaration of human rights*. Retrieved from http://www.un.org/en/ga/search/view_doc.asp?symbol=A/RES/217(III)

United Nations. (1968). *United Nations final act of the international conference on human rights*. Teheran, Iran. Retrieved January 28, 2017, from http://www.cfr.org/human-rights/un-international-conference-human-rights-1968-final-outcome-document/p25933

United Nations. (2000). *Millennium Summit (6–8 September 2000)*. Retrieved January 20, 2017, from http://www.un.org/en/events/pastevents/millennium_summit.shtml

United Nations. (2015). *United nations sustainable development goals. 17 goals to transform our world*. Retieved January 27, 2017, from http://www.un.org/sustainabledevelopment/sustainable-development-goals/

WHO. (1992). *The prevention and management of unsafe abortion*. Report of a Technical Working Group. Geneva, 12–15 April 1992. WHO/MSM/92.5. Geneva: WHO. Retrieved December 21, 2016, from http://whqlibdoc.who.int/hq/1992/WHO_MSM_92.5.pdf

WHO. (2011). *Unsafe abortion: Global and regional estimates of the incidence of unsafe abortion and associated mortality in 2008* (6th ed.). Geneva: WHO.

WHO. (2012). *Safe Abortion: Technical and policy guidance for health systems* (2nd ed.). UNDP/UNFPA/WHO/World Bank Special Programme of Research. ISBN: 978 92 4 154843 4. Retrieved Decemeber 28, 2016, from http://apps.who.int/iris/bitstream/10665/70914/1/9789241548434_eng.pdf?ua=1

World Bank. (2016a). *Guatemala panorama general*. Retrieved January 4, 2017 from http://www.bancomundial.org/es/country/guatemala/overview

World Bank. (2016b). *Latinoamérica Indígena en el siglo XXI*. Retrieved January 3, 2017, from http://www.bancomundial.org/es/region/lac/brief/indigenous-latin-america-in-the-twenty-first-century-brief-report-page

28 Maternal Care in Guatemala: Problematizing Discourses of Development, Transnational Advocacy, and Indigeneity

Briana Nichols and Lisette Farias

28.1 Introduction

In this chapter, we will focus on the impact of development discourses of biomedical care and transnational approaches (e.g., biomedical programming) to maternal care on the lives of the indigenous Maya in Guatemala. This focus is particularly crucial because indigenous Mayan communities have disproportionally high rates of maternal mortality in comparison with the Guatemalan nonindigenous population, and also because solving the "problem" of indigenous birth practices and maternal mortality has been a governance priority both for the international community and for the Guatemalan state since the early 1970s (Berry 2010; Goldman and Glei 2003; Santiso-Galvez and Bertrand 2004). In order to better understand the context that frames maternal mortality in Guatemala, this chapter is organized into six sections. First, we examine the historical relationship between the Guatemalan State, *Ladino*, and indigenous populations, followed by a description of the role of traditional midwives (i.e., *comadronas*) and the significance of traditional birth practices for Mayan communities. Subsequently, we introduce the Guatemalan Health system, highlighting specific structural barriers that prevent indigenous Guatemalan women from seeking medical care. Then, we introduce the historical influence of transnational agencies on Guatemalan health provision, followed by an examination of how the role of traditional midwives has been repositioned through the implementation of national policy and international recommendations. Finally, we conclude by describing how the influence of development discourses and transnational advocacy has resulted in naturalization of biomedical care as the only "good" care in Guatemala, shifting moral responsibility for maternity outcomes to individuals (i.e., *comadronas*, women and their families) which renders indigenous Maya as both

B. Nichols, Ph.D. (✉)
Department of Anthropology, University of Pennsylvania,
Philadelphia, PA, USA
e-mail: brianan@gse.upenn.edu

L. Farias, BSc(OT), MSc(OT), OT Reg, PhD
Graduate Program of Health and Rehabilitation Sciences,
Western University, London, ON, Canada

D. A. Schwartz (ed.), *Maternal Death and Pregnancy-Related Morbidity Among Indigenous Women of Mexico and Central America*, Global Maternal and Child Health: Medical, Anthropological, and Public Health Perspectives, https://doi.org/10.1007/978-3-319-71538-4_28

immoral and barriers to national progress. This ultimately results in the marginalization of indigenous women, and exacerbates persistently high rates of maternal mortality despite numerous interventions.

Before moving on to the examination of the historical relationship between the Guatemalan State, *Ladino*, and indigenous populations, we situate this chapter by clarifying the use of the terms "biomedicine" and "recipients of care." We employ the term biomedicine (also biomedical) to denote the medical profession in Western nations and to indicate the profession's emphasis on biology, pathology, and the scientific method (Gibson 2016). This term is also used throughout this chapter because of the fact that its underpinning assumptions (e.g., the individual seen as independent from his/her sociocultural context, the positivistic notions of "right" and "wrong" care) have been criticized in favor of more holistic or humanistic approaches to care that consider the "whole person" rather than physical pathology (Gibson 2016). Similarly, we employ the term recipients of care instead of the terms "patient," "client," "service user," or "consumer" to avoid promoting assumptions that neglect the social, political, cultural, and personal aspects that shape health care. In particular, we prefer to not use the term patient because of its association with paternalistic assumptions that perpetuate power imbalances between health professionals and recipients of care (Hammell 2006). Similarly, we avoid using the terms client, service user, or consumer since these terms are usually underpinned by the assumption that health care is a form of service provision embedded within a neoliberal discourse that promotes particular values such as individualism, autonomy, and self-efficiency (Gibson 2016). This emphasis on personal and economic freedom is problematic from a critical stance since it shifts the responsibility for prosperity onto individuals instead of on the system, structures, and practices that perpetuate (social) disadvantage and inequities (Bhaskar 2011; Harvey 2007; Wright 2010). Thus, we use the terms recipients of care, women, or people in this chapter to emphasize the importance of considering the context in which care is provided and the assumptions that shape the relationships between health professionals and indigenous populations in Guatemala.

28.2 Histories of Violence: The Guatemalan State, *Ladinos*, and Indigenous Guatemalans

In Guatemala, the term "*Ladino*" refers to Guatemalans who are Spanish speaking, of mixed indigenous and European heritage, and generally do not practice indigenous Mayan customs. *Ladinos* are structurally privileged, occupying positions of power within the government and controlling disproportionate amounts of land and wealth in the country. *Ladinos* tend to live in urban areas, have more formal education and higher incomes than indigenous Mayans. These disparities are both caused by, and result from, widespread racial prejudice against indigenous populations who are often viewed as "backwards," "brutish," and as threats to progress in the modern nation-state (Berry 2010; Cosminsky 2001; McCalister and Nelson 2013; Metz 2001).

While discrimination against the indigenous populations is embedded in Guatemalan history, it reached unprecedented levels of violence during the 36-year-long Guatemalan civil war. After the 1954 overthrow of the democratically elected president, and the military takeover of the Guatemalan government that followed, the Guatemalan state embarked on a "counter-insurgency" campaign largely targeting indigenous Mayan communities. State and state-related actors murdered over 200,000 Guatemalans during the conflict. Most of the victims were indigenous Maya, believed to be left-wing sympathizers (Nelson 2009; Sanford 2003). The Guatemalan military practiced a "scorched earth" campaign in which over 440 indigenous villages were completely annihilated (Ishida et al. 2012). In addition to the systematic murder of indigenous Maya during the war, the Guatemalan state also instituted practices of Mayan population control, including the forced sterilization of Mayan women (Metz 2001). These extreme examples of historical physical violence perpetrated against indigenous people by the predominately *Ladino* Guatemalan state exist alongside countless examples of the everyday violence indigenous Guatemalans have suffered.

As a result of these histories of violence and contemporary experiences of discrimination, indigenous Maya are often wary of state sponsored health programs. Family planning initiatives instituted by state actors are viewed with skepticism by Mayan communities, and thus are largely ineffective (Metz 2001; Santiso-Galvez and Bertrand 2004; Shiffman and Garces Del Valle 2006). The Guatemalan population has increased significantly from 3 million in the 1950s to over 15 million today, with most of this population increase being driven by indigenous and rural Guatemalans (World Bank 2015). In parallel, maternal mortality in Guatemala has remained one of the highest in the Americas (140 per 100,000) with a mortality risk for indigenous women three times greater than for nonindigenous women (PAHO 2007; UNICEF 2015). Despite the expanding needs resulting from Guatemala's population growth and maternal mortality rates, services provided by the Guatemalan health care system remain woefully inadequate, especially for rural indigenous populations. Many factors undoubtedly stand behind this inadequacy of services, including decades of neglect during the civil war that left Guatemala's health system seriously underfinanced with very little coverage of health services outside of urban areas, and a lack of consensus about intervention strategies that often promote practices that are condescending and discriminatory towards indigenous populations (Berry 2010; Cosminsky 1982; Goldman et al. 2001; Rööst et al. 2004; Ruiz et al. 2013; Shiffman 2007). In the following sections, to help destabilize the taken-for-granted "problem" of indigenous practices, we provide an analysis of the complex Guatemalan health system and structural barriers that shape the personal experiences of indigenous Guatemalans, often resulting in an avoidance of state-provided biomedical care. But first, in order to understand the discrepancies between indigenous and biomedical approaches to birth, we provide an overview of the role of traditional midwifes or *comadronas*, the most common traditional practices and values related to pregnancy and birth within Guatemalan indigenous communities, and the sociocultural roles of home birth for Mayan women.

28.3 Traditional Birthing Practices: The Role of *Comadronas* and Home Births

Indigenous Maya birthing practices are heterogeneous, varying widely both within and between indigenous communities. Two traditional practices often viewed most skeptically by biomedical service providers are the tendency to prefer homebirths over births in a medical setting, and to seek the assistance of a *comadrona,* a traditional midwife, during pregnancy and labor (Berry 2010; Cosminsky 2012; Walsh 2006). In addition to homebirth and the use of a *comadrona*, which shall be discussed in depth, many indigenous women also prefer to give birth in a traditional squatting position rather than a supine position, receive therapeutic massages from the *comadrona* throughout their pregnancy and as labor approaches, and use a traditional *temascal*, or sweat lodge, during labor (Ruiz et al. 2013).

The role of the *comadrona* has been written about extensively both in literature describing indigenous Guatemalan birth practices and in the attempts to explain persistently high maternal mortality rates (Berry 2005, 2010; Hallowell 2014; Goldman et al. 2003) with midwives often being held accountable for the death of women in their care (Cosminsky 2012). In government and transnational programming targeted towards reducing maternal mortality in Guatemala, *comadronas* are alternately positioned as unskilled, ignorant, backwards and harmful to pregnant women, or as low-skilled potential allies in a biomedical service provision network (Berry 2005, 2010). From a public health policy perspective, *comadronas* are in a unique position to either refer or dissuade pregnant women from seeking biomedical care in the event of an emergency. However, this positioning of the *comadrona* as a health care "referee" misinterprets the role of midwives for pregnant women and their communities (Berry 2010), understands seeking biomedical care as the ultimate moral and rational choice women can make, and obscures the structural barriers (e.g., distance from care, cost of care, confusing structure of care provision, experiences of discrimination, linguistic barriers, and disrespect for indigenous cultural values) preventing indigenous Guatemalan women from seeking medical care (Hallowell 2014). It is worth noticing that the term "structural barriers" is used in this chapter to denote those systemic features of the health care system and society that are beyond one person's control, and that actively obstruct people's access to services, producing marginalization of specific groups (Angus et al. 2013), and a perception of "us" and "them" between *Ladino* and indigenous communities.

While frequently misinterpreted as biomedical proxies, the role of *comadronas* for indigenous Mayan communities is that of a spiritual guide rather than a medical caretaker (Berry 2010; Walsh 2006). As Berry (2005) explains, the main role of a midwife is to birth babies using spiritual guidance, not intervene in birthing problems. In interviews, *comadronas* clarify that becoming a midwife is a spiritual calling. Their position as a birth attendant is a ritual one, charged with creating a sacred space for the birth, helping the mother feel comfortable, working to instantiate critical familial bonds during the birthing process and using spiritual guidance to help deliver the new baby (Walsh 2006). While midwives can and do look for signs of distress in the birthing process, their primary role is not a medical one, and electing to refer recipients of care to biomedical care is a choice informed by factors beyond the biomedical. Thus, even when referred by a midwife, indigenous women and their families often elect to not seek medical services at a hospital for a myriad of reasons including extensive structural barriers (discussed in the next section), cultural values, and fears around surgical procedures that may result in the infertility or death of the mother—fears informed at least in part by extensive mistrust of the state (Berry 2005, 2010; Glei et al. 2003; Goldman et al. 2003; Metz 2001).

In her seminal text on maternal mortality in Guatemala, Berry (2010) reminds us that both biomedical and indigenous belief systems are ultimately cultural. Biomedical practices naturalize the notion of individual patients seeking individualized care for physical pathologies; thus, under this cultural system, a woman giving birth at home who is experiencing medical difficulty should seek biomedical care to ensure her individual safety and the safety of her child. However, within Mayan communities, the significance of birth is not just measured by the physical health of the mother and child, instead, birth becomes a site through which social relationships are made and strengthened, specifically relationships between the pregnant woman, her partner, and her affinal family (Berry 2010). Birth as a site to make meaning of social relationships is often completely obscured within a biomedical paradigm.

During a Mayan homebirth, women are most often in the home of their partner's family. They are attended to and cared for by their partner, their partner's mother, and other females in the household. The mother-in-law is frequently tasked with finding a suitable *comadrona* and preparing the birthing space, a job that is taken seriously, and represents the care and intentions of the mother-in-law towards her daughter-in-law. The older women in the household oversee the birthing process both materially and emotionally. A successful birth is able to strengthen ties of obligation between the recent mother and her affinal family through their participation in the process. Birthing provides an opportunity for each family member to occupy their ascribed roles within the family unit, and a moment in which the pregnant woman can display her physical and spiritual strength as well as deference to her mother-in-law. When problems arise during labor, these problems are not seen as biomedical instantiations of a pathological nature, but rather as evidence of relational strife (the evil wishes of an outsider, familial neglect, etc.). Thus, for the pregnant woman, her partner, and her partner's family, there is a lot riding on the ability to have a successful home birth (Berry 2010). Berry reminds us that in communities already struggling from structural disenfranchisement and intense poverty, any weakening of social ties and thus support is incredibly meaningful and must be taken seriously because these supports are relied upon for survival. Shifting a birth from the home to a hospital necessarily creates a shift in how both the mother and their kin make meaning of their relational roles. In a hospital birth, many of the meaningful cultural elements of birth, such as the presence of the woman's partner and family, are prohibited. Kinship ties are critical in decision-making processes around birth. In moments of medical emergency, it is often the family, not the *comadrona*, who decide when and if to seek biomedical care. These decisions are predicated not just on perceived risks to the mother, structural barriers, and distrust of the medical system, but also on the social ramifications of moving the birth outside of the home.

28.4 Health Care System: Lack of Coordination and Structural Barriers

The health care system in Guatemala is often characterized as pluralistic because of the coexistence of traditional, biomedical, and popular practices (Goldman et al. 2001). However, these practices become blurred as biomedical or "modern" care and a reliance on Western pharmaceuticals increases in Guatemala, a trend occurring across the developing countries (Goldman et al. 2001). Currently, Guatemala's health care system is difficult to navigate even for its own inhabitants, since it encompasses highly fragmented levels, operating independently and with minimal coordination (Avila et al. 2015). The main actors in the public sector are the Ministry of Health and Social Assistance (Ministerio de Salud Pública y Asistencia Social or MSPAS), the Guatemalan Institute of Social Security (Instituto Guatemalteco de Seguridad Social or IGSS), and the Military Health Service (Sanidad Militar). The MSPAS is the main regulatory agency, theoretically responsible for governance of the health sector and for providing services to the uninsured population (75% of the population) (Avila et al. 2015) (see Table 28.1).

At the central level of the public health system, there are 29 MSPAS health care offices that, in theory, should serve as an intermediary between the central level and local health facilities in order to supervise and evaluate the execution of health policies and distribution of drugs and other health commodities (Avila et al. 2015). Thus, these offices oversee the district health offices, which in turn manage and supervise the health centers and health posts within their respective district (Bossert et al. 2003). As such, the MSPAS Service Delivery Network can be divided into three levels of care (see Table 28.2). Tertiary health facilities or hospitals are staffed by physicians, nurses, and specialists. Secondary facility staffs usually consist of physicians, nurses, and in some cases, specialists. At the

Table 28.1 Guatemalan health system (Adapted from Becerril-Montekio and Lopez-Davila, 2011)

Sector	Public			Private	
Sources	General taxes	Mandate members contributions (usually salary-related)	Employer contributions, members contributions (usually salary-related), general taxes	Voluntary private insurance payment, out-of-pocket payment	Donor contributions
Main actors	MSPAS	Military Health Service	IGSS	IGSS, for-profit providers	Not-for-profit organizations
Providers	MSPAS Health centers, clinics and hospitals	Military clinics and hospitals	IGSS health center, clinic and hospitals	Private providers	Not-for-profit organizations
Users	Uninsured population	Military and police beneficiaries	IGSS Beneficiaries	IGSS beneficiaries, population able to pay	Uninsured population
%	75%	0.5%	17.5%	<5%	

Table 28.2 MSPAS levels of care and health infrastructure (Adapted from Avila et al. 2015)

Level	Type of establishment	Number of establishments
Primary	Converge centers[a]	2220
	Health posts	1302
Secondary	Health centers	902
	Health centers with specialists	21
	Mobile clinics	379
Tertiary	Hospitals	51

[a]The Convergence Centers were closed by the cancellation of the PEC program in 2014

primary level, health posts or community centers are staffed by one or two auxiliary nurses supported by a team of community volunteers including community facilitators and *comadronas* (Hernández et al. 2014). Although the primary level of care is meant to be the point of entry into the health system, Guatemalans often need to bypass health posts and secondary facilities (Avila et al. 2015) to seek services directly in the few hospitals (51) that are supposed to provide specialized services to the entire population. This situation is partly due to the lack of physicians and nurses available at the primary level, as well as the complexity of the system that is managed without coordination across the three levels of care. For instance, health district offices should theoretically coordinate efforts between the different levels, but in practice, the primary and secondary levels run without coordination with the tertiary level, with the latter facilities typically running by "themselves" with budgetary autonomy and reporting directly to the central instead of the district health office (Avila et al. 2015). It is worth noticing that this lack of coordination between levels of care is not a minor issue when considering that Guatemala is the most populous nation in Central America with 16.3 million habitants, more than one-half of whom live below the national poverty line, are uninsured, and in need of public health services (World Bank 2015).

This lack of coordination implies that referrals between levels are weak or nonexistent in practice, and that recipients of care have consultations at different times and places, making access to health care more difficult for women who need to travel great distances to seek care and have children who require different kinds of medical services (Gragnolati and Marini 2003). A weak system of referrals also suggests that the tertiary level, which has fewer facilities than the secondary and primary levels (see Table 28.2), receives more people than it can handle. As a result, since the cost of a visit to a hospital is four times as great as the cost of a visit to a health center, and is almost eight times as high as a visit to a health post, the cost of health care is higher for the Guatemalan state and its citizens (Gragnolati and Marini 2003).

In addition to this highly fragmented system, health facilities are often out of stock of essential medicines. This prevents health centers and posts from meeting people's demands, instead sending them to seek care at hospitals, which also often experience shortages of supplies (Berry 2006; Goldman et al. 2001). For example, when conducting fieldwork in 2015, the authors visited Chimaltenango's hospital and a health post outside of the city (see Fig. 28.1) and found that both facilities had been missing essential supplies for several weeks. This lack of supplies is a common reality in rural and urban facilities since, as the authors observed, hospitals will often place a sign outside their entrance announcing the list of stockouts (e.g., acetaminophen, saline (*suero*), gauze, and pads). The drugs that people are in need of, and that should be available at a subsidized price at the hospital pharmacy, are often only obtainable from private pharmacies in town centers, increasing the cost of a visit (Gragnolati and Marini 2003; Hallowell 2014). These drugs can cost the equivalent of several days' wages, and recipients of care report feeling unable to challenge doctors' prescriptions. As such, many families may not be able to afford medicines prescribed at health centers and posts, which are supposed to be sources of free supplements such as iron and folate for undernourished

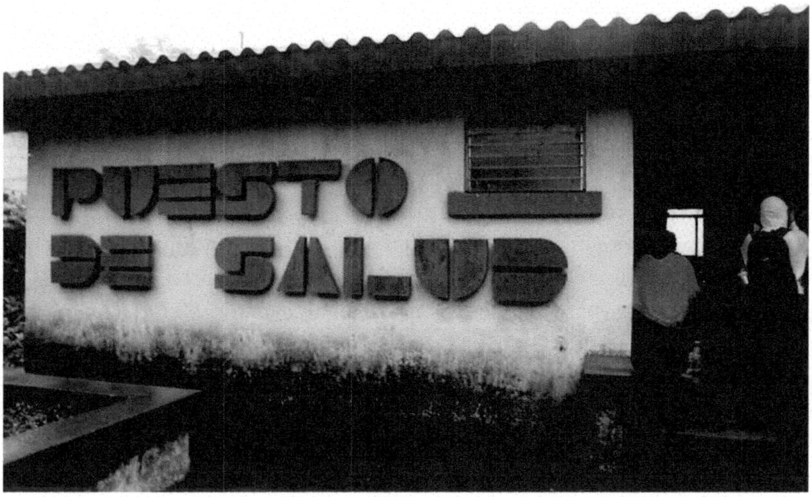

Fig. 28.1 Health Post outside of Chimaltenango city 2015. *Source*: Photo taken by Lisette Farias

pregnant women (Berry 2006). What is more, even if doctors have free medicines or vitamins in stock, the results of the Family Health Survey (Encuesta Guatemalteca de Salud Familiar) show that almost all doctors charge for them (Goldman et al. 2001). Thus, given the lack of a reliable supply in health facilities and cost associated to doctors' prescriptions, Guatemalans take a highly agentive role and frequently go directly to the pharmacy for treatment or rely on traditional medicines (Berry 2006; Goldman et al. 2001).

Distance and transportation to health care facilities are also major structural barriers for accessing health services. For example, secondary and primary levels do often not have an ambulance to transport critical recipients of care from their home or health post to hospitals. There are also no call centers or coordinated systems for facilities that do not have an ambulance (Avila et al. 2015). This means that possibilities for transferring women with obstetric emergencies or complications are limited as recipients of care are responsible for providing their own transport regardless of their health condition, socioeconomic status, or distance to a health facility (PAHO 2012). This lack of transportation disproportionately affects people in rural areas since they have to travel greater distances to reach a public hospital, increasing their travel time, the cost of transportation, and the risks associated with accessing medical care. For example, the travel time on average for reaching a public hospital can range from approximately 1 h up to 90 min for people in rural areas, twice the time compared to people in urban areas (Gragnolati and Marini 2003). For many of the women we spoke with, the circumstances are even more extreme, with some having to travel many hours, at least partially by foot, to access medical care. In particular, according to the results of the Qualitative Poverty and Exclusion Study (QPES) conducted in ten rural communities (Gragnolati and Marini 2003), the most important cause of death for women in some rural villages in Guatemala is the lack of ambulances for transportation. Other structural barriers to health facilities include the poor quality of the roads making travel more difficult and time consuming, made worse during inclimate weather, and the fact that facilities are sometimes closed when they are supposed to be open (Gragnolati and Marini 2003; Shiffman and Garces del Valle 2006).

The cost of health care for pregnant women is another structural barrier that prevents indigenous and rural women from accessing health care. This implies that even when referred by a midwife, indigenous women and their families often elect to not seek biomedical services because the costs associated with pre- and postnatal checks and delivery are higher for the rural population. The cheapest alternative for Mayan pregnant women is to have prenatal checks and delivery performed at home, often with the help of family members, followed by assistance from a traditional midwife, who often accept payments in kind from people that do not have money. In general, *comadronas* charge less per visit than any other group of health practitioners (Goldman et al. 2001). Other affordable alternatives are public hospitals where births may be attended by doctors or nurses. However, as public hospitals may be located at greater distance from women's villages, because of transportation and housing needs this option is often not ultimately cost-effective. It is worth noting that in rural areas, nurses tend to charge more than doctors although they might not have formal training or licensure/certification to practice as a nurse midwife (Chary et al. 2013; Gragnolati and Marini 2003). The most expensive option for indigenous women is to have prenatal checks and delivery in a private hospital which has an average cost of 750 Quetzals in urban areas and 350 Quetzals in rural areas, more than twice as much as the average monthly household consumption (140 Quetzals) (Goldman et al. 2001).

In addition to costs and distance, indigenous pregnant women in Guatemala also have to be content with health care facilities which are staffed predominately by *Ladino* personnel who speak only Spanish, even when serving Mayan communities (Goldman et al. 2001; Ishida et al. 2012). This language barrier can create power imbalances by positioning indigenous women as less knowledgeable with respect to health professionals, who tend to evaluate the knowledge of the recipients of care based on biomedical approaches to reproduction and their ability to communicate about their health concerns (Berry 2006; Ishida et al. 2012). In addition, a rapid rotation of staff in health facilities impedes fluent communication and establishment of a rapport between indigenous women and health professionals (Gragnolati and Marini 2003; Goldman et al. 2001). Thus, this combination of structural barriers (e.g., the high cost of visits to health facilities, lack of possibilities for transportation, and a perceived discrimination by recipients of care related to their indigenous ethnicity and/or inability to speak Spanish) makes it very difficult for indigenous women to seek biomedical health care and trust in the knowledge and services provided by health staff.

28.5 Transnational Advocacy: Shifting to Biomedical Providers

Maternal mortality reduction has been an international priority since 1987 when three United Nations (UN) agencies—the UN Population Fund (UNFPA), the World Bank, and the World Health Organization (WHO)—sponsored what is referred to as the Nairobi Conference. These agencies, together with two other important international organizations (Planned Parenthood International and the Population Council) launched the Safe Motherhood Initiative (SMI) to lower global maternal deaths by at least 50% by the year 2000 (Berry 2010). This initiative was followed by a series of UN-sponsored international conferences throughout the 1990s that reaffirmed a global commitment to reducing maternal mortality (Shiffman 2007). However, despite these efforts to position maternal mortality on the international agenda, SMI had little progress with regard to lowering maternal mortality rates during its first decade (Berry 2010).

More recently, maternal mortality was addressed by the international community in 2000 when it was included as one of the eight Millennium Development Goals (MDGs) aimed at ending extreme poverty by the year 2015 (World Bank 2009). Following these initiatives, the government of Guatemala was pushed to prioritize safe motherhood by donor agencies such as the American branch of the WHO, the Pan American Health Organization (PAHO), the United States Agency for International Development (USAID), the Inter-American Development Bank, the UN Children's Fund (UNICEF), and UNFPA, who invested in improving provisions of basic maternal and infant health care (Shiffman and Garces del Valle 2006). It is worth noting that maternal mortality was a neglected issue in Guatemala until the year 2000, when transnational influence materialized in financial and technical resources to address maternal mortality (e.g., USAID provided $50 million for a global project entitled MotherCare that focused on midwife training and prenatal care, implemented in Guatemala in 1999) (Shiffman 2007).

In practice, to expand maternal and infant care health centers, not-for-profit organizations such as faith-based organizations (FBOs) and nongovernmental organizations (NGOs) have, over the past 20 years, been contracted by MSPAS to provide health services in rural areas throughout the country. This outsourcing began with the signing of the Peace Accords of 1996, mandating an increase of public expenditure for health to specifically extend health services to marginalized rural areas (PAHO 2012). Following this international request, MSPAS elected to contract NGOs to expand coverage more rapidly through the Extension of Coverage Program (Programa de Extensión de Cobertura or PEC). The PEC's basic package provided 26 services, including maternal services in a broad mix of facilities ranging from rooms in houses of local leaders to actual PEC facilities mostly built by local government municipalities and community members, and a few built by the government (Avila et al. 2015). Visits to the community were scheduled once a month, and a nurse or doctor provided maternal care, immunizations, nutritional supplementation, and growth monitoring to children under 5 years of age (Avila et al. 2015). With additional funding from the international donor community, this program expanded rapidly to cover approximately 2.9 million people by 2000 (Pena 2013). However, a growing dissatisfaction with what was perceived as lower quality health services provided to indigenous communities, together with accusations of inefficiency and a lack of transparency, led to legislation prohibiting the outsourcing of health care services and the cancellation of most of MSPAS' contracts with NGOs in the fall of 2014 (Avila et al. 2015). This cancellation is also associated with the fact that, despite efforts to expand health care, maternal mortality in Guatemala has not improved significantly and still falls short in comparison with other countries in the region (World Bank 2003).

By prioritizing the transnational agenda behind the safe motherhood initiative, Guatemala has experienced international donor encouragement followed by national studies that have heavily drawn on quantitative health services and demographic data to identify determinants of maternal mortality and provide recommendations for addressing them (Shiffman and Garces del Valle 2006). However, these studies have focused almost exclusively on determinants that keep women at the center of maternal mortality by holding women responsible for maternal health outcomes while neglecting socioeconomic and cultural barriers that extend beyond the control and choice of pregnant women and their families (e.g., lack of reliable supply in health facilities, high cost associated to visits and drugs prescriptions, discrimination). As Shiffman and Garces del Valle (2006) summarize, these determinants tend to emphasize "biomedical causes, such as hemorrhaging and eclampsia" (p. 57), as well as that contact with traditional midwives or *comadronas* is a key determinant for seeking traditional instead of biomedical health care (Glei and Goldman 2000; Sibley et al. 2004). Thus, it is not surprising that most policy efforts, influenced by transnational norms and international-funded research, have focused on ensuring that pregnant women seek biomedical health services and that skilled attendants are present at all births (Chary et al. 2013; Shiffman and Garces del Valle 2006; Berry 2010). Often these programs are structured with the assumption that *comadronas* can and should serve as medical proxies and the first line of defense against unsafe births.

28.6 Repositioning of Traditional Midwives or *Comadronas*

Given the configuration of the determinants of maternal mortality, and in keeping with the directive of the SMI and MDGs, the Guatemalan government has championed traditional midwife training initiatives. While there are no formal training or licensure requirements for nurses that attend births, the Ministry of Health has granted licenses to practice as traditional birth attendants (TBAs) to those individuals who demonstrate consistent attendance at continuing education activities, typically 15-day training sessions held at regional or local Health Posts. Although most sessions are taught by auxiliary nurses who have little experience in delivery, professional nurses are officially responsible for this training (Goldman et al. 2001). Traditional midwives who have not received training and licences are legally prohibited from practicing. These training and licencing requirements have primarily been enforced by refusing to grant birth certificates to parents who contract non-licensed midwives (Chary et al. 2013; Goldman et al. 2001). As such, midwives have been positioned as actors under supervision who risk everything (e.g., license) by not referring their recipients of care to biomedical facilities (Hallowell 2014). This biomedical supervision has been evident during their training and through the implementation of Emergency Plans (planes de emergencia) which are based on the general assumption that the practice of traditional midwives is related to poor pregnancy outcomes (Berry 2010; Hallowell 2014). The Emergency Plans are cardboard posters that depict the steps midwifes and a woman must take during pregnancy and in case of a potential obstetrical emergency. According to these plans, midwives are responsible for planning with women and their families, so that a pregnant woman can anticipate how much money she will need to pay for food and transport, and who will take care of her children while she leaves to give birth. Similarly, during an emergency, it is expected that the pregnant woman and her midwife take the "appropriate" actions outlined in the Emergency Plan, all which should lead to getting the woman to a hospital as quickly as possible. Thus, although traditional midwives are largely held responsible for planning and executing the emergency plans, their role as spiritual guides and use of traditional practices have been increasingly discredited in favor of "skilled" attendants (i.e., individuals with biomedical credentials) (Berry 2010). This tendency to antagonize the spiritual role of traditional midwives against biomedical care has resulted in positioning "skilled" professionals as the "sole" experts in maternal health, disempowering midwives and women in general (Berry 2006).

Not surprisingly, TBA programs have been largely criticized for their strong reliance on Western or biomedical models of training, and for being unnecessarily complicated and culturally inappropriate (e.g., failing to take local context into account and employing a top-down approach) (Chary et al. 2013; Goldman et al. 2001; Hallowell 2014). For example, the programs usually rely on advanced literacy skills and use of Spanish; this is a language many *comadronas* do not speak or understand. Additionally, traditional midwives have reported feeling discouraged, or sometimes condemned for utilizing traditional practices that are unlikely to have negative effects and may well benefit delivery (e.g., promoting upright delivery instead of supine position). Midwives have also argued that TBA training has been utilized to restrict or eliminate traditional practices by presenting indigenous ways of thinking and acting as "backwards" or even "harmful" to pregnant women (Berry 2005, 2010; Chary et al. 2013).

Following this criticism and poor results with regard to maternal mortality reduction, transnational advocacy and the Guatemalan state have shifted the focus of safety motherhood from midwife training to improving skilled attendance at all births (Berry 2010). To support this shift, the Guatemalan government has redirected funding away from TBA programs to strengthen emergency obstetric care in district health services, emphasizing a near universal referral of pregnant women to district facilities (Chary et al. 2013). This new emphasis has further undercut and restricted the role of traditional midwives as autonomous spiritual guides to the health care "referrers" of pregnant women to biomedical care (Berry 2005, 2010; Chary et al. 2013). Thus, although traditional midwives have attempted to collaborate with this biomedical approach by recommending women to seek care in hospitals, midwives are often poorly treated by medical personnel when accompanying pregnant women to health facilities (Goldman et al. 2001). For instance, midwives describe experiences of humiliation by not being allowed to accompany women into the delivery room, or to stay in the facility even though they have traveled long distances (Shiffman an Garces del Valle 2006).

Despite these efforts to reduce the role of traditional midwives, most indigenous and rural women do not seek biomedical services at any point during their pregnancy or delivery (Goldman et al. 2001). Furthermore, there is no significant evidence that undermining and controlling traditional midwife's practices have decreased maternal mortality in Guatemala (Berry 2010). The explicit expectation is that individual women should choose to seek biomedical birthing services in district facilities in order to reduce perceived risks. This expectation shifts the moral responsibility for maternity outcomes to "individuals" (i.e., midwives and pregnant women) and positions biomedical birth as the only "good" possible action.

28.7 Implications and Further Questions

Despite efforts by the Guatemalan government and collaboration with international advocates, indigenous Maya maternal mortality rates remain a significant concern. Approaches taken to resolving persistently high maternal mortality have centered on increased access to biomedical care through the introduction of birthing centers where high-risk mothers can stay overnight in anticipation of going into labor, integrating *comadronas* into the biomedical referral process, along with training *comadronas*, nurses, and community health workers through certification programs to be "skilled attendants" at birth. These approaches have been supported by both international and national initiatives focused on "safe motherhood," and often involve, as we have demonstrated, a complex assemblage of caregivers who span both state run and NGO-based programming. This structure is incredibly complicated to navigate, often forces women and their families to incur hidden costs associated with transportation, medication, and supplies, serves to reproduce discourses that place indigenous practices in contrast with "modernity," and ultimately neglects the critical social role of successful home birth for Mayan women. Moving forward, when considering the implications of development discourses and transnational advocacy in relation to maternal health, we argue it is necessary to shift the focus beyond that of access to biomedical care. As both practitioners and researchers, we suggest that effective reduction of maternal mortality among indigenous women in Guatemala necessitates problematizing three aspects of current programming: (1) the manner in which health-related policy ideas and norms take social form; (2) how forms of expertise enable and shape forms of collaboration among care providers; and (3) how discourses of modernity and the modern subject serve to reinstantiate discriminatory practices at the expense of Maya women and families.

The "Safe Motherhood Initiative," and other programs that followed, was conceived at an international level to be implemented within a national context. International initiatives, such as this one, are often grounded in beliefs around care and care provision that influence policy creation and implementation. In the Guatemalan context, the overwhelming orientation is towards birthing as an individual process necessitating biomedical care. Thus, the approaches to resolving persistently high maternal mortality rates have focused on getting women and their families to choose biomedical care throughout the pregnancy and during labor. However, policies written to encourage access to biomedical care among indigenous women take specific, and often unanticipated, social forms on the ground. The policies promoting safe motherhood in Guatemala have served to further a neoliberal individuation of Mayan women and restructure both safety networks and the performance of kinship. The social forms of these policies are significant not only because they have lasting impacts on the social relations within Mayan communities but also because they obscure significant structural barriers to care, and often work against the state objective of reducing maternal mortality. Promoting policies that focus on the decision-making of individual mothers and/or *comadronas* places at risk already established networks of care within the family. Rather than integrating the potentially beneficial aspects of biomedical care into indigenous practices and kinship structures, programming often places the two in opposition—either women can opt to enrich their social connections through traditional birthing practices, or they can choose biomedical care. Expecting women to choose biomedical care only privileges a worldview in which the health of each individual mother supersedes other considerations (the financial burden biomedical care places on families, the inability for mothers to be near their other children, the social bonds created and maintained through home birth, etc.), producing social forms which can be detrimental to both the mother and her community.

The proliferation of NGO health service providers and an increased focus on orienting *comadronas* towards biomedical care have encouraged notions of expertise that privilege Western medicine and biomedical techniques. Positioning NGO actors and doctors as experts informs the possibilities for collaboration with non-biomedical caregivers. Frequently this privileging of expertise leads *comadronas* to integrate Western medical practices into their midwifery without adequate training or concerns for the environment of care provision (Goldman and Glei 2003). These adaptations are not malicious but rather come from a dynamic in which collaboration between midwives, NGOs, and doctors are structured by power imbalances. Each actor does not bring equal value to the interaction when the knowledge of biomedical care providers is systemically privileged. Within this asymmetrical collaboration, it is understandable that *comadronas* would adopt biomedical practices positioned as "superior" in an effort to provide the "best" possible care to the women they are working with and maintain their own relevancy. A collaborative framework where *comadronas*, doctors, nurses, NGO service providers, and families were each valued as producers of legitimate knowledge could be advantageous to the medical, social, and spiritual health of Mayan mothers, allowing for the integration of biomedical care when necessary without significant subjective restructuring of the actors.

Finally, it is essential to understand that in addition to hierarchies of collaboration and social forms produced by policies attempting to reduce maternal mortality, the discourses of development these policies are derived from also reaffirm a world in which specific notions of modernity and modern subjects are constructed. In Guatemalan contexts, these notions of modernity are particularly insidious because they align with already extant social divisions between Mayan and *Ladino* populations in which *Ladinos* are considered subjects of a "modern" and progressive Guatemala while the Maya act as a regressive force in Guatemala's attempts to develop. Maternal mortality is a critical element of the Human Development Index, and thus persistently high maternal mortality rates impacts the ability of a country to be considered "developed" within the international sphere. When the onus of reducing maternal mortality is placed not just on individual women, but on individual indigenous women, these women are rendered culpable for not "choosing" biomedical. While this "choice" might appear self-evident within a transnational advocacy framework, those who develop policy often fail to consider the social, cultural, financial, and personal dignity implications of birthing at a hospital. The naturalization of childbirth in Western medical settings moralizes this practice as self-evidently correct, thus positioning those who do not go to the hospital as immoral actors. Constructing Mayan women as not only uniformed but also immoral does not serve the goal or reduce maternal mortality. Rather, as we have shown, it reinstantiates discriminatory practices towards indigenous women and the alienation of indigenous communities who are written outside of the narratives of modern "progress."

References

Angus, J., Lombardo, A., Lowndes, R., Cechetto, N., Ahmad, F., & Bierman, A. (2013). Beyond barriers in studying disparities in women's access to health services in Ontario, Canada: A qualitative metasynthesis. *Qualitative Health Research, 23*(4), 476–494. https://doi.org/10.1177/1049732312469464

Avila, C., Bright, R., Gutierrez, J. C., Hoadley, K., Manuel, C., Romero, N., et al. (2015). *Guatemala health system assessment*. Bethesda, MD: Health Finance & Governance Project, Abt Associates.

Becerril-Montekio, V., & Lopez-Davila, L. (2011). [The health system of Guatemala]. Salud Publica Mex, *53*(Suppl 2), s197–208.
Berry, N. S. (2005). *Incorporating cultural diversity into health systems: An example of midwives teaching midwives*. East Lansing: Women and International Development, Michigan State University.
Berry, N. S. (2006). Kaqchikel midwives, homebirths, and emergency obstetric referrals in Guatemala: Contextualizing the choice to stay at home. *Social Science & Medicine, 62*, 1958–1969.
Berry, N. S. (2010). *Unsafe motherhood: Mayan maternal mortality and subjectivity in post-war Guatemala*. New York: Berghahn Books.
Bhaskar, R. (2011). *Reclaiming reality: A critical introduction to contemporary philosophy*. London, England: Routledge.
Bossert, T., Bowser, D., Amenyah, J., Copeland, R., & GETSA. (2003). *Decentralization and integration in the health logistic system in Guatemala*. Final report. Boston: Harvard School of Public Health. Arlington, VA: JSI/DELIVER, for USAID.
Chary, A., Díaz, A. K., Henderson, B., & Rohloff, P. (2013). The changing role of indigenous lay midwives in Guatemala: New frameworks for analysis. *Midwifery, 29*(8), 852–858.
Cosminsky, S. (1982). Knowledge and body concepts of Guatemalan midwives. In M. Kay (Ed.), *Anthropology of human birth* (pp. 233–252). Philadelphia: F.A. Davis.
Cosminsky, S. (2001). Maya midwives of southern Mexico and Guatemala. In B. R. Huber & A. R. Sandstrom (Eds.), *Mesoamerican healers* (pp. 179–210). Austin: University of Texas Press.
Cosminsky, S. (2012). Birth and blame: Guatemalan Midwives and reproductive risk. In L. Fordyce & A. Maraesa (Eds.), *Risk, reproduction, and narratives of experience* (pp. 81–101). Nashville, TN: Vanderbilt University Press.
Gibson, B. E. (2016). *Rehabilitation: A post-critical approach*. Boca Raton, FL: Taylor & Francis.
Glei, D. A., & Goldman, N. (2000). Understanding ethnic variation in pregnancy-related care in rural Guatemala. *Ethnicity and Health, 5*(1), 5–22.
Glei, D. A., Goldman, N., & Rodríguez, G. (2003). Utilization of care during pregnancy in rural Guatemala: Does obstetrical need matter? *Social Science & Medicine, 57*(12), 2447–2463.
Goldman, N., Glei, D., Pebley, A., & Delgado, H. (2001). *Atención Prenatal en Áreas Rurales de Cuatro Departamentos de Guatemala: Resultados de la Encuesta Guatemalteca de Salud Familiar, 1995*. Guatemala City: Instituto de Nutrición de Centro América y Panamá.
Gragnolati, M., & Marini, A. (2003). *Health and poverty in Guatemala*. Policy Research Working Paper 2966. The World Bank—GUAPA 1. Retrieved from https://www.researchgate.net/publication/2354951 3_Health_and_Poverty_in_Guatemala
Hallowell, E. (2014). "Between the wall and the sword": Reproductive governance and the technology of emergency in Guatemalan maternity care. *Feminist Formations, 26*(3), 100–121.
Hammell, K. W. (2006). *Perspectives on disability & rehabilitation: Contesting assumptions, challenging practice*. Amsterdam: Elsevier Health Sciences.
Harvey, D. (2007). *A brief history of neoliberalism*. Oxford, UK: Oxford University Press.
Hernández, A. R., Hurtig, A.-K., Dahlblom, K., & San Sebastián, M. (2014). More than a checklist: A realist evaluation of supervision of mid-level health workers in rural Guatemala. *BMC Health Services Research, 14*(1), 112. https://doi.org/10.1186/1472-6963-14-11
Ishida, K., Stupp, P., Turcios-Ruiz, R., William, D. B., & Espinoza, E. (2012). Ethnic inequality in Guatemalan women's use of modern reproductive health care. *International Perspectives on Sexual and Reproductive Health, 38*(2), 99–108.
McAllister, C., & Nelson, D. M. (Eds.). (2013). *War by other means: Aftermath in post-genocide Guatemala*. Durham, NC: Duke University Press.
Metz, B. (2001). Politics, population, and family planning in Guatemala: Ch'orti'Maya experiences. *Human Organization, 60*(3), 259–271.
Nelson, D. M. (2009). *Reckoning: The ends of war in Guatemala*. Durham, NC: Duke University Press.
PAHO (Pan American Health Organization). (2007). *Health in the Americas: Guatemala*. Retrieved from http://ais.paho.org/hia_cp/en/2007/Guatemala%20English.pdf
PAHO (Pan American Health Organization). (2012). *Health in the Americas: Guatemala*. Retrieved from http://www.paho.org/saludenlasamericas/index.php?option=com_docman&task=doc_view&gid=132&Itemid=
Pena, C. L. (2013). *Guatemala—Improving access to health care services through the expansion of coverage program (PEC): The case of Guatemala*. Universal Health Coverage (UNICO) studies series; no. 19. Washington, DC: World Bank. Retrieved from http://documents.worldbank.org/curated/en/967411468039876158/Guatemala-Improving-Access-to-Health-Care-Services-through-the-Expansion-of-Coverage-Program-PEC-The-Case-of-Guatemala
Rööst, M., Johnsdotter, S., Liljestrand, J., & Essén, B. (2004). A qualitative study of conceptions and attitudes regarding maternal mortality among traditional birth attendants in rural Guatemala. *BJOG: An International Journal of Obstetrics & Gynaecology, 111*(12), 1372–1377.

Ruiz, M. J., van Dijk, M. G., Berdichevsky, K., Munguía, A., Burks, C., & García, S. G. (2013). Barriers to the use of maternity waiting homes in indigenous regions of Guatemala: A study of users' and community members' perceptions. *Culture, Health & Sexuality, 15*(2), 205–218.

Sanford, V. (2003). *Buried secrets: Truth and human rights in Guatemala*. Berlin: Springer.

Santiso-Galvez, R., & Bertrand, J. T. (2004). The delayed contraceptive revolution in Guatemala. *Human Organization, 63*(1), 57–67.

Shiffman, J. (2007). Generating political priority for maternal mortality reduction in 5 developing countries. *American Journal of Public Health, 97*(5), 796–803.

Shiffman, J., & Garcés del Valle, A. L. (2006). Political history and disparities in safe motherhood between Guatemala and Honduras. *Population and Development Review, 32*(1), 53–80.

Sibley, L., Sipe, T. A., & Koblinsky, M. (2004). Does traditional birth attendant training improve referral of women with obstetric complications: a review of the evidence. *Social Science & Medicine, 59*(8), 1757–1768.

UNICEF. (2015). *The state of the world's children 2015 country statistical tables*. Guatemala. Retrieved from http://www.unicef.org/infobycountry/guatemala_statistics.html

Walsh, L. V. (2006). Beliefs and rituals in traditional birth attendant practice in Guatemala. *Journal of Transcultural Nursing, 17*(2), 148–154.

World Bank. (2003). *Poverty in Guatemala*. Washington, DC: World Bank.

World Bank. (2009). *Guatemala—Poverty assessment: Good performance at low levels*. Washington, DC: World Bank. Retrieved from http://documents.worldbank.org/curated/en/803331468254934801/Guatemala-Poverty-assessment-good-performance-at-low-levels

World Bank. (2015). *GNI per capita, Atlas method*. Guatemala. Retrieved from http://data.worldbank.org/indicator/NY.GNP.PCAP.CD?order=wbapi_data_value_2014+wbapi_data_value+wbapi_data_value-last&sort=desc

Wright, E. O. (2010). *Envisioning real utopias*. London, England: Verso.

"The Mosquito Brings the Sickness": Local Knowledge, Stigma, and Barriers to Zika Prevention in Rural Guatemala

29

Michaela E. Howells and Michelle M. Pieters

29.1 Introduction: The Emergence of Zika: Global Crisis, Local Challenge

The emergence of the Zika virus has resulted in a major global public health problem, and resulted in significant distress to individuals, families, health care systems, and entire countries. According to the Centers for Disease Control and Prevention (CDC), Zika virus infection poses the greatest health risks to pregnant women and their unborn fetuses (CDC 2016c). Countries in South and Central America have experienced the highest rates of Zika and associated newborn microcephaly (CDC 2017a). This has produced a critical need for information regarding the economic, cultural, environmental, and educational pressures influencing Zika risk in these communities. Here, we take an ethnographic approach to examine preventative barriers to the Zika crisis in rural Guatemala.

The Zika virus was originally identified in 1947 from a rhesus macaque by a team of Rockefeller Foundation investigators while researching yellow fever in the Zika Forest of Uganda. Following its isolation in 1948 from mosquitoes in the same location, it was given the name Zika virus. A serological survey performed in Uganda in 1952 revealed that approximately 6% of sera were positive for neutralizing antibodies. No human disease was associated with Zika virus until 1954, when a 10-year-old Nigerian girl with fever and headache was believed to be infected (MacNamara 1954). Following this, several additional cases of symptomatic infection were reported from Africa (Schwartz 2017a, b). The first large outbreak of Zika virus occurred in humans in the Pacific Island of Yap in the Federated States of Micronesia—before this, no outbreaks and only 14 cases of human Zika virus disease had been documented anywhere in the world. During 2013 and 2014, a large outbreak of Zika virus spread through the islands of Oceania including French Polynesia, New Caledonia, Easter Island, Vanuatu, and the Cook Islands, infecting many thousands of inhabitants. A retrospective analysis of this epidemic revealed that there had been cases of fetal infection and microcephaly as a result of maternal infection (Cauchemez et al. 2016). In early 2015, a widespread illness characterized by

M. E. Howells, Ph.D. (✉) · M. M. Pieters, B.A.
Department of Anthropology, University of North Carolina Wilmington, Wilmington, NC, USA
e-mail: howellsm@uncw.edu; mmp8296@uncw.edu

D. A. Schwartz (ed.), *Maternal Death and Pregnancy-Related Morbidity Among Indigenous Women of Mexico and Central America*, Global Maternal and Child Health: Medical, Anthropological, and Public Health Perspectives, https://doi.org/10.1007/978-3-319-71538-4_29

skin rash and fever was reported to be occurring in several states of northeastern Brazil. Originally believed to be caused by dengue virus, on April 29, 2015, the Bahia State Laboratory reported that patient samples tested positive for Zika virus (Schwartz 2017a). In October and November of 2015, Brazil reported the occurrence of a large increase in the incidence of fetuses and infants with congenital microcephaly and other malformations, leading the World Health Organization (WHO) to declare in February 2016 that the recent association of Zika infection with clusters of microcephaly and other neurologic disorders constituted a Public Health Emergency of International Concern (WHO 2016a). After many months of investigation, on April 13, 2016, the United States Centers for Disease Control and Prevention (CDC) issued a statement that Zika virus was a cause of microcephaly and other severe fetal brain defects (Rasmussen et al. 2016).

Significant public attention has focused on microcephalic infants who are born with abnormally small heads and limited brain growth (CDC 2017b; Schwartz 2017c), which has been termed the congenital Zika syndrome. This syndrome has also been associated with other congenital abnormalities including vision and hearing deficits, seizures, epilepsy, permanent brain damage, developmental delays, malformations including arthrogryposis and craniosynostosis, and spontaneous abortion and perinatal death (Alvarado and Schwartz 2017; CDC 2017b).

Transmission of the Zika virus is novel in that it can not only be spread by the same mosquitoes (*Aedes aegypti*) that carry other pathogenic flaviviruses, such as chikungunya, dengue, and yellow fever, but can also be transmitted through sexual contact. Zika is the first identified disease that is both arthropod-borne and sexually transmitted. As a result, Zika prevention combines the challenges associated with other mosquito-borne viruses (e.g., dengue, yellow fever) and sexually transmitted infections (e.g., human immunodeficiency virus (HIV), syphilis, chlamydia) (Tambo et al. 2016). Further complicating Zika prevention is the fact that the majority of individuals infected (80%) are asymptomatic, and that the disease may be spread up to 6 months after infection through sexual fluids (CDC 2016a).

The CDC has responded by recommending preventative measures to reduce exposure to the virus. These recommendations include avoiding mosquito bites by wearing long-sleeved shirts and pants, using bed nets, insect repellent, and window screens, and removing standing water. Additionally, because Zika virus has been identified in semen and vaginal fluids up to 6 months after infection, it is recommended that men wear condoms when having sex with women of reproductive age (CDC 2016b).

Although these recommendations are practical in affluent communities, they can be nearly impossible to follow for women who face long-term systematic barriers to education, health care, and reproductive justice in rural areas. In other words, these responses fail to take into account the realities of women's tenuous control over their reproductive choices and access to other preventative measures in impoverished communities where individuals lack the economic or social capital needed to prevent Zika infection. These factors are especially prevalent among indigenous women living in resource-poor countries.

Zika-related microcephaly, combined with the associated neurological complications, have triggered strong responses by the public health infrastructures of affected countries. The human cost of the congenital Zika syndrome is high (e.g., pregnancy loss, disabled children). Furthermore, there are significant and as yet uncalculated monetary costs in terms of special education, lifetime health care needs, and therapy for the affected children.

In 2016, 3231 cases of Zika infection were reported to health authorities in Guatemala, of which at least 319 were pregnant women. As of April 6, 2017, there have been 3598 suspected and 921 confirmed autochthonous cases of Zika virus infection since the start of the pandemic; 59 confirmed cases of Zika congenital syndrome have occurred (Pan American Health Organization 2017; Pocasangre and Orozco 2016).

Financial deficits in the Guatemalan public health system severely limit its capabilities. Although the Guatemalan Constitution guarantees health care to all of its citizens, the government spends only $233 USD per capita annually (compared to $9990 USD in 2015 in the United States) on public health care (Banco Mundial 2016; National Health Expenditure 2015). These funds are particularly strained by the need to combat other mosquito-borne epidemics, including dengue, chikungunya, and malaria (Hayes 2009). As a result, the government has become dependent on nongovernmental organizations (NGOs) and other external agencies for Zika virus education, prevention, and attempts at eradication.

Without the unified public health response required to cover all aspects of Zika exposure, there may be lapses or inconsistencies in coverage across the country. For instance, in this primarily Catholic nation, religious aid organizations may provide incomplete family planning information in respect to church doctrine. Indeed, informational health posters found around the country from these organizations have opted to leave out information about sexual transmission of Zika, and exclude listing condoms as a preventative measure.

29.2 "When a Woman is Pregnant, It Is Worrisome": Top-Down Zika Prevention Recommendations Meet Reality in Rural Guatemala

To prevent Zika virus infection, the WHO and CDC have recommended limiting exposure to mosquito bites and sexual transmission. These recommendations include restricting time spent outdoors while mosquitoes are active, wearing protective clothing (long sleeves and pants), and using insect repellant. They also recommend sleeping under bed nets, using window screens (or glass window panes), staying in air-conditioning when possible, and draining standing water containers (to interrupt the mosquitoes' life cycle). Finally, they recommend using condoms during sexual intercourse with women who are pregnant or likely to become pregnant.

These recommendations represent ideal measures, but are challenging to achieve in impoverished rural conditions where people's livelihoods rely on working outdoors, infrastructure is poor, and there are severe financial constraints. Quantitative methods, including knowledge attitude and practices (KAP) surveys, are valuable methods used in the social sciences to reveal misconceptions or misunderstandings that may represent obstacles to the implementation of activities and potential barriers to behavior change, including those related to the Zika virus epidemic (WHO 2016b). The challenges raised by the threat of Zika infections necessitate engaged research into the barriers to prevention in local communities. Our research represents a first step in better understanding how these challenges are experienced by a rural Guatemalan community and may help identify similar challenges in other South and Central American populations.

We focused our study in the rural municipality of Nueva Concepción, Escuintla (henceforth Escuintla) (Fig. 29.1) in South Central Guatemala. The region begins 148 km southwest of the capital of Guatemala City and extends to the Pacific Ocean. Its temperature (annual range 19.1–31.9 °C), tropical climate (3516 mm of yearly rainfall), rich volcanic soil, and topographic diversity make it a prime location for agriculture, livestock farming, and horticulture (INSIVUMEH 2016). Although the population of Escuintla comprises three different ethnic groups of *mestizo* descent, the majority of the population speaks Spanish (Información Socioeconómica de Guatemala 2015). We conducted interviews at two family-owned farms that employ nonfamily workers.

In these areas, we combined data from participant observation and 40 semi-structured interviews among a *mestizo* community primarily composed of Jehovah's Witnesses. Both women and men were included in this study. Our goal was to assess this rural, low-literacy population's understanding of and gaps in knowledge associated with Zika. All interviews were conducted in Spanish by a member of our team (MMP), who is a native speaker from the region.

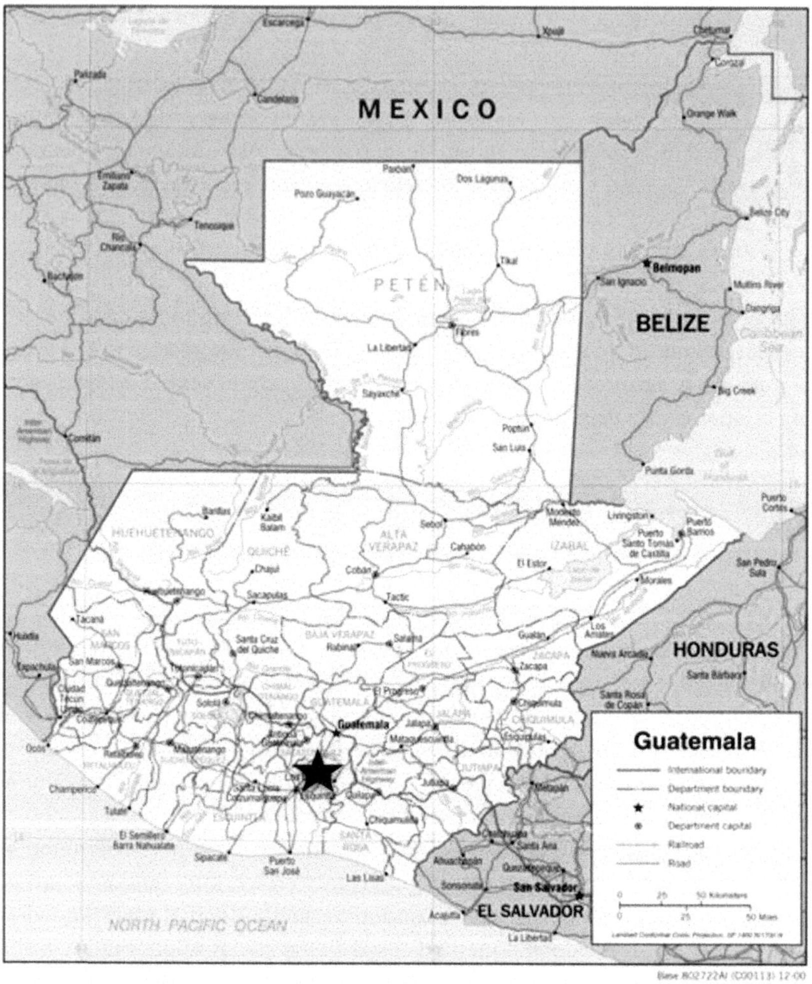

Fig. 29.1 Map of Guatemala. A star marks the approximate location of our fieldwork. Map courtesy of Central Intelligence Agency. Available from: https://www.cia.gov/library/publications/resources/cia-maps-publications/map-downloads/Guatemala_Transportation.jpg/image.jpg

Table 29.1 Characteristics of the participating Escuintla farms

Products	Cashews, rubber, bamboo, teak, cattle
Number of residents	91
Literacy level (Escuintla region of Guatemala)[a]	88.2%
Number of houses	21
Size of houses	34.1–44.76 m^2
Housing materials	Wood/concrete walls, dirt/concrete floors, tin roofs
Window screens or glass panes?	No
Open water containers?	Yes

[a]Literacy level expected to be lower specifically on the farms

In addition to probing knowledge about Zika, the questionnaires included demographic information such as age and education level. Our interviews included open-ended questions such as "What are some ways of avoiding Zika infection?", true/false items, and Likert-scale questions. The 40 participants ranged between 21 and 83 years old (mean 40.8 ± 16.0), and were predominantly female ($n = 24$, 60%).

The two farms at the center of our study are family-owned, with outside employees and their families living permanently on-site. Both farms produce rubber, wood (teak and bamboo), cashews, and beef. These farms are adjacent to each other and are separated only by a dusty road. The similarities of these farms outweigh the differences, and we have chosen to combine them for our analyses (Table 29.1).

29.3 Zika Virus in Rural Guatemala: "Fight the Bite" and Other Well-Meant Advice

Employees of the farms are *mestizo* (individuals of mixed Spanish and indigenous descent). Men are employed as day laborers, cowboys, mechanics, managers, and administrators. Day laborers prune trees, collect the rubber, pick the cashews, fix fences, and perform other maintenance duties. Cowboys move the cattle from pasture to pasture to ensure the best grazing, while monitoring the health of the animals. Mechanics drive and fix the tractors. Managers assign duties to the day laborers and mechanics, contact buyers when products are ready, and manage workers' payments. Finally, the administrators ensure the overall successful running of the farm and provide updates to the landlord. Those men who work as laborers, cowboys, mechanics, and managers spend the majority of their day outdoors (8+ hours in the field), increasing their possible exposure to mosquitoes.

The employees' families also live on the farms. Much like their husbands, partners, brothers, and fathers who are working on the farm, women work in open-air conditions that expose them to mosquitoes throughout the day. Women's labor centers on domestic support of their households, although girls are also seasonally employed to pick cashews. Women are household managers who take care of their children, wash clothes, clean their homes, prepare meals, and perform other domestic duties. Women included in our study reported spending less than 3.3 years in school, with the majority leaving before completing primary school (approximately achieving a second-grade education by United States standards). This is not significantly different from men's education levels in this region (4.4 years, $p = 0.7$). Many of these women are illiterate and reported dropping out of school to support their families' domestic needs. As a result, the women who are most at risk of acquiring Zika virus infection are unable to read informational posters meant to alert them to these risks (Fig. 29.2).

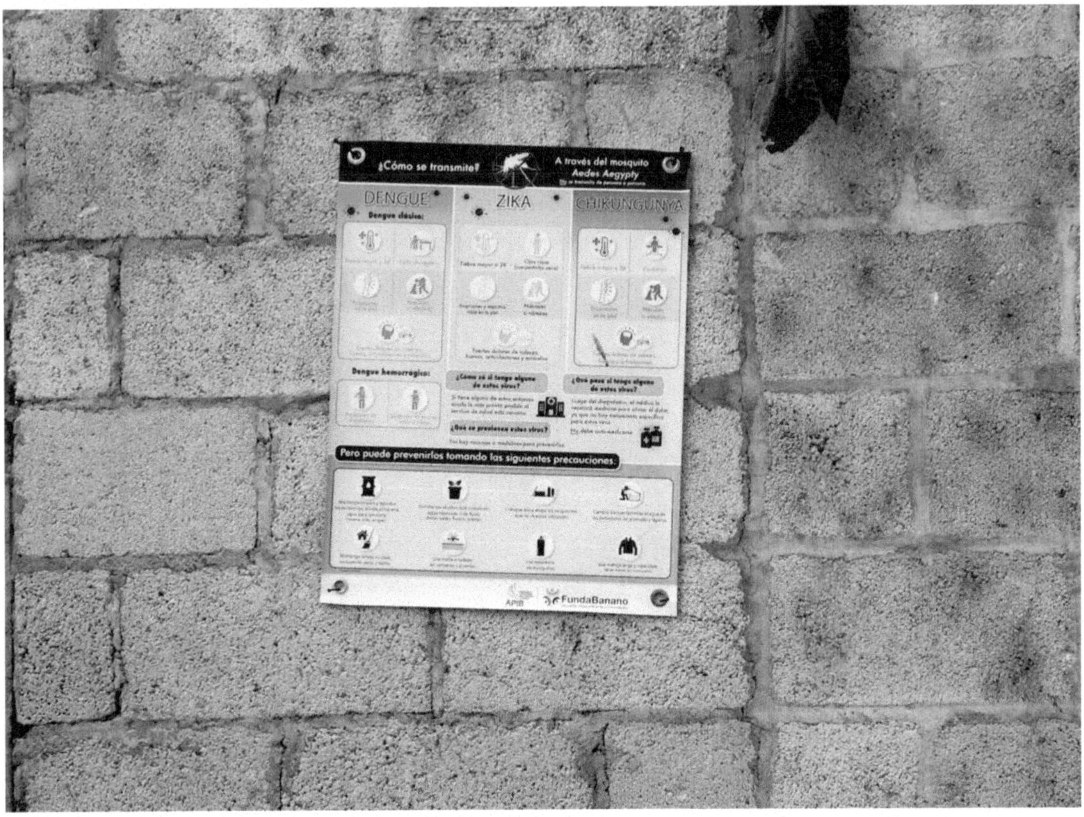

Fig. 29.2 An informational poster discussing mosquito-borne diseases—dengue, Zika, and chikungunya. It does not address sexual transmission or condom use as a preventative measure

Although the majority of the women at the farms are not paid laborers, they fulfill vital, time-consuming, economically driven tasks that expose them to mosquitoes throughout the day. In order to stay comfortable in the sometimes-oppressive heat, women dress in knee-length skirts and short-sleeved shirts. Although this helps them keep cool, it also results in additional skin being exposed to mosquitoes.

In addition to food preparation and the majority of child-rearing tasks, women spend a significant amount of time walking to the nearby river that flows through the farms to wash clothes and socialize. They also attend to all of the household shopping at the open-air market that is 20 km away by public minibus. Finally, women reported spending an additional 3.4 h per day socializing with their neighbors and friends in the shade. While all of these behaviors are essential for community connections, they also increase exposure to mosquitoes and arthropod-borne viral infections (arboviruses).

We asked participants 12 true/false questions associated with prevention of Zika exposure through both mosquito transmission and sexual activity. These questions focused on clothing, bed nets, and insect repellant. The majority of participants (95–100%) were able to answer these questions accurately (90% response rate). However, all but one participant declined to answer any of the true/false questions association with prevention of Zika exposure through condom use. We also asked five open-ended questions meant to elicit knowledge of prevention and risk (Figs. 29.3 and 29.4).

Although participants were able to articulate the *need* to prevent mosquito bites, their actual *ability* to prevent these bites is limited. For instance, none of those interviewed had the WHO- and CDC-recommended glass window panes or access to air-conditioning. A minority of participants (15%) had screens on their windows, with one-half of these individuals reporting rips in their screens. Approximately one-half of the participants reported sleeping under bed nets, and less than 30% used insect repellant more than once a week (Table 29.2).

The majority of houses on the farm consist of a single open living space, with areas separated by cloth curtains. The kitchen and its open-fire stove can be separated by a concrete wall, a thin wooden board, or included as part of the single room. Average household occupancy is 4.5. None of the windows have glass panes or screens. However, they do have wooden covers that are closed at

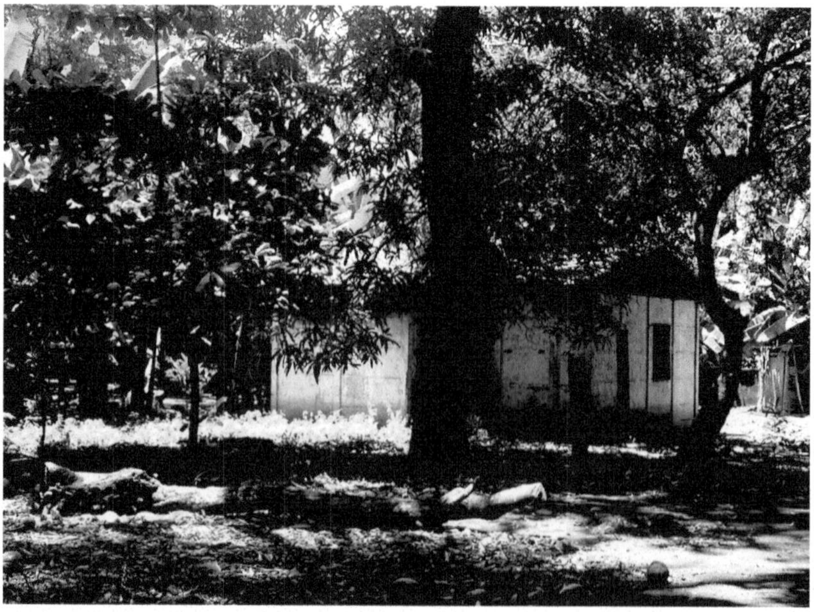

Fig. 29.3 Typical housing in the region of Escuintla

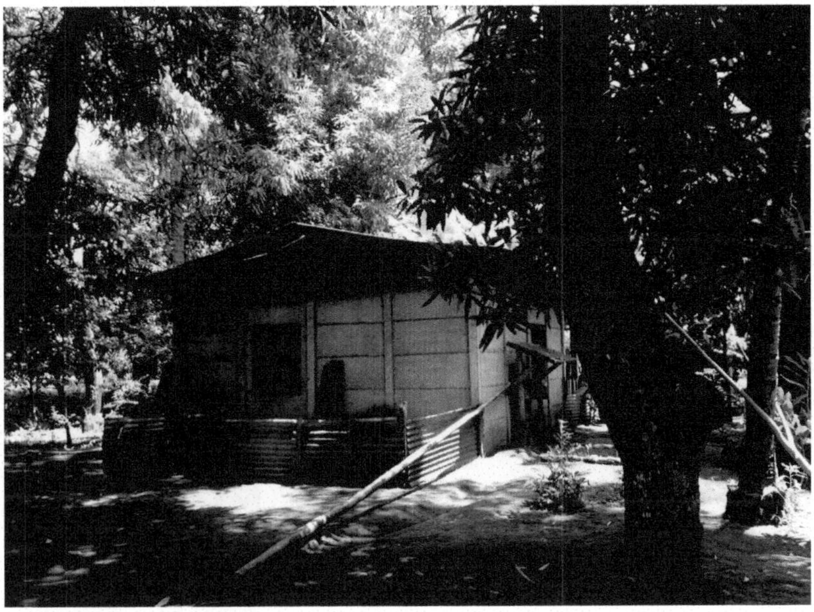

Fig. 29.4 Another house in Escuintla. These houses have many locations where standing water can accumulate, leading to mosquito breeding

Table 29.2 Prevalence (%) of women ($N = 24$) and men ($N = 16$) with access to preventative measures

	Yes		No	
Preventative measure	Women	Men	Women	Men
Air-conditioning in house	0 (0)	0 (0)	24 (100)	16 (100)
Glass window panes in house	0 (0)	0 (0)	24 (100)	16 (100)
Screens on windows	4 (17)	2 (13)	19 (83)	14 (88)
Sleep under a bed nets	11 (46)	9 (56)	13 (54)	7 (44)
Use insect repellant >once/week	7 (29)	3 (19)	17 (71)	13 (81)

night. The lack of a window barrier allows mosquitoes to fly freely into the house throughout the day, increasing the risk of exposure to Zika for the individuals inside. In addition, participants complained that mosquito nets, when combined with the closed windows, make the room stifling (Figs. 29.5 and 29.6).

There is no running water or plumbing in the employees' homes. Instead, families draw water from the local well and use 42-gallon plastic barrels to store water. These containers are stored close to the house for convenience, are not covered, and quickly become a nursery for mosquito larvae. Although the Guatemalan Ministry of Public Health and Social Assistance sporadically provides larvicide to homeowners, these interventions usually occur less frequently than the recommended three-month schedule, allowing for larval growth (Fig. 29.7).

Next to most of the houses are elongated washing basins or *pilas*, where the families shower, brush their teeth, and clean their dishes (Fig. 29.8). There is no plumbing. Instead, families use latrines, located in small wooden sheds usually about 10 m away from the houses. During the rainy season, the fields can become very humid and damp, which attracts mosquitoes and puts people working on the fields at a higher risk of contracting the virus. In addition, abandoned cattle troughs near the houses accumulate water, making them a perfect breeding site for mosquitoes. Although some public health campaigns have visited the family farms and fumigated, many of the participants resisted these campaigns, thinking that fumigating meant poisoning their environment (Figs. 29.9 and 29.10).

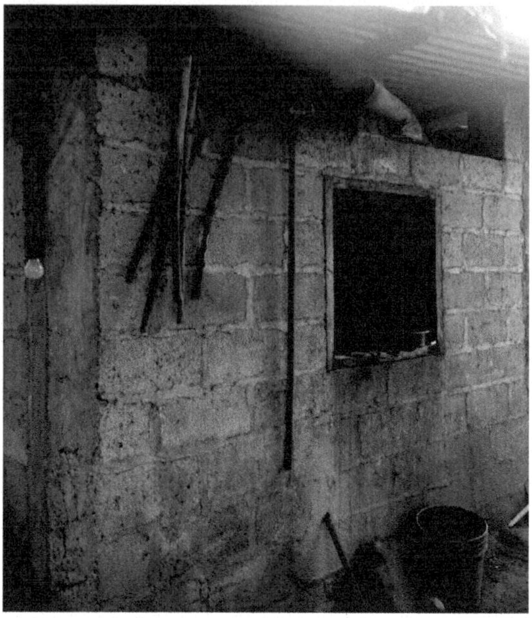

Fig. 29.5 Typical farm home in Escuintla with unscreened windows and bucket filled with standing water

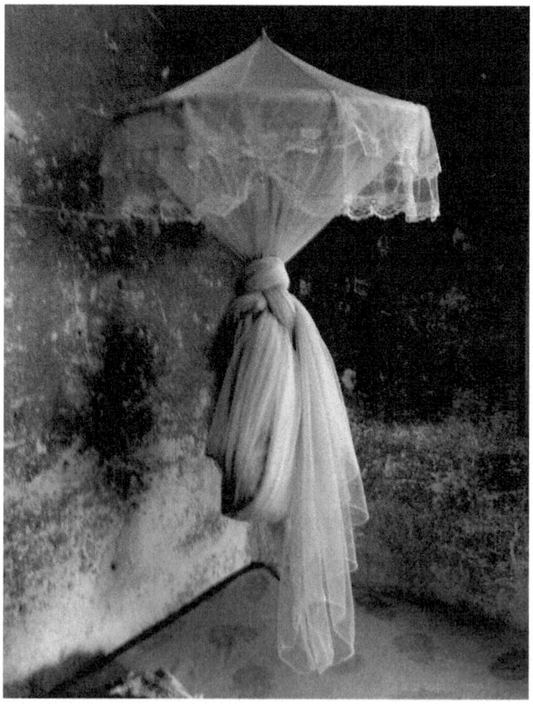

Fig. 29.6 A bed net used to keep out mosquitoes. They are often not used due to the heat

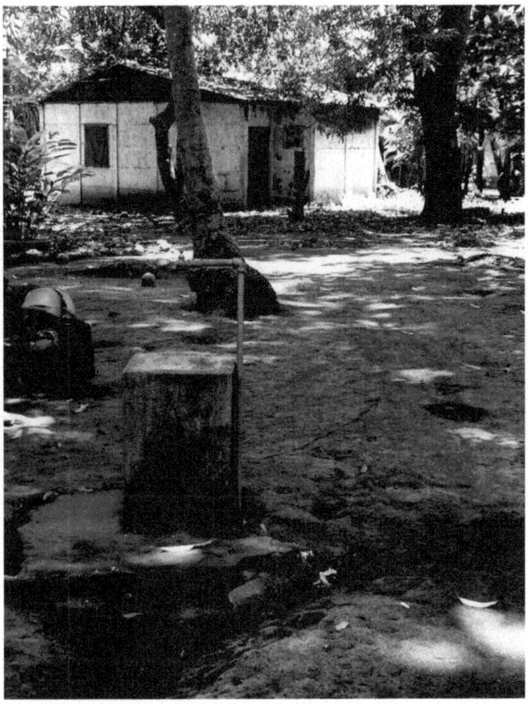

Fig. 29.7 A farm home in Escuintla with house well in the foreground

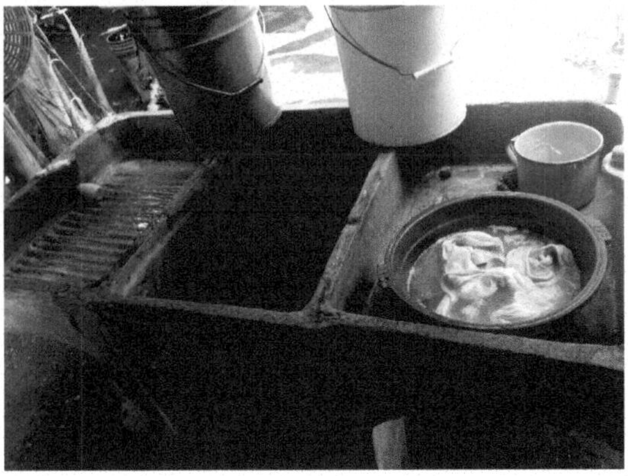

Fig. 29.8 A washing basin or pila where the families shower, brush their teeth, and clean their dishes. They are also potential mosquito breeding grounds

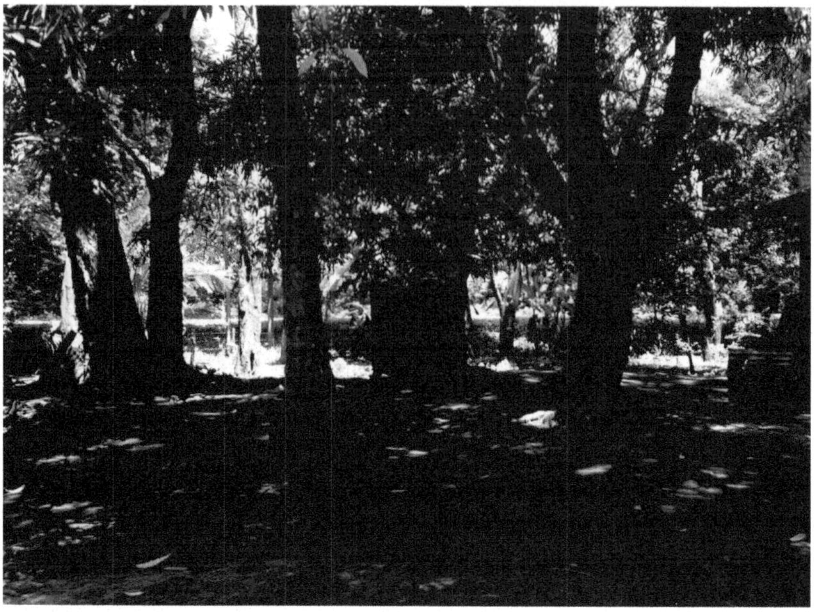

Fig. 29.9 A latrine outside of the house. Inhabitants are exposed to mosquitoes when accessing the latrine

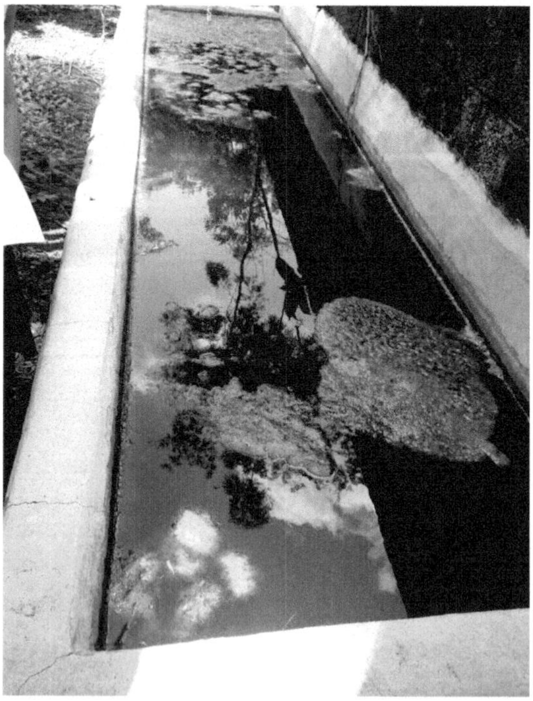

Fig. 29.10 Abandoned cattle troughs are frequent sources of standing water

29.4 Private Cost of Prevention, Public Burden of Risk

Participants associated the lack of preventative measures with the high cost or discomfort of these measures (Table 29.3). For instance, the CDC recommends using insect repellent to avoid being bitten by mosquitoes (CDC 2016b). However, some participants reported being unable to afford the $5 cost (1.2% of the average monthly income in Escuintla) of a 6-ounce bottle of insect repellent, which would last for approximately a week (Table 29.3). Others reported avoiding bed nets because they were thought to reduce ventilation and were considered a nuisance (Fig. 29.10).

The Guatemalan Ministry of Public Health and Social Assistance tours the rural areas offering lectures on a variety of health topics. However, only men were included in these outreach events, since the Ministry took advantage of the men gathering at the beginning of their work day when they receive their assignments. As a result, women were forced to depend on their husbands and male family members for secondhand health information. The farms where we conducted our study were not included in government-funded anti-Zika programs. Instead, they relied on private organizations to fill this need. However, these private organizations frequently provided incomplete health information. For instance, they discussed the importance of avoiding mosquito bites, but did not mention the risk of contracting Zika through sexual transmission.

These educational challenges extend to printed materials, such as posters, which although prominently displayed around the farm, focused on mosquito transmission of Zika but excluded sexual transmission. None of the posters listed condoms as a way of preventing transmission of the virus. In addition, the images can be confusing and misleading, creating an additional health barrier for illiterate and low literacy individuals (Figs. 29.2 and 29.11).

Taken together, this community is reflective of the environmental realities of people living in the tropics. The livelihoods of these individuals include constant exposure to mosquitoes and the diseases they carry. As a result, the well-intentioned recommendations from public health specialists can be challenging if not impossible to comply with for those in lower economic statuses. Wearing protective clothing against mosquitoes can lead to overheating, insect repellent is expensive, bed nets are stifling, and screens on windows are nonexistent. As a result, although people were exceptionally well educated about the risk of mosquito transmission, they were unable to follow these recommendations. In

Table 29.3 Financial and geographic availability of preventative measures against Zika virus transmission in Escuintla, based on \$385.76 monthly income (*Source*: Ministerio de Trabajo y Provision Social 2017)

Preventative measure	Price ($US)	Average monthly income (%)	Availability (distance from farms in Escuintla)
Condom	\$0.58–\$1.19	0.2–0.3	5 km away, 10 min bus ride
Condom	FREE	n/a	20 km away, 40 min bus ride
Insect repellent	\$5 (per can)	1.2	20 km away, 40 min bus ride
Bed nets (72″)	\$45 (minimum)	11.0	20 km away, 40 min bus ride

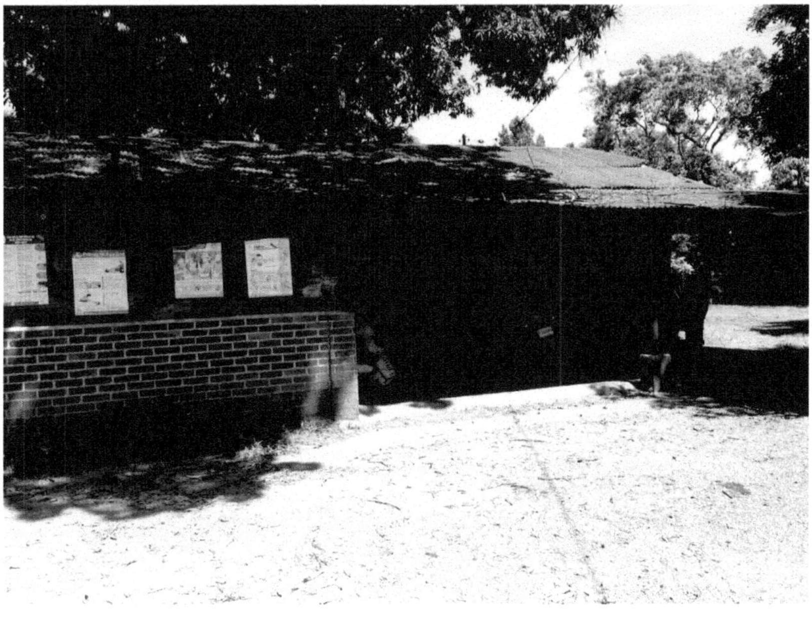

Fig. 29.11 A tool shed where male workers gather every morning to receive assignments. Informational posters on different health issues, some related to Zika virus, hang from the shed. Unfortunately, they cannot be read by the illiterate villagers

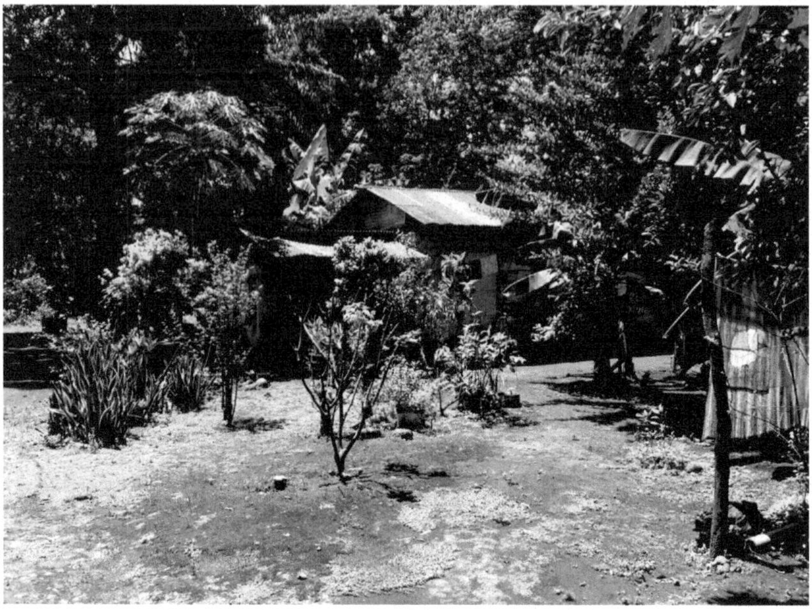

Fig. 29.12 Garden behind a house—there are many damp areas where mosquitoes can breed

comparison, the lack of education surrounding family planning and the role of condoms in protecting against Zika is not being clearly communicated. This, combined with the lack of comprehensive sexual health education and access to condoms, can paralyze the efforts to combat the spread of Zika (Fig. 29.12).

29.5 "They Feel Women": Women's Empowerment and Access to Family Planning

Zika virus can be sexually transmitted for up to 6 months after infection. In response, the CDC has recommended using condoms during sexual intercourse with pregnant women or women who may become pregnant. Some South and Central American countries (not including Guatemala) have gone as far as issuing recommendations against becoming pregnant until the crisis has passed. Frequently, family planning decisions are framed as the sole responsibility of the individual. However, the ability to make these decisions depends on the larger cultural systems the individual is a part of. Religious, political, health care, educational, and legal systems can all play a substantial role in influencing access to family planning resources (Howells and Pieters 2016).

Although Zika virus can be transmitted sexually, this mode of transmission is widely ignored by the government and private organizations fulfilling rural public health needs. This issue is further exacerbated by the lack of resources plaguing the public health system, and the stigma cultural restrictions placed on birth control. By law, access to birth control and family planning in Guatemala is free and public, and every government health post is mandated to have condoms, birth control pills, and contraceptive injections (Depo-Provera) available. However, the demand frequently outpaces the supply, especially in rural areas like the farms we studied in Escuintla (Colom, personal communication). Physical distance from health posts can also be a limiting factor. For instance, our participants needed to travel 20 km by mini bus to access the nearest health post, with no guarantee that these centers would be stocked with the desired family planning resources. Young women (age 15–24 years) are likely to be most heavily impacted by these limitations, since they are usually the ones seeking family planning options.

Cultural factors further add to the burden of strained family planning resources. Guatemalan women reported attempting to conceal their visits to family planning offices at health posts and their use of birth control from partners and family members to avoid conflict (Colom, personal communication). In Escuintla, women rely on men to buy condoms at the local pharmacy (a 5 km mini bus ride away), although participants reported that it was rare for women to ask men to purchase or use them. This may reflect the perceived role of distrust and infidelity associated with condom use, and the fact that condoms are rarely re-introduced in a relationship (Abraham et al. 2011).

Female ignorance of sexual matters, especially in Guatemala, is often viewed as a sign of purity and good virtue (Weiss et al. 2000). In a study focusing on sexual decision-making in Guatemala, both males and females indicated that men should be more knowledgeable of and more experienced in sexual matters than women. Male respondents also indicated that they should be the women's teachers (Weiss et al. 2000). This ideology can lead to coercive behaviors and inadvertently condone non-consensual sexual behaviors (Sunday and Obioha 2016). Alternatively, as a family planning specialist in Guatemala put it, when women have access to family planning information and are able to make decisions about their bodies, they feel empowered—"they feel women" (Colom, personal communication).

During our interview process, both women and men were visibly uncomfortable with questions associated with sexual transmission. Of the 40 participants we interviewed, only one was willing to answer true/false statements regarding the role of condoms in prevention (compared to a 95% + response rate for mosquito-based questions). When asked in open-ended questions to explain how one contracts Zika, only two (5%) people listed sexual transmission ("intimate relations") as a risk factor (in comparison, 87% listed mosquitoes) and no one listed condoms as a preventative measure. This lack of response does not necessarily indicate a lack of knowledge regarding Zika, but instead reflects the tabooed nature of these conversations. However, this taboo may extend to condom use as a preventative measure against Zika, and presents a significant challenge to public health programs.

Jehovah's Witnesses, such as the participants in our study, are permitted to use contraception when they are married. In this light, the hesitancy to discuss family planning—even in the framework of Zika—in this community was initially surprising. However, this may indicate larger cultural pressures associated with living in a predominantly Catholic nation. As discussed above, this pressure is reflected by the exclusion of condoms as a preventative measure and sexual activity as a transmission factor on health messaging posters. It may also be reflected in the lack of resources allocated to family planning (Colom, personal communication).

The intersection of politics and religion is also reflected in Guatemala's surgical abortion laws. Guatemalan law permits abortion only if the life of the mother is in danger (Singh et al. 2006). Due to this law, many women seek abortions under unsanitary and unsafe conditions. Unsafe abortions contribute to the high rates of maternal mortality and morbidity in the country (Schwartz 2015; Singh et al. 2006). Combined with the inadequate access to other family planning options, these laws may put Zika-infected women who wish to terminate their pregnancies at high risk. Inadequate access to other family planning options, contraceptive services and information limits Guatemalan women's safety when considering pregnancy in a Zika-affected environment.

Taken together, these public health realities are particularly sobering with the recognition that the communities with the highest exposure to Zika-carrying mosquitoes are also least likely to have access to preventative measures. As a result, these communities face restricted access to preventative and long-term health care, and limited access to special education and disability services for children. Therefore, the burden of care for disabled children is likely to fall on the affected mothers and other women of the community.

29.6 Conclusion: Local Context and Structural Barriers to Zika Prevention

The reemergence of Zika has taken significant human and financial tolls on communities in South and Central American, with pregnant women and their unborn fetuses facing the greatest burden of risk. For this study, we took an ethnographic approach to examining preventative barriers to combating the Zika crisis in rural Guatemala. We reviewed the WHO and CDC recommendations for Zika prevention and found that although these recommendations are practical in affluent communities, they can be nearly impossible to follow for people who face long-term systematic barriers to education, health care, and reproductive justice in rural areas. The realities of working long hours outdoors in paid or unpaid labor, combined with the punitive financial and social costs of prevention, challenge the ability of individuals to protect themselves from this reemerging virus.

Although the majority of individuals in this study were able to list avoiding mosquitoes as a way to prevent Zika, none listed condoms as a protective measure. This may reflect the stigmatization against family planning associated with a predominantly Catholic polity and its effects on reducing access to comprehensive care. This produces a critical need for information regarding the economic, cultural, environmental, and educational pressures influencing Zika risk in high-risk communities.

Acknowledgments We would like to extend our sincere thanks to the participants of the Escuintla farm communities who shared their lives with us. We would also like to extend our thanks to Richard Bender, Carolyn Robinson, Christopher Dana Lynn, Samantha Fernando, Holly Wood, Katherine Woolard, Mallory Walker, Santiago Ortiz, David A. Schwartz, and Uli Howells-Loudon for feedback on drafts. Additionally, we would like to acknowledge Katherine Pieters, Nicole De Nes, Jacobo Pieters, Ruth Escobar, Barbara Arroyo, and Amadeo Garcia for their support throughout the field work. Funding was provided by University of North Carolina Wilmington's Center for the Support of Undergraduate Research and Fellowships (CSURF) and the Summer Undergraduate Research and Creativity Awards (SURCA).

This study was approved by the University of North Carolina Wilmington Internal Review Board (protocol number 16-0340).

References

Abraham, T., Macauda, M., Erickson, P., & Singer, M. (2011). "And let me see them damn papers!" The role of STI/AIDS screening among urban African American and Puerto Rican youth in the transition to sex without a condom. *AIDS and Behavior, 15*, 1359–1371. https://doi.org/10.1007/s10461-0109811-z

Alvarado, M. G., & Schwartz, D. A. (2017). Zika virus infection in pregnancy, microcephaly, and maternal and fetal health: What we think, what we know, and what we think we know. *Archives of Pathology & Laboratory Medicine, 141*(1), 26–32.

Banco Mundial. (2016). *Gasto en salud per capita (US$ a precios actuales)*. Retrieved March 7, 2017, from www.datos.bancomundial.org/indicator/SH.XPD.PCAP

Cauchemez, S., Besnard, M., Bompard, P., Dub, T., Guillemette-Artur, P., Eyrolle-Guignot, D., et al. (2016). Association between Zika virus and microcephaly in French Polynesia, 2013–2015: A retrospective study. *Lancet, 387*(10033), 2125–2132.

Centers for Disease Control and Prevention. (2016a). *Clinical evaluation and disease*. Retrieved March 7, 2017, from https://www.cdc.gov/zika/hc-providers/preparing-for-zika/clinicalevaluationdisease.html

Centers for Disease Control and Prevention. (2016b). *Protect yourself and others*. Retrieved March 7, 2017, from https://www.cdc.gov/zika/prevention/protect-yourself-and-others.html

Centers for Disease Control and Prevention. (2016c). *What we know about Zika*. Retrieved March 7, 2017, from https://www.cdc.gov/zika/about/index.html

Centers for Disease Control and Prevention. (2017a). *All countries and territories with active Zika virus transmission*. Retrieved March 7, 2017, from https://www.cdc.gov/zika/geo/active-countries.html

Centers for Disease Control and Prevention. (2017b). *Microcephaly and other birth defects*. Retrieved from https://www.cdc.gov/zika/healtheffects/birth_defects.html

Hayes, E. B. (2009). Zika virus outside Africa. *Emerging Infectious Diseases, 15*(9), 1347–1350. Retrieved April 3, 2017, from https://www.ncbi.nlm.nih.gov/pmc/articles/PMC2819875/

Howells, M. E., & Pieters, M. M. (2016). *Zika's frightening stranglehold.* Sapiens. 8 April 2016. Retrieved April 3, 2017, from http://www.sapiens.org/body/zika-and-family-planning/

Información Socioeconómica de Guatemala. (2015). *Gobierno de la República de Guatemala.* Retrieved March 22, 2017, from http://dae.mineco.gob.gt/mapainteractivo/index.php?controller=crm&action=detalles&id=6

INSIVUMEH. (2016). *Gobierno de la Republica de Guatemala.* Retrieved March 22, 2017, from http://www.insivumeh.gob.gt/meteorologia/ESTADISTICAS.html

MacNamara, F. N. (1954). Zika virus: A report on three cases of human infection during an epidemic of jaundice in Nigeria. *Transactions of the Royal Society of Tropical Medicine and Hygiene, 48*(2), 139–145.

National Health Expenditures. (2015). *Highlights.* Centers for Medicare & Medicaid Services. Retrieved March 21, 2017, from https://www.cms.gov/research-statistics-data-and-systems/statistics-trends-and-reports/nationalhealthexpenddata/downloads/highlights.pdf

Pan American Health Organization. (2017). *Zika cases and congenital syndrome associated with Zika virus reported by countries and territories in the Americas, 2015–2017. Cumulative cases.* Data as of 6 April 2017. Retrieved April 6, 2017, from http://www2.paho.org/hq/index.php?option=com_content&view=article&id=12390&Itemid=42090&lang=en

Pocasangre, H., & Orozco, A. (2016). Nacieron 36 niños con microcefalia asociada al Zika. *Prensa Libre.* 6 January 2017. Retrieved April 3, 2017, from http://www.prensalibre.com/guatemala/comunitario/nacieron-36-nios -con-microcefalia-por -zika-el-2016

Rasmussen, S. A., Jamieson, D. J., Honein, M. A., & Petersen, L. R. (2016). Zika virus and birth defects reviewing the evidence for causality. *New England Journal of Medicine, 374*(20), 1981–1987.

Schwartz, D. A. (2015). Unsafe abortion: A persistent cause of maternal death and reproductive morbidity in resource-poor nations. In D. A. Schwartz (Ed.), *Maternal mortality: Risk factors, anthropological perspectives, prevalence in developing countries and preventive strategies for pregnancy-related death* (pp. 425–439). New York: Nova Science Publishers.

Schwartz, D. A. (2017a). The origins and emergence of Zika virus, the newest TORCH infection: What's old is new again. *Archives of Pathology & Laboratory Medicine, 141*(1), 18–25.

Schwartz, D. A. (2017b). *Searching for yellow fever: The Rockefeller Foundation, Haddow towers, monkeys, and the discovery of the Zika virus.* First International Conference on Zika Virus, Washington, DC February 22, 2017.

Schwartz, D. A. (2017c). Autopsy and postmortem studies are concordant: Pathology of Zika virus infection is neurotropic in fetuses and infants with microcephaly following transplacental transmission. *Archives of Pathology & Laboratory Medicine, 141*(1), 68–72.

Singh, S., Prada, E., & Kestler, E. (2006). Induced abortion and unintended pregnancy in Guatemala. *International Family Planning Perspectives, 32*(3), 136–145. Retrieved from http://www.jstor.org/stable/4147623

Sunday, E. A., & Obioha, E. E. (2016). Partner communication and decision-making regarding sexual issues among students in a South African University. *Journal of Sociology and Social Policy, 7*(2), 103–124. https://doi.org/10.14267/CJSSP.2016.02.05

Tambo, E., Chuisseu, D. P., Ngogang, Y., & Khater, E. I. M. (2016). Deciphering emerging Zika and dengue viral epidemics: Implications for global maternal–child health burden. *Journal of Infection and Public Health, 9*(3), 240–250. https://doi.org/10.1016/j.jiph.2016.02.005

Weiss, E., Whelan, D., & Gupta, G. R. (2000). Gender, sexuality and HIV: Making a difference in the lives of young women in developing countries. *Sexual and Relationship Therapy, 15*(3), 233–245. Retrieved from http://www.tandfonline.com/doi/abs/10.1080/14681990050109836

World Health Organization. (2016a). *WHO Director-General summarizes the outcome of the Emergency Committee regarding clusters of microcephaly and Guillain-Barre Syndrome.* Retrieved from www.who.int/mediacentre/news/statements/2016/emergency-committee-zika-microcephaly/en/

World Health Organization. (2016b). *Knowledge, attitudes and practice surveys Zika virus disease and potential complications.* Resource pack. WHO reference number: WHO/ZIKV/RCCE/16.2.

Maternal Morbidity and Mortality in the Rural Trifinio Region of Southwestern Guatemala: Analysis of the Problems, Strategic Successes, and Challenges

30

Gretchen Heinrichs

30.1 Introduction

The causes of maternal mortality and morbidity are most often viewed through the Three Delay framework (Thaddeus and Maine 1994). The first delay, a deferral in the decision to seek care, occurs at the household level. It is often caused by a lack of understanding of pregnancy complications and risk factors during labor. This can occur on the side of the family or a minimally trained birth attendant. The second delay, reaching an adequate health care facility, is caused by long distances to hospitals, expense of transport, poor roads and infrastructure, or direct patient costs associated with medical care (admission fees, food and living expenses away from home, required tests, or medications). The third delay, receiving timely and adequate life-saving care, is due to poorly resourced medical facilities, a lack of medical supplies, inadequately trained medical staff, and/or inadequate referral systems.

In Guatemala, maternal mortality is one of the highest in the Latin American region. In 2010 the World Health Organization (WHO) estimated a maternal mortality ratio of approximately 120 per 100,000 live births, while more recent estimates from 2011 to 2015 hover between 88 and 109/100,000 live births (WHO 2015). The prevalence of contraceptive use (at 54%) is also one of the lowest in Latin America (UN Data 2013). Within the country, rural and indigenous populations experience disproportionately high maternal mortality, child mortality, and malnutrition as compared to urban, nonindigenous populations.

Life is especially difficult in the coastal lowlands of southwestern Guatemala near the border with Chiapas, Mexico. This region is named the southwest Trifinio (triangle) for the confluence of the three departments (states) of San Marcos, Quetzaltenango, and Retalhuleu (Fig. 30.1). Decades ago these pasturelands were transformed into large agro-business enterprises to cultivate crops for export, namely bananas and palm oil. Due to the opportunity for unskilled laborers to find steady work in a country

G. Heinrichs, M.D., F.A.C.O.G.
University of Colorado, Aurora, CO, USA

Denver Health, Denver, CO, USA

Center for Global Health, Colorado School of Public Health, Aurora, CO, USA
e-mail: Gretchen.heinrichs@ucdenver.edu

D. A. Schwartz (ed.), *Maternal Death and Pregnancy-Related Morbidity Among Indigenous Women of Mexico and Central America*, Global Maternal and Child Health: Medical, Anthropological, and Public Health Perspectives, https://doi.org/10.1007/978-3-319-71538-4_30

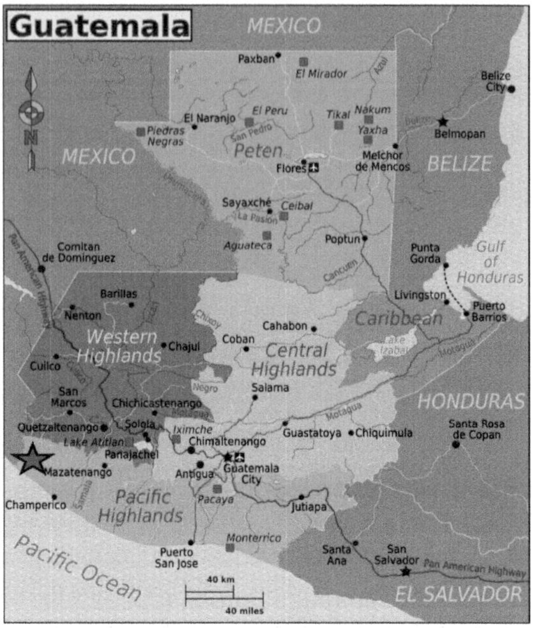

Fig. 30.1 Map of the Guatemala and neighboring counties. The SW Trifinio region is marked with a red star (Adapted from Wikimedia Commons, author: Burmesedays, available at: https://commons.wikimedia.org/wiki/File:Guatemala_Regions_map.png)

recovering from a prolonged and bloody civil war, many people migrated to this region, which is now home to approximately 25,000 people. Given that these individuals migrated from all over the country, they represent a diverse group of Ladinos–Spanish-speaking persons who are partly indigenous, Amerindian or mestizo. However, given their lack of common familial and ethnic roots, these small communities lack the cohesion, shared tradition, and culture of older communities such as those in the Guatemalan highlands. Combined with prevalent poverty and corruption, such community dynamics lead to lack of trust in leaders, inconsistent participation in public health efforts, and a lack of neighborly assistance among residents. Thus, when an emergency arises in the community, there is no easily accessible public emergency system in place and "Good Samaritan" actions of individuals are mistrusted. For example, neighbors may not feel willing to use their own limited resources to assist in saving a nonrelative because that favor will not be repaid—e.g., loaning out their car or giving money to a neighbor to take a pregnant woman to the hospital. Others may feel they will be blamed for their involvement if something goes wrong, e.g., attending a birth when there is a poor outcome. Governmental infrastructure, specifically roads and health services, are scarce because this population spans the three departments. This results in each department viewing the people living in these areas as "border" populations, and may try to pass the responsibility to other departments for furnishing road infrastructure and health services. In addition to the complex political structure, the region is susceptible to natural disasters such as hurricanes and flooding. The region has areas at or below sea level, and battles the seasonal rains and runoff from Guatemala's high mountains to the northeast. Flooding causes damage to the already weak road infrastructure, increasing the barriers to accessing adequate health care. Because most families use pit latrines for waste disposal and shallow wells as their source of water, flooding can contaminate the water supply, spreading gastrointestinal disease. The low elevation and flooding also promote mosquito-borne infections such as dengue (DENV), chikungunya (CHIKV), and Zika (ZIKV) virus infections. This, in return, increases the types and severity of health complications experienced by mothers and their babies.

In 2011, there was no access to physician care in the Trifinio community and a trip to the nearest city, Coatepeque, to see a doctor was 1 h away with emergency travel costing more than a month's wages (Asturias et al. 2016). One of the largest employers in the southwest Trifinio is Agro-America, a private family-owned Guatemala agro-business that operates banana and palm oil plantations in the region (Fig. 30.2). Recognizing the urgent health needs of the families and communities in the area,

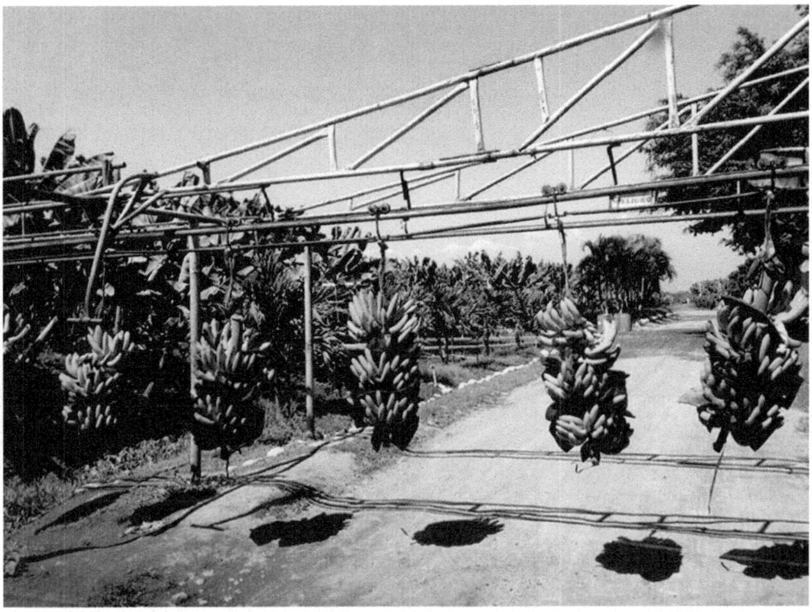

Fig. 30.2 Bananas at harvest heading to the packing plant. Banana cultivation is an important part of the local economy

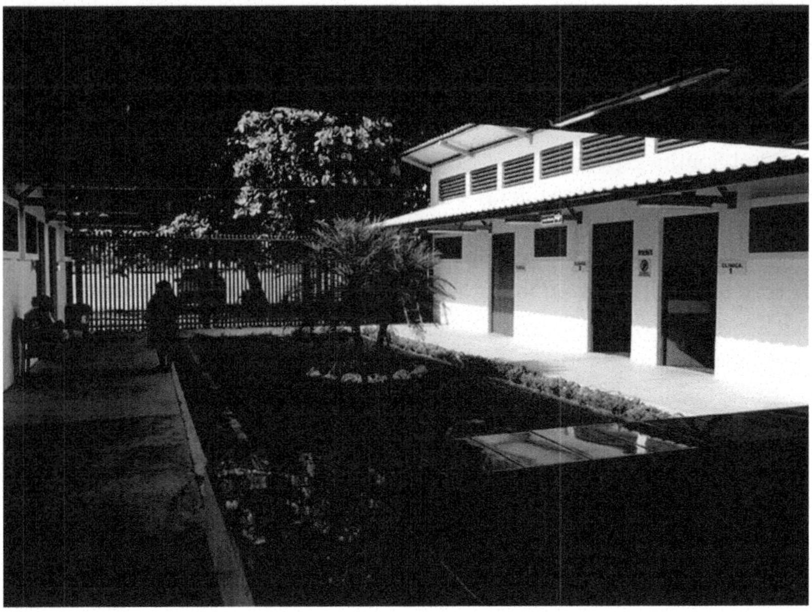

Fig. 30.3 Inside of Trifinio CDH clinic with patients waiting

Agro-America partnered with the Center for Global Health (CGH) at the Colorado School of Public Health, one of two WHO Collaborating Centers for Family and Child Health in the Americas, to design a health intervention program for its workers and the surrounding communities. The CGH, Children's Hospital Colorado (a University-affiliated hospital) and Agro-America's Foundation "Jose Fernando Bolaños Menendez" (FJFBM) signed a memorandum of understanding (MOU) in July 2011 to "promote the development of scientific and technical activities, research and projects in the field of public health sciences, that promote the comprehensive improvement of health and human development and mitigate the impact of disasters in the area of influence in Guatemala" (Asturias et al. 2016). With this partnership in place, an assessment of the communities' health began in order to better target program priorities for health interventions (Figs. 30.3 and 30.4).

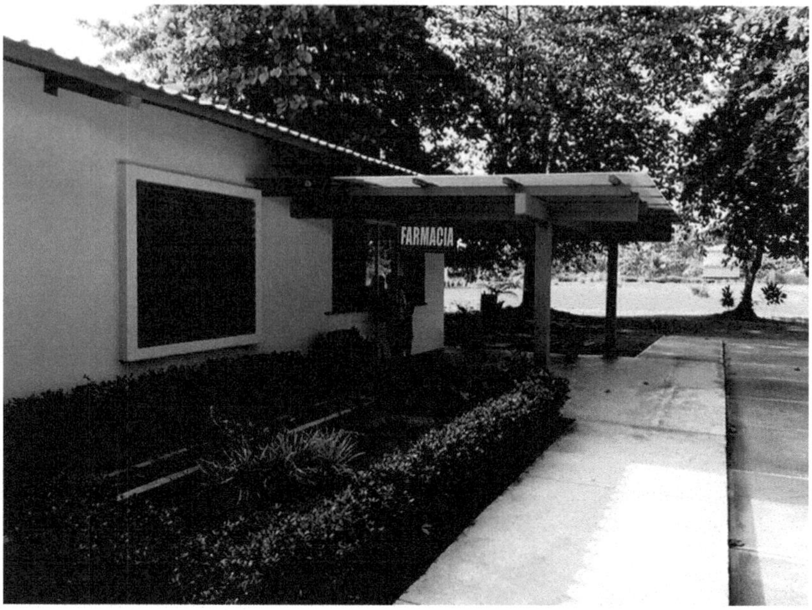

Fig. 30.4 Pharmacy on outside of Trifinio CDH clinic

30.2 Understanding the Reproductive Health Context

In rural Southwest Guatemala, we conducted multiple inquiries into the communities' health to better understand how the three delays model of maternal mortality affected maternal, neonatal, and child health in this region. The initial community-based health assessment conducted in 2011 revealed low rates of education and literacy, high parity, high rates of adolescent pregnancy, and significant numbers of women using traditional birth attendants (TBAs) for their sole delivery provider. Additionally, women reported high rates of pregnancy complications, and alarming levels of perinatal, neonatal, and childhood mortality (Table 30.1).

Subsequent assessments of the SW Trifinio population, using open-ended interviews, surveys, on-site observation, and focus group methodology revealed a maternal health system facing significant challenges. Deliveries occurred either at the hospital, a 45–60 minutes' distance from the community, attended by physicians or nurses or at home in the community attended by traditional birth attendants (TBAs). TBAs were minimally or untrained women who provided the bulk of maternity and neonatal care in the community. Skilled health care workers (nurses, doctors, or trained midwives) were largely nonexistent in the region. In fact, a professional midwifery-training program was initiated by the Guatemalan government only in 2015. Thus, training and educational issues of providers and families were deemed a significant cause of the first delay. With regard to the second delay, people reported transportation issues, cost barriers, and ideological and cultural differences (e.g., crowding, fear of episiotomy, lack of ability to have family support while in labor at hospital) that prevented women from accessing the regional hospital services. Significant human resource and supply deficiencies were also apparent at the regional hospitals, preventing optimal, timely provision of obstetric care in some cases, contributing to the third delay.

Table 30.1 Baseline reproductive health characteristics from initial needs assessment of 287 women (2011)

Category	Characteristic	*N* (%)
Maternal	Literacy	186 (65)
	Education >6th grade	22 (7.5)
	Parity >5	56 (20)
	Age at first pregnancy <18	145 (51)
	TBA only prenatal care provider	198 (69)
	TBA delivering provider of youngest child	129 (45)
	Report significant complications at time of delivery	86 (30)
Neonatal/infant	Death of child prior to age 5	40 (14)
	Death occurring in first 2 months of life	22 (56)

Households/mothers interviewed = 287, *TBA* Traditional Birth Attendant

30.3 Applying Global Health Evidence to Create Solutions in the SW Trifinio

The SW Trifinio region clearly suffered outcomes caused by risk factors described in the Three Delays Model. This model allows a means for identifying the specific problems that cause maternal mortality, which permits the creation of targeted solutions that can change the outcome of pregnancy and childbirth for women. Systematic solutions addressing these delays from the household to referral facility levels have been described in the global health literature (Kerber et al. 2007). Thus, our approach in the SW Trifinio region was designed to identify the individual problems impacting our patients within each of the three delays, in order to try to improve maternal mortality from the community to the referral level.

30.3.1 Targeting the First Delay: Household-Level Problems, Solutions, and Challenges

One need only meet with TBAs or any obstetric provider, especially in low resource settings, before a few stories of real tragedies emerge. When we began to meet with the TBAs in our communities, one volunteered the story of a woman she was caring for who developed prolonged labor in the pushing phase. The woman was obese, and because the situation began to make the TBA very nervous, she recommended that the family go to the hospital. The family was concerned about the cost of transport in the middle of the night and declined to go. Following another hour or more of pushing, the TBA once again recommended transport to the hospital since no delivery had occurred. The family once more declined. Finally, after employing other family members and continuing to push, the baby's head delivered but the body did not follow. The TBA pulled on the baby's head, but they could not accomplish delivery. The family then recognized the emergency and called a truck. The family and the TBA went to the hospital an hour away, where the baby was delivered stillborn. This tragic case still haunts this family as well as the TBA. Sadly, the outcome could have been prevented.

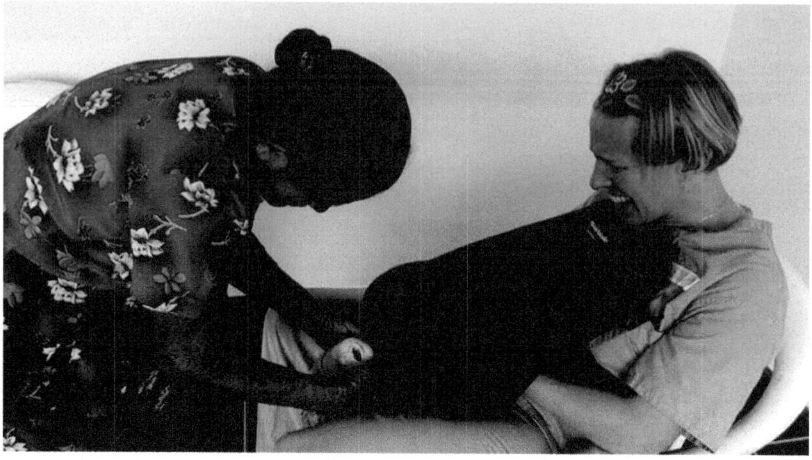

Fig. 30.5 The author conducting MommaNatalie® training with a traditional birth attendant. The MommaNatalie® is a birthing simulator that is worn by the person playing the role of the pregnant woman, and which can create realistic simulations of normal or complicated deliveries. These include obstetrical hemorrhage, breech delivery, delivery of the placenta, vacuum-assisted delivery, fetal heart sounds, and others

Our initial community assessments identified (1) a lack of TBA training to manage obstetric emergencies and (2) the lack of patient/family recognition of the signs of serious complications as contributing factors to many of the reported cases of morbidities and mortalities. In order to address these issues, we proposed the following: (1) to improve TBA knowledge and skills in the recognition of pregnancy complications, (2) the provision of rapid life-saving management of obstetric emergencies, and (3) the rapid referral to a higher level of care. To support these changes we sought to increase the number of pregnant women who receive the WHO recommended four prenatal visits to ensure adequate family and patient education on pregnancy and its complications. Given the lack of health care workers in this geographic area, we understood that we would need to "train up" any health care providers. Since there were no skilled birth attendants (SBAs) we adopted the approach suggested by Byrne and Morgan, to incorporate TBAs into the formal health system, supervised by a physician or nurse, in order to improve skilled birth attendance (Byrne and Morgan 2011) (Fig. 30.5).

After 4 years of program implementation, we have noted the following successes in programs targeting improved TBA knowledge and skills:

1. We have gained the partnership of respected women leaders (the TBAs) in the birth center planning and maternal health program roll-out.
2. We continue to have excellent TBA attendance at community level trainings (Fig. 30.6).
3. The Emergency Obstetric Care (EmOC) skills of the TBAs have significantly improved. Increased skill levels have been demonstrated consistently with repeat educational testing for the following emergencies: shoulder dystocia, postpartum hemorrhage, and eclampsia.
4. Our programs have not denigrated the culturally valued antepartum/postpartum care given by the TBAs with nearly one-third of pregnant women still delivering at home with a TBA.

The following have presented challenges to increasing TBA knowledge and skills:

1. Low TBA literacy/educational level compounded by older age (average TBA age of 56 years) is a barrier to training, especially in those skills requiring complex algorithmic decision-making (e.g., postpartum hemorrhage management.)

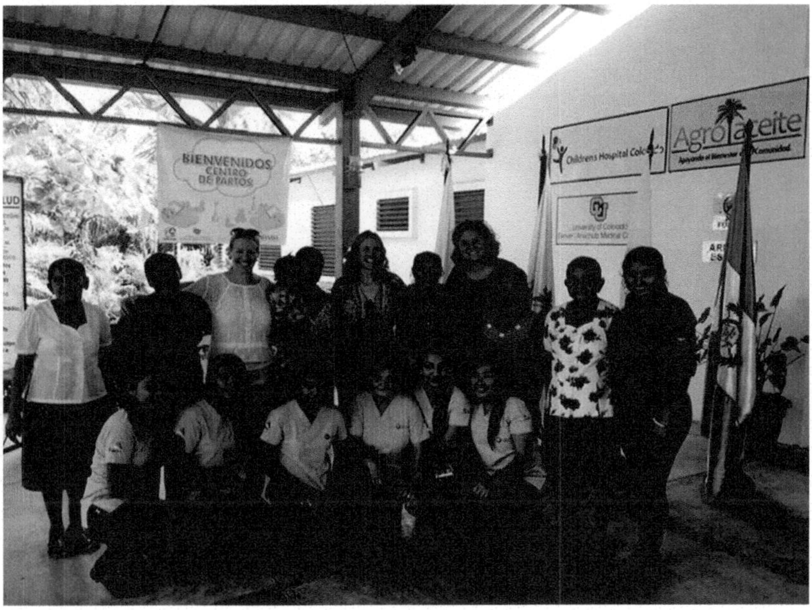

Fig. 30.6 Centro de Partos (Birth Center) team: Skilled birth attendants (SBAs) and traditional birth attendants (TBAs) with CGH trainers

2. The implementation of the skilled birth attendant—TBA partnership model requires intensive supervision, extensive training of SBAs, and ongoing mentorship of both groups to have a successful partnership.

To decrease morbidity resulting from the first delay, we also had to improve patient and family education. Since transportation is such a problem in the region, a model of household delivery of prenatal care was developed to minimize barriers to patient education and prenatal care access. These prenatal visits utilize the topics endorsed by the Guatemalan Ministry of Health for routine prenatal care, including education about the danger signs of pregnancy, and also promote the importance of skilled birth attendance at delivery. In addition, the visits provide a means to track maternal and neonatal outcomes in the community where no prior community level surveillance data existed. Strategic successes in our attempts to minimize the first delay include:

1. Education is conducted during prenatal home visits. Using visual aids led by a trained nurse/community health worker, patients and families participate in facilitated discussions of pregnancy danger signs and normal prenatal preventive care, including family planning. Since the group prenatal care model was introduced in 2015, 44.8% of women have received at least one group prenatal visit. Health workers favor this model, as it is more efficient than individual visits and pregnant women find it more fun and educational, as they learn through games and from their peers. The home-based care model has helped to improve communication and trust between community members and our community nurses (Figs. 30.7 and 30.8).
2. Implementation of a mobile technology quality improvement database which allows for remote data collection by community health workers during prenatal home visits. Weekly or biweekly data analysis is conducted by supervising physicians of important clinical outcomes. This allows for an ongoing educational process with the community nurses where clinical signs are reviewed by the physician and acute issues communicated back to the nurses on the ground for action. In addition, we can track our reach as well as pregnancy and neonatal outcomes, to better assess the effect of our programs. Home-based individual or group prenatal care with postpartum follow-up in the

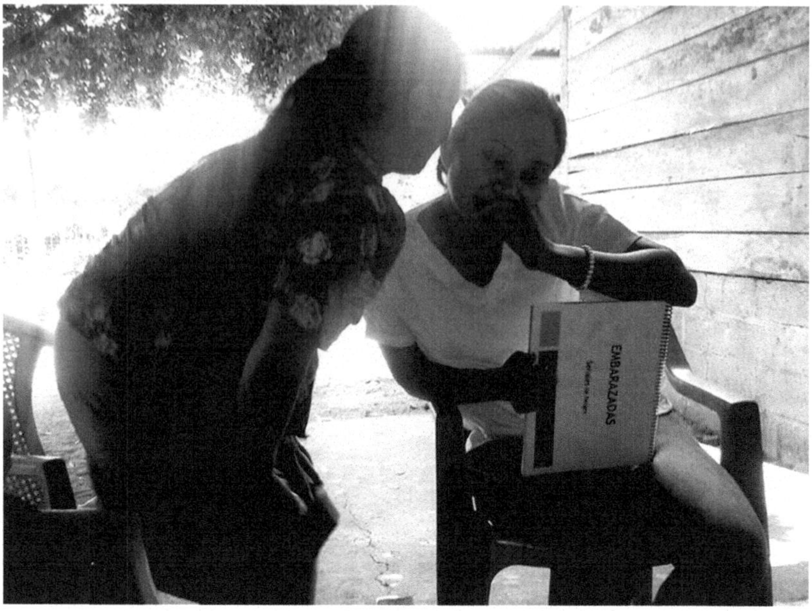

Fig. 30.7 A community nurse and group prenatal care participant play the game "telephone" using messages related to pregnancy danger signs during a home visit

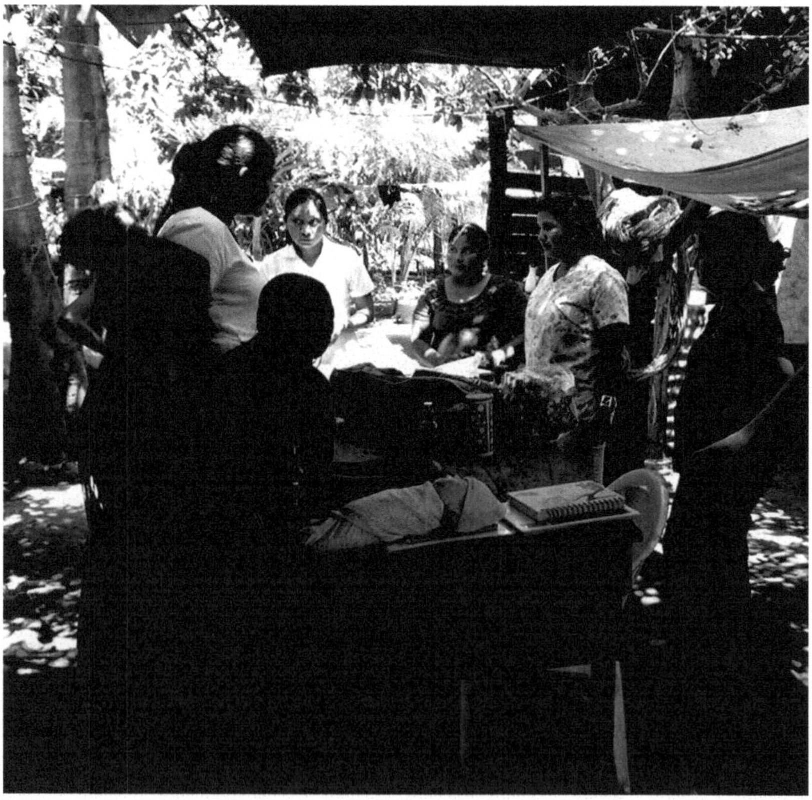

Fig. 30.8 Nurses preparing for a group prenatal care visit in the community

communities has reached 344 women since June 2015. In total, 664 women have been reached with at least one visit, but of those completing postpartum care, 38% of participants had four prenatal visits, 31% had three visits, and 61% had at least one visit with our program during pregnancy, in addition to the Ministry of Health (MoH) and TBA care visits. The programs have also improved rates of modern contraceptive uptake postpartum, even though we have not expanded contraceptive access within our programs.

3. A pilot program targeting male community members with education on pregnancy and childhood danger signs and the importance of a father's role during pregnancy and early childhood was well received and generated increased interest in family planning and saving for familial medical expenses.

Our providers have been called for assistance in multiple life-threatening instances. Examples of the impact of our programs in decreasing the first delay can be seen in the following cases from the field. These included being called in the setting of a home birth where a woman's family brought the pregnant woman to our clinic for a retained placenta, and where her condition was successfully managed without complication. In another case, a father delivered his own child at home, and then subsequently called for assistance because of signs of respiratory distress in the infant after delivery. The nurses responded and brought the infant to the clinic, where he was assessed by the physician, stabilized, and subsequently transferred via ambulance to the hospital for further care (Fig. 30.9).

Despite these successes on a household level, challenges to improving prenatal care and increasing family and patient awareness included:

1. Difficulties in data completeness, accuracy, and real-time access to data for those in the field from the Quality Improvement database.
2. Persistent inability to achieve four prenatal visits in >75% of participants after 2 years of fully implemented programming, although the program was able to improve the rate of three prenatal visit completion.
3. Stable rates of TBA-attended or -unattended home birth remaining at 30% since the program onset.

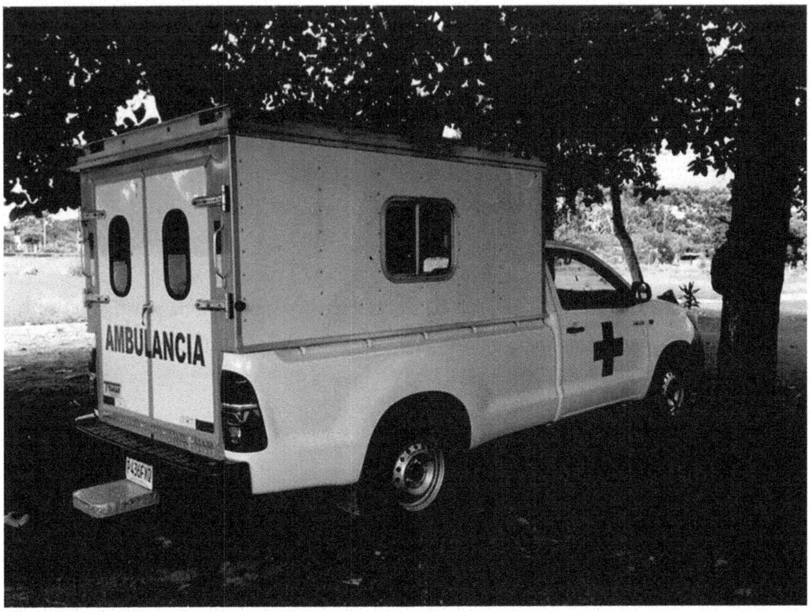

Fig. 30.9 Clinic ambulance supplied by the funder and outfitted in Guatemala

4. Inability to expand access to modern contraceptives within our program structure because of limitations to access, MoH supply, and political barriers.
5. Initial attempts to "train up" community health workers failed and prenatal care delivery succeeded only when Nurse Assistants and Nurses were employed instead to deliver the community-based prenatal education and clinical care. This raised human resource costs within the program, but ultimately allowed for improved community relations and improved job satisfaction for staff.

30.3.2 Targeting the Second Delay: Identifying the Financial, Physical, Cultural, or Logistical Barriers Between Pregnant Women and Proper Care, Implementing Solutions, and Facing Challenges

The concept is simple—if you can't reach a facility or access its care due to a barrier such as cost, it will prevent or delay your ability to receive quality medical care at critical moments. To minimize such financial barriers, Guatemalan maternity care is often provided at no/low/at-cost to women for pregnancy-related care and delivery. The Guatemalan government provides a no-cost delivery at public hospitals. However, for many who live in the SW Trifinio region, the costs associated with accessing that care are insurmountable. These costs are often related to food, laboratory or radiological tests that the hospital lacks, or the need to purchase medications, surgical or delivery supplies due to government-related supply chain shortages. Cultural barriers also exist in people's attitudes toward their care—this is especially true when providing care for indigenous women. If a patient is going to have to pay for equipment and transport to access the public sector, many patients choose instead to deliver at private hospitals, even though these facilities charge two to three times the amount needed to deliver at the public facilities. It is the perception that the care is superior and the facility safer than the public hospital, although our program outcomes demonstrate a higher Cesarean section rate among those women delivering their infants in the private facilities. Interestingly, the workers at the Agro-America plantation pay into the Guatemalan social security system and therefore can access the social security hospital. However, due to cost and administrative barriers, many choose not to seek care at the social security hospital. Many marriages in the SW Trifinio are informal, so even though her partner may be an insured agro-worker, an informally married woman may not be able to access care in the Social Security hospital for herself and her child without first jumping through administrative hoops. Thus, one-third of women in our database continue to deliver their infants at home.

In addition to cost, transportation to and from the hospital and its related cultural issues are significant causes of the second delay in the Trifinio region. Many patients elect to take low cost public transportation to routine appointments, requiring an hour travel time each way. However, when labor has begun, there are cultural concerns regarding the entrance of "*aire*" or bad air into the woman's body that are believed to cause complications for her delivery, so private transport such as an ambulance is necessary. As only one fee-for-service ambulance was in circulation, it could cost 1 month's wage for the trip. The option for most patients was transport via a private vehicle. Vehicles are a precious commodity, so drivers can charge what they want. Transport in the middle of the night for a woman in labor could cost the equivalent of one or even 2 week's wages. In addition to these challenges, and similar to women in some other resource-poor regions of the world (Schwartz 2015), women in this region rarely have access to their own money, as men are usually the wage-earner, decision-maker, and the keeper of the family resources. This limits women's ability to choose and pay for health care-related expenses when they arise. One such instance occurred when a woman with a 35-week pregnancy was found in our clinic to have ruptured membranes and had a breech presentation. We called the ambulance, and they were willing to come and transport the patient, but she had no money to pay for the ride. Her husband was in the fields and after a short delay we were able to call him via cell phone, but when we

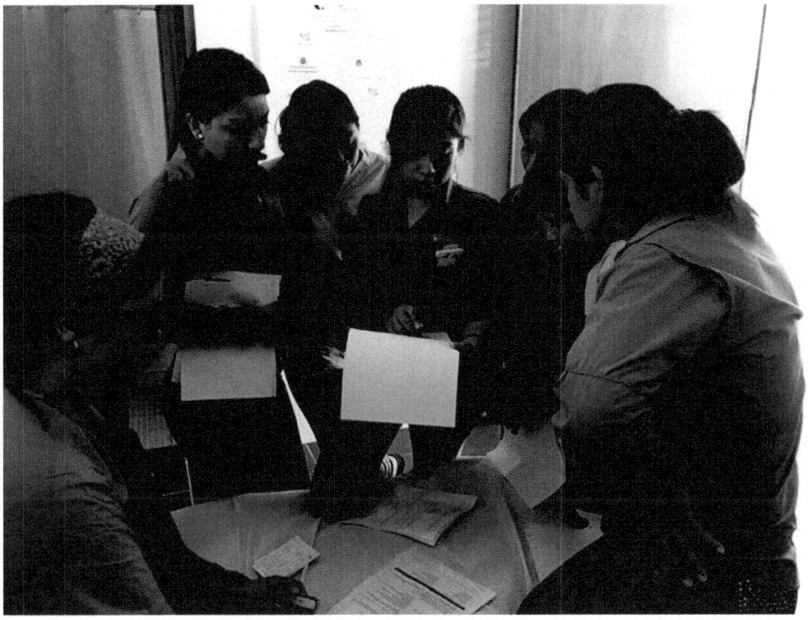

Fig. 30.10 Community nurses practicing labor admission process using a modified WHO Safe Childbirth checklist

reached him, he told her he had no money to give her to pay for transportation. In the end, we took her to the hospital ourselves in our own vehicle on our way home from clinic. Our nurses gave the family money from their own pocket for food and expenses at the public facility where she was safely delivered with a good maternal and fetal outcome. However, this is not a sustainable option.

Strategic successes in addressing the financial, physical, and cultural barriers include:

1. We have brought safe birth closer to the community by opening a low risk, low cost birth center (Fig. 30.10).
2. A delivery at the birth center costs one-third less than the costs of transport and supplies at the public facility. Costs are one-fourth the amount of delivery at a private hospital and can be paid in arrears or in advance through a savings plan.
3. We have purchased and outfitted an ambulance with a driver that is available to the clinic for any patients requiring referral to the hospital for half the cost of the fee-for-service ambulance (Fig. 30.9). In those cases which are emergent, care is free or can be paid in arrears.
4. To diversify the male dominated control of resources, we have held pilot education sessions at work with men about the importance of saving money for family health care costs, such as birth, and responsible family spending.

Strategic challenges have remained, however, which are mostly related to the cost of any health care expenditure in an impoverished community such as Guatemala.

1. Since opening the birth center several months ago, we have yet to achieve a major change in the number of home births. This is likely due to the patients choosing home delivery because they prefer/can only access a no- or extremely low-cost delivery, despite the risks, some even choosing not to involve a TBA. Ongoing work on promotion and clarification of care provision at the birth center is needed in the future (Fig. 30.11).
2. Obtaining access to men in order to educate them on family topics such as health care needs, expenditures, and the importance of monetary savings is difficult. The majority of men in the community

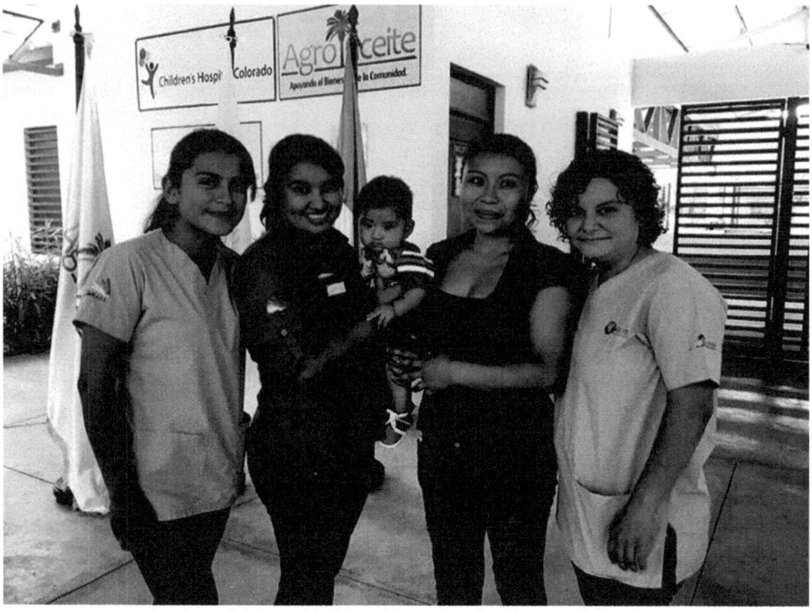

Fig. 30.11 Delivering nurses together with mother and baby. He is the second baby born at the Center for Human Development Birth Center which opened in 2016

work long hours all days except Sunday. Work-time sessions in our pilot program were required to be extremely early (5 a.m.) and for very short periods of time (5–10 min), which limited scalability of that intervention. When the idea of a Sunday "school" for parents was proposed, it met with a lukewarm response since most of the women believe that their partners would be unlikely to attend on their day off. Additional media methods are being explored for implementation in the communities or in the workplace to maximize communication with family decision-makers.

30.3.3 Targeting the Third Delay: Supply, Process, or Knowledge Issues at the Facility Level That Prevent Quality Care Delivery, Solutions, and Ongoing Challenges

Multiple problems potentially affecting maternal mortality and morbidity were identified within the SW Trifinio region on the referral facility level. Additional challenges were found in the continuum between home and facility that contributed to suboptimal outcomes at the facility level. Most of these issues were related to dysfunctional processes and limited resources, including a lack of health care workers themselves. For the most part people at the facility level did their best to provide good care for patients, to the extent allowed by a rigid medical culture and health system with limited resources. As an example of a suboptimally organized system, it became immediately apparent that we needed to establish contact with the chief physicians at the regional public facility to ensure a functioning referral chain. Since there are no centralized emergency services, in order to refer a patient to the hospital you must call the physician you personally know, or alternatively contact the hospital directly, to find out who is on call. After doing this, you can then give a direct report to the resident or attending physician, who may then receive your obstetric patient in the emergency room. A referral letter is also sent with the patient, but this is met with less priority than direct personal contact. Such a person-to-person dependent system is fraught with potential for miscommunication, but it has worked surprisingly well most of the time in our experience. It is a classic example of people doing the best for patients, and for their colleagues, despite a system that does not support them. Additionally, for the majority of time that we have been working in Guatemala, the hospitals have been in "crisis." This is the term that the country uses to denote a chronic lack of supplies, shipments that never arrive, and a political culture of corruption where government officials skim off the top, causing those at the terminal end of the supply chain to suffer. This has resulted in patients needing to buy their own sutures, cross the street to pay out of pocket for lab tests due to lack of reagents in the hospital lab, or to purchase medications that were out of supply in the hospital pharmacy. It also is a system that cannot adequately pay its physician staff, so they round on patients with residents (physicians in postgraduate training) and nurses and perform surgeries in the morning, but go to their own fee-for-service private clinics in the afternoon, where they are available to residents or nurses via phone for the remainder of the day. This is the standard for most of Latin America and the developing world, and is a way the system can provide low cost care in the public sector. However, this system contributes to a lack of knowledge affecting optimal patient care, when residents and nurses are left to find their own way through the clinical presentations of complicated patients with little access to internet resources and no one with full certification immediately present to help recognize emergencies and assist trainees in maintaining a wide differential diagnosis and treatment plan. It also leads to sporadic learning for the residents, who then graduate having learned only from what they have already done, and not necessarily to the best medical standards. A lack of oversight and communication can be especially problematic in the largely male dominated and hierarchical medical establishment that can make it difficult for nurses or those in training to question the judgment of their superiors, even when the patient's best interests are at stake, leading to inevitable delays in appropriate care. These system deficiencies are clearly recognized to cause needless death and disability.

Any successes we have had in tackling these difficult systems, supplies, and human resources issues were due to the personal relationships that we established with local physicians, and using professional relationships in our Center for Global Health's network to ameliorate conditions wherever possible.

1. On a systems level, we networked with the staff physicians in the hospital through meetings, supply and hospital needs assessments, and joint educational conferences, so that referrals for emergency or ongoing care not offered in our clinic could be provided to our patients at the hospital without excessive delays.
2. From a resource level, our Center raised money to send a shipping container of hospital-requested medical equipment, donated through *Project Cure* to the regional public hospital.
3. In addition, we attempted, through participation in their yearly physician's conference, to bring additional interdisciplinary, collaborative, evidence-based practice standards to their area. We also provided faculty lectures to the residents (schedule permitting), including a simulation-based Emergency Obstetric Care (EmOC) skills workshop for management of shoulder dystocia, and training on appropriate use and interpretation of electronic fetal monitoring for the high-risk patient. Partnerships with people in decision-making positions on ground were integral to our successes.

Ongoing challenges to the causes of the third delay are:

1. The chronic undersupply in the system due in part to high-level government corruption and complex administrative processes. Such duplicative and indirect processes create a lack of accountability in the public sector, which results in chronic supply shortages of essential medications, lab equipment, and overtasked infrastructure and human resources.
2. There is an overall sense of abandonment by the government, and people feel they are left to their own devices. Public systems are already overburdened with many more patients than their hospitals

are equipped or registered to handle, and supply shortages only worsen morale and quality of care. On many occasions health workers have reported purchasing necessary equipment or medications for their patients themselves, or even going without them, hoping for an optimal outcome in spite of the resources and evidence suggesting the contrary.

3. When health care workers face chronic stress and resource depletion, they are at risk for providing poor quality care and developing "compassion fatigue." Such chronic stress may cause health workers to be less productive, adopt bad habits, pay less attention to detail, and over time could even impair a health worker's ability to recognize critical illnesses in their patients, leading to delays in care and poor clinical outcomes (Fig. 30.10).

Such chronic abandonment and lack of governmental functioning and accountability can translate to real public dissatisfaction as evidenced in the 2015 presidential ousting in Guatemala and call for new elections. Eventually, a health care system that can't provide for its populace, or its patients, has to change. Our hope is that the medical system can change before more mothers and their children die unnecessarily (Fig. 30.12).

As our efforts in partnership with Agro-America and the communities of the SW Trifinio region move forward, we will continue to work on implementation of evidence-based interventions to improve maternal, neonatal, and childhood health by targeting the three delays. We are fostering a

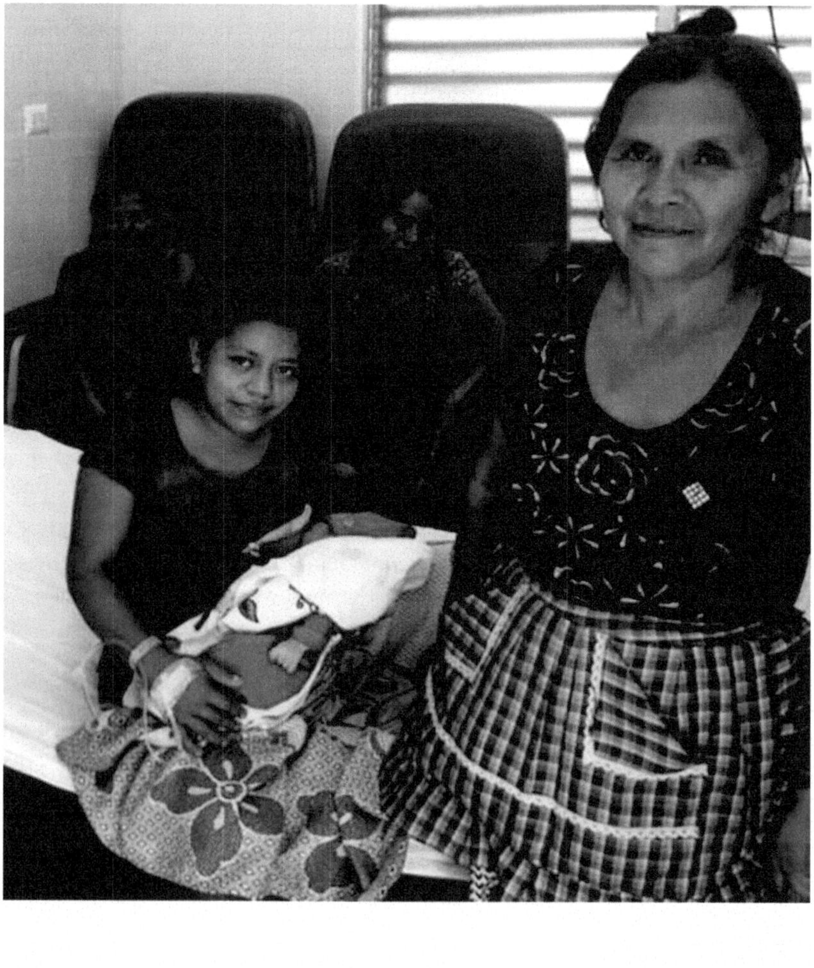

Fig. 30.12 First Center for Human Development Birth Center delivery in 2016. Patient and child with family members and her traditional birth attendant

new approach to extend prenatal care coverage using a home-based, group-care model. We are extending access to safe birth by offering low risk labor and delivery closer to the communities of these rural families by training-up nurses as midwives and skilled clinicians. This approach has the potential to extend safe and effective maternity services to rural and indigenous areas, where the number of physicians are limited. Finally, we are continuing to partner with clinicians at the referral center level to improve patient transport and the quality and timeliness of treatment when advanced care is needed. The SW Trifinio region is a land of "endless needs" but our partnership will continue to demonstrate the endless promise of lives saved and families growing toward a common goal, better health.

References

Asturias, E., Heinrichs, G., Domek, G., Brett, J., Shick, E., Cunningham, M., et al. (2016). The Center for Human Development in Guatemala: An innovative model for global population health. *Advances in Pediatrics, 63*(1), 357–387. https://doi.org/10.1016/s0065-3101(16)30001-9

Byrne, A., & Morgan, A. (2011). How the integration of traditional birth attendants with formal health systems can increase skilled birth attendance. *International Journal of Gynecology & Obstetrics, 115*(2), 127–134. https://doi.org/10.1016/s0020-7292(11)00389-4

Kerber, K., de Graft-Johnson, J., Bhutta, Z., Okong, P., Starrs, A., & Lawn, J. (2007). Continuum of care for maternal, newborn, and child health: From slogan to service delivery. *Lancet, 370*, 1358–1369. https://doi.org/10.1016/S0140-6736(07)61578-5

Schwartz, D. A. (2015). Interface of epidemiology, anthropology and health care in maternal death prevention in resource-poor nations. In D. A. Schwartz (Ed.), *Maternal mortality: Risk factors, anthropological perspectives, prevalence in developing countries and preventive strategies for pregnancy-related death*. New York: Nova Science Publishers.

Thaddeus, S., & Maine, D. (1994). Too far to walk: Maternal mortality in context. *Social Science & Medicine, 38*(8), 1091–1110.

UN Data (2013). *Contraceptive prevalence rate (CPR) Guatemala 2007–2012. United Nations Children's Fund.* Retrieved September 13, 2016, from http://data.un.org/Data.aspx?q=guatemala+contraceptive+prevalence&d=SOWC&f=inID%3a34%3bcrID%3a451

WHO. (2015). *Maternal mortality in 1990–2015: Guatemala*. WHO, UNICEF, UNFPA, World Bank Group, and United Nations Population Division Maternal Mortality Estimation Inter-Agency Group. Retrieved September 12, 2016, from http://www.who.int/gho/maternal_health/countries/gtm.pdf?ua=1

31 The Emerging Role of the *Comadrona* as a Broker Between Ancient Cultural Beliefs and Modern Biomedicalization to Improve Maternal Health Care in Guatemala

Sobaata Chaudhry, Jessica Oliveira, and Taraneh Shirazian

31.1 Maternal Mortality and the Status of Women

Guatemala still has one of the highest maternal mortality ratios (MMRs) in Central America. Between 2010 and 2015, an estimated 88/100,000 expectant women die each year from pregnancy or childbirth-related causes (WHO 2012). This is a significant reduction from the MMR in 2007 of 140/100,000 (WHO 2013). Since these approximations are based on documented cases, the MMR is in reality likely to be much higher. In fact, in the 2007 National Maternal Mortality Study, maternal death in Guatemala was found to be underreported by 40.7% (PAHO 2012). This study also recognized that the majority of the women who died were indigenous (70%), and almost one-half (46%) of the indigenous women died while in their homes. These findings are congruent with the results of a baseline study conducted by the Ministry of Health (MOH) that states the MMR for indigenous women is estimated to be three times higher than that of nonindigenous women. Furthermore, the outcomes of a maternal mortality study conducted in 2013 using the Reproductive Age Mortality Study (RAMOS) methodology also revealed the large gaps in healthcare between indigenous and nonindigenous women. In Guatemala, of the 452 maternal deaths in 2013, 68% were indigenous women (USAID 2015a, b). Illustrated in Fig. 31.1 are the leading causes of death in Guatemala for 2013, which were hemorrhage, eclampsia, and preeclampsia; all were potentially treatable conditions that demonstrate the need for access to skilled birth attendants in rural areas. The same baseline study revealed that women face discriminatory barriers of access to health services such as the absence of financial means

S. Chaudhry, M.S. · J. Oliveira, M.S.P.A.
Saving Mothers, New York, NY, USA

T. Shirazian, M.D., F.A.C.O.G. (✉)
Saving Mothers, New York, NY, USA

Department of Obstetrics and Gynecology, New York University School of Medicine and NYU Langone Medical Center, New York, NY, USA
e-mail: tshirazian@savingmothers.org

D. A. Schwartz (ed.), *Maternal Death and Pregnancy-Related Morbidity Among Indigenous Women of Mexico and Central America*, Global Maternal and Child Health: Medical, Anthropological, and Public Health Perspectives, https://doi.org/10.1007/978-3-319-71538-4_31

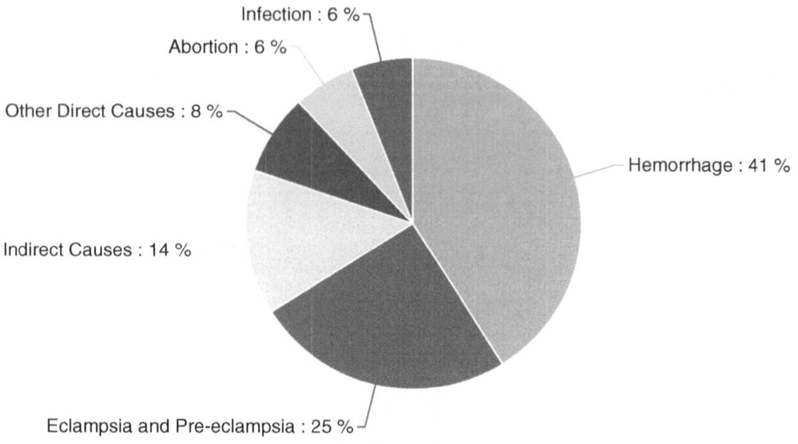

Fig. 31.1 Causes of maternal mortality in Guatemala in 2013, $n = 452$ (USAID 2015a, b)

for transport and care (47%) or the lack of decision-making power to seek care by the woman or her family (33%) (MSPAS 2000). In Guatemala, men are intrinsically entitled to more resources, higher salaried positions, and an overall higher socioeconomic and educational status than women. When a doctor from the health center in Retalhuleu was confronted on hiring mostly male health promoters instead of females, he responded with the statement, "It is because of the custom. Men first, men second, men third, women last, which is a Guatemalan tradition" (Cosminsky 1987). For these reasons, it is customary for the husband or husband's family to determine whether or not his wife may seek medical care. Overall, and in common with neighboring countries with indigenous populations, indigenous women in Guatemala have the most precarious living conditions, highest fertility rates, highest illiteracy rates, and smallest percentage of births attended by doctors, nurses, or skilled birth attendants than the rest of the country, making this population extremely vulnerable to disease, poverty, and death.

To make matters worse, Guatemala is faced with a significant number of pregnancies as a result of child marriages or rape. According to the country's Human Rights Office, thousands of children are sexually abused by relatives each year. Eighty-nine percent of rapists are immediate family members, and 30% are parents (COHA 2015). Forty-five percent of women in Guatemala have reported experiencing sexual harassment. In 2015, 4431 girls between the ages of 10–14 became pregnant in Guatemala (OSAR 2015). Latin America is the only region in the world where birthing rates are increasing for girls under the age of 15 (UNFPA 2013). In the professional opinion of Dr. Carlos Vasquez, chief of the Gynecology Department at a hospital in Sayaxche, Peten, "Thirteen is too young. The pelvis is still not fully developed and they (girls) have neither the physical or mental capacity. It's sad. The babies that grow up are rarely healthy." Acknowledging the severity of underage pregnancies, the Guatemalan government introduced the Law Against Sexual Violence, Exploitation, and Trafficking of People, which criminalizes sexual relations with girls under 14 (Congreso de la Republica de Guatemala 2009). It included strict directives for sentencing, assisting victims of sexual violence, and stipulations requiring all hospitals and maternity centers to report pregnancies and births in girls under the age of 14.

Previously, the legal age of marriage was 14 for girls and 16 for boys, but over 4354 underage girls gave birth in 2013 (UNICEF 2014). In 2015, the Guatemalan government increased the legal age of marriage to 18 years in order to reflect international standards. This has exacerbated the consequences of underage pregnancies by discouraging girls from seeking facility-based maternity care during childbirth, since the staff is required by law to report all cases of underage sex and the male perpetrators involved. In many cases, the perpetrator is the husband or romantic interest, further complicating the decision to pursue care in which case the husband will be arrested or forced to flee. Between January 2012 and March 2015, over 21,000 cases of rape had been registered, with only 974 guilty verdicts (Forsell and Lyche 2015). With a limited set of options for care, underage girls will often give birth at home without any professional supervision, resulting in a higher likelihood of complications and, at worst, maternal or infant mortality.

Since one-half of all women are married by the age of 20, 44% become mothers by the same age, with much higher proportions of young mothers among indigenous (54%) and uneducated women (68%). By the age of 30, many of these women have had up to eight children, almost twice the national fertility rate of 3.8 (WHO 2013). Despite a federal mandate that provides reproductive health education and family planning services, only 5% of women in Guatemala consistently use an effective method of birth control. This is mainly due to cultural norms and the impact of the Catholic Church's ban on contraceptive use (COHA 2015). In Guatemala, these cultural practices, lack of education, widespread poverty, endemic sexual violence, and strong Catholic influence over decisions on reproductive health make women vulnerable to early pregnancy and its consequences.

31.2 *Comadrona* Prenatal Care, Delivery, and Afterbirth

The Mayan highlands of Guatemala are home to the culturally esteemed *comadronas*, spiritually selected women that serve as ritual and obstetric providers for expectant mothers in these indigenous communities (Paul and Paul 1975). *Comadronas*, also known as Mayan midwives or Mayan traditional birth attendants (TBAs), subscribe to a cultural set of beliefs that are primarily based on "El Don," a destiny determined by God. Superstitions and practices are highly variable and dependent on locale. Generally, *comadronas* are selected on the basis of symbolic dreams, omens, illness, and signs believed to be sent by God and usually interpreted by a shaman (Cosminsky 1982). One *comadrona* from Chuchexic reported envisioning the reflection of a white-haired woman on a red and white mirror, later concluded to embody Santa Ana. She is the patroness of childbirth, and the red color symbolizes the fire of the sweat bath, a common *comadrona* preparation for the mother after childbirth. To reject this destiny would result in a cursed life, so *comadronas* are profoundly serious about their responsibilities and regularly pray to God and the spirits of dead *comadronas* for guidance. These forces are thought to regularly interact with the *comadronas* through bodily movements, dreams, and throughout the labor and delivery process. *Comadronas* believe these forces confer sacred knowledge and messages apropos differing maternal states and treatments such as perceiving complications, administering herbs, fetal repositioning, the sex of the baby, etc. (Cosminsky 1982). This intercession between the living world and the spirit world legitimizes the role of the *comadrona* as a cultural authority figure and, as such, commands a high level of respect from the community.

In the department of Solola, the heart of the western highlands, it is well known that women in indigenous communities rely almost exclusively on *comadronas* for prenatal care and the birthing process. Solola (the Hispanicized version of its pre-Columbian name *T'zolojy'a*) has an urban center of almost 14,000 inhabitants as well as surrounding villages on a mountainside overlooking Lake Atitlán, and almost all persons of *Kaqchikel* are of Mayan heritage. The ordinarily untrained *comadronas* there presume all skills and knowledge are God-given, rendering major disparities between the skills of individual *comadronas*. It is also known that culturally there is a strong preference for family-centered home birth, and hospitals are often seen as a last resort, as illustrated in Fig. 31.2. Research has shown that most women in indigenous communities prefer to give birth in a familiar home environment with people whom they know and trust (Foster et al. 2004; Berry 2006). Not only are Mayan communities entrenched in poverty, which already severely limits access to facility-based care, but as a result are often mistreated and stigmatized in facilities by medical personnel. Patients from poor

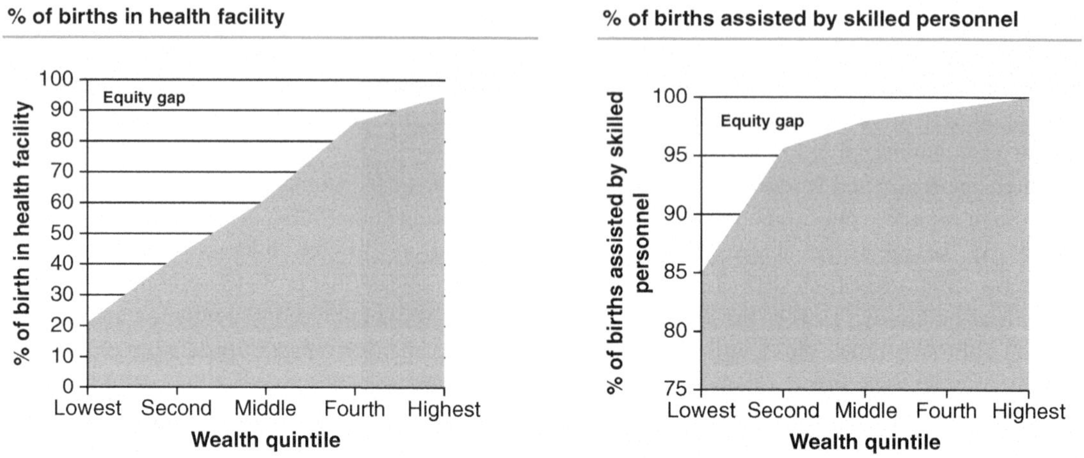

Fig. 31.2 Utilization of services by wealth quintile in Guatemala (WHO 2013)

backgrounds are often reprimanded for not seeking care sooner and are subject to neglectful tendencies during care at facilities (Cosminsky 1987). As biomedicine increasingly collides with traditional care, interpersonal relationships between *comadronas* and healthcare professionals function as necessary cultural bridges to reduce maternal mortality through proper referral, training, and support.

Prenatal care is initiated toward the end of the second trimester by the husband or the mother-in-law of the expectant mother, sometimes in a ritualized manner by presenting the midwife with various gifts or money to be used later for the mother (Cosminsky 1982). The *comadrona* usually visits once a month until the final month and then once a week until delivery. Conventional visits commence in the inspection of the breasts and abdomen size, color, and shape followed by abdominal massage thought to promote uncomplicated birthing. Some *comadronas* use the position of the baby to determine the sex; others use skin pigmentation or markings. Once, a *Quiche*-speaking *comadrona* determined the sex of baby to be male due to the dark facial markings on the mother's face, which she stated was an indication of strong fetal blood (Cosminsky 1982). Some Mayan cultures have certain beliefs that affect pregnant women and the growing fetus. One such Mayan belief is that solar and lunar eclipses are believed to cause infant deformities (Lang and Elkin 1997). Many linkages between moods and nature are linked to the well-being of the child in Mayan culture.

Another deeply rooted concept in Mayan spiritual health is that the body's proportions of hot and cold must balance one another or illness will develop. Food, drinks, and bodily symptoms such as feeling sweaty or feverish are classified into either hot or cold categories. Treatment is centered on restoring the balance (Cosminsky 1976). Pregnancy is a very hot condition due to the excess blood in the body which is consequently treated with cold foods including beans, pork, avocados, greens, sodas, and occasionally eggs (Cosminsky 1982). This practice is commonly criticized by health training programs which encourage the mother to eat all nourishing foods, regardless of hot or cold associations. Interestingly, Guatemala has the highest chronic malnutrition rate in Latin America and the third highest in the world, which is a particularly serious issue for pregnant women as this can lead to severe fetal complications (UNICEF 2009). In the event of a stillbirth, the mother may blame the hot-and-cold diet or other unfulfilled cravings, while the family unit tends to blame the mother for not controlling her emotions and provoking the stillbirth. In this scenario, the role of the *comadrona* is to mitigate this blame by providing interventions designed to restore the body to a neutral state and normalize social relations which will ultimately protect the well-being of the mother and child.

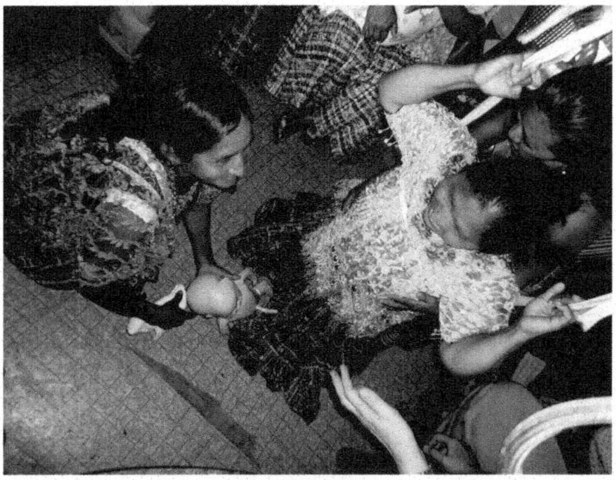

Fig. 31.3 A Mayan woman demonstrates the traditional birthing position of hanging from a rope

Since many basic medical supplies are unavailable to the *comadronas*, patient examinations and deliveries are often performed with bare hands and household items (Lang and Elkin 1997). The *comadrona* may provide herbal teas or massages to alleviate pain and discomfort. Delivery usually takes place in the mother's home, so the midwife is summoned at the onset of labor. *Comadronas* do not distinguish between the stages of labor and may have women push too early, usually in a kneeling or squatting position. Preferred birthing positions range from squatting on the dirt floor to semi-reclined on a bed to hanging from a rope (Fig. 31.3).

The leading cause of death during childbirth for women globally is postpartum hemorrhage, which is defined as losing approximately 500 mL of blood or more within 24 h after birth (Schwartz 2015; WHO 2012). When bleeding starts during or after birth, it is crucial to stop the bleeding, but some *comadronas* believe it is better to get rid of all the blood as fast as possible to cleanse the mother (Lang and Elkin 1997). Beliefs like this can often result in maternal death, caused by hypovolemia and shock. Poor clinical outcomes of both the mother and the newborn are attributed to the will of God or are blamed on the mother for arbitrary behaviors such as being lazy, being too emotional, eating too many hot foods, or leaving the house during an eclipse. After the baby is born, the *comadronas* usually refuse to cut the umbilical cord until the placenta is delivered in fear that the placenta will rise up within the mother and choke her (Lang and Elkin 1997). Many *comadronas* cut the placenta with non-sterile scissors or cauterize it with a candle. If the baby needs to be resuscitated, a variety of techniques are employed including rubbing alcohol over the body, swinging the baby in the air, placing the baby in a hot bath, turning the baby upside down and shaking it, placing an onion in front of the baby's nose, and blowing on the baby's face or fontanels (Lang and Elkin 1997). In the Lake Atitlan region, it is customary to bathe neonates, or newborns, in water and rose petals as soon as the cord has been cut to bless and cleanse the baby (Fig. 31.4). The cord is then sometimes examined by the *comadronas* to predict various prophecies for the mother and child based on texture and shape (Cosminsky 1982).

After the birth, the *comadronas* often wash the clothes and the sheets of the mother who will remain in the home for the next 20 days (confinement period) to heal and bond with the baby (Cosminsky 1982). The *comadrona* will continue to visit the mother throughout this time to provide massages and change the dressings on the baby. Since the mother is considered to be in a "hot" state during the pregnancy, she is considered to be in a "cold" state postpartum. To balance this, the mother keeps her head and shoulders covered and takes baths to warm her breast milk. Near the end of the confinement period, the *comadrona* may provide a bed cleaning ritual and a final bath for the mother. The final bath occurs in the *temazcal*, a Mayan sauna where volcanic rock is heated. Water is poured over the rocks to produce steam, and buckets of hot water are then used to bathe the mother while in the sweat lodge. After the confinement period, some families will hold a ritual feast termed *Elesan Xe Chat* which marks the termination of *comadrona* services.

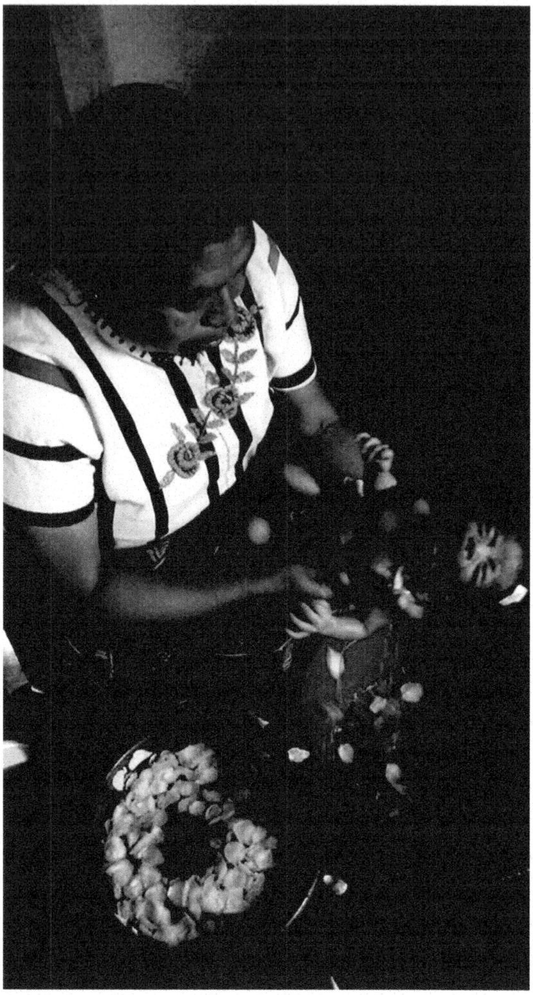

Fig. 31.4 Customary *Tzutujil* rose petal bath given to newborns

In Guatemala, the minimum wage has been set to $250 a month, equating to less than $9 a day. One US dollar is equivalent to 7.47 Guatemalan quetzals. Wages for rural indigenous workers are 34% lower than their nonindigenous counterparts, and even less for women, equating to approximately $5 a day, a salary regarded as high for indigenous populations who comprise 72% of the extremely poor sector in Guatemala (PAHO 2012). Transport and medical fees vary by region but usually amount to roughly 3 days of labor wages (Cosminsky 1987). Services offered at local public health posts tend to fluctuate, and the staff limits the number of patients seen per day. Upon reaching health facilities, indigenous women frequently report being met with condescending and inattentive staff and long waits and being often turned away with no treatment at all if the facility has reached maximal capacity (Cosminsky 1987). This creates tension between indigenous communities and healthcare facilities. Mayan women are very conservative and prefer to be fully clothed, but when seeking facility-based care, they are often required to change into gowns that are culturally inappropriate. Another common issue is that physicians at rural health posts are often male, so Mayan women tend to avoid seeking treatment there for gynecological problems and will instead visit the *comadrona*, a female, who will provide herbal treatments, massage, or baths while the patient is fully clothed (Cosminsky 1987). This indicates a demand for more female examiners and confirms the vital community role of the *comadrona* as the preferred health professional. *Comadronas* charge very little for the services offered

Table 31.1 Average cost of maternal healthcare services during pregnancy and delivery in Guatemala (after Goldman and Glei 2003)

Midwives ($n = 66$)	Average charged for pregnancy and delivery[a,b]	Q40	
	If patient has no money	Accepts payment in kind (%)	77.3
		Does not charge (%)	4.5
Private doctors ($n = 26$)	Average charge for prenatal exam[a,c]	Q16	
	Average charge for delivery[a,d]	Q350	
	If patient has no money	Accepts payment in kind (%)	19.2
		Does not charge (%)	57.7

[a]At the time of the survey, one quetzal (Q) was worth about 20 cents in the USA
[b]Two midwives report the charge per visit and are excluded from the calculation of charges for pregnancy and delivery
[c]One doctor did not report charges for prenatal exams and is excluded from descriptive statistics
[d]Only 12 doctors offer delivery care. Average charges are based on these 12 providers

(Table 31.1), complete home visits at the mother's convenience, and fully acknowledge the values of Mayan culture. The direct accessibility and meaningful impact of the *comadronas* on indigenous women are key to optimizing their role as community healthcare providers and ensuring the best possible outcomes for the mother and child.

31.3 Maternal Healthcare for Indigenous Women

The recent problematic history of Guatemala has principally contributed to the current pauperized conditions and marginalized status of indigenous Mayans, in particular, Mayan women. The 36-year civil war that began in 1960 culminated in the mass genocide of the Mayans. The Commission for Historical Clarification (CEH) suggests the total victim count is over 200,000 since many victims were reported missing or abducted; 83% were Mayan (1994). Today, Guatemala is a country of 22 regions with over 16 million people, more than half of which are Mayan (World Bank Group 2016). The Mayans, despite a significant population drop during the civil war, still represent the largest and the poorest demographic in Guatemala, while *ladinos*, the descendants of European colonists, maintain the wealthiest. The absence of education, healthcare, and employment opportunities in Mayan communities has taken the largest toll in the postwar era on women and children (USAID 2015a, b). These groups are typically uneducated and illiterate and have had scarce opportunities to develop adequate technical skills. Mayan communities, often located in extremely remote areas, are well below the poverty line (World Bank Group 2016). Additionally, the national language of Guatemala is Spanish, although over 22 native Mayan languages are spoken and preserved in Mayan communities (UNICEF 2014). Despite the government's attempts at reconciling the status of Mayans through recent funding of targeted programs, access and communication with indigenous communities remain a few of the largest setbacks.

Guatemala's public healthcare system had a strong and stable institutional legacy resulting from a well-established regulatory framework and experienced, dedicated health workers until a few decades ago. Within recent decades, several matters have seriously compromised the public health sector's effectiveness, including recent high-profile scandals of alleged corruption throughout the national administration. The result is a profoundly fragmented, inefficient healthcare system, as well as widespread skepticism from the general public who distrust their government. Within the public sector, there is the Ministry of Health and Public Assistance (MSPAS), which is responsible for implementation of national healthcare policies and provision of all services, and the Guatemalan Institute of Social Security (IGSS), which offers free health insurance to employees with fixed positions within government ministries.

Those in the armed forces are provided with healthcare coverage through Sanidad Militar, another public-sector entity. The private sector covers only 5% of the population, which includes many diverse players, including both not-for-profit and for-profit institutions. Approximately 25% of Guatemalans have some form of health insurance as indicated in Table 31.2. The remaining population is supposed to be covered by the MSPAS; however, nongovernmental organizations (NGOs) provide services to roughly 18% of the population (USAID 2015a, b). This leaves an alarmingly large portion of the population without proper insurance coverage. Many who are not provided with coverage reside within indigenous communities which are known for the highest maternal mortality rates and the fewest amount of healthcare services in the country (PAHO 2012). Those willing and able to seek healthcare face common barriers which include finances to cover both the transport and services required, the amount of time and energy to reach the facility, unpleasant experiences in facilities, and an innate disconnection to western medical practices. Additionally, the stark contrast between urban and rural health professional densities (25.7 health workers per 10,000 population in urban areas compared to only 3.0 per 10,000 in rural areas), the dearth of clinicians fluent in the various indigenous languages, and the disparities in accessing skilled birth attendants (SBAs) (73% among ladinas but only 36% among indigenous women) all exacerbate access to care among rural indigenous populations in Guatemala (USAID 2015a, b). The sheer lack of obstetricians, gynecologists, female physicians, and other women's health specialists in rural regions is both deeply reflective of the country's priorities in regard to maternal health and demonstrates the demand for *comadronas*, who fill this critical role for women in their communities. According to the USAID's Health System Assessment of Guatemala in 2015, service utilization patterns highlight the fragmentation of the Guatemalan health system and reveal that the Guatemalan population regularly turns to the private sector for health services, particularly for the treatment of chronic conditions and preventative screening services such as Pap tests (smears). Furthermore, utilization rates among women reinforce the important role of the private sector in providing access to family planning services. In particular, the nonprofit International Planned Parenthood Federation's affiliate in Guatemala (Asociaci6n Pro-Familia or APROFAM) provides 16% of family planning commodities for the population and 20% of Pap tests, indicated in Table 31.3 (MSPAS 2016).

The signing of the Peace Accords in 1996 was a catalyst to improve the health system and extend health services to marginalized rural populations. Since then NGOs were contracted to provide these services and have had a major role in the expansion and improvement of health services nationally. This extended coverage began with the Ministry of Health's implementation of the Extension of Coverage Program (*Programa de Extension de Cobertura*, PEC) which provided coverage of basic health services to 46% of the country's population in rural indigenous communities by contracting

Table 31.2 National insurance coverage in Guatemala

IGSS	Sanidad Militar	Private insurance	Uninsured population
17.5%	0.5%	<5%	75%

Table 31.3 Source of care for females ages 15–49 (%)

	Public[a]	IGSS	Private clinic or hospital	APROFAM	TBA/home	Other
Family planning	51	9	22	16	–	2
Place of delivery	35	8	7	1	48	–
C-section	59	17	21	3	–	–
Pap test	39	6	32	20	–	3

[a]Public sources consist primarily of MSPAS facilities but also include other publicly funded facilities, such as those funded by municipalities

NGOs to provide basic health services (primarily mother and child care and immunizations) to underserved communities. The program rapidly expanded and by 1999 had extended basic health services to 3.5 million people, an estimated 76.8% of the previously unserved population at that time (USAID 2015a, b). However, in 2014, all contracts with NGOs were canceled, and the outsourcing of health services became prohibited by legislation resulting in suspension of all healthcare services provided by the PEC to the majority of Guatemala's rural population. A growing dissatisfaction with perceived inferior health services for the indigenous communities under the PEC, accusations of inefficiency, and a lack of transparency in award of PEC contracts to NGOs led to the passing of this legislation in 2013 (USAID 2015a, b). Since then, there has been no official program to replace these services provided to such a large and underserved community in rural Guatemala, leaving millions without coverage again.

Healthcare practices in Guatemala have frequently been characterized as pluralistic, because of the coexistence and concurrent use of traditional, biomedical, and popular practitioners. Pregnancy-related care in rural Guatemala is primarily provided by *comadronas* who offer care during pregnancy and childbirth and in the postpartum period. The most common sources of biomedical maternal care are the MSPAS-supported health centers or posts and from private medical doctors. Health centers located in municipal capitals are typically directed by a physician and sometimes have in-patient facilities. In contrast, health posts located in small communities are usually managed by an auxiliary nurse, rural health technician, or medical student and offer limited services (Goldman and Glei 2003). Auxiliary nurses are actually nurse assistants who graduate from a national program officially recognized by the MSPAS. After successfully completing didactic and practical training requirements, they are recruited into the nursing staff and maintained under the supervision of a professional nurse (*Enfermera Profesional*, EP). Auxiliary nurses provide direct and individualized care to the patient, as well as promote health to the family and community. They have no specialized training in women's health or pediatrics. Delivery services are free at specific health centers designated as Centers of Permanent Attention (CAP) or in government-operated hospitals. The health centers are very often difficult to access due to lack of transportation and poor conditions of the roads leading to these more rural communities. Some health centers, primarily those in communities with high maternal health needs, are designated as CAPs, functioning similar to a 24-h urgent care center also offering prenatal consults during the day. Biomedical health services and health professionals tend to be concentrated in urban areas, leaving rural populations with scarce public resources. Figure 31.5 shows a map of San Martin, a predominantly indigenous community (88%) comprised of 1 small town, 5 small villages, 21 small settlements, and 14 farms with a total population of 22, 635 inhabitants. There is only 1 CAP, open 24 h, that provides prenatal care and birthing services. This CAP is staffed by one doctor and at least one auxiliary nurse at all times. There are two health centers (*puestos de salud*) in the more remote surroundings generally staffed by 1–2 auxiliary nurses who serve populations of 1500–3000 people (Chomat et al. 2014). Sadly, the distressing ratio of 1 doctor to a population of over 22, 000 is surprisingly common, and health provisions in San Martin are representative of health provisions available in most rural communities in Guatemala. This also emphasizes the need to incorporate *comadronas* and other traditional healers into its healthcare system. According to Guatemala's Ministry of Planning and Programming of the Presidency (SEGEPLAN), 87% of births in San Martin Sacatapequez were attended by a *comadrona*. There are many more midwives (210 per 100,000 population) than medical doctors (17 per 100,000) in Guatemala who are able to provide specialized care (Hurtado and Saenz de Tejada 2001). Traditional community-based organizations among indigenous peoples, as well as the local health committees, Community Development Councils (*Consejos Comunitarios de Desarrollo* or COCODES), and networks of community health facilitators and *comadronas* constitute an important element of the country's health system, yet they have not been successfully integrated into the national health system (USAID 2015a, b).

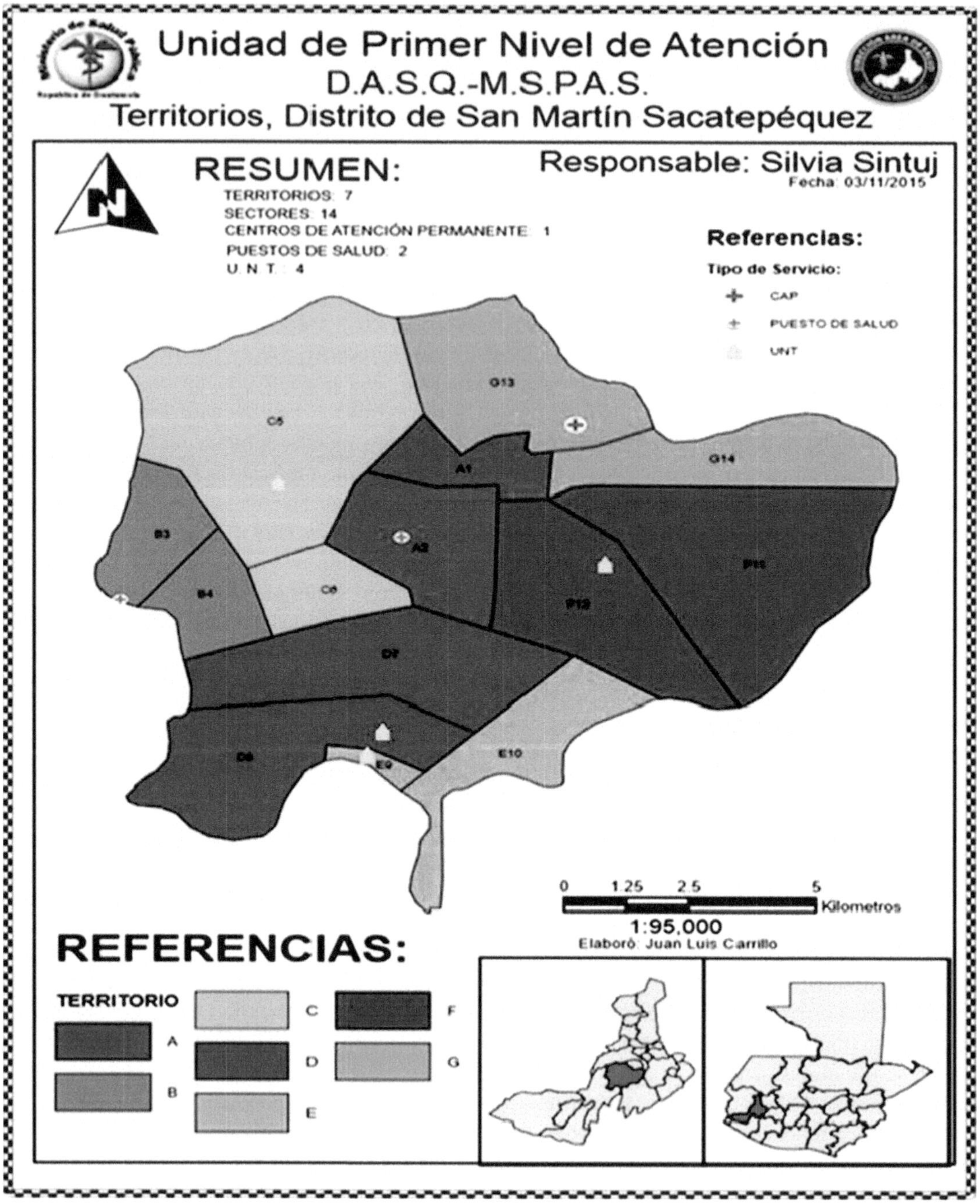

Fig. 31.5 Map of the district of San Martin in the department of Quetzaltenango in the western highlands of Guatemala. There is only one CAP (red cross) and two health posts (blue cross) in all of San Martin, serving a population of 22,635 (MSPAS 2016)

31.4 Long-Term Solutions

Systemic deficiencies are deeply rooted in the organization and management of the public health sector. Health sector financing, organization of health service delivery, citizen participation, and oversight within health services are some of the most recent issues that must be addressed as components of an integrated national healthcare strategy in order to achieve sustainable improvement for all of Guatemala (USAID 2015a, b). In April of 2015, the MSPAS met with regional health directors to create a new primary healthcare strategy, which emphasized service on the community level, an approach previously implemented by NGOs through the PEC program. The program is intended to strengthen and develop primary healthcare services with a focus on promotion, prevention, epidemiological disease surveillance, nutritional deficiencies, prioritization of pregnant, lactating women, and children under 2 years, without neglecting the family and community (USAID 2015a, b). The new strategy borrows heavily from two successful community-based models that have been implemented in Guatemala over the past decade. These have demonstrated improved access to services and health outcomes: the Inclusive Health Model (*Modelo Incluyente de Salud* or MIS) and the NGO *TulaSalud*'s public-private partnership and mHealth approach in Alta Verapaz (USAID 2015a, b).

The MIS pilot program, created in the early 2000s, was a collaboration with three MOH districts in response to the need for improved healthcare for the rural indigenous population. The MIS model was created by a coalition of grassroots organizations like NGOs, cooperatives, health promoters, *comadronas*, and other social organizations collectively called the INS (Instancia Nacional en Salud, Petition in National Health) and was specifically designed for Guatemala. Currently, the INS is not active, but it was created to conduct research and to develop proposals that would help to achieve an improved public health system in Guatemala. In 2002, after conducting an investigation which took into account many different perspectives, the INS published a paper presenting the Model for Inclusive Health (MIS). The purpose of this proposal was to implement and strengthen the first national primary healthcare (PHC) system in Guatemala, which incorporated the *comadrona* as one of many fundamental figures. The MIS is based on four perspectives: the right to health, gender equality, intercultural relevance, and the environment. It differs from the government's standard of care which covers a quarter of the nation's population and, instead, aligns with the position of the Pan American Health Organization which offers services through programs that integrate the individual, family, and community. Primary healthcare has been established as a key component of successful health systems and is tremendously adaptable to cultural context, making MIS an excellent model for Guatemala (Macinko et al. 2007). Coverage, quality of care, and utilization measures increased significantly during the 5-year period after the service delivery model was initially implemented (Fort et al. 2011).

Another NGO, TulaSalud, implemented an mHealth project in the department of Alta Verapaz which started in 2012. This department has 1.2 million inhabitants (78% living in rural areas and 89% from indigenous communities) and, in 2012, had a maternal mortality ratio of 273 for every 100,000 live births (Martinez-Fernandez et al. 2015). This mHealth initiative is based on the provision of a cell phone to community facilitators (CFs). CFs are community volunteers that receive basic training in health prevention, promotion, and care. The CFs receive a small stipend from the MSPAS and a kit of essential drugs to serve a population of 1500 inhabitants. The intervention CFs (tele-CFs) were given cell phones to be able to consult healthcare professionals during patient exams, send full epidemiological reports and clinical information, receive continuous training, and perform activities for the prevention and promotion of community health in the *Q'eqchí* and/or *Poqomchi'* languages. As a result of the telemedicine initiative, the intervention areas, which were selected for their high maternal and infant mortality rates, showed significantly lower maternal and child mortality indicators than the control areas and the provincial average (Martinez-Fernandez et al. 2015).

The new Guatemalan PHC strategy will incorporate key components of both the MIS and TulaSalud initiatives and is expected to reach coverage of more than 5 million people nationwide. Health areas are undergoing a reorganization of territories to ensure that each health post has a catchment area of no more than 5000 inhabitants (USAID 2015a, b). These health areas are to be further divided into two sectors of approximately 2500 inhabitants, which will be directly supported by CFs and *comadronas*. Auxiliary nurses will be expected to divide their time between the health facilities and community conducting outreach visits in both sectors. Each health post is expected to be supported by two auxiliary nurses, six CFs, and ten *comadronas*—a far higher number of health workers than is currently supporting health posts under the MSPAS (USAID 2015a, b). Telemedicine is a new, important aspect of the health strategy. Auxiliary nurses and community health facilitators will be equipped with mobile phones that utilize a system platform which includes WhatsApp, video chat, photo messaging, direct messaging, and Internet capabilities to improve the flow of information between the community facilitators and health workers based in the facilities (USAID 2015a, b). The use of mobile technology to identify, track, and refer patients to health facilities has contributed to a reduction in maternal deaths in communities in Alta Verapaz (Martinez-Fernandez et al. 2015).

31.5 Strengthening the Role of the *Comadrona*

The importance of traditional birth attendants (TBAs) for years has been denied by allopathic medical practitioners and other scientists until the late 1980s, when the World Health Organization discovered that TBAs have a significant role in reducing maternal and newborn mortality. The Safe Motherhood Initiative found that most of developing countries had limited medical personnel and health facilities for provision of healthcare in rural areas. The next option was to utilize existing resources such as the TBAs who are already present in rural communities (Kayombo 2013). To reduce maternal mortality and severe morbidity, either there must be an increase in TBAs' detection of obstetric complications or referral for them, or women must recognize danger signs and go to a hospital on their own (Bailey et al. 2002). Hospitals in Guatemala reportedly have a capacity to provide services to only 20% of women giving birth. In contrast to this limited capacity of institutions, there are as many as 20 TBAs per 10,000 inhabitants, with some 70% of those TBAs having received some formal training, according to published and unpublished reports (Bailey et al. 2002). Government facilities in rural areas, particularly health centers and posts, usually lack critical equipment, medical supplies, and personnel adequately trained in maternal health. Hospital environments also need to be more welcoming to indigenous women and their *comadronas*. Indigenous women often fear hospitals and associate them with death, surgery, or sterilization. Interactions between traditional and biomedical providers are often tense, in part due to social, ethnic, and cultural differences between providers (Goldman and Glei 2003). *Comadronas* or TBAs have enough influence in their communities to help break the sociocultural barriers that currently prevent expectant women from seeking facility-based care. Guatemala has an indigenous culture rooted in traditional practices that are based on ancestral beliefs expressed in the oral tradition, ideograms, symbols, and abstract ideas that are solid and profound. Traditional healers and *comadronas* possess Mayan ancestral medical lore, and their legitimacy is rooted in the trust placed in them by their indigenous community. The success of any primary health program depends on the integration of these cultural practitioners through trust, transparency, and tolerance in order to manifest a willingness to learn and begin to bridge the gap between allopathic and traditional practitioners.

Currently, there is no official midwife training program in Guatemala. The training program created for the *comadronas* has changed frequently within the past few decades. It emphasizes aseptic techniques such as hand washing, disinfecting medical instruments, the horizontal delivery position, and when to refer patients to the nearest hospital. These trainings largely condemned the traditional practices of herb usage, sweat bath, and delivery in the squatting or kneeling position (Cosminsky 1978). The MOH sponsors continuing education activities, which are typically 1-day training sessions held on a monthly basis at regional or local health facilities, granting a license to *comadronas* that consistently attend (Chary et al. 2013). The monthly training sessions additionally serve as a data collection period for the MOH, who request information from the *comadronas* regarding births, referrals, and active patients. In the past, each *comadrona* received a small monetary incentive for participation, but this is no longer in effect due to a lack of funds. Licensing and training requirements are enforced primarily by local health authorities who refuse to grant a birth certificate to parents who deliver the baby with a non-licensed midwife (Chary et al. 2013). The MOH recently created a new manual for training of the *comadronas* which began its implementation in select communities in January 2016. The preparation of this new manual was based on the most recent (2006) version of the manual "Intervencion Corta" (Short Intervention), which focuses on strengthening knowledge, skills, and practices of the *comadronas*. By applying an educational program that has been contextualized for indigenous communities, the new training program favors personalized teaching and promotes an exchange of knowledge and practices (MOH 2016). The new program consists of nine modules covering topics such as prenatal care, labor, delivery, family planning, and newborn care. The manual also focuses on preventative care with emphasis on prenatal care. It includes recognition and referral of emergencies for patients, thereby integrating *comadrona* care into the health facilities. Under the new training program, *comadronas* will be expected to shadow the doctors and auxiliary nurses in the local CAPs. The *comadronas* must show proficiency in basic history taking, clinical skills, and labor and delivery care listed in the required checklist used for evaluation, prior to receiving a license. Unfortunately, the new program is not being implemented in all departments, and there are no criteria for the amount of time a new *comadrona* must participate in the monthly trainings and shadowing before being given a license.

Most projects targeting TBAs tend to be short-term, pilot programs that test various training modules. Unfortunately, many of these training models have failed to be integrated into the national health system due to cumulative undermining effects of the already problematic health system, marginalization, cultural and linguistic barriers, and poorly designed programming (Goldman and Glei 2003). Currently, two ongoing programs in Guatemala are showing promise of success in training and incorporating *comadronas* into the biomedical healthcare system. Curamerica and Saving Mothers are NGOs that have both collaborated with the MOH and recognize the critical importance of *comadrona* training and referral. Curamerica has been successful in strengthening maternity care in isolated indigenous mountain communities through *Casa Maternas* (birthing facilities). There are three *Casa Maternas* in the isolated municipalities of the northwestern highlands, in the department of Huehuetenango where the MMR is 338 deaths per 100,000 live births (Stollak et al. 2016). The project integrates three key methodologies (Fig. 31.6).

The *comadronas* are encouraged to refer their patients to the birthing facilities and are welcomed into the labor and delivery process, unlike heath centers or hospitals where care is primarily administered by doctors or nurses. Families are also encouraged to stay and are even provided with sleeping arrangements. The *Casa Maternas* are staffed with a trained auxiliary nurse and assistants who act as support for the *comadrona* and patient. Since 2002, Curamericas has established a relationship of respect and collaboration with *comadronas*, through a culturally sensitive approach to the strong relationship between families and *comadronas* (Stollak et al. 2016). The purpose of the case study was to examine whether *Casas Maternas* have contributed to increasing facility-based deliveries and to evaluate what factors impact decision-making in relation to birthing outside the home. Findings clearly indicate there was a relatively high rate of utilization of the *Casas Maternas*, and by 2014, 54% of women living in the Calhuitz and Santo Domingo partner communities were giving birth at the respective *Casas Maternas*. These findings are particularly impressive in light of the low percentage of births (21%) taking place at facilities in the overwhelmingly indigenous department of

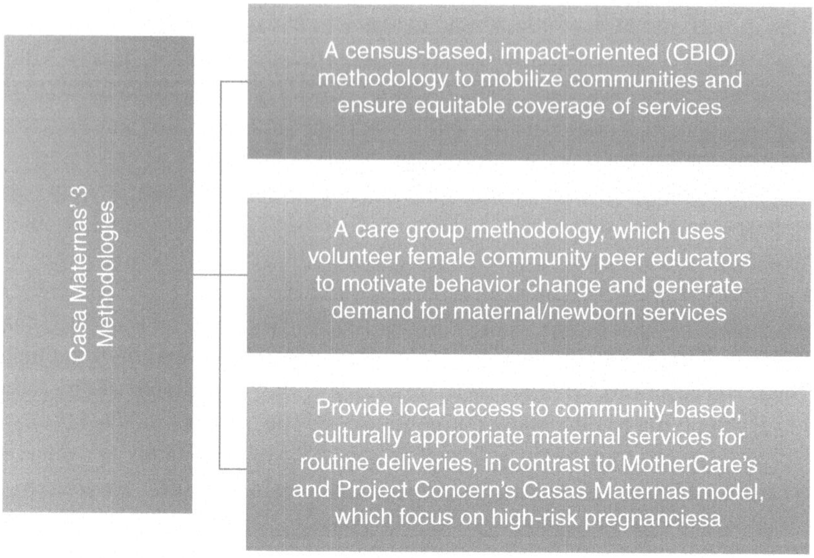

Fig. 31.6 Curamerica's effective Casa Maternas model strategies (Stollak et al. 2016)

Huehuetenango and the low percentage of facility births (29%) among indigenous women in the country as a whole (Stollak et al. 2016). *Casa Materna* is an extremely successful model and will continue to expand to other departments.

Curamerica is currently launching the fourth *Casa Materna* in the department of San Marcus in collaboration with the Ministry of Health as part of their new outreach program. This is the first *Casa Materna* that has received direct support from the national government.

Saving Mothers is an international NGO dedicated to eradicating preventable maternal deaths and birth-related complications in the developing world. In May 2016, Saving Mothers established its sister chapter, *Salvando Madres Guatemala*, a local NGO based in Santiago Atitlan. Saving Mothers has been working in the western highlands department of Solola since 2009, providing education and training to local MOH providers and *comadronas* on maternal and reproductive health. In 2014, Saving Mothers launched the first *Comadrona* School of POWHER (Providing Outreach in Women's Health and Educational Resources) training program in Santiago Atitlan. The curriculum was designed for 22 women, consisting of 12 new *comadronas*, 4 elder *comadronas*, 3 CFs, and 3 auxiliary nurses, who all successfully completed the program. The school of POWHER is a 14-week intensive care course based on a two-pronged approach. The first approach is comprised of a 28-module didactic portion, and the second approach is a separate clinical component designed to incorporate all literacy levels. Two afternoons each week are dedicated to 4-h intercultural didactics which have an emphasis on prenatal care, recognizing high-risk signs of referral for mother and baby, and initial management of postpartum complications. The clinical arm of the school ensures that the *comadronas* refine their traditional midwifery skills while learning to incorporate newer skills such as measuring blood pressure, using a fetal Doppler monitor, and correctly estimating delivery date. A minimum of 15-recorded prenatal visits, 3–5 supervised births, and 3 postpartum visits are required of each student. The entire program is operated and overseen by a licensed physician or physician's assistant specializing in women's health. This school created a new model of *comadrona* recruitment and training which instills the values of sharing knowledge, apprenticeship, and partnerships with local health facility providers. This model also directly addresses at least two out of the four aspects (recognizing complications and deciding to seek care) that contribute to complicated labor. Since its 2014 conception, the School of POWHER has had 3 classes in 2 different departments within Guatemala (Sololá and Quetzaltenango) which has trained 45 *comadronas*. Graduates from the school have demonstrated an

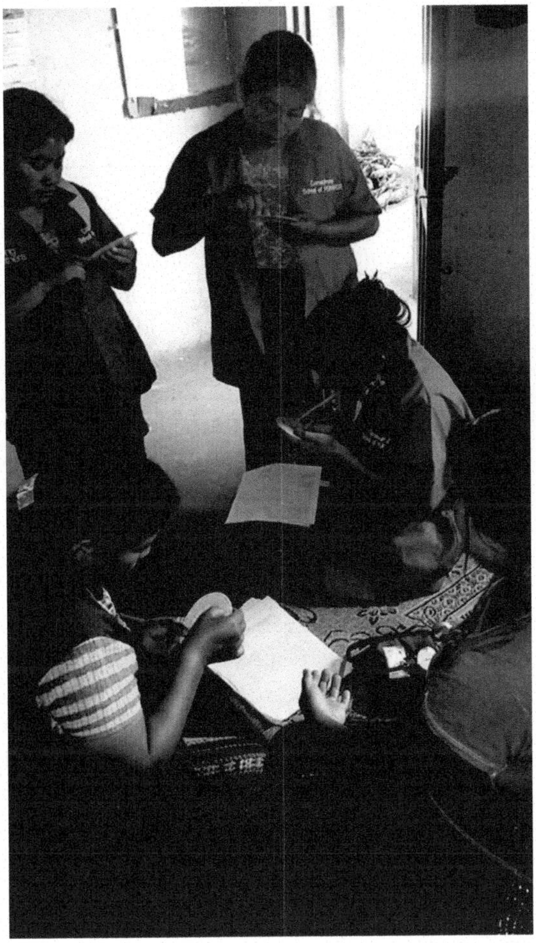

Fig. 31.7 Three School of POWHER *comadrona* graduates (red coats) and a community facilitator (left) are using pregnancy wheels to identify the due date of the patient (right) during a prenatal care visit

improvement in multiple basic knowledge areas such as anatomy, physiology, and pregnancy management. Figure 31.7 illustrates four graduates of the School of POWHER 2014 in Santiago—3 *comadronas* and 1 community facilitator—using the tools and training provided by the school to determine the due date of a patient. This program has additionally strengthened knowledge in the areas of newborn assessment and care, labor, delivery, and family planning. Results of the program revealed that the culturally adapted, formal training produced a measurable increase in knowledge retention and care (Rana et al. 2015).

Over the past few years, the School of POWHER has been well received by the *comadronas*, the local health departments, and the Guatemalan Ministry of Health. In light of these changing attitudes toward traditional birth attendants and their role in the healthcare system, the School of POWHER will launch a new model in March of 2017 in collaboration with the MSPAS department of Solola. In this model, the teaching facilitators will be School of POWHER graduates of the 2014 class who have continued their training with Saving Mothers since graduation. Two head *comadronas*, who are also licensed auxiliary nurses, have been identified as the lead educators. They will deliver the didactic portion of the school in the local Mayan dialect, reducing the linguistic barrier encountered in the past. Five other *comadrona* graduates have been identified as clinical preceptors that will oversee the new students during prenatal home visits and will teach the clinical component. Two of these *comadrona* preceptors also work as community facilitators for the MOH. The recruitment of students for this new school will also be modified. In the past, the *comadronas* were selected based on proximity to the school, which prevented *comadronas* from farther and more remote regions from attending. The new school in 2017 has received enough support to enroll students from outside regions who will stay on campus for the duration of the program. A major goal of this training model designed for *comadronas* is that it will eventually be independently operated by *comadronas* and community facilitator graduates. Integrating *comadronas* as leaders and educators reinforces their emerging role as credible healthcare professionals and escalates their status within the healthcare infrastructure (Chary et al. 2013). Additionally, after consulting Curamerica, *Salvando Madres Guatemala* is launching its first *Casa Materna* in San Juan la Laguna in November of 2016. *Casa Materna* is a collaborative effort of the local municipality and the School of POWHER graduates, who will provide healthcare services at the center. The new School of POWHER and *Casa Materna* will further fortify the pivotal role *comadronas* hold as both educators and providers helping to improve maternal morbidity and mortality.

To help reduce the high rates of maternal mortality in these populations, it is essential to reduce the cultural barriers that hinder cooperation between *comadronas* and biomedical healthcare professionals, a change that cannot be achieved without promoting mutual recognition and assessment of health practices between both systems. The biomedical model of pregnancy views the condition as a disease with symptoms to be treated. In Mayan culture, pregnancy is tied to a natural, spiritual, and more holistic perspective that is centered on balancing the forces between the body and the environment. The Mayan perspective and practices have been largely condemned by biomedical healthcare professionals who embolden western practices without recognizing the value of cultural literacy (Cosminsky 1982). Biomedical practitioners also assume a more legitimate status within the formal healthcare system of Guatemala, leaving the cultural expertise and credibility of *comadronas* largely unrecognized and often undermined. The MOH is fully aware that facility capacity is reached at just 20% of annual births, so the country must rely on *comadronas* for home deliveries, while only referring patients with complications to the hospital (Hurtado and Saenz de Tejada 2001). Progress has been substantial within the past 2 years through NGO- and government-supported rigorous *comadrona* training programs. These efforts are shaping a future that places the critical role of the *comadronas* and the severity of maternal mortality as a priority on the national healthcare agenda. Though the *comadronas* are already experts in Mayan culture, by providing effective clinical training, their role is transformed to one that is recognized and legitimized both by their communities and within the formal healthcare system of Guatemala. This is expected to reduce maternal mortality by increasing referrals, reducing the delay in seeking care, and improving diagnoses.

References

Bailey, P. E., Szaszdi, J. A., & Glover, L. (2002). Obstetric complications: Does training traditional birth attendants make a difference? *Revista Panamericana de Salud Publica, 11*(1). https://doi.org/10.1590/s1020-49892002000100003

Berry, N. S. (2006). Kaqchikel midwives, home births, and emergency obstetric referrals in Guatemala: Contextualizing the choice to stay at home. *Social Science & Medicine, 62*(8), 1958–1969. https://doi.org/10.1016/j.socscimed.2005.09.005

Chary, A., Díaz, A. K., Henderson, B., & Rohloff, P. (2013). The changing role of indigenous lay midwives in Guatemala: New frameworks for analysis. *Midwifery, 29*(8), 852–858. https://doi.org/10.1016/j.midw.2012.08.011

Chomat, A. M., Solomons, N. W., Montenegro, G., Crowley, C., & Bermudez, O. I. (2014). Maternal health and health seeking behaviors among indigenous Mam mothers from Quetzaltenango, Guatemala. *Revista Panamericana de Salud Pública, 35*(2), 113–120.

Congreso de la República de Guatemala. (2009). *Directo Número 9–2009*. Resource document. Retrieved May 25, 2016, from https://www.unicef.org/guatemala/spanish/LeyContraViolenciaSexual_Explot_y_Trata.pdf.

Cosminsky, S. (1976). Birth rituals and symbolism: A Quiche Maya-Black Carib comparison. In P. Young & J. Howe (Eds.), *Ritual and symbol in native central America* (pp. 105–117). Eugene: University of Oregon Press.
Cosminsky, S. (1978). Midwifery and medical anthropology. In B. Belimrovic (Ed.), *Modern medicine and medical anthropology in the united states Mexico border population* (pp. 116–126). Washington, DC, Pan American Health Organization.
Cosminsky, S. (1982). Childbirth and change: A Guatemalan study. In C. MacCormack (Ed.), *Ethnography of fertility and birth* (pp. 205–229). New York, NY: Academic Press.
Cosminsky, S. (1987). Women and health care on a Guatemalan plantation. *Social Science & Medicine, 25*(10), 1163–1173. https://doi.org/10.1016/0277-9536(87)90358-3
Council on Hemispheric Affairs (COHA). (2015, June 17). *Why is Guatemala's teen pregnancy rate so high?* Retrieved May 25, 2016, from http://www.coha.org/why-is-guatemalas-teen-pregnancy-rate-so-high/.
Forsell, L., & Lyche, K. (2015, August 27). Rape, ignorance, repression: Why early pregnancy is endemic in Guatemala. *The Guardian*.
Fort, M. P., Grembowski, D. E., Verdugo, J. C., Morales, L. C., Arriaga, C. A., Mercer, M. A., & Lim, S. S. (2011). Implementation and progress of an inclusive primary health care model in Guatemala: Coverage, quality, and utilization. *Revista Panamericana de Salud Pública, 30*(3), 217–224. https://doi.org/10.1590/s1020-49892011000900005
Foster, J., Anderson, A., Houston, J., & Doe-Simkins, M. (2004). A report of a midwifery model for training traditional midwives in Guatemala. *Midwifery, 20*(3), 217–225. https://doi.org/10.1016/j.midw.2004.01.004
Goldman, N., & Glei, D. A. (2003). Evaluation of midwifery care: Results from a survey in rural Guatemala. *Social Science & Medicine, 56*(4), 685–700. https://doi.org/10.1016/s0277-9536(02)00065-5
Hurtado, E., & Saenz de Tejada, E. (2001). Relations between government health workers and traditional midwives in Guatemala. In B. Huber & A. Sandstrom (Eds.), *Mesoamerican healers*. Austin, TX: University of Texas Press.
Kayombo, E. J. (2013). Impact of training traditional birth attendants on maternal mortality and morbidity in Sub-Saharan African countries. *Tanzania Journal of Health Research, 15*(2). https://doi.org/10.4314/thrb.v15i2.7
La Comisión para el Esclarecimiento Histórico (CEH). (1994). *Guatemala Memory of Silence Tz'inil Na'tab'al*. Resource document. Retrieved May 25, 2016, from https://www.aaas.org/sites/default/files/migrate/uploads/ mos_en.pdf.
Lang, J. (1997). A study of the beliefs and birthing practices traditional midwives in rural Guatemala. *Journal of Nurse-Midwifery, 42*(1), 25–31. https://doi.org/10.1016/s0091-2182(96)00069-9
Macinko, J., Montenegro, H., Adell, C., & Etienne, C. (2007). La renovación de la atención primaria de salud en las Américas. *American Journal of Public Health, 21*, 73–84.
Martínez-Fernández, A. C. A., Lobos-Medina, I., Díaz-Molina, C. A., Chen-Cruz, M. F., & Prieto-Egido, I. (2015). TulaSalud: An m-health system for maternal and infant mortality reduction in Guatemala. *Journal of Telemedicine and Telecare, 21*(5), 283–291. https://doi.org/10.1177/1357633x15575830
Ministerio de Salud Pública y Asistencia Social (MSPAS). (2000). *Línea basal de mortalidad materna para el año 2000*. Guatemala City: MSPAS.
Ministerio de Salud Pública y Asistencia Social (MSPAS). (2016). *Operative plan for healthcare model at the primary level for the municipal health district San Martin Sactatepequez, Quetzaltenango*. Guatemala City: MSPAS.
Ministry of Health of Guatemala (MOH). (2016). Manual Para Capacitar Comadronas en Atencion Materno Neonatal. *Programa Nacional de Salud Reproductiva*. Departmento de Regulación de Los Programas de Atención a Las Personas.
Observatorio en Salud Sexual y Reproductiva (OSAR). (2015). *Embarazadas de 10 a 14 anos*. Retrieved May 25, 2016, from http://www.osarguatemala.org/embarazo.php?id=243.
Pan American Health Organization (PAHO). (2012). *Guatemala: The maternal mortality challenge*. Resource document. Retrieved May 25, 2016, from http://www.paho.org/hq/.
Paul, L., & Paul, B. D. (1975). The Maya midwife as sacred specialist: A Guatemalan case. *American Ethnologist, 2*(4), 707–726. https://doi.org/10.1525/ae.1975.2.4.02a00080
Rana, R., Shirazian, T., & Oliveira, J. (2015). Culturally adapted obstetrics course for traditional Mayan birth attendants. *Obstetrics & Gynecology, 125*. https://doi.org/10.1097/01.aog.0000463208.33901.fe
Schwartz, D. A. (2015). The pathology of maternal death—the importance of accurate autopsy diagnosis for epidemiologic surveillance and prevention of maternal mortality in developing countries. In D. A. Schwartz (Ed.), *Maternal mortality: Risk factors, anthropological perspectives, prevalence in developing countries and preventive strategies for pregnancy-related death* (pp. 215–253). New York, NY: Nova Science Publishers.
Stollak, I., Valdez, M., Rivas, K., & Perry, H. (2016). Casas maternas in the rural highlands of Guatemala: A mixed-methods case study of the introduction and utilization of birthing facilities by an indigenous population. *Global Health: Science and Practice, 4*(1), 114–131. https://doi.org/10.9745/ghsp-d-15-00266
United Nations Children's Fund (UNICEF). (2009). *State of the world's children*. Retrieved May 25, 2016, from https://www.unicef.org/sowc/.
United Nations Children's Fund (UNICEF). (2014). *Guatemala country programme document 2015–2019*. Retrieved May 25, 2016, from https://www.unicef.org/about/execboard/files/2014-PL14-Guatemala_CPD-Final_approved-EN.pdf.

United Nations Population Fund (UNFPA). (2013). *Motherhood in childhood: Facing the challenge of adolescent pregnancy*. Resource document. Retrieved May 25, 2016, from http://kyrgyzstan.unfpa.org/sites/default/files/pub-pdf/motherhood-in-childhood-_en.pdf.

United States Agency for International Development (USAID). (2015a). *Guatemala Health System Assessment 2015*. Retrieved May 25, 2016, from https://www.usaid.gov/sites/default/files/documents/1862/Guatemala-HSA%20_ENG-FULL-REPORT-FINAL-APRIL-2016.pdf..

United States Agency for International Development (USAID). (2015b). *Bread brings hope to the Guatemala highlands*. Retrieved May 25, 2016, from https://www.usaid.gov/results-data/success-stories/bread-brings-hope-guatemala-highlands.

World Bank Group. (2016). *Guatemala*. Retrieved May 25, 2016, from http://www.worldbank.org/en/country/guatemala.

World Health Organization (WHO). (2012). *WHO recommendations for the prevention and treatment of postpartum haemorrhage*. Retrieved May 25, 2016, from http://apps.who.int/iris/bitstream/10665/75411/1/9789241548502_eng.pdf.

World Health Organization (WHO). (2013). *Guatemala: Maternal and perinatal health profile*. Retrieved May 25, 2016, from http://www.who.int/maternal_child_adolescent/epidemiology/profiles/maternal/gtm.pdf.

32 Poverty, Local Perceptions, and Access to Services: Understanding Obstetric Choices for Rural and Indigenous Women in Guatemala in the Twenty-First Century

Alejandra Colom and Marcela Colom

32.1 Introduction

Obstetric choice in Guatemala mirrors the country's historical challenges to guaranteeing the well-being of its citizens, as well as the continuing disparities in access to services between rural and urban and indigenous and nonindigenous populations. It also reflects the coexistence of two different paradigms regarding maternal health: one that looks at the issue through the lens of public health and biomedicine and one that looks at pregnancy and birth from the perspective of traditional midwives (or traditional birth attendants, TBAs), local indigenous cultures, and women themselves. Both operate in a context that is characterized by endemic poverty.

This chapter offers an overview of obstetric choice in Guatemala from both perspectives, with the goal of illustrating the frequent non-amicable relationship between the two. It also presents recent attempts at a compromise that encompasses wider aspects of women's lives within the limitations of a national budget that is yet to prioritize health. Finally, this chapter addresses the challenges and questions still to be answered in order to speak about true choices for women during pregnancy, childbirth, and postpartum.

Differences in access to healthcare have their roots in Guatemala's medical and political history, and reflect the country's investing priorities, or lack thereof (ICEFI and UNICEF 2016, p. 36; ACCESA 2015). Government efforts to address disparities in access to health, including prenatal and postpartum care, have been characterized by a series of starts and stops that began during the

A. Colom, Ph.D., M.A. (✉)
Population Council in Guatemala,
Guatemala City, Guatemala

Department of Anthropology, Universidad del Valle de Guatemala,
Guatemala City, Guatemala
e-mail: acolom@popcouncil.org

M. Colom, M.D.
Wuqu' Kawoq | Maya Health Alliance,
Santiago, Sacatepéquez, Guatemala

D. A. Schwartz (ed.), *Maternal Death and Pregnancy-Related Morbidity Among Indigenous Women of Mexico and Central America*, Global Maternal and Child Health: Medical, Anthropological, and Public Health Perspectives, https://doi.org/10.1007/978-3-319-71538-4_32

liberal governments that predominated during the late 1940s and early 1950s. These, and subsequent efforts, assumed a discourse of modernization, in which traditional practices not aligned with biomedical understandings of pregnancy and birth should eventually disappear through health education (Berry 2010). What we know about obstetric choice from those initial decades comes mostly from anthropological literature that described community dynamics, practices, and belief systems, with midwives as the principal characters. Very few national statistics exist from that period, so understanding the evolution of maternity care and options can only be gathered by examining these studies and by looking at what was not there. For example, the absence of community health posts, proper infrastructure, and means of transportation during the time period studied complements the context described by anthropologists of rural women, mostly all indigenous, relying on traditional midwives and female relatives to support them during pregnancy, birth, and the postpartum period. Literature from that period depicts contexts of poverty as de facto status for most Guatemalan women. The first publications on the issue, described later in this chapter, lacked critique of the structures that perpetuated the precarious economic conditions in which midwives and women interacted. They also offered very limited descriptions of gender and generational dynamics within households. In most of these narratives, pregnant women have "nonspeaking roles." Despite the limitations of existing data, it is possible to piece together a history of little to no public investment on adolescent girls and women. From a public health perspective, this could be seen as "planned poverty" (Bruce 2016), a condition of persistent disinvestment that limits opportunities and choices for most Guatemalans.

As in other parts of the world, proposed public health solutions to the diverse challenges associated with improving care for women can be aligned across a spectrum that expands from full to no inclusion of women's preferences and needs (Davis-Floyd and Sergant 1996, p. 111). It is important to highlight that Guatemala differs from other Latin American countries in that, during the 1990s and 2000s, it transitioned from public universal or almost universal coverage to increased privatization of healthcare. Rather, most regions in Guatemala went from no publicly financed healthcare coverage to a mixture of health options which were mostly privatized (Rolhoff and Chary 2015).

Understanding women's choices today requires reflecting critically on the history of power dynamics and tensions between a centralized Ministry of Health, shaped according to Western medical standards, and lay care providers, culture-specific concepts of birth, and local knowledge in rural and mostly indigenous areas. In this chapter, the history of obstetric care and choice in Guatemala is reviewed through an ecological approach[1] that focuses on past and present-day conditions that influence why and how women, their families, and health providers make certain choices regarding obstetric care. While the chapter looks at the entire public health system, its services, and policies, it gives special attention to its relationship with rural Maya communities because poor, indigenous women continue to face the most disadvantages, discrimination, and stigmatization when attempting to access health services in Guatemala.

Persistent high rates of maternal[2] and neonatal[3] mortality in Guatemala have challenged practitioners, researchers, and public officials since the first reliable national indicators began to be

[1]An ecological approach or paradigm views individuals as part of a wider social context that influences their behavior and perceptions. Context includes family and peer groups and other spaces where individuals interact such as school, the workplace, church, public institutions, etc. This analytical approach requires that all elements mentioned above are considered when assessing an issue (Schensul and LeCompte 1999).

[2]Maternal death is defined as the death of a woman while she is pregnant or within the 42 days following the conclusion of the pregnancy, independently of its duration and state of the pregnancy, due to any cause related or worsened by the pregnancy or its care, excluding accidents or incidentals (OPS 1995, p. 139).

[3]The neonatal period begins at birth and ends 28 days after birth (OPS 1995, p. 136).

Table 32.1 Millennium and sustainable development goals: current status for Guatemala[a]

MDG	Status by 2015	SDG
Reduce by three fourths, between 1990 and 2015, maternal mortality. Goal for Guatemala: 55	113 per 100,000 live births. Highest MMR: 232.6 (Huehuetenango) lowest MMR: 23.4 (El Progreso) (MSPAS 2015)[b]	By 2030, reduce the global MMR ratio to under 70 per 100,000 live births
Reduce by two thirds, between 1990 and 2015, under-five mortality. Goal for Guatemala: 37	Neonatal mortality: 17 per 1000 live births (MSPAS et al. 2017)[c] Under-five mortality: 35 per 1000 live births (national). 30 per 1000 live births (urban) and 44 per 1000 live births (rural)[d] (MSPAS et al. 2017)	By 2030, end preventable deaths of newborns and children under 5 years of age, with all countries aiming to reduce neonatal mortality to at least as low as 12 per 1000 live births and under-five mortality to at least as low as 25 per 1000 live births
Achieve, by 2015, universal access to sexual and reproductive healthcare services	Unmet need (urban): 10.2% Unmet need (rural): 16.6% Unmet need (nonindigenous): 10.8% Unmet need (indigenous): 17.4 (MSPAS et al. 2017, pp. 169–70)	By 2030, ensure universal access to sexual and reproductive healthcare services, including for family planning, information and education, and the integration of reproductive health into national strategies and programs

[a]All data from 2015, unless otherwise noted
[b]Data from 2013
[c]Indigenous: 19 per 1000 live births. Nonindigenous: 16 per 1000 live births (MSPAS et al. 2017, pp. 186–188)
[d]Indigenous: 43 per 1000 live births. Nonindigenous: 35 per 1000 live births (MSPAS et al. 2017)

collected—in 1987—when the first maternal and infant health survey took place.[4] This period also coincides with the United Nations-led worldwide efforts to engage countries in setting goals to improve the lives of their citizens. In September of 2000, 189 countries, including Guatemala, agreed to work toward the Millennium Development Goals (MDGs) (SEGEPLAN 2015, p. 11). The MDGs sparked a series of analyses that compared indicators across countries, drawing attention to Guatemala's poor ranking in the Latin American region. For example, Guatemala's under-five mortality rate in 2015 (35 per 1000 live births) was higher than the 1990 rate of 17 Latin American countries (Cecchini and Azócar 2007, p. 61). Guatemala's score vis-à-vis the Millennium Development Goals (MDGs) and, more recently, the Sustainable Development Goals (SDGs) illustrates that, while progress has been made, the country continues to rank among the lowest performers in the region (SEGEPLAN 2015). Table 32.1 summarizes the original MDG, the status as of 2015 (target year), and the new SDG for the same indicators.

As Table 32.1 illustrates, some MDGs were achieved at a national scale but important disparities between urban and rural and nonindigenous and indigenous groups persisted. Because national surveys began around the time most present-day health policies were created, very little is known about national-level patterns prior to 1987. The absence of official information on certain populations prior to that date can be in part compensated with anthropological literature which, from the 1950s onward, included studies on medical issues in rural communities (Adams and Hawkins 2007, p. 4). Most of this research, however, did not include the generation of large-scale statistics, so information can seldom be compared to current demographic data.

In this chapter, efforts were made to provide a balance between the Western, biomedical data, and information generated from anthropological approaches. This combination will, hopefully, allow readers to look at the issue from more than one angle, including present-day medical practitioners, community level actors, and the public sector. It combines diachronic and synchronic approachesto evaluate change and persistence over time as documented in government documents,

[4]Many other indicators continue to be a cause of concern. However, for the purposes of highlighting issues associated with obstetric choice, this chapter will focus on the three more closely associated to the topic: maternal and neonatal mortality and access to reproductive health services.

medical and anthropological literature, and other sources. Regardless of the perspective, existing data lacks, in many cases, the perspective of pregnant women concerning factors that affect their choices or lack thereof.

Existing literature is as relevant to analysis as are the gaps in information encountered during the research process. The lack of mention of Guatemala's cultural diversity in early official documents, and the apparent reinvention of approaches to service over time, reveals patterns of neglect and discrimination that, despite recent efforts to improve care, persist today. Medical anthropological literature helps explain the complexities which are seldom addressed in government reports. Information generated by nongovernmental organizations (NGOs) that focus on maternal health has been useful because they filled some gaps regarding this complex, multidimensional issue. Additional documents reviewed included the various iterations of Guatemala's public policies concerning maternal and child care.

The chapter is divided into five sections. The first one focuses on the history of obstetric care in Guatemala and the challenges the country has faced reducing maternal morbidity and mortality. It includes the most recent data available on national indicators addressing deliveries assisted by skilled birth attendants (SBAs)[5] and differences associated with women's ethnicity, income, place of residence, and education. It describes the types of public services available to pregnant women and the principal actors involved in service provision, including lay birth attendants. Perspectives in this section come mostly from a biomedical, public health standpoint.

In the second section, the focus shifts to the past, in an attempt to provide some answers as to why Guatemala historically lags behind most Latin American countries in many of the SDGs. It follows the chronology of the development of services, including the creation of laws that addresses the cultural and linguistic needs of roughly one half the population of women who seek obstetric services.

Section 32.4 focuses on the individual, family, and community levels and is mostly based on anthropological literature that describes and contextualizes cultural practices around pregnancy and birth among indigenous women in rural Guatemala. This section includes historical as well as current and applied contributions to the analysis of gaps in access to services, highlighting present-day engaged positions (Ginsburg and Rapp 1991, p. 317) of medical anthropologists.

Section 32.5 shifts back to medical literature and the factors associated with decision-making at the community level. It contains descriptions of common services provided to women in rural communities in Guatemala, as well as the limitations faced by women and their families when faced with "choices" that are not accessible to them. The authors analyze the views of local nurses and biomedical practitioners of challenges and opportunities related to obstetric care and choice. These are contrasted with the experiences of lay midwives who navigate and adapt to the changing landscape of policies and services with the women they care for.

The chapter ends with Section 32.6, "Can We Talk About "Choice"?," where we wrap up the analysis of the different levels of decisions and barriers associated to women's exercising their choices. It includes the identification of gaps in information in the different levels of the ecological framework. Conclusions included in this section are presented under the light of a possible third alternative to look at obstetric choice and how services can strengthen agency and access.

[5] According to Guatemala's public health policies, "skilled birth attendants" include medical doctors and nurses (MSPAS et al. 2017). The terminology used to refer to midwives is more confusing because the ministry of health sometimes refers to "trained midwives" to identify "traditional" birth attendants that have received some form of training on public health standards. Because these standards have changed and been redefined and challenged over time, it is difficult to establish what "trained" means today and how midwives' roles differ from those of other health extension workers trained in the different iterations of expansion of coverage plans. Additionally, the term "traditional" masks the heterogeneity found among Maya and Ladino midwives. For the purpose of this study, the term "lay midwife" will be used to refer to them, following King et al. (2015), p. 126, 141 recommendation.

32.2 Maternal Care Services in Guatemala and Present-Day Indicators

Healthcare services in Guatemala are provided through public and private systems. The public system includes the Ministry of Health (Ministerio de Salud Pública y Asistencia Social), Social Security (Instituto Guatemalteco de Seguridad Social), which provides coverage for people with formal employment, and the Military Health System, which serves the armed forces and operates as a private hospitals for civilian patients. The private sector is composed of for-profit and nonprofit providers, as well as alternative and traditional health practitioners (Ávila et al. 2015). The Ministry of Health is responsible for providing free, universal healthcare coverage and services about 70.0% of the population (OPS 2007). Social Security provides coverage to 17.5%, and an additional 5% of the population has private health insurance (MSPAS 2010). The proportion of the population that depends on services provided by the Ministry of Health is higher in rural areas, where fewer people have formal employment or can afford private coverage. Additionally, it is estimated that 18.0% of the population receive services from nongovernmental organizations (Becerril-Montekio and López-Dávila 2011). Even though only a small percentage of Guatemalans pays for private insurance, as of 2015, 22.0% of health services were provided by private providers and institutions (MSPAS et al. 2017, p. 4). This means that a good proportion of Guatemalans who sought these services payed full price for them.

The public health system is divided into three levels of care facilities managed by 29 administrative areas (Areas de Salud). First-level facilities correspond to health posts and community centers. They offer prenatal and postpartum care, usually provided by an auxiliary nurse,[6] with the help of community volunteers. A total of 1167 first-level facilities were operational in 2016 (MSPAS 2017). Health centers located in municipal seats, maternal and child services, district hospitals, and peripheral clinics are all considered secondary level facilities (MSPAS 2017). These centers are equipped with delivery rooms for attending noncomplicated deliveries and have a few inpatient units that can be utilized for postpartum women. Secondary level facilities also include maternal and child centers that have an emergency, delivery, and operative rooms for women in need of caesarian sections. A total of 346 secondary level facilities were operational in 2016. Third level facilities total 44. They offer full obstetric services (MSPAS 2017). Of these, only two are referral hospitals (Roosevelt and San Juan de Dios hospitals, both in Guatemala City).

Data from the 2014 to 2015 National Maternal and Child Health Survey (Encuesta National de Salud Materno Infantil) reveals that 93.7% of urban and 89.9% of rural women received prenatal care during their last pregnancy. The difference between types of residency is only 3.8%. However, the type of care received indicates a difference in access—while 81.5% of urban women received prenatal care from a medical doctor, only 53.3% of rural women did (MSPAS et al. 2017, p. 209). Rural women received prenatal care from nurses (36.5%) and trained midwives (5.1%) in higher proportions than urban women (MSPAS et al. 2017). The difference between indigenous and nonindigenous women is also worth of note. While 54.0% of indigenous women received prenatal care from a medical doctor, 74.0% of nonindigenous did (MSPAS et al. 2017, p. 207). Important gaps are also observed by level of income and education. Additionally, 97.7% of women at the highest level of income received prenatal care. This was true for only 86.4% of women at the lowest level. Almost all women with a college degree of more received prenatal care (99.6%) versus women without education (84.0%) (MSPAS et al. 2017). Figures 32.1, 32.2, and 32.3 illustrate how, despite increased efforts to improve maternal care services, access is still determined by the demographic factors cited above.

While there is a trend toward increasing utilization of healthcare facilities and seeking skilled birth attendants, there are still important differences in rates between women who live in rural areas and

[6]Auxiliary nurses have a secondary education level and have received 1 year of training as nurses (MSPAS et al. 2017, p. 3).

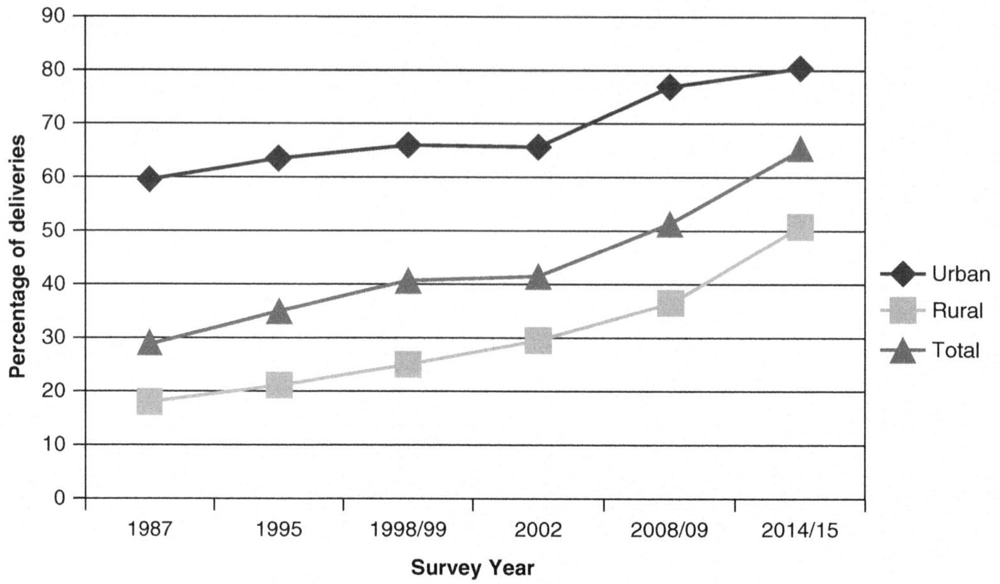

Fig. 32.1 Use of skilled birth attendants by place of residence of the mother, 1987–2015. Data from MSPAS 2010, 2015

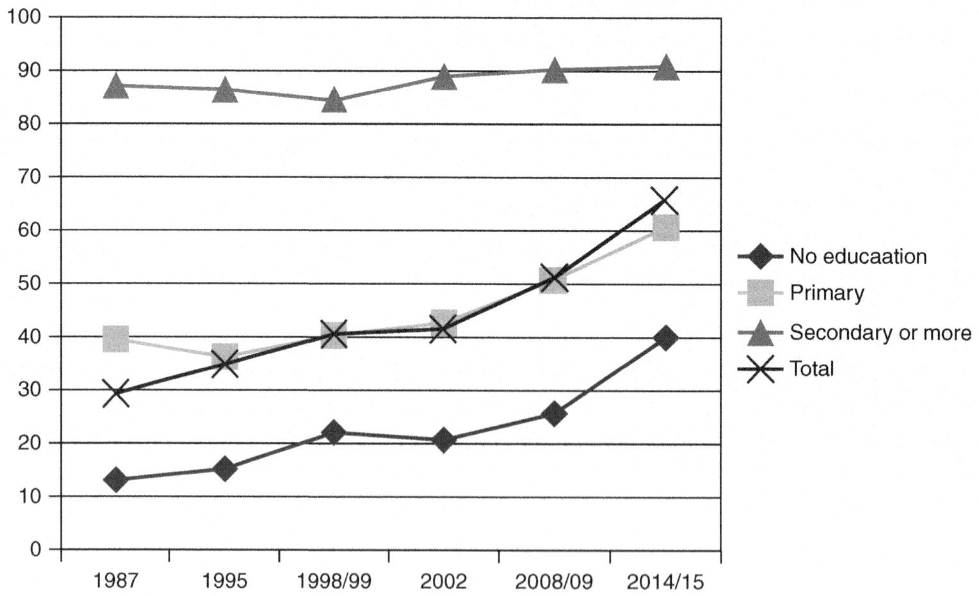

Fig. 32.2 Use of skilled birth attendants by level of education of the mother, 1987–2015. Data from MSPAS 2010, 2015

those who live in urban areas, between indigenous and nonindigenous women, and across groups with different socioeconomic and wealth status (MSPAS et al. 2017). This leads to the question of which factors influence Guatemalan women's decisions regarding their desired type of care during pregnancy and birth. The complex dynamics of contemporary "choice" are addressed in Sects. 32.3 to 32.6. Before focusing on the community-, family-, and individual-based factors, it is important, however, to contextualize recent trends by looking at the history of public obstetric services in Guatemala.

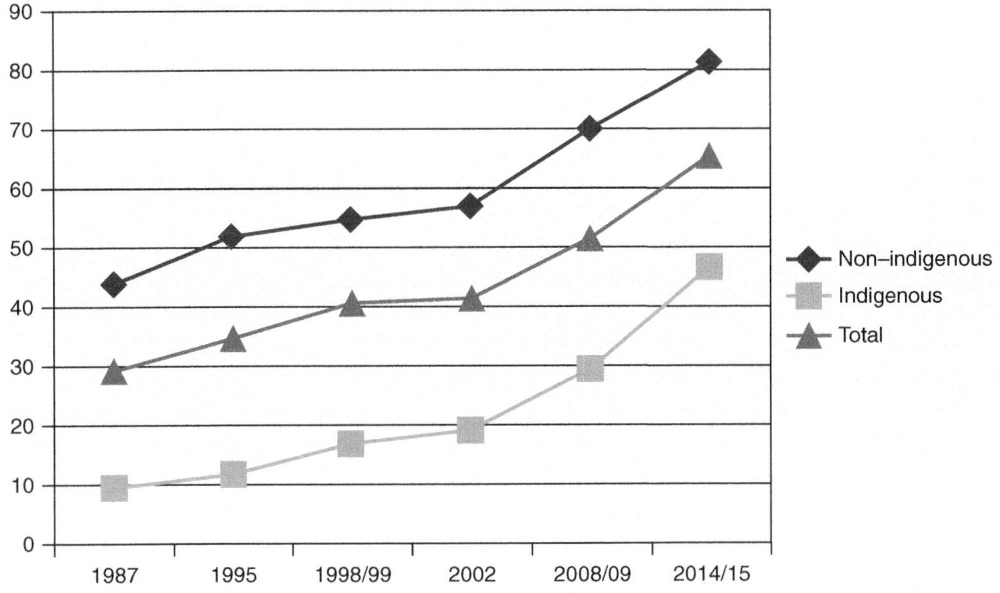

Fig. 32.3 Use of skilled birth attendants by ethnicity of the mother, 1987–2015. Data from MSPAS 2010, 2015

32.3 A Brief History of Public Services and Birth Attendants in Guatemala

The first public policy of the twentieth century concerning the role of lay midwives was published on April 16, 1935 (Governmental Decree, articles 98 and 99). The two articles provide a rare glimpse into the type of public services available to Guatemalans at the time, as well as the challenges to provide coverage in areas outside the capital. Article 98 explains how, in the absence of enough "professional midwives" to cover the needs of the population, "traditional but trained midwives" would be permitted to attend births. The article goes on to clarify that "traditional midwives" needed to be certified by the local sanitation delegation, the municipal mayor, and the governor of the department. Article 99 declares that all "traditional midwives" must respond to the government's summons to be trained. Noncompliance would result in a revocation of authorization to practice their craft (Guatemalan Government 1935, articles 98 and 99, fully cited in Sacayon Sapón 2015). These articles are also relevant because they clearly illustrate how Western-based medicine perceives traditional knowledge. The pressure to "professionalize" lay midwives has persisted through time and, as it is described later in this chapter, continues to be one of the central issues affecting obstetric choice in rural Guatemala today.

The construction of the first public maternity ward began 9 years after the midwives decree was issued. It was planned as part of Hospital Roosevelt, on which construction began in 1944, and at the end of the 13-year dictatorship of Jorge Ubico. The newly elected liberal government of Juan José Arévalo expanded the planned capacity of the hospital. It was completed in 1955, and the maternity ward opened in December of the same year (Prensa Libre 2015).

The period between 1954 and 1985 saw very few changes in terms of expansion of services, quality of care, or considerations to the population's cultural and linguistic diversity (Cazali Avila 2002, p. 108; Becerril-Montekio and López-Dávila 2011, p. 201; Rolhoff and Chary 2015, p. xv). Additionally, very little quantitative data was gathered during the period, leaving considerable gaps in terms of patterns of access and other indicators prior to the mid-1980s. The first Maternal and Child Health Survey took place a year after the first civilian government took office, in 1986, after 15 years of military regimes (Fuentes et al. 2003, p. 2). The change toward a democratic, if weak, regime brought hope to many Guatemalans and promises of expanded coverage for both education and health.

The Peace Accords signed in 1996 specifically addressed the need for reforming the public health sector and emphasized that health services should be available to the entire population. At that time, the Guatemalan government committed to increasing the percentage of the national budget allocated to public health, and in particular, to allocate more resources for preventive services and for strategies aimed to reduce maternal and child mortality (Wikisource 1996). The reforms that were brought about after the signing of the Peace Accords were included in the new Health Code that was established by the National Congress in 1997. The Health Code placed upon the Ministry of Health (MSPAS) the responsibility of ensuring that all of the population had access to health services. In 2003, it was established that these services should be free (Ávila et al. 2015) (Decreto 90–97 1997). The Peace Accords also include agreements about the use of indigenous languages in all public services, recognizing the need to serve the population in their native tongue. This process began in 2000 with the establishment of the Traditional and Alternative Medicine Program, charged with formulating and promoting policies, norms, strategies, and lines of action to value, acknowledge, and respect the knowledge, resources, methods, and practices of traditional and alternative medicine, highlighting the need of developing an intercultural approach to health.

In 2009, the MSPAS created the Unit of Indigenous Populations' Healthcare and Interculturality, the objectives of which were, among others: "To develop the health of Indigenous Populations in Guatemala; To value, recognize, and respect the knowledge, therapeutic elements, methods and practices of indigenous populations' health systems; The modification and evaluation of current health services in order for them to be adapted to indigenous cultures; The strengthening and promotion of indigenous health practices, and; propitiating cultural appropriateness in health at the national level" (Acuerdo Ministerial No. 1632–2009).

The right of a woman to receive culturally appropriate services during her pregnancy, labor, and delivery is included in the Norm for Cultural Appropriateness in Health Services issued by the MSPAS in 2009 (MSPAS 2012b). The norm states, for example, that a woman should be allowed to walk around during labor, if she so wishes; be informed of her choices regarding birthing position; be accompanied by a family member or by a midwife if she so desires; and take the food and beverages that are culturally accepted and that are determined harmless for the mother and the child. Overall, according to the Norm and the Law for Healthy Motherhood, biomedical practitioners at all levels of care should respect every aspect of an indigenous culture—especially those related to the provision of health services. This includes, importantly, acknowledging and respecting the role of indigenous health providers and lay midwives. The rationale for this is that if current health services are not adapted to local cultures and local populations' practices, women are unlikely to trust public health institutions and seek care in these places. This adaptation should include the provision of services in a woman's preferred language. As Fig. 32.4 demonstrates, the Mesoamerican region, including Guatemala, still has large populations of Maya speakers. In Guatemala, there are smaller numbers of speakers of the *Xinca* and *Garifuna* indigenous languages.

The Law for Healthy Motherhood which was issued in 2010 establishes that, among other things, the MSPAS, IGSS, and NGOs hired by MSPAS must guarantee access to maternity and neonatal health services of quality, with cultural appropriateness and without discrimination. It also states that attention by qualified providers is mandatory during prenatal care, delivery, and postpartum care. This same law states that secondary level health centers specialized for providing obstetric care need to be officially incorporated into the public health system. These specialized centers are staffed with physicians, nurses, and auxiliary nurses, and it is mandated by the law that midwives are allowed to participate in deliveries at these facilities.

Increased visibility of these issues resulted in a flurry of activities to implement and operationalize the new norms and policies. Workshops and collaborative interactions with public health services in countries where inclusion policies existed allowed personnel from the Ministry of Health to learn about

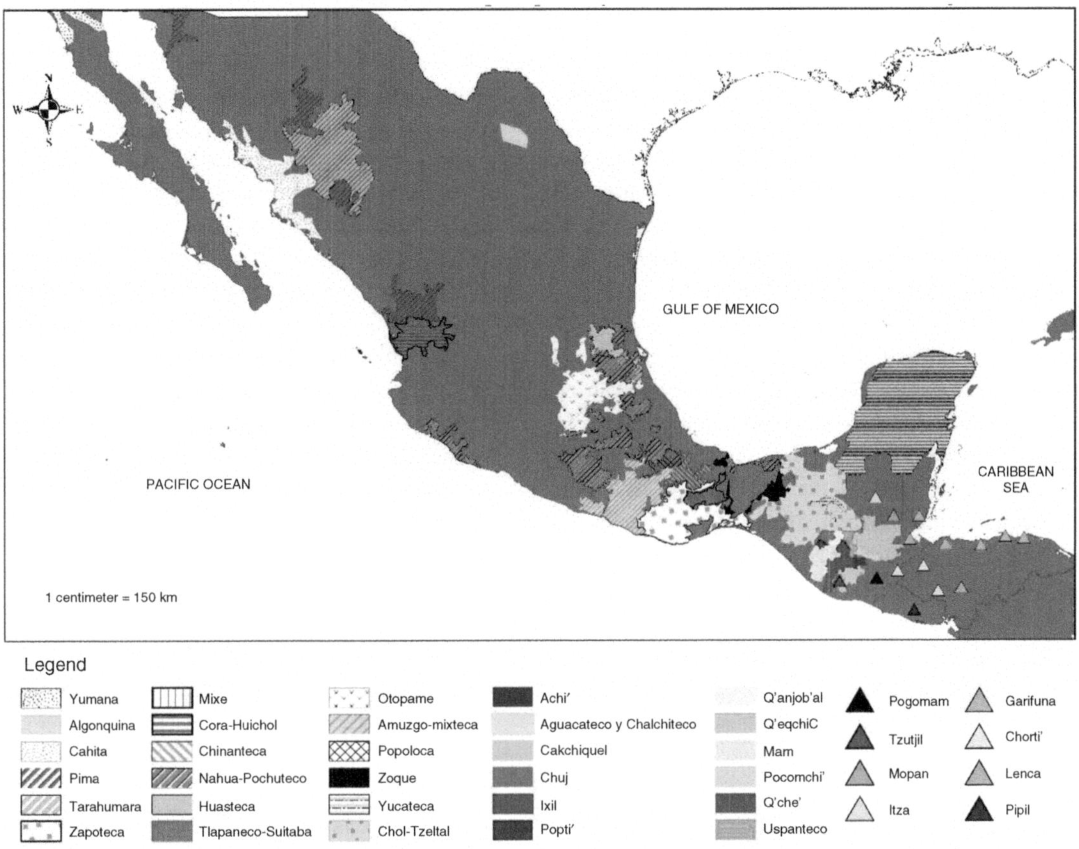

Fig. 32.4 Mesoamerican languages spoken today. Source: Kayayan 2017

these practices and work toward implementing the new mandates (Population Council 2010a). Public medical personnel were expected to attend these training courses and then to ensure that the new norms were implemented in the establishments under their supervision. One of the authors had the opportunity to observe several of these training sessions. The responses from physicians and nurses varied greatly—some recognized the need to make services friendlier and less intimidating to women. Unfortunately, there were those who thought the training sessions were a waste of time, that these norms simply represented more work for the overburdened, understaffed public hospitals and clinics and that indigenous women and midwives should "modernize." Efforts to sensitize service providers and address racism, stigmatization, and discrimination toward indigenous women continue to aim at reducing women's fears of mistreatment as a barrier to health services (see, e.g., Hemmings et al. 2007).

The trend of increasing the use of skilled birth attendants (SBAs) and healthcare facilities for deliveries reflected in the data from ENSMI (Encuesta Nacional de Salud Materno Infantil) was also noticed in a study by (Garcés et al. 2015) that took place in the Chimaltenango area from 2010 to 2013. They found decreases in perinatal mortality, stillbirth rate, and neonatal mortality during that period. There was a rise in use of services which coincided with efforts at the Chimaltenango hospital to subscribe to the new cultural appropriateness norm. According to the authors, there were also improvements in the quality of services provided at the only referral public hospital in that area of the country. This last observation could explain why more indigenous women sought care at that particular facility.

These changes also exemplify complex dynamics noticed in other countries where midwives continue to play an important role in obstetric services (Ginsburg and Rapp 1991, p. 322) despite World's Health Organization (WHO) push to increase the number of births in medical facilities. In Guatemala, 29.1% of deliveries were attended by "trained" midwives (per live births in 5 years previous to the last ENSMI) (MSPAS et al. 2017, p. 218). The number of reported home births was even higher, at 34.4% (MSPAS et al. 2017). As the following section illustrates, the relationship between public services and lay midwives varies and is dependent on factors beyond the existence of laws. For example, midwives are still not counted as "qualified" personnel. The arguments of the 1935 laws therefore speak to realities that have somewhat changed in form but have remained structurally true: the government of Guatemala is yet to achieve universal coverage of services, and the reasons why women choose to give birth at home are informed by different factors including culturally specific concepts of birth (Berry 2010). From a biomedical and public health perspective, it is assumed that these limits in coverage constitute challenges that can be solved by involving midwives and aligning their practices with the approach espoused by the MSPAS. While recognizing its gaps and shortcomings, the same system that proposes the incorporation of midwives depends on the will and capacity of medical practitioners to accept the presence of midwives in the public health arena. Midwives are then expected to promote the use of public services among rural women, receive training from the Ministry, and yet accept that their services will continue to be considered less desirable than Western-based ones. This dissonance is developed in the next section.

32.4 Local Knowledge, Cultural, and Economic Aspects Affecting Obstetric Choices

The contribution of anthropology as a discipline to understanding pregnancy and birth around the world began with a focus on cross-cultural studies focusing on beliefs and practices. Only later studies began to address issues of power dynamics within and beyond the household (Ginsburg and Rapp 1991, p. 312). In Guatemala, anthropological studies evolved in a similar pattern, with older studies highlighting cross-cultural comparisons that focused on specific practices, to later give preference to a more critical approach to the issue in the wider context of public policy, discrimination, power relations, the role of development organizations, and multinational corporations (Ginsburg and Rapp 1991) including the continuing expansion of different forms of privatized medical practices (Rolhoff and Chary 2015; Chary and Rohloff 2015) and the different ways in which authoritative knowledge impacts the exercise of obstetric choice in rural, indigenous communities (Cosminsky 2016)

The history of medical anthropology in Guatemala is also characterized by a strong applied focus, beginning in the 1950s, and led by Professor Richard N. Adams, a Professor of Anthropology at the University of Texas at Austin. Engaging anthropologists to understand traditional beliefs was considered necessary to design programs to "modernize" indigenous populations and is aligned with the wider, regional "indigenismo" movement of the time. Monographs and papers published in the 1950s and 1960s included brief descriptions of public services available in communities under study at the time. These present a picture which is not unlike current descriptions of existing services in rural Guatemala. For example, Solien de Gonzalez (1963) work in San Antonio la Paz, el Progreso, in 1957, describes a town without public or private health services and a population that did not access those nearby but preferred to travel to Guatemala City to obtain care in public hospitals when conditions deemed it necessary (Solien de Gonzalez 1963, p. 413). The application of anthropological methods to improve provision of services is still relied on today in some programs aimed at improving access to services and quality of care. One example is the Pan-American Social Marketing Organisation (PASMO[7]) PEER study. Their PEER study (Participatory Ethnographic Evaluation and Research)

[7]PASMO is an NGO dedicated to social marketing of HIV prevention and FP products and services.

among young indigenous men and women (Hemmings et al. 2007) is a recent example of this continuing relationship between anthropologists and public health experts.

Not all medical anthropological research of the 1950s through the 1970s included details on pregnancy, birth, and midwifery and its relation to the public health system (Paul and Paul, The Maya Midwife as Sacred Specialist: A Guatemalan Case, 1975), so existing knowledge of the time is partial. The work of Lois and Benjamin Paul helps fill some of the gaps left by public and official documents regarding the role of midwives in the period between the establishment of the national health system and the various efforts of the two last decades to improve maternal and child health (Paul 1975; Paul and Paul 1975). Their work presents a context far wider and more complex than the depictions of midwives and their roles given in government or public health documents. It describes a wider spectrum of responsibilities, including spiritual ones (Paul and Paul 1975, p. 708). It is through their work that we know that the 1935 law of midwives passed at a time when midwives in San Pedro la Laguna, the location where the Pauls conducted their fieldwork through the years, prenatal and postnatal visits totalled approximately 18 per pregnancy. Their estimates, based on participant observation and their own community census, indicated that midwives worked almost part-time serving pregnant women and their newborns. The level of effort invested by Pedrano midwives continued to be very high in the following decades, with some of them seeing over 100 women per year (Paul and Paul 1975, p. 713). Their studies included comparisons to data from other ethnographers who worked in rural Guatemala from the late 1930s until the 1960s. Based on these studies, it is possible to see partial pictures of what pregnancy and birth looked like, including the already heterogeneous nature of midwifery in Guatemala. While the Pauls documented very specialized practices and a favorable social status of midwives in San Pedro, studies from other areas of Guatemala and Chiapas pointed to different dynamics, including the social standing of midwives (respected members of the community versus feared or pitied women), their sources of knowledge (divine revelation versus practical experience), their spiritual tasks (leader of birth rituals versus none), their average workload (almost part-time to a few cases per year), and their age (late 30s versus mid-50s and older) (Paul and Paul 1975, pp. 714–6). These studies demonstrated that while practices varied, practically all women in rural communities were served by midwives or female relatives. These monographs and papers, however, did not include much on how women and their families decided on who would care for them during pregnancy and birth. A few studies mention some women delivering in public hospitals (Solien de Gonzalez 1963, p. 413) to reduce the risk of maternal death (Solien de Gonzalez 1963), so it is possible to assume that some midwives referred women or families of pregnant women made the decision to opt for hospital care. None of the authors of the time provide specific numbers regarding maternal and child death in their areas of work nor did they interview women regarding their perceptions of risk during pregnancy or other decision-making factors. Therefore, it is impossible to ascertain whether the changes brought by the different attempts to include midwives as "collaborators" of the public health services had an impact vis-à-vis maternal and child mortality rates from the 1950s to the 1980s.

Medical anthropological studies of pregnancy and birth in Guatemala evolved to include more ecological approaches to understanding the issue (see, e.g., Mosquera and Paredes Marín 2008; Mosquera Saravia 2006; Berry 2010), as well as analyses of the growing medicalization of birth even in remote rural communities (Cosminsky 2016). Some of these studies have added elements of analysis such as national and regional statistics to contextualize ethnographic data. For example, Berry (2010) explains how municipal-level indicators, calculated based on populations of 100,000, look very differently vis-à-vis the actual numbers of maternal deaths in a given year in a specific area. Several current anthropological studies are complemented by some demographic analyses that, while relying mostly on national survey data, do focus on levels of choice at the individual, household, and community level (Pembley et al., 1996) to illustrate the complexities of choice.

Relevant recent additions to the knowledge base regarding choice include the analysis of agency among midwives as they navigate present-day opportunities and challenges vis-à-vis public health expectations and demands and other competing services (King et al. 2015). The dynamics between midwives and the state are also pointed out by Mosquera Saravia (2006) in her study of midwives in Rabinal. She illustrates how current conceptions of what a midwife is and does have changed over time to encompass elements associated with public health. For example, they are expected to carry a MSPAS identification to demonstrate they are registered with the ministry and have gone through official training. Notions of certification also affect women's choice because symbols of authority and validation, like an officially issued ID, are more prevalent now and may influence how younger generations, including pregnant women, decide on a midwife to provide them care. Changes in preferences around pregnancy and birth can be appreciated by looking at the most recent ENSMI (MSPAS et al. 2017) where trends in preferences vary across generations.

Gender roles continue to differentiate how indigenous men and women interact with public institutions, information, and people outside their family and neighbors. Puberty reduces girls' mobility (Population Council 2010b), and marriage and childbearing change the status of women. Fertility is still valued (Hemmings et al. 2007) even though the desired number of children has decreased consistently since reproductive health services became available in public facilities in the 1990s.While the role of men in choice and decision-making is absent from most studies (Ginsburg and Rapp 1991, p. 328), research by some authors including Berry (2010) and (Pebley et al. 1996) constitute important contributions to understanding the multilayered factors affecting how women and their newborns are cared for. Additionally, over the years, ENSMI has included more questions regarding women's decision-making processes thus providing an additional, though indirect, source of information on how the husband and his family participate in these events. The role of men in making decisions related to health is also linked to control of economic resources. Men control family finances, and cost is taken into account when deciding whether to seek services in public clinics and hospitals or not.

Finally, regarding the involvement of family members, generational dynamics give mothers-in-law an important role in the decision-making processes affecting the couple (Hemmings et al. 2007) and who cares for their pregnant daughter-in-law (Berry 2010). Understanding the extended family context among indigenous people and its influence in the health decision-making context is important to comprehend why choosing one type of service over another is more complex than simply accepting the messages promoted by the health center.

Regarding the choice about where to give birth, there is an increasing trend toward using healthcare facilities. This is illustrated in Figs. 32.1, 32.2, and 32.3 in the first section of the chapter, represented by the use of skilled birth attendants (almost all births attended by skill personnel are attended in a healthcare facility and not at home). There is still, however, a proportion of the population that prefers to give birth at home. According to data from the latest ENSMI (MSPAS et al. 2017), more indigenous women gave birth at home than non-indigenous (49.7% versus 17.9%), and the proportion was also higher for rural areas compared to urban areas (44.3% versus 16.6%). Figure 32.5 shows that a higher proportion of women over 40 years of age chose to have a home birth, compared to women in younger age groups. This difference might be explained by the fact that women who have had previous positive experiences with giving birth at home prefer to do so again and that obstetric choice is not only influenced by external factors (education campaigns, promotion of health services utilization) but also by women's prior experiences (Berry 2010). Vertical birth, while a right, is still discouraged by medical professionals during training sessions with midwives (Mosquera Saravia 2006, p. 58), and vertical birth techniques are not routinely taught to physicians. This might explain why, although it is encouraged by maternal health policies, the rate of vertical birth is still low.

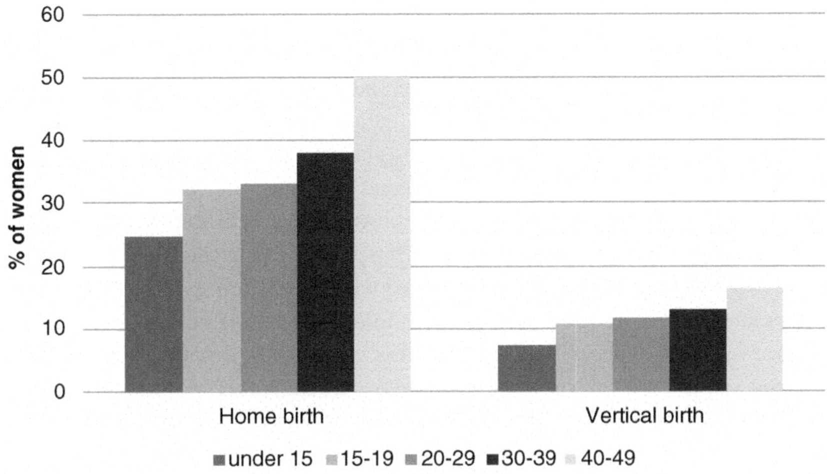

Fig. 32.5 Select characteristics of birth by age of women. Data from ENSMI 2014–2015 (MSPAS et al. 2017)

32.5 "Choice" at the Community Level: Biomedical Views on Barriers to Services

Obstetric choices were presented in the previous section from the perspectives of women, family members, and midwives. The view "from the community" is now contrasted to public health views as manifested in public policy, arguments, and analysis by biomedical professionals charged with improving Guatemala's indicators associated to pregnancy, birth, and postpartum care of women and newborns.

The obstetric referral route states that a patient should enter the public health system through a first-level facility and, if warranted, be referred to a center of higher complexity. There are, however, multiple factors that limit the functionality of the referral system. It is often complicated to get transportation from a community to a healthcare facility. Ambulances are not available at primary level health posts, so patients have to travel there by their own means, or seek help from their families or from members of their community. The situation at secondary level health centers is not much better, as there is not always an ambulance available at every clinic (Ávila et al. 2015). Even when transportation is available, traveling to a healthcare facility where there is a skilled attendant with adequate equipment can take hours. In 2015, it was estimated that more than 20% of the Guatemalan population lived more than 5 km away from any MPSAS healthcare facility (Ávila et al. 2015); this proportion increases when the distance from a facility staffed and equipped for delivery attention is considered. All these limitations lead not only to potentially significant delays in care but also represent additional expenses for patients, who often need to cover the costs of transportation.

A review of determinants of delivery service use in low- and middle-income countries by Gabrysch and Campbell (2009) identified 20 such determinants grouped in four different categories: sociocultural factors, perceived benefit/need of skilled attendance, economic accessibility, and physical accessibility. Within the economic accessibility category, there are almost always moderate to large differences in seeking service from skilled birth attendants between women who reside in urban or rural areas. Gabrysch and Campbell's proposed hypothesis is that in rural areas, services may be of lower quality, there is more poverty, and there are more traditional beliefs. In Guatemala in 2014, the percentage of indigenous households experiencing multidimensional poverty was 69.8%, significantly higher than that of "mestizo" and "other" (41.9%) (ICEFI 2012, p. 36). This difference in income might explain why there is a lower utilization of healthcare facilities among rural, indigenous populations.

In one of the authors' experience from performing rotations at a clinic in the rural area, women would give several reasons why they preferred not giving birth at a public healthcare facility. From the author's point of view, women and their families often understood the need for being referred to a higher-level facility when the clinical situation mandated it. Traditional midwives working in the area and who were familiar with the clinic's staff would bring in the women in a timely way and help explain the patient's situation and the need for transfer. Even in those complicated cases where the women and their families understood the importance of getting more specialized care, they would express their concerns about going to a hospital. Among the reasons they mentioned more frequently were that they would not be allowed to be with their families, they feared being mistreated by the hospital's staff, and they would be in an unfamiliar and hostile environment without personalized attention. Also, even though the clinic is in an area close to the Spanish-speaking capital, a good part of the women spoke only their indigenous language, *Kaqchikel*. Although the law (MSPAS 2012a, 2012b) states that it is mandatory to provide health services in the patient's native language, this is thought to rarely occur. The language barrier is also frequently mentioned as a reason why indigenous women don't seek care in hospitals. Similar forms of mistreatment were documented in a qualitative study about discrimination toward indigenous people in public healthcare facilities (Cerón et al. 2016).

There were cases, however, when attention would be sought too late or not at all. The reasons for this would be the previously mentioned physical access barriers such as lack of transportation or living too far from any healthcare facility. Also, noted by the author and mentioned in the literature, the decision of seeking care for a pregnant woman is not always hers but depends on what her husband or other family members think is best. These are several of the classic factors involved in the Three Delays Model of maternal mortality. A report on the use of healthcare facilities for obstetric emergencies in the department of Izabal mentions: "Within this barrier (referring to a cultural barrier) it is important to include the persistence of machismo as a prejudicial element in women's health. Decision making about how to respond to emergencies during delivery is strongly affected by two factors: the cost of transportation and the value that is placed on the woman. These two factors cannot be addressed separately, because during the interviews, participants always proposed a very tight link between one and the other: the husband decides to take the risk of having the woman die during birth, because the elevated cost of transportation to a hospital puts the family in a difficult position" (PRRAC 2004, unpublished document).

Guatemalan-trained medical doctors usually have little or no knowledge about non-biomedical healthcare practices, even though they are exposed to patients who come from very diverse cultural backgrounds. Discrimination toward indigenous patients and their health practices is prevalent among physicians (Ginsburg and Rapp 1991, p. 323). It is fair to say that healthcare practitioners often feel frustrated when they face resistance from their patients regarding therapeutic actions that make more sense from a biomedical point of view. Not being aware of language and cultural differences makes communication difficult and often leads physicians and other healthcare providers to believe that indigenous patients are stubborn or are not interested in improving their health. From the patients' point of view, this creates an environment of mistrust toward state institutions, mistreatment of women, and absence of care providers who speak women's languages when it is not Spanish (Shiffman and Garcés del Valle 2006, p. 65)

32.6 Can We Talk About "Choice"?

It is risky to talk about obstetric choice without specifying the context and conditions under which most Guatemalan women give birth nowadays. Additionally, as previous sections have illustrated, the analysis of choice is incomplete when studies miss important units of analysis, like the family or individual women themselves. Studies like Berry's (2010) and Pebley's (1996) are very important contributions to the issue because of their inclusion of the complexities of household level decisions in their research. Also, importantly, these and a few other studies highlight the importance of acknowledging that choice is also happening in a context of social and economic change (Pebley et al. 1996, p. 231). Midwives, still the principal providers of care in many rural indigenous communities in Guatemala, remain today a heterogeneous group of women representing a range of knowledge, community-level standing, and responsibilities. Midwives themselves are exercising choice by rejecting, adopting, interpreting, and adapting resources and information offered by the public and nongovernmental entities interested in reducing maternal and child mortality (King et al. 2015).

Applied anthropological literature of the 1950s already recommended that cultural practices be taken into account in healthcare service provision. Recent applied ethnographic studies confirm the importance of understanding aspects beyond the specific health issues addressed when analyzing how both women and men make health-related decisions and when it comes to providing viable choices for them. For example, issues like confidentiality and the preference for discretion and anonymity can make the difference between gaining women's trust and perpetuating feelings of misunderstanding and mistreatment (Hemmings et al. 2007; Berry 2008).

It is necessary not only to make services and information accessible to the entire population but also make sure that they are offered in ways that encourage agency and allow women to understand them and take advantage of opportunities. Increasing the number of healthcare facilities and trained medical personnel should be accompanied by efforts in improving the understanding and acceptance of traditional or indigenous practices by biomedical practitioners. It is important to keep in mind that barriers are not all addressed by improving technology and availability of more modernized services. Some traditional practices continue to provide more comprehensive care than even that received by women with higher education and those who belong to the higher income strata. While respecting communities' and families' practices, it is also important to remain critical of those barriers that limit choice making at the different individual, family, community, and wider public levels.

References

ACCESA. (2015). *El acceso universal a la salud, algunos elementos para la discusión*. Guatemala: Serviprensa. Retrieved from http://icefi.org/sites/default/files/el_acceso_universal_a_la_salud.pdf.

Adams, W. R., & Hawkins, J. P. (2007). *Health care in Maya Guatemala: Confronting medical pluralism in a developing country*. Norman, OK: University Oklahoma Press.

Ávila, C., Bright, R., Gutiérrez, J. C., Hoadley, K., Manuel, C., & Romero, N. (2015). *Guatemala, Análisis del Sistema de Salud 2015*. Bethesda, MD: Proyecto Health Finance and Governance, Abt Associates Inc..

Becerril-Montekio, V., & López-Dávila, L. (2011). Sistema de Salud en Guatemala. *Salud Pública de México, 53*(2), S197–S208.

Berry, N. S. (2008). Who's judging the quality of care? Indigenous Maya and the problem of "not being attended.". *Medical Anthropology, 27*(2), 164–189. https://doi.org/10.1080/01459740802017413.

Berry, N. S. (2010). *Unsafe motherhood. Mayan maternal mortality and subjectivity in post-war Guatemala*. New York, NY: Berghahn Books.

Bruce, J. (2016). The difficulties of "living while girl". *Journal of Virus Eradication, 2*(3), 177–182.

Cazali Avila, A. (2002). *Los militares en el poder: el gobierno de Carlos Arana Osorio*. Universidad San Carlos de Guatemala, Dirección General de Investigación. Guatemala: Universidad San Carlos de Guatemala.

Cecchini, S., & Azócar, I. (2007). *Indicadores de los Objetivos de Desarrollo del Milenio en América Latina y el Caribe: una comparación entre datosnacionales e internacionales*. Santiago de Chile: CEPAL/ONU.

Cerón, A., Ruano, A. L., Sánchez, S., Chew, A. S., Díaz, D., Hernández, A., et al. (2016). Abuse and discrimination towards indigenous people in public health care facilities: Experiences from rural Guatemala. *International Journal for Equity in Health, 15*(1), 77. https://doi.org/10.1186/s12939-016-0367-z

Chary, A., & Rohloff, P. (2015). *Privatization and the new medical pluralism*. Lanham, MD: Lexington Books.

Cosminsky, S. (2016). *Midwives and mothers. The medicalization of childbirth on a Guatemalan plantation*. Austin, TX: University of Texas Press.

Davis-Floyd, R., Sergant, C. (1996). Introduction: The social production of authoritative knowledge in pregnancy and childbirth. Medical Anthropology Quarterly, 10(2), 111–120. Retrieved September 4, 2016, from http://www.jstor.org/stable/649323.

Fuentes, J. A., Balsells, E., & Arriola, G. (2003). *Guatemala: Human development progress towards the MDGs at the sub National Level. United Nations development programme*. Guatemala: UNDP.

Garces, A., Mcclure, E. M., Hambidge, K., Krebs, N. F., Figueroa, L., Aguilar, M., et al. (2015). Trends in perinatal deaths from 2010 to 2013 in the Guatemalan Western Highlands. *Reproductive Health, 12*(Suppl 2), S14. https://doi.org/10.1186/1742-4755-12-S2-S14

Gabrysch, S., & Campbell, O. M. (2009). Still too far to walk: Literature review of the determinants of delivery service use. *BMC Pregnancy and Childbirth, 9*(1), 34. https://doi.org/10.1186/1471-2393-9-34.

Ginsburg, F., & Rapp, R. (1991). The politics of reproduction. *Annual Review of Anthropology, 20*, 311–343.

Hemmings, J., Nieto-Andrade, B., Rivas, J. R., & Longfield, K. (2007). *Bajo el poncho-Pillow talk: Relationships and sexuality among indigenous peoples in Guatemala. Results from a PEER/FoQus study*. Guatemala: Options Consultancy Services Ltd and PASMO Guatemala.

ICEFI. (2012). ¡Quiero crecer con mamá! *Boletín Contamos* (9), ICEFI, Guatemala.

ICEFI, UNICEF. (2016). *Pobreza multidimencional infantil y adolescente en Guatemala: privaciones a superar*. Guatemala: ICEFI.

Kayayan, V. (2017). *Principales idiomas mesoamericanos hablados hasta el siglo XXI*. Proyecto Mesoamérica (poner aquí el nombre oficial del proyecto). Population Council, Guatemala [not yet published].

King, N., Chary, A., & Rohloff, P. (2015). Leveraging resources in contemporary Maya midwifery. In A. Chary & P. Rohloff (Eds.), *Privatization and the new medical pluralism* (pp. 125–141). Lanham, MD: Lexington Books.

Prensa Libre. (2015, November 11). El entonces resplandeciente Hospital Roosevelt. *Prensa Libre*.

Ministerio de Salud Pública y Asistencia Social (MSPAS). (2010). Encuesta Nacional de Salud Materno Infantil 2008 (ENSMI-2008/09). Ministerio de Salud Pública y Asistencia Social (MSPAS)/Instituto Nacional de Estadística (INE)/Centros de Control y Prevención de Enfermedades (CDC). Guatemala.

Ministerio de Salud Pública y Asistencia Social (MSPAS). (2012a). *Diagnóstico Nacional de Salud*. Guatemala: MSPAS.

Ministerio de Salud Pública y Asistencia Social (MSPAS). (2012b). *Normas con Pertinencia Cultural*. Guatemala: MSPAS.

Ministerio de Salud Pública y Asistencia Social (MSPAS). (2015). *Situación de la mortalidad materna: informe de país 2013*. Retrieved from http://www.osarguatemala.org/Archivos/PDF/201510/255_3.pdf.

Ministerio de Salud Pública y Asistencia Social (MSPAS). (2017). *Ministerio de Salud Pública y Asistencia Social*. Retrieved January 29, 2017, from http://www.mspas.gob.gt/index.php/institucional/acerca-del-mspas.

Ministerio de Salud Pública y Asistencia Social (MSPAS), Instituto Nacional de Estadística (INE), & Segelpán. (2017). *VI Encuesta nacional de salud materno infantil 2014–2015. Informe final*. Guatemala: MSPAS INE ICF.

Mosquera, M. T., Paredes Marín, V. H. (2008). Legislación de la medicina alternativa en Guatemala. Criterios de "validez" y "cientificidad" desde la perspectiva de los grupos étnicos en Guatemala. Universidad de San Carlos de Guatemala, Dirección General de Investigación, Instituto de Estudios Interétnicos, Programa de Investigación: Cultura, Pensamiento y Sociedad Guatemalteca, Guatemala. Obtenido de Retrieved from http://digi.usac.edu.gt/bvirtual/informes/cultura/INF-2008-052.pdf.

Mosquera Saravia, M. T. (2006). *Lógicas y racionalidades: entre comadronas y terapeutas traditionales*. Guatemala: IDEI-USAC Serviprensa S.A.

Pan American Health Organization (OPS). (1995). *Clasificación estadística internacional de enfermedades y problemas relacionados con la salud*. Washington, DC: OPS.

Pan American Health Organization (OPS) (2007, February). *Health systems profile Guatemala, 2007* (3rd ed.). Washington, DC: PAHO Retrievied from http://new.paho.org/hq/dmdocuments/2010/Health_System_Profile-Guatemala_2007.pdf.

Paul, L. (1975). Recruitment to a ritual role: The midwife in a Maya community. *Ethos, 3*(3), 449–467.

Paul, L., & Paul, B. D. (1975). The Maya midwife as sacred specialist: A Guatemalan case. *American Ethnologist, 2*(4), 707–726.

Pebley, A. R., Goldman, N., & Germán, R. (1996). Prenatal and delivery care and childhood immunization in Guatemala: Do family and community matter? *Demography, 33*(2), 231–247.

Population Council. (2010a). *Mejora de la salud materna de mujeres indígenas y garífunas a través de políticas públicas con enfoque de derechos e interculturalidad*. Guatemala: Population Council.

Population Council. (2010b). *Guatemala rising one girl at a time: Findings from the 2009–2010 evaluation*. Guatemala: Population Council.

Rolhoff, P., & Chary, A. (2015). Introduction. In A. Chary & P. Rolhoff (Eds.), *Privatization and the new medical pluralism* (pp. xiii–xxxi). Lanham, MD: Lexington Books.

PRRAC 2004 (Proyecto Salud). (2004). *Informe de Avances*. Preparado por: Alejandra Colom. Guatemala, Guatemala.

Sacayon Sapón, C. A. (2015). *Condiciones de ingreso de pacientes referidas por comadronas*. Tesis Presentada ante las autoridades de la Escuela de Estudios de Postgrado de la Facultad de Ciencias Médicas Maestría en Ciencias Médicas con Especialidad en Ginecología y Obstetricia.

Schensul, J. J., & LeCompte, M. D. (1999). *Ethnographer's toolkit*. Walnut Creek, CA: Altamira Press.

Segeplan. (2015). *Informe final de cumplimiento de los Objetivos de Desarrollo del Milenio*. Guatemala: Segeplan.

Shiffman, J., & Garcés del Valle, A. L. (2006). Political history and disparities in safe motherhood between Guatemala and Honduras. *Population and Development Review, 32*(1), 53–80.

Solien de Gonzalez, N. (1963). Some aspects of child-bearing and child-rearing in a Guatemalan Ladino community. *Southwestern Journal of Anthropology, 19*(4), 411–423.

Wikisource. (1996). *Acuerdo sobre Aspectos Socieconómicos y Situación Agraria*. Guatemala. Retrieved from https://es.wikisource.org/wiki/Acuerdo_sobre_aspectos_socioecon%C3%B3micos_y_situaci%C3%B3n_agraria.

Family Planning Methods Among Mayan Women in Guatemala and the Challenges Facing the Indigenous Population

33

Julia Festa and Taraneh Shirazian

33.1 Guatemala's Population

As of 2013, there were more than 15 million people living in Guatemala, making it the most populous country in Central America (UNICEF 2015; MSPAS 2011). Out of the population of 15 million, 40–50% are indigenous Mayan, and 3.9 million are women between the reproductive ages of 15 and 49 years (Haub and Gribble 2011).

It has been suggested that Guatemala's ever-increasing population is a result of the country's high fertility rate and reduction in general mortality (MSPAS 2011). Guatemala's rate of maternal mortality, however, remains the highest in Central America as 1 out of every 170 women die due to preventable childbirth complications (Haub and Gribble 2011). This statistic, however, has been shown to differ among different ethnicities in Guatemala.

There are two major ethnic identities in Guatemala: the *Ladinos* and the Mayans. The *Ladino* population is made up of those who have full or partial descent from European and/or African populations and those from Mayan descent who have abandoned traditional indigenous language and culture in favor of a more western outlook (Matthew 2006). The indigenous or Mayan population is composed of those individuals who have ancestral connections to the precolonial Maya or *Xinca* groups and still practice indigenous language and culture (Matthew 2006) (Fig. 33.1). It is estimated that maternal mortality rate is three times greater among the indigenous community where many women choose to give birth at home with the aid of an unskilled traditional birth attendant (TBA) (Schooley et al. 2009; Chomat et al. 2014; Lemus 2016).

As governments from developing nations and global health nongovernment organizations (NGOs) continue to combat maternal mortality through interventions that focus on the preventable causes of

J. Festa, B.A. (✉)
Warren Alpert Medical School, Brown University, Providence, RI, USA

Saving Mothers, New York City, NY, USA
e-mail: julia_festa@brown.edu

T. Shirazian, M.D., F.A.C.O.G.
Saving Mothers, New York, NY, USA

Department of Obstetrics and Gynecology, New York University School of Medicine and NYU Langone Medical Center, New York, NY, USA

D. A. Schwartz (ed.), *Maternal Death and Pregnancy-Related Morbidity Among Indigenous Women of Mexico and Central America*, Global Maternal and Child Health: Medical, Anthropological, and Public Health Perspectives, https://doi.org/10.1007/978-3-319-71538-4_33

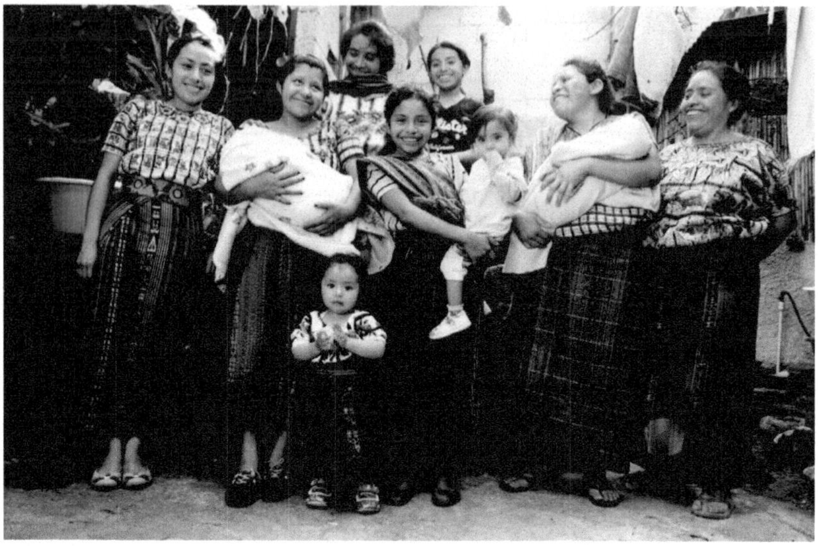

Fig. 33.1 Indigenous women and children in traditional attire

maternal death during labor, there is evidence that indicates the increased use of family planning methods and proper birth-spacing could also help lower maternal mortality rates (Norton 2005; MSPAS 2011; Kestler et al. 2011; Chomat et al. 2014). Given this connection, it is not surprising that indigenous Mayan women, who statistically are using contraceptives less and giving birth more, are experiencing higher rates of maternal mortality when compared to their nonindigenous *Ladino* counterparts in Guatemala (MSPAS 2011).

As with many aspects of health and health care, sociological factors often play a prominent role in the health decisions and outcomes of an individual (Marmot et al. 2008). In order to fully understand the disparities that exist between contraceptive use and maternal mortality rates among Mayan and *Ladino* women, it is imperative to first understand the different sociological environments of these respective populations.

33.2 Socioeconomic Environment and Education Levels of Mayan Women

Guatemala's landscape can be divided into eight major regions. Indigenous groups are concentrated in the more rural areas such as the Northern (2), Central (5), Southwest (6), and Northwest (7) regions of the country (Fig. 33.2). In contrast, *Ladinos* are prevalent in the more metropolitan areas such as Guatemala City (1), as well as the Northeastern (3) and Southeastern (4) regions of the country. Petén (8) is a highly rural region of the country that is equally populated by both ethnicities (MSPAS 2011).

In Guatemala, there is a correlation between areas of residence and wealth. Those individuals who live in rural regions are more likely to be found in the lower wealth quintiles, which are composite measures of a person's living standard based on that individual's assets, expenditures, and access to basic necessities (MSPAS 2011; Demographic and Healthy Surveys Program 2016). Indigenous women, who are more concentrated in these impoverished rural regions, have higher rates of poverty, illiteracy, and infant and maternal mortality when compared to their *Ladino* counterparts (Lindstrom and Muñoz-Franco 2005, Figs. 33.3 and 33.4). A national study conducted in 2009 by the Guatemalan Ministry of Health revealed that 64% of sexually active indigenous women lived in rural areas, compared to only 38% of sexually active *Ladino* women (Ishida et al. 2012; MSPAS 2011). In the same year, 32% of sexually active indigenous women were in the lowest household wealth quintile, com-

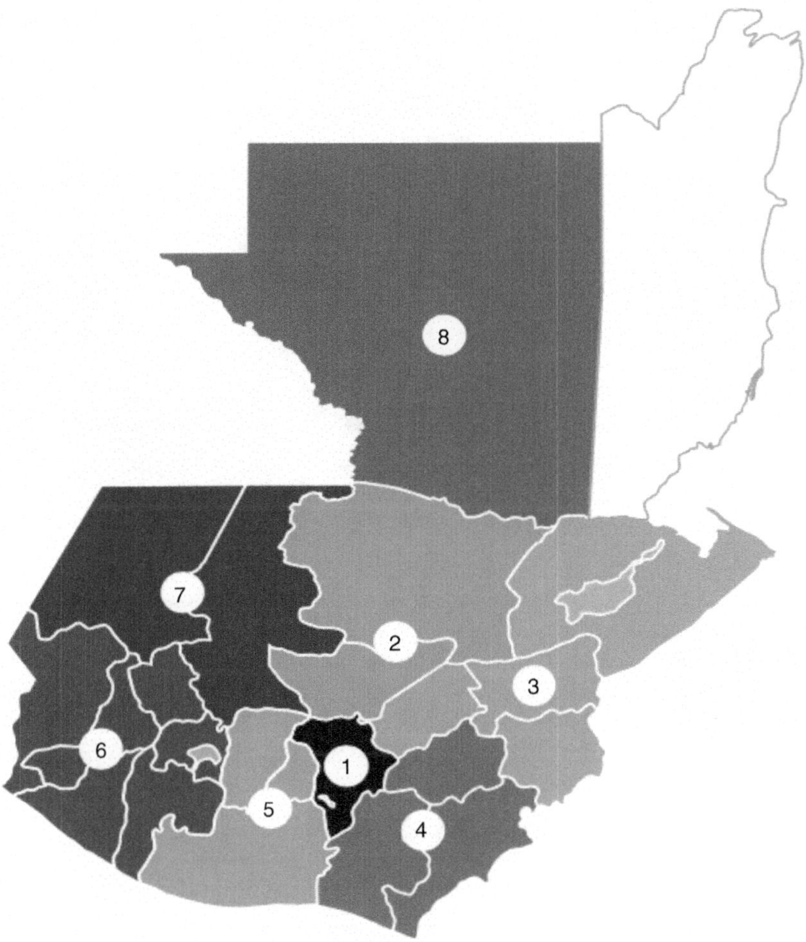

Fig. 33.2 Guatemala numerically divided into its eight regions (MSPAS 2011)

pared to only 8% of *Ladino* women. In fact, in 2006 it was found that 75.7% of the indigenous population was living in poverty, and 27.6% of the indigenous population was living in extreme poverty which is almost double the national average (World Bank 2009). To put these percentages into perspective, in the same year, the World Bank defined extreme poverty as living on $1.25 or less per day. That number has increased to $1.90 per day by the year 2015 (World Bank 2015). While poverty has decreased among nonindigenous groups, poverty levels among the indigenous population have remained the same (World Bank 2009) (Figs. 33.3 and 33.4).

These differences in residence and wealth among the Mayan and *Ladino* populations seem to be highly correlated with rates of contraceptive use. A Guatemala Ministry of Health study found that only 25.8% of women in the lowest wealth quintile use a form of modern contraception compared to 61.8% of women in the highest wealth quintile (MSPAS 2011) (Fig. 33.5). According to the World Health Organization (WHO), contraception methods that are considered to be modern include oral hormonal pills, intrauterine devices (IUDs), male and female condoms, hormonal injections, implants, male and female sterilization, lactational amenorrhea method, emergency contraception, standard days method, basal body temperature method, TwoDay Method, and Sympto-Thermal Method (World Health Organization 2015). Contraceptive methods that are considered traditional include the rhythm method and the coitus interruptus method (World Health Organization 2015).

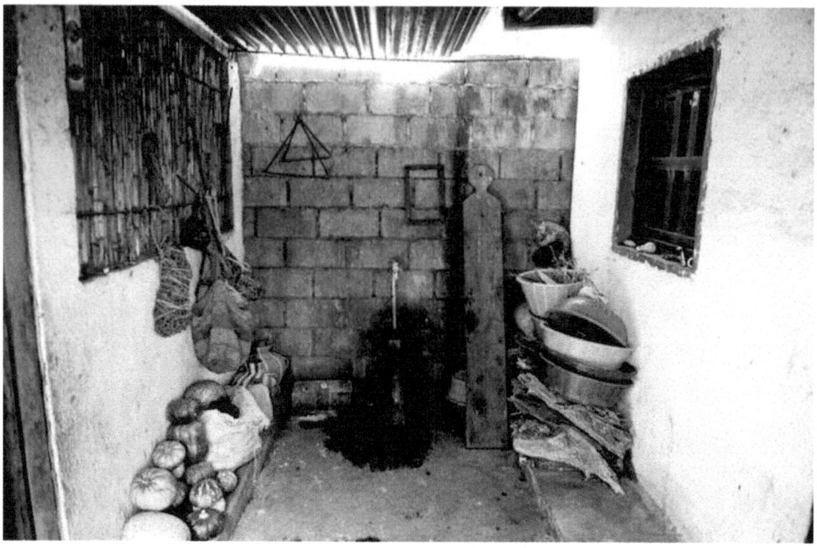

Fig. 33.3 Traditional Mayan kitchen (Saving Mothers 2012)

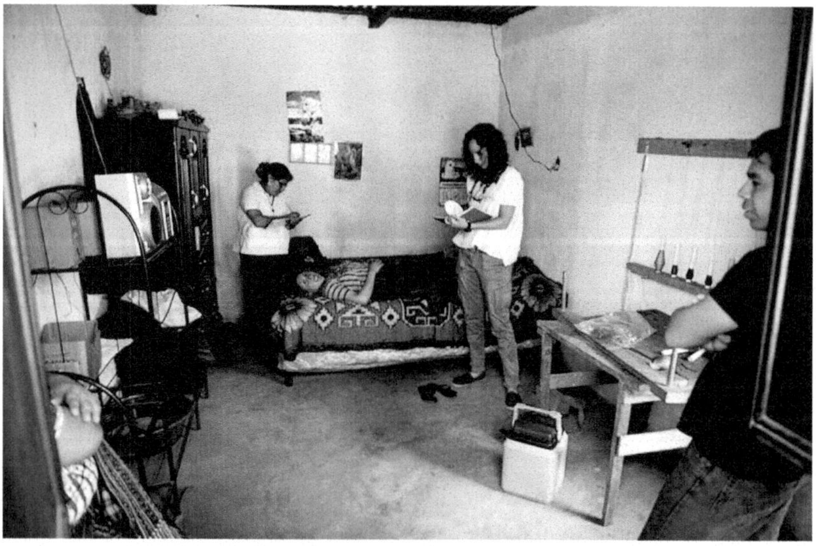

Fig. 33.4 Traditional Mayan home (Saving Mothers 2012)

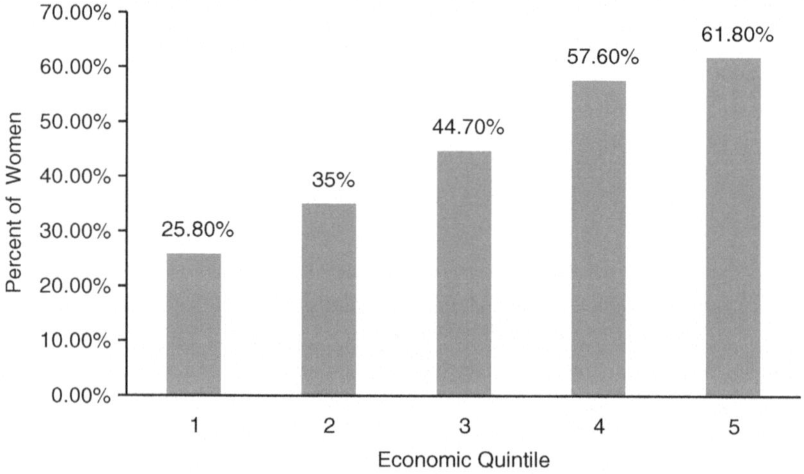

Fig. 33.5 Percent of women using a modern method of contraception based on economic quintile (Adapted from MSPAS 2011)

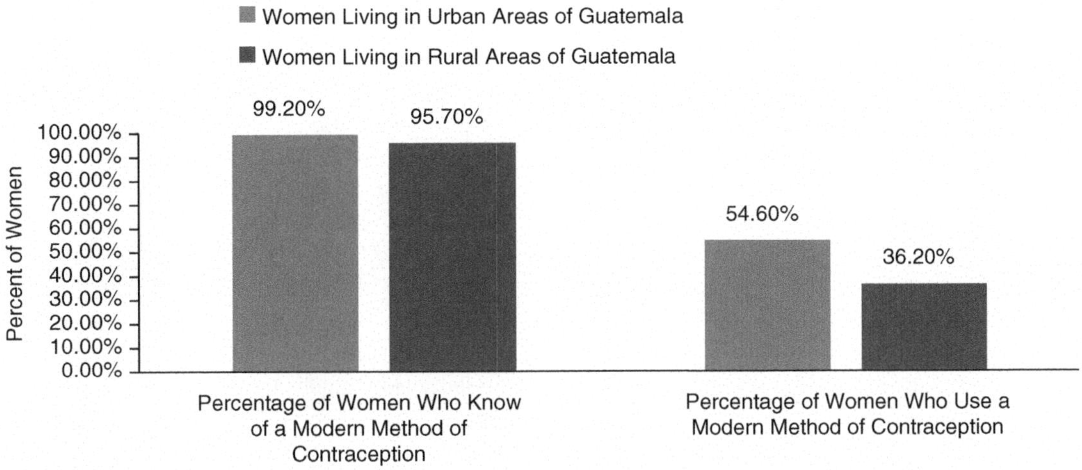

Fig. 33.6 Percentage of women who know of a modern method of contraception or use a modern method of contraception based on their place of residence (MSPAS 2011)

Place of residence was also found to be correlated with contraception use. In 2009, 54.6% of women in urban areas use a modern contraceptive method compared to only 36.2% of women in rural areas (MSPAS 2011) (Fig. 33.6). Studies have even found that migration to urban areas from rural areas, as well as having relatives who live in urban settings, are correlated with an increase in contraceptive knowledge and use (Lindstrom and Muñoz-Franco 2005).

In conjunction with poverty rates and area of residence, differences in education have also been shown to correlate with contraceptive use. High illiteracy rates among Mayan women can be explained by the fact that 34.7% of indigenous women are without schooling. This number is considerably greater than the 11.1% of *Ladino* women who have not attended school (MSPAS 2011). Among those without an education, only 46.4% of married women have used a modern contraceptive method at least once, compared to 89% of women with the highest level of education. Among the uneducated subset of the population, however, only 40% of indigenous women used modern contraceptives compared to 58% of *Ladinas*. This discrepancy among ethnicities with the same level of education suggests that education level is not the only factor influencing contraception use (MSPAS 2011; Ishida et al. 2012).

Although the correlation between sociological factors and contraceptive use is strong, it is equally important to understand how these factors compound with the Guatemalan political landscape surrounding family planning funding and access.

33.3 Government Funding of Family Planning Initiatives and Guatemalan Politics

The three major providers of reproductive health care and family planning distribution in Guatemala are the national government's Ministerio de Salud Pública y Asistencia Social (MSPAS), Instituto Guatemalteco de Seguridad Social (IGSS), and the national nongovernment organization Asociación Pro Bienestar de La Familia (APROFAM) (Cisek et al. 2015). In 2002, APROFAM distributed 32% of the contraceptives used in the country, while MSPAS provided 32% and IGSS provided 6%. In 2008 this dynamic shifted with 50% of all contraceptives being distributed by MSPAS, 9% by IGSS, and only 16% by APROFAM (Cisek et al. 2015) (Fig. 33.7).

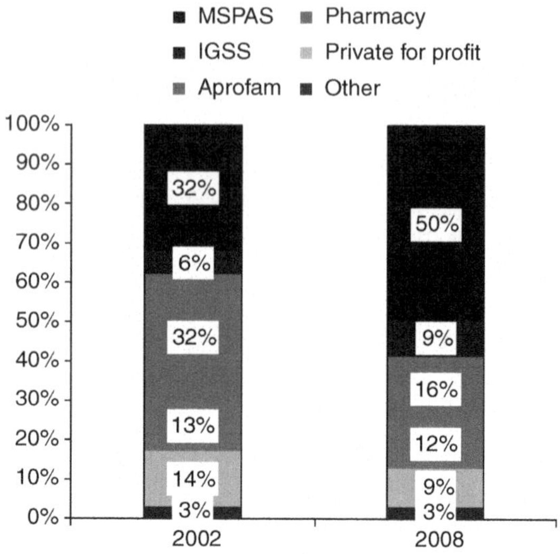

Fig. 33.7 Percentage of market share for family planning products in 2002 and in 2008 (after Cisek et al. 2015)

Those seeking to purchase contraceptive options from MSPAS or IGSS can go to many locations in the country ranging from major urban hospitals to smaller community health centers. For populations that live far away from major public health centers, MSPAS has opened smaller health posts called *centros de atención permanente* (CAPS). These health posts are capable of providing contraceptive services to those in the surrounding community (Fig. 33.8).

Smaller nongovernment organizations also play a role in distributing reproductive health services and information. Some nongovernment organizations that distribute family planning services and information among predominately indigenous communities include *Manos Abiertas*, *Wuqu' Kawoq*, and Wings. Among these three organizations however, only Wings focuses primarily on sexual and reproductive health. It is also the only organization out of the three listed that has published data on its impact and distribution of family planning services. For example, in 2015 Wings distributed 16,624 injectable hormones, 2396 hormonal pills, and 8835 condoms at subsidized costs to a total of 7796 patients. Additionally, the organization claims that it provided its patients with 1783 implants, 291 IUDs, 92 vasectomies, and 472 tubal ligations (Wings 2015). It is important to note, however, that although these numbers seem significant, the sum of nonprofit family planning efforts only constitutes 3% of the market (Cisek et al. 2015) (Fig. 33.7).

Although there is an expansive market for contraception, many indigenous women are restricted by their limited financial resources. In 2006, 35% of indigenous families stated that lack of money was a major barrier to seeking medical attention (World Bank 2009). Additionally, in 2009 it was found that only 7.2% of indigenous women and 12.2% of indigenous men had a form of health insurance, compared to 24.2% of *Ladino* women and 39.2% of *Ladino* men (MSPAS 2011).

Due to greater rates of poverty and limited insurance coverage, indigenous women tend to be more dependent on public health facilities (Ishida et al. 2012; World Bank 2009). In fact, in 2008 it was found that over 80% of persons in the lowest wealth quintile used government-based health facilities to receive contraceptive services (Cisek et al. 2015) (Fig. 33.9). As indigenous women use government-based health-care services more often, they are disproportionately affected by government involvement and spending on health-care and family planning initiatives (Ishida et al. 2012; World Bank 2009).

In 2014, only 17.83% of all government expenditure was spent on public health endeavors, representing only 6.2% of the country's gross domestic product (World Health Organization 2014). It appears as though most of the financial backing for health programs in Guatemala come from private nongovernment organizations. When factoring total expenditure on health in the same year, the

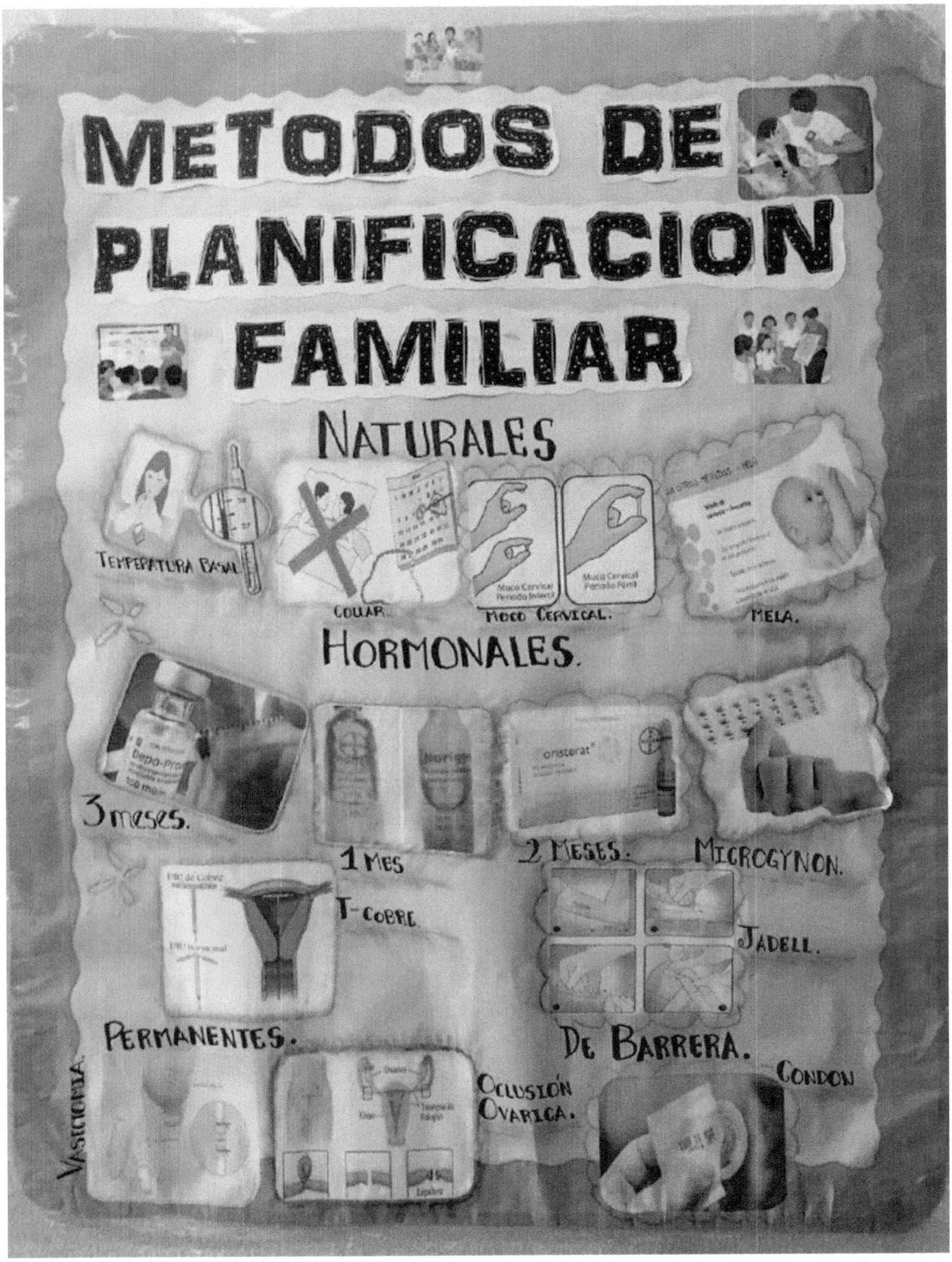

Fig. 33.8 A poster found in the *centro de atención permanente* of San Martin, a rural and predominately indigenous community, displaying available family planning options

Guatemalan government accounted for only 37.8% of total health expenditure, while the private sector spent approximately 62.2% on health (World Health Organization 2014). Despite the small amount of funds being dedicated toward health care, the Guatemalan government has recognized the importance of family planning and formed the National Commission for Contraceptive Security in 2009. This program is led by administrators from MSPAS and intends to develop mechanisms to obtain

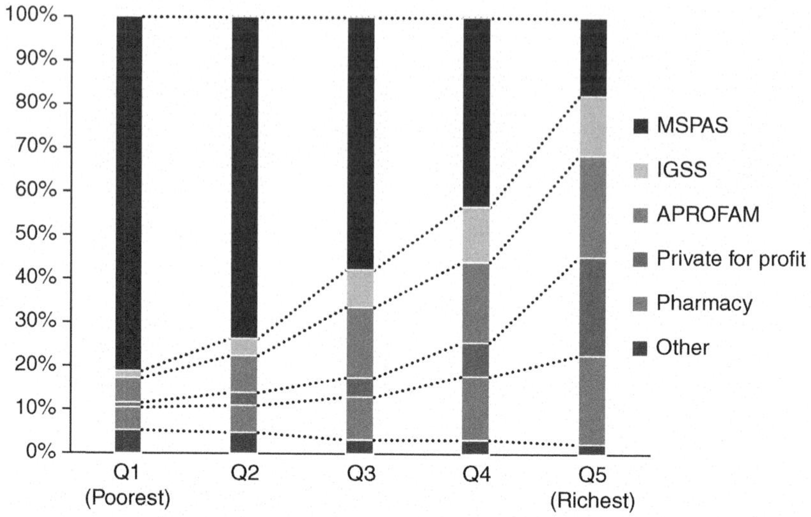

Fig. 33.9 Consumer's source of modern contraception methods based on their wealth quintile (after Cisek et al. 2015)

affordable contraceptives for women and to allocate incoming government funding toward family planning resources (Cisek et al. 2015). Although the creation of this commission is a step in the right direction, continual mismanagement of funds and inefficient use of resources have so far inhibited this initiative from reaching its full potential (Cisek et al. 2015).

Lack of government expenditure has not greatly affected the quantity of public health facilities, as studies have shown that there is little difference in the physical access to facilities offering contraception between Mayan and *Ladino* populations, but it may be contributing to the quality of services found in these locations (Seiber and Bertrand 2002). Studies have shown that many local health-care facilities offer family planning methods at inconvenient times of the day and require indigenous women to wait long periods of time to receive contraception (Netzer and Mallas 2008). Additionally, there have been reports of deficient supplies of contraception methods at all levels of government-based care from major hospitals to smaller community health centers such as CAPS (Cisek et al. 2015).

The quality of service is so poor in many public facilities that those women who can afford it travel further to visit private APROFAM locations (Seiber and Bertrand 2002). A study in 2002 found that APROFAM was the nearest facility for only 7% of respondents, but 48% of participants used APROFAM as their primary family planning source (Seiber and Bertrand 2002). The researchers suggested that APROFAM's modern environment, access to electricity and running water, and counseling services may be influencing this trend. Due to declining donor support and the need to generate funding, however, APROFAM may not be a financially accessible or a stable source of family planning for indigenous women (Aguilar et al. 2001). Possible price increases in APROFAM's contraceptive services have been shown to influence women's decisions regarding their reproductive health choices. In a field study conducted in 2001, 50% of APROFAM's clients claimed that they would be unwilling to pay a higher price for their Depo-Provera hormonal shots. When questioned as to what they would do if the price of their hormonal shots increased, 40% of clients responded that they would try and change to a different form of birth control or would give up using contraception all together (Aguilar et al. 2001).

Competing ideologies in the political realm have also hindered the Guatemalan government's attempt at increasing contraception use and access through public health initiatives (Cisek et al. 2015). The Catholic Church, for example, holds a significant amount of power in the political landscape and often condones family planning outreach as it does not align with the church's religious tenets.

In 2005 the Guatemalan government passed the "Law on Universal and Equitable Access to Family Planning Services" which required increased access to contraceptives, increased funding to those efforts that provide family planning methods, and mandatory reproductive health education in all schools (Manos Abiertas 2013; Netzer and Mallas 2008). Political opposition to this law by the Catholic Church in Guatemala, however, delayed its official implementation to the Fall of 2009 (Valladares 2009). During this time, the Archbishop of Guatemala City, the Most Reverend Rodolfo Quezada, encouraged his constituents to disallow their children from attending classes as an act of civil disobedience in order to protest the implementation of this public health intervention (Valladares 2009). This incidence is not the first time the Catholic Church has influenced public health policies in Guatemala as there has been a long history of the church opposing large-scale family planning efforts in the country (Metz 2001). Given the controversy it has created and the Catholic Church's strong opposition to its implementation, the "Law on Universal and Equitable Access to Family Planning Services" has yet to fulfill its goal of increasing equity to reproductive health services, and contraception is still being underutilized among poor, indigenous women (Manos Abiertas 2013; Netzer and Mallas 2008).

Lack of government expenditure on health services, deficiencies of physical and financial access to family planning services, and conflicting political ideologies surrounding the issue of contraception use all disproportionately affect the indigenous female population of Guatemala who are more dependent on public health facilities (Ishida et al. 2012; Cisek et al. 2015). A long history of ethnic unrest and tension between the Mayan people and the politically empowered *Ladino* populations, however, is impacting provider-patient relationships and ultimately the quality of services found in public health facilities.

33.4 Political History of Guatemala and Lack of Culturally Sensitive Care

Guatemala's long history of civil unrest between the indigenous and *Ladino* people, a 36-year conflict that left hundreds of thousands of indigenous men and women dead, continues to negatively impact relations between poor rural Mayan communities and politically empowered *Ladino* communities (Santiso-Galvez and Bertrand 2000; Terborgh et al. 1995). Although peace accords were signed in 1996 to end the civil unrest and violence between the two ethnic populations, in 2002 the United Nations stated that racism continued to govern the attitudes of authorities and that Mayans were still being discriminated against on a social, political, and economic level (O'Neill et al. 2006).

This history is not far from the minds of the Mayan population, many of who view the family planning efforts of foreign- or *Ladino*-based organizations as being akin to predetermined elimination or reduction of the indigenous population (Santiso-Galvez and Bertrand 2000; Terborgh et al. 1995; Ward et al. 1992).

This historically based distrust between ethnicities in Guatemala has carried over into the healthcare setting where many providers and hospitals are supervised by *Ladinos*. Many indigenous women express that they feel as though their *Ladino* providers treat them poorly because of their ethnicity and their inability to speak fluent Spanish (Netzer and Mallas 2008). They feel as though their providers are not sensitive or aware of their needs and therefore lack confidence in the services and information that they provide (Netzer and Mallas 2008).

Unfortunately, these feelings are not misplaced. A recent study showed that many *Ladino* providers do hold biased views of indigenous women as they feel that they are less intelligent and are less able to understand and properly use contraceptive methods. Many *Ladino* providers admitted to withholding information about certain contraceptive methods from indigenous women as they felt they would not be able to use it properly (Netzer and Mallas 2008). These discriminatory (or stigmatizing) practices in the health-care setting are a major deterrent to indigenous women seeking care at public health facilities and can be attributed to the poorer health outcomes seen among indigenous population (Castro et al. 2015).

Many family planning clinics do not provide culturally sensitive services that take into account the unique viewpoints and needs of indigenous women with regard to their reproductive health. Some health clinics that are physically accessible to the Mayan women lack private, closed-off areas for consultation, and this causes many women to feel uncomfortable about sharing their reproductive health history or asking about contraceptive methods. As a result, many women leave these clinics without information regarding their reproductive health and family planning options (Netzer and Mallas 2008).

More practically, some indigenous women visiting their local clinics do not speak Spanish, and a translator is often needed to communicate between patient and provider. Instead of using a trained and designated translator, many providers ask another family member, another client, a security guard, or a facility maintenance person to assist with the translation (Netzer and Mallas 2008). Although not directly stated by research participants, one can imagine the privacy issues that may arise when asking a patient to reveal sensitive information to an unknown third party, and how this may inhibit some women from revealing their full sexual history or reproductive health questions to their physician or nurse.

Delivery of culturally appropriate care continues to be an issue, and it has been suggested that increasing the presence of Mayan-speaking staff that are sensitive to indigenous norms and practices could increase the use of formal health services by Mayan women (Chomat et al. 2014). In 2009, the Guatemalan Ministry of Health along with other international health partners put forth recommendations for the incorporation of Mayan beliefs and practices into the care of pregnant women (Chomat et al. 2014; Cabrera et al. 2009). Although this guide is a step in the right direction in making reproductive health services more culturally sensitive, it lacks a section on cultural sensitivity and awareness surrounding contraception and therefore fails to enhance the cultural sensitivity of family planning services in this area.

The implementation of culturally sensitive and nondiscriminatory care is vital as there is a high prevalence of non-biomedical beliefs and misconceptions about contraception among the Mayan community. Without the trust and communication that develops as a result of culturally sensitive care, there will continue to be barriers toward eradicating misconceptions and reeducating the community on the benefits of various family planning methods.

33.5 Non-Biomedical Mayan Beliefs, Sociocultural Barriers, and Unsafe Abortion

Mayan culture espouses the idea that fertility, number of children, place of residence, death, and occupation are predetermined by God (Metz 2001). It is believed that each woman is born carrying the exact number of children she will eventually conceive (Ward et al. 1992). Utilization of family planning methods can be seen as resisting God's predetermined plan by preventing the creation of children that God had endowed them with (Metz 2001).

The Catholic Church's influence in the Mayan community and its stance on pronatalism also reinforces Mayan's belief that fate plays a role in childbearing (Terborgh et al. 1995). The Catholic Church, preaching that family planning methods are sinful and harmful, plays a large role in influencing the Mayan community's understanding of reproductive health (Ward et al. 1992; Netzer and Mallas 2008). When asked in a 1992 qualitative study what they thought about family planning, many Mayans replied that they felt it was a sin and that it was akin to murder (Ward et al. 1992).

Statistical analysis at the local level in Mayan-concentrated communities continues to be more revealing about sociocultural barriers to contraceptive use. In 2012 a medical nonprofit organization, Saving Mothers, conducted a survey of 155 Mayan women in the province of Santiago, Lago Atitlán. Among the participants, 20.7% of the women have had five or more pregnancies, and 16.4% of pregnancies were unplanned. In this community, 63.7% of the population surveyed had never tried contraceptives, and 55% of women reported that they were not currently using a contraceptive method (Saving Mothers 2012). When queried what factors acted as obstacles to them using contraceptives, 55.6% of women reported that the main obstacles to contraceptive use were their cultural and religious beliefs. In conjunction with this statistic, approximately one-fifth of the study participants felt that they could not talk openly about reproductive health with health-care providers or with their spouses.

A USAID study found similar sociocultural barriers to contraceptive use—indigenous women listed opposition from mothers, mothers-in-law, community elders, and spouses as major factors limiting their autonomy to make contraceptive decisions (Netzer and Mallas 2008). The study also found that there is a sentiment among the Mayan community that those who use family planning methods are or will be unfaithful to their spouses, and many women fear the possible community criticism and ostracism that comes with family planning use (Ward et al. 1992; Netzer and Mallas 2008). It appears clear that the cultural, social, and religious environments of Mayan communities in Guatemala play a major role in promoting stigma surrounding contraceptive use and ultimately act as a barrier to accessing family planning knowledge and services.

A high prevalence of misconceptions surrounding contraception can also be seen as impeding indigenous women's ability to make informed family planning choices. Among the Mayan population, there seems to be a notion that "chemical" family planning methods have adverse side effects (Ward et al. 1992). In qualitative studies, it has been shown that Mayans believe that the pill can cause rapid weight gain and/or weight loss. Many women worried that this obvious physical change would reveal their contraception use, which would in turn result in criticism from the community. Others suggested that the pill can cause cancer, that it can act as an abortifacient, that it was toxic, and that it can cause a woman to become severely ill or die. Indigenous women justified these assumptions by recounting stories of women they knew who were hospitalized or died after using modern contraceptive methods (Ward et al. 1992).

Despite the incompatibility of medicinal contraception and Mayan culture, there seems to be a strong need among Mayan women to control their fertility. In 2009, it was found that 18.8% of women without education already had more children than their ideal size compared to only 4.5% of women with the highest level of education (MSPAS 2011). In fact, at the time of the study, 41.7% of married indigenous women expressed that they no longer desired to have any more children, and 31% of married women who were not currently using contraception expressed the desire to postpone or avoid pregnancy (MSPAS 2011; Haub and Gribble 2011).

Many Mayans recognize the danger of having children beyond their capacity to provide suitable care (Metz 2001). To manage their fertility, while avoiding the stigma associated with modern methods of contraception, many Mayans have resorted to the rhythm method. However, this method is unreliable, and most Mayans use it incorrectly (Metz 2001; Ward et al. 1992).

As a result of poor contraception use, unintended pregnancy and resultant unsafe abortion continue to be a major killer of women in Guatemala where abortion is illegal unless it is used to save a woman's life (Singh et al. 2006). Mayan women in desperate situations have resorted to dangerous and unreliable traditional abortifacient such as insertion of objects into the vaginal canal or postpartum neglect of the child to maintain the number of children they want (Metz 2001). Other known abortifacients in the Mayan community include swallowing an avocado pit, inserting aspirin into the vaginal canal, drinking lemon mixed with vervain herb, and ingesting soot leftover from cooking (Ward et al. 1992). Although many

Mayans condone the use of natural abortifacients, researchers have suggested that the widespread knowledge about their use indicates that it may be a more common practice than recognized (Ward et al. 1992).

More recent data confirms this suspicion as between July 2003 and December 2004, 13,928 incomplete induced abortions were treated at 22 public hospitals (Singh et al. 2006). Although this sample included both *Ladino* and Mayan women, the study goes on to say that from 49 to 63% of poor and indigenous women utilized unskilled traditional birth attendants to perform their abortion, and suggesting that the majority of these cases may have been from the Mayan community. The prominence of unsafe abortions can be seen as a reflection of the failure of the Guatemalan government and health infrastructure to meet the family planning needs of women at risk for unintended pregnancies (Warriner and Shah 2006).

33.6 Gender Inequality and the Potential of Gender-Transformative Approaches in the Mayan Community

Socioeconomic environment, education level, government spending, political ideologies, ethnic tensions, culturally insensitive care, and traditional Mayan beliefs have all been shown to play a role in limiting an indigenous women's access to family planning methods, thus contributing to the reproductive health disparities seen among the indigenous female population. One particular aspect of Mayan culture, however, is beginning to be recognized by public health officials as one of the most restrictive but malleable obstacles facing indigenous women and their ability to make family planning decisions: patriarchy.

In patriarchal Mayan culture, the man is responsible for most of the decision-making that happens within a household, including those decisions regarding his wife's reproductive health (Martinez 2003; Netzer and Mallas 2008). The most unfortunate part of this marital dynamic is that the men who make these reproductive decisions are often quite uninformed about contraception themselves (MSPAS 2011). In 2009, only 29.1% of indigenous men knew about the IUD, 22.8% knew of the female condom, 64.2% knew of male sterilization, and only 10% knew of the female contraceptive ring (MSPAS 2011). Although in the same year greater than 80% of indigenous men knew about the pill and the male condom, many indigenous men hold negative perceptions and non-biomedical beliefs about the effect of using these respective methods. For example, many men feel that male condoms can cause genital cancer in women (Ward et al. 1992). It is not surprising that when surveyed in 2009, only 2.5% of indigenous married men said that they use condoms (MSPAS 2011).

In addition to their unfamiliarity and underutilization of modern contraceptive methods, indigenous men are equally unaware about the correct use of natural family planning methods. When using the rhythm method, it is vitally important to know when one's partner is ovulating, but when surveyed, 81.3% of indigenous men could not correctly state the time when their partner would be most fertile (MSPAS 2011).

Despite the authoritative role that Mayan men play in making reproductive health decisions for their wives, it seems as though indigenous men rarely communicate with their wives about family planning options. When asked how often they talk with their partners about family planning, only 19.6% of indigenous men responded frequently, 41.4% of men responded once or twice, and 39.1% of men responded that they never engaged in such discussions (MSPAS 2011).

Patriarchal culture severely limits the autonomy of women to decide on family planning methods. As a result, the majority of women choose not to make reproductive health decisions on their own at the threat of facing verbal, physical, or financial abuse from their partner (Lemus 2016). Common misconceptions among the Mayan community about the safety of family planning methods influence this power dynamic. Men feel as though their wives do not have the intellectual or verbal capacity to communicate effectively with health-care providers and may end up with a contraceptive method that is harmful to their physical well-being (Terborgh et al. 1995; Ward et al. 1992).

Given the significant role that men play in the reproductive health of their wives, together with the limited and misinformed knowledge they have on contraceptive methods, many public health interventions in low-income countries with dominant patriarchal cultures have begun to look at the effectiveness of including men in family planning discussions and programs.

In a 2007 analysis of 58 programs that engaged men and boys in women's health issues, the World Health Organization found that these programs were able to (1) increase the use of contraception; (2) decrease intimate partner violence; (3) increase spousal communication and shared decision-making on child health, contraception, and reproductive health; (4) increase the use of sexual and reproductive health services; (5) increase condom use; (6) decrease rates of sexually transmitted infections; and (7) increase social support of their respective spouses (World Health Organization 2007). Although almost all the programs that engaged men and boys were effective, the World Health Organization found that those programs with a gender-transformative approach had a higher rate of effectiveness in changing health behaviors and attitudes of men. A gender-transformative approach is one that promotes gender equality by actively challenging normative gender roles, or socially constructed expectations of male or female behavior, and encouraging more gender-equitable relationships between men and women (World Health Organization 2007).

It has been shown that male gender roles and male perception of the female gender roles can impact the health decisions that a man makes as well as how he interacts with his spouse on reproductive health issues (Cohen and Burger 2000; World Health Organization 2007; Croce-Galis et al. 2015). In many cultures, gender norms dictate how many sexual partners a woman or a man is allowed to have, the power to control when and how often intercourse is had, and if and when contraceptive methods are used (Schuler and Ramírez 2012; Brown et al. 2005). Although the idea of using gender-transformative approaches to better reproductive health outcomes is relatively well-established in other low- to middle-income countries, the idea of implementing this approach to increase contraception use and better reproductive health outcomes among the indigenous population in Guatemala is relatively new (World Health Organization 2007; Muralidharan et al. 2015). Those few initiatives that have engaged indigenous men and women in gender-transformative interventions, however, have already seen tremendous success in creating more equitable relationships between Mayan men and women and increasing shared decision-making on family planning use (Schuler and Ramírez 2012; Lemus 2016).

In 2012 C-Change, FHI360, and USAID published the results of a field test in which they aimed to test the hypothesis that promotion of gender equity in the context of family planning among rural Guatemalan men and women would lead to greater contraception use and more equitable gender attitudes. The study was conducted in 30 indigenous-concentrated communities in the rural Western Highlands. Indigenous men and women attended workshops that aimed to engage participants to think actively about gender and power through role-play, practice of nonviolent communication between men and women on sexual health issues, and practice of open communication and shared decision-making on family planning use. They found that their intervention created more gender-equitable attitudes in men and women and increased knowledge of contraceptive methods among them. The authors suggested that given their promising results, more work should focus on implementing gender-transformative programs in the context of reproductive health in Guatemala (Schuler and Ramírez 2012).

In 2016, both the USAID and PSI supported a gender-transformative program termed the Support for International Family Planning Organization (SIFPO), which is being implemented in the Western Highlands of Guatemala. This program is working to create new masculinity roles and promote more equitable gender relations in the context of family planning. The program is working with men, women, youth, and traditional birth attendants to think critically about gender norms in the context of family planning, as well as how these norms impact the well-being of their community members. In addition to directly engaging with the community, this program is running a local media campaign that emphasizes the shared responsibility of men and women in management of household finances, children's health, children's education, and family planning (Lemus 2016). A more formal analysis of the impact of this work, however, has yet to be published.

While gender-transformative programming is becoming increasingly popular due to rates of success, it is also important to understand the possible limitations and problems with this approach. Some potential problems and limitations include an overemphasis of the role masculinity plays in complicated social health issues while ignoring the structural, economic, and cultural tenets that also contribute to this issue; the difficulty of having men who feel disempowered due to economic, cultural, or social disadvantages embracing a new more empowered status of women; and how to maintain new healthy behaviors and attitudes in men after the program is finished (Dworkin et al. 2015).

Ultimately when analyzing the reasons why Mayan women underutilize family planning methods and experience worse reproductive health outcomes when compared to *Ladino* women in Guatemala, it becomes clear how intricately connected an indigenous woman's reproductive health is to her unique sociocultural and economic environment. It is promising, then, that for an issue that is so multifaceted and complicated, rapid change can be achieved by engaging the community to think critically about their gender norms. Given the proven success of gender-transformative programming, the Guatemalan government should focus its family planning funding and efforts on integrating gender-transformative programs into government-based reproductive health facilities. By increasing equity between the indigenous man and woman, there is hope for bettering the reproductive health outcome of Mayan women, eliminating the reproductive health disparities among indigenous and nonindigenous groups and lowering high maternal mortality rates that have plagued indigenous communities for decades.

References

Aguilar, Z., Duarte, T., Bratt, J., Brambila, C., & Foreit, J. (2001). *Willingness to pay for reproductive health services among APROFAM clients Guatemala*. USAID. Retrieved March 20, 2016, from http://pdf.usaid.gov/pdf_docs/Pnacn826.pdf.

Brown, J., Sorrell, J., & Raffaelli, M. (2005). *An exploratory study of constructions of masculinity, sexuality and HIV/AIDS in Namibia, Southern Africa*. Faculty Publications, Department of Psychology at University of Nebraska-Lincoln, Paper 54.

Cabrera, L., Rosales, P., Echeverría, G., Palma, S., López, S., Haeussler, R., et al. (2009). *Normas con pertinencia cultural hacia la interculturalidad*. MSPAS. Retrieved July 20, 2016, from http://www.mspas.gob.gt/files/Descargas/UNIDADES/pueblosindigenas/documentos/Normas%20Pertinencia%20Cultural%20en%20Servicios%20de%20Salud.pdf.

Castro, A., Savage, V., & Kaufman, H. (2015). Assessing equitable care for Indigenous and Afrodescendant women in Latin America. *Revista Panamericana de Salud Pública, 38*(2), 96–109.

Chomat, A. M., Solomons, N. W., Montenegro, G., Crowley, C., & Bermudez, O. I. (2014). Maternal health and health-seeking behaviors among indigenous *Mam* mothers from Quetzaltenango, Guatemala. *Revista Panamericana de Salud Pública, 35*(2), 113–120.

Cisek, C., Revuz, C., & Kramer, C. (2015). *Guatemala health system assessment 2015: Private sector assessment of family planning, antenatal care, and delivery*. USAID. Retrieved May 30, 2016, from https://www.usaid.gov/documents/1862/guatemala-health-system-assessment-2015-private-sector-assessment-family-planning.

Cohen, S., & Burger, M. (2000). *Partnering: A new approach to sexual and reproductive health*. UNFPA. Retrieved August 20, 2016, from https://www.unfpa.org/sites/default/files/pub-pdf/partnering_eng.pdf.

Croce-Galis M., Gay, J., & Hardee, K. (2015). Gender considerations along the HIV treatment cascade: An evidence review with priority actions. Retrieved August 20, 2016, from http://evidenceproject.popcouncil.org/wp-content/uploads/2015/09/WWA-Treatment-Brief.pdf.

Demographic and Healthy Surveys Program. (2016). *Wealth Index*. Retrieved February 20, 2016, from http://www.dhsprogram.com/topics/wealth-index/Index.cfm.

Dworkin, S. L., Fleming, P. J., & Colvin, C. J. (2015). The promises and limitations of gender-transformative health programming with men: Critical reflections from the field. *Culture, Health & Sexuality, 17*(2), S128–S143.

Haub, C., & Gribble, J. (2011). *The world at 7 billion*. Population Reference Bureau. Retrieved January 20, 2016, from http://www.prb.org/Publications/Reports/2011/The-World-at-7-Billion.aspx.

Ishida, K., Stupp, P., Turcios-Ruiz, R., William, D. B., & Espinoza, E. (2012). Ethnic inequality in Guatemalan women's use of modern reproductive health care. *International Perspectives on Sexual and Reproductive Health, 38*(2), 99–108.

Kestler, E., Orozco, M. R., Palma, S., & Flores, R. (2011). Initiation of effective postpartum contraceptive use in public hospitals in Guatemala. *Revista Panamericana de Salud Pública, 29*(2), 103–107.

Lemus, H. (2016). *New masculinity and family planning: A gender transformative approach to SBCC in rural Guatemala*. Social and Behaviour Change Summit. Retrieved February 20, 2016, from http://www.comminit.com/sbcs2016/content/new-masculinity-and-family-planning-gender-transformative-approach-sbcc-rural-guatemala.

Lindstrom, D. P., & Muñoz-Franco, E. (2005). Migration and the diffusion of modern contraceptive knowledge and use in rural Guatemala. *Studies in Family Planning, 36*(4), 277–288.

Manos Abiertas. (2013). *Overview*. Retrieved January 20, 2016, from http://asociacionmanosabiertas.org/en/about-us/overview.html.

Marmot, M., Friel, S., Bell, R., Houweling, T. A., & Taylor, S. (2008). Closing the gap in a generation: Health equity through action on the social determinants of health. *The Lancet, 372*(9650), 1661–1669.

Martinez, J. (2003). *Guatemala report*. Reproductive health rights. Retrieved January 20, 2016, from http://www.reproductiverights.org/sites/default/files/documents/guatemala.pdf.

Matthew, L. (2006). Mexicanos and the meanings of Ladino in colonial Guatemala. *Journal of Colonialism and Colonial History, 7*(1).

Metz, B. (2001). Politics, populations and family planning in Guatemala: Chorti Maya experiences. *Human Organization, 60*(3), 259–271.

MSPAS. (2011). *Encuesta nacional de salud materno infantil 2008 (ENSMI-2008/09)*. Retrieved January 30, 2016, from http://www.ine.gob.gt/sistema/uploads/2014/01/22/LYk4A1kGJAO7lvfS0Aq6tezcUa9tQh35.pdf.

Muralidharan, A., Fehringer, J., Pappa, S., Rottach, E., Das, M., & Mandal, M. (2015). *Transforming gender norms, roles, and power dynamics for better health: Evidence from a systematic review of gender-integrated health programs in low and middle income countries*. Retrieved August 20, 2016, from http://www.healthpolicyproject.com/index.cfm?ID=publications&get=pubID&pubID=381.

Netzer, S., & Mallas, L. (2008). *Increasing access to family planning among indigenous groups in Guatemala*. USAID. Retrieved January 20, 2016, from http://www.popline.org/node/206721.

Norton, M. (2005). New evidence on birth spacing: Promising findings for improving newborn, infant, child, and maternal health. *International Journal of Gynecology & Obstetrics, 89*, S1–S6.

O'Neill, J., Bartlett, J., & Mignone, J. (2006). *Best practices in intercultural health*. Inter-American Development Bank. Retrieved January 20, 2016, from http://www.iadb.org/wmsfiles/products/publications/documents/1484415.pdf.

Santiso-Galvez, R., & Bertrand, J. T. (2000). The stymied contraceptive revolution in Guatemala. *Human Organization, 63*(1), 57–67.

Saving Mothers. (2012). *Family planning survey-abstract draft part II*. Santiago. Saving Mothers 501(c)3, https://www.savingmothers.org New York, NY.

Schooley, J., Mundt, C., Wagner, P., Fullerton, J., & O'Donnell, M. (2009). Factors influencing health care-seeking behaviours among Mayan women in Guatemala. *Midwifery*, 25, 411–421

Schuler, S., and L. Ramírez. (2012). Interactive Workshops to Promote Gender Equity and Family Planning in Rural Guatemalan Communities: Results of a Field Test. Washington, DC: C-Change/FHI 360. from https://www.c-changeprogram.org/sites/default/files/Guatemala-report-workshops-on-FP-genderequity.pdf

Seiber, E., & Bertrand, J. (2002). Access as a factor in differential contraceptive use between Mayans and Ladinos in Guatemala. *Health Policy and Planning, 17*(2), 167–177.

Singh, S., Prada, E., & Kestler, E. (2006). Induced abortion and unintended pregnancy in Guatemala. *International Family Planning Perspectives, 32*(3), 136–145.

Terborgh, A., Rosen, J. E., Santiso-Gálvez, R., Terceros, W., Bertrand, J., & Bull, S. E. (1995). Family planning among indigenous populations in Latin America. *International Family Planning Perspectives, 21*, 143–9 & 166.

UNICEF. (2015). *State of the world's children 2015 country statistical information*. Retrieved January 20, 2016, from http://data.unicef.org/resources/the-state-of-the-worlds-children-report-2015-statistical-tables/.

Valladares, D. (2009). *Guatemala: Sex education, family planning finally available*. Inter Press Service News Agency. Retrieved January 20, 2016, from http://www.ipsnews.net/2009/11/guatemala-sex-education-family-planning-finally-available/.

Ward, V. M., Bertrand, J. T., & Puac, F. (1992). Exploring sociocultural barriers to family planning among Mayans in Guatemala. *International Family Planning Perspectives, 18*(2), 59–65.

Warriner, I. K., & Shah I. H. (2006). *Preventing unsafe abortion and its consequences: Priorities for research and action*. WHO. Retrieved March 20, 2016, from http://www.who.int/reproductivehealth/publications/unsafe_abortion/0939253763.pdf.

Wings. (2015). *Wings 2015 annual report*. Retrieved March 20, 2016, from http://www.wingsguate.org/our-work/#our-impact.

World Bank. (2009). *Guatemala—Poverty assessment: good performance at low levels*. Retrieved March 20, 2016, from http://documents.worldbank.org/curated/en/803331468254934801/Guatemala-Poverty-assessment-good-performance-at-low-levels.

World Bank. (2015). *FAQS: Global poverty line update*. Retrieved July 20, 2016, from http://www.worldbank.org/en/topic/poverty/brief/global-poverty-line-faq.

World Health Organization. (2007). *Engaging men and boys in changing gender-based inequity in health: Evidence from programme interventions*. Retrieved August 20, 2016, from http://www.who.int/gender/documents/Engaging_men_boys.pdf.

World Health Organization. (2014). *Global health observatory date repository: Health expenditure ratios, by country, 1995–2014, Guatemala*. Retrieved January 20, 2016, from http://apps.who.int/gho/data/view.main.HEALTHEXPRATIOGTM?lang=en.

World Health Organization. (2015). *Family planning/contraception*. Retrieved February 20, 2016, from http://who.int/mediacentre/factsheets/fs351/en/.

34 Toward an Understanding of Placentas, Umbilical Cords, and Cauls Among *Kaqchikel* Maya Midwives of Guatemala

Servando Z. Hinojosa

34.1 Introduction

For Maya midwives of Guatemala, organs like placentas, umbilical cords, and cauls are anything but ordinary. Midwives handle these body parts as they must, and when they must, and look to see that they are intact and functioning when they first emerge. But when midwives behold them, they see more than just the agglomerations of tissues, vessels, and blood that clinical workers reduce these materials to. When a midwife squints at the wet contours of the afterbirth, the cord, and the amniotic shroud, she sees the outcomes of both physical growth processes and of fetal animation, as surely as the newborn warms her hands. She knows that at the moment these body parts emerge, nothing will be the same again for the woman whose body produced them, nor for the small wiggling being breathing air for the first time. For this reason, a Maya mother entrusts her midwife with the sacred duty of not only helping deliver her child but of ensuring that the future of both mother and child are better protected. The midwife is uniquely qualified to do both.

I began learning about the Maya midwives' way of being in 1992 when I was beginning my graduate fieldwork and living in San Juan Comalapa, a *Kaqchikel* Maya community in the central Guatemalan highlands. Though I did not know it at the time, this town was to become my second home in the dozen or so years that were to follow. Comalapa's inhabitants would walk me through their ideas of health and sickness and of spirit and body, in the many ways that these intersected with their lives. During my months there, including when I was doing my doctoral research, I sought out as many midwives as I could, thinking that these women would have insights into processes of human gestation and ensoulment that no one else might. When I did get to speak with them, sitting in their family spaces, they indeed came across as knowledgeable about pregnancy and childbirth. I expected this. What I did not expect, though, was that their work had many more features than I had supposed and that many of these features were invisible to clinical eyes.

In this chapter I will walk through some of the contours of the Maya midwives' experiences that often go unnoticed or undervalued by researchers and health workers. I will specifically discuss what

S. Z. Hinojosa, Ph.D.
Department of Sociology and Anthropology, University of Texas Rio Grande Valley, Edinburg, TX, USA
e-mail: Servando.hinojosa@utrgv.edu

D. A. Schwartz (ed.), *Maternal Death and Pregnancy-Related Morbidity Among Indigenous Women of Mexico and Central America*, Global Maternal and Child Health: Medical, Anthropological, and Public Health Perspectives, https://doi.org/10.1007/978-3-319-71538-4_34

placentas, umbilical cords, and cauls mean for Mayas and what they entail in the larger context of the midwife's vocation. Since much has already been written about the type of care that Maya midwives give their clients, especially relating to uterine massage and palpation, I will not repeat that here (Cosminsky 1982a, 2016; Hinojosa 2004, 2015; Jordan 1993). Needless to say, the midwives' handling of placentas, umbilical cords, and cauls is an extension of their already very manual work, and I expect that the reader is already familiar with this work. This chapter, then, centers on what these placental organs and tissues mean according to Maya outlooks, bringing together the experiences of 15 *Kaqchikel* Maya midwives whose views have shaped my research. One of these midwives is shown in Fig. 34.1, appearing in her home patio, the kind of space where most of my interactions with midwives took place. By considering commonalities and variations in the views of midwives like her, I hope to both summarize and explore what we know and do not know about Maya pregnancy and childbirth and in the process try to fill in some of these gaps of knowledge.

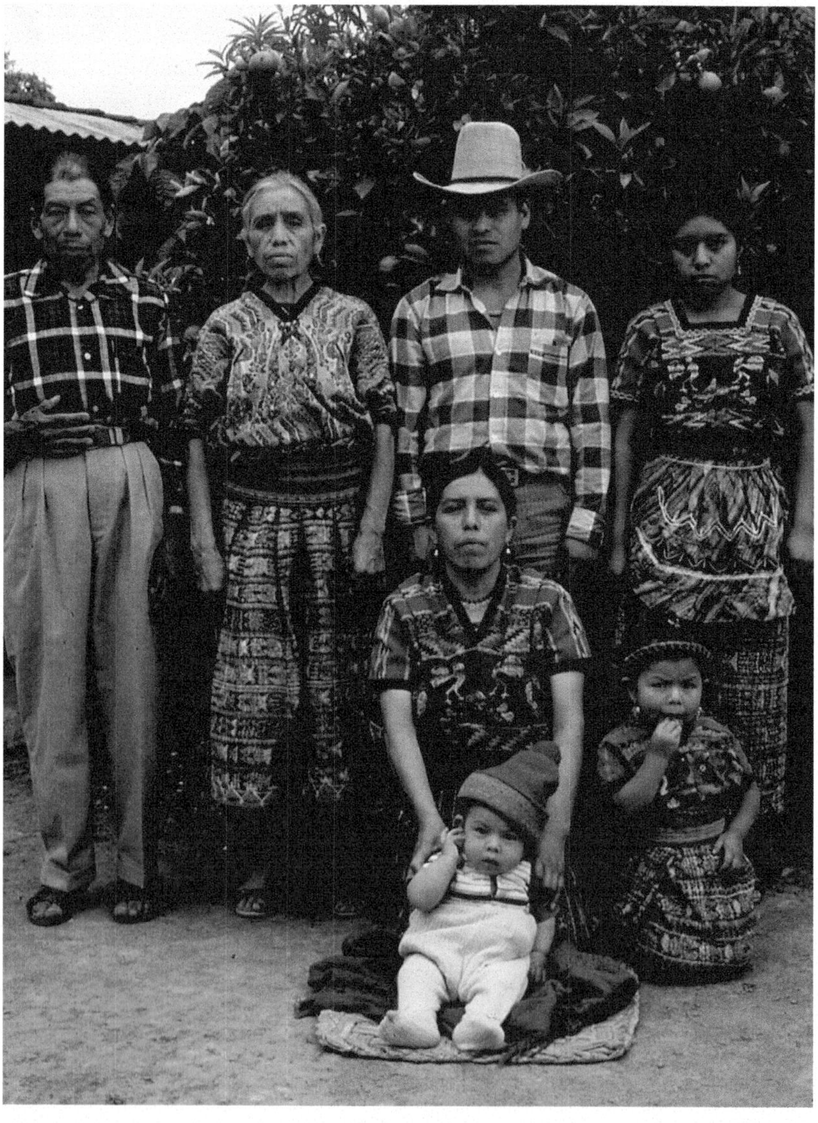

Fig. 34.1 A *Kaqchikel* Maya midwife kneels with her grandson and niece. Standing behind her are (left to right) her father, mother, brother, and daughter. San Juan Comalapa, Guatemala, 1995

34.2 Placentas

If a midwife does her job well in the months before the birth and if the pregnancy is normal, the child will pass easily through the birth canal. This leaves the midwife, following her necessary treatment of the umbilical cord, to await the placenta. Most of the time, it emerges shortly after the birth, within a half-hour, but if she needs to she will carefully massage the uterus to ease the process along, ever careful not to apply traction to the umbilical cord. When the afterbirth does arrive, the midwife must carefully examine it and verify that it is intact or else decide that its incomplete state signals a risk of hemorrhage for which she must seek emergency help (Klein 1995, p. 200). She also makes sure that as the placenta emerges, it does not remain adhered to the uterine lining, risking an inverted uterus, a condition that all midwives know about but that only some have had to deal with directly.

Following most births, though, once the placenta has moved fully out of the mother's body and onto the midwife's hands, this specialist must then set a necessary procedure into motion. After the midwife tends to the newborn, she must either burn or bury the placenta. *Kaqchikel* Maya families usually want to have this done quickly, but most midwives recommend against simply burying it. Midwives caution that burying the placenta might expose it to too much "coldness" in the ground, especially during the rainy months of the year. They prefer to treat it in a ritually "hot" way, and this usually involves placing humorally "hot" plants, such as lavender, parsley, and cumin, on the placenta and then wrapping it in newspaper or old rags. The placental bundle is then burned in the *tuj* or *temascal*, the family sweatbath and space where childbirth traditionally takes place. This small structure is also where many Maya midwives later enact important postpartum cleansing and prayer rituals as shown in Fig. 34.2. If the *Kaqchikel* family does not have a *tuj* in which to burn the placenta, they can burn it in a fire built in the house patio or in their main cooking fire, the hearth. One midwife explained to me that it is better to burn the placenta in the hearth because, "There is (found) the heat of the mother." For other midwives, meanwhile, the act of burning the placenta matters more than where this burning is done.

The main reason the placenta must be burned is to prevent any potential physical problems in the mother after the delivery. One midwife warns that if the organ is not burned, the mother might develop lasting facial blemishes. Another says not burning the placenta can rob a mother of her appetite. For most midwives, though, the placenta is burned, "So that the woman won't have any stomach pains," as one midwife puts it. She, like many others, argues that if the placenta is not burned, the mother's uterus or stomach can remain swollen and distended, possibly for the rest of the mother's life, connoting how an inordinately "cold" body part can exhibit edema and pain. In this sense, burning the placenta ensures that the "heat" borne by this organ is conveyed instantly to the mother's womb, which retains affective ties with the placenta. The burning thus offsets any latent coldness in each organ and the swelling it can cause.

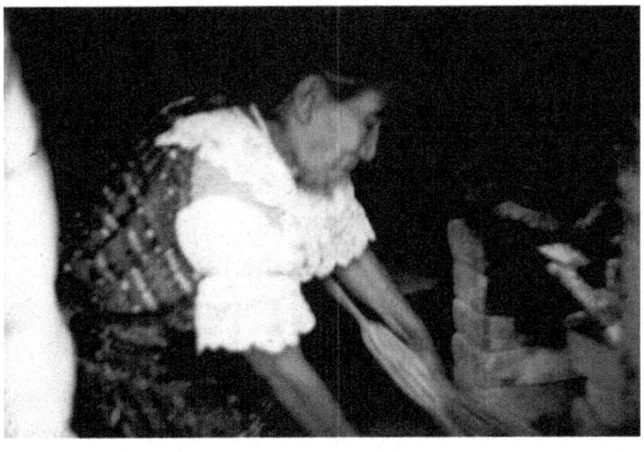

Fig. 34.2 A *K'iche'* Maya midwife performs a ritual in a *tuj* at the end of the 20-day postnatal period. After giving the mother a sweatbath, the midwife cleans the ashes from the hearth where she will then light candles and place incense and white roses. The midwife then recites various prayers. Santa Lucía Utatlán, Guatemala, 1974. Photo courtesy of Sheila Cosminsky, PhD

One midwife who strongly advocates for ritual and actual heating of the afterbirth says that, "Since it was fire that burned the placenta, the womb shrivels up rapidly," speeding up the mother's recovery. Proper burning of the placenta is also said to protect the mother's ability to bear more children. For this to be assured, a midwife tells me, hot herbs are applied to the placenta, and then the ash in which the placenta will be burned is arranged into a circle. The placenta is then placed in the circle, "mouth up," and this ashen womb is then burned, becoming singularly heated. In the view of *Kaqchikel* Mayas, the fact that placentas are not burned when delivery takes place in clinical settings amounts to poor care, even negligence. A midwife cautions that when women give birth in a hospital and the placentas are simply thrown away, "Women's stomachs look like they're very…[making an obese gesture], they look as if they're expecting."

Midwives keep foremost in mind that whatever happens to the mother's uterus also affects her other organs, especially the stomach. A family that neglects to burn the placenta may thus be endangering more than just the mother's figure; it may also be triggering problems with her stomach and all that that entails. Although midwives do not necessarily think of the stomach and uterus as a paired organ system, they know that mishandling of the placenta will affect both organs.

Despite admonitions about needing to burn the placenta, though, some midwives show uncertainty about it. This is especially the case among midwives who have received much of the official clinical "training" that the Guatemala state requires indigenous midwives to receive or at least sit through. One young midwife dismisses the idea that one should put culinary herbs on the placenta. Another says that while burning the placenta might help the mother avoid stomach pains, the burning might itself cause the child's teeth to rot when he grows older. She thus raises questions about the burning's efficacy but using a native line of reasoning. According to her, strong connections persist between both the mother and the placenta and between the child and the placenta. And since this organ was bound to both of them, they will each bear the lasting imprint of that connection, even if it is physically severed.

Still, Mayas generally regard the placenta as having a more enduring connection with the mother, at least in terms of the affective relationships recognized by ritual. We also see this recognition at work throughout the larger region where Mayas live. *K'iche'* Mayas of Santa Lucía Utatlán, for example, are among those Mayas who burn their placentas (Cosminsky 1982a, p. 243), as are *Yucatec* Mayas of Chan Kom, Yucatán, who say that placentas can be buried or burned but who favor burying them under the hearthstones of an unoccupied house (Redfield and Villa Rojas 1971, 182). The hearthstones there and their "warm" ashes will convey warmth to the mother. *Tzotzil* Mayas of Chiapas, similarly, prefer to burn or bury the placenta somewhere near the home (Fabrega and Silver 1973, p. 42; Guiteras Holmes 1961b, p. 165; Vogt 1969, p. 181) or even inter it inside the house (Holland 1961, p. 218). The afterbirth's connection with the mother and its kinship with the child must be enacted in these ways.

Other protective practices have also been observed. Guiteras-Holmes (1961b, p. 165) reported that *Tzotzil* and *Tzeltal* Mayas try to keep placentas away from individuals who might use them to ritually afflict the child; they protect the children by throwing their placentas into a river. In a Guatemalan setting, *Q'anjob'al* Mayas also try to dispose of the placenta and cord either by burning, burying, or throwing it into a river (La Farge 1947, p. 40). Their practices are motivated as much by fears of witchcraft as by a general sense that these organs are somehow unclean (La Farge 1947). In Eastern Guatemala and Western Honduras, *Chorti'* Maya parents have also acted out of a fear of witchcraft. Wisdom (1940, p. 288) reported that the child's father would insert the placenta into a gourd which was then wrapped in a banana leaf. He then buried the gourd in a secret place in the home compound. Taken together, while these accounts point to many fears of witchcraft, they nonetheless hinge on the idea that there exists an enduring connection between the child and its maternal nexus, whether placenta or umbilical cord or both. Because of this, these body parts must be ritually shielded from harm.

Mayas recognize such a strong connection between the placenta and child that the placenta is sometimes called "the second child." This designation, found among *K'iche'* Mayas of Santa Lucía Utatlán, clearly originates from the sequential appearance of the placenta after the child (Cosminsky 1982a, p. 243). Jordan (1989, p. 931), meanwhile, pointed out how *Yucatec* Mayas called the placenta the "companion" of the child. These Mayas also feel strongly that how one treats the placenta will affect the child's well-being and safety, so *Yucatec* fathers make certain to bury the "companion" of their newborn in a hidden place. In San Juan Comalapa, only the oldest midwife in the sample, an 83-year-old woman, refers to the afterbirth as a second body or child. She calls the placenta "its second," noting the order of its appearance. This woman's advanced age, together with her working vocabulary, is suggestive of how midwives of earlier generations may have voiced a clearer recognition of the affinal ties between placenta and child. But the way most local *Kaqchikel* Maya midwives refer to the placenta is no less profound.

Most local midwives refer to the placenta as *ruk'u'x ak'wal* or *ruk'u'x ti ni ne'y*, the "*k'u'x*/heart of the child." The word common to both designations, *k'u'x*, has long encased different meanings in colonial and modern *Kaqchikel* (Hinojosa 2002). Depending on its usage, it can refer to "heart," "center," or even "soul." When a *Kaqchikel* person says, "niq'axon pa nuk'u'x," she is saying that "my heart is pain" or, more figuratively, "my soul aches." But it is quite telling that when it is incorporated into the phrase, "ruk'u'x kaj, ruk'u'x ulew," it is referring not only to "the heart of the sky, the heart of the earth" but to the godhead invoked by this in the *K'iche'* Maya text, the *Pop wuj*. We can thus see how *k'u'x* enfolds a broad range of realities including a life source, a divinity, or even an animistic center (López Austin 1988). This is very much the case when Mayas talk about the human placenta.

Using very succinct phrasing, one midwife says that the placenta is, "that which gave life to the child, it gave suckle to the child from the inside, that's why they call it the *k'u'x*, that's why they say it is the child's heart, also." Her statement is revealing of how the placenta is not just a mere organ: it engenders the child, nurses it, and kindles the very heartbeat allowing the child to grow and develop. Together with the womb itself (which some *Kaqchikel* Mayas also regard as an expression of *k'u'x*), the placenta enables the fetal growth, heartbeat, movement, and even awakening of desire that midwives perceive as evidence of ensoulment. Since so much depends on the placenta, it is hardly surprising that this singular organ receives such near-reverential care among Mayas of so many places and cultural settings. As an embodiment of procreative forces, it cannot be taken lightly.

34.3 Umbilical Cords

Just as Maya midwives go to great lengths to handle placentas properly, they pay much physical and ritual attention to umbilical cords. They must of course be handled carefully when a child is born. Most local midwives take care to cut the umbilical cord about two finger-widths or 2 inches from the newborn's abdomen, making sure to cut the cord only after it has stopped pulsing and after they have tied it in two places with a strong, commercially available ribbon. Some midwives, though, may indicate the need to cut the cords of boys and girls differently. One *Kaqchikel* Maya midwife, for instance, stresses that a boy's cord should be cut 4 in. from his belly while a girl's cord should be cut 3 in. from her belly. This is because, she says, a man has authority over a woman, voicing a sentiment otherwise rarely heard among women in Comalapa. One explanation for this differential counting of inches may tie into early claims that the numbers three and four correspond with female and male numerical associations found throughout the Maya area (Thompson 1990, p. 166). For the most part, though, local midwives find 2 inches to be the right length to cut a baby's cord.

Before the cutting can happen, though, there is something that midwives are often asked to do for the woman and her family. The midwife is often asked to take a close look at the drops of blood in the umbilical cord. The parturient might tell the midwife, "tatz'eta' ri ru k'u'x jampe ak'wala' e k'o chiri'," "look at the placenta/cord for how many children are there." With this prompting the midwife will count the drops of blood still visible in the cord, drops that are considered to be the woman's future children. The midwife might see no blood drops at all, meaning that mother will have no future pregnancies, or she might see many drops, in which case the woman will become pregnant many more times.

There is more information that a midwife can deduct from the blood drops, including the sex of the children to come. Some midwives insist that a red drop portends and boy and a white drop portends a girl. Still other midwives say that the differences in color signal different body temperatures of the corresponding babies. For those subscribing to this diagnostic reasoning, yellow and green drops of blood foretell a child with abnormal body temperature, whereas white drops of blood foretell a child with healthy body temperature.

We find similar kinds of attention to the umbilical cord in other Maya settings. Cosminsky (1982a, p. 243, 1977, p. 86) finds that in the *K'iche'* region, and on a coastal plantation, Maya midwives pay close mind to what they see in the cord. Different features of the cord will reveal the number of children to come, their sex, and their chronological spacing in a particular mother's case. Even the shapes of the features matter, with round lumps portending girls and long lumps portending boys (Cosminsky 1982b, p. 215). Maya midwives of other groups also find the umbilical cord very revealing of a mother's fertility future, as we see with *Tz'utujil* Mayas of San Pedro la Laguna, *K'iche'* Mayas of Totonicapán, *Mam* Mayas of San Marcos, and *Tzotzil* Mayas of San Pedro Chenalhó (Paul and Paul 1975, p. 708; Greenberg 1982, p. 1604; Guiteras Holmes 1961a, pp. 108–109). Among *Kaqchikel* Mayas of Comalapa, the umbilical blood drops are said to reveal not only how many children a woman will have and their sex, but also whether she will ever abort a fetus. For one *Kaqchikel* midwife, yet another umbilical sign can foretell the mother's future fertility: if the child's umbilicus dries up and falls off within 3 or 4 days following birth, the parturient will become pregnant again soon. Other umbilical conditions are predictive of certain sexual outcomes among some *K'iche's*. According to these Mayas, the longer the umbilical cord is tied before being cut, the more libido that child will have when it reaches adulthood (MacKenzie 2016, p. 96).

Of all the information that the umbilical cord reveals, perhaps none is as important to a *Kaqchikel* mother as that concerning whether or not she will have a twin pregnancy in the future, something that local women wish to preclude. Comalapan women dread this kind of pregnancy because, as taxing as a single-child pregnancy is in Guatemala, a pregnancy with twins would be far more difficult, complicated, and potentially dangerous. It is basically not worth the risk. But with the right handling of the umbilical cord, Maya women can feel assured that they are doing everything possible to forestall such a pregnancy.

What a *Kaqchikel* midwife must do is examine the drops of blood in the umbilical cord and check to see whether any of them appear in pairs, as if they were joined together. Any blood drops that appear in pairs are said to show twins. In order to keep the twins from ever taking full physical form, she will cut the umbilical cord between the twinned drops of blood. By separating the two drops, the twins are separated. This cutting action expresses a practical application of contiguous magic in that since the blood drops were in contact with the womb, the action applied to the drops will directly affect the future activity of the womb. So meticulously have some women espoused this procedure that it is not uncommon for a parturient to ask her midwife to *aplastar*, or "crush," not only blood twins but other blood "children" in the cord so that they do not develop into fetuses down the road.

To be clear, not all midwives say that they subscribe to these procedures. But all of them know about these procedures. Those who disavow them dismiss them as old beliefs, and say they have only heard about them from others, while still showing remarkably detailed knowledge of the practice. We are left to wonder to what degree this ostensible native contraception method still features in delivery practices today. One midwife who appears very knowledgeable about reading the umbilical cord and intervening in it waxes skeptical about the blood twin cutting procedure. People must do this because of ignorance, she reasons, since the manipulated part of the umbilical cord and the placenta are burned and do not go back into the woman's body where they might otherwise have some effect. She, like other midwives, has received clinical orientations, and this might account for her skepticism. But at the same time, she strongly avows the need to burn the placenta, a practice which her current line of reasoning might also dismiss as unsupportable.

Another midwife also takes the cord-cutting procedure to task, even though women still ask her to cut blood twins and to count how many male and female children they will have. As she ponders why these beliefs persist, she reasons that people must think the blood drops in the cord are actually a woman's ova and that these will develop into fetuses. Even if this were the case, she argues, it would still make no sense to try to manipulate the ova by manipulating the cord, since the cord will not reenter the woman and affect her reproductive organs. Those who believe in these practices, she says, tend to be older women. Younger women express more doubts about them and come right out and ask the midwife if local ideas about the cord are actually true.

Midwives still want to know what to make of all the drops of blood in the umbilical cord, and this has led some midwives to surmise that the blood drops are not actually children; they are the *ruway ri ak'wal*, the "food of the child." One midwife says she knows this is the case because, when a child is born and there is no blood in the cord, that child will immediately want to nurse and will look for the breast. "They say that (the child) is hungry," she says, because "the child eats through the navel." When he has eaten everything in the umbilical pathway, leaving it clean, he is born ready to eat some more.

Viewing blood drops as fetal food largely makes sense to another midwife, who cautions that if the umbilical cord is cut before the child has finished "eating" through it, there is a high risk of hemorrhage. If food is still flowing through the cord, it is very likely to bleed when cut, and this can really endanger the newborn. She recommends that midwives not cut the cord immediately but to wait 5 min so that the child can finish "eating." Significantly, this view aligns with Jordan's (1993, p. 86) observation that the umbilical cord should not be cut too soon after delivery, as often occurs in obstetric practice. She points out that if cutting occurs prematurely, the newborn might be deprived of up to 25% of its requisite blood supply (Jordan 1993). Cosminsky (2016, p. 122) reiterates that the kind of delayed cord clamping practiced by Maya midwives has been shown to make more oxygen and iron available to the newborn.

To the extent that Maya midwives see the umbilical blood drops as food or as blood that the child still needs, they sometimes frame the cord as a kind of conduit that carries the child's strength or energy, a potency known as *chuq'a'*. For this reason, midwives liken the child's blood to the child's *chuq'a'*, something that can be spilled and irreparably lost if the cord bleeds too much. Underlining the gravity of such a situation, a *Kaqchikel* Maya soul healer states that when an umbilical cord bleeds out, "The *chuq'a'* of the baby is being lost." As among other Mayas who understand blood to be closely interwoven with and even synonymous with soul, *Kaqchikels* see heavy bleeding as spiritually perilous. Blood is considered so spiritually charged that many midwives say that any blood that issues from the umbilical cord should be burned. One midwife adds that this blood should be burned along with the placenta, as if to stress that these detached drops of spiritual energy and their source must both be heated.

Clearly, at the moment the cord is exposed, a final burst of life-sustaining energy is moving from placenta to child. It is at this moment that midwives can catch a glimpse of the procreative life force in the mother. Since the life force is embodied in the moving, multicolored clusters of drops, the mother can have the midwife examine, count, and even permanently separate them. And because the umbilical cord makes the generative *chuq'a'* available to the child, the cord will play an ongoing role in the child's future development.

Kaqchikel Mayas perform different procedures with the child's umbilicus, procedures that are meant to impact the child's life course. When the umbilicus, the part of the cord that stays attached to the newborn's navel, dries up and falls off in the week following birth, Mayas must attend to it ritually depending on whether the child is male or female. If the child is female, the usual practice is to wrap her umbilicus in a cloth, place this cloth in a small pouch, and then hang this pouch in the kitchen. Smoke from the stove or kitchen fire should hit the pouch and in this way ensure that the girl will be good at kitchen work. In line with this, one midwife recommends that the girl's umbilicus should be placed behind the *comal*, "griddle," so that she will know how to make tortillas, that is, provide for her family as a good cook. Another midwife, meanwhile, extends the girl's vocational space out to the *tuj*, saying that her umbilicus should be placed there since the girl will later have an important connection with this structure.

If a boy is born, his father must take the child's umbilicus to the forest and place it in the forking branches of a young tree. Comalapans say this is done so the boy will not be afraid of climbing trees nor of going to the hills to work. The tree should be young, many say, so that as it grows, so will the boy grow strong. Recalling the gendered toolkits of the community, one midwife says that some people will hang the boy's umbilicus among men's agricultural tools, like the hoe and gourd, so that "he can be a cultivator man." We can observe the same principle at work in the advice of another midwife who recommends that the boy's placenta be buried in the *tuj*, so that from an early age, he will be able to build fires.

Practices like these are known throughout the Maya highlands. We see among the *Tzotzil* Mayas of Larraínzar, Chiapas, for instance, that when a girl is born, her midwife cuts her cord over a grinding stone. This sets her on the path of knowing how to grind maize. A boy's umbilical cord, meanwhile, is cut over the head of an axe so that he can cut trees well in the future (Holland 1961, p. 218; see Guiteras Holmes 1961a, p. 108). In this refraction of Maya thinking, grinding stones and axes shape women and men into what society needs for them to be to function as basic providers.

According to Maya midwives in Comalapa, if umbilical rituals go unperformed, the mother or her child might have some very unpleasant experiences, though generally nothing as severe as what might occur if placental ritual gets neglected. What reports exist suggest simply that if a child's umbilicus goes untreated, he or she can become timid, fearful, and even weak. As a midwife explained, if a child's umbilicus is not treated ritually, the child will also experience swelling of his navel. His stomach might swell up, too, and cause a lot of pain. Many Comalapans feel that instead of leaving a child's health to chance, parents should simply give the umbilicus its ritual due.

34.4 Cauls

As part of every delivery, the Maya midwife will handle the amniotic sac, which normally emerges with the placenta. *Kaqchikel* Maya midwives pay a lot of attention to this membrane because if the newborn moves through the birth canal covered partially or completely by it, the child is believed to have a special destiny. The caul or amniotic shroud will certainly catch her attention, but at the moment of its appearance, even before she can ponder its meaning, she must act quickly to ensure it poses no physical danger to the child.

Kneeling at her backstrap loom, a midwife explains to me that if a child emerges with the caul completely covering its head, she has to swiftly remove this obstruction. To show me how she does this, she reaches into a nearby basket to grab a clear plastic bag holding balls of thread. She grips one ball from outside of the bag and says that a newborn's head in the sac resembles this. Then she pinches a section of plastic bag and pulls it away from the ball, motioning how she would have to pinch the slippery sac and pull it away from the head and neck, at which point she would cut the sac with a pair of scissors. They have to be strong scissors since this membrane is very strong, she says. Once she makes the incision, she would carefully uncover the newborn's head, allowing it to breathe. She would next use a squeeze bulb to clear the mouth and nose of mucus, making sure the breathing continues. The rest of the body can be uncovered after this.

When a newborn emerges covered in its *bolsita*, "little sack," midwives might remark that "petenaq xti ru q'uj xti ru tzyaq," "it is emerging/nearing covered up in its clothes." And because rather few children are born wearing any such "clothes," these births get noticed. *Kaqchikel* Maya midwives say that a special vocation awaits a child born with such a covering. For instance, if a boy is born with his head and body enclosed in the sac, he will one day become an *aq'omanel*, a "physician." A girl born covered by the sac is predestined to be a *k'exelon*, a "midwife." At the moment of birth, something of the child's future temperament can also be revealed, especially by the condition of the umbilical cord. For instance, if the child is born with the umbilical cord encircling his neck, he is said to be very *listo*, "clever and troublesome," and this disposition will likely remain part of his character. The midwife, being the first person to see such portents (and in some cases, the one who burns the amniotic sac along with the placenta in the *tuj*), must tell the child's parents what probably lies in store for the child. Midwives of other Maya communities shoulder similar responsibilities.

In San Pedro la Laguna, Guatemala, for example, the midwife is expected to divine what different caul configurations mean for newborns (Paul and Paul 1975). A boy born with an amniotic tissue resembling the shoulder bag of a shaman is thus said to be a future shaman. If a girl is born with a white mantle-like head covering, meanwhile, she has the calling of a midwife. In this *Tz'utujil* Maya community, though, the midwife is also tasked with identifying other kinds of ritual specialists. If a child is born balled up and enclosed in an unbroken amniotic sac, for example, it is said he or she might become a transforming witch. Being born with a sort of cap or cape is the sign of a rainmaker. Lastly, a child born holding "worms" or "flies" in his fist is fated to become a sorcerer (Paul and Paul 1975, pp. 708–9).

While few parents in either San Juan Comalapa or San Pedro la Laguna would probably seek out an ominous future for their child, parents nonetheless want to get their children on a favorable vocational path. Some parents might be disappointed if their children are not born with a caul, but they can still try to bring about a desired vocational future by other means. These means can include magical contiguous procedures of the kind a *Kaqchikel* Maya midwife describes. She says that some people want to give their child's dried umbilicus to a physician so that the child can become a physician. This manipulation of birth organs to affect the child's future working life is mirrored in the practices of some Ladinos, culturally non-Maya Guatemalans. A midwife in Comalapa says that, because some Ladinos toss their sons' placentas into a river, their sons leave the town for work and never come back. This reminds her that for Mayas, how one reads the caul and how one handles other birth organs can have a lasting effect on what a child's future holds.

34.5 Closing Observations

For the most part, *Kaqchikel* Mayas of Comalapa find good reason to handle different birth organs ritually. To ritually handle the placenta, for instance, is seen as involving little risk to the mother and as probably supplying something very beneficial to her. There is thus widespread support for this handling. Mayas express both certainty and ambivalence about how the umbilical cord should be handled, though, largely because competing worldviews converge in the domain of Maya midwifery like never before. Still, when it comes to umbilicus ritual, Mayas generally approve of it, whether or not they individually admit to practicing it. They see umbilicus ritual as more than just a way to ensure the child's health. This kind of ritual speaks to enduring Maya concerns about properly gendering children and about setting children on the paths laid out by generations of working people. And even though gendered roles have been undergoing rapid change, there still exists the view that all children should be socialized into a larger community of norms and mores, one that still leaves room for gendered vocational expression. This is where the caul or amniotic shroud becomes such a potent catalyst for specialized vocations. Midwives and parents know that this membrane does more than just envelope the fetus; it can imprint the child with the touch of destiny left by unseen forces of germination in the womb.

What are clinicians to make of these Maya views? Since Maya midwives know that health workers, who are usually non-Maya, reject and often sharply criticize Maya ways of thinking, clinicians should be mindful of a few things. Local people usually weigh the benefits of disclosing their beliefs to health workers, and this is particularly the case with Maya midwives who may be attending obligatory training sessions. The fact that many training sessions are conducted in Spanish, which many Maya midwives do not speak fluently (Chary et al. 2013), further precludes the free sharing of beliefs and assumptions between session participants who already stand on either side of a deep cultural divide. Clinicians should know that, even if Maya midwives do not talk freely about birth organ practices, Maya midwives and mothers still might consider these practices crucial for the well-being of the mother and child, including for the child's vocational well-being. And whether one examines Maya lives in Guatemala or in surrounding countries, it is important to bear in mind that considerable variation exists in the ways midwives think about birth organs and how they enact this thinking in ritual. Certain midwives might not even give credence to native ideas about birth organs, but these ideas can still affect their work and how they maintain trust among their neighbors. So being aware of and respectful of these practices goes a long way toward building trust in rural areas where the health stakes are highest.

It is also important to remember that the way clinicians treat native peoples will impact not only whether those clinicians can actually improve the physical lives of those people, it will also impact how those people might later accept or reject future clinicians or hold in them suspicion. How a single health worker treats indigenous people in a state health center or in private practice can leave a very lasting impression, one that might be talked about over the course of an entire generation. These enduring impressions are revealing of how perceived lapses in care or respect affect how later individuals size up visiting health workers and the system they come from. Midwives can quickly see whether the clinicians assigned to their towns are competent and can be trusted or whether they conform to a worldview that has marginalized their work in the past. These native health specialists are thus in a position to either share their knowledge of birth organs with respectful and open-minded counterparts or continue to keep their experiences concealed from medical eyes.

References

Chary, A., Kraemer Diaz, A., Henderson, B., & Rohloff, P. (2013). The changing role of indigenous lay midwives in Guatemala: New frameworks for analysis. *Midwifery, 29*(8), 852–858.

Cosminsky, S. (1977). Childbirth and midwifery on a Guatemalan finca. *Medical Anthropology, 1*(3), 69–104.

Cosminsky, S. (1982a). Knowledge and body concepts of Guatemalan midwives. In M. Artschwager (Ed.), *Anthropology of human birth* (pp. 233–252). Philadelphia, PA: F.A. Davis Company.

Cosminsky, S. (1982b). Childbirth and change: A Guatemalan study. In C. P. MacCormack (Ed.), *Ethnography of fertility and birth* (pp. 205–229). London and New York: Academic Press.

Cosminsky, S. (2016). *Midwives and mothers: The medicalization of childbirth on a Guatemalan plantation*. Austin, TX: University of Texas Press.

Fabrega, H., & Silver, D. B. (1973). *Illness and shamanistic curing in Zinacantan: An ethnomedical analysis*. Stanford, CA: Stanford University Press.

Greenberg, L. (1982). Midwife training programs in highland Guatemala. *Social Science & Medicine, 16*(18), 1599–1609.

Guiteras Holmes, C. (1961a). *Perils of the soul: The world view of a Tzotzil Indian*. New York, NY: The Free Press of Glencoe.

Guiteras Holmes, C. (1961b). La magia en la crisis del embarazo y parto en los actuales grupos mayances de Chiapas. *Estudios de Cultura Maya, 1*, 159–166.

Hinojosa, S. Z. (2002). *K'u'x* como vínculo corporal en el cosmos. *Estudios de Cultura Maya., 22*, 185–197.

Hinojosa, S. Z. (2004). Authorizing tradition: Vectors of contention in highland Maya midwifery. *Social Science & Medicine, 59*(3), 637–651.

Hinojosa, S. Z. (2015). *In this body: Kaqchikel Maya and the grounding of spirit*. Albuquerque, NM: University of New Mexico Press.

Holland, W.R. (1961). *Highland Maya folk medicine: A study of culture change*. Doctoral dissertation, Department of Anthropology, University of Arizona.

Jordan, B. (1989). Cosmopolitical obstetrics: Some insights from the training of traditional midwives. *Social Science & Medicine, 28*, 925–944.

Jordan, B. (1993). *Birth in four cultures: a crosscultural investigation of childbirth in Yucatan, Holland, Sweden, and the United States*. Fourth edition. Revised and expanded by R. Davis-Floyd. Prospect Heights, IL: Waveland Press.

Klein, S. (1995). *A book for midwives: A manual for traditional birth attendants and community midwives*. Palo Alto, CA: The Hesperian Foundation.

La Farge, O. (1947). *Santa Eulalia: The religion of a Cuchumatán Indian town*. Chicago, IL: University of Chicago Press.

López Austin, A. (1988). *The human body and ideology: concepts of the ancient Nahuas*. Translated by T. Ortiz de Montellano & B. Ortiz de Montellano. Salt Lake City, UT: University of Utah Press.

MacKenzie, C. J. (2016). *Indigenous bodies, Maya minds: Religion and modernity in a transnational K'iche' community*. Boulder, CO: University Press of Colorado.

Paul, L., & Paul, B. D. (1975). The Maya midwife as sacred specialist: A Guatemalan case. *American Ethnologist, 2*(4), 707–726.

Redfield, R., & Villa Rojas, A. (1971). *Chan Kom: a Maya village. Fourth edition, abridged*. Chicago, IL: University of Chicago Press.

Thompson, J.E.S. (1990). *Maya history and religion*. Forward by D.M. Pendergast & E. Graham. Norman and London: University of Oklahoma Press.

Vogt, E. Z. (1969). *Zinacantan: A Maya community in the highlands of Chiapas*. Cambridge, MA: Harvard University Press, Belknap Press.

Wisdom, C. (1940). *The Chorti Indians of Guatemala*. Chicago, IL: University of Chicago Press.

Part VI

Costa Rica

From Dengue to Zika: Environmental and Structural Risk Factors for Child and Maternal Health in Costa Rica Among Indigenous and Nonindigenous Peoples

35

Gabriela Alvarado and Jorge Benavides-Rawson

35.1 Introduction

The news of a possible association between Zika virus and fetal malformations in 2015 shifted the traditional paradigms in women's health. Until that point in time, no vector-borne diseases had ever been found to be associated with teratogenicity (Steele 2016). The widespread increased incidence of microcephaly and neurologic damage in fetuses and newborns with a history of maternal exposure to Zika in Brazil forced international authorities to act quickly and investigate the causes and implications of this disease (Torjesen 2016). Following the confirmation of the causative link between congenital fetal malformations and the Zika virus (CDC 2016), public health authorities across Latin America and other countries in the Western Hemisphere raced to strengthen their national infrastructures to minimize the threats and impact of Zika virus infections (Chan et al. 2016). Because the *Aedes* mosquito, the vector responsible for Zika virus transmission, is widely spread throughout Latin America (Petersen et al. 2016), it created extensive fear and concerns regarding the "inevitable" impact of the virus on newborn babies across the Americas (Bell et al. 2016).

Costa Rica is situated in Central America between Panama and Nicaragua. In Costa Rica, the *Aedes* mosquito is quite prevalent, and commonly causes ailments such as dengue fever and chikungunya (Tilak et al. 2016). Yellow fever, another disease transmitted by this mosquito, had previously been eradicated from the country. Since the arthropod vector was already present in the country, national health authorities began to prepare themselves for what seemed to be an imminent Zika outbreak on Costa Rican soil (Benavides Lara et al. 2016). Costa Rica has a well-developed health system in place,

G. Alvarado, M.D., M.S.P.H., M.A. (✉)
Department of Anthropology, Georgia State University, Atlanta, GA, USA
e-mail: gabriela@alvaradomd.com

J. Benavides-Rawson, M.D., M.A.
Department of Anthropology, The George Washington University, Washington, DC, USA

D. A. Schwartz (ed.), *Maternal Death and Pregnancy-Related Morbidity Among Indigenous Women of Mexico and Central America*, Global Maternal and Child Health: Medical, Anthropological, and Public Health Perspectives, https://doi.org/10.1007/978-3-319-71538-4_35

and boasts among the highest health indicators in the region (Morgan 1993). However, national indicators do not reflect the underlying disparities that are present in the country, especially among the rural and impoverished indigenous populations. Indigenous groups account for approximately 2% of Costa Rica's population, yet they have the highest unemployment rates, poverty rates, adolescent pregnancy rates (18.6%), teenage marriage (22% versus the national average of 4.6%), and lowest investment in infrastructure and health (Fallas Hidalgo et al. 2006). Moreover, in the event of a Zika outbreak, there could be a disproportionately higher risk for indigenous populations due to structural inequalities, health disparities, and the inability for indigenous people to contend with the medical and financial aspects of needs for children with developmental disabilities due to the congenital Zika syndrome.

Costa Rica implemented a series of measures and epidemiological procedures in response to the impending Zika epidemic. Among the first was the creation of a task force composed of members of the Ministry of Health, the national health service (CCSS—Caja Costarricense del Seguro Social), and the national health research institute (INCIENSA—Instituto Costarricense de Investigación y Enseñaza en Nutrición y Salud) (Benavides Lara et al. 2016). Detailed procedures and guidelines were created for the notification and management of Zika virus infections, airport and border security were heightened (Fig. 35.1), training for health professionals was implemented, and weekly bulletins with reports and cases were published (Benavides Lara et al. 2016; Hernandez Chaves et al. 2016; Ministerio de Salud de Costa Rica 2017). As Costa Rica braced for impact—the epidemic that was expected did not strike. How

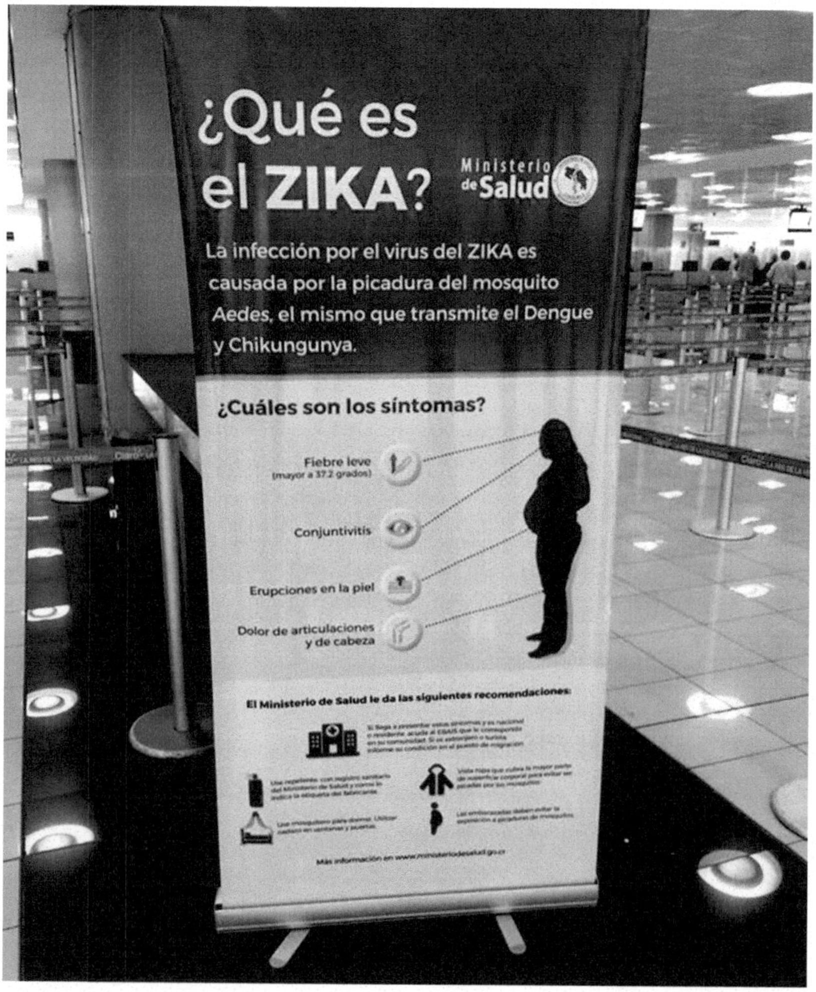

Fig. 35.1 "What is ZIKA? (Qué es el ZIKA?)" at Juan Santamaria Airport, Costa Rica. Photo by Jorge Benavides, June 2016

is it that a country with all the ingredients in the recipe for an infectious disease disaster could walk away at the end of the year reasonably unscathed? This unexpected outcome, and the potential vulnerability of the country's indigenous populations, are the topics of this chapter, where we draw from multiple disciplines such as medicine, public policy, public health, and anthropology to analyze this case study.

35.2 Explaining Change

A classic approach to understanding change in public policy is through Kingdon's Three Streams Model (Buse et al. 2012). The model proposes that change occurs during "windows of opportunity" when three separate streams align or meet. The problem stream is when attention is drawn to a particular issue, the policy stream is when there is a potential solution available for the said problem, and the politics stream is when there is an incentive and motivation to convert the potential solution into a concrete policy (Cairney and Jones 2016). In Brazil, the streams that aligned for the Zika epidemic were (1) the problem stream; (2) ecological factors; and (3) lack of treatment or solution to the problem (see Fig. 35.2). In the case of Brazil, the problem stream was created when a newly imported virus initially entered the country. The ecological factors included the presence of a mosquito vector to transmit the virus, climate and specific weather conditions that favored arthropod-borne transmission, and nonimmune vulnerable populations exposed to the mosquito vector (particularly due to socioeconomic conditions of poverty and overcrowding). Finally, the lack of treatment or solution to the problem developed with the nonrecognition between maternal Zika infection and congenital fetal malformations. Furthermore, as there is no treatment for Zika, there were no measures in place at the time to prevent Zika infection from occurring.

In Costa Rica, several conditions existed that had the result of these three streams escaping convergence in 2016. Fortunately, the level of epidemic seen in Brazil that had been feared throughout the Costa Rican region was ultimately avoided (Fig. 35.2). The "protective" ecological factors included geographic location and conditions of certain populations, including indigenous communities, the way that the Costa Rican health system is structured, regional efforts for vector control, existence of

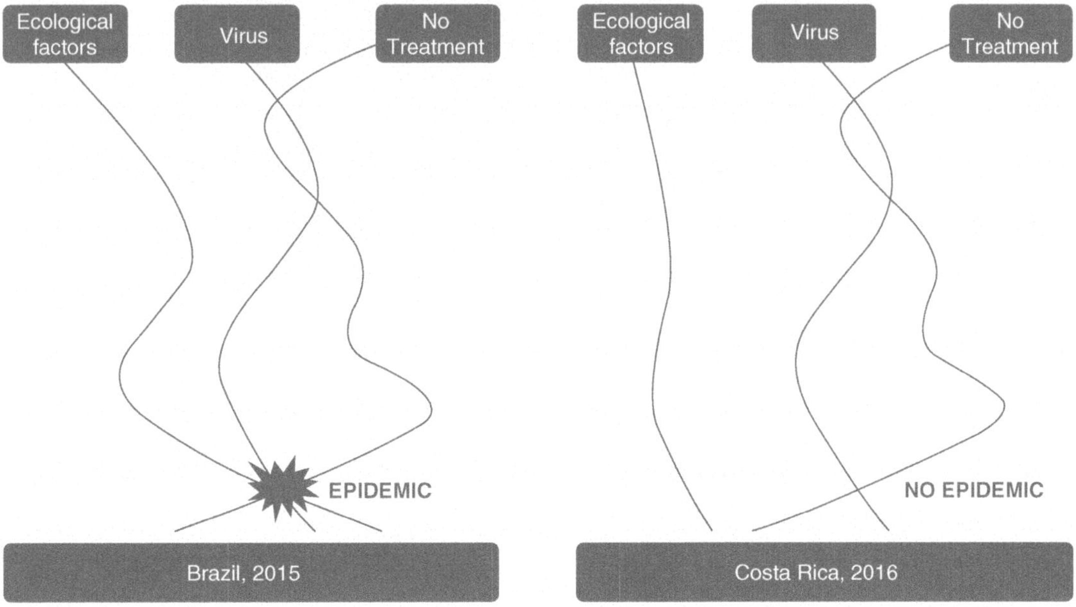

Fig. 35.2 Model based on Kingdon's Three Stream Model outlining conditions in Brazil in 2015 and Costa Rica in 2016

other flaviviruses in the region, and the seasonal timing of the Zika virus threat. This meant that even if the *virus* and *no treatment* streams met, the *ecological factors* stream did not permit the conditions for an infectious disease disaster on the national level.

35.3 Indigenous Communities in Costa Rica

Costa Rica is the second smallest country in Central America, with 50,990 km^2 and a population of 4,301,712 in the most recent census (INEC 2013; Low 1985). Over one-half of the population lives in the Central Valley, greater than 90% of the population self-identify as having Hispanic descent (being "white"), and 2% are Black (located mainly along the Caribbean coast). In 2016, indigenous people made up approximately 2.5% of the population, numbering 104,143 persons, of whom 78,703 identify as being a member of one of the eight indigenous groups recognized by the government (IWGIA 2016; Low 1985). In the 1550s Costa Rica had not yet been conquered, and the exploration of the Spanish was confined to the northern Nicoya peninsula and the coastal regions (Perez 1997). Because Costa Rica did not have minerals that were considered valuable to Europeans, it was largely ignored during the initial periods of Spanish conquest and colonialization (Cofresi 1994). When the Spaniards began to settle in the Central Valley, the *Chibchan* indigenous group that lived in the area were completely eliminated as they resisted colonization. The first assessment of indigenous peoples in Costa Rica was conducted by Perefán de Rivera, in what he called "repartimiento," which means "to divide up" in a form of indentured servitude closely resembling slavery (Perez 1997). Estimates and projections state that between the years 1500 to 1524 the indigenous population of Costa Rica may have numbered approximately 337,000, declining to 120,000 in 1550, 54,000 in 1580, and decreasing even further to only a few thousand between the 1600s–1800s, followed by a gradual increase in population from the 1900s until the present (Perez 1997).

Following the initial conquest by the Spanish, indigenous populations retreated and were forced outside of the Central Valley. As agriculture became the main economic activity of the country, lands were seized for coffee and banana plantations, pushing indigenous communities further out into inaccessible and "hostile" environments (Cofresi 1994). All over the world there is a history of repression by the political majorities; slowly, marginalized communities realized that this type of exploitation between nation-states and indigenous people was "part of a global pattern" (Hodgson 2011, p. 29). These patterns of exploitation and repression included, but were not limited to, land alienation, forced settlement, linguistic discrimination, economic marginalization, disparities in health and education, and cultural disparagement (Hodgson 2011). There were calls from communities and activists from all over the world to protect people's rights to "cultural, social, economic, and political self-determination within the framework of the nation states in which they reside" (Hodgson 2011, p. 39). The international response to these calls was the creation of a working group within the United Nations, from which the Indigenous and Tribal Peoples Convention 169 resulted in 1989, termed the "Convention Concerning Indigenous and Tribal Peoples in Independent Countries," which was later adopted by the International Labor Organization (International Labour Organization, n.d.). It was after the United Nations declaration that the Costa Rican government created 24 official indigenous territories, which covered a total of 3344 km^2, or 5.9% of the land. Here, eight different indigenous groups reside, autonomous from the state (Schliemann 2012). These groups and the regions they inhabit are: the *Teribe* (Térraba), *Guatuso* (north-central areas), *BriBri* (Salitre, Cabagra, Talamanca Bribri and Kekoldi), *Huetar* (Quitirrisí and Zapatón), *Chorotega* (Matambú), *Ngöbe* (Abrojos Montezuma, Coto Brus, Conte Burica, Altos de San Antonio and Osa), *Cabecar* (Alto Chirripó, Tayni, Talamanca Cabécar, Telire and China Kichá, Bajo Chirripó, Nairi Awari and Ujarrás), and *Brunca* (Boruca and Rey Curré). Most of these indigenous groups maintain a traditional language in addition to Spanish (except for *Huetar* and *Chorotega* populations who are monolingual Spanish speakers exclusively). The majority of indigenous territories in the country are southeast of the Central Valley, in areas with very poor infrastructure and difficult access (see Fig. 35.3).

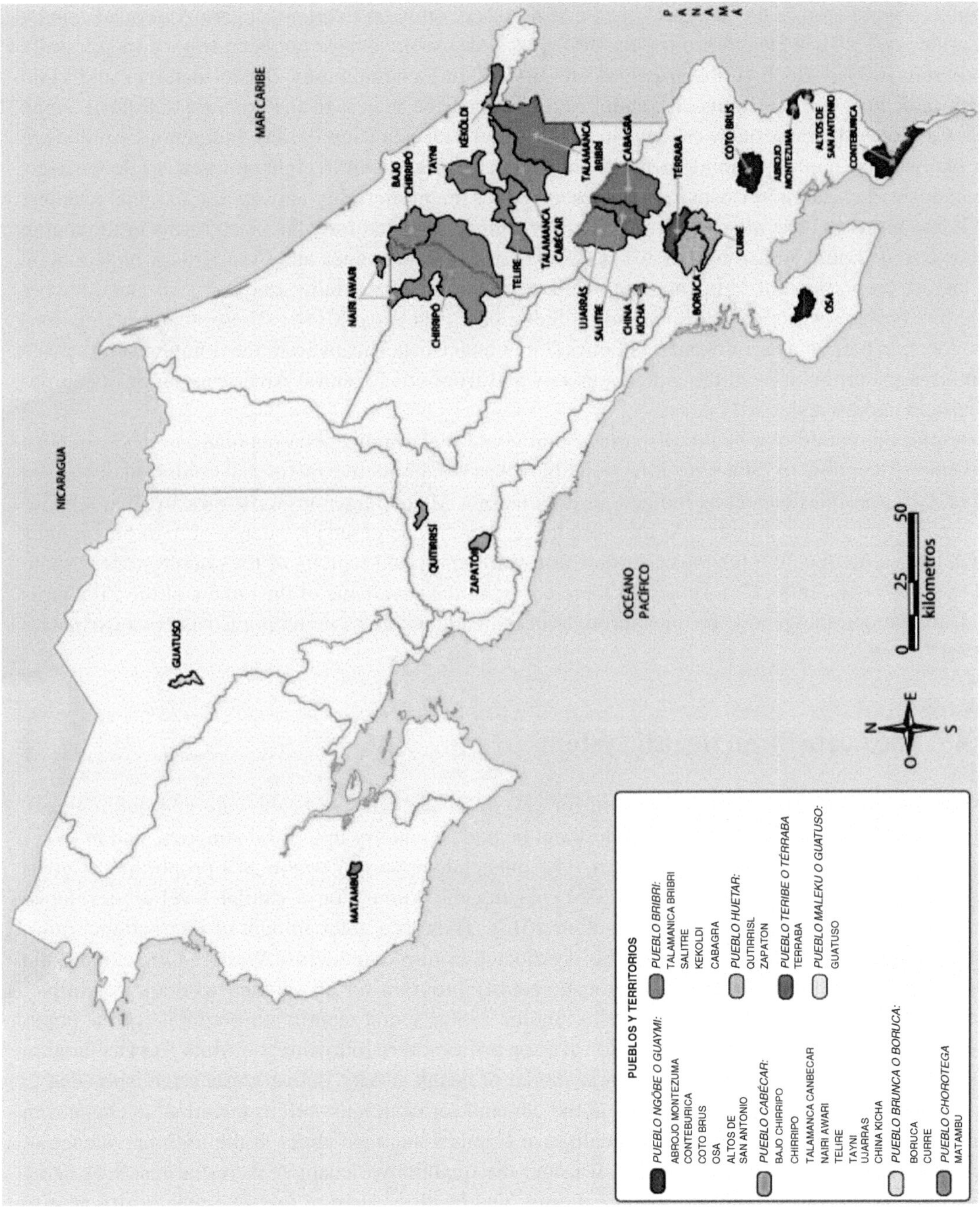

Fig. 35.3 Indigenous territories of Costa Rica. Source: INEC 2013

Health in indigenous communities is a result of competing medical ideologies, marginalization, women's rights issues, poverty, lack of education, language incompatibility, stigmatization, and poor infrastructure. Mainstream approaches to health fail to understand and consider the cultural diversity and local customs of indigenous communities, which in turn leads to mistrust on behalf of the communities when it comes to "Western" medical models (Comision Economica para America Latina y el Caribe et al. 2010). Health promotion strategies and discourse have not been framed in culturally appropriate ways, which further marginalizes indigenous communities. Thus, maternal and child health indicators in indigenous communities are among the lowest in the country, similar to some other Central American countries (Ministerio de Salud de Costa Rica 2014a). Indigenous women are less likely to use family planning methods and have on average four to eight children, while the average number of children in Costa Rica is closer to two. Infant mortality is twice the national average, and home births in the *Cabecar* territory have recently accounted for 71% of all births in the region (Ministerio de Salud de Costa Rica 2014a). The regions of Talamanca and Coto Brus, which contain the largest proportions of indigenous populations, have infant mortality rates of 15.6 and 13.7 per 1000 live births, respectively (Ministerio de Salud de Costa Rica 2014b). These health inequalities have roots, in part, in a narrative of "whiteness" in which Costa Ricans from the dominant culture see themselves as different from the indigenous few and from other Central American nations (Campo-Engelstein and Meagher 2011).

Despite the underlying health disparities that could make indigenous populations in Costa Rica markedly susceptible to Zika virus infection, there was one protective factor that conferred decreased risk of Zika transmission among indigenous populations. Most indigenous territories are in mountainous regions and at high altitudes. As a consequence, there is decreased prevalence of *Aedes* mosquitos which have a predilection for lower altitude and warmer coastal regions of the country (Mena et al. 2011; Troyo et al. 2008). Unfortunately, there are scant data available of the effects of the Zika virus pandemic among indigenous peoples throughout the endemic areas including Costa Rica (Schwartz 2017a).

35.4 The Costa Rican Health System

Costa Rica has an international reputation for very high standards of health care and public health (Morgan 1993). Costa Rica is the wealthiest and healthiest country in Central America, and has very high spending on social welfare programs. The financial support of health as a proportion of gross domestic product (GDP) was 9.3% in 2014, placing the country on a similar level as developed European nations (World Health Organization 2017). There is a great amount of international influence on Costa Rican health models, and this is reflected in current models of Western biomedicine and approaches to public health. In 1941 a social security program for all salaried workers was implemented that covered for health and disability; by the 1980s, social security covered 85% of the population of Costa Rica and was redesigned to focus on primary care following the Alma Ata Declaration of 1978 (Morgan 1993). In the 1990s a new model of health service delivery was established due to reforms of the State, qualitative changes in the demand for health, as well as quantitative changes in demand (Vargas Gonzalez 2006). The qualitative changes included shifts in the high prevalence of infectious diseases toward chronic illnesses, and the quantitative changes were the result of aging population, urbanization, and migration patterns. The health system at the time was insufficient to cope with these changes, and so the model of Integrated Health Services was created (Vargas Gonzalez 2006). Following the implementation of the new model, health indicators in Costa Rica have soared, with maternal mortality ratios (MMRs) decreasing from 390 per 100,000 live births in 1994, to 330 in 2003, and to 250 in 2015 (INEC 2015; Vargas Gonzalez 2006; World Bank 2016). Infant mortality

(IM) has also significantly improved, going from 15.7 per 1000 live births in 1994, to 10.1 in 2003, and 7.95 in 2014 (INEC 2016; Vargas Gonzalez 2006). Even though Costa Rica has achieved extraordinary success in health indicators, there has been relatively little scientific interest in studying the Costa Rican model. A model that has health expenditures per capita of around one-tenth of those in the United States, yet has similar infant mortality rates and higher life expectancy than the richest country in the American continent (Unger et al. 2008).

The new Integrated Health Services model was based on three basic principles: (1) universality, where the national health system would provide health coverage for all citizens, regardless of geographic location, socioeconomic status, or culture; (2) solidarity, which created the need for a mandatory contribution regime; and (3) equity, by aiming to reduce differences in health levels in various regions of the country and populations, as well as securing equal access to health services of good quality to all users. To achieve this, the health system was broken down into levels of attention. A first level of attention would offer basic health services through health posts called EBAIS (Equipo Básico de Atención Integral en Salud), which stands for basic team for integrated health services. The second level supports the first level through ambulatory procedures and through the five main specialties (internal medicine, pediatrics, obstetrics-gynecology, psychiatry, and general surgery). At the third level, highly specialized services are available, as well as inpatient services. The emphasis of the model was placed on the first level, which was characterized by holistic and continuous care, assigning families to health teams, continuous education, information systems, regionalization, administrative decentralization, new financing mechanisms, and social participation (Vargas Gonzalez 2006). The financing mechanisms for the social security system are employer-based, and constructed on the principle of solidarity. Employers match and contribute 12% of their employees' salaries, employees provide 9% of their salary, and the state supplies an undisclosed amount (Vargas Gonzalez 2006).

Social participation was envisioned as a change in attitude toward health on behalf of communities, based on self-care and health promotion, implementation of activities, and management of health services (Vargas Gonzalez 2006). Between the 1970s and 1980s the concept of community participation was a key feature of the government's primary health programs. These programs were cut back following the economic crisis in the country, and reinstated in recent years to "revamp" current public health programs and strategies. However, community participation can be a double-edged sword. There are different degrees of community participation ranging from spontaneous, to induced, to coerced, and participation is ultimately transformed into another way of exerting power (Morgan 1993). The concept of community participation has been promoted in indigenous populations, with little success in the past. This is because these initiatives have not been spontaneous and have been either induced or imposed. True community participation comes from the community spontaneously and cannot be rushed or forced. The following section in this chapter details further efforts conducted in an indigenous territory of Costa Rica to create an inclusive model of health care.

35.5 Bridging the Health Gap—Maternal and Child Health

Despite the monumental advances Costa Rica has made in the area of population health, the principle of equity established in the Integrated Health Services model has yet to be fully achieved. There are significant gaps in access to health services in indigenous populations, as well as lagging health indicators, including higher maternal and infant mortality than the national average. Nonetheless, there is a success story that is proving there is a way to bridge these gaps: the Coto Brus health care area.

Even with the history of neglect suffered by indigenous communities in Costa Rica and the rest of Central America, there is a model of inclusive health services and community participation in the *Ngöbe* territory located in Coto Brus county in the south of Costa Rica. In this impoverished county that shares a border with Panama, a new model of primary care was established in 2010 (Ortiz et al. 2009). This model not only invites the participation of the community but also includes traditional medicine in its model of service provision, making it the first multicultural primary care project in Costa Rica. Even though the building for the new clinic was opened in 2010, the new approach began at least 5 years earlier with the creation of the figure of "cultural advisor." These advisors are members of the *Ngöbe* indigenous group who serve as liaisons between the community and the local health authorities (Area de Salud). Their roles include translating health policies, consulting in the creation and validation of health programs, and serving as health promoters that educate their own communities (Area de Salud de Coto Brus 2012). The project hinges on two fundamental structures. The first one is physical, the primary care clinic which includes traditional knowledge even in its architecture (see Fig. 35.4); and the second is technical structure, which is a document detailing good practices in the maternal and child health delivery system. This new model is currently fully implemented in Coto Brus, one of the poorest counties in the country; therefore, it is paramount to understand how it came to fruition.

The *Ngöbe* (also known as *Ngöbe-Bügle*) are the largest indigenous community in the southern part of Central America. Their territory is located in Costa Rica and Panama, with the majority of it in the latter. The *Ngöbe* migrate back and forth between both countries to work on the coffee plantations (*fincas*) of Costa Rica during harvest season. Because of this constant movement, there is usually a sub-register of the population on both sides of the border. Although many travel as complete family units, including their small children, the majority of those who migrate are men of working age. The *Ngöbe* are a highly vulnerable population from many perspectives. Poverty is generalized throughout the community, as the economy is either subsistence farming or working on plantations for very low daily wages. The birth rates of the *Ngöbe* are four children per woman, which is twice the national rate. Access to health care is difficult, in many cases because of geographic barriers. There are also several cultural barriers to improved health care, including language (not everyone speaks Spanish), male dominated patterns of behavior, and low education status (Area de Salud de Coto Brus 2012).

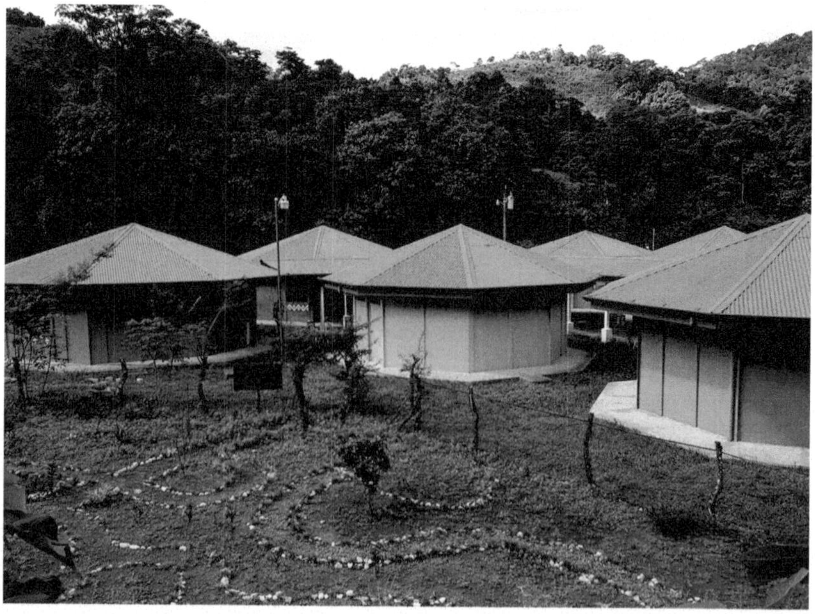

Fig. 35.4 Traditional building style incorporated into the construction of the local health care facility, EBAIS La Casona, Coto Brus, Costa Rica. Source: Jorge Benavides, May 2015

In the 1990s and 2000s the childhood and maternal health indicators were disheartening. Women rarely had access to or utilized birth control, even though it is freely provided by the Costa Rican health care system. This was the result of a combination of factors—the clinic was not close to everyone, services were only available certain days of the month, and cultural norms required a female doctor (who was not always available) to do the physical examination of female patients. The permanence of children in primary and secondary education was also low, even with free education. Many had to work with their families to provide daily food, and the schools are not always geographically accessible.

Driven by the severe inequalities found in this community and inspired by principles of interculturality and inclusion, the head of the Coto Brus health care office, Dr. Pablo Ortiz, began to include different small projects in the indigenous communities in the last two decades. These initiatives were eventually compiled in a document titled "Systematization of good practices developed for the promotions of healthy lifestyles and the delivery of maternal and child healthcare in the Ngöbe population." This document was published in 2012 and was partly funded by UNICEF and the Spanish Cooperation Agency for International Development. One of the major impacts that this document had is in the role that the local community and its leaders play in the creation and execution of health care plans. The figure of the "cultural advisor" is a spin-off from a previous project called *Finca Sana* (Healthy Farm), which trained *Ngöbe* individuals to act as educators, translators, and advisors for different health delivery projects such as use of birth control, hand washing, oral health, and prevention of sexually transmitted diseases (STDs). The good practices initiative also recruits and trains local midwives and trains them to participate as aids for pregnant women during their prenatal attention visits. This resulted in a significant increase in prenatal care coverage, decrease in maternal mortality, and a drop in the child mortality rates from 17.1/1000 live births in 2001, to fewer than 10/1000 live births by the end of the same decade (Area de Salud de Coto Brus 2012).

Parallel to the development of the previously mentioned guidelines, the local health administration proposed the creation of a culturally appropriate primary care clinic. Up to that point, the clinic was run out of an old house that was refurbished to host a team of one doctor, one nurse, one records technician, one pharmacist, and two primary care technicians. In 2009, the leadership of the local health care administration submitted a proposal for less than $250,000 for the funding of a brand new clinic that would be built from the ground up (Ortiz et al. 2009). The project was successfully funded by the Spanish Cooperation Agency for International Development. The design of the buildings followed local patterns of construction, including the painting of the walls. The clinic was created with a space that would not only host a physician, but also a traditional healer; and included a medicinal plant garden in the back of the clinic (see Fig. 35.4). The ongoing functions of the clinic are funded by the national health care system (CCSS), and the clinic has had a large impact in the participation of the community in health care delivery. The local population not only has a clinic that is culturally sensitive, but because they were consulted in the design stages, they also have a sense of ownership of the project (Area de Salud de Coto Brus 2012).

While this community is not affected by the Zika virus, it has been affected by other infectious diseases, such as diarrheal disease. The establishment of an ongoing project that creates successful partnerships between the community and the health care system creates an effective barrier for the control of new infectious threats. In the specific case of Zika virus, any potentially affected mothers and children will have access to improve prenatal control, child and development consults, and referral to higher levels of specialized medicine, when needed, that will ameliorate the potential impacts of this new viral infection if it arrives.

35.6 From Dengue to Zika

35.6.1 Dengue

Dengue fever is a disease caused by a Flavivirus, transmitted by a mosquito vector of the genus *Aedes*, and is the arbovirus causing the greatest morbidity and mortality worldwide (Mena et al. 2011). Estimates range from 50 to 100 million cases each year and 12,000–24,000 deaths annually (Troyo et al. 2009). In Costa Rica the vector had been eradicated in the 1960s, but became a problem again after reinsertion of *Aedes* in the 1990s. By 2005 Costa Rica became the country with the highest incidence of dengue fever in Latin America, and has maintained high levels ever since (Mena et al. 2011). The vector breeds in both urban and suburban environments where there is poor garbage collection and water deposits in artificial containers such as old tires, flower pots, and buckets (Troyo et al. 2009). The infection is usually self-limited and asymptomatic. In cases where symptoms occur, the most common manifestations are an acute febrile illness, headache, myalgia, arthralgia, vomiting, and a maculopapular rash that may be confused with other exanthematic conditions, such as measles, rubella, enterovirus, adenovirus, and influenza (Simmons et al. 2012). The severe manifestation of dengue fever is dengue hemorrhagic fever (DHF), characterized by a systemic vascular leakage syndrome and thrombocytopenia. As there is no known cure for dengue fever, treatment remains supportive, and focuses on fluid management and control (Simmons et al. 2012).

Attempts to control dengue have focused on two main fronts: vector control and vaccination. Vector control has been promoted throughout Latin America by encouraging garbage collection, and educating the public on frequent breeding sites for mosquitos (Troyo et al. 2009). New approaches to vector control have also included the release of genetically modified mosquitos that will sterilize the female mosquito population (Simmons et al. 2012). Development of vaccines has been a priority for many pharmaceutical companies; however, the complexity of immune interactions between the four serotypes of dengue have made the development of the vaccine problematic and slow (Simmons et al. 2012). Emphasis on vector control over vaccination has risen in the past years with the emergence of chikungunya, and now Zika, which are both transmitted by the same mosquito (Tilak et al. 2016). The high incidence of dengue in Costa Rica was the factor that instigated such a coordinated response on behalf of Costa Rican authorities, as there was a great concern that because of the wide prevalence of the mosquito, Zika would be spread rapidly throughout the nation.

35.6.2 Zika

The Zika virus was first isolated in 1947 from a Rhesus monkey, in the Zika Forest of Uganda, where studies were being carried out for yellow fever (Schwartz 2017b; Tilak et al. 2016). Zika is an arthropod-borne virus (arbovirus) and is part of the Flavivirus family, which includes dengue, yellow fever, West Nile fever, and Japanese encephalitis (Ladhani et al. 2016; Panchaud et al. 2016; Tilak et al. 2016). The virus had never been associated with microcephaly until 2015, and had been usually limited to sporadic and confined outbreaks (Culjat et al. 2016; de Fatima Vasco Aragao et al. 2016). The announcement by Brazilian authorities that Zika virus was being investigated as causal agent of microcephaly cases in Brazil came as a shock to the international community, as the virus was considered to be of limited public health importance. During the months of July to September 2015, physicians in Brazil noted during routine ultrasound screenings an increase in fetuses with congenital malformations, which included severe cerebral atrophy, ventriculomegaly, and intracranial calcifications (Costa et al. 2016). Following the unprecedented increase in microcephaly cases in Brazil, the World Health Organization (WHO) declared a Public Health Emergency of International Concern on

February 1, 2016 (Costello et al. 2016). Subsequent evidence and case studies were published, including retrospective data from the French Polynesia outbreak in 2014, all of which led the Centers for Disease Control and Prevention (CDC) to formally declare in April of 2016 that there was a causal relationship between prenatal Zika virus infection and microcephaly/brain abnormalities (Panchaud et al. 2016). Autopsy studies of stillborn fetuses and neonates with Zika virus infection confirmed that Zika virus was neurotropic, resulting in a spectrum of gross and microscopic neuropathological abnormalities in addition to microcephaly (Schwartz 2017c).

Zika virus infection usually presents itself as a self-limited illness, with an average duration of 4–7 days. The majority of patients are asymptomatic; those who do manifest symptoms have such nonspecific symptoms as low-grade fever, maculopapular rash, arthralgia, headache (or retro-orbital headache), conjunctivitis, and myalgia (Tilak et al. 2016). During maternal infection, the virus has been proven to be neurotropic, generating malformations in the central nervous system of fetuses that lead to microcephaly (Alvarado and Schwartz 2017; Culjat et al. 2016; Schwartz 2017c). Microcephaly is defined as an occipito-frontal circumference below the third percentile or below two standard deviations (2SD) from the normal curve (Panchaud et al. 2016). Microcephaly and most other congenital abnormalities have very complex causal mechanisms, and often have multifactorial causes (de Oliveira et al. 2016). These causes can be divided into prenatal and postnatal, depending on whether the microcephaly was present at birth, and can be further categorized into genetic or acquired (Nunes et al. 2016).

Careful differential diagnosis should be conducted when analyzing microcephaly cases associated with Zika virus. Other infections in pregnancy, which also have mild or imperceptible clinical manifestations, are known to cause congenital abnormalities in the fetus; these infections are collectively known as TORCH (Toxoplasmosis, Other, Rubella, Cytomegalovirus, Herpes simplex virus) (Culjat et al. 2016; Schwartz 2017b). As part of confirming that a case of microcephaly is due to Zika, exclusion of other TORCH infections should be performed. The presence of microcephaly is the most emphasized aspect in most descriptions of congenital Zika syndrome, yet there are a wide range of clinical and radiological manifestations that have been described in recent case studies such as severe cerebral atrophy, ventriculomegaly, and extensive intracranial calcifications (Costa et al. 2016). The majority of case reports focus on the effect of Zika on the central nervous system, nevertheless there have been reported instances of ocular abnormalities and malformations of the limbs (de Paula Freitas et al. 2016; de Miranda et al. 2016; Perez et al. 2016; Alvarado and Schwartz 2017). There has been no documented evidence of direct Zika virus cytotoxicity in liver, lungs, heart, bone marrow, or skin (Culjat et al. 2016; Schwartz 2017c). Table 35.1 summarizes the most important and current findings in congenital Zika syndrome.

Shortly after the announcement of the emergency of international concern related to Zika virus, Costa Rican health authorities began tracking Zika in February 2016, with weekly updates published into 2017. In the initial report of Zika virus infections there were eight new cases described; by December 2016, a total of 1614 cases had been reported. The peak of incidence of Zika virus infection was approximately from week 31 to week 35, which coincided with the peak of dengue incidence which had been forecast at the beginning of 2016 (Ministerio de Salud de Costa Rica 2016). The peak in incidence of pregnant women with positive Zika serology was a few weeks after the peak in weekly new cases. By the end of 2016, 150 women who were pregnant had serologic evidence of Zika virus infection. In the same year, only one case of microcephaly associated with maternal Zika virus infection in Costa Rica had been confirmed (Ministerio de Salud de Costa Rica 2017). Considering the magnitude of the epidemic in Brazil, and the widespread presence of the *Aedes* mosquito vector in Costa Rica, having just one case of microcephaly associated with maternal Zika virus infection was a true public health victory. Figure 35.5 describes in a single graph the number of new cases reported in the weekly bulletins published by the Costa Rican Ministry of Health.

Table 35.1 Manifestations of the congenital Zika syndrome

Categories of malformations associated with congenital Zika syndrome	
Category	Examples
Neurologic	• Microcephaly
	• Hydrocephalus
	• Micrencephaly
	• Lissencephaly
	• Polymicrogyria
	• Pachygria
	• Agyria
	• Holoprosencephaly
	• Ventriculomegaly
	• Corpus callosum abnormalities
	• Intracerebral calcifications
	• Destructive brain lesions
Ocular	• Chorioretinal atrophy
	• Optic nerve abnormalities
	• Maculopathies
	• Vascular abnormalities
Musculoskeletal	• Arthrogryposis
	• Craniofacial abnormalities (craniosynostosis)
	• Clubfoot
	• Acetabular dysplasia
Genitourinary	• Cryptorchidism
	• Hypospadias
Other	• Intrauterine growth restriction
	• Anasarca
	• Pulmonary hypoplasia
	• Single umbilical artery

Source: Alvarado and Schwartz (2016)

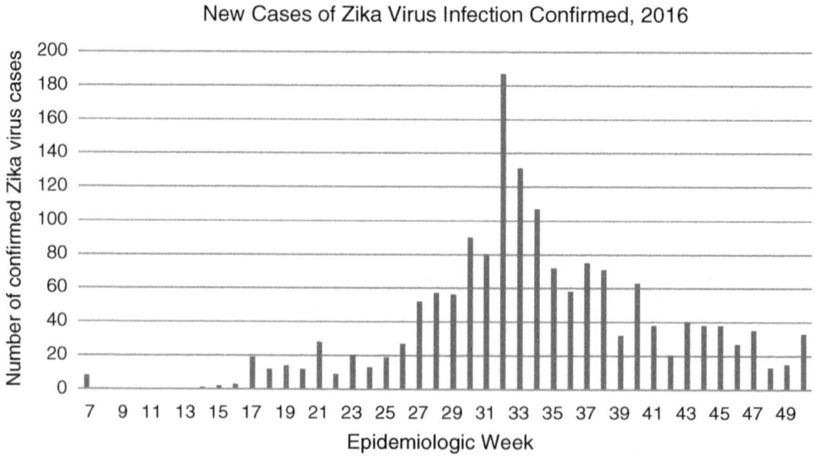

Fig. 35.5 Trends in new cases of Zika Virus in Costa Rica. Source: Data collected from Ministry of Health bulletins 2016

Surveillance for Zika virus infections in Costa Rica has continued into 2017, alongside routine dengue and chikungunya reporting. The first quarter of 2017 demonstrated a significantly higher incidence of Zika virus in Costa Rica in comparison to 2016. This could be due to underreporting in the initial stages of the epidemiologic vigilance, or it could mean a true increase in the prevalence of the virus in mosquito vectors. During the first quarter of 2017, 16 cases of pregnant women with Zika virus infection were confirmed, and no cases of microcephaly secondary to Zika. In 2016 the impact of Zika virus on maternal and child morbidity in Costa Rica was close to nonexistent; however, it remains a very real threat, especially when reports are significantly higher than the previous year during the traditionally "low" season.

35.6.3 The Overlap

Both dengue and Zika viruses are members of the Flavivirus family, transmitted through the mosquito vector *Aedes aegypti*. The sharing of a vector suggested that Zika would spread quickly and easily as the vector was already in place. The peak incidence of dengue virus infections in Costa Rica occur during the rainy season of Costa Rica, and incidences are extremely high along the coasts. Public health authorities assumed that Zika transmission would be as common as dengue, and fortunately it was not. Is there a reason why Zika did not spread like wildfire in Costa Rica? A possible explanation could be related to underreporting. It is possible that the virus was occurring at low levels among the mosquito vectors, and that 2017 will present much higher incidences of Zika infection in Costa Rica. An alternate theory lies in immunologic responses to dengue and Zika.

Recent immunologic studies researching the association and impact of Zika and dengue infection in the same organism have suggested possible mechanisms in which dengue fever might confer a level of protection against Zika virus infection. A study of epitopes examined Zika virus and dengue virus cross-reactive CD8+ T cells and found CD8+ T cell responses in dengue that reduced Zika virus levels (Wen et al. 2017). A separate mechanism involving envelope dimer epitopes found a class of human monoclonal antibody from dengue can neutralize Zika virus and have a protective effect (Swanstrom et al. 2016). These results could suggest that due to the high incidence of dengue in Costa Rica, this generated lower than expected Zika virus incidence due to still poorly understood cross-protection mechanisms. However, these theories have yet to be confirmed in vivo, and there are other in vitro studies that have proven just the opposite—suggesting that dengue virus antibodies actually enhance Zika virus infection (Paul et al. 2016).

35.7 Ecological Factors

Regional and global climate trends created favorable conditions for the spread of the *Aedes* mosquito, which in turn favored the rapid spread of Zika in Brazil. Transmission risk modeling has shown that the risk for transmission in South America was at its highest for 60 years in 2015 due to favorable temperature coupled with low mosquito mortality rates and short incubation periods (Caminade et al. 2016). In addition to these warming trends due to the El Niño phenomenon, there are also seasonal variations that depend on such variables as temperature, humidity, and rainfall. Adult mosquito prevalence is low during the winter, and high during the summer, especially when average temperatures are above 18 °C, and there is increased rainfall (da Cruz Ferreira et al. 2017; Escobar et al. 2016).

In addition to climate, other external and ecological factors influence the spread of Zika virus infections. The proportions of local *Aedes* mosquitos of different species could also have significant impact on the spread of Zika due to differences in feeding behaviors among different species. *Aedes aegypti* feeds exclusively on human blood, which means it is an effective vector for Zika; on the other hand, *Aedes albopictus* has a range of hosts in addition to humans, which means it is a less effective vector for transmitting the virus to humans (Caminade et al. 2016). *A. albopictus* was introduced into the Americas in the late 1990s, and has slowly expanded through the continent. In some areas, due to direct competition for breeding sites, *A. albopictus* has displaced *A. aegypti*, while in other areas they coexist. Surveys of mosquito species distribution have found that *A. aegypti* tends to be more prevalent in urban settings, while *A. albopictus* is more common in rural settings (Rey and Lounibos 2015). This could explain why Zika transmission in Costa Rica has been lower than expected. Coastal areas of Brazil that present altitude and temperature favorable for high mosquito prevalence are highly urbanized, which means they most likely will have larger *A. aegypti* populations. On the other hand, the coastal areas of Costa Rica are rural, which presents a higher likelihood of larger *A. albopictus* proportions, which are less effective vectors for Zika. A final factor related to urbanization is that a high human population density is a risk factor for Zika transmission (Santos and Meneses 2017). Costa Rica has very scarcely populated coastal areas in comparison to Brazil, which could have served as an added protective feature.

35.8 Waiting for the Epidemic

Although 2016 was a good year for Costa Rica and most of Central America, public health authorities must remain vigilant. Vector control initiatives must be maintained and intensified, and protection against mosquito bites, especially for pregnant women, is crucial. At the height of the Brazilian epidemic, the World Health Organization recommended women delay pregnancy until risks were lower (Costello et al. 2016). However, as postponing pregnancy in all women in at risk regions is unrealistic, some authors propose using windows of opportunity for conception that align the first trimester of pregnancy with seasons of low vector prevalence (Martinez et al. 2016).

Additional strategies could also be implemented to monitor vector trends in order to effectively predict future transmission risks for Zika. Monitoring vectors has currently been proposed as a strategy for dengue virus, yet it could also serve as an effective measure for the Zika virus. The surveying, monitoring, and quantification of mosquitos can serve as short-term indicators of the risk for infection. When values of the Mean Female *Ae. aegypti* Index (termed the MFAI, an entomological index of the mean number of female Ae. aegypti mosquitos caught per trap) increases by an average of 0.1 per week, the probability of dengue transmission to humans is increased by 25% (da Cruz Ferreira et al. 2017). Another model that uses sea surface temperature from El Niño Southern Oscillation and indices derived from the Moderate Resolution Spectrometer from the Terra Satellite has been able to predict dengue outbreaks 40 weeks in advance (Fuller et al. 2009). This technology could potentially be used for the prediction of Zika.

Conclusions

The factors that were pivotal in minimizing the effects of Zika in Costa Rica were global and local climate trends, geographic distribution of vector species, the strong and integrated health system, and potential immunologic interactions with dengue virus. Additionally, the most impoverished communities in Costa Rica, the indigenous populations, unlike in Brazil, were protected due to their geographic location in mountainous regions. These external and ecological factors did not align with the other two streams to generate a public health emergency in Costa Rica.

There are significant efforts by governmental and private agencies to develop and test a vaccine for Zika virus in a number of countries, including Costa Rica (National Institutes of Health 2017). However, until that time, health authorities in all *Aedes* prevalent regions must remain vigilant. Zika virus is a very real threat to child and maternal health, and must remain high on the public health agenda until concrete treatments or vaccines are available to the general public. In the case of vulnerable populations such as the indigenous peoples of Costa Rica, the health system can expand the model initiated in Coto Brus with the *Ngöbe* community. This model considers the cultural characteristics of the population, making them part of the effective implementation of maternal and child health programs. Such an approach can minimize the impact of an eventual Zika outbreak in these communities.

References

Alvarado, M. G., & Schwartz, D. A. (2016). Zika virus infection in pregnancy, microcephaly, and maternal and fetal health—What we think, what we know, and what we think we know. *Archives of Pathology & Laboratory Medicine, 141*(1), 26–23. https://doi.org/10.5858/arpa.2016-0382-RA. Retrieved from http://www.archivesofpathology.org/doi/full/10.5858/arpa.2016-0429-ED

Alvarado, M. G., & Schwartz, D. A. (2017). Zika virus infection in pregnancy, microcephaly, and maternal and fetal health: What we think, what we know, and what we think we know. *Archives of Pathology & Laboratory Medicine, 141*(1), 26–32.

Area de Salud de Coto Brus. (2012). *Sistematización de buenas prácticas: Desarrolladas para la promoción de estilos de vida saludables y la atención de la salud materno-infantil en la población indígena Ngöbe*. Caja Costarricense del Seguro Social. Coto Brus.

Bell, B. P., Boyle, C. A., & Petersen, L. R. (2016). Preventing Zika virus infections in pregnant women: An urgent public health priority. *American Journal of Public Health, 106*(4), 589–590. https://doi.org/10.2105/AJPH.2016.303124

Benavides Lara, A., María de la Paz Barboza Arguello, Hernandez de Mezerville, M., Gonzalez Elizondo, M., Prevencion y Control de Infecciones Hospital Nacional de Ninos. (2016). *Protocolo de vigilancia de microcefalia en el marco de vigilancia del virus del Zika en Costa Rica*. San Jose. Retrieved from https://www.ministeriodesalud.go.cr/index.php/vigilancia-de-la-salud/normas-protocolos-y-guias/2995-protocolo-de-vigilancia-microcefalia-en-rn-el-marco-de-la-vigilancia-del-virus-del-zika-en-costa-rica/file

Buse, K., Mays, N., & Walt, G. (2012). *Making health policy (understanding public health)* (2nd ed.). London: Open University Press.

Cairney, P., & Jones, M. D. (2016). Kingdon's multiple streams approach: What is the empirical impact of this universal theory? *Policy Studies Journal, 44*(1), 37–58. https://doi.org/10.1111/psj.12111

Caminade, C., Turner, J., Metelmann, S., Hesson, J. C., Blagrove, M. S. C., Solomon, T., et al. (2016). Global risk model for vector-borne transmission of Zika virus reveals the role of El Niño 2015. *Proceedings of the National Academy of Sciences, 114*(1), 119–124. https://doi.org/10.1073/pnas.1614303114

Campo-Engelstein, L. & Meagher, K. (2011). Costa Rica's 'White legend': how racial narratives undermine its health care system. *Developing World Bioethics, 11*(2), 99–107.

CDC (Centers for Disease Control and Prevention). (2016). *CDC concludes Zika causes microcephaly and other birth defects*. Retrieved April 19, 2017, from http://www.cdc.gov/media/releases/2016/s0413-zika-microcephaly.html.

Chan, J. F. W., Choi, G. K. Y., Yip, C. C. Y., Cheng, V. C. C., & Yuen, K. Y. (2016). Zika fever and congenital Zika syndrome: An unexpected emerging arboviral disease. *Journal of Infection, 72*(5), 507–524. https://doi.org/10.1016/j.jinf.2016.02.011

Cofresi, I. M. (1994). *Migration and health in Talamanca, Costa Rica: An applied medical anthropology approach*. Georgia State University.

Comision Economica para America Latina y el Caribe, Organizacion Panamericana de la Salud, UNFPA, & Naciones Unidas. (2010). *Salud materno infantil de pueblos indigenas y afrodescendientes de America Latina: una relectura desde el enfoque de derechos*. Santiago. Retrieved March 17, 2017, from http://www.cepal.org/publicaciones/xml/8/41668/lcw346.pdf.

Costa, F., Sarno, M., Khouri, R., de Paula Freitas, B., Siqueira, I., Ribeiro, G. S., et al. (2016). Emergence of congenital Zika syndrome : Viewpoint from the front lines. *Annals of Internal Medicine, 164*(10), 689–691. https://doi.org/10.7326/M16-0332

Costello, A., Dua, T., Duran, P., Gülmezoglu, M., Oladapo, O. T., Perea, W., et al. (2016). Editorial: Defining the syndrome associated with congenital Zika virus infection. *Bulletin of the World Health Organization, 94*(6), 406–406A. https://doi.org/10.2471/BLT.16.176990

Culjat, M., Darling, S. E., Nerurkar, V. R., Ching, N., Kumar, M., Min, S. K., et al. (2016). Clinical and imaging findings in an infant with Zika embryopathy. *Clinical Infectious Diseases, 63*(6), 805–811. https://doi.org/10.1093/cid/ciw324

da Cruz Ferreira, D. A., Degener, C. M., de Almeida Marques-Toledo, C., Bendati, M. M., Fetzer, L. O., Teixeira, C., et al. (2017). Meteorological variables and mosquito monitoring are good predictors for infestation trends of Aedes aegypti, the vector of dengue, chikungunya and Zika. *Parasites & Vectors, 10*(1), 78. https://doi.org/10.1186/s13071-017-2025-8. Retrieved from http://parasitesandvectors.biomedcentral.com/articles/10.1186/s13071-017-2025-8

de Fatima Vasco Aragao, M., van der Linden, V., Brainer-Lima, A. M., Coeli, R. R., Rocha, M. A., Sobral da Silva, P., et al. (2016). Clinical features and neuroimaging (CT and MRI) findings in presumed Zika virus related congenital infection and microcephaly: retrospective case series study. *British Medical Journal, 353*. https://doi.org/10.1136/bmj.i1901

de Oliveira, W. K., Cortez-Escalante, J., Gonçalves Holanda De Oliveira, W. T., Ikeda do Carmo, G. M., Pessanha Henriques, C. M., Coelho, G. E., et al. (2016). Increase in Reported prevalence of microcephaly in infants born to women living in areas with confirmed Zika virus transmission during the first trimester of pregnancy—Brazil, 2015. *MMWR: Morbidity & Mortality Weekly Report, 65*(9), 242–247. https://doi.org/10.15585/mmwr.mm6509e2

de Paula Freitas, B., de Oliveira Dias, J. R., Prazeres, J., Almeida Sacramento, G., Icksang Ko, A., Maia, M., et al. (2016). Ocular findings in infants with microcephaly associated with presumed Zika virus congenital infection in Salvador, Brazil. *Journal of the American Medical Association Ophthalmology, 134*(5), 529–535.

Escobar, L. E., Romero-Alvarez, D., Leon, R., Lepe-Lopez, M. A., Craft, M. E., Borbor-Cordova, M. J., et al. (2016). Declining prevalence of disease vectors under climate change. Scientific Reports, 6, 39150. doi:https://doi.org/10.1038/srep39150. . Retrieved from https://www.nature.com/articles/srep39150

Fallas Hidalgo, G., Quiros Valverde, M., Gamboa Quesada, M., Viales Araya, E. (2006). *Diagnostico Socioeconomico region Brunca*. San Jose. Retrieved from http://www.infoagro.go.cr/Inforegiones/RegionBrunca/Documents/Planes, Proyectos, Programas/DIAGNÓSTICO REGION BRUNCA 2006 VERSION FINAL.pdf.

Fuller, D. O., Troyo, A., & Beier, J. C. (2009). El Niño Southern Oscillation and vegetation dynamics as predictors of dengue fever cases in Costa Rica. *Environmental Research Letters, 4*(1), 14011. https://doi.org/10.1088/1748-9326/4/1/014011

Hernandez Chaves, O. N., César Gamboa, P., Daniel Salas, P., Rafael Salazar, P., Porras, H., & Griselda Ugalde, U. (2016). *Lineamientos nacionales para el abordaje integral de la mujer embarazada y el recién nacido, relacionado con la infección Zika*. San Jose. Retrieved from https://www.ministeriodesalud.go.cr/index.php/biblioteca-de-archivos/3054-lineamientos-nacionales-para-el-abordaje-integral-de-la-mujer-embarazada-y-el-recien-nacido-relacionado-con-la-infeccion-del-zika/file

Hodgson, D. L. (2011). *Being Maasai, becoming indigenous. Postcolonial politics in a neoliberal world*. Bloomington, IN: Indiana University Press.

INEC. (2013). *Territorios indígenas principales indicadores demográficos y socioeconómicos 2011*. San Jose. Retrieved from http://www.inec.go.cr/sites/default/files/documentos/inec_institucional/estadisticas/resultados/repoblaccenso2011-02.pdf.pdf

INEC. (2015). *Mortalidad materna y su evolucion reciente*. San Jose. Retrieved from http://www.inec.go.cr/sites/default/files/documentos/poblacion/mortalidad/publicaciones/mmerd14.pdf

INEC. (2016). *Mortalidad infantil y su evolucion reciente*. San Jose. Retrieved from http://www.inec.go.cr/sites/default/files/documetos-biblioteca-virtual/repoblaciodef-is2016.pdf

International Labour Organization. (n.d.). *C169—Indigenous and tribal peoples convention, 1989 (No. 169)*. Retrieved from http://www.ilo.org/dyn/normlex/en/f?p=NORMLEXPUB:12100:0::NO::P12100_ILO_CODE:C169

IWGIA (International Work Group for Indigenous Affairs. (2016). *Indigenous peoples in Costa Rica*. Retrieved from http://www.iwgia.org/regions/latin-america/costa-rica

Ladhani, S. N., O'Connor, C., Kirkbride, H., Brooks, T., & Morgan, D. (2016). Outbreak of Zika virus disease in the Americas and the association with microcephaly, congenital malformations and Guillain–Barré syndrome. *Archives of Disease in Childhood, 101*(7), 600–602. https://doi.org/10.1136/archdischild-2016-310590

Low, S. (1985). *Culture, politics and medicine in Costa Rica. An anthropological study of medical change*. Bedford Hills, NY: Redgrave.

Martinez, M. E., Cortez-Escalante, J., Tenório, W., Holanda, G., Madeleine, G., & Eyrolle-Guignot, D. (2016). Preventing Zika virus infection during pregnancy using a seasonal window of opportunity for conception. *PLoS Biology, 14*(7), e1002520. https://doi.org/10.1371/journal.pbio.1002520

Mena, N., Troyo, A., Bonilla-Carrión, R., & Calderón-Arguedas, O. (2011). Factors associated with incidence of dengue in Costa Rica. Revista Panamericana de Salud Publica, 29(4), 234–242. Retrieved March 17, 2017, from http://www.ncbi.nlm.nih.gov/pubmed/21603768.

Ministerio de Salud de Costa Rica. (2014a). *Aproximación a la condición de salud los pueblos indígenas de Costa Rica*. San Jose. Retrieved March 17, 2017, from https://www.ministeriodesalud.go.cr/ops/documentos/docEpidemiologi del Pueblos Indigenas de Costa Rica.pdf.

Ministerio de Salud de Costa Rica. (2014b). *Analisis de situacion de salud Costa Rica*. San Jose. Retrieved from https://www.ministeriodesalud.go.cr/index.php/vigilancia-de-la-salud/analisis-de-situacion-de-salud/2618-analisis-de-situacion-de-salud-en-costa-rica/file

Ministerio de Salud de Costa Rica. (2016). *Boletín epidemiológico No 1—2016 Zika, Chikungunya y Dengue*. San Jose. Retrieved from https://www.ministeriodesalud.go.cr/index.php/vigilancia-de-la-salud/analisis-de-situacion-de-salud/2861-chikungunya-2016/file

Ministerio de Salud de Costa Rica. (2017). *Resumen 2016 de la situacion Zika, Chikunguya y Dengue*. San Jose. Retrieved from https://www.ministeriodesalud.go.cr/index.php/biblioteca-de-archivos/3189-resumen-de-la-situacion-en-america-del-zika-chikungunya-y-dengue-para-el-ano-2016/file

de Miranda, H. A., Costa, M. C., Frazão, M. A. M., Simão, N., Franchischini, S., & Moshfeghi, D. M. (2016). Expanded spectrum of congenital ocular findings in microcephaly with presumed Zika infection. *Ophthalmology, 123*(8), 1788–1794. https://doi.org/10.1016/j.ophtha.2016.05.001

Morgan, L. M. (1993). *Community participation in health*. Cambridge: Cambridge University Press.

National Institutes of Health. (2017, March 31). *Phase 2 Zika vaccine trial begins in U.S., Central and South America*. Retrieved from https://www.nih.gov/news-events/news-releases/phase-2-zika-vaccine-trial-begins-us-central-south-america

Nunes, M. L., Carlini, C. R., Marinowic, D., Neto, F. K., Fiori, H. H., Scotta, M. C., et al. (2016). Microcephaly and Zika virus: A clinical and epidemiological analysis of the current outbreak in Brazil. *Jornal de Pediatria, 92*(3), 230–240. https://doi.org/10.1016/j.jped.2016.02.009

Ortiz, P., Fernandez, W., & Tropper, E. (2009). *Proyecto Dotacion De Infraestructura Nueva Para Un Ebais: "Construcción De Un Ebais Modelo En El Territorio La Casona Coto Brus*. Coto Brus.

Panchaud, A., Stojanov, M., Ammerdorffer, A., & Vouga, M. (2016). Emerging role of Zika virus in adverse fetal and neonatal outcomes. *Clinical Microbiological Reviews, 29*(3), 659–694. https://doi.org/10.1128/CMR.00014-16. Address

Paul, L. M., Carlin, E. R., Jenkins, M. M., Tan, A. L., Barcellona, C. M., Nicholson, C. O., et al. (2016). Dengue virus antibodies enhance Zika virus infection. *Clinical & Translational Immunology, 5*(12), e117. https://doi.org/10.1038/cti.2016.72

Perez, H. (1997). Estimates of the indigenous population of Central America (16th to 20th Centuries). In A. R. Pebley & L. Rosero-Bixby (Eds.), *Demographic diversity and change in the Central American isthmus* (pp. 95–115). Santa Monica: RAND.

Perez, S., Tato, R., Cabrera, J. J., Lopez, A., Robles, O., Paz, E., et al. (2016, March). Confirmed case of Zika virus congenital infection, Spain. *Euro Surveillance, 21*(24). https://doi.org/10.2807/1560-7917.ES.2016.21.24.30261

Petersen, L. R., Jamieson, D. J., Powers, A. M., & Honein, M. A. (2016). Zika virus. *New England Journal of Medicine, 374*(16), 1552–1563. https://doi.org/10.1056/NEJMra1602113

Rey, J. R., & Lounibos, P. (2015). Ecología de Aedes aegypti y Aedes albopictus en América y transmisión enfermedades. *Biomédica, 35*, 177–185.

Santos, J., & Meneses, B. M. (2017). An integrated approach for the assessment of the Aedes aegypti and Aedes albopictus global spatial distribution, and determination of the zones susceptible to the development of Zika virus. *Acta Tropica, 168*, 80–90. https://doi.org/10.1016/j.actatropica.2017.01.015

Schliemann, C. (2012). La autonomía de los pueblos indígenas de Costa Rica una contrastación del estándar internacional con la legislación nacional y su implementación. *Revista Latinoamericana de Derechos Humanos, 23*(1), 145–185.

Schwartz, D.A. (2017a, March 20). What do we know about Zika virus in indigenous populations? Interview by Sarah Anwar, Washington, DC. *Contagion Live*. Retrieved from http://www.contagionlive.com/videos/what-do-we-know-about-zika-virus-in-indigenous-populations

Schwartz, D. A. (2017b). The origin and emergence of Zika virus, the newest TORCH infection—What's old is new again. *Archives of Pathology & Laboratory Medicine, 141*(1), 18–25. Retrieved from http://www.archivesofpathology.org/doi/full/10.5858/arpa.2016-0429-ED

Schwartz, D. A. (2017c). Autopsy and postmortem studies are concordant: Pathology of Zika virus infection in neonates and stillborn fetuses with microcephaly following transplacental transmission. *Archives of Pathology & Laboratory Medicine, 141*(1), 68–72. Retrieved from http://www.archivesofpathology.org/doi/full/10.5858/arpa.2016-0343-OA

Simmons, C. P., Farrar, J. J., van Vinh Chau, N., & Wills, B. (2012). Dengue. *New England Journal of Medicine, 366*(15), 1423–1432. https://doi.org/10.1056/NEJMra1110265

Steele, R. W. (2016). Zika Virus: An explosive pandemic and a new TORCH agent. *Clinical Pediatrics, 55*(8), 698–700.

Swanstrom, J. A., Plante, J. A., Plante, K. S., Young, E. F., McGowan, E., Gallichotte, E. N., et al. (2016). Dengue virus envelope dimer epitope monoclonal antibodies isolated from dengue patients are protective against Zika virus. *mBio, 7*(4), e01123-16. https://doi.org/10.1128/mBio.01123-16

Tilak, R., Ray, S., Tilak, V. W., & Mukherji, S. (2016). Dengue, chikungunya … and the missing entity – Zika fever: A new emerging threat. *Medical Journal Armed Forces India, 72*(2), 1–7. https://doi.org/10.1016/j.mjafi.2016.02.017

Torjesen, I. (2016). Zika virus outbreaks prompt warnings to pregnant women. *British Medical Journal, 352*, i500. https://doi.org/10.1136/bmj.i500

Troyo, A., Calderón-Arguedas, O., Fuller, D. O., Solano, M. E., Avendaño, A., Arheart, K. L., et al. (2008). Seasonal profiles of Aedes aegypti (Diptera: Culicidae) larval habitats in an urban area of Costa Rica with a history of mosquito control. *Journal Of Vector Ecology: Journal Of The Society For Vector Ecology, 33*(1), 76–88. Retrieved from http://ezproxy.gsu.edu/login?url=http://search.ebscohost.com/login.aspx?direct=true&db=mnh&AN=18697310&site=eds-live

Troyo, A., Fuller, D. O., Calderón-Arguedas, O., Solano, M. E., & Beier, J. C. (2009). Urban structure and dengue incidence in Puntarenas, Costa Rica. *Singapore Journal of Tropical Geography, 30*(2), 265–282. https://doi.org/10.1111/j.1467-9493.2009.00367.x

Unger, J., De Paepe, P., Buitron, R. & Soors, W. (2008). Costa Rica: achievements of a heterodox health policy. *American Journal of Public Health, 98*(4), 636–643.

Vargas Gonzalez, W. (2006). *Atencion primaria de salud en accion*. San Jose: EDNASSS.

Wen, J., Tang, W. W., Sheets, N., Ellison, J., Sette, A., Kim, K., & Shresta, S. (2017). Identification of Zika virus epitopes reveals immunodominant and protective roles for dengue virus cross-reactive CD8+ T cells. *Nature Microbiology, 2*, 17036. https://doi.org/10.1038/nmicrobiol.2017.36

World Bank. (2016). *Maternal mortlaity ratio*. Retrieved from http://data.worldbank.org/indicator/SH.STA.MMRT

World Health Organization. (2017). World Health Organization. *Costa Rica*. Retrieved from January 1, 2017, http://www.who.int/countries/cri/en/

Part VII

Panama

Improving Maternal Health Status in Indigenous Communities of Panama: Community-Based Participatory Research and Interventions Among the *Ngäbe-Buglé* People of Panama

36

Arlene Calvo and Arturo Rebollón

36.1 Introduction

Indigenous communities perform poorly in global health indicators, when compared to other populations. Reports from the World Health Organization (WHO) indicate that indigenous groups have higher rates of maternal and child mortality, lower access to health services, and more people living under extreme poverty conditions and as a result have a shorter lifespan (Rosenstock et al. 2013; Zhao et al. 2013). This common scenario occurs in Panama, where indigenous groups have limited access to basic health services, health education, and clean drinkable water. A complex combination of social, demographic, and educational factors impacts their health status (Contraloria Nacional de la República 2000; Ministerio de Economía y Finanzas 2003). Collaborative efforts guided by the academic community, government and non-governmental organizations (NGOs), and community members resulted in a community-based educational intervention aiming to improve health literacy in the *Comarca Ngäbe-Buglé* (*Comarca* is the equivalent to an autonomous indigenous reservation in Panama). Figure 36.1 illustrates the geographical location of the *Comarca Ngäbe-Buglé*.

Starting in 2010, and funded through the Panamanian National Secretariat of Science, Technology, and Innovation (SENACYT), a public health educational intervention in the *Ngäbe-Buglé* region, following participatory processes, identified that health educators yearned for culturally appropriate

A. Calvo, Ph.D., M.P.H. (✉)
Department of Community and Family Health, Global Health, Panama Program at the City of Knowledge, University of South Florida, Tampa, FL, USA
e-mail: acalvo@health.usf.edu

A. Rebollón, M.D., M.P.H., C.P.H.
Department of Global Health, University of South Florida, Tampa, FL, USA
e-mail: arebollo@health.usf.edu

D. A. Schwartz (ed.), *Maternal Death and Pregnancy-Related Morbidity Among Indigenous Women of Mexico and Central America*, Global Maternal and Child Health: Medical, Anthropological, and Public Health Perspectives, https://doi.org/10.1007/978-3-319-71538-4_36

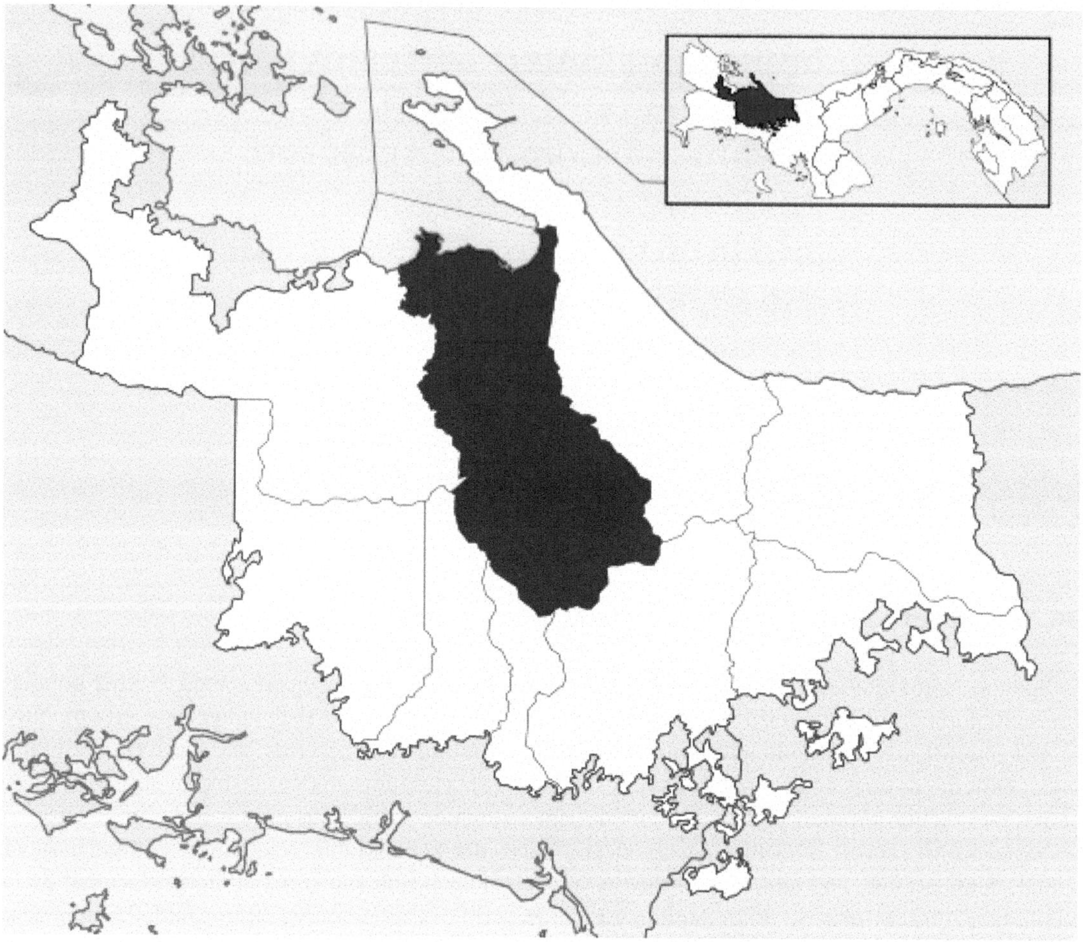

Fig. 36.1 Map of Panama highlighting the *Comarca Ngäbe-Buglé* (red shading)

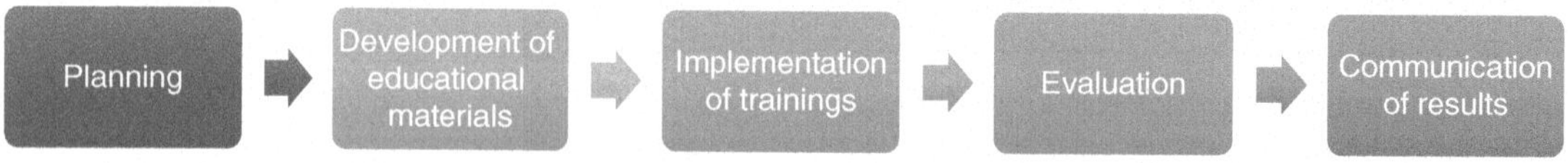

Fig. 36.2 The project phases

materials. This project aimed to develop these materials using evidence-based references and also involving community members in the process (Fig. 36.2). The project followed social marketing and community-based participatory research processes (Lefebvre and Rochlin 1997) to develop the health education intervention that includes training of health promoters and development of educational materials. The intervention had four phases: (1) planning, design, and selection of *Promotores* (local community health promoters); (2) formative research; (3) development of culturally appropriate material; (3) training and implementation; and (4) evaluation and sustainability. This chapter describes each of these four phases, barriers for its implementation, and the lessons learned focusing on the pregnancy and reproductive health aspects of the project.

36.2 The *Ngäbe-Buglé* People

Panama is a small country, located in Central America, with an estimated population of four million people, 13% of which are indigenous. There are eight indigenous groups in Panama that include the *Guna*, *Ngäbe* (previously known as *Guaymi*), *Buglé*, *Teribe/Naso*, *Bokotá*, *Emberá*, *Wounaan*, and *Bri Bri*. These indigenous groups are dispersed throughout the country, but the majority lives in indigenous reservations called *Comarcas*. The *Comarcas* are autonomous indigenous reservations with distinct geopolitical borders, local governments, and political authorities and national representation at the Panamanian national legislative congress (Fig. 36.3).

The *Ngäbe* and the *Buglé* people live in the *Comarca Ngäbe-Buglé*, merging into one mixed group with similar languages and residing in the northwestern side of the country, close to the Costa Rican border. The Ngäbe-Buglé used to be known as *Guamí* by Panamanians. /However, during the 1990s as the Comarca became a more distinct organizational culture, the indigenous groups requested to be known as the Ngäbe-Buglé. Historic records show that indigenous groups lived in the region since the 1500s, making them one of the oldest indigenous groups in America. These groups share cultural aspects, diet, and traditional medicine (Fig. 36.3).

The *Comarca Ngäbe-Buglé*, which encompasses three Panamanian provinces—Veraguas, Chiriquí, and Bocas del Toro—is a mountainous region occupying 2700 square miles, and it is divided into nine districts (Kankintú, Kusapín, Jirondai, Calovébora, Besikó, Mironó, Nule Düima, Müna, Ñürüm). The total population of the *Comarca Ngäbe-Buglé* is approximately 203,185 people, although some reports count greater than 280,000 residents. Life expectancy in the *Comarca* is 69.6 years, significantly lower than the country average of 77.8 years. The fertility rate is 98.3 per 1000 women, which is 30 times greater than the fertility rate of 2.33 in 2016 for rest of Panama (Index Mundi 2016). The main causes of death include malnutrition, diarrhea, and pneumonia. Maternal and child deaths are also observed, mostly due to lack of access to prenatal care and proper health services. The poverty index in the *Comarca* is above 90%, with the Ngäbe-Buglé living in extreme levels of poverty. Main sources of income include small-scale sustainable agriculture, handcraft sales, informal work, and government subsidies. Most males work on coffee farms (*fincas*), where they migrate during cropping

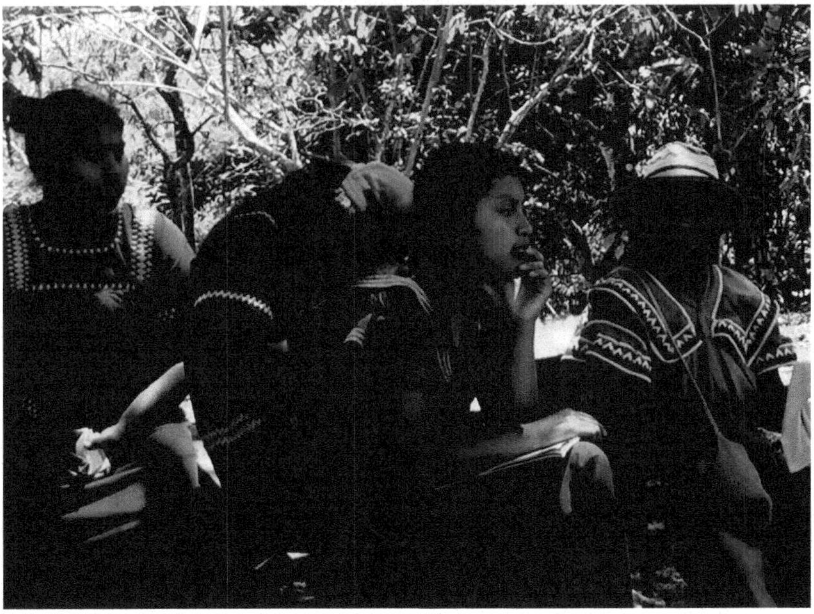

Fig. 36.3 *Ngäbe-Buglé* women dressed in their typical attire, the enagua

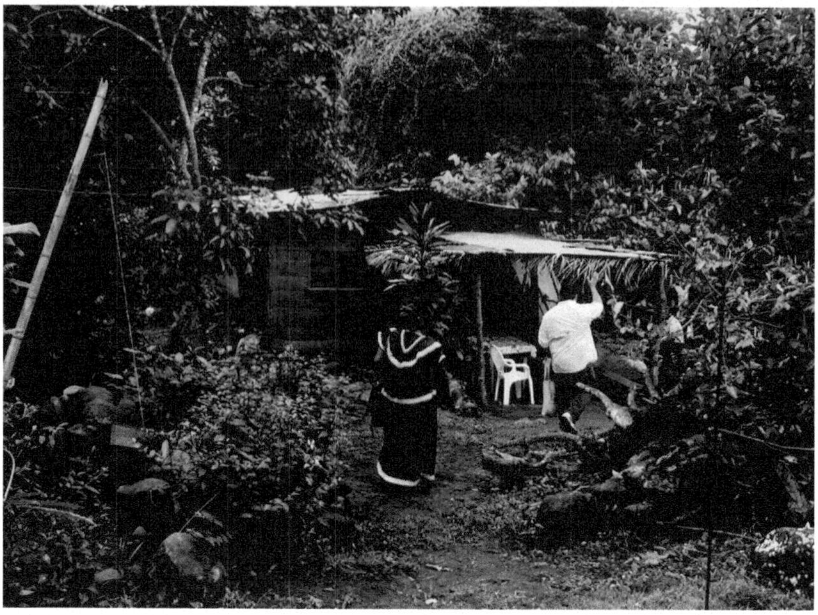

Fig. 36.4 A typical *Ngäbe-Buglé* household in the *Comarca*

seasons. The families tend to migrate together, making it difficult for healthcare delivery and follow-up. Figure 36.4 shows a typical Ngäbe-Buglé household in the *Comarca*.

36.3 Planning the Intervention

The *Comarca Ngäbe-Buglé* is located 400 km from the capital of Panama City, Panama. Because the distance, cost of travel, and difficult terrain are major barriers for implementation of health interventions, thus, detailed planning preceded the implementation phase of the project. Planning processes involved hiring of qualified staff, identification of key partners, definition of the overall scope of the project, determining the costs and potential barriers of implementation, and communication of results (Keyonzo et al. 2015; Wright et al. 2015; Kaur et al. 2013). Each of these steps is described in Table 36.1.

36.4 Development of Educational Materials

Health education consists of a continuous iterative process and a combination of learning techniques to improve health in the population. It must be a continuous process because new information is available constantly. However, evidence-based materials for health education at the community level are scarce, especially for indigenous populations of Panama. Our goal was to develop culturally and linguistically appropriate educational materials for the *Ngäbe-Buglé* population. One of the first steps was to organize a community advisory board (CAB), represented by local leaders, traditional doctors, and community health promoters. The CAB identified the health topics, the intervention format, the type of material to be developed, and the trainer profile. The CAB assisted the research team in guiding the process iteratively and to maintain the cultural appropriateness of the project (see Fig. 36.5).

Table 36.1 Sample processes included in the planning phase

Process	Description
Hiring qualified staff	Multidisciplinary projects are complex interventions by design. Therefore, hiring adequate staff is the first step. The project started with a limited staff that included a team leader, educational advisor, a medical advisor, a project coordinator, a community liaison, and administrative staff (e.g., accountings, auditors)
Identification of key partners	Selected partners included health education specialists from the Ministry of Health, community organizations, academic partners, and local *Promotores*. A community advisory board (CAB) guided the process
Scope of the project	Objectives of the intervention included development of culturally appropriate educational materials, implementation of a "train-the-trainer" educational intervention for community *Promotores*, and implementation of community-based training by *Promotores*
Costs of the project	The project had a budget of approximately USD $400,000 and a duration of 2 years. These costs included staff salary; frequent travel to the community; design and production of educational materials; implementation of train-the-trainer intervention; follow-up trainings at the community level; data analysis; and communication of results in newspapers, scientific journals, conferences, and policy-makers' meetings
Identification of barriers	This is a unique intervention for the country, and it had multiple barriers at every stage of the project, from sociocultural complications (e.g., closing of roads due to demonstrations), unexpected expenses (e.g., price surges in airline tickets, transportation stipends for community speakers), and extensive iterative processes to develop educational materials in constant consultation with community members and the CAB
Communication of results	Selected channels for communication of results included local and international conferences, press releases, social media, and presentations to community partners

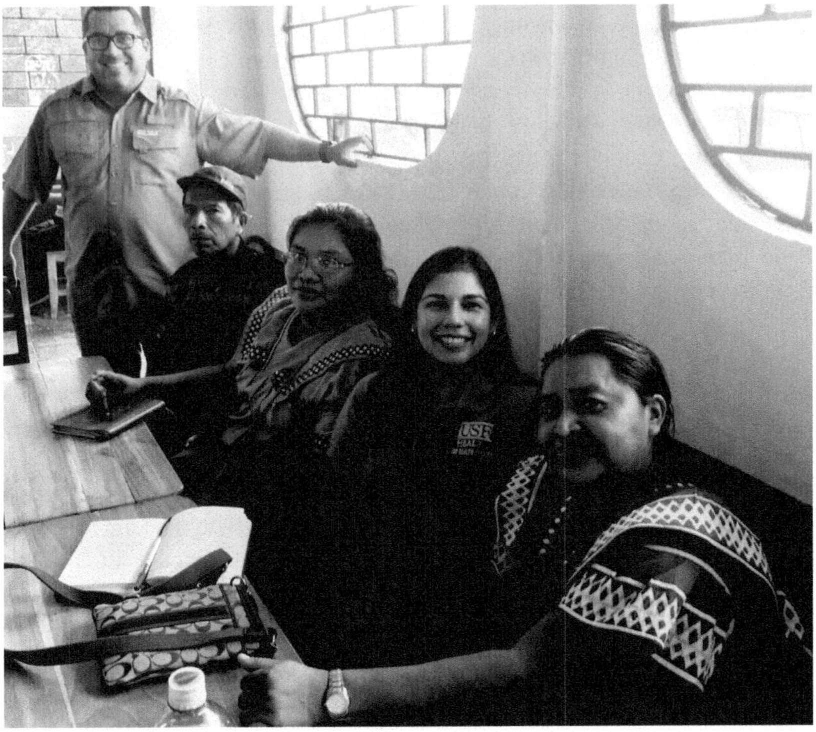

Fig. 36.5 The community advisory board (CAB) and research team members

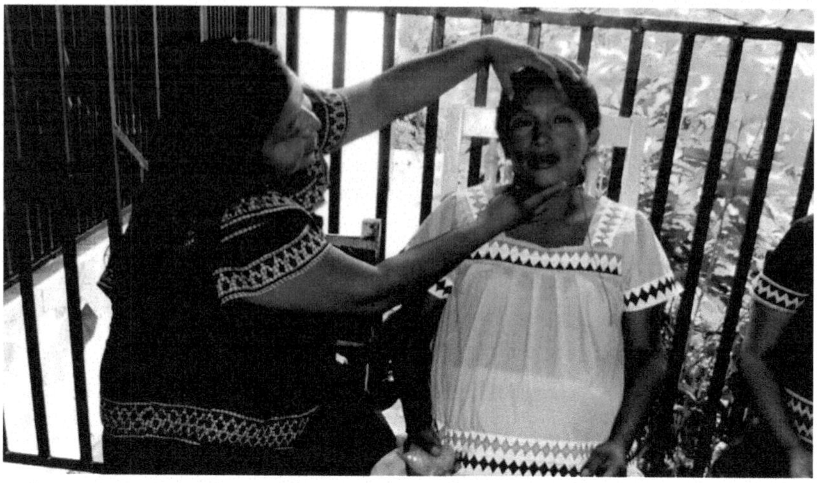

Fig. 36.6 Cover of the lay midwife section of culturally appropriate flipchart

Our team conducted four semi-structured focus groups onsite with community members to analyze in great depth their health priorities. Focus group participants identified target populations consisting of men and women, aged 18–54, including every district of the *Comarca Ngäbe-Buglé*. Participants decided that their health priorities were (1) hygiene, (2) nutrition, (3) environment, (4) role of the lay midwife in the community, (5) healthy pregnancy, and (6) domestic violence.

Through the CAB and focus groups, the participants identified the use of flipcharts as an ideal way of reaching the community with health messages (Fig. 36.6). Based on these priorities, our team selected the Hesperian Health Guide's[1] *Where There is No Doctor* (*Donde no hay doctor*) to provide a scientific baseline (Conant and Fadem 2008; Klein et al. 2013; Werner and Bower 2010; Werner et al. 2010). Identification of relevant information using text guided the selection of messages. Each of these messages was later matched with local pictures to capture the participant's attention and improve their understanding of the material. Afterwards, these messages and pictures were mounted in a flipchart as a method to deliver these messages. These messages underwent a thorough iterative process to validate their cultural and language adequacy. The process had both an internal phase (with team members) and an external phase (with community members) and was executed during a 24-month period.

36.4.1 Internal Phase

The purpose of the internal phase was to develop short messages based upon evidence-based sources, match them with pictures, and convert them into digital slides for easy management. Also, based on CAB feedback, our team decided that using flipcharts would be the best method to deliver community health training (McKay et al. 2015; Chi et al. 2014; Caniza et al. 2007). This phase of the process lasted 6 weeks.

[1] Hesperian is a nonprofit organization that works on health education since the 1970s. Since then, the organization has published more than 50 books in 20 different languages on health training, health education, community empowerment, international health, and women's health. For more information visit http://hesperian.org.

36.4.2 External Phase

The goal of the external phase was to field test the materials with community members, a form of pretesting. Our team traveled to several *Ngäbe-Buglé* communities, seeking representation throughout the *Comarca*, to discuss educational materials with community members and *Promotores* using participatory processes. The participative processes included several focus groups to evaluate texts and images. Our team collected perceptions and recommendations to tailor the educational materials (Reed et al. 2014; Bryan et al. 2014; Revere et al. 2014).

During this phase, *Promotores* also shared their concerns about the weather and the long walking distances that were required to travel to communicate these messages. Their proposed solution was to use waterproof flipcharts with detachable pages and a comfortable bag to carry the material. This was an unexpected feedback for the team, only obtained through participatory processes.

36.5 Implementation

The implementation phase of the project included the *train-the-trainer* aspect of the intervention for *Promotores* and a 6-month follow-up period to measure the reach of the project.

36.5.1 Training the Trainers

A *train-the-trainers* intervention is based on a basic premise—the transfer of knowledge from experienced trainers to less, or naïve, trainers who, in turn, train their peers or implement an educational intervention. If successful, the trainees gain additional skills, become experienced trainers, and continue the training process (Sarli 2016; Pearce et al. 2012; Murphy et al. 2008; Mintjes et al. 2001).

Prior to the initial training, extensive logistics planning was undertaken to ensure maximum participation from the selected *Promotores*:

- Identification of speakers (trainers)
- Development of the training agenda
- Development of educational materials (slides, practices)
- Transportation stipends
- Adequate lodging and meals
- Centrally located meeting area that could accommodate the group

Experienced trainers prepared a comprehensive agenda that included material from the flipchart, physical language, effective teaching methods, community-gathering techniques, practice skits, reporting of results, and evaluation. The training period used a hands-on approach to identify weaknesses while delivering the community trainings and empowering participants with teaching tips to overcome possible issues in the field.

A total of 78 *Promotores*—consisting of lay midwives, traditional medicinal doctors, and community health promoters—participated in the training and received a training kit that included a 75-page sturdy and waterproof flipchart, a bag, and evaluation report forms. The training the *Promotores* received lasted 3 days at a time. At the end of their training, the *Promotores* signed a contract agreeing to reach a minimum of 20 people in their own community. Each *Promotor* prepared a training agenda (e.g., a document describing the communities, proposed dates for trainings, and topics to be discussed) and made commitments to deliver ten community trainings and submit a monthly report to the project team members (see Fig. 36.7).

36.5.2 Follow-up

At the end of their training, *Promotores* were highly motivated and ready to deliver training to their communities. The implementing team randomly selected some communities along the *Comarca* and visited these communities bi-weekly. The purpose of the follow-up was to evaluate *Promotores* in the field, while delivering the educational intervention, to provide support to the community members, and to evaluate difficulties while delivering the trainings (Fig. 36.8). This phase lasted 6 months.

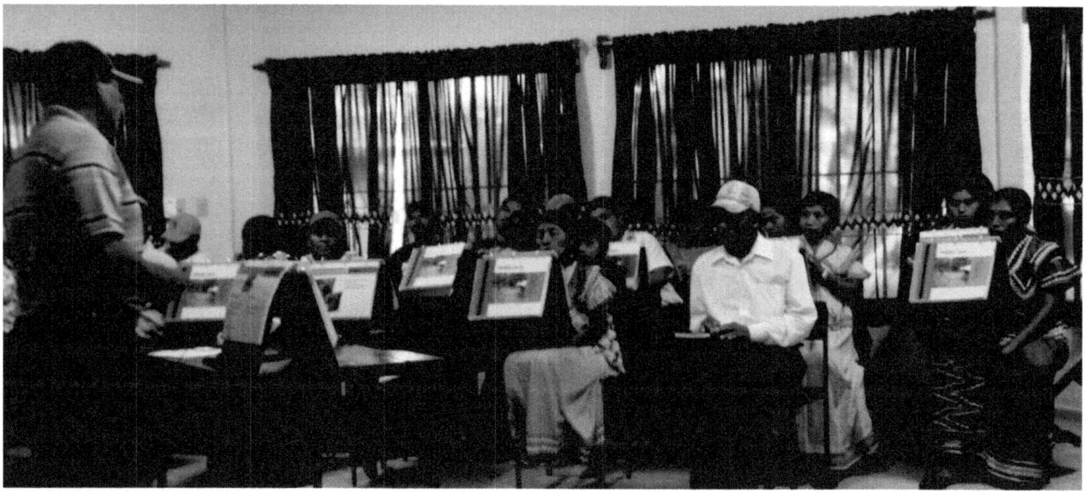

Fig. 36.7 Training the Trainers

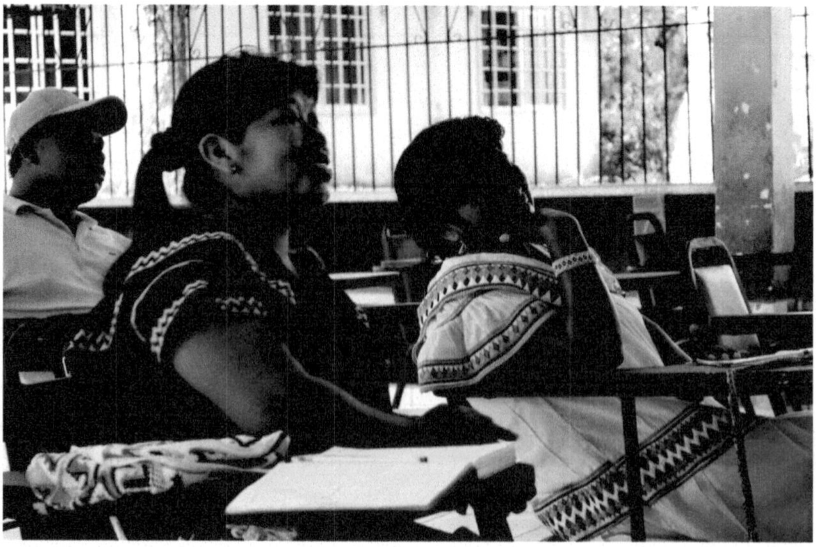

Fig. 36.8 Follow-up of training in the field in the *Comarca*

Table 36.2 Baseline, process, and result evaluation

	Baseline evaluation	Process evaluation	Result evaluation
Purpose	To identify feasibility of the intervention and understand needs from the community member's perspective	To assess completion of activities of the project	To describe the overall result of the project and measure if objectives were completed
Moment of implementation	Beginning of the project	Entire duration of the train-the-trainers intervention	End of project
Method of implementation	Semi-structured focus groups and interviews of key stakeholders	Observational using predesigned forms	Intention measurements Knowledge evaluations Report forms
Results	*Gathering preference*: 67% of community trainings included individuals or small groups *Target population*: 81% of the lectures are oriented to adults, women less than 33%, children and adolescents 44% *Health priorities*: personal hygiene (78%), food-related (41%), environment (44%)	*Number of trainings*: 3 (2 days each session) *Number of people trained*: 78 *Topics*: role of the community promoter, use of flipchart, delivering reports	*People trained*: 6876 people during the project (an additional 12,460 people were trained after a 1-year follow-up) *Number of community trainings*: 651 trainings in every district of the indigenous reservation

36.6 Evaluation

Measuring impact of any intervention is a difficult task, even for experienced teams. For this project, the team developed an extensive evaluation process that included a baseline evaluation (needs assessment), process evaluation (program monitoring), and a result evaluation (Waqa et al. 2013; Rawat et al. 2013; Crawford and Garrard 2013). Table 36.2 describes briefly each of these evaluation processes.

36.7 Communication of Results

To be sustainable over time, community health education must be firmly anchored in the health system. If leaders successfully guide and promote effective health practices, the health status of the indigenous population should improve. Effective communication of results is as important as using a thorough implementation process and analysis of results.

Selected channels of communication included meeting with health authorities, community organizations, public health conferences in Panama and the United States, scientific journals, radio shows, newspaper publications, and social media. Each of these targeted a different population and improved communication of the results.

36.8 Application of Training to Maternal Health Among the *Ngäbe-Buglé*

As mentioned before, the CAB and community members selected six main health topic areas: hygiene, nutrition, healthy environments, prenatal care, the role of the lay midwife in the community, and domestic violence. Most of these topics are consistently related to disease burden and mortality rates, mainly pregnancy issues in poor rural settings. Women and children in the *Comarca Ngäbe-Buglé* tend to present the most disease burden. The Ministry of Social Development and the National Institute of Women in Panama had been working toward reaching the millennium development goals (MDGs) and sustainable development goals of the United Nations (https://www.un.org/sustainabledevelopment/sustainable-development-goals/) of decreasing maternal and child mortality among indigenous groups in Panama, where maternal and child mortality occurred at higher rates than in the rest of the country.

The educational intervention presented in this chapter is part of the initiative of the Panamanian government, coupled with the research team from the University of South Florida Panama Program at the City of Knowledge in Panama, to provide relevant health information to the largest indigenous group in the country. The health topics identified by the community reflect the needs of reproductive-aged indigenous women during pregnancy. Also, the community members identified the need to gain access to better health services for prenatal care, delivery, and postnatal care of these women. The evaluation and improvement of health service delivery are beyond the scope of this project; however, information on prenatal care, proper nutrition during pregnancy, working with lay midwives in the community, domestic violence, and environmental health all relate to pregnancy outcomes in the *Comarca*. For example, cases of domestic violence tend to increase during pregnancy. Thus, incorporating the health topics into maternal health was a main objective of the project (Figs. 36.9 and 36.10).

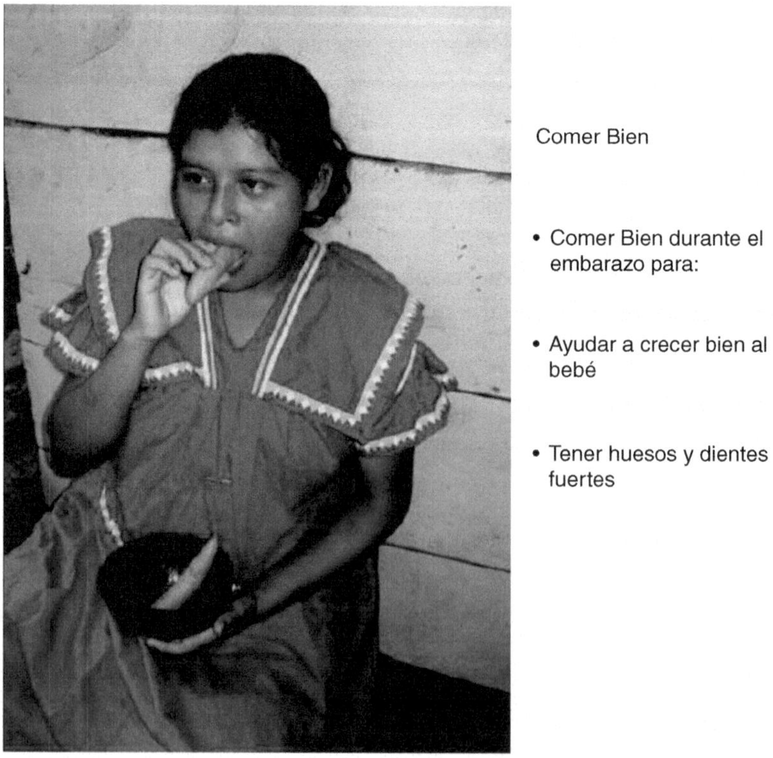

Fig. 36.9 Flipchart sections explaining the importance of nutrition (comer bien) during pregnancy and what constitutes a healthy pregnancy (embarazada sana)

Fig. 36.10 Flipchart sections explaining the importance of nutrition (comer bien) during pregnancy and what constitutes a healthy pregnancy (embarazada sana)

Embarazada Sana

- La embarazada debe tener buen estado de salud
- Tiene piel sana
- Se siente con energía
- Se mueve con fácil
- Piensa y habla con claridad
- Está contenta
- Proyecta seguridad

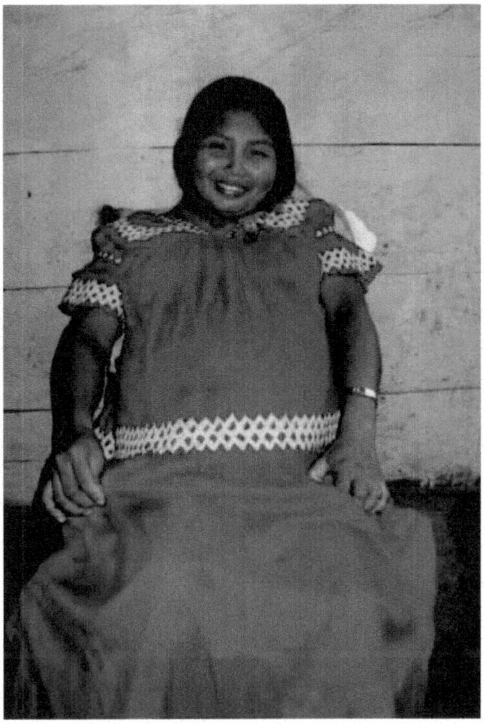

Conclusions

Creating a community advisory board (CAB) and incorporating the community into the decision-making, implementation, educational, and evaluation processes proved to be important techniques to follow when working in international community settings with indigenous groups. Several important conclusions can be drawn from this process. It was clearly that empowerment of community participants occurred. When the project was first initiated, the *Promotores* were timid and quiet; by the end of the project, the same group of *Promotores* were outspoken and handled the health information expertly.

The community members are specialists on their own community needs and identified health topics that the research team had not considered incorporating into this training project. Domestic violence was one of such topics selected by participants as an important problem. Although the research team had been well aware of the issues of domestic violence occurring in the communities of *Comarca Ngäbe-Buglé* (Calvo et al. 2014), this topic had not been expected to be identified in the participatory process. Nonetheless, during iterations, the domestic violence issues sparked much reaction and acceptance by community members, despite the associated stigma.

Finally, community participation resulted in the acceptance of the project. Community members eagerly participated in focus group discussions, shared their insights, accepted information, took ownership of the project, and continued the sustainability of the project after it was finalized. The initial goal of community participation was to have the participation of 800 community members. This proved to be unexpectedly conservative—through outreach and participatory processes, over 6000 community members were reached during the active phase of the project. Once the project finalized, the *Promotores* continued performing outreach and education, reaching over 12,000 people upon last report. Based upon our results, we can conclude that working closely with community members, gaining their trust, respecting their cultural beliefs, and including them in the process provide positive outcomes when working with indigenous groups in international settings.

References

Bryan, V., Brye, W., Hudson, K., Dubose, L., Hansberry, S., & Arrieta, M. (2014). Investigating health disparities through community-based participatory research: Lessons learned from a process evaluation. *Social Work in Public Health, 29*(4), 318–334. https://doi.org/10.1080/19371918.2013.821356

Calvo, A. E., Hess-Holtz, M., Rebollón Guardado, A., Alguero, L., & Vega, S. (2014). Participatory processes applied to developing culturally appropriate educational material among the Ngäbe-Buglé women of Panama for domestic violence prevention. *Journal of Cognitive Psychotherapy: An International Quarterly, 28*(3), 238–248.

Caniza, M. A., Maron, G., Moore, E. J., Quintana, Y., & Liu, T. (2007). Effective hand hygiene education with the use of flipcharts in a hospital in El Salvador. *Journal of Hospital Infection, 65*(1), 58–64. https://doi.org/10.1016/j.jhin.2006.08.011

Chi, D. L., Ko, A., & Kim, J. Y. (2014). Bilingual flipcharts help improve oral health-related knowledge and self-efficacy of Korean-American caregivers of preschoolers. *Journal of Public Health Dentistry, 74*(4), 261–265. https://doi.org/10.1111/jphd.12073

Conant, J., & Fadem, P. (2008). *A community guide to environmental health*. Berkeley: Hesperian.

Contraloria Nacional de la República. (2000). *Censo Nacional*. Panama: Contraloria Nacional de la República.

Crawford, S., & Garrard, J. (2013). A combined impact-process evaluation of a program promoting active transport to school: Understanding the factors that shaped program effectiveness. *Journal of Environmental and Public Health, 2013*, 816961. Retrieved from https://www.hindawi.com/journals/jeph/2013/816961/.

Index Mundi. (2016). *Panama total fertility rate*. Retrieved from http://www.indexmundi.com/panama/total_fertility_rate.html.

Kaur, B., Roberton, D. M., & Glasgow, N. J. (2013). Evidence-based medical workforce planning and education: the MSOD project. *Medical Journal of Australia, 198*(10), 518–519.

Keyonzo, N., Nyachae, P., Kagwe, P., Kilonzo, M., Mumba, F., Owino, K., et al. (2015). From project to program: Tupange's experience with scaling up family planning interventions in urban Kenya. *Reproductive Health Matters, 23*(45), 103–113. https://doi.org/10.1016/j.rhm.2015.06.010

Klein, S., Miller, S., & Thomson, F. (2013). *Un libro para parteras. Atención del embarazo, el parto y la salud de la mujer*. Berkeley: Hesperian.

Lefebvre, R. C., & Rochlin, L. (1997). Social marketing. In K. Glanz (Ed.), *Health behavior and health education*. San Francisco: Josey-Bass Inc. Publishers.

McKay, C. C., Chang, A. B., Versteegh, L. A., & McCallum, G. B. (2015). Culturally appropriate flipcharts improve the knowledge of common respiratory conditions among Northern Territory Indigenous families. *Health Promotion Journal of Australia, 26*(2), 150–153. https://doi.org/10.1071/HE14100.

Ministerio de Economía y Finanzas. (2003). *Economía, Nivel de Vida (D. d. P. Sociales, Trans.)*. Panama: Dirección de Políticas Sociales. Ministerio de Economía y Finanzas.

Mintjes, J., Boldewijn, W., Aerts, G., & Sparnaay, M. (2001). Train the trainers course on infection control and hospital hygiene in Bangladesh. *Tropical Doctor, 31*(1), 36–37.

Murphy, M. A., Neequaye, S., Kreckler, S., & Hands, L. J. (2008). Should we train the trainers? Results of a randomized trial. *Journal of the American College of Surgery, 207*(2), 185–190. https://doi.org/10.1016/j.jamcollsurg.2008.02.032

Pearce, J., Mann, M. K., Jones, C., van Buschbach, S., Olff, M., & Bisson, J. I. (2012). The most effective way of delivering a train-the-trainers program: a systematic review. *The Journal of Continuing Education in the Health Professions, 32*(3), 215–226.

Rawat, R., Nguyen, P. H., Ali, D., Saha, K., Alayon, S., Kim, S. S., et al. (2013). Learning how programs achieve their impact: embedding theory-driven process evaluation and other program learning mechanisms in alive & thrive. *Food and Nutrition Bulletin, 34*(3 Suppl), S212–S225.

Reed, H., Langley, J., Stanton, A., Heron, N., Clarke, Z., Judge, S., et al. (2014). Head-Up; An interdisciplinary, participatory and co-design process informing the development of a novel head and neck support for people living with progressive neck muscle weakness. *Journal of Medical Engineering & Technology, 39*(7), 404–410. https://doi.org/10.3109/03091902.2015.1088092

Revere, D., Dixon, B. E., Hills, R., Williams, J. L., & Grannis, S. J. (2014). Leveraging health information exchange to improve population health reporting processes: lessons in using a collaborative-participatory design process. *EGEMS (Washington DC), 2*(3), 1082. https://doi.org/10.13063/2327-9214.1082.

Rosenstock, A., Mukandi, B., Zwi, A. B., & Hill, P. S. (2013). Closing the gaps: competing estimates of indigenous Australian life expectancy in the scientific literature. *Australian and New Zealand Journal of Public Health, 37*(4), 356–364. https://doi.org/10.1111/1753-6405.12084

Sarli, L. (2016). The need to train trainers. *Acta Biomédica, 87*(Suppl 2), 5–6.

Waqa, G., Moodie, M., Schultz, J., & Swinburn, B. (2013). Process evaluation of a community-based intervention program: Healthy Youth Healthy Communities, an adolescent obesity prevention project in Fiji. *Global Health Promotion, 20*(4), 23–34. https://doi.org/10.1177/1757975913501909

Werner, D., & Bower, B. (2010). *Aprendiendo a promover la salud.* Berkeley: Hesperian.

Werner, D., Thurman, C., & Maxwell, J. (2010). *Where there is no doctor. A villa health care handbook.* Berkeley, CA: The Hesperian Foundation.

Wright, M. T., Killian, H., Block, M., von Unger, H., Brandes, S., Ziesemer, M., et al. (2015). Participatory quality development: Engaging Community members in all phases of project planning and implementation. *Bundesverband der Ärzte des Öffentlichen Gesundheitsdienstes (Germany), 77*(Suppl 1), S141–S142. https://doi.org/10.1055/s-0033-1,347,268

Zhao, Y., Wright, J., Begg, S., & Guthridge, S. (2013). Decomposing indigenous life expectancy gap by risk factors: a life table analysis. *Population Health Metrics, 11*(1), 1. https://doi.org/10.1186/1478-7954-11-1

37 Clinicians Working Alongside the Traditional *Ngäbe-Buglé* Lay Midwives of Panama

Arlene Calvo, Arturo Rebollón, and Rodrigo Arosemena

37.1 Panama: A Land of Contrasts

Panama is a country occupying a small isthmus in Central America, located between Costa Rica and Colombia, which links it with South America. With a population of approximately 4.1 million inhabitants (Focus Economics 2016), the distribution of income in Panama places it as the second most unequal income distribution in Latin America (Central Intelligence Agency—CIA 2016). Panama has a thriving dollar-based economy, focusing mostly on the service sector. Services such as the Panama Canal, with its recent expansion, international logistics, banking, insurance, the Colon Free Trade Zone, marine container ports, a demanding flagship registry, and tourism, provide important sources of income to this small but important Central American country. Nonetheless, the affluence that the country observes does not translate to all sectors of society.

About one-fourth of the country's general population lives in poverty (Central Intelligence Agency—CIA 2016), which in turn affects access to social programs such as education and health services, especially among the indigenous populations. Education and inclusion, flexibility and technology, democratic values, and social entrepreneurship are the paths to a modern and humane society (World Economic Forum 2013). Indigenous groups in Panama live in extreme poverty, starkly contrasting with the economic prosperity observed in other sectors of the country, mainly in the larger cities (Dirección de Asuntos Sanitarios Indígenas 2016; MINSA 2015) (Fig. 37.1).

A. Calvo, Ph.D., M.P.H. (✉)
Department of Community and Family Health, Global Health, Panama Program at the City of Knowledge, University of South Florida, Tampa, FL, USA
e-mail: acalvo@health.usf.edu

A. Rebollón, M.D., M.P.H., C.P.H.
Department of Global Health, University of South Florida, Tampa, FL, USA

R. Arosemena, M.D.
Ministry of Health, Panama City, Panama

D. A. Schwartz (ed.), *Maternal Death and Pregnancy-Related Morbidity Among Indigenous Women of Mexico and Central America*, Global Maternal and Child Health: Medical, Anthropological, and Public Health Perspectives, https://doi.org/10.1007/978-3-319-71538-4_37

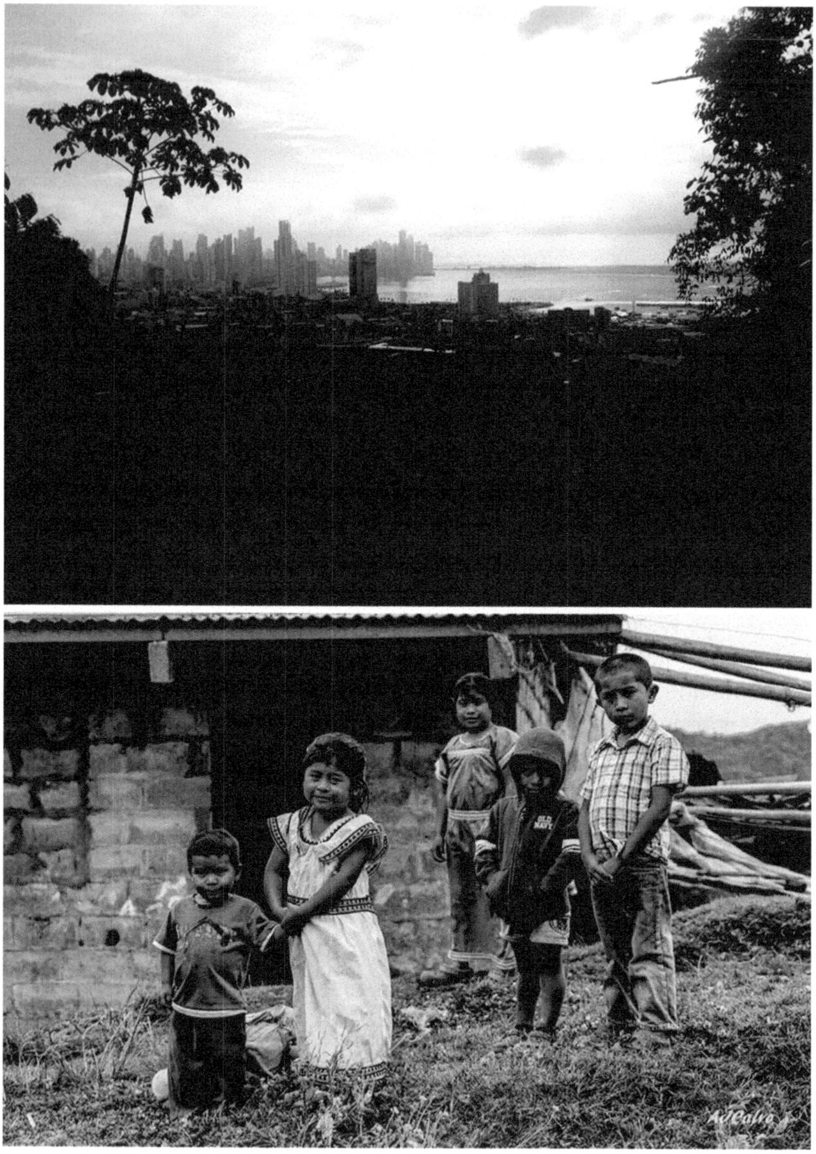

Fig. 37.1 Panama, a land of contrasts: cosmopolitan Panama City (top) compared to a *Ngäbe-Buglé* home in the *Comarca* (bottom)

37.2 Indigenous Groups in Panama and the Ngäbe-Buglé

Panama houses several different indigenous groups, the *Guna*, *Ngäbe* (previously known as *Guaymí*), *Buglé*, *Teribe/Naso*, *Bokotá*, *Emberá*, *Wounaan*, and *Bri Bri*, encompassing about 12.3% of the total population of the country (UNDP—United Nations Development Programme 2010). The largest indigenous group in Panama is composed of the *Ngäbe* and the *Buglé* (Fig. 37.2). In 1997, the previously known *Guaymí* were merged into one *Comarca* (autonomous indigenous territory) by the Panamanian government and named the *Ngäbe-Buglé* for their original traditional moniker. And, the political subdivisions of districts and *corregimientos* (smaller townships) were legally created by the

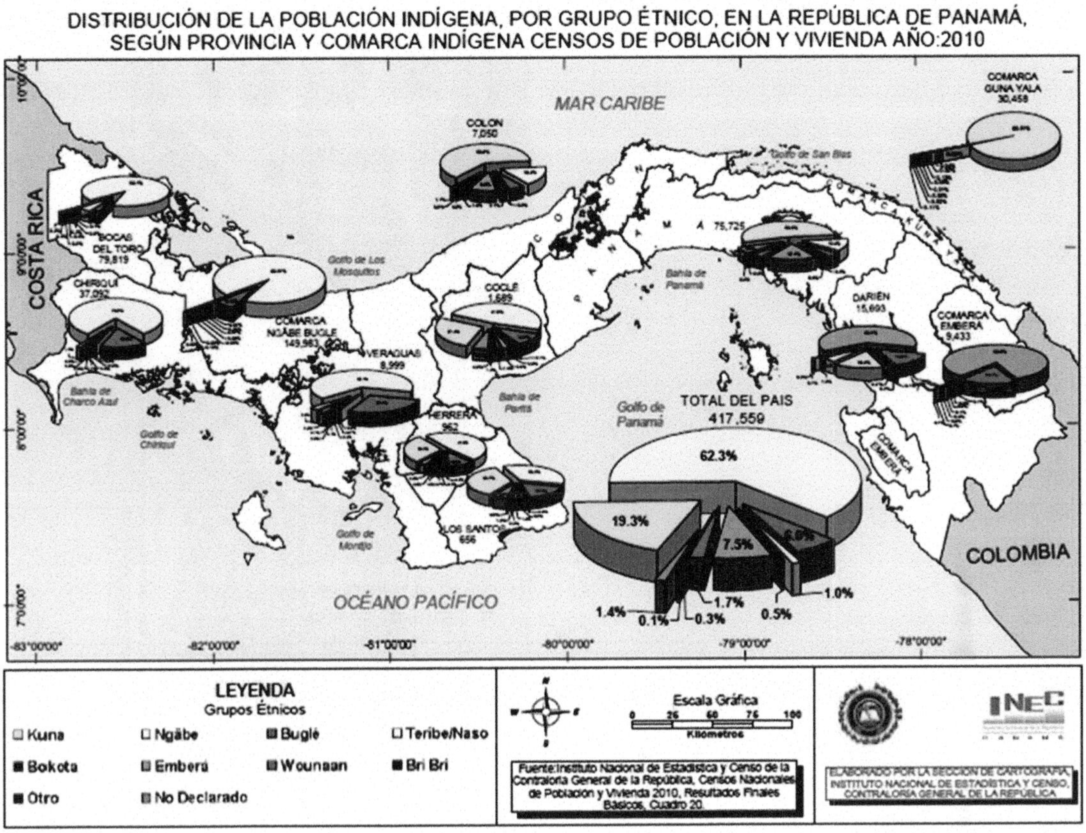

Fig. 37.2 The distribution of the indigenous populations of Panama

government of Panama in the year 2012 (Asamblea Nacional 2012). Before then, the tribe lived dispersed in the countryside, but through time, the Spanish conquistadores, Latino farmers, and US-owned banana plantations propelled them to the mountainous region. Currently, over 280,000 people are estimated to live in the *Comarca*. Of those, approximately 260,058 are *Ngäbe* and 24,912 are *Buglé*, according to the national comptroller's office (INEC 2012). The UNDP (2010) reports that among all of the indigenous groups of Panama, 46% are composed of women in the reproductive age groups (10–49 years of age), creating important public health and reproductive health challenges (UNDP—United Nations Development Programme 2010).

The *Ngäbe-Buglé Comarca* is a highly mountainous region of Panama with difficult terrain, encompassing three provinces: Bocas del Toro, Veraguas, and Chiriquí. The environment is not conducive to systematic large-level agriculture, other than small areas of sustainable family farming. The difficult topography, travel distances, lack of appropriate health services and personnel, limited educational opportunities and attainment, and absence of employment and job opportunities in the *Comarca* result in poor health outcomes for the *Ngäbe-Buglé*. Due to these conditions, the *Ngäbe-Buglé* live in extreme levels of poverty, which negatively impacts their health outcomes, resulting in an unacceptably high prevalence of pregnancy-related results (Instituto Nacional de Estadísticas y Censo-INEC 2010; Valeggia 2016; World Bank 2016) (Fig. 37.3).

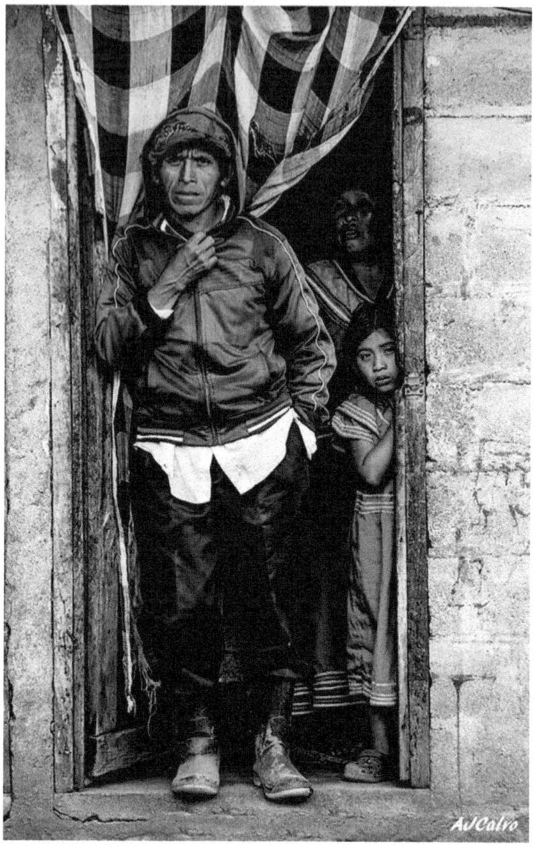

Fig. 37.3 People of the *Ngäbe-Buglé Comarca*

37.3 Health Conditions and Pregnancy Outcomes

Indigenous groups have poorer health outcomes as compared to nonindigenous populations, including decreased life expectancy at birth, higher infant and maternal mortality and morbidity, increased low birth weight infants, and poorer nutritional status, educational attainment, and economic status (Anderson et al. 2016). Maternal mortality continues to claim the lives of thousands of women in Latin America, mostly among indigenous populations (Llamas and Mayhew 2016; Castro et al. 2015; Locklear et al. 2013). In Panama, the low birth weight rate among indigenous populations, including the *Ngäbe-Buglé*, tends to be at least six times higher than in the nonindigenous population (Anderson et al. 2016). Reasons for these poor health outcomes among indigenous groups include poverty, discrimination, and marginalization due to profound social inequities (Santos Preciado and Paredes 2011; Valeggia 2016). As a result, indigenous women in Latin America have poorer maternity and reproductive health consequences, including high rates of adolescent fertility (Wurtz 2012; Torri 2010). The Ministry of Health of Panama (2016) reports that the *Ngäbe-Buglé* have a 31 percent proportion of pregnant individuals who are adolescent, one of the highest in the country. The case for maternity-related educational, public health, and other interventional programs among indigenous groups is a reality, and among the *Ngäbe-Buglé*, they are a necessity (Ministerio de Salud 2016).

Since 1972, the Ministry of Health has supervised a small health post in the rural area where the *Ngäbe-Buglé* people have settled (Bletzer 1998). There is no evidence that any form of Westernized biomedical care existed in the area prior to 1899, when the United Fruit Company entered the region. Based on the United Nations Declaration on the Rights of Indigenous Peoples (2007), the Millennium

Development Goals (MDGs) (Sachs 2012; United Nations 2007; Instituto Interamericano de Derechos Humanos 2006), and the plethora of supporting evidence of the health needs of indigenous groups, the Ministry of Health of Panama created the Direction of Indigenous Health Issues (Dirección de Asuntos Sanitarios Indígenas 2016). Their mission is *to protect and conserve the ancestral knowledge and fundamental rights of indigenous health, promoting health, preventing disease, and guaranteeing integral health care to this population* (Ministerio de Salud 2014). The direction of indigenous issues includes the departments of health development, of research, and of traditional medicine of indigenous people. Within the different programs, they conduct regular training for traditional lay community midwives (traditional birth attendants or TBAs) of the *Ngäbe-Buglé* to decrease maternal and infant mortality.

37.4 Working Alongside Traditional Midwives or *Parteras*

Since the 1960s, a movement of self-identity began among the indigenous groups of Panama. However, the legal significance and human rights of indigenous populations are a recent occurrence. The Panamanian constitution version of 2004 recognizes and respects the ethnic identity of national indigenous communities (INEC 2010). In June 2016, the Panamanian government approved a decree to establish the protection of the knowledge, the use, and practice of traditional ancestral indigenous medicine (Asamblea Nacional 2016). The decree included the establishment of a commission of government agencies representing environmental and agricultural research, University of Panama Departments of Pharmacy and Medicine, and Ministry of Health representatives to work alongside traditional medicinal doctors and midwives or *parteras* in health issues of their populations.

Since the 1990s, the Ministry of Health of Panama initiated a policy to support the training of traditional lay community midwives or *parteras* of the *Ngäbe-Buglé*. Through the years, international organizations such as the United Nations Children's Development Fund (UNICEF 2006) and the Pan American Health Organization (PAHO) have worked in concert with the Ministry of Health's nurses in primary care settings to train traditional midwives. The overall *National Program of Traditional Midwives (Programa Nacional de Parteras Tradicionales)* consists of training, coordination, follow-up, and evaluation of traditional *Ngäbe-Buglé* midwives. Topics include health promotion, clean and aseptic labor and birthing practices, timely recognition of high-risk pregnancies, and the timely referral to a healthcare setting (UNICEF—United Nations Children's Development Fund 2006). The program, organized as a 40-hour course, consists of 7 modules structured in 38 topics (Table 37.1).

The arduous work that these nurses conduct in performing their fieldwork in the *Comarca* includes community visits (in difficult mountainous terrain) to meet with groups of *Ngäbe-Buglé* midwives, presentations of reports, and maintaining registries. Overall, approximately 500 indigenous midwives of all tribes are trained annually throughout the country (Dirección de Asuntos Sanitarios Indígenas 2016). Of these, at the *Ngäbe-Buglé* region, approximately 75–80 *parteras* and the same number of medical doctors are trained annually. The utilization of labor and birthing simulators has been recently introduced (Dominguez 2015). The community health workers have evolved since the 1990s into a local nonprofit association named ASASTRAN (Association for the Support of Traditional Medicine and Knowledge). Their *parteras*, medical doctors, and health promoters work alongside the Ministry of Health to support traditional cultural beliefs and applications into Westernized medicine. The 40-h training includes a certification by the Ministry of Health, which is required to work in the program.

Structural factors, including housing, are also provided for high-risk pregnant women through the *Nuestra Vírgen del Camino* Foundation, managed by Jesuit priests. The program began in 2006 with 6 women receiving benefits, increasing to 445 recipients in 2012. By the sixth year of operation, a total of 2109 women had received care, housing, transportation to medical facilities, meals, and other

Table 37.1 Content of the *National Program of Traditional Midwives* training program

Modules	Topics
1. How does pregnancy occur?	• Characteristics of men and women, difference • How is a new life made? • How to identify pregnancy? Signs and symptoms Child's growth during pregnancy
2. Why is prenatal care important?	• Calculating the approximate birth date • Nutrition of the pregnant woman • Immunization, preparation for breastfeeding • Identification of risks of pregnant woman. Height, age, multiparity, anemia, malnutrition, pregnancy of twins, transverse presentation • Birth preparation • Data capture and registration of pregnancy • STI/HIV/AIDS prevention
3. Birthing and asepsis	• Beginning the birthing process • Cervical dilation and pushing indication • The midwife equipment for birthing care • Hand washing and care • Hygiene of birthing mother • Normal birthing attention • Placenta expulsion and revision • Identification of high-risk pregnancy and what to do • Immediate postpartum surveillance • Patient reference and birth registry • Care and deep cleaning of materials and birthing equipment
4. Newborn assistance	• Maintaining body heat • Cleanliness and care of newborn • Umbilical cord care • Baby's weight, using the string balance • Importance of breastfeeding and immediate attachment
5. Puerperium attention, family planning, sexual and reproductive rights	• Mother care during puerperium immediate and tardy • Complications and signs of danger • Mother's nutrition during puerperium • Initiation of sexual relations • Importance of spacing between pregnancies
6. Health promotion and social participation	• Community organization for emergency transports • Family orientation for baby's name registration in the legal civil registry • Importance of registration and notification of maternal and perinatal deaths • Utilization of midwife guide and manual • Healthy environment for mother and child
7. Coordination, follow-up, and evaluation	• Midwife identification • Midwife census • Coordination, follow-up, and evaluation of the work of the midwife

benefits. It is estimated that through this program, 10,215 people have been benefitted, either directly or indirectly. The program is also subsidized by the Ministry of Health, providing clinician assistance and a budget for meals (Fundación Nuestra Señora del Camino 2013; Icaza 2005).

In addition to support from the Ministry of Health and biomedical clinicians, traditional healers have contributed their knowledge and experience using traditional plant medicines—a local laboratory in the rain forest was built for this purpose. Working together as a team, approximately 350 traditional doctors, *parteras,* and biomedical clinicians have been providing skilled prenatal care, birthing, and postpartum follow-up to *Ngäbe-Buglé* women in the *Comarca* (Arcia 2006). About one-half of births

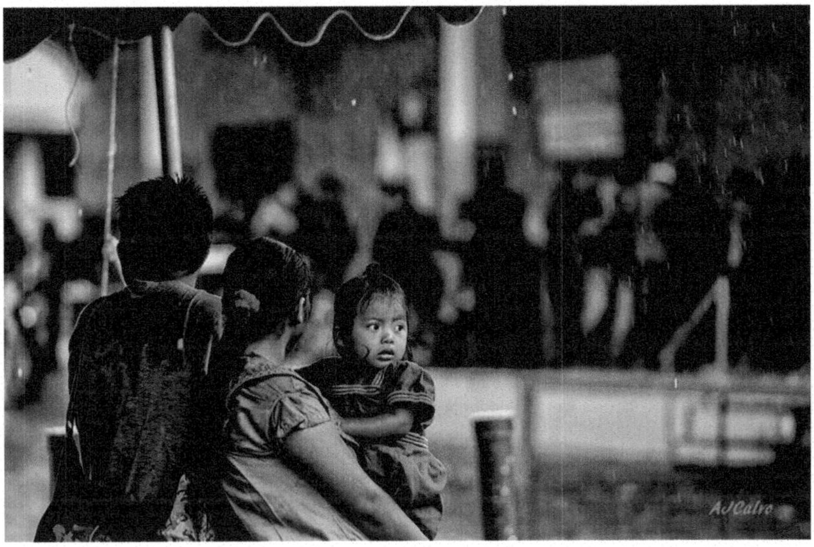

Fig. 37.4 A Ngäbe-Buglé family at a health installation at the *Comarca* on a rainy day

in the *Ngäbe-Buglé Comarca* are attended by biomedical clinicians (INEC 2014), who are working with traditional *parteras.* This team approach plays an important role in maternity care outreach to the one-half of indigenous women who give birth in isolated conditions at home due to factors including distance, difficult terrain, and costs. The traditional healers are proud that for over 600 years, their ancestors strove for the recognition of their knowledge, and now it is up to the newer generations to demonstrate the benefit of their tradition and culture upon working together with the clinicians (Fig. 37.4).

Conclusions

The alarming conditions of extreme poverty, quality of life, and social vulnerability that the *Ngäbe-Buglé* people of Panama face daily are reflected in the dangerous pregnancy and birth outcomes that are observed. Although exact data is unavailable, only one-half of births are performed by certified professionals. The rest are performed in unsafe conditions that put at risk the lives of young women and their children. Numerous attempts for a number of years have been made by local and international agencies, and from both the public and private sectors, to improve maternal health outcomes for the *Ngäbe-Buglé* on the *Comarca*. Unfortunately, the poor maternity and birth outcomes continue despite all the efforts.

Working together with local medicinal healers and *parteras* is a last attempt to improve maternity outcomes. Structural factors have been addressed as well, offering transportation, food and nutrition, and housing for high-risk pregnant women closer to healthcare facilities. Qualitative data show that women in general value the attention they receive from the numerous programs (Fundación Nuestra Señora del Camino 2013; Calvo et al. 2014). Nonetheless, maternity outcomes of the largest indigenous group in Panama are still at a suboptimal level.

The continued training of local indigenous healers and lay healthcare workers (*promotoras*) needs to be sustained, encouraged, and financially supported. Inclusion of private agencies and production of research and evaluation information including clinical outcome data on reproductive health parameters are necessary to continue improvement. Community involvement is a key to the success of the programs, promoting further awareness and consciousness building among the *Ngäbe-Buglé* people. Systematic documentation of programs is necessary to seek additional sources of funding, because government-run programs alone are not sustainable. Local leaders must become involved with the projects in order to maintain the traditional cultural aspects of care and to ensure that agencies are providing culturally appropriate services that respond to the real needs of the *Ngäbe-Buglé* community.

Acknowledgments A special thanks to the Panama Ministry of Health Department of Indigenous Health Issues (Departamento de Asuntos Indígenas) and to the Department of Sexual and Reproductive Health, especially to Drs. Raúl Bravo and Rodrigo Arosemena for all of their information and support; to the *parteras* of ASASTRAN for helping us understand the *Ngäbe-Buglé* health culture, especially Rosmery Pascacio; and to Arturo Calvo, MD, for providing the beautiful pictures for this chapter.

References

Anderson, I., Robson, R., Connolly, M., Al-Yaman, F., Bjertness, E., King, A., et al. (2016). Indigenous and tribal peoples' health (The Lancet-Lowitja Institute Global Collaboration): A population study. *Lancet, 388*(10040), 131–157. https://doi.org/10.1016/S0140-6736(16)00345-7

Arcia, O. (2006). *Cerca de 350 médicos tradicionales y parteras*. Panamá América. Retrieved May 4, 2017, from www.panamaamerica.com.pa.

Asamblea Nacional. (2012). Ley 33, Que crea dos distritos y seis corregimientos en la Comarca Ngäbe-Buglé. *Gaceta Oficial, 27032B*, 2–19, 3–7.

Asamblea Nacional. (2016). Decreto Ejecutivo No. 174, que establece la protección de los conocimientos de la medicina tradicional indígena. *Gaceta Oficial, 28063-B*, 3–7, 3–7.

Bletzer, K. (1998). *Health care among the Ngawbere in Panama*. Cultural Survival Quaterly Magazine. Retrieved May 4, 2017, from https://www.culturalsurvival.org/publications/cultural-survival-quarterly/health-care-among-ngawbere-panama.

Calvo, A., Hess-Holtz, M., Rebollon, G. A., Alguero, L., & Vega, S. (2014). Participatory processes applied to developing culturally appropriate educational material among the Ngäbe-Buglé women of Panama for domestic violence prevention. *Journal of Cognitive Psychotherapy, 28*(3), 238–248. https://doi.org/10.1891/0889-8391.28.3.238

Castro, A., Savage, V., & Kaufman, H. (2015). Assessing equitable care for indigenous and Afrodescendant women in Latin America. *Revista Panamericana Salud Publica, 38*(2), 96–109.

Central Intelligence Agency—CIA. (2016). *World Factbook*. Central America and the Caribbean: Panama. Retrieved November 2016, from https://www.cia.gov/library/publications/the-world-factbook/geos/pm.html.

Dirección de Asuntos Sanitarios Indígenas. (2016). *Dirección de Asuntos Sanitarios Indígenas*. Retrieved March 2016, from minsa.gob.pa.

Dominguez, Y. (2015). *Parteras de Vida*. El País edición América, Panamá. Retrieved April 2017, from www.elpais.com.

Focus Economics. (2016). *Economic forecasts from the world's leading economists*. Panama economic outlook. Retrieved November 21, 2016, from http://www.focus-economics.com/countries/panama.

Fundación Nuestra Señora del Camino. (2013). *Evaluación cualitativa del impacto de los programas sociales de la fundación nuestra señora del camino en San Félix y la Comarca Ngabe-Buglé*. Panama: Fundación Nuestra Señora del Camino.

Icaza, M. (2005). Strengthening of the family and improvement of the sexual and reproductive health of the Ngöbe indigenous people. In *Indigenous women and the United Nations system: Good practices and lessons learned*. New York City: United Nations.

Instituto Nacional de Estadística y Censo-INEC. (2010). *National Census 2010 [Censos Nacionales 2010]*. Panama: Contraloría General de la República. Retrieved from http://estadisticas.contraloria.gob.pa/inec/cgi-bin/RpWebEngine.exe/PortalAction?&MODE=MAIN&BASE=LP2010&MAIN=WebServerMain_censos.inl.

INEC. (2010). *Distribución de la población indígena, por grupo étnico, en la república de Panamá, según provincia y comarca indígena censos de población y vivienda año: 2010 (pp. Appendix. Table 20)*. Panama: Contraloría General de la República.

INEC. (2012). *Cuadro 20. Población indígena en la república de Panamá, por sexo, según provincia, comarca indígena, grupo indígena al que pertenece y grupos de edad*. Panama: Contraloría General de la República.

INEC. (2014). *Cuadro 77. Resumen de la estimación y proyección de la Población total de la república según provincia, comarca indígena y sexo: Años 2010-20*: Contraloría General de la República.

Instituto Interamericano de Derechos Humanos. (2006). In O. P. d. l. Salud (Ed.), *Medicina indígena tradicional y medicina convencional* (p. 44). Costa Rica: Organización Panamericana de la Salud.

Llamas, A., & Mayhew, S. (2016). The emergence of the vertical birth in Ecuador: An analysis of agenda setting and policy windows for intercultural health. *Health Policy and Planning, 31*(6), 683–690. https://doi.org/10.1093/heapol/czv118

Locklear, T. D., Perez, A., Caceres, A., & Mahady, G. B. (2013). Women's health in Central America: The complexity of issues and the need to focus on indigenous healthcare. *Current Women's Health Reviews, 9*(1), 30–40. https://doi.org/10.2174/1573404811309010002

Ministerio de Salud-MINSA. (2014). *Indicadores de Salud Básicos*. Panamá: MINSA.

MINSA. (2015). *Análisis de situación de Salud de Panamá*. Panama: Ministerio de Salud de Panamá.

Ministerio de Salud Panamá. (2016). Tabla 1. Proporción de adolescentes embarazadas, según región de salud y comarca indígena. Enerodiciembre 2016. *Sistema de Información Estadística en Salud*, Panamá: MINSA.

Sachs, J. D. (2012). From millennium development goals to sustainable development goals. *Lancet, 379*(9832), 2206–2211. https://doi.org/10.1016/S0140-6736(12)60685-0

Santos Preciado, J. I., & Franco Paredes, C. (2011). Health initiatives in Latin America: A historical assessment from the inception of the Pan American Sanitary Bureau to the Mesoamerican Health Initiative. *Revista de Salud Publica Mexicana, 53*(Suppl 3), S289–S294.

Torri, M. C. (2010). Health and indigenous people: Intercultural health as a new paradigm toward the reduction of cultural and social marginalization? *World Health & Population, 12*(1), 30–41.

United Nations. (2007). Declarations of the rights of indigenous peoples. UN General Assembly, December 2007. New York.

United Nations Childrens Development Fund-UNICEF. (2006). *Manual de enfermería: el trabajo con parteras tradicionales en Panamá*. Panama: Ministerio de Salud.

United Nations Development Programme- UNDP. (2010). *La población en Panamá. Censo de población y vivienda 2010*. Panama: Instituto Nacional de Estadística y Censo.

Valeggia, C. (2016). The global and the local: Health in Latin American indigenous women. *Health Care for Women International, 37*(4), 463–477. https://doi.org/10.1080/07399332.2014.954704

World Bank. (2016). Indigenous health in the Latin American golden decade. *Lancet, 387*(10021), 818. https://doi.org/10.1016/S0140-6736(16)00552-3

World Economic Forum. (2013). *World Economic Forum on Latin America Delivering Growth, Strengthening Societies* (pp. 1–36). Geneva, Switzerland: World Economic Forum.

Wurtz, H. (2012). Indigenous women of Latin America: Unintended pregnancy, unsafe abortion, and reproductive health outcomes. *Pimatisiwin, 10*(3), 271–282.

Part VIII

Nicaragua

Overcoming Barriers to Reducing Adolescent Pregnancy and Improving Maternal Health in Nicaragua

38

Katherine E. Bliss

38.1 Introduction

Compared to women in other countries in Central America, including Belize, Costa Rica, El Salvador, Guatemala, Honduras, and Panama, Nicaraguan women are more likely to die during childbirth. The average maternal mortality ratio (MMR), a statistical measurement of maternal death, among Nicaragua's neighboring countries is 70 maternal deaths per 100,000 live births; however, in 2015, Nicaragua's MMR was 150 maternal deaths per 100,000 live births (World Bank 2017b). This is down from 212 deaths per 100,000 live births in 1995, when studies showed that within the Latin America and Caribbean region, Nicaragua had the fewest women giving birth with a skilled birth attendant (SBA) present (WHO 2015). Nicaragua has made progress in raising the number of women who seek prenatal care and facility-based delivery services, and Nicaraguan women now bear an average of 2.2 children over their lifetimes, a total fertility rate (TFR) that is comparable to the regional average of 2.3 (World Bank 2017a). Indeed, with less violence and insecurity associated with drug trafficking than in the countries of the Northern Triangle (El Salvador, Guatemala, and Honduras), Nicaragua might be expected to have a more favorable climate for protecting the health of its mothers.

38.2 Adolescent Pregnancy

One factor that distinguishes Nicaragua from its regional counterparts is the high rate of pregnancy among adolescents. In 2015, the adolescent fertility rate was 88 births per 1000 girls between the ages of 15 and 19, a figure that was down from 118 births per 1000 girls between the ages of 15 and 19 in 2000 but still higher than the other countries in the Central American region (World Bank 2017a). According to a report issued by CODENI (Colectivo Pro Derechos de la Niñez), a federation of nongovernmental organizations working to protect the rights of children and adolescents, approximately one-quarter of all births each year in Nicaragua are to girls between the age of 15 and 19 (CODENI 2017a).

K. E. Bliss, Ph.D.
Principal, Girasol Global Policy Consulting, Dallas, TX, USA

Formerly Global Health Policy Center, Center for Strategic and International Studies, Washington, DC, USA
e-mail: kbliss@girasolglobal.com

D. A. Schwartz (ed.), *Maternal Death and Pregnancy-Related Morbidity Among Indigenous Women of Mexico and Central America*, Global Maternal and Child Health: Medical, Anthropological, and Public Health Perspectives, https://doi.org/10.1007/978-3-319-71538-4_38

And one-half of all women in Nicaragua have delivered a baby before reaching the age of 20 (Guttmacher Institute 2006). Although Nicaragua's annual gross national income (GNI) per capita of US$1940 makes it a lower-middle-income country under World Bank criteria; there is considerable income inequality, and nearly 30% of the population lives in poverty (World Bank 2017c). Many of the country's youngest mothers live in peri-urban or remote rural areas, such as along the country's remote Caribbean coast, which is home to several autonomous indigenous groups, and are among the poorest of the poor, with limited or no formal education.

There are several obstacles adolescent girls in Nicaragua face in avoiding unwanted pregnancy. The first is a lack of awareness about sexuality and human reproduction. Surveys show that up to one-half of adolescent girls (15–19 years) and young women (20–24 years) have never had any sex education (Guttmacher Institute 2006). In a recent publication, one woman, now in her 30s, recalled her first sexual experience at age thirteen: "Neither in my family, not at school, had I learned about sexual education, and at the time it was seen as bad for parents to talk to their children about sexuality, to the point that I didn't even know what a condom was." Not understanding that she was at risk of becoming pregnant, the young woman bore two children with her boyfriend, who was 6 years older than her, by the time she was 16 years old (Red de Empresarias de Nicaragua 2017).

A second challenge faced by young Nicaraguan women who wish to avoid becoming pregnant is accessing family planning services. Eighty-six percent of sexually active girls under the age of 19 reported to CODENI that they did not wish to have a child within the next 2 years, yet unmarried adolescents who are aware of contraceptive methods nevertheless encounter difficulties securing access to them without the consent of their parents (CODENI 2017a). Cost appears to be a factor for economically dependent adolescents, as well. A 2006 study in which vouchers for free sexual and

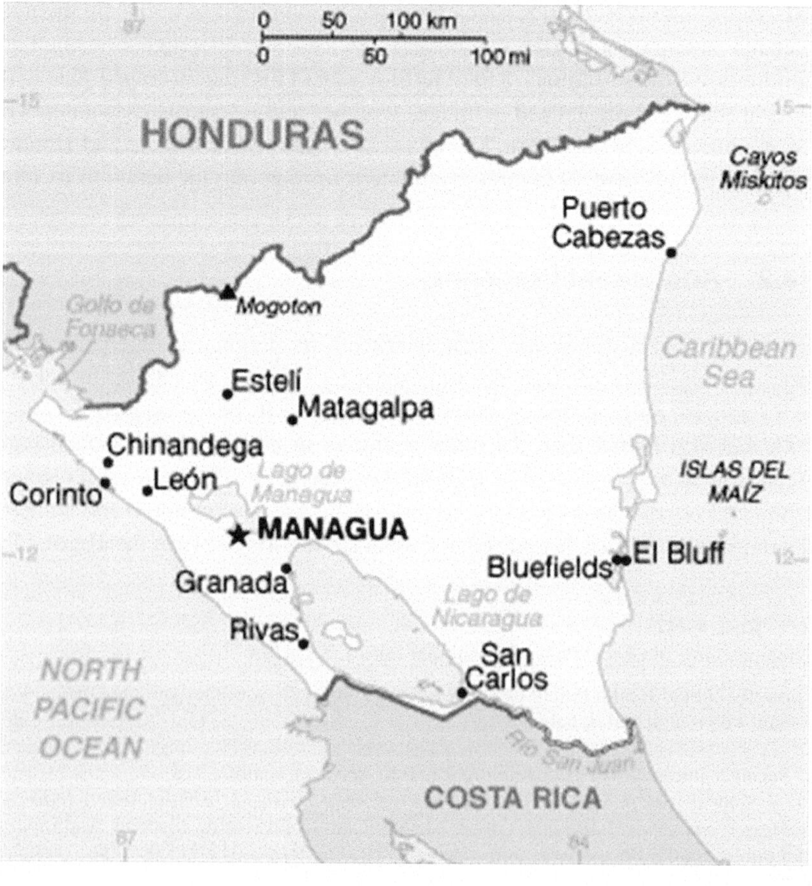

Fig. 38.1 Map of Nicaragua and neighboring countries. Photo source: Central Intelligence Agency. Available from: https://www.cia.gov/library/publications/the-world-factbook/graphics/maps/nu-map.gif

reproductive health care were distributed to adolescents living in impoverished areas of Nicaragua's capital, Managua (Fig. 38.1), showed that the recipients of the vouchers were more likely to use contraception than their non-recipient peers (Meuwissen et al. 2006).

A compounding factor is that many young women in Nicaragua become pregnant because a man in their household has raped them. Nearly 50% of children and adolescents report having experienced sexual abuse, and seven of ten formal reports of sexual abuse are by girls younger than 17 years old, with the household as the most commonly reported site of the violations (CODENI 2017b). Between 2009 and 2012, Nicaragua's Ministry of Health reported that 6404 girls between the ages of 10 and 14 had become pregnant due to sexual violence (CODENI 2017b). Since 2008 abortion has been illegal in Nicaragua under all circumstances, including in cases of rape and to protect the health of the mother. Pregnant girls who seek abortions, as well as the health-care providers who perform them, can face lengthy prison sentences (Amnesty International 2009; Zeka and Kahn, 2014).

38.3 Legal and Institutional Context

Although the Nicaraguan government recognizes the problems of adolescent pregnancy and maternal mortality, reversing the trends through laws and policies alone has proven difficult. National legal codes to protect the rights of children and adolescents have been in place since the mid- to late-1990s, bringing Nicaragua into compliance with its obligations under the United Nations Convention on the Rights of the Child, which it ratified in 1990 (Law Library of Congress 2007). Article 195 of the Nicaraguan Penal Code defines rape as sexual contact with a girl under the age of 14, with maximum penalties reserved for those convicted of raping a girl under the age of 10 (OAS 2007). The National Population Policy, released in 1996, recognized the problem of adolescent pregnancy and set forth a set of specific goals to reduce fertility rates among adolescents, particularly unmarried adolescents (Guttmacher Institute 2006). Policies promoting the dissemination of information about pregnancy and contraception have been in place since at least 2009, when the Ministry of Education introduced a new sexual education curriculum at the national level (Altamirano et al. 2016).

However, the government's implementation of the population and sexual education policies has been uneven. In large cities, such as Managua, adolescents may access some youth-friendly reproductive health services to procure contraception or prenatal care in a non-stigmatizing environment, but such services are not widespread and are almost entirely absent from rural areas (Guttmacher Institute 2006). Although the Ministry of Education, with support from UNFPA, developed several guides to help educators teach about sexuality in the classroom following the release of the 2009 policy, a 2013 study showed that only 18% of primary and secondary schools had actually used official texts in educating students (Altamirano et al. 2016).

And when it comes to addressing intrafamilial sexual abuse, child welfare advocates note that even where there are good laws in place, victims often fail to report episodes of sexual abuse, and officials can be reluctant to intervene in family affairs. A 2010 Amnesty International report found that police frequently failed to adequately protect those who came forward to denounce family members for rape and that there were few efforts to ensure victims received counseling and emotional support (Amnesty International 2010). Some experts have described research showing that law enforcement officials, who are often men and themselves heads of households, fail to respond effectively to girls' reports that they have been raped by a family member, leaving these young women vulnerable to repeated episodes of abuse and unwanted pregnancy.[1] A study of men who admitted to having had sexual relations with girls under the age of 15 showed that those with the greatest education or income levels were least concerned about the possibility of being arrested, suggesting that when it comes to rape charges, bribing authorities to look the other way may not be uncommon (CODENI 2005).

[1] Author interviews with health providers and advocacy groups, Managua, Nicaragua, January 20–22, 2016.

Gendered assumptions regarding acceptable behavior for men and women may also frame the lens through which young women in Nicaragua perceive their options in life and complicate efforts to prevent adolescent pregnancy and protect maternal health. With high rates of gender-based violence and family expectations, particularly in rural areas, that young women who are not in school will contribute to the upkeep of the household, adolescents who are unhappy at home because of violence or what they view as unreasonable demands for their contributions to housework may decide to embark on a sexual relationship with an older male in order to leave the family setting (Quintanilla 2014). Furthermore, interviews suggest that among girls living in the most impoverished rural settings, "young women who are poor and have little schooling may see entering into union and motherhood as their best options, if they believe that they have few better prospects" (Guttmacher Institute 2006).

But evidence shows that early unions and childbearing can have deadly consequences for young women in Nicaragua. In 2010, according to the Pan American Health Organization, 20% of all maternal deaths in Nicaragua were among adolescents (PAHO 2012). The majority of deaths among adolescent mothers in Nicaragua take place in impoverished rural areas where indigenous people and ethnic minorities are concentrated. The principal causes of maternal death include hemorrhage, hypertensive diseases of pregnancy such as preeclampsia and eclampsia, and sepsis. One study of national health data from 2003 to 2005 showed that young women who died during childbirth were unlikely to have sought adequate prenatal care and had elected to give birth at home with a midwife and family members in attendance, rather than at a health facility (Hernández 2007). Surveys among women living in indigenous communities in Nicaragua's Region Autónoma Atlántica Norte (RAAN), located along the country's Caribbean coast, suggest that young, pregnant Miskito women who do seek health care frequently experience racial discrimination within the clinic setting, where health workers treat them roughly or speak disparagingly to them (Organización Indigena Wangki Tangni Mairin Asla takanka tah upla et al. 2012). According to the 2003–2005 national health data, children born to young, rural mothers face death and long-term health complications, with the newborn's health closely linked to the adolescent mother's educational attainment and nutritional status. These observations are consistent with findings in other countries in the region (Hernández 2007; Conde-Agudelo et al. 2005).

38.4 Programmatic Efforts

In recent years the government of Nicaragua has worked through health programs to address the institutional and cultural factors that lead to the country's high rates of adolescent pregnancy and maternal mortality. Recognizing that young women were failing to receive adequate prenatal care, the government redoubled its efforts to encourage their attendance at all recommended prenatal visits. A recent study by the Fundación Nicaraguense para el Desarrollo Economico y Social (FUNIDES) showed that these efforts have paid off but that they come with a high cost (Altamirano et al. 2016). According to the FUNIDES study, the vast majority of the 35,000 adolescents between the ages of 15 and 19 believed to give birth each year now seek services in public clinics. Nine out of ten pregnant adolescents pay nothing for prenatal care, and 30% of those who give birth in publicly funded facilities receive the services of skilled birth attendants free of charge (Altamirano et al. 2016). The program costs an estimated $US 5.1 million per year (Velázquez 2016).

The government has also worked with nongovernmental organizations to strengthen a system of *casas maternas*, where expectant mothers living in remote areas can spend the last few days of their pregnancies and first few weeks after giving birth close to health-care services (Cortez et al. 2008). Situated in rural areas where the risk of dying in childbirth is especially high, the *casas* are meant to be available to all pregnant women regardless of civil status or income level. According to the 2012 National Strategy for Maternity Homes, the number of casas and women served has risen over the years, thanks to the fact that services are provided free or charge and the women can have their family members stay with them while they receive care (Ministerio del Poder Ciudadano para la Salud 2012). Women who stay in the *casas* can access a basic level of food and lodging, medical attention, and health education, services that can be essential for pregnant girls who have little education or access to resources (UNICEF 2013).

But there are obstacles to young women's utilization of the *casas*, including that they may lack the means to get to them, much less pay for the services of a skilled attendant at the time of delivery. The administration of President Daniel Ortega has publicly committed to expanding women's access to the *casas maternas*, but in recent years budget support for constructing new *casas* has been erratic, with fewer funds spent than allocated and some years in which there was no construction budget at all (Bárcenas 2015). Acknowledging that the number of women delivering babies without a skilled attendant is still high, in January 2016 MINSA announced plans to train 700 additional midwives for deployment to the existing *casas maternas*, and other remote communities (*El nuevo diario* 2016).

Positively engaging men in women's experience of pregnancy, birth planning, and child rearing can also benefit mothers and their children. Some studies have suggested that fathering children with many different women is frequently seen by men in Nicaragua as an expression of their masculinity and strength, while taking responsibility for providing for children is viewed to be a feminine responsibility. (Zelaya et al. 1997; Lancaster 1992). In Nicaragua, as elsewhere in Central America, men make many of the household decisions around access to health care and can determine when partners or daughters may seek antenatal, as well as labor and delivery, services. Through a 2009–2012 USAID-funded project carried out in the remote Matagalpa area by Catholic Relief Services, behavior change agents counseled men whose wives were pregnant to sensitize them regarding their participation in the women's visits to a health-care provider and to appreciate the importance of seeking timely care for labor and delivery (USAID 2014). Evaluations of the project revealed that the men who received counseling were more likely to support their wives in obtaining antenatal care, as well as labor and delivery services, and to help with the care of newborns, as well. While this project's results may offer hope for future efforts to reform gender dynamics within stable partnerships, focusing exclusively on married couples may not enhance the access of unmarried pregnant adolescents to health care and support.

The engagement of civil society groups focused on health may improve the outlook for adolescent mothers and their children. In the 1980s, during the period of social revolution, the Sandinista regime placed special emphasis on popular education, and on health education in particular, creating a cadre of community health workers known as the *Brigadistas Populares en Salud*. These volunteers supported the Ministry of Health by working in rural and peripheral urban areas to bring information about health and health services to the population (Howe 2007). Over the course of considerable political changes since the 1990s, the *brigadista* model of community outreach has remained, but their role has shifted. They do less to facilitate public engagement on health topics and focus more on going door-to-door to gather information about family health conditions to share with MINSA. Finding ways to use the *brigadistas* to encourage isolated pregnant adolescents or young mothers to engage with the health system may help them better understand how to care for themselves and their newborns.

More recently, a women's group known as the Mujeres de Liderazgo (MdL) in Nicaragua has launched a program called "Lo que debe ser penoso" in order to raise awareness about the challenge of adolescent pregnancy in Nicaragua. With funding from the US-based National Democratic Institute (NDI), the group seeks to create cultural change with respect to the understanding of adolescent pregnancy in Nicaragua and uses popular media outlets, including fashion websites and video, to draw attention to the issues (Red de Empresarias de Nicaragua 2017).

Conclusions

Since the early 2000s, Nicaragua has made progress in reducing maternal mortality and the related challenge of adolescent pregnancy, although the country's maternal mortality ratio and adolescent fertility rates remain higher than those of regional counterparts. Nicaragua's total fertility rate is consistent with the regional average, and the country does not currently face many of the security and migration challenges afflicting populations in some of the other Central American countries. However, adolescents in Nicaragua have children at a higher rate than those in neighboring countries and face a greater risk of pregnancy-related complications, including death, as well as a greater risk of poverty for themselves and their children. While legal and educational program have led to mixed results, health programs focused on improving the access of the most remote and disadvantaged groups to low-cost care during the prenatal period have proven effective, but the need is still great.

Like other countries throughout the hemisphere, in 2016 Nicaragua confirmed local transmission of the mosquito-borne Zika virus, which has been shown to be associated with congenital problems, including microcephaly and other neurological disorders, among children born to women infected with Zika while pregnant (Schwartz 2017). As of the end of February 2017, Nicaragua had reported a total of 2055 confirmed cases of Zika virus infection, with 1117 pregnant women confirmed to have been infected with the virus, underscoring the urgency of improving the access of Nicaragua's most vulnerable women and girls to contraception (PAHO 2017).

As recent history shows, it is important to have laws, education policies, and health programs in place to protect the health of Nicaragua's young women and future mothers. But official initiatives may not be enough to further reduce rates of adolescent pregnancy and maternal death in Nicaragua. Engaging civil society through advocacy campaigns and the media may help change entrenched cultural assumptions about the roles of young women and men vis-à-vis education, work, and family formation. Finding a way to empower Nicaragua's youngest mothers to participate in civic activities and public discussion about family health and their own well-being should be a priority.

References

Altamirano, A., Pacheco C., Huelva L., Sáenz, M., López, A. (2016). *Embarazo adolescente en Nicaragua: Causas y consecuencias económicas y sociales del embarazo adolescente en Nicaragua*. Serie de documentos de trabajo Número 7. FUNIDES. Retrieved April 21, 2017, from http://funides.com/embarazo-adolescente-en-nicaragua/.

Amnesty International. (2009). *The total abortion ban in Nicaragua: women's lives and health endangered, medical professionals criminalized*. London: Amnesty International Publications. Retrieved May 3, 2017, from http://www.amnestyussa.org/sites/default/files/pdfs/nicaragua_abortion_ban_report__english.pdf.

Amnistía Internacional. (2010). *Escucha sus voces y actúa: no más violación y violencia sexual contra niñas en Nicaragua*. Editorial Amnistía Internacional (EDAI). Retrieved May 4, 2017, from https://doc.es.amnesty.org/cgi-bin/ai/BRSCGI/NO%20MÁS%20VIOLACIÓN%20Y%20VIOLENCIA%20SEXUAL%20CONTRA%20NIÑAS%20EN%20NICARAGUA?CMD=VEROBJ&MLKOB=29281302222.

Bárcenas, J. (2015). Reformas presupuestarias: un balance después de la crisis. In *Qué sucedió con las casas maternas, los subsidios a las viviendas de interés social, y el bono productivo alimentario?* Managua: Instituto de Estudios Estratégicos y Políticas Públicas.

CODENI. (2005). *Así piensan y actúan los abusadores y explotadores sexuales: una visión masculina de la violencia sexual*. Managua: CODENI. Retrieved April 3, 2017, from http://www.poderjudicial.gob.ni/genero/documentos/11_asi_piensan_y_actuan.pdf.

CODENI. (2017a). *Situación de los embarazos en las adolescentes*. Retrieved April 3, 2017, from http://www.codeni.org.ni/situacion-los-embarazos-las-adolescentes/.

CODENI. (2017b). *Violencia sexual*. Retrieved April 3, 2017, from http://www.codeni.org.ni/proteccion-especial/violencia-intrafamiliar/violencia-sexual/.

Conde-Agudelo, A., Belizán, J. M., & Lammers, C. (2005). Maternal-perinatal morbidity and mortality associated with adolescent pregnancy in Latin America: Cross-sectional study. *American Journal of Obstetrics and Gynecology, 192*, 342–349. https://doi.org/10.1016/j.ajog.2004.10.593

Cortez, R., García Prado, A., Kok, H., Largaespada, C. (2008). *Las casas maternas en Nicaragua*. Washington, DC: Banco Mundial and Banco Interamericano de Desarrollo (BID). Retrieved April 3, 2017, from http://siteresources.worldbank.org/INTLACREGTOPGENDERINSPA/Resources/Cuaderno4casas_maternas.pdf.

El Nuevo Diario. (2016). *Capacitarán a 500 bachilleres en salud ya 700 parteras*. El nuevo diario. Retrieved April 3, 2017, from http://www.elnuevodiario.com.ni/nacionales/381419-capacitaran-500-bachilleres-salud-700-parteras/.

Guttmacher Institute. (2006). *Early childbearing in Nicaragua: A continuing challenge*. In Brief, 2006 Series, No. 3. Retrieved May 4, 2017, from https://www.guttmacher.org/sites/default/files/report_pdf/rib_nicaragua2006-09en_0.pdf.

Hernández, M. (2007). *Mortalidad materna en adolescentes y mortalidad infantil en hijos de madres adolescentes en Nicaragua*. Organización Panamericana de la Salud (OPS). Retrieved May 4, 2017, from http://www.paho.org/nic/index.php?option=com_docman&task=doc_view&gid=234&Itemid=235.

Howe, C. (2007). Gender, sexuality, and revolution: Making histories and cultural politics in Nicaragua, 1979–2001. In W. E. French & K. E. Bliss (Eds.), *Gender, sexuality and power in post-independence Latin America* (pp. 230–260). Lanham, MD: Rowman and Littlefield.

Lancaster, R. (1992). *Life is hard: Machismo, danger, and the intimacy of power in Nicaragua*. Berkeley, CA: University of California Press.

Law Library of Congress. (2007). *Nicaragua: children's rights: international and national laws and practices*. Retrieved April 3, 2017, from http://www.loc.gov/law/help/child-rights/pdfs/childrensrights-nicaragua.pdf.

Meuwissen, L., Gorter, A., & Knottnerus, A. (2006). Impact of accessible sexual and reproductive health care on poor and underserved adolescents in Managua, Nicaragua: A quasi-experimental intervention study. *Journal of Adolescent Health, 38*, 56e1–56e9.

Ministerio de Salud, Dirección General de Extensión y Calidad de la Atención. (2012). *Estrategia Nacional Casasa Maternas Porla reducción de la mortalidad materna y perinatal*. Retrieved May 3, 2017, from http://www.minsa.gob.ni/index.php/repository/Descargas-MINSA/Dirección-General-de-Servicios-de-Salud/Estrategia-Nacional-de-Casa-Materna/.

Organización Indigena Wangki Tagni Mairin Asla tajanka tah upla, FIMI, CADPI, Alianza de Mujeres Indigenas de Centroamerica y Mexico, ONU Mujeres. (2012). *Estudio de caso: Violencia contra mujeres Miskitus*. Comunidades del Wangki. Retrieved May 4, 2017, from http://www.fimi-iiwf.org/archivos/84fa5f31561e5fed22bf79a917110fb4.pdf.

Organization of American States (OAS). (2007). *Red hemisférica de intercambio de información para la asistencia mutua en materia penal y extradición*. Código Penal de la República de Nicaragua. Retrieved May 4, 2017, from https://www.oas.org/juridico/mla/sp/nic/sp_nic-int-text-cp.html.

Pan American Health Organization (PAHO). (2012). *Health in the Americas, 2012*. Country volume: Nicaragua. Retrieved April 3, 2017, from http://www.paho.org/salud-en-las-americas-2012/index.php?option=com_docman&task=doc_view&gid=140&Itemid=.

Pan American Health Organization/World Health Organization (PAHO/WHO). (2017). *Zika- epidemiological report Nicaragua*. PAHO/WHO. Retrieved May 2, 2017, from http://www2.paho.org/hq/index.php?option=com_docman&task=doc_view&gid=35217&Itemid=270&lang=en.

Quintanilla, M. (2014). *Adolescent pregnancy in Nicaragua: More than just an issue about adolescent women*. Unpublished manuscript. Retrieved May 3, 2017, from http://www.academia.edu/7415620/Más_allá_de_las_adolescentes_otras_dimensiones_del_embarazo_adolescente_en_Nicaragua.

Red de empresarias de Nicaragua (REN). (2017). *Lo que debe ser penoso*. Retrieved May 5, 2017, from https://ren.org.ni/lanzamiento-campana-lo-que-debe-ser-penoso/.

Schwartz, D. A. (2017). Autopsy and postmortem studies are concordant. Pathology of Zika virus infection is neurotropic in fetuses and infants with microcephaly following transplacental transmission. *Archives of Pathology & Laboratory Medicine, 141*(1), 68–72. Retrieved from http://www.archivesofpathology.org/doi/full/10.5858/arpa.2016-0343-OA.

UNICEF. (2013). *Casas maternas: Refugios de vida*. Nicaragua. Retrieved May 3, 2017, from http://en.unicef.org.ni/prensa/37/.

USAID and Catholic Relief Services (CRS). (2014). *An innovative approach to involving men in maternal and newborn health care: Program experiences in the Department of Matagalpa, Nicaragua*. Operations Research Brief. Retrieved from https://www.usaid.gov/sites/default/files/documents/1864/CRSORBrief.pdf.

Velázquez, U. (2016). *País gasta US$5,1 millones en atender a madres adolescentes*. Diario metro. Retrieved April 17, 2017, from http://diariometro.com.ni/nacionales/101465-pais-gasta-us51-millones-en-atender-a-madres-adolescentes/.

World Bank. (2017a). *Adolescent fertility rate (births per 1,000 women ages 15–10)*. Belize, Costa Rica, El Salvador, Guatemala, Honduras, Nicaragua, Panama. Retrieved May 4, 2017, from http://data.worldbank.org/indicator/SP.ADO.TFRT?locations=BZ-CR-GT-SV-HN-NI-PA&view=chart.

World Bank. (2017b). *Maternal mortality ratio (modeled estimate, per 100,000 live births)*. Belize, Costa Rica, El Salvador, Guatemala, Honduras, Nicaragua, Panama. Retrieved May 2, 2017, from http://data.worldbank.org/indicator/SH.STA.MMRT?locations=BZ-CR-SV-GT-HN-NI-PA&view=chart.

World Bank. (2017c). *Nicaragua: Poverty headcount ratio at national poverty lines (% of population)*. Retrieved April 10, 2017, from http://data.worldbank.org/indicator/SI.POV.NAHC?locations=NI.

World Health Organization, UNICEF, UNFPA, World Bank Group, and United Nations Population Division Maternal Mortality Estimation Inter-Agency Group. (2015). *Maternal mortality in 1990–2015: Nicaragua*. Retrieved April 3, 2017, from http://www.who.int/gho/maternal_health/countries/nic.pdf.

Zeka, A., Kahn, H.S. (2014). *A quiet inquisition*. Documentary film. Film website. Retrieved May 6, 2017, from https://www.facebook.com/aquietinquisitionthefilm/.

Zelaya, E., Marín, F., García, J., Berglund, S., Liljestrand, J., & Persson, L. (1997). Gender and social differences in adolescent sexuality and reproduction in Nicaragua. *Journal of Adolescent Health, 21*, 39–46. https://doi.org/10.1016/S1054-139x(96)00277-7

Part IX

Aids for Epidemiological, Anthropological, and Biomedical Studies of Reproductive and Maternal Health Among Indigenous Women of Mexico and Central America

39 A Lexicon for Anthropological, Epidemiological, and Biomedical Research of Reproductive and Maternal Health

David A. Schwartz

39.1 Introduction

According to the Chinese philospher Confucius, "If language is incorrect, then what is said is not meant. If what is said is not meant, then what ought to be done remains undone." The lexicon of specialists working in the areas of reproductive and maternal health can be highly specific and often complex. The three major groups of viewpoints contained in this present volume—anthropologists and social scientists, physicians and nurses, and public health specialists and epidemiologists—may all have a specific technical vocabulary that they employ in their day-to-day analysis and evaluation of issues regarding complications of pregnancy among indigenous women. Unfortunately, that vocabulary may not, and often is not, shared by experts in different specialties working among the same people and societies. Too often, miscommunications can develop between specialists—statistical terms may be confusing; diagnostic criteria may vary; rates, ratios, prevalence, frequency, and incidence may be mistakenly interchanged; and so forth.

This brief glossary is not meant to be either exhaustive or encyclopedic. It does, however, attempt to highlight and define some of the most important terms and concepts which are in everyday usage by specialists dealing with maternal morbidity and mortality, as well as selected terms that deal with reproductive health and maternal-child health.

Unfortunately, having two sets of criteria for the same term or concept can be confusing. Because that situation exists for several frequently used terms in maternal morbidity and mortality analysis, wherever possible both terms have been stated.

39.2 The Lexicon

Abortifacient—a drug or other medication, herb, or device that can cause an abortion.

Abortion—the termination and expulsion of the products of a pregnancy before birth. Also, the termination of a pregnancy by removal of the embryo or fetus prior to its viability outside of the uterus.

D. A. Schwartz, M.D., M.S. Hyg., F.C.A.P.
Department of Pathology, Medical College of Georgia, Augusta University, Augusta, GA, USA

D. A. Schwartz (ed.), *Maternal Death and Pregnancy-Related Morbidity Among Indigenous Women of Mexico and Central America*, Global Maternal and Child Health: Medical, Anthropological, and Public Health Perspectives, https://doi.org/10.1007/978-3-319-71538-4_39

If it is caused intentionally, it is referred to as an induced abortion. If the abortion occurs because of natural processes, it is termed a spontaneous abortion.

Abortion rate—the number of abortions per 1000 women ages 15–44 or 15–49 in a given year.

Abortion ratio—the number of abortions per 1000 live births in a given year.

Abstinence—not having sex with a partner.

Achieved status—refers to a status that is acquired in a group or society by doing something. For instance, someone acquires a criminal status by committing a crime. Likewise, the status of mother is attained by having a baby.

Adolescence—The period of emotional and physical changes which occur between the beginning of puberty and early adulthood.

Adolescent pregnancy—a pregnancy in girls aged 19 years and under. About 16 million girls aged 15–19 and some 1 million girls under 15 give birth every year—most in low- and middle-income countries. Complications during pregnancy and childbirth are the second leading cause of death for 15–19-year-old girls globally.

Adrenarche—the period in early puberty when secondary sex characteristics begin to develop.

Adult lifetime risk of maternal death—the probability of dying from a maternal cause during a woman's reproductive lifespan. The adult lifetime risk of maternal mortality can be derived using either the maternal mortality ratio, MMR, or the maternal mortality rate, MMRate.

Advanced maternal age—pregnant women 35 years of age and older. Women of advanced maternal age have a higher risk for poor obstetrical outcomes than do younger women.

Adverse pregnancy outcome—clinical outcomes of pregnancies or births that result in either a non-healthy pregnancy or the birth of a non-healthy infant; these can include neonatal, infant and maternal morbidity and mortality, low and very low birth weight babies, premature births, or the development of acute or chronic conditions during pregnancy.

Afterbirth—the lay term for the placenta and associated tissues.

Age-adjusted mortality rate—a mortality rate statistically modified to eliminate the effect of different age distributions in the different populations.

Agent—refers to a factor, such as a microorganism, chemical substance, or form of radiation, whose presence, excessive presence, or (in deficiency diseases) relative absence is essential for the occurrence of a disease.

Age sets—age grades that are clearly recognized in a culture as distinct identifiable groups of people. They consist of people of similar age and usually of the same gender who share a common identity and maintain close ties throughout their lives. They also pass through age-related statuses together as a group. The transition between these statuses is usually marked by a rite of passage.

Age-specific mortality rate—refers to a mortality rate limited to a particular age group. The numerator is the number of deaths in that age group; the denominator is the number of persons in that age group in the population.

Analytic study—refers to a comparative study intended to identify and quantify associations, test hypotheses, and identify causes. Two common types of analytic studies are a cohort study and case-control study.

Androgynous – refers to the characteristic of having a blend of both masculine and feminine personality characteristics but not strongly either one.

Antenatal care—health care, including screening tests and counseling, provided to women during pregnancy. Also referred to as prenatal care.

Antenatal care coverage—the percentage of women who have given birth who received antenatal care from a skilled attendant at least once during their pregnancy.

Arranged marriage—refers to the practice in which both parties consent to marriage with the assistance of their parents or a third party (matchmaker) to identify a spouse.

Attack rate—is a variant of an incident rate, applied to a narrowly defined population observed for a limited period of time, such as during an epidemic.

Attributable proportion—refers to the measure of the public health impact of a causative factor; proportion of a disease in a group that is exposed to a particular factor which can be attributed to their exposure to that factor.

Attributable risk—is a measure of association in cohort studies and experimental studies. The attributable risk is a difference measure and calculated as the difference between the incidence of the outcome in the exposed group (or intervention) and the incidence of the outcome in the unexposed group (or control).

Balanced reciprocity—a term that applies to exchanges between people who are more distantly related than are members of the same band or household.

Band—the basic unit of social organization among foragers that includes fewer than 100 persons.

Barrier methods of birth control—those contraceptives that prevent sperm from entering the uterus. These include the condom, female condom, diaphragm, cap, spermicide, and sponge.

Basal body temperature (BBT) method—a method for natural family planning in which the basal body temperature is charted to estimate the time of ovulation. A woman's hormone levels during her menstrual cycle cause her BBT to fall 1–2 days before she ovulates. It will then rise a day or two after she ovulates. This is used to calculate the timing of avoidance of sexual intercourse.

Basic emergency obstetric and newborn care (BEmONC)—is defined as seven essential medical interventions, or "signal functions," that treat the major causes of maternal and newborn morbidity and mortality: (1) antibiotics to prevent puerperal infection, (2) anticonvulsants for treatment of eclampsia and preeclampsia, (3) uterotonic drugs (e.g., oxytocics) administered for postpartum hemorrhage, (4) manual removal of the placenta, (5) assisted or instrumental vaginal delivery, (6) removal of retained products of conception, and (7) neonatal resuscitation.

Basic reproductive rate—is the average number of people directly infected by an infectious case during its infectious period, when the case enters a completely susceptible population. The basic reproductive rate is the theoretical potential of an infection to spread in an entirely susceptible population.

Bias—the deviation of results or inferences from the truth or processes leading to such systematic deviation. Any trend in the collection, analysis, interpretation, publication, or review of data that can lead to conclusions that are systematically different from the truth.

Birth rate—the number of births during a given period of time, typically 1 year, expressed as a percentage of the total population or the total number of women of childbearing age in a region.

Body mass index (BMI)—also referred to as the Quetelet index. It is a value derived from the weight and height of an individual. The BMI is defined as the body weight divided by the square of the body height and is universally expressed in units of kg/m^2, resulting from mass in kilograms and height in meters. See also Ponderal Index.

Caesarean (Cesarean) section—the use of surgery to deliver a baby (babies) through an intra-abdominal incision. See also emergency cesarean section.

Case—as used in epidemiology, a countable instance in the population or study group of a particular disease, health disorder, or condition under investigation. Sometimes, an individual with the particular disease.

Case-control study—a type of observational analytic study. Enrollment into the study is based on presence ("case") or absence ("control") of disease. Characteristics such as previous exposure are then compared between cases and controls.

Case definition—a set of standard criteria for deciding whether a person has a particular disease or health-related condition, by specifying clinical criteria and limitations on time, place, and person.

Case fatality rate (CFR)—the proportion of persons contracting a disease who die from it during a specified time period.

Case reports—describe the experience gained from one single patient, participant, or client. Case reports may identify unusual features of a disease or an individual.

Case series—are usually based on a very small group of patients, participants, or clients who have similar signs, symptoms, diagnoses, histologies, experiences, or behaviors. Case series identify unusual features of a disease or of individuals and may lead for example to the formulation of new etiological hypotheses, the identification of a new disease identity, or the identification of adverse effects to a certain exposure.

Cause-specific death rate—the number of deaths attributable to a specific cause per 100,000 population in a given year.

Census—the enumeration of an entire population, usually with details being recorded on residence, age, sex, occupation, ethnic group, marital status, birth history, and relationship to head of household.

Child marriage—considered by international organizations to be a formal marriage or informal union in which one or both of the partners are less than 18 years of age.

Childbearing years—the reproductive age span of women, assumed for statistical purposes to be 15–44 or 15–49 years of age.

Class interval—a span of values of a continuous variable which are grouped into a single category for a frequency distribution of that variable.

Clinical audit—entails a systematic review or audit of the obstetric care provided to pregnant women against established protocols or criteria aimed at improving the quality of care. Protocols for the management of obstetric complications have to be established beforehand in order to ascertain whether cases are properly being managed at health facilities. If well implemented, it leads to standardized and improved care across health facilities.

Closed cohort—is a cohort in which membership begins at a defined time or with a defining event and ends only with the observed study outcome, the end of eligibility for membership, or the end of the study period.

Cluster—refers to an aggregation of cases of a disease or other health-related condition, particularly cancer and birth defects, which are closely grouped in time and place. The number of cases may or may not exceed the expected number; frequently the expected number is not known.

Coding—is the process of assigning numbers to the categories of a categorical variable for statistical analysis (e.g., for the categorical variable gender: 0 = female; 1 = male). Coding is not required for numerical variables, as they are already documented in numbers (e.g., age in years).

Cohort—a well-defined group of people who have had a common experience or exposure, who are then followed up for the incidence of new diseases or events, as in a cohort or prospective study. A group of people born during a particular period or year is called a birth cohort.

Cohort study—A type of observational analytic study. Enrollment into the study is based on exposure characteristics or membership in a group. Disease, death, or other health-related outcomes are then ascertained and compared.

Community midwife—see traditional birth attendant.

Comprehensive emergency obstetric and newborn care (CEmONC)—also includes blood transfusions, surgery (e.g., cesarean section), neonatal intubation, and advanced resuscitation (intubation and respirator available). These advanced care components require access to advanced supplies and trained personnel, which may be burdensome for resource-poor health systems.

Confidential enquiries into maternal deaths—a national or subnational multidisciplinary committee that meets periodically to systematically investigate a representative sample of (or all) maternal deaths to identify the causes and associated factors; the committee then gives written guidelines to health personnel and administrators on how to prevent similar deaths in the future. The investigation is carried out in a confidential manner. It requires a complete and functioning civil registration or health management information system. A subnational or district-level panel might be more appropriate in countries with high mortality, so that the guidelines issued can be tailored to local situations.

Confounding bias—is one of the three main types of bias. Confounding may occur if the effect of the study factor on the outcome is mixed in the data with the effect of another variable (= confounder). Whether confounding truly exists in a study can only be assessed during data analysis.

Continuum of care—an approach to maternal, newborn, and child health that includes integrated service delivery for women and children from before pregnancy to delivery, the immediate postnatal period, and childhood.

Contraception—the intentional prevention of pregnancy or conception through hormones, technologies, sexual practices, or surgical procedures.

Contraceptive prevalence rate (CPR)—the percentage of women of reproductive age (15–49) who are practicing, or whose sexual partners are practicing, any form of contraception.

Contragestion—occurs when an agent (for example RU-486) interrupts or prevents the gestation of a fertilized egg.

Control—in the setting of a case-control study, comparison group of persons without disease.

Convenience sampling—is a form of non-probability sampling. A convenience sample is a sample of "conveniently" available participants such as "patients from a hospital" or "woman on the street" sampling.

Critical interventions—interventions that are required for the management of life-threatening and potentially life-threatening obstetric conditions. These include blood transfusion, laparotomy including hysterectomy and abdominal surgery but excluding cesarean section, and interventional radiology.

Cross-sectional study—is one of the three basic observational study designs. Cross-sectional studies can be purely descriptive or analytical. In cross-sectional studies, the presence or absence of disease and study factor(s) (or their amount if they are quantitative) is determined for each individual participant at one particular point in time. A cross-sectional study is nondirectional.

Crude mortality rate—refers to the mortality rate from all causes of death for a population.

Cultural colonialism—a term that refers to internal domination by one group and its culture or ideology over others.

Cumulative frequency—refers to a frequency distribution, the number or proportion of cases or events with a particular value or in a particular class interval, plus the total number or proportion of cases or events with smaller values of the variable.

Cumulative frequency curve—a plot of the cumulative frequency rather than the actual frequency for each class interval of a variable. This type of graph is useful for identifying medians, quartiles, and other percentiles.

Cumulative incidence—is the number of new cases (i.e., people newly acquiring a disease or an attribute) occurring over a specified period of time divided by the total number of people in the population at risk of becoming a new case at the beginning of the time period.

Death in pregnancy, childbirth, and the puerperium—the death of a woman while pregnant or within 42 days of termination of pregnancy, irrespective of the cause of death (obstetric and non-obstetric). The term "death in pregnancy, childbirth, and the puerperium" replaces the earlier term "pregnancy-related deaths."

Death rate (or crude death rate)—the number of deaths per 1000 population in a given year.

Death-to-case ratio—the number of deaths attributed to a particular disease during a specified time period divided by the number of new cases of that disease identified during the same time period.

Demographic and Health Surveys (DHS) Program—is responsible for collecting and disseminating accurate, nationally representative data on health and population in developing countries.

Demographic information—refers to the "person" characteristics—age, sex, race, and occupation—of descriptive epidemiology used to characterize the populations at risk.

Dependent variable—in a statistical analysis, the outcome variable(s) or the variable(s) whose values are a function of other variable(s) (called independent variable(s) in the relationship under study).

Determinant—refers to any factor, whether event, characteristic, or other definable entity, that brings about change in a health condition or in other defined characteristics.

Direct estimation of maternal deaths—a method which relies on asking questions about maternal deaths in a household during a recent interval of time, for example, 1 to 2 years. These questions can be asked in the context of a household survey or a census of all households, although as yet experience with the latter is fairly limited.

Direct obstetric case fatality rate—the percent of women admitted to a hospital or an emergency obstetric care (EmOC) facility with major direct obstetric complications, or who develop such complications after admission, and die before discharge.

Direct obstetric deaths—those deaths resulting from obstetric complications of the pregnant state (pregnancy, labor, and puerperium); from interventions, omissions, and incorrect treatment; or from a chain of events resulting from any of the above.

Direct transmission—the immediate transfer of an agent from a reservoir to a susceptible host by direct contact or droplet spread.

Discrimination—a term that refers to policies and practices that harm a group and its members.

Diseases of poverty—refer to a group of abnormal health conditions, disabilities, and diseases that are more prevalent among poor than among wealthy people. In many of these conditions, poverty is a leading risk factor for the development of the condition. Diseases of poverty are frequently comorbid with other diseases and disabilities, including infection, malnutrition, and psychological disturbances.

Distribution—in epidemiology, refers to the frequency and pattern of health-related characteristics and events in a population. In statistics, the observed or theoretical frequency of values of a variable.

Dynamic cohort—is a cohort that gains and loses members throughout its existence. Most cohorts in epidemiology are dynamic.

Early fetal death—a fetal death occurring between 20 and 27 weeks' gestation.

Early neonatal death (END)—the death of a live newborn in the first 7 days (i.e., 0–6 days) of life.

Embryo—in the human conceptus, the stage of development between the 5th and 11th weeks following fertilization, after which it is termed a fetus.

Emergency cesarean section—an unscheduled and unanticipated cesarean section performed in an urgent manner for a maternal or fetal emergency. See also cesarean section.

Emergency newborn care (EmNC)—a package of lifesaving measures for newborns (e.g., clean cord care and neonatal resuscitation).

Emergency obstetric care (EmOC)—is a package of medical interventions that includes urgent services to prevent maternal death (e.g., access to essential pharmaceuticals, including antibiotics, anticonvulsants, and uterotonics). EmOC has been the primary focus of international research and program development.

Emergency obstetric and newborn care (EmONC)—is a package of medical interventions to treat life-threatening complications during pregnancy and childbirth. Multiple forms of EmONC appear in clinical and public health literature, classified by type and breadth of services.

Endemic disease—the constant presence of a disease or infectious agent within a given geographic area or population group; may also refer to the usual prevalence of a given disease within such area or group.

Equality of opportunity—see gender equality.

Ethnic group—refers to a group that shares certain customs, beliefs, values, habits, and norms because of their common background.

Ethnocide—occurs when a dominant group tries to destroy the cultures of certain ethnic groups.

Evidence-based practice—is an approach to health care where health professionals use the best currently available evidence possible. Evidence-based practice uses the most appropriate and most current information available to make optimal clinical decisions for individual patients.

Experimental studies—constitute one of the two major branches of analytical research (observational studies form the second branch). In experiments, the study factor—usually an intervention—is actively and deliberately managed by the investigator. The researcher intentionally alters one or more factors under controlled conditions in order to study the effects of doing so. For example, one group is given the new drug while the control group receives the standard treatment.

Exposed—an individual or group whose members have been brought into contact with a supposed cause of disease or health state of interest, or possess a characteristic that is a determinant of the health outcome of interest.

Exposure odds ratio—is a measure of association used in case-control studies. The exposure odds ratio compares the odds of exposure in the cases with the odds of exposure in the controls.

Facility-based maternal death review—an in-depth investigation of the causes of and associated factors in maternal deaths that occur in health facilities. It entails interviews of health personnel who attended to the deceased. Can also be extended to interviews of family members who accompanied the deceased. The review is nonjudgmental to encourage the cooperation of the health workers involved. It provides information for improving obstetric care.

Family balancing—see sex selection.

Female empowerment—refers to a process by which women and girls acquire the power to act freely, exercise their rights, and fulfill their potential as full and equal members of society. While empowerment often comes from within, the individual, cultures, societies, and institutions create conditions that facilitate or undermine the possibilities for empowerment.

Fetal death—Death before the complete expulsion or extraction from the mother of a product of human conception, irrespective of the duration of pregnancy, that is not an induced termination of pregnancy. The death is indicated by the fact that, after such expulsion or extraction, the fetus does not breathe or show any other evidence of life such as beating of the heart, pulsation of the umbilical cord, or definite movement of voluntary muscles. Heartbeats are to be distinguished from transient cardiac contractions; respirations are to be distinguished from fleeting respiratory efforts or gasps.

Fetus—a prenatal stage of human development which occurs between the embryonic period and birth. According to some, it begins at approximately the 9th week or, according to others, the 12th week, after fertilization.

Filicide—the deliberate act of a parent murdering his/her own child.

Fixed cohort—is a cohort in which membership is fixed by being present at some defining event; often the start of the study period.

Forced marriage—refers to the practice of marriage in which one or both of the parties are married against his or her will.

Frequency distribution—a complete summary of the frequencies of the values or categories of a variable; often displayed in a two-column table: the left column lists the individual values or categories, and the right column indicates the number of observations in each category.

Frequency polygon—a graph of a frequency distribution with values of the variable on the *x*-axis and the number of observations on the *y*-axis; data points are plotted at the midpoints of the intervals and are connected with a straight line.

Gender—a term which signifies the socially constructed characteristics of women and men—these include norms, roles, and relationships of and between groups of women and men. It varies from society to society and can be changed. When individuals or groups do not "fit" into the established gender norms within their society, they often face stigmatization, discriminatory practices, or social exclusion—all of which can adversely affect health.

Gender-based division of labor—refers to where, how, and under what conditions women and men work (for or without pay) based on gender norms and roles.

Gender analysis—Gender analysis identifies, assesses, and informs actions to address inequality that come from (1) different gender norms, roles, and relations, (2) unequal power relations between and among groups of men and women, and (3) the interaction of contextual factors with gender such as sexual orientation, ethnicity, education, or employment status.

Gender-based violence—Any act of aggression that results in, or is likely to result in, physical, sexual, or psychological harm or suffering to women, including threats of such acts, coercion, or arbitrary deprivations of liberty, whether occurring in public or in private life. It is a violation of human rights and a form of discrimination. It is estimated that one of every three women worldwide will experience gender-based violence in her lifetime.

Gender blind—a term which refers to Level 2 of the WHO Gender Responsive Assessment Scale: Ignores gender norms, roles, and relations and very often reinforces gender-based discrimination. By ignoring differences in opportunities and resource allocation for women and men, such policies are often assumed to be "fair" as they claim to treat everyone the same.

Gender equality—a term referring to equal chances or opportunities for groups of women and men to access and control social, economic, and political resources, including protection under the law (such as health services, education, and voting rights). It is also known as equality of opportunity—or formal equality. Gender equality is often used interchangeably with gender equity, but the two refer to different, complementary strategies that are needed to reduce gender-based health inequities.

Gender equity—gender equity refers more than formal equality of opportunity—it addresses the different needs, preferences, and interests of women and men. This may mean that different treatment is needed to ensure equality of opportunity. This is often referred to as substantive equality (or equality of results) and requires considering the realities of women's and men's lives. Gender equity is often used interchangeably with gender equality, but the two refer to different, complementary strategies that are needed to reduce gender-based health inequities.

Gender equity in health—refers to a process of being fair to women and men. It has the objective of reducing unjust and avoidable inequality between women and men in health status, access to health services, and their contributions to the health workforce.

Gender imbalance—a disparity between the numbers of males and females in a population.

Gender mainstreaming—A term which refer to the process of assessing the implications for women and men of any planned action, including legislation, policies, or programs, in all areas and at all levels. It is a strategy for making women's as well as men's concerns and experiences an integral dimension of the design, implementation, monitoring, and evaluation of policies and programs in all political, economic, and societal spheres so that women and men benefit equally and inequality is not perpetuated.

Gender norms—a term used to signify the dominant social expectations and standards related to the roles, attributes, and behaviors associated with being "male" or "female" within a given culture.

Gender Parity Index (GPI)—a socioeconomic indicator, used by UNESCO and other international organizations, to measure the relative access to education by males and females. The GPI is calculated as the quotient of the number of females by the number of males enrolled in a given stage of education (primary, secondary, etc.).

Gender roles—a term which refers to what males and females are expected to do (in the household, community, and workplace) in any given society.

Gender sensitive—a term which refers to Level 3 of the WHO Gender Responsive Assessment Scale: Indicates gender awareness, although no remedial action is developed.

Gender specific—a term which refers to Level 4 of the WHO Gender Responsive Assessment Scale: Considers women's and men's specific needs and intentionally targets and benefits a specific group of women or men to achieve certain policy or program goals or meet certain needs. Such policies often make it easier for women and men to fulfill duties that are ascribed to them based on their gender roles, but do not address underlying causes of gender differences.

Gender stereotypes—refers to images, beliefs, attitudes, or assumptions about certain groups of women and men. Stereotypes are usually negative and based on assumed gender norms, roles, and relations.

Gender stratification—Unequal distribution of rewards (socially valued resources, power, prestige, and personal freedom) between men and women, reflecting their different positions in a social hierarchy.

Gender transformative—a term referring to Level 5 of the WHO Gender Responsive Assessment Scale: Addresses the causes of gender-based health inequities by including ways to transform harmful gender norms, roles, and relations. The objective of such programs is often to promote gender equality and foster progressive changes in power relationships between women and men.

Gender unequal—a term which refers to Level 1 of the WHO Gender Responsive Assessment Scale: Perpetuates gender inequality by reinforcing unbalanced norms, roles, and relations and often leads to one sex enjoying more rights or opportunities than the other.

Gendericide—the targeted and systematic killing of members of a specific gender in a population.

General fertility rate (GFR)—is the number of live births per 1000 women aged 15–49 years in a given year. Data calculated from average births and female population over the PM or MMR time interval using data from the UN Population Division.

Generalized reciprocity—refers to the principle that characterizes exchanges between closely related individuals.

Genocide—is the deliberate elimination of a group through mass murder.

Gestational age—the age of a human conceptus. There are several methods for estimating the gestational age. A common method is to calculate the number of days since the first day of the last menstrual period. It can also be estimated using obstetrical ultrasound.

Gestational diabetes—an abnormal condition in which a woman who did not have diabetes prior to pregnancy develops high blood sugar levels while pregnant. It occurs from 3 to 9% of pregnancies worldwide and can be associated with poor obstetrical outcomes including necessity for cesarean section, unusually large birthweight fetuses, neonatal hypoglycemia, congenital fetal malformations, and stillbirth.

Gestational hypertension—the occurrence of new-onset elevated blood pressure developing after 20 weeks gestation, and often beginning near term, in the absence of proteinuria.

Gestational weight gain—refers to the amount of weight gained by a pregnant women from conception to the birth of the baby. An important metric as a risk factor for poor obstetrical outcomes.

Grand multipara—a woman who has experienced five or more live births at a gestational age of 24 or more months. Grand multiparous women are considered to have a higher risk for poor obstetrical outcomes.

Gravida (gravidity)—a pregnant woman; used to indicate the number of times the woman has been pregnant, regardless of whether these pregnancies were carried to term.

Habitual abortion—a condition in which a woman has three or more successive pregnancy losses consisting of spontaneous abortions or miscarriages. Also termed recurrent pregnancy loss (RPL).

Health indicator—a measure that reflects, or indicates, the state of health of persons in a defined population, e.g., the maternal mortality rate.

High-risk group—refers to a group in the community with an elevated risk of disease.

Host—the person or other living organism that can be infected by an infectious agent under natural conditions.

Host factor—an intrinsic factor (age, race, sex, behaviors, etc.) which influences an individual's exposure, susceptibility, or response to a causative agent.

Human Development Index (HDI)—a composite statistic of life expectancy, education, and income indices used to rank countries into four tiers of human development. The Human Development Index accounts for between 82 and 85% of the maternal mortality rates among countries.

Human sex ratio—a demographic term describing the ratio of males to females in a given population.

Hyperendemic disease—a disease that is constantly present at a high incidence and/or prevalence rate.

Independent variable—an exposure, risk factor, or other characteristic being observed or measured that is hypothesized to influence an event or manifestation (the dependent variable).

Indirect obstetric deaths—those deaths resulting from previous existing disease or disease that developed during pregnancy and which was not due to direct obstetric causes, but which was aggravated by physiologic effects of pregnancy.

Indirect transmission—transmission of an agent carried from a reservoir to a susceptible host by suspended air particles or by animate (vector) or inanimate (vehicle) intermediaries.

Individual data—data that have not been put into a frequency distribution or rank ordered.

Infant death—a live birth that results in death within the first year (<365 days).

Infant mortality rate (IMR)—the number of deaths of infants below the age of 1 year of age per 1000 live births. The infant mortality rate is often used as a measure of the overall health of a country and its economic development. From a global perspective, the IMR of the world is 32 according to the World Health Organization.

Infanticide—the intentional killing of infants. In many past societies, certain forms of infanticide were considered permissible. In some countries, female infanticide is more common than the killing of male offspring, due to sex-selective infanticide.

Inference—in statistics, the development of generalizations from sample data, usually with calculated degrees of uncertainty.

Interquartile range—The central portion of a distribution, calculated as the difference between the third quartile and the first quartile; this range includes about one-half of the observations in the set, leaving one-quarter of the observations on each side.

Intersex—a term which refers to a person having variation in any variation of sexual characteristic, including gonads, sex hormones, genitalia, or chromosomes that do not fit the typical definitions of male or female bodies.

Intrapartum period—the period extending from the beginning of contractions that cause cervical dilation to the first 1–4 h after delivery of the newborn and placenta.

Intrauterine fetal demise (IUFD)—a fetal death occurring after the 20th week of pregnancy.

Intrauterine growth restriction (IUGR)—refers to the abnormal chronic intrauterine process of pathological fetal growth and development prior to delivery. IUGR has two major forms—symmetrical (the frequent) and asymmetric (the most frequent). It is associated with poor obstetrical outcomes.

Late fetal death—a fetal death occurring at or later than 28 weeks' gestation.

Late maternal death—the death of a woman from direct or indirect obstetrical causes more than 42 days, but less than 1 year, after termination of pregnancy.

Late neonatal infant death—death of an infant occurring at from 7 to 27 days after birth.

Late termination of pregnancy—an induced ending of pregnancy occurring after the 20th week of gestation according to most authors, but also after 16 weeks' gestation by a minority of authors, and even following 27 weeks in some sources. Because it results in a fetus which would be viable outside of the uterus (hence the term "post-viability abortion"), this procedure is more controversial that the standard first-trimester abortion procedure.

Latency period—refers to the period of subclinical or inapparent pathologic changes following exposure, ending with the onset of symptoms of chronic disease.

Lay midwife—see traditional birth attendant.

Lethality rate—the ratio of maternal deaths to all obstetric patients admitted for treatment or surveillance to an intensive care unit or the closest equivalent surgical or medical resuscitation or critical care unit in the region.

Life expectancy at birth (LEB)—the average number of years a newborn is expected to live if mortality patterns at the time of its birth remain constant in the future.

Lifetime risk of maternal death—refers to the probability that a 15-year-old female will die eventually from a maternal cause if she experiences throughout her lifetime the risks of maternal death and the overall levels of fertility and mortality that are observed for a given population.

Majority groups—refers to the superordinate, dominant, or controlling group in a society or population.

Malaria Indicators Surveys (MIS)—provides data on bed net ownership and use, prevention of malaria during pregnancy, and prompt and effective treatment of fever in young children. In some cases, biomarker testing for malaria and anemia are also included.

MamaNatalie—The MamaNatalie is a birthing simulator that is worn by the person playing the role of the pregnant woman and which can create realistic simulations of normal or complicated deliveries. These include obstetrical hemorrhage, breech delivery, delivery of the placenta, vacuum-assisted delivery, fetal heart sounds, and others.

Matching—is a design feature in analytical observational studies. Matching is a technique that tries to create comparable groups (i.e., cases and controls in case-control studies or the exposure groups in cohort studies) with respect to extraneous factors (e.g., matching for gender in a case-control study means that for each case a gender-matched control is included in the study).

Maternal death—the death of a woman while pregnant or within 42 days of termination of pregnancy, irrespective of the duration and site of the pregnancy, from any cause related to or aggravated by the pregnancy or its management, but not from accidental or incidental causes.

Maternal death audit—an in-depth systematic review of maternal deaths to delineate their underlying health social and other contributory factors. The lessons learned from such an audit are used in making recommendations to prevent similar future deaths.

Maternal health—the health of women during pregnancy, childbirth, and the postpartum period.

Maternal morbidity—includes physical and psychological conditions that result from or are aggravated by pregnancy and have an adverse effect on a woman's health. Also defined as any health condition attributed to and/or aggravated by pregnancy and childbirth that has a negative impact on the woman's well-being.

Maternal morbidity—defined by the World Health Organization as "the death of a woman while pregnant or within 42 days of termination of pregnancy, irrespective of the duration and site of the pregnancy, from any cause related to or aggravated by the pregnancy or its management but not from accidental or incidental causes.".

Maternal mortality rate (MMRate)—the number of maternal deaths in a population divided by the number of women of reproductive age, usually expressed per 1000 women.

Maternal mortality ratio (MMR)—the ratio of the number of maternal deaths during a given time period from any cause related to or aggravated by pregnancy or its management (excluding accidental or incidental causes) per 100,000 live births during the same time period.

Maternal near miss (MNM)—an event in which a pregnant woman comes close to maternal death, but does not die—a near miss. Defined by the WHO as "a woman who nearly died but survived a complication that occurred during pregnancy, childbirth or within 42 days of termination of pregnancy." This category includes those women who have had a serious adverse event that only failed to result in a maternal death by luck or by adequate management.

Maternal neonatal program index (MNPI)—this indicator is a score (ranging from 0 to 100) that measures the strength of the national maternal and neonatal health program of a given country based on five main areas: policy and support services, facility capacity, access to services, care received, and family planning (FP).

Mean, arithmetic—refers to the measure of central location commonly called the average. It is calculated by adding together all the individual values in a group of measurements and dividing by the number of values in the group.

Mean, geometric—refers to the mean or average of a set of data measured on a logarithmic scale.

Measure of association—the quantified relationship between exposure and disease; includes relative risk, rate ratio, odds ratio.

Measure of central location—the central value that best represents a distribution of data. Measures of central location include the mean, median, and mode. Also called the measure of central tendency.

Measure of dispersion—the measure of the spread of a distribution out from its central value. Measures of dispersion used in epidemiology include the interquartile range, variance, and the standard deviation.

Median—the measure of central location which divides a set of data into two equal parts.

Medical abortion—a safe option for terminating a pregnancy using medications (e.g., mifepristone and misoprostol or misoprostol alone).

Menarche—the first menstrual period of a woman. From both an anthropological and biomedical perspective, it is considered to be the sentinel event of "coming of age" and beginning of puberty and the reproductive cycle.

Met need for EmOC—the percent of all women with major direct obstetric complications who are treated in a health facility providing emergency obstetric care (EmOC) in a given reference period. This indicator is calculated as: (number of women treated for direct obstetric complications at EmOC facilities, over a defined period/estimated number of women who would have major obstetric complications (or 15% of expected births), during the same defined period) × 100.

Millennium Development Goals (MDGs)—a series of eight broad development goals established in 2000 by the United Nations and adopted by countries around the world, which encompass issues of poverty, education, and health. They were set to be achieved by 2015.

Millennium Development Goal (MDG) 5—the goal developed by the United Nations to improve maternal health; targets for achieving this goal include the reduction of maternal mortality by 75% between 1990 and 2015 and the assurance of universal access to reproductive health by 2015.

Miscarriage—a fetal death occurring in the first 20 weeks of gestation.

Misclassification of maternal deaths—occurs when a maternal death is inaccurately classified to causes not used for the purpose of identifying maternal deaths (according to ICD-10 convention, maternal deaths are identified primarily using codes from Chap. 15) and/or where no indication of the temporal nature to pregnancy is indicated on the death certificate to flag this potential misclassification.

Mistimed pregnancy—a pregnancy that occurred earlier than desired.

Mode—a measure of central location, the most frequently occurring value in a set of observations.

Morbidity—the frequency of disease, illness, injuries, and disabilities in a population.

Mortality—deaths as a component of population change.

Mortality index—the number of maternal deaths divided by the sum of maternal deaths and near misses. The higher the index, the more women with life-threatening conditions die (low quality of care).

Multiculturalism—the view of cultural diversity in a country as something good and desirable.

Multigravida—is a woman who has been pregnant more than one time.

Multiple Indicator Cluster Surveys (MICS)—surveys run under the program developed by the United Nations Children's Fund (UNICEF) to provide internationally comparable, statistically rigorous data on the situation of children and women.

Near miss—see maternal near miss.

Near miss/maternal mortality ratio—the numerical relationship between the number of maternal near-miss cases and the number of maternal deaths or the number of near misses for every case of maternal death.

Necessary cause—a causal factor whose presence is required for the occurrence of the effect (of the disease).

Negative predictive value—of a diagnostic or screening test is the probability that a person with a negative test result will actually be disease free.

Neonatal death—the death of a baby in the first 28 days of life.

Neonatal mortality rate (NMR)—the number of neonatal deaths per 1000 live births.

Neonaticide—the practice of killing infants within the first 24 h of the child's birth.

Nomadism, pastoral—refers to the movement throughout the year by the whole pastoral group with their animals.

Non-obstetrical maternal deaths—maternal fatalities during but unrelated to a pregnancy. They are also termed accidental or incidental maternal deaths.

Normal curve—is a bell-shaped curve that results when a normal distribution is graphed.

Normal distribution—refers to the symmetrical clustering of values around a central location. The properties of a normal distribution include the following: (1) It is a continuous, symmetrical distribution; both tails extend to infinity; (2) the arithmetic mean, mode, and median are identical; and (3) its shape is completely determined by the mean and standard deviation.

Nulligravida—a woman who has never been pregnant.

Observational study—an epidemiological study in situations where nature is allowed to take its course. Changes or differences in one characteristic are studied in relation to changes or differences in others, without the intervention of the investigator.

Obstetric fistula—a pathologic condition in which a communicating defect (hole or fistula) develops between either the rectum and vagina, a ureter and the vagina, or the urinary bladder and the vagina, as a result of pregnancy and/or childbirth. It is a frequent complication of unsafe abortion practices.

Obstetric hemorrhage—also known as maternal hemorrhage and obstetrical bleeding, is a pathological condition of maternal bleeding as a result of pregnancy. It can occur during pregnancy, labor, or the puerperium. It is the major cause of maternal death in most resource-poor countries. Obstetric hemorrhage has many causes, including placental abruption, uterine atony, coagulation abnormalities, obstructed labor, placenta previa, miscarriage, and disorders of clotting (coagulopathy).

Obstetric transition—a reproductive health concept used to describe the secular trend of countries gradually shifting from a pattern of high maternal mortality to low maternal mortality, midwifery, from direct obstetric causes of maternal mortality to indirect causes, aging of maternal population, and moving from the natural history of pregnancy and childbirth to institutionalization of maternity care, medicalization, and over medicalization.

Obstructed labor—an abnormal delivery condition in which the pregnant uterus is contracting normally but is physically blocked from exiting the birth canal. The causes include a large baby, mispositioning of the baby such as shoulder dystocia, problems with the birth canal, and an abnormally small pelvis as occurs in some adolescents or with malnutrition. It is an important cause of maternal death in some resource-poor countries.

Odds ratio—a measure of association which quantifies the relationship between an exposure and health outcome from a comparative study; it is also known as the cross-product ratio.

Oxytocin—a medication that is used to initiate labor contractions, to increase the speed of labor, or to treat obstetrical hemorrhage. It is naturally produced by the hypothalamus and released by the posterior pituitary gland. Oxytocin is on the World Health Organization's *List of Essential Medicines*, the most important medications needed in a basic health system.

Paired statistical test—is a version of a statistical test suitable for paired data, i.e., situations where the same individuals were measured twice (or more often) resulting in multiple measurements of the same characteristic in the identical individuals.

Pap test—also termed a Pap smear, is a diagnostic screening procedure performed by entering the vaginal canal using a speculum and collecting surface cells at the outer opening of the transformation zone of the cervix (where the outer squamous cervical cells meet the inner glandular endocervical cells). These collected cells are then placed on a glass slide (smear), stained, and examined microscopically by a pathologists or cytologist for such abnormalities as precancerous cells, malignant cells, inflammation, and other conditions.

Parity—or "para" indicates the number of greater than 20-week gestation births (including viable and nonviable, i.e., stillbirths). Pregnancies consisting of multiples, such as twins or triplets, count as one birth for the purpose of this notation.

Pastoralists—those groups or people who use a food-producing strategy of adaptation based on care of herds of domesticated animals.

Patrilineal-patrilocal complex—consisting of patrilineality, patrilocality, warfare, and male supremacy.

Perinatal mortality rate—the number of fetal deaths after 28 weeks of pregnancy (late fetal deaths) plus the number of deaths to infants under 7 days of age per 1000 live births.

Period prevalence—the amount a particular disease present in a population over a period of time.

Person-time rate—refers to a measure of the incidence rate of an event, e.g., a disease or death, in a population at risk over an observed period to time, that directly incorporates time into the denominator.

Plural society—a society combining ethnic contrasts, ecological specialization, and the economic interdependence of these groups.

Point prevalence—is the amount of a particular disease present in a population at a single point in time.

Ponderal Index (PI) –as used in pregnancy, it is a measure of the leanness of a newborn infant, also referred to as Rohrer's Index. It is the standard statistic used in obstetrics, neonatology, and perinatal pathology to diagnose the asymmetrical type of intrauterine growth restriction (IUGR) of a newborn. It is calculated by dividing the birth weight in grams times 100 by the birth length in centimeters cubed. A Ponderal Index below the tenth percentile adjusted for gestational age is diagnostic of asymmetrical IUGR. The most frequent cause of an abnormally low Ponderal Index is chronic placental insufficiency. The Ponderal Index is utilized by both neonatologists and perinatal pathologists to assess the presence of asymmetrical intrauterine growth restriction and its causes. See also body mass index.

Population at risk—are all people under observation who initially do not have the disease or the attribute but are "at risk" of acquiring the disease or the attribute.

Positive predictive value—of a diagnostic or screening test is the probability that a person with a positive test result will actually have the disease.

Postneonatal infant death—an infant death occurring at from 28 to 364 days of life.

Postpartum period—is commonly defined as the 6 weeks after childbirth.

Postterm—Also termed post-term, a pregnancy that is greater than 42 weeks gestation.

Postterm labor—labor that begins after the 42nd week of pregnancy.

Potentially life-threatening conditions (PLTC)—obstetrical conditions which can result in maternal death but are less likely to than those in the category of life-threatening conditions (LTC) which include maternal near misses and maternal deaths.

Preconception health—refers to the health of women and men during their reproductive years and, specifically, focuses on steps that women can take to protect the health of a baby in the future.

Pregnancy-associated death—the death of a woman while pregnant or within 1 year of termination of pregnancy, irrespective of cause.

Pregnancy-related death—the death of a woman while pregnant or within 1 year of termination of pregnancy, irrespective of the duration and site of the pregnancy, from any cause related to or aggravated by her pregnancy or its management, but not from accidental or incidental causes. Another commonly used definition is the death of a woman while pregnant or within 42 days of termination of pregnancy, irrespective of the cause of death.

Pregnancy-related mortality rate—death from obstetric causes within 1-year postpartum, per 100,000 live births.

Prejudice—the act of devaluing a group because of its assumed behavior, values, capabilities, or attributes.

Prenatal care—see antenatal care.

Prenatal period—the time between conception and birth.

Preteen pregnancy—a pregnancy occurring in a girl before the start of her teen years.

Preterm—a pregnancy that is earlier than 37 weeks' gestation.

Preterm labor—labor that begins prior to the 37th week of pregnancy.

Prevalence—the number or proportion of cases or events or conditions in a given population.

Prevalence odds ratio—is a measure of association used in cross-sectional studies. The prevalence odds ratio compares the odds of the prevalence of the outcome in the exposed group with the odds of the prevalence of the outcome in the unexposed group.

Prevalence rate—The proportion of persons in a population who have a particular disease or attribute at a specified point in time or over a specified period of time.

Primigravida—a woman who is pregnant for the first time or has been pregnant one time.

Primip—see primagravida.

Prolective data—are specifically collected for the purpose of a particular study. Prolective data collection can be adapted to the specific needs of a study; the researcher is able to decide on the type and format of the required data. Prolective data collection allows control over the quality of the data and is the preferred option for research.

Propagated outbreak—refers to an outbreak that does not have a common source, but instead spreads from person to person.

Proportion—is a type of ratio in which the numerator is included in the denominator. The ratio of a part to the whole, expressed as a "decimal fraction" (e.g., 0.2), as a fraction (1/5), or, loosely, as a percentage (20%).

Proportion—refers to a type of ratio in which the numerator is included in the denominator. The ratio of a part to the whole, expressed as a "decimal fraction" (e.g., 0.2), as a fraction (1/5), or, loosely, as a percentage (20%).

Proportion maternal (PM)—is the proportion maternal among deaths of females of reproductive age and is calculated as the number of maternal deaths divided by the total deaths among females aged 15–49 years.

Proportionate mortality—the proportion of deaths in a specified population over a period of time attributable to different causes. Each cause is expressed as a percentage of all deaths, and the sum of the causes must add to 100%. These proportions are not mortality rates, since the denominator is all deaths, not the population in which the deaths occurred.

Public health surveillance—refers to the systematic collection, analysis, interpretation, and dissemination of health data on an ongoing basis, to gain knowledge of the pattern of disease occurrence and potential in a community, in order to control and prevent disease in the community.

Puerperium—the period extending from the delivery of the placenta after childbirth to 6 weeks postpartum during which time the maternal organs return to their nonpregnant condition. This is considered the most critical and neglected phase in the lives of mothers and babies; most deaths occur during this period.

***p*-value**—is the result of a statistical hypothesis test. The *p*-value gives the probability of obtaining in a sample a difference as large as the actually observed one (or an even larger one) if in reality (i.e., in the wider population) there is no such difference. Thus the *p*-value is the probability that an observed difference is attributable to chance alone. The smaller the *p*-value, the less likely that an observed difference occurred by chance alone. If the *p*-value is less than a set alpha level (usually less than 0.05), then the result of the statistical hypothesis test is called statistically significant.

Race—a potentially controversial concept; an ethnic group that is assumed to have a biological basis.

Race-specific mortality rate—a mortality rate limited to a specified racial group. Both numerator and denominator are limited to the specified group.

Racism—the act of discrimination against a race.

RAMOS (reproductive age mortality surveys)—studies which seek to identify all female deaths in the reproductive period, using a combination of approaches, such as cross-sectional household surveys, continuous population surveillance, hospital and health center records, and key informants.

Random error—is a type of error that is governed by chance. The smaller the random error in a study, the more reliable are the results of the study. Random error occurs in every epidemiological study due to natural or biological variation. Random error is assessed during the statistical analysis of the data collected in a study.

Random sample—a sample derived by selecting individuals such that each individual has the same probability of selection.

Randomized controlled trial (RCT)—is a specific type of experimental study. In a RCT participants are randomized to an intervention or a control group. The control group of a randomized controlled trial is concurrent.

Range—in statistics, the difference between the largest and smallest values in a distribution. In common use, the span of values from smallest to largest.

Rate—an expression of the frequency with which an event occurs in a defined population.

Rate ratio—a comparison of two groups in terms of incidence rates, person-time rates, or mortality rates.

Reciprocity—refers to one of the three principles of exchange that governs exchange between social equals.

Redistribution—is the major exchange mode of chiefdoms, many archaic states, and some states with managed economies.

Relative risk—the comparison of the risk of some health-related event such as disease or death in two groups.

Representative sample—a sample whose characteristics correspond to those of the original population or reference population.

Reproductive health—the state of complete physical, mental, and social well-being in all matters relating to the reproductive system, its functions, and processes.

Reservoir—refers to the habitat in which an infectious agent normally lives, grows, and multiplies; reservoirs include human reservoirs, animal reservoirs, and environmental reservoirs.

Risk—is the probability that an event will occur, e.g., that an individual will become ill or die within a stated period of time or age.

Risk factor—an aspect of personal behavior or lifestyle, an environmental exposure, or an inborn or inherited characteristic that is associated with an increased occurrence of disease or other health-related event or condition.

Risk ratio—refers to a comparison of the risk of some health-related event such as disease or death in two groups.

Safe motherhood—encompasses a series of initiatives, practices, protocols, and service delivery guidelines designed to ensure that women receive high-quality gynecological, family planning, prenatal, delivery, and postpartum care, in order to achieve optimal health for the mother, fetus and infant during pregnancy, childbirth, and postpartum.

Sample—a selected subset of a population. A sample may be random or nonrandom, and it may be representative or nonrepresentative.

Sample size—in quantitative epidemiological research, it is important for a study to have an adequate sample size to allow estimations and comparisons with some predefined statistical confidence. Sample size calculation ensures optimal sample size in the sense that a study has sufficient power to detect an existing difference with statistical confidence—without wasting resources to collect too large a sample.

Sampling frame—is the source entity from which the sample will be drawn. Examples of sampling frames include the telephone book or a list of hospital patients.

Scatter diagram—A type of graph in which each dot represents paired values for two continuous variables, with the x-axis representing one variable and the y-axis representing the other; used to display the relationship between the two variables; also called a scattergram.

Seasonality—refers to the change in physiological status or in disease occurrence that conforms to a regular seasonal pattern.

Secondary attack rate—refers to a measure of the frequency of new cases of a disease among the contacts of known cases.

Secular trend—refers to changes over a long period of time, generally years or decades.

Secundogravida—refers to a woman who has had two pregnancies.

Selection bias—is one of the three main types of bias. Selection bias refers to a distortion in the effect measure resulting from the manner in which the people are selected for the sample. For example, selection bias may be introduced if sampling techniques are inappropriate. If selection bias occurs, the sample(s) do not represent the target population.

Sensitivity—refers to the proportion of persons with disease who are correctly identified by a screening test or case definition as having disease.

Severe acute maternal morbidity (SAMM)—is defined as "A very ill pregnant or recently delivered woman who would have died had it not been that luck and good care was on her side." This concept is relatively new in maternal care but is increasingly becoming important in areas with low maternal mortality ratios or where the geographic area is small. See also maternal near miss.

Severe maternal complications—consist of "potentially life-threatening conditions." This is an extensive category of clinical conditions that includes diseases that can potentially threaten a woman's life during pregnancy and labor, as well as after termination of pregnancy. A summary list of potentially life-threatening conditions has been produced by the WHO Working Group on Maternal Deaths and Morbidity Classifications. For example, severe postpartum hemorrhage, severe pre-eclampsia, eclampsia, ruptured uterus, and sepsis/severe systemic infection.

Severe maternal morbidity—potentially life-threatening maternal disease, complication, or condition. See also maternal near miss.

Severe maternal outcome (SMO)—a category which includes both maternal deaths and maternal near misses.

Severe maternal outcome ratio (SMOR)—the number of cases of severe maternal outcome (maternal near misses + maternal deaths) per 1000 live births (MNM + MD/LB).

Sex selection—refers to the attempt to control the sex of the offspring to achieve a desired sex. It can be accomplished in several ways, both pre- and postimplantation of an embryo, as well as at childbirth.

Sex-selective abortion—the practice in some societies of electively terminating a pregnancy based upon the predicted sex of the infant.

Sex-selective infanticide—the practice of killing an infant based upon the sex of the infant.

Sexual and reproductive rights—A series of rights related to sexual and reproductive health, including the rights to freely and responsibly decide on the number, spacing, and timing of children; to receive the highest standard of sexual and reproductive health; to make decisions about reproduction free from discrimination, coercion, and violence; and to pursue a safe, satisfying, and consensual sex life.

Sisterhood methods (direct)—direct sisterhood methods obtain information by interviewing respondents about the survival of all their siblings (the age of all living siblings, age at death and year of death of those dead, and among sisters who died when at least 12 years of age, how many died during pregnancy, delivery, or within 2 months of the end of the pregnancy). This approach identifies all deaths in pregnancy, childbirth, and the puerperium, rather than maternal deaths. The direct sisterhood method generally produces estimates referring to a 7-year period preceding the survey, and these estimates are subject to substantial uncertainty (wide confidence intervals), making it difficult to monitor changes over time. This is the standard approach currently used in Demographic and Health Surveys (DHS) and Multiple Indicator Cluster Surveys (MICS).

Sisterhood method (indirect)—asks respondents four simple questions about how many of their sisters reached adulthood, how many have died, and whether those who died were pregnant around the time of death. This method relies heavily on a number of assumptions about the relationships between fertility and age-specific maternal mortality. This approach is no longer commonly used, although before 2007 it was incorporated into some MICS surveys.

Skewed—refers to a distribution that is asymmetrical.

Skilled attendant at birth (SAB) percentage—percentage of births attended by skilled health personnel (doctor, nurse, or midwife).

Skilled birth attendant (SBA)—is a midwife, physician, obstetrician, nurse, or other health-care professional who provides basic and emergency health-care services to women and their newborns during pregnancy, childbirth, and the postpartum period. WHO defines an SBA as someone "trained to proficiency in the skills needed to manage normal (uncomplicated) pregnancies, childbirth and the immediate postnatal period, and in the identification, management and referral of complications in women and newborns."

Specificity—refers to the proportion of persons without disease who are correctly identified by a screening test or case definition as not having disease.

Sporadic—refers to a disease that occurs infrequently and irregularly.

Spot map—is a map that indicates the location of each case of a rare disease or outbreak by a place that is potentially relevant to the health event being investigated, such as where each case lived or worked.

Standard Days Method (SDM)—a method of natural family planning (NFP) devised by Georgetown University in which the couple abstains from sexual intercourse on days 8 through 19 of the woman's menstrual cycle. SDM is 95% effective when used properly.

Standard deviation—is the most widely used measure of dispersion of a frequency distribution, equal to the positive square root of the variance.

Standard error (of the mean)—the standard deviation of a theoretical distribution of sample means about the true population mean.

Stereotypes—preformed or fixed ideas about what the members of a group are like.

Stillbirth—the death of a fetus in the uterus after 20 weeks' gestation. Another definition is the death of a fetus weighing 500 g or more or of 22 weeks' gestation or more if weight is unavailable.

Sufficient cause—refers to a causal factor or collection of factors whose presence is always followed by the occurrence of the effect (of disease).

Survey of severe morbidity—an in-depth investigation of the factors that led to a near-miss maternal event. It evaluates what worked well in the treatment of the life-threatening complications and the lessons learned. Unlike the other approaches, in this one the pregnant woman herself is also interviewed, creating the opportunity to obtain more insight into the circumstances. This survey is less threatening to health personnel than the others, since the women have survived.

Survival curve—refers to a curve that starts at 100% of the study population and shows the percentage of the population still surviving at successive times for as long as information is available. May be applied not only to survival as such but also to the persistence of freedom from a disease or complication or some other endpoint.

Systematic error—is a type of error which acts on the results of a study in a systematic way. The smaller the systematic error in a study, the more valid are the results of the study. Systematic error occurs in every epidemiological study. Study design features such as randomization, blinding, and matching are used to minimize systematic error.

Taboo—A behavior that is outside the moral limits of cultural norms for a society.

Task shifting—involves the rational redistribution of tasks among cadres of health workers and has become an important strategy in the field of maternal health care. Task shifting increases the skill sets of associate clinicians, nurses, and midwives to assume tasks previously undertaken only by other cadres.

Teenage pregnancy—a teenage girl, usually within the ages of 13–19, becoming pregnant. A pregnancy can take place after the start of the puberty before first menstrual period but usually occurs after the onset of periods.

Temperature method—A fertility awareness-based method for predicting fertility in which women chart when ovulation occurs by taking their temperature every morning before getting out of bed. It can be used for contraception or for planning pregnancy.

Therapeutic abortion—refers to the termination of a pregnancy because of fetal abnormality or to protect a woman's physical or mental health or her life.

Third trimester—the last 3 months of pregnancy.

Threatened miscarriage—refers to an abnormal condition in which a woman bleeds, with or without mild cramps, but the cervix has not yet begun to dilate. One-half of threatened miscarriages end in pregnancy loss; in the other half, the bleeding stops, and the pregnancy continues normally.

Three delays model—the "three delays" model proposes that pregnancy-related mortality is overwhelmingly due to delays in (1) deciding to seek appropriate medical help for an obstetric emergency, (2) reaching an appropriate obstetric facility, and (3) receiving adequate care when a facility is reached.

Traditional birth attendant (TBA)—is a pregnancy and childbirth care provider. Traditional birth attendants provide the majority of primary maternity care in many developing countries and may function within specific communities in developed countries. They are sometimes referred to as a traditional midwife, community midwife, or lay midwife.

Traditional midwife—see traditional birth attendant.

Transhumance—one of two variants of pastoralism; part of the population moves seasonally with the herds while the other part remains in home villages.

Trend—is a long-term movement or change in frequency, usually upward or downward.

Two-day method—a form of natural family planning that identifies the fertile days in a woman's cycle by using the presence of secretions as an indicator of fertility. It is 96% effective in preventing pregnancy with correct use and 86% with typical use.

Under-five mortality rate (U5M)—the probability per 1000 that a newborn baby will die before reaching age five, if subject to age-specific mortality rates of the specified year. In 2016 the U5M was 41 deaths per 1000 live births globally. In the WHO African Region, the U5M is 76.5, approximately 8-times higher than in the WHO European Region where the metric is 9.6.

Underreporting of maternal deaths—may occur due to misclassification or if the death was never reported.

Unintended pregnancy—refers to a pregnancy that was either mistimed or unwanted. Unintended pregnancies occur most frequently among poor and low-income women, teenagers and women up to 24 years of age, and minorities. It is estimated that approximately 87 million women each year have unintended pregnancies.

Univariate—an adjective used in statistics to describe situations or procedures where one single variable only is considered or involved.

Unmet need—the family planning needs of sexually active fecund women who do not use contraceptives and have a desire to delay or limit childbearing. Unmet need for family planning is a useful measurement for identifying and targeting women at high risk of unwanted pregnancy.

Unmet obstetric need—women who require obstetric care and have not received it.

Unpaired statistical test—is a version of a statistical test suitable for unpaired data, i.e., situations where different groups of individuals are measured once only resulting in a single measurement (per assessed characteristic) for the individuals.

Unplanned pregnancy—one that occurred when the woman used a contraceptive method or when she did not desire to become pregnant but did not use a method.

Unsafe abortion—is the termination of a pregnancy by people lacking the necessary skills or in an environment lacking minimal medical standards or both. According to WHO, unsafe abortion is "a procedure for terminating an unintended pregnancy carried out either by persons lacking the necessary skills or in an environment that does not conform to minimal medical standards, or both."

Unsafe motherhood—consists of maternal mortality or morbidity due to preventable pregnancy and childbirth-related causes.

Unwanted/unintended pregnancy—a pregnancy that a woman or girl decides, of her own free will, is undesired.

Validity—the degree to which a measurement actually measures or detects what it is supposed to measure.

Variable—any characteristic or attribute that can be measured.

Variance—is a measure of the dispersion shown by a set of observations, defined by the sum of the squares of deviations from the mean, divided by the number of degrees of freedom in the set of observations.

Vector—is an animate intermediary in the indirect transmission of an agent that carries the agent from a reservoir to a susceptible host.

Vehicle—is an inanimate intermediary in the indirect transmission of an agent that carries the agent from a reservoir to a susceptible host.

Verbal autopsy—a community-based maternal death review, also known as a verbal autopsy. An in-depth nonjudgmental investigation of the causes and the associated factors of maternal deaths that occur outside health facilities. It entails interviews of family members who cared for the deceased. This requires a community informant to let local authorities know whenever there is a death of a reproductive-age female in the community. The interviewer, who is usually not a health worker, should be sensitive when probing the circumstances leading to the maternal death. In some cultures, the interview is done after the mourning period. A team of physicians then examines the interview notes to determine the cause of death. When this is combined with the facility-based review described above, it gives a more complete picture of maternal deaths in a given local jurisdiction. The findings of verbal autopsy studies cannot be extrapolated to obtain national MMRs.

Virulence—refers to the proportion of persons with clinical disease, who after becoming infected, become severely ill or die.

Vital statistics—refers to systematically tabulated information about births, marriages, divorces, and deaths, based on registration of these vital events.

Years of potential life lost—is a measure of the impact of premature mortality on a population, calculated as the sum of the differences between some predetermined minimum or desired life span and the age of death for individuals who died earlier than that predetermined age.

A Glossary for Anthropological Research Referring to Indigenous Peoples of Mexico and Central America

40

David A. Schwartz

40.1 Introduction

Mexico and the countries of Central America are rich with the traditions, cultures, and languages of their indigenous peoples. In many parts of the globe, indigenous peoples have disappeared or, if they survived, have had their cultures and languages assimilated into that of their colonizers or conquerors. Following contact with Europeans in the early sixteenth century, the total number of indigenous people inhabiting Mexico and Central America plummeted by 8% or more. Despite this, the indigenous peoples and their cultures in these countries have stubbornly survived in spite of conquest, hundreds of years of colonization, newly introduced diseases, and even attempts at genocide. In Mexico alone, over 25 million people self-identify as indigenous, representing approximately 21% of the population and 62 officially recognized indigenous languages. In Guatemala, almost 40% of the population is indigenous, with 23 recognized indigenous languages. The other countries—Honduras, El Salvador, Nicaragua, and Belize—have variable number of surviving indigenous peoples, cultures, and languages. This glossary attempts to briefly introduce the large number of indigenous languages and ethnic groups in this region, together with additional terms and concepts that may be useful in conducting anthropological research and related studies in Mexico and Central America.

40.2 The Glossary

Abejones Zapotec language—an indigenous Zapotec language of Oaxaca, Mexico.

Achi language—a Mayan language spoken by Achi people of Guatemala. There are two Achi dialects, Rabinal Achi (also known as Rab'ina:l, Rabinal Quiché, Rabinal K'iche', or Chicaj Achi) and Cubulco Achi (also known as Kubul, Kub'u:l, or Cubulco Quiché). Achi is the people's own name for both themselves and their language. Because the Achi language is closely related to the Quiché Maya language, many linguists consider it as a dialect of Quiché. However, the two groups have distinct ethnic and historical identities.

D. A. Schwartz, M.D., M.S. Hyg., F.C.A.P.
Department of Pathology, Medical College of Georgia, Augusta University, Augusta, GA, USA

D. A. Schwartz (ed.), *Maternal Death and Pregnancy-Related Morbidity Among Indigenous Women of Mexico and Central America*, Global Maternal and Child Health: Medical, Anthropological, and Public Health Perspectives, https://doi.org/10.1007/978-3-319-71538-4_40

Achi people—are a Mayan ethnic group numbering approximately 100,000 persons who live in Guatemala and speak the Achi language. Achi deities include Ajaaw (the divine), *uk'u'x kaaj* and *uk'u'x uleew*, to whom they ask for permission to perform their traditional dances.

Acculturation—the process by which a culture is transformed due to the massive adoption of cultural traits from another society. It is what happens to a culture when alien traits diffuse in on a large scale and substantially replace preexisting traditional cultural patterns.

Acephalous society—a society in which political power is diffused to the degree that there are no institutionalized political leadership roles such as chiefs and kings. Bands and tribes are acephalous. Most foragers and simple horticulturalists have highly egalitarian, acephalous societies. The word "acephalous" is Greek for "without a head."

Akatek language—a Mayan language spoken by the Akatek people of Guatemala and belonging to the Q'anjob'alan branch of Mayan languages. Akatek is closely related to two other Mayan languages, Jakaltek and Q'anjob'al. These three languages constitute the Q'anjob'al–Jakaltek subbranch, which together with the Mocho' language form the Q'anjob'alan subbranch. This subbranch, together with the Chujean languages, Chuj and Tojolab'al, form the Q'anjob'alan–Chujean branch of the Mayan languages.

Akatek people—an indigenous Maya people from Guatemala, most of whom live in San Miguel Acatán and San Rafael La Independencia, in the Department of Huehuetenango. Numbering approximately 40,000 people, they speak the Akatek language.

Albarradas Zapotec language—also termed Santo Domingo Albarradas Zapotec, is a Zapotec language of Oaxaca, Mexico. It is spoken by approximately 5500 individuals in the towns of Santa María Albarradas, Santo Domingo Albarradas, and San Miguel Albarradas. The language in the neighboring towns of Santa Catarina Albarradas and San Antonio Albarradas is not mutually intelligible.

Aldea—Spanish term for a small settlement or hamlet, usually smaller than a village.

Aloápam Zapotec language—is an indigenous Zapotec language of Oaxaca, Mexico, with approximately 3400 speakers.

Ambilineal descent—a form of cognatic descent in which individuals can select to trace descent either through matrilineal or patrilineal lines. The decision may be made each generation based on the relative wealth and/or importance of the father's and the mother's family lines.

Ambilocal residence—the residence pattern in which a newly married couple has the choice of living with or near the groom's or the bride's family.

Amuzgo language—is an indigenous language of Mexico. It is an Oto-Manguean language spoken in the Costa Chica region of the Mexican states of Guerrero and Oaxaca by approximately 44,000 speakers, many of whom are monolingual.

Amuzgo people—an indigenous people residing in a region along the Guerrero/Oaxaca state border in southwest Mexico. Most of the Amuzgo people reside in the area of four municipalities—Xochistlahuaca, Tlacoachistlahuaca, Ometepec in Guerrero, and San Pedro Amuzgos in Oaxaca. The origin of the Amuzgo people is not known, but their language is similar to the Mixtec, and their territory overlaps that of the Mixtec region. The Mixtecs call them "*Ñuuñama*" which means "people of *totomoxtle* (dried corn leaves)." The Aztecs referred to them as Amoxco, believed to be the origin of the term Amuzgo.

Ancestral spirits—refers to souls or ghosts of ancestors. A belief in ancestral spirits is consistent with the widespread belief that humans have at least two parts—a physical body and some kind of nonphysical spirit. The spirit portion is generally believed to be freed from the body by death and continues to exist. Ancestral spirits are often seen as retaining an active interest and even membership in their family and society.

Antequera Zapotec language—is the dialect of Zapotec written in post-contact sixteenth-century colonial documents such as Córdova 1578. "Antequera" is an old name for the city of Oaxaca.

Apache people—are an indigenous group of Native American people from the Southwestern United States. They have traditionally lived in Eastern Arizona, Northern Mexico (Sonora and Chihuahua), New Mexico, West Texas, and Southern Colorado. Together, these areas are collectively known as Apacheria. They developed several differing languages and cultures. The contemporary postcolonial division of Apache groups includes Western Apache, Chiricahua, Mescalero, Jicarilla, Lipan, and Plains Apache (also known as the Kiowa–Apache). Many Native American Indians stayed in present-day Mexico in the State of Chihuahua near the Sierra Madre Occidental, where they are termed the "Sierra Tarahumara."

Asunción Mixtepec Zapotec—also termed North Central Zimatlan Zapotec, is a nearly extinct Oto-Manguean language of western Oaxaca, Mexico, last known to have only 100 speakers. It is a divergent Zapotec language, 22% intelligible with Ayoquesco Zapotec, the most similar other language.

Awakatek people—also termed the Aguacateco, they are an indigenous Mayan ethnic group primarily residing in the municipality of Aguacatán (Huehuetenango) of Guatemala and in Chiapas, Mexico. Their native language is also called Awakatek and is related to the Ixil language. They number approximately 11,000–18,000 persons.

Awakatek language—the language of the Awakatek people, an indigenous Mayan ethnic group. The Awakatek people themselves refer to their language as *qa'yol*, which means *our word*. The language is closely related to Ixil, with the two languages forming the Ixilean subbranch. This subbranch, together with the Mamean languages, Mam and Tektitek, form a sub-branch termed Greater Mamean.

Ayoquesco Zapotec language—also referred to as Western Ejutla Zapotec and Zapoteco de Santa María Ayoquezco, is a Zapotec language spoken by approximately 800 persons in Oaxaca, Mexico.

Aztec people—a term referring to indigenous peoples of Central Mexico, particularly those groups who spoke the Nahuatl language and who dominated large parts of Mesoamerica from the fourteenth to sixteenth centuries during the Postclassic period of Mesoamerican chronology. The Nahuatl words *aztecatl* [asˈtekat͡ɬ] (singular) and *aztecah* [asˈtekaʔ] (plural) mean "people from Aztlan," a mythological place for the Nahuatl-speaking culture of the time, and later adopted as the word to define the Mexica people. The term "Aztec" can refer, in particular, to the Mexica, the ethnic group that had a leading role in establishing the hegemonic empire based at Tenochtitlan. The term can also be extended to additional ethnic groups associated with the Aztec Empire such as the Acolhua and Tepanec and others that were incorporated into the empire. In the field of ethnolinguistics, the term Aztec refers to the branch of the Uto-Aztecan languages (also sometimes called the Yuto-Nahuan languages) that includes the Nahuatl language and its closest relatives Pochutec and Pipil.

Barrida—a Nahua term for the ritual cleansing (or literally, sweeping) by which the body is purged of disease-causing spirits.

Belize Kriol language—also referred to as Kriol or Belizean Creole. It is an English-based creole language closely related to Miskito Coastal Creole, Bocas del Toro Creole, Colón Creole, Rio Abajo Creole, Jamaican Patois, San Andrés–Providencia Creole, and Limón Coastal Creole. It is estimated that there are approximately 150,000 speakers of the Belize Kriol language, with all of the 70,000 Creoles in Belize speaking the language.

Bokota people—also termed the Bogotá or Bugleres, are an indigenous group of approximately 1000 people residing in Panama, predominantly in Bocas del Toro and north of Veraguas. They speak the Bogota language, a member of the Chibchan group of languages.

Bonesetter—also termed a huesero, is a Mayan healer who receives their sacred calling from the gods. The bonesetter's bone is considered to be a sacred object. It is surrounded by taboos and credited with miraculous abilities. It is a repository of supernatural power, a potent cultural symbol binding patient and practitioner in a bond of faith. The bonesetter's medicine works because his bone is a conductor of supernatural forces. The Mayan bonesetters use the innate skills of their hands to diagnose and treat lesions and injuries, using a combination of intuition and experience. They use sacred objects in their work called "*baq*," which can be bones from small animals, obsidian, pieces of old ceramic, or pieces of antique jade. The bonesetter uses these objects to realign the bones and then uses his hands on the area to finish the treatment.

Boruca people—also referred to as the Brunca or Brunka, are a group of approximately 2660 indigenous people living in Costa Rica, most of whom live on a reservation, the Reserva Indígena Boruca, in the Puntarenas Province in southwestern Costa Rica, a few miles away from the Pan-American Highway where it follows the Rio Terraba. In past times, the ancestors of the modern Boruca were composed of chiefdoms that ruled most of Costa Rica's Pacific coast, from Quepos to what is now the Panamanian border, including the Osa Peninsula. The Boruca people spoke the Boruca language, which is now nearly extinct.

Bribri language—the indigenous language of the Bribri people of Costa Rica. It is an SOV (subject-object-verb) language belonging to the Chibchan language group, with approximately 11,000 remaining indigenous speakers remaining.

Bribri people—the Bribri are an indigenous people of Costa Rica. They were the autochthonous people of the Talamanca region, living in the mountains and Caribbean coastal areas of Costa Rica and, formerly, northern Panama. They now live in the Talamanca (canton) in Limón Province of Costa Rica. They speak the Bribri language and Spanish. There are varying estimates of the population of the tribe, which reach up to a maximum of 35,000. Many of the Bribri people are isolated, which has allowed them to maintain their indigenous culture.

Buglere language—an indigenous language, also known as Murire or Muoy, spoken by approximately 18,000 Guaymi people residing in Panama and Costa Rica. It is a Chibchan language and consists of two dialects, Sabanero and Bokotá (Bogota).

Cabécar language—is an indigenous language belonging to the Chibchan language family which is spoken by the Cabécar people in Costa Rica. It is spoken in the inland Turrialba Region of the Cartago Province, where 80% of speakers are monolingual.

Cacaopera people—an indigenous people from El Salvador, also known as the Matagalpa or Ulua, speaking the Cacaopera language, a Misumalpan language.

Cahitan languages—are indigenous languages that are a branch of the Uto-Aztecan language group and include the Yaqui and Mayo languages of Northern Mexico.

Cajonos Zapotec language—also termed Southern Villa Alta Zapotec and Zapoteco de San Pedro Cajonos, is an indigenous Zapotec language of Oaxaca, Mexico. Cajonos Zapotec is spoken in several towns named Cajonos, as well as, San Pedro Cajonos, San Pablo Yaganiza, and Santo Domingo Xagacía.

Changuena language—is an extinct indigenous Chibchan language that was once spoken in Costa Rica and Panama and is closely related to the living language Bribri.

Chatino language—the indigenous language of the Chatino people of Oaxaca. It belongs to branch of the Zapotecan language family within the Oto-Manguean language family. The Chatino people call their language *ChaqF TnyaJ*, which means "difficult word,". The Chatino languages consist of a group of three languages. Zenzontepec Chatino is spoken in approximately 10 communities in the district of Sola de Vega, Tataltepec Chatino is spoken in Tataltepec, and a group of languages called the Eastern Chatino languages are spoken in approximately 15–17 communities.

Chatino people—an indigenous people living in the southeastern region of Chiapas in Mexico. Numbering approximately 23,000 people, they speak the Chatino language and refer to themselves as *qne-a tnya-e*. They have close linguistic and cultural ties with the Zapotec people.

Chibchan languages—also referred to as Chibchano, refer to an indigenous language family from the Isthmo-Colombian Area, extending from eastern Honduras to northern Colombia. It includes indigenous populations in these countries as well as Nicaragua, Costa Rica, and Panama. Although previously believed to have originated near Bogota in Colombia, it is currently thought that the Chibchan languages and Chibchan-speaking peoples may not have been in Colombia at all but in the area of the Costa Rica–Panama border where the greatest variety of Chibchan languages exist.

Chichicapan Zapotec language—also termed Eastern Ocotlán Zapotec and Zapoteco de San Baltazar Chichicápam, is an indigenous Zapotec language of Oaxaca, Mexico, spoken by approximately 2700 persons. The town's name is spelled as both Chichicápam and Chichicapan.

Chichimeca people—a name used historically by the Nahua people of Mexico for the numerous tribes and bands of nomadic and seminomadic peoples of Northern Mexico. The term was used in a similar context to that of "barbarian" used by the Romans to describe people living outside of settled areas.

Chichimeca Jonaz people—a modern day group of indigenous peoples living in Guanajuato and San Luis Potosí, where in Guanajuato State the Chichimeca Jonaz people live mostly in a community of San Luis de la Paz municipality. There are approximately 83,000 members of this indigenous group.

Chichimeca language—the indigenous language of the Chichimeca people of Mexico. It is a member of the Pamean subbranch of the Oto-Pamean branch of the Oto-Manguean language family. The closest relative of the Chichimeca Jonaz language is the Pame language. There are 2600 speakers of this indigenous language.

Chinamita people—also termed the Tulumkis (Nahuatl *chinamitl*, Mopan *tulumki)* were an indigenous ethnic group of Mopan Maya people inhabiting a territory in the eastern Petén Basin and western Belize between the Itza of Nojpetén, within the borders of modern Guatemala, and their allies at Tipuj, now in Belize.

Chinantec languages—a group of 14 mutually unintelligible indigenous languages spoken by approximately indigenous 130,000 people residing mostly in Oaxaca and Veracruz, Mexico. It is a tonal language and is part of the Oto-Manguean family of languages.

Chinanteco people—the Chinantecs are an indigenous people of Mexico residing in Oaxaca and Veracruz, concentrated in the districts of Cuicatlán, Ixtlán de Juárez, Tuxtepec, and Choapam. Their language, Chinantec, belongs to the Western Oto-Mangue group. There are approximately 130,000 speakers of the Chinantec language.

Choápam Zapotec language—also termed Zapoteco de Choápam and, in Veracruz, Zapoteco de San Juan Comaltepec, is an indigenous Zapotec language of Oaxaca, Mexico.

Chocho language—an indigenous Mexican language spoken by approximately 770 members of the Chocho people of Oaxaca.

Chocho people—formerly termed the Chochones (Chocho: *Ngiwa*), are an indigenous group of people residing in the Mexican state of Oaxaca. They have an indigenous language, Chocho, that is a member of the Popolocan branch of the Oto-Manguean language family. The Mixtec term for the Chochos is *tay tocuii* (also spelled *tocuij* or *tocuiy*).

Choco language family—are a small group of indigenous languages spoken in Colombia and Panama. Choco consists of half a dozen known languages, all but two of them extinct: the Emberá languages (also known as Chocó proper, Cholo), Noanamá (also known as Waunana, Woun Meu), Anserma, Arma, Sinúfana (Cenufara), and Caramanta. Anserma, Arma, and Sinúfana are all extinct languages.

Ch'ol people—are an indigenous people of southeastern Mexico, mainly located in the northern Chiapas highlands in the state of Chiapas. They speak the indigenous language Ch'ol, a member of the Mayan language family. There are approximately 140,000 speakers of Ch'ol in Chiapas, including 40,000 who are monolingual.

Ch'ol language—an indigenous Mayan language spoken by the Ch'ol people of Chiapas. In Ch'ol, the word for their language is *Lak ty'añ* meaning "our speech." The Ch'ol language consists of three branches: Sabanilla, Tilá, and Tumbalá.

Ch'olan languages—a group of indigenous Mayan languages, also termed the Cholan–Tzeltalan languages, spoken in Mexico. This group is divided into two languages—Cholan and Tzeltalan. Cholan is broken into Western Cholan and Ch'olti'an; Tzeltalan is also broken into two sections—Tzendal (colonial Tzeltal), Tzotzil, and Wastekan.

Ch'olti' language—an extinct Mayan language which is a member of the Cholan–Tzeltalan language branch and was spoken by the Manche Ch'ol people of eastern Guatemala and southern Belize. Although extinct, Ch'olti' is of archeological significance in the investigation of Mayan hieroglyphs because it is believed that most of the glyphic texts are written in an ancient variety of Ch'olti' called Classic Ch'olti'an or Classic Maya by epigraphers.

Chontal Maya language—is an indigenous language belonging to the Cholan family of Mayan languages. It is spoken by approximately 37,000 Chontal Maya people of the state of Tabasco in southeastern Mexico. Chontal Maya is also referred to as *Yoko ochoco* and *Acalan.*

Chontal Maya people—are an indigenous people of the Mexican state of Tabasco. "Chontal" is derived from the Nahuatl word *chontalli*, which means "foreigner." The Chontal refers to themselves as the *Yokot'anob* or the Y*okot'an*, meaning "the speakers of Yoko ochoco." The Yokot'an inhabit 21 towns in a large area known as "la Chontalpa," extending across five municipalities of Tabasco. They consider themselves to be descendants of the Olmec people.

Chorotega people—the most powerful group of indigenous people in northwest Costa Rica at the time of the Spanish contact. Spread through Honduras, El Salvador, Nicaragua, and Costa Rica, the Chorotega people numbered approximately 10,000 in 1981. The indigenous language of Chorotega (Mangue) was an Oto-Manguean language which is extinct - Chorotega-speaking peoples included the Mangue and Monimbo; dialects included Chorotega proper, Diria, Nagrandan, Nicoya, Orisi, and Orotiña.

Ch'orti' language—a Mayan language spoken by the indigenous Ch'orti' people. This language is a survival of the classic Choltian language, which is the language of the inscriptions in the Late Classic Maya era site of Copán. Approximately 51,000 persons speak Ch'orti', mostly in Guatemala, with much fewer numbers in Honduras and El Salvador. Ch'orti' is the modern version of the ancient Mayan language Ch'olan, which was actively used between the years of 250 and 850 CE.

Ch'orti' people—an indigenous group of people of Mayan origin living in small communities and towns in southeastern Guatemala, northwestern El Salvador, and southwestern Honduras. There are approximately 51,000 speakers of their indigenous language, Ch'orti'. Because the Ch'orti' people belong to the Meridional Mayan group, they are closely related to the Mayans in Yucatán, Belize, and northern Guatemala.

Chuj language—an indigenous Mayan language spoken by approximately 40,000 people belonging to the Chuj ethnic group in Guatemala and approximately 10,000 Chuj people in Mexico. It belongs to the Q'anjob'alan branch of the Mayan languages, together with the languages of Tojolab'al, Q'anjob'al, Akateko, Popti', and Mocho'. These languages, together with the Ch'olan branch, form the Western branch of the Mayan family of languages. The Chujean branch is believed to have emerged approximately 2000 years ago. Chuj has been heavily influenced by the Spanish language, and Chuj speakers tend to borrow words from Spanish, termed code-mix.

Chuj people—an indigenous Maya people numbering approximately 68,000 persons residing in Guatemala and Mexico. The large majority of Chuj people live in Guatemala, mostly in the department of Huehuetenango and in the municipalities of San Mateo Ixtatán and San Sebastián Coatán.

The Chuj people and their ancestors are believed to have lived in this area for over 4000 years and, following their first contact with the Spanish conquestidores in the 1530s, were not subdued by the colonial administration until the 1680s.

Coatecas Altas Zapotec language—is a Zapotec language spoken by approximately 5000 individuals in southern Oaxaca, Mexico, around the town of Coatecas Altas in the Ejutla District, south of Oaxaca City. It is 83% intelligible with Ozolotepec Zapotec and similar to Miahuatlán Zapotec. Some communities of Coatecas Altas speakers can also be found in Soconusco, Chiapas, San Bernardino, Oaxaca, and in the areas surrounding San Quintín, Baja California.

Cochimí people—were the original inhabitants of the central part of the Baja California peninsula in Mexico, from El Rosario in the north to San Javier in the south.

Cocopah language—is a member of the indigenous Delta–California branch of the Yuman language family spoken by the Cocopah people. The language was endangered as it was spoken by fewer than 400 people at the turn of the twenty-first century; however, Cocopah language lessons are currently being offered in an effort to maintain its use.

Cocopah people—an indigenous group of approximately 1000 persons residing in Baja California and Sonora, Mexico, and in Arizona in the United States. The Cocopah language belongs to the Delta–California branch of the Yuman family. The Spanish term for Cocopah is *Cucapá*. Their self-designation is *Xawiɬ kwñchawaay*, which can be translated as "Those Who Live on the River."

Cora language—the indigenous language of the Cora people of Jalisco, in West Central Mexico. It is a member of the Corachol languages branch of the Uto-Aztecan language family.

Cora people—an indigenous ethnic group residing in Western Central Mexico and numbering approximately 24,000 people. They live in the municipality El Nayar in the Mexican state of Nayarit and in a few settlements in the neighboring state of Jalisco. They call themselves *náayerite* (plural; *náayeri* singular), from which the name of the present-day Mexican state of Nayarit is derived.

Comadrona—midwife (Spanish).

Comarca—term used in some countries to represent a local traditional region, municipality, or administrative district. It is used in Panama, Nicaragua, and Brazil in the Western Hemisphere and in Portugal and Spain in Europe.

Complex societies—refers to large and populous societies with social stratification and central governments.

Cosmovision—a collection of presumptions and assumptions (i.e., myths, religion, ideas, symbols) that a group sustains, practices, and maintains on the world and how it was, is, and will be—how a cultural group sees, explains, and interprets the world around them.

Creole language—a term referring to any one of many stable natural languages developed from a mixture of different languages.

Creole peoples—a poorly defined term referring a group of widely divergent peoples in different countries and through differing times that are descended from a mixture of colonial settlers of Caucasian European origin with non-European peoples including indigenous peoples, people of African origin, slaves, and others.

Cuicatec language—is an indigenous Oto-Manguean language of Mexico, spoken by the Cuicatec people of Oaxaca. It belongs to the Mixtecan branch together with the Mixtec languages and the Trique language. There are two major dialects of Cuicatec. Similar to other Oto-Manguean languages, Cuicatec is tonal.

Cuicatec people—an indigenous people residing in the Mexican state of Oaxaca, who closely related to the Mixtecs. They inhabit two towns—Teutila and Tepeuxila—in western Oaxaca and number approximately 23,000 individuals, of whom an estimated 65% are speakers of their indigenous language. The name Cuicatec is a Nahuatl exonym, from [ˈk^w*ika*] "song" [ˈ*teka*] "inhabitant of place of".

Cultural assimilation—a process by which a person or a group's language and/or culture come to resemble those of another group. The process of cultural assimilation can be rapid or gradual, forcible, or spontaneous. Full or complete assimilation occurs when new members of a society become indistinguishable from those members of the other group.

Cultural hegemony—a Marxist philosophy in which a culturally diverse society is dominated by the ruling class who manipulate the culture of that society. In this philosophy, the worldview imposed by the ruling class becomes the accepted cultural norm and the dominant ideology.

Cuarentena—literally quarantine, is a tradition among many indigenous and mestizo peoples of Mexico and other Latin American countries of 40 days of rest for a mother following the delivery of her infant.

Cultural capital—refers to those social assets of a person, including education, intellect, style of speech and dress, etc., that promote social mobility in a stratified society.

Curanderismo—literally translated as "healing" from the Spanish word curar, it consists of a set of traditional beliefs, rituals, and practices that address the physical, spiritual, psychological, and social needs of the people who use it. The Spanish verb curar means to heal. Therefore, curanderismo is translated as a system of healing. In Mexico, it is also known as Mexican traditional medicine, "medicina del campo," and traditional folk medicine.

Curandero—a traditional native healer, shaman or witch doctor. The curandero is found in indigenous peoples and other societies throughout parts of Latin America. The curandero practices administration of remedies for mental, emotional, physical, and spiritual illnesses based on their evaluation. In addition to healing of physical ailments; they can also have the role of a psychiatrist or mental health worker. The powers of the curandero are believed to be supernatural, as it is commonly believed that many illnesses are caused by lost malevolent spirits, a curse, or a lesson from God. The curandero often employs Catholic elements, such as holy water and pictures of saints. The use of Roman Catholic prayers and other elements of the church is often utilized together with native religious elements.

Daughter languages—refers to those languages that descend from the same parent language and that have been changing separately for hundreds or thousands of years.

Dead language—occurs when a language is no longer in current use as the native language of any community. A dead language may still be in use and have speakers—a well-known example of a dead language is Latin.

Descriptive linguistics—the scientific study of a spoken language.

Dialect—a term which refers to a variety of a language that is a characteristic of a particular group of the language's speakers. Typically, dialects of the same language are mutually intelligible.

Dialect continuum—refers to the process of the diffusion of language varieties which are spoken across some geographical area such that each differs only slightly from its neighbors, but the differences accumulate over distance so that widely separated varieties are not mutually intelligible. It is also termed a dialect chain.

Diaspora—a term which refers to the occurrence of a scattered population whose origin lies within a smaller geographic locale. Diaspora can also refer to the movement of the population from its original homeland. Labor migrations, as occur with indigenous peoples of Mexico and Central America, can form a diaspora.

Diglossia—refers to the situation in which two languages (or two varieties of the same language) are used under different conditions within a community, typically by the same speakers.

Dorasque language—is an extinct indigenous Chibchan language of Panama. It had the dialects Chumulu, Changuena (Changuina), and Gualaca.

Dzadzac—also *x-dzadzac*, referred to Maya male or female herbalists. Often the h-mens' wife was a *dazdzac*, also known as a medicine man or woman. Unlike the h-men, the *dzadzac* could not perform religious ceremonies or act as an intermediary between humans and gods.

Ehecatl—the Nahua term for the most common of disease-causing spirits, which can enter a person's body and bring disease, misfortune, and death.

Ejective consonants—a characteristic form of speech of all Mayan languages, also termed glottalized consonants. They are usually voiceless consonants that are pronounced with a glottalic egressive airstream and contrast with aspirated, tenuis, and voiced consonants. In the Mayan languages, ejective consonants are written using an apostrophe after the letter (e.g., /p'/, /t'/, /k'/) to distinguish them from plain consonants (/p/, /t/, /k/).

El Alto Zapotec language—also known as Zapoteco de San Pedro el Alto and South Central Zimatlan Zapotec, is a Zapotec language of Oaxaca, Mexico, spoken by approximately 900 persons in the towns of San Pedro el Alto, San Antonino el Alto, and San Andrés el Alto. It has 20% intelligibility with the most similar variety of Zapotec, Totomachapan Zapotec.

Elotepec Zapotec language—also termed Zapoteco de San Juan Elotepec, is a small Zapotec language spoken by approximately 200 persons in the single village in western in the Municipio of Villa Sola de Vega. It is one of several Zapotec languages called Papabuco and has 68% intelligibility of Zaniza Zapotec.

Emberá languages—also termed *ẽberá bedéa*, are a group of mutually intelligible indigenous languages spoken by the Emberá people throughout Panama and Colombia. Along with Wounmeu, they are the only extant members of the Chocó language family and not known to be related to any other language family of Central or South America.

Emberá people—also known as the Chocó or Katío Indians, are an indigenous people of Panama and Colombia. There are approximately 33,000 Emberá people living in Panama and 50,000 in Colombia.

Embera–Wounaan people—an indigenous group of seminomadic people living in Darién Province in Panama, on the shores of the Chucunaque, Sambú, and Tuira rivers and water ways. The Embera–Wounaan people consist of approximately 9000–10,000 Embera and 6000 Wounaan, and were formerly and widely known by the name Chocó. They speak the indigenous Embera and Wounaan languages, part of the Chocó language family.

Endangered language—connotes a language that is at risk of falling out of use, generally because its speakers have shifted to using another language or are themselves undergoing reduction in living members. It generally refers to indigenous languages. If there are no remaining speakers of the language, it becomes an extinct language.

Ethnic group—a term used in the social sciences to refer to a group of people who identify with each other based on such shared similarities as common ancestral, language, social, cultural, or national experiences. Membership in an ethnic group tends to be defined by a shared cultural heritage, ancestry, origin myth, history, homeland, language or dialect, symbolic systems such as religion and spiritual beliefs, physical appearance, mythology, ritual, cuisine, customs of clothing, self-adornment, and art.

Ethnocentric—used to denote the evaluation of other peoples and cultures according to the standards of one's own culture.

Ethnolect—a term used in linguistics which refers to a variety of a language associated with a specific ethnic or cultural subgroup.

Extinct language—a language with no remaining living speakers.

Femifocal—a term used to represent types of women-led kinship structures and household patterns that move beyond the strict relationship of a mother to her child.

Finca—Spanish term for a ranch, plantation, or country estate.

Focal vocabulary—a specialized set of terms and distinctions that is particularly important to a certain group: those with a particular focus of experience or activity.

Garifuna people—mixed-race descendants of Central African, West African, Arawak, and Island Carib people. They are referred to as *Garinagu* in the Garifuna language. They have resided in Central

America since the early 1700s, mostly along the coast of Honduras but also in Belize, Nicaragua, and Guatemala.

Garifuna language—spoken by the Garifuna people, it is an offshoot of the Island Carib language. It is an Arawakan language with influences from French, English, and Spanish, containing a large number of loan words. The language is of linguistic interest because parts of the Garifuna vocabulary are divided between men's speech and women's speech. In addition, some concepts have two words to express them, one for women and one for men. Those terms which are used by men are generally loanwords from Carib, while those used by women are of Arawak derivation.

Greater Mamean language family—a branch of the Eastern Mayan languages group. It includes the Mam, Tektiteko, Ixil, and Awakatek languages.

Guarijío people—an indigenous people of Mexico concentrated in 17 villages near the West Sierra Madre Mountains in Chihuahua and the Sonoran border. They are mostly monolingual and speak their indigenous language, Huarijio (Guarijío).

Guatemalan Civil War—a war waged during the years 1960–1996 between the government of Guatemala and the rural poor of Guatemala, including various leftist rebel groups and supported chiefly by ethnic Maya indigenous people and Ladino peasants. The government of Guatemala at that time has been widely condemned for committing genocide against the indigenous, primarily Maya, population of Guatemala during the civil war and for widespread human rights violations against civilians. Although the exact numbers will never be known, it has been estimated that between 140,000 and 200,000 Guatemalans perished or were missing during the war, mostly indigenous people.

Guatuso people—also known as the Maleku people, are an indigenous people of located in the Guatuso Indigenous Reserve near the town of Guatuso (San Rafael de Guatuso). Around 600 people live on the reserve, making this the smallest ethnic group in Costa Rica. They speak an indigenous language, Maleku, which is a Chibchan language.

Guevea Zapotec language—also termed Guevea de Humboldt Zapotec (Northern Isthmus Zapotec), is an indigenous Zapotecan language spoken by approximately 4700 individuals in the isthmus of Mexico.

Güilá Zapotec language—also referred to as Zapoteco de San Pablo Güilá and Zapoteco de San Dionisio Ocotepec, is an indigenous Zapotec language of Oaxaca, Mexico. It is spoken by approximately 9500 persons in the town of San Pablo Güilá, Tlacolula District, Oaxaca, Mexico. A closely related but not identical form of Zapotec is spoken in the adjacent town of San Dionisio Ocotepec in Oaxaca.

Hechicero—Spanish term for shaman.

Hegemony—see cultural hegemony.

Historical linguistics—refers to the longer-term change of contemporary variation in speech.

H-man—refers a traditional male Maya priest who diagnosed illnesses and also performed healing ceremonies, a shaman-priest. He led religious rituals, made offerings to the gods, and said prayers. In order to perform his healing, he used a looking glass, called the *zaz-tum*; rattlesnake fangs; porcupine quills; henequen thorns and other vegetables; obsidian leaves (volcanic rock) or glass, with which they bled the patients; and some gourds called *homa*, which were used during the ceremonies to hold the sacred wine, termed *balche*.

Huarijio language—also termed Guarijío, Varihío, Warihío, and, in Spanish, Huarijío, is an indigenous Uto-Aztecan language which is spoken in the states of Chihuahua and Sonora in northwestern Mexico by approximately 5000 Huarijio people, most of whom are monolingual. The Huarijio (Guarijío) language has two variants, known as Mountain Guarijío (Guarijío de la sierra) and River Guarijío (Guarijío del río).

Huastecan languages—a family of indigenous Mayan languages of Mexico. Including the Wastek (Huastec) and Chikomuseltek (Chicomuceltec) languages, they are believed to be the most divergent branch of the Mayan language family.

Huastec language—also termed Wasteko language, an indigenous Mayan language of Mexico spoken by the Huastec people. It is estimated that there are approximately 200,000 current speakers of the Huastec language. The language and its speakers are also called Teenek. It is a member of the Huastecan language family of the Mayan languages, which includes the now extinct Chikomuseltek language.

Huastec people—contraction of *Te' Inik*, "people from here"; also known as Huaxtec and Wastek people, are an indigenous group living in Mexico, and concentrated in the La Huasteca region. This includes the states of Hidalgo, Veracruz, San Luis Potosí, and Tamaulipas concentrated along the route of the Pánuco River and along the coast of the Gulf of Mexico. Based upon archeological evidence, the Huastec civilization is one of the ancient pre-Columbian Mesoamerican cultures, believed to date back to approximately the tenth century BCE, although their most productive period of civilization is usually considered to be the Postclassic era between the fall of Teotihuacan and the rise of the Aztec Empire.

Huave language—an indigenous language spoken by the indigenous Huave people in four villages on the Pacific Coast of the Isthmus of Tehuantepec, in the southeast part of the Mexican state of Oaxaca. It is spoken by approximately 18,000 people. Genetic relationships between the Huave language and several language families have been proposed, but none has been substantiated, and as a result Huave continues to be considered a language isolate.

Huave people—an indigenous people of Mexico, also referred to as the Huavi or Wabi. The term used by the Huave to refer to themselves is *Ikoots* or *Kunajts* (the first-person inclusive pronoun, thus meaning "us") or *Mareños* (meaning "sea people" in Spanish). They preceded the Zapotec people in settling in the Isthmus of Tehuantepec more than 3000 years ago. The approximately 30,000 Huave people speak four languages, some of which are mutually intelligible.

Huesero—in the Mexican curanderismo, they are bone/muscle therapists who emphasize physical ailments. See also Bonesetter.

Huichol people—an indigenous ethnic group in Mexico. They reside in the Sierra Madre Occidental range in the Mexican states of Nayarit, Jalisco, Zacatecas, and Durango. Although they are best known to the world as the Huichol, they refer to themselves as the Wixáritari ("the people") in the indigenous Huichol language.

Huichol language—an indigenous language of the Uto-Aztecan language family spoke by the Huichol people of Mexico. Together with the indigenous Cora language (whose territories are contiguous), it constitutes the Coracholan language subgroup of the Uto-Aztecan languages. The Huichol language is currently considered a "vulnerable" language by UNESCO. The majority of the Huichol people retain their traditional pre-Columbian belief systems and are resistant to changes—this includes four principal deities: the trinity of Corn, Blue Deer, Peyote, and the Eagle, all descended from their Sun God, "*Tao Jreeku*." Similar to other indigenous peoples, they have traditionally used the peyote (*hikuri*) cactus in religious rituals. These rituals involve singing, weeping, and contact with ancestor spirits. They interact with the primal ancestor spirits of fire, deer, and other elements of the natural world.

Huipil—also huipal, the most common traditional garment worn by indigenous women in Mexico and Central America. The word is derived from the Nahuatl word *huīpīlli*.

INALI—refers to the Instituto Nacional de Lenguas Indígenas (*National Indigenous Languages Institute*), a governmental agency in Mexico attached to the Secretariat of Public Education. INALI promotes and protects the use of Mexico's indigenous languages, which it divides into 68 living "linguistic groups" and hundreds of "linguistic varieties."

Indian—a historical and traditional term to refer to the indigenous peoples of the Americas, most commonly of the United States

Indigenous people—in the setting of Mexico and Central America, pre-Columbian people and their descendants. They are often referred to as *pueblos indígenas* or *indígenas* in Spanish-speaking countries and as *povos indígenas* in Portuguese. Other terms for the indigenous peoples of the Americas include *amerindio* (in Spanish) and *ameríndio* (in Portuguese).

Isihuayo—an ethnomedical category of illness and is the Nahua term for a fallen or displaced uterus. Organ displacements are common conditions among some indigenous peoples of Latin America, which are caused by a general imbalance on the body.

Isthmus Zapotec language—also known as Juchitán Zapotec and termed *diidxazá* by its speakers and Zapoteco del Istmo in Spanish, is a Zapotecan language spoken by approximately 85,000 persons in Tehuantepec and Juchitán de Zaragoza, in the Mexican state of Oaxaca.

Itza' language—one of the four branches of the Yucatecan Mayan language family, originally spoken in the Petén region of Guatemala. The government of Guatemala banned the use of the Itza' language in the 1930s, after which two generations of the Itza' Mayan people spoke only Spanish. Currently, the language is almost extinct and is spoken by only a few elderly persons in communities to the north of Lake Petén Itzá in northern Guatemala, such as San José.

Itza people—an ethnic Mayan group of people numbering approximately 2000 individuals who retain some elements of their indigenous culture. They reside in the Petén department of Guatemala, in and around the city of Flores on the Lake Petén Itzá. In archeology, the Itza were descended from the *Ah Itzá* Yucatecan Maya people and were an important Mesoamerican group who dominated the Yucatán peninsula in the Postclassic Maya period.

Ix Chel—also Ixchel, Mayan: [iʃˈt͡ʃel], the ancient Mayan jaguar goddess of midwifery and medicine. She is the approximate Mayan equivalent to *Toci Yoalticitl*, an Aztec earth goddess inhabiting the sweatbath.

Ixcatec language—or Xwja, is an indigenous language spoken by approximately 190 people of the Mexican village of Santa María Ixcatlan, in the northern part of the state of Oaxaca. The Ixcatec language belongs to the Popolocan branch of the Oto-Manguean language family.

Ixcatec people—a small group of indigenous people residing in the northern part of the Mexican state of Oaxaca. They have an indigenous language, Ixcatec. There were approximtely 10,0 00 Ixatec people in pre-contact times; now there are only 200 surviving. Their culture and language are similar to their neighbors, the Chocho.

Ixil language—a Mayan language spoken by the Ixil people of Guatemala and belonging to the Greater Mamean group of Mayan languages. It is believed to have originated in approximately 500 CE.

Ixil people—an indigenous Maya people residing in Guatemala. Numbering approximately 95,000 persons, thousands of Ixil were systematically killed during a genocide operation in the 1980s during the Guatemalan Civil War. They live in three municipalities in the Cuchumatanes mountains, located in the northern region of the Quiché Department. The majority speak their indigenous Ixil language.

Ixil triangle—also termed the Ixil Community, refers to an area bounded by three neighboring towns in the Quiché Department in the western highlands of Guatemala – Santa Maria Nebaj, San Juan Cotzal, and San Gaspar Chajul – which form a triangle on a map. The population is mostly of indigenous origin and speaks the Ixil language. The Ixil Community has remained mostly isolated from the rest of the world because of its location in the Cuchumatanes mountains, and the inhabitants have maintained their traditional culture, unaffected by influences of the outside world. During the Guatemalan Civil War, villagers of the Ixil Community were caught in the cross fire, and thousands of civilians were killed, tortured, or vanished.

Ixtlán Zapotec language—is an indigenous Zapotec dialect cluster of Oaxaca, Mexico.

Jakaltek language—also referred to as *Popti',* is an indigenous Mayan language of Guatemala spoken by approximately 9000 people in the department of Huehuetenango and approximately 500 people in the adjacent part of Chiapas in southern Mexico.

Jakaltek people—an indigenous Mayan group of people who have resided in the foothills of the Cuchumatán Mountains in the department of Huehuetenango in northwestern Guatemala since pre-conquest times. Most live in the area of the town of Jacaltenango, referred to in their language as *Xajlaj*, or "place of the big white rock slabs." The Jakaltek people are relatively isolated, preserving many traditional customs which have been lost among other ethnic groups—they still use the blow-gun for hunting birds and small animals, for example.

Jicaquean languages—also termed Tolan, is a small indigenous language family in Honduras. There are two Jicaquean languages, Tol (Eastern Jicaque) and the now extinct Western Jicaque. These two languages were mutually intelligible.

Kaqchikel language—the indigenous language of the Kaqchikel people of the highlands of Guatemala which is spoken by approximately 400,000 persons. It is a member of the Quichean–Mamean branch of the Mayan languages family and is closely related to the K'iche'(Quiché) and Tz'utujil languages.

Kaqchikel people—also called Kachiquel, Cakchiquel, Cakchiquel, Kakchiquel, Caqchikel, and Cachiquel, are an indigenous group of Mayan people residing in the midwestern highlands of Guatemala. Numbering over 800,000 individuals, they speak their indigenous language, Kaqchikel. Their history can be traced to the Postclassic Maya period, when their capital was Iximché. Iximché was conquered by the Spanish conquistador Pedro de Alvarado in 1524.

Kejache people—also termed Kehache, Quejache, Kehach, Kejach, or Cehache, are an extinct group of Mayan people who inhabited the southern Yucatán Peninsula at the time of Spanish contact in the seventeenth century.

K'iche' language—or Quiché, is the language of the K'iche' people, termed by its speakers in Guatemala *Qatzijob'al* or "our language." Approximately 7% of the population of Guatemala, numbering greater than one million persons, speak K'iche'. The majority of K'iche' speakers have at least a working knowledge of Spanish.

K'iche' people—are an indigenous group of Maya people. The K'iche' people living in the highlands during pre-Columbian times were associated with the Maya civilization. The Nahuatl translation of Quiché, *Cuauhtēmallān*, means "place of the many trees (people)" and is the origin of the word Guatemala. The large majority of K'iche' people live in the highlands of Guatemala and account for 11% of the country's population or approximately 1,610,013 persons. Several regions of Guatemala are predominantly composed of K'iche' people, including the Quiché Department, which is 65.1% K'iche' and has a total K'iche' population of 622,163; Totonicapán, which is 95.9% K'iche' and has a total K'iche' population of 453,237; Quetzaltenango, which is 25.9% K'iche' and has a total K'iche' population of 205,228; and Sololá, which is 35.3% K'iche' and has a total K'iche' population of 151,992. The majority of K'iche' people speak their indigenous language, also termed K'iche'.

Kiliwa language—the indigenous language spoken by the Kiliwa people of Baja California, Mexico. It is a member of the Yuman language group and is spoken by approximately 50 persons.

Kiliwa people—are indigenous people of northern Baja California, Mexico. They occupied a territory lying between the Cochimí to the south and the Paipai to the north and extending from San Felipe on the Gulf of California to San Quintín on the Pacific coast. Their indigenous language is the Kiliwa language, in which they call themselves the *K'olew*.

Kumeyaay people—also known as Tipai-Ipai, formerly Kamia or Diegueño, are Native American indigenous people of the extreme southwestern United States extending into northwest Mexico. They number approximately several thousands of people, residing in the states of California in the United States and Baja California in Mexico.

Kuna people—also referred to as the Guna and Cuna, are an indigenous group of approximately 50,000 people residing in Panama and Colombia. In the Kuna language, they refer to themselves as *Dule* or *Tule*, meaning "people," and the name of the language in Kuna is *Dulegaya*, literally "people-mouth."

Lacandon language—an indigenous Yucatecan Mayan language spoken by all (less than 1000) Lacandon people of Chiapas. They refer to their language as *Jach t'aan* or *Hach t'an.*

Lacandon people—an indigenous Mayan people of Mexico living in the jungles of the state of Chiapas. They are one of the most isolated and culturally conservative of the indigenous people of Mexico and by 1943 were almost extinct. Currently their population has increased yet remains small, with approximately 650 speakers of the Lacandon language.

Lachiguiri Zapotec language—also termed Northwestern Tehuantepec Zapotec and Zapoteco de Santiago Lachiguiri, is a Zapotecan language spoken by approximately 5000 persons in the isthmus of Mexico in Oaxaca.

Lachixío Zapotec language—is a Zapotec language of Oaxaca, Mexico. It is spoken by approximately 3000 persons in the Sola de Vega District in the towns of Santa María Lachixío and San Vicente Lachixío. Lachixío is part of the West Zapotec language branch, which is considered the earliest divergent branch of the Zapotec family and adjacent to the Chatino language family. Although many other Zapotec languages have undergone significant language shifts to Spanish, most children in these towns are raised with Zapotec and learn Spanish at an early age.

Lakandon Ch'ol people—are an extinct people who were Ch'ol-speaking Maya people inhabiting the Lacandon Jungle in what is now lowland Chiapas in Mexico and the bordering regions of northwestern Guatemala, along the tributaries of the upper Usumacinta River and the foothills of the Sierra de los Cuchumatanes.

Ladino people—people with mixed ancestry referring principally to inhabitants of Mexico and Central America. It has several meanings, including persons of a mixed mestizo or hispanicized ancestry, but in some areas also includes persons with a mixed mestizo and indigenous background. In Guatemala, it can also refer to westernized Amerindians. It is also used to refer to the mestizo class or to indigenous people who have obtained upward social mobility or have Western lifestyles and manner of dress.

Language attrition—refers to the process of losing a native, or first, language. It is generally the result of isolation from speakers of the first language and the acquisition and use of a second language, which interferes with the correct production and comprehension of the first.

Language death—a term used in linguistics, also referred to as language extinction, linguistic extinction or linguicide, and rarely also glottophagy, which refers a situation of a language losing its last native speaker. See also extinct language.

Language revitalization—is also referred to as language revival or reversing language shift. It is an attempt to halt or reverse the decline of a language or to revive an extinct language.

Language shift—also referred to as language transfer, language replacement, and language assimilation, is a process in which a speech community of a language shifts to speaking another language. A language shift has occurred among the majority of the indigenous peoples of Mexico and Central America, typically to the Spanish language.

Lapaguía Zapotec language—also referred to as Lapaguía-Guivini Zapotec, is a Zapotec language spoken by approximately 4200 individuals in southern Oaxaca, Mexico.

Lenca languages—a small extinct family of indigenous languages from El Salvador and Honduras. There were two identified Lenca languages. Salvadoran Lenca was spoken in Chilanga and Potó. Lencans had arrived in El Salvador about 2000 years ago, founding the site of Quelepa—there is reportedly only one speaker remaining. Honduran Lenca was spoken with minor dialect differences in Intibuca, Opatoro, Guajiquiro, Similatón (modern Cabañas), and Santa Elena.

Lenca people—an indigenous group residing in southwestern Honduras and eastern El Salvador. The Lenca people previously spoke their indigenous language, Lenca, which is now extinct. The Lenca are the largest indigenous group in Honduras, numbering approximately 100,000. El Salvador's Lenca population is estimated at about 37,000. Lenca culture developed for centuries preceding the Spanish conquest, and they had frequent contact with various Maya groups as well as other indigenous peoples of Mexico and Central America. It has been suggested that the Lenca migrated to the region from South America around 3000 years ago.

Lingua franca—refers to a language or dialect that is systematically (as opposed to occasionally or casually) used to make communication possible between people who do not share a native language or dialect, particularly when it is a third language that is distinct from both native languages.

Linguistic anthropology—a branch of anthropology that studies language in its social and cultural context, across space and over time.

Linguistic imperialism—also termed language imperialism, refers to a process in which there has been the transfer of a dominant language to other people. The transfer is for the most part a demonstration of power—traditionally, military power but also, in the modern world, economic power—and aspects of the dominant culture are usually transferred along with the language.

Linguistic productivity—refers to the use of rules of a language to produce entirely new expressions that are comprehensible to other native speakers.

Living language—refers to a language that has at least one living speaker for whom it is their first language.

Machismo—a term which refers to an expression of masculinity that celebrates displays of hypersexuality, physical strength, and aggressiveness, as well as violence, especially against women. It is prevalent in both indigenous and non-indigenous cultures in Mexico and Central America.

Macro-Chibchan language macrofamily—refers to a proposed grouping of the languages of the Lencan, Misumalpan, and Chibchan families into a single large phylum (macrofamily). Previously, the Lencan and Misumalpan languages had been included in the Chibchan language family proper but were excluded pending further evidence as that family became well established.

Macrofamily—also called a superfamily or phylum, is a term used in historical linguistics referring to a proposed genetic relationship grouping together language families (also isolates) in a larger-scale classification.

Mam language—is a widely spoken indigenous Mayan language with approximately one-half million speakers in the Guatemalan departments of Quetzaltenango, Huehuetenango, San Marcos, and Retalhuleu and 10,000 in the Mexican state of Chiapas. It is also spoken by immigrants in some areas of the United States, notably Washington, DC, and California. The Mam language is closely related to the Tektitek language. These two languages together form the Mamean subbranch, which together with the Ixilean languages, Awakatek and Ixil, form the Greater Mamean subbranch of the Mayan language tree. Together, Greater Mamean and the Greater Quichean languages (consisting of ten Mayan languages, including K'iche') form the Quichean–Mamean branch. There are three major dialects of the Mam language—Northern Mam, Southern Mam, and Western Mam. The Mam language has 10 vowels—5 short and 5 long—and 27 consonants.

Mam people—an indigenous Maya people numbering approximately 617,000 in Guatemala and 23,000 in Mexico. In the pre-Columbian period, the Mam were a part of the Maya civilization and had their capital Zaculeu. The modern city of Quetzaltenango or Xela was originally Mam. Today, the majority of Mam people reside in Guatemala, in the departments of Huehuetenango, San Marcos, and Quetzaltenango. The Mam people of Mexico live mostly in the Soconusco region of Chiapas.

Mangue language—also known as Chorotega, was an indigenous Oto-Manguean language spoken by the Mangue and Monimbo peoples in Honduras, Costa Rica, El Salvador and Nicaragua. The ethnic population numbered around 10,000 in 1981, but the language is now extinct. In Western Nicaragua the dialect was termed Mangue proper which was subdivided into Nagrandan and Dirian; the Choluteca dialect in the area of the Bay of Fonseca in Honduras; and Orotiña in the Nicoya Peninsula of Costa Rica.

Matagalpa language—was a Misumalpan language, closely related to the Cacaopera language, formerly spoken in the central highlands of Nicaragua. The language became extinct in the nineteenth century, and there only a few short wordlists that remain. The ethnic group, which numbers approximately 20,000 persons, now speaks Spanish.

Matlatzincan languages—are two closely related indigenous Oto-Manguean languages of the Oto-Pamean branch that are spoken in Central Mexico: Tlahuica/Ocuiltec and Matlatzinca. The name of the language in the language itself is *pjiekak'joo*. Because of the extremely small population and the unfavorable age structure, the Matlatzincan languages are considered to be highly endangered indigenous languages. In the year 2000, Matlatzinca was spoken by approximately 650 persons in San Francisco Oxtotilpa, and in 2011 Ocuiltec/Tlahuica was spoken by approximately 100 persons in the municipality of Ocuilan de Arteaga in the villages San Juan Atzingo and Santa Lucía del Progreso.

Matlatzinca people—is a name referring to various indigenous ethnic groups in the Toluca Valley in the state of Mexico, located in the central highlands of Mexico. The term is applied to the ethnic group inhabiting the valley of Toluca and to their language, Matlatzinca. Matlatzinco was the Aztec (Nahuatl) term for the Toluca Valley.

Matrilineal—an anthropological term referring to a society in which individuals trace their descent through the female line. From a societal perspective, it describes a culture in which each person is described by their matriline ("mother's line") and which can influence the inheritance of titles, names, rights, and property. See also patrilineal.

Matrilocal—a social system in anthropology whereby a married couple resides with or nearby the wife's parents. As a result, the female children of the wife remain living near or in the mother's house, forming large multi-generational clan–families living in the same location.

Maya people—an indigenous group of people found throughout Mesoamerica. They reside predominantly in Guatemala and Mexico and are also present in Belize and Honduras, with scattered groups in other areas. Approximately 30 Mayan languages are spoken by greater than five million people. They constitute the largest indigenous ethnic group in Mexico and Central America, with the greatest numbers of contemporary Maya residing in Guatemala, Belize, and the western portions of Honduras and El Salvador, as well as large segments of population within the Mexican states of Yucatán, Campeche, Quintana Roo, Tabasco, and Chiapas. The ancient Maya civilization is well-known, with archeological evidence for its protodevelopment extending to the Archaic period prior to 2000 BCE, which subsequently developed into the Preclassic Period (2000 BCE to 250 CE), and with the origins of cities by 750 BCE and hieroglyphic writing by the third century BCE. Currently it has been estimated that approximately seven million Maya people live throughout the region.

Mayan languages—the languages of the indigenous Maya people of Mexico and Northern Central America (Mesoamerica). Guatemala formally recognized 21 Mayan languages, and Mexico recognizes eight additional ones. The Mayan languages are spoken by an estimated six million persons living predominantly in Mexico, Belize, Guatemala, and Honduras. The contemporary Mayan languages are descended from the Proto-Mayan language (or, in K'iche' Maya, *Nab'ee Maya' Tzij* ("the old Maya Language"), believed to have been spoken up to 5000 years ago.

Mayangna people—an indigenous group of people living on the eastern coats of Nicaragua and Honduras, often termed the Mosquito Coast. Although they are also known as the Sumo people, this term is considered to be a derogatory term used to refer to them by the Miskito people. Historical evidence resulting from linguistic analysis of the Misumalpan language family, which includes not only the Mayangna languages but also the Miskitu as well as the extinct Matagalpan and Cacaopera languages once spoken in the Nicaraguan highlands and southern El Salvador, indicates the continuous presence of these groups in the region from around 2000 BCE. Presently, the Mayangna people are divided into the Panamahka, Tawahka, and Ulwa ethnolinguistic subgroups.

Mayangna languages—a group of indigenous languages spoken in Nicaragua and Honduras and part of the Misumalpan language family. They are divided into the northern Mayangna, composed of the Tawahka and Panamahka dialects, and southern Ulwa languages.

Mayo people—an indigenous group of approximately 40,000 people residing in the Mexican states of Southern Sonora, Northern Sinaloa, and small settlements in Durango. In their own language, they call themselves the Yoreme. The term *Mayo* means "the people of the river bank" and is derived from the Mayo River. They speak their indigenous language, Mayo.

Mazahua language—an indigenous language of Mexico spoken by approximately 116,000 persons. It belongs to the Oto-Pamean languages branch of the Oto-Manguean languages family, related to such indigenous languages as Otomi, Pame, Matlatzinca, and others. The number of speakers of Mazahua is decreasing. The Mazahua language is currently the sixth most commonly language spoken in Mexico City as a result of migration of the indigenous speakers.

Mazahua people—an indigenous people inhabiting the northwestern portion of the State of Mexico and small parts of Michoacán and Querétaro. The Mazahua people refer to themselves as *Tetjo ñaa jñatjo*, meaning "those who speak their own language." The word Mazahua probably comes from Nahuatl term for "deer-foot," which refers to those who track deer for hunting. They speak Mazahua, which is an indigenous Mesoamerican language.

Mazatec people—an indigenous group of people living predominantly in the Sierra Mazateca in the state of Oaxaca in southern Mexico and also in some communities in the adjacent states of Puebla and Veracruz. Mazatec means "people of the deer," which is derived from the Nahuatl word for deer, *mazatl*.

Mazatecan languages—a group of closely related indigenous languages spoken by approximately 200,000 people living in the define La Sierra Mazateca in the northern part of the Mexican state of Oaxaca, as well as in Puebla and Veracruz. There are eight languages belonging to this language group, some of which are mutually unintelligible to speakers of other Mazatecan languages. The Mazatecan languages are part of the Oto-Manguean language family and belong to that family's Eastern branch where they belong to the Popolocan subgroup together with the Popoloca, Ixcatec, and Chocho indigenous languages.

Medicocentric—a term used to describe viewing a person's well-being (or lack of it) by focusing on disease, including signs and symptoms, rather than by the patient's perception of the problem. Often referring to care provided by a physician, the medicocentric viewpoint utilizes a reductionist model, in which a diagnosis is made by reducing (or narrowing) the problem down to medically explained phenomena. It is also sometimes used in reference to the belief in the superiority of Western biomedical teachings and practices, including the role of the physician (doctor) over indigenous or traditional methods of healing.

Mesoamerica—is both a geographic region as well as a cultural area which extended from central Mexico to include Honduras, Guatemala, El Salvador, Belize, and northern Costa Rica. It is one of the six regions in the world which represent the "cradle of civilization" and where ancient civilization arose independently. It contained numerous indigenous cultures which developed their own languages and which shared a number of cultural traits and close cultural and historical connections.

Mesoamerican language (linguistic) area—an area of linguistic convergence (also termed a diffusion area, language crossroads, or *sprachbund*) consisting of the native or indigenous languages spoken in the cultural area of Mesoamerica (see also Mesoamerica). The existence of this *sprachbund* is based upon analysis by ethnolinguists of the similarities of syntactic, lexical, and phonological traits as well as a number of ethnolinguistic traits found in the indigenous languages of Mesoamerica. As a result, it is believed that their origins were the result of diffusion rather than inheritance, the standard criteria for defining a *sprachbund*.

Mexicanero people—an indigenous people of Mexico, residing predominantly in Durango and Nayarit. They speak the Mexicanero language, an indigenous Nahuatl dialect. As of 2011, there were approximately 1300 persons speaking the Mexicanero language. The Mexicanero people have incorporated various elements of Catholicism into their religion and have also retained their indigenous worship practices of the sun and moon, Venus, the eagle, and the deer. The Mexicanero people reside in three communities—Santa Cruz in Nayarit, and San Agustín de San Buenaventura, and San Pedro Jícoras in southern Durango.

Miahuatlán Zapotec language- also known as Cuixtla Zapotec, is a Zapotec language spoken by approximately 1000 individuals in southern Oaxaca, Mexico.

Miskito (Miskitu) people—an indigenous ethnic group made up of persons of Native American, African, and English descent. The majority of Miskito people reside in Honduras and Nicaragua.

Miskito language—an indigenous language spoken by the Miskito people of Nicaragua and Honduras. It is part of the Misumalpan group of languages, which also include Sumo and the now extinct Matagalpan languages. In addition to many elements borrowed from other Misumalpan languages, Miskito has a large number of loanwords from English through creole languages. There are believed to be approximately 200,000 speakers of the Miskito language.

Misumalpan languages—a small group of indigenous languages spoken in the eastern coast of Nicaragua. It was given the name "Misumalpan" by John Alden Mason (who was the author of this chapter's mentor), which is derived of syllables from the names of the family's three members Miskito, Sumu, and Matagalpan. The languages of the Matagalpan branch are now extinct; however, the Miskito and Sumu languages are still spoken. Miskito has nearly 200,000 speakers and remains a second language for speakers of other Indian languages on the Miskito Coast, and the majority of speakers of the Sumu language also speak Miskito.

Mitla Zapotec—referred to as *Didxsaj* by native speakers, is an Oto-Manguean language spoken by approximately 20,000 persons in the Mitla Valley of Oaxaca, Mexico. The related language Guelavia Zapotec is reported to be 75% intelligible, but the reverse is apparently not the case.

Mixe languages—indigenous languages belonging to the Mixean branch of the Mixe–Zoquean language family spoken in Oaxaca in southern Mexico.

Mixe people—an indigenous group residing in the eastern highlands of the Mexican state of Oaxaca and speaking the Mixe language. The Mixe name for themselves is *ayuujkjä'äy* meaning "people who speak the mountain language," and the term Mixe is probably derived from the Nahuatl word for cloud, *mīxtli*. There is linguistic evidence that connects the Mixe with the Olmecs, but the Mixe people themselves do not associate themselves with the Olmec. According to Mixe legend, their forefathers arrived in Mexico by boat from the South American Andes and settled at the holy mountain Cempoaltepetl, where they were led by the legendary king Condoy and built a successful kingdom.

Mixe–Zoque languages—an indigenous language family spoken in the region of the Isthmus of Tehuantepec, Mexico. The Mexican government officially recognizes that there are three distinct Mixe–Zoquean languages: Mixe or *ayook* with 188,000 speakers, Zoque or *o'de püt* with 88,000 speakers, and the Popoluca languages of which some are Mixean and some Zoquean with 69,000 speakers.

Mixed language—refers to a language that develops through fusion of two or more source languages, normally in situations of thorough bilingualism. Typically, it is not possible to classify the resulting language as belonging to either of the language families that were its sources.

Mixtec languages—are a group of indigenous Mexican languages spoken by greater than one-half million people. The Mixtec languages are members of the Otomanguean language family of Mexico and are closely related to the Trique and Cuicatec languages. The name "*Mixteco*" is a Nahuatl exonym, from [miʃ] "cloud" [teka] "inhabitant of place of." The historical distribution of the Mixtec languages is the region known as La Mixteca, which is shared by the states of Oaxaca, Puebla, and Guerrero. However, the languages have now expanded into many urban areas.

Mixtec people—an indigenous people of Mexico inhabiting the region known as La Mixteca of Oaxaca and Puebla as well as the state of Guerrero's Región Montañas and Región Costa Chica, which includes parts of the Mexican states of Oaxaca, Guerrero, and Puebla. In the pre-Columbian period, a number of Mixtecan city states competed with each other and with the Zapotec kingdoms. The major Mixtec polity was Tututepec which rose to prominence in the eleventh century under the leadership of Eight Deer Jaguar Claw, the only Mixtec king who ever united the highland and lowland polities into a single state. The Mixtec region and the Mixtec peoples consist of approximately 830,000 people and have traditionally been divided into three groups, two based on their original economic caste and one based on the region they settled. High Mixtecs or "mixteco alto" were of the upper class and generally wealthier; the Low Mixtecs or "mixteco bajo" were generally poorer. The third group is the Coastal Mixtecs, termed "mixteco de la costa," whose language is closely related to that of the Low Mixtecs. They currently reside on the Pacific slope of Oaxaca and Guerrero. The Mixtec languages form a major branch of the Otomanguean language family. The term Mixtec (*Mixteco* in Spanish) comes from the Nahuatl word *mixtecah* [miʃˈtekaʔ], meaning "cloud people."

Mixtepec Zapotec language—also termed San Juan Mixtepec Zapotec and Eastern Miahuatlán Zapotec, is an Oto-Manguean language spoken by approximately 7000 individuals in Oaxaca, Mexico. It has 80% intelligibility with Lapaguía Zapotec but with only 45% intelligibility in the other direction.

Mocho' language—also termed Mototzintleco, is an indigenous and is a Mayan language which is a survival of the western branch of Mayan languages spoken in the Mexican state of Chiapas. Mocho' speakers refer to this language as *qatô:k* (also spelled "Cotoque" in some older literature), which means "our language." As there are fewer than 30 current speakers known, it is now considered a moribund language.

Modern language—a term which refers to any human language that is currently in use.

Mopan language—an indigenous language belonging to the Yucatecan branch of the Mayan languages and spoken by the Mopan people who live in the Petén Department of Guatemala and in the Maya Mountains region of Belize. Mopan is spoken in towns which include San Luis, Poptún, Melchor de Mencos, and Dolores in Guatemala, and also in San Antonio in the Toledo District of Belize.

Mopan people—one of the Maya peoples in Belize and Guatemala. Their indigenous language is also called Mopan and belongs to the Yucatec Mayan languages. There are approximately 10,500 Mopan people in Belize and 2800 in Guatemala.

Motozintlecos people—also referred to as the Mochós, are an indigenous Mexican people residing in Chiapas. They speak the Mocho' language, part of the western branch of Mayan languages. There are believed to be only about 100 speakers; the Mocho' language is in danger of extinction.

Movconspicuous people—also called Movere, Western Guaymi, or Ngäbere, are a Chibchan (Dorasque–Guaymi) speaking people in Panama (150,000) and Costa Rica (4300).

Mulatto—a largely outdated and controversial term which used to refer to persons born of one white parent and one black parent or to persons born of a mulatto parent or parents. In modern English, the term is generally confined to historical contexts.

Nahua people—an indigenous group residing primarily in central Mexico, with some living in El Salvador. Their language, Nahuatl, was historically referred to as Aztec. There are approximately 1.5 million speakers of Nahuatl, which is in the Uto-Aztecan language family. The name Nahua is derived from the Nahuatl root word *nāhua*, meaning "audible, intelligible, clear" with several differing derivations. They have also been referred to as Mēxihcatl [meːˈʃiʔkat͡ɬ] (singular), Mēxihcah [meːˈʃiʔkaʔ] (plural), or in Spanish Mexicano(s) "Mexicans," after the Mexica, the Nahua tribe which founded and predominated in the Aztec Empire.

Nahuan languages—also termed the Aztecan languages, they are the languages in the Uto-Aztecan language family. These languages have undergone a sound change, referred to as Whorf's law. Whorf's law is a sound law in Uto-Aztecan linguistics proposed by the linguist Benjamin Lee Whorf, in which he explained the origin in the Nahuan languages of the phoneme /tɬ/ which is not found in any of the other languages of the Uto-Aztecan family. As of 2008, the government of Mexico recognizes 30 distinct varieties that are spoken as distinct indigenous languages. The differences between these varieties can be profound, resulting in some cases little or even no intelligibility between speakers of differing Nahuan languages.

Nahuatl—the indigenous language of the modern Nahua people and formerly the Aztec civilization. It is a member of the Uto-Aztecan language group and is spoken by approximately 1.5 million persons in Mexico. Classical Nahuatl was the language of the Aztec Empire, where it was used as a lingua franca in much of Mesoamerica from the seventh century CE until the Spanish conquest in the sixteenth century. It was originally written in a pictographic script. The modern dialects of Nahuatl spoken in the Valley of Mexico most resemble Classical Nahuatl.

Necaxantle—also termed "the weakening disease," is a term used by the Nahua of Mexico to represent a disease of reproductive health in which a postpartum woman develops a wasting syndrome. It is generally considered to result from insufficient rest after giving birth. It is similar to a condition among indigenous Andean people termed *sobreparto*.

Ngäbe people—formerly termed the Guaymi people, are an indigenous group residing in Panama and Costa Rica. Guaymí is an outdated name which was derived from the Buglere term for them (*guaymiri*). The Ngäbe people reside mostly within the Ngäbe-Buglé comarca in the Western Panamanian provinces of Veraguas, Chiriquí, and Bocas del Toro. They speak an indigenous language, Ngäbere.

Ngäbere language—also referred to as Valiente, Movere, and Chiriquí, is an indigenous language spoken by the Ngäbe people living in Panama and Costa Rica. The people refer to themselves as Ngäbe and to their language as Ngäbere. The Ngäbere language belongs to the Chibchan language family, which is indigenous to an area extending from eastern Honduras to northern Colombia. Ngäbere is one of two languages classified under a group called Guaymí; the other language is related but is mutually unintelligible language and is termed Buglere. This language is spoken by the Buglé people within the Comarca Ngäbe-Buglé.

Ocotlán Zapotec language—also referred to as San Antonio Ocotlán Zapotec, Ocotlán Oeste Zapotec, and Zapoteco del Poniente de Ocotlán, is a Zapotec language of Oaxaca, Mexico with approximately 15,000 speakers.

Oluta Popoluca language—also termed Olutec, refers to a moribund Mixe–Zoquean language of the Mixean branch spoken by a few elderly people in the town of Oluta in Southern Veracruz, Mexico.

O'odham language—also termed Papago-Pima, is an indigenous language and member of the Uto-Aztecan language of southern Arizona and northern Sonora, Mexico, where the Tohono O'odham (formerly called the Papago) and Akimel O'odham (traditionally called Pima) reside.

Opata language—also termed Teguima, Eudeve, Heve, Dohema, refers to either of two closely related Uto-Aztecan languages, *Teguima* and *Eudeve*, spoken by the Opata people of northern central Sonora in Mexico. Thought to be extinct in the early twentieth century, a handful of persons were located that self-identify as being speakers of the language. The INALI (National Indigenous Languages Institute) does not count Opata among the currently extant indigenous languages of Mexico.

Opata people—are three indigenous peoples native to the northern Mexican border state of Sonora. As an identifiable ethnic group, the Opata and their language are now either extinct or nearly extinct.

Oracionista—in Mexican curanderismo, a healer or curandero who works through the use of prayer and prayer songs (oraciones) to heal people's ailments. As with other methods of modern curanderismo, this form of prayer healing is markedly influenced by Roman Catholicism as well as the indigenous traditions of a given region. The ability of the oracionista to heal is believed to result from a spiritual gift known as "*el don*." The oracionista is thought to have received his/her healing gift through an apprenticeship, family lineage, or visionary experience.

Oto-Manguean languages—one of the world's primary language families which consists of several subfamilies of indigenous languages of the Americas. All of the Oto-Manguean languages that are remaining and still spoken are indigenous to Mexico. However, the extinct Manguean branch of the family was spoken as far south as Nicaragua and Costa Rica. The Oto-Manguean language family is the most diverse and most geographically widespread language family represented in Mesoamerica. The internal diversity of this indigenous language family can be considered to be comparable with that of the Indo-European language family. The Proto-Oto-Manguean language is believed to have been spoken some time before 2000 BCE. Thus, for at least the past 4000 years, the Oto-Manguean languages have coexisted with the other languages of Mesoamerica, where they developed many shared traits and features, to the extent that they believed to be a *sprachbund* called the Mesoamerican linguistic area. The Oto-Manguean language family is the only language family in North America, Mesoamerica, and Central America whose members are all tonal languages.

Oto-Pamean languages—are a branch of the Oto-Manguean languages family that includes languages of the Otomi-Mazahua, Matlatzinca, and Pamean language groups, all of which are spoken in central Mexico. Like all of the Oto-Manguean languages, the Oto-Pamean languages are tonal languages, though most have relatively simple tone systems.

Otomi language—the indigenous language of the Otomi people. It is one of the Oto-Pamean languages family, which also includes Chichimeca Jonaz, Mazahua, Pame, Ocuilteco, and Matlatzinca, which belong to the Oto-Manguean language group (Amuzgoan, Chinantecan, Mixtecan, Oto-Pamean, Popolocan, Tlapanecan, and Zapotec language families).

Otomi people—an indigenous ethnic group inhabiting the central altiplano (Mexican Plateau) region of Mexico. The term Otomi is an exonym and is derived from the Nahuatl term *otomitl*, which is possibly derived from an older word *totomitl* "shooter of birds." Currently numbering over 300,000 people, the Otomi are one of the early complex cultures of Mesoamerica and were likely the original inhabitants of the central Mexican altiplano before the arrival of Nahuatl speakers ca. 1000 CE. They were gradually replaced and marginalized by Nahua peoples. They speak the Otomi language.

Ozolotepec Zapotec language—is an indigenous Zapotec language spoken by approximately 6500 individuals residing in southern Oaxaca, Mexico. It is partially intelligible with Cuixtla Zapotec and Loxicha Zapotec. There are towns named Ozolotepec where the residents speak Xanaguía Zapotec or Xanica Zapotec.

Paipai people—an indigenous group of approximately 100 people of northern Baja California in Mexico. At the present time, they are concentrated primarily at the multiethnic community of Santa Catarina in Baja California's Sierra de Juárez.

Pame language—the indigenous language of the Pame people of San Luis Potosí in Mexico. It belongs to the Oto-Pamean branch of the Oto-Manguean language family.

Pame people—calling themselves the Xi'úi, an indigenous people of Central Mexico residing in the state of San Luis Potosí. It i s believed that the Pame people were a part of the Chichimeca peoples, a group of nomadic hunters of northeastern Mexico. They were never fully colonized by either the Spanish military or missionaries.

Papabuco languages—a group of Zapotec languages spoken by the indigenous Zapotec people of Oaxaca, Mexico.

Partera—midwife (Spanish).

Partería—midwifery (Spanish).

Patrilineal—an anthropological term referring to a society in which individuals trace their descent through the male line. It is a common kinship system that uses a patriline ("father's line") to trace descent of an individual through generations of male relatives. The patriline can dictate the inheritance of property, names, rights, or titles by persons related through male kin.

Patrilocal—a cultural anthropology term referring to a social system in which a married couple resides with or near the husband's parents. See also matrilocal.

Pech people—an indigenous people living in northeastern Honduras. They are also known as the Paya people. The *Pech language* is in danger of extinction in the near future—it is a member of the *Chibchan* family of languages and is mostly spoken by the older people.

Petapa Zapotec language—also referred to as *Zapoteco de Santa María Petapa*, is a Zapotecan language spoken by approximately 8000 persons in the isthmus of Mexico.

Peyote—a small, spineless cactus with psychoactive alkaloids, particularly mescaline which is known for its psychoactive properties when ingested. Peyote is used as an entheogen and supplement to various transcendence practices, including meditation, psychonautics, and psychedelic psychotherapy. Peyote has a long history of ritualistic and medicinal use by indigenous Americans. The term comes from the Nahuatl name *peyōtl* [ˈpejoːt͡ɬ]. Its usage by native North Americans is ancient—they probably have used peyote for spiritual purposes for at least 5500 years.

Peyotero—in Mexican curanderismo, a healer or *yerbero* who works with peyote to heal people's ailments.

Phoneme—a term used in linguistics to represent a sound contrast that makes a difference.

Pima Bajo people—are an indigenous people residing in the mountainous region along the border between the states of Chihuahua and Sonora in Northern Mexico. The Pima Bajo people are related to the Pima and Tohono O'odham of Arizona and northern Sonora, speaking a similar but distinct language. The major communities in the Pima Bajo region include Maycoba and Yécora on the Sonoran side of the border, Yepáchic on the Chihuahuan side.

Piman languages—refers to an indigenous language group belonging to the Uto-Aztecan family that are spoken by ethnic groups (including the Pima) spanning from Arizona in the north to Durango, Mexico, in the south.

Pipil language—referred to as *Nawat* by the remaining 11,000 indigenous speakers in El Salvador, is an Uto-Aztecan language which is similar to Nahuatl and which was spoken in several parts of present-day Central America before the Spanish conquest. The varieties of *Nawat* which were formerly spoken in Guatemala, Honduras, and Panama are now extinct. In El Salvador, *Nawat* is an endangered language.

Placental encapsulation—the traditional practice of ingesting the placenta after it has been steamed, dehydrated, ground, and placed into pills. It is ingested by the mother and is believed to have numerous health benefits including recovery during the postpartum period.

Pochutec language—refers to a now extinct Uto-Aztecan language belonging to the Nahuan (or Aztecan) branch which was spoken in and around the town of Pochutla on the Pacific coast of Oaxaca, Mexico.

Popoluca people—is a Nahuatl term (meaning "gibberish, unintelligible speech") for various indigenous peoples of southeastern Veracruz and Oaxaca. Approximately 30,000 of them speak languages of the Mixe–Zoque family, while others speak the Mazatecan languages. "Popoluca" is the

Castilian alteration of the Nahuatl word *popoloca*, meaning "barbarians' or "people speaking a foreign language."

Poqomam language—an indigenous Mayan language spoken by approximately 50,000 people residing in several departments of Guatemala, the largest of which is the department of Jalapa. It is a member of the closely related to the Poqomchi' language.

Poqomam people—an indigenous Mayan ethnic group living in Chinautla (Guatemala Department), Palín (Escuintla Department), and in San Luis Jilotepeque (Jalapa Department). They practice a mix of Catholic, Evangelical, and Mayan religions.

Poqomchi' language—an indigenous Mayan language spoken by the Poqomchi' people of Guatemala and which is related to the *Quichean–Poqom* branch. It has two main dialects, eastern and western, and is spoken by approximately 90,000 people living in Chicamán, Purulhá, Baja Verapaz, and in the following municipalities of Alta Verapaz—Santa Cruz Verapaz, Tactic, Tamahú, San Cristóbal Verapaz, and Tucurú. It has close similarities with the Mayan language Poqomam.

Poqomchi' people—also termed Pocomchi, Poconchi, Pokomchi, Pokonchi, Poqomchi, are an indigenous Maya people of Guatemala numbering approximately 115,000 people. They speak the Poqomchi' language. Similar to other Mayan peoples, they have incorporated some elements of Christianity into their belief system but still maintain indigenous Mayan rituals and religious elements.

Pre-Columbian—the period prior to the advent of significant European influences in the American continents (New World). It spans the time from the Upper Paleolithic period to the waves of European colonization in the early modern period. Because there is confusion of this term with the arrival of Christopher Columbus to the New World following his voyage of 1492, pre-Columbian generally refers to the entire history of indigenous peoples of the Americas until their cultures were conquered, vanquished, destroyed, or extensively changed by European contact. Because of this, additional terms include Precontact Americas, Pre-Colonial Americas, Pre-Hispanic Americas, or Prehistoric Americas.

Precontact—a term referring to the period before the Spanish arrival in the New World. See also pre-Columbian.

Protolanguage—a term used in ethnolinguistics to refer to a language, usually hypothetical or reconstructed and unattested, from which a number of attested, or documented, known languages are believed to have descended by evolution or slow modification of the protolanguage into languages that form a language family.

Proto-Mayan language—a term used to refer to the ancestral common language of the 30 contemporary Mayan languages which are still spoken, as well as the Classic Mayan language.

Proto-Mixe–Zoque language—refers to an indigenous precontact language that linguists and historians believe it was spoken on the isthmus of Mexico during the Initial Formative Period (c. 2000–1200 BC).

Pulyah—refers to a Mayan black magician, sorcerer, or "witch doctor," who has exceptional powers of healing. According to some, a pulyah can be a man or a woman.

Purépecha language—also referred to as P'urhépecha, is an indigenous language spoken by approximately 140,000 people living in the northwestern region of the Mexican state of Michoacán and mostly in the areas of the cities of Cherán and Pátzcuaro. Purépecha has long been classified as a language isolate, unrelated to any other known language.

Purépecha people—also known as the Tarascan people, are indigenous people living northwestern region of the Mexican state of Michoacán, predominantly in the area of the cities of Cherán and Pátzcuaro. The Purépechas established the Tarascan state in the fourteenth century, which was one of the major pre-Columbian civilizations of Mesoamerica. Their capital city was Tzintzuntzan, and they constructed step pyramids in the shape of the letter "T." Historically, Purépechas occupied most of Michoacán's territory, but they also occupied some of the lower valleys of both Guanajuato and Jalisco.

Q'anjob'al—also termed Kanjobal, is a Mayan language spoken by approximately 78,000 indigenous people in Guatemala and 9000 in Mexico. It is a member of the Q'anjob'alan branch of the Mayan language family, which also includes Chuj, Akatek, and Jakaltek, all of which are spoken in Guatemala.

Q'anjob'alan languages—also termed the Kanjobalan–Chujean languages, are a branch of the Western Mayan language family. It includes the Mayan languages of Chuj, Akatek, Q'anjob'al and Jakaltek. They are among the most conservative of all traditional Mayan languages.

Q'eqchi' language—also referred to as Kekchi, K'ekchi', or kekchí, is one of the Mayan languages, spoken within Q'eqchi' communities in Guatemala and Belize.

Q'eqchi' people—also termed K'ekchi' or Kekchi, are an indigenous Maya people numbering approximately 900,000 persons, residing in Guatemala and Belize.

Quiatoni Zapotec—also termed San Pedro Quiatoni Zapotec and Eastern Tlacolula Zapotec, is a Zapotec language spoken by approximately 15,000 individuals in Oaxaca, Mexico.

Quiavicuzas Zapotec language—also referred to as Northeastern Yautepec Zapotec and Zapoteco de San Juan Lachixila, is an indigenous Zapotecan language spoken by approximately 400 persons in Oaxaca in the isthmus of Mexico.

Quiché people—see K'iche' people.

Quichean–Mamean languages—a branch of the Eastern Mayan languages which includes the indigenous languages of Mam and Tektitek.

Quiegolani Zapotec—also referred to as Western Yautepec Zapotec, is a Zapotec language spoken by approximately 2000 individuals in Oaxaca, Mexico.

Quioquitani Zapotec language—also termed Quioquitani–Quierí Zapotec, Zapoteco de Quioquitani y Quierí, and *Tiits Së* by native speakers, is a Zapotec language of Oaxaca, Mexico. San Pedro Leapi Zapotec is divergent and perhaps a separate language.

Rama language—a severely endangered indigenous language spoken by the Rama people on the island of Rama Cay and south of lake Bluefields on the Caribbean coast of Nicaragua. It is a member of the Chibchan family of indigenous languages.

Rama people—an indigenous group living on the eastern coast of Nicaragua. Although their population has declined precipitously as a result of loss of territory, disease, and conflict, in recent times, it has increased to approximately 2000 persons. The majority of the Rama resides on the island of Rama Cay. Their language, the Rama language, is a part of the Chibchan family and is becoming extinct—there are less than 30 elderly speakers.

Ramon—breadfruit, a dietary staple among some groups.

Rarámuri language—The Rarámuri language is an indigenous language belonging to the Uto-Aztecan language family and is spoken by approximately 85,000 indigenous people in the Mexican state of Chihuahua. It is also referred to as the Tarahumara language and *Rarámuri ra'ícha* and means "people language." The speakers of this language reside in an area dominated almost entirely by the Sierra Madre Occidental, a mountain range in western Mexico. The Rarámuri language had been believed to be a member of the Taracahitic group of the Uto-Aztecan languages. However, this concept is not considered correct, and currently it is has been placed in the Tarahumaran group together with its closest linguistic relative, the Guarijío language (Varihío, Huarijío), which is also spoken in the Sierra Madre Occidental.

Rarámuri people—also termed the Tarahumara, are an indigenous people of northwestern Mexico. In the indigenous language, the term *rarámuri* refers specifically to the men, and the women are referred to as *mukí* (individually) and as *omugí* or *igómale* (collectively). The Rarámuri are believed to be descended from people of the Mogollon culture. The Rarámuri repulsed and were never conquered by the Spanish conquistadors or fully converted by the Jesuit missionaries. They continue to practice transhumance and share with other Uto-Aztecan tribes a veneration of peyote.

Reboso (rebozo)—a 4–5-foot-long scarf or shawl of Mayan origins, traditionally used in Mexico, which has multiple functions during and after pregnancy, including assisting a pregnant women in labor to find a more comfortable position and to carry the baby following delivery.

Rincón Zapotec language—also termed Northern Villa Alta Zapotec (Nexitzo) is a Zapotec language of northern Oaxaca, Mexico. The Temaxcalapan dialect may be distinct enough to be considered a separate language. The next closest language is Choápam Zapotec, with 65% intelligibility.

Sakapultek language—also termed Sacapulteco, is an indigenous Mayan language spoken in Guatemala by approximately 15,000 people, residing mostly in Sacapulas, Quiché Department and in Guatemala City. Sakapultek belongs to the Quichean–Mamean language group and is very closely related to K'iche' (Quiché).

Sakapultek people—a group of approximately 10,000 indigenous people residing in the Sacapulas municipality of Guatemala. They speak the Sakapultek language, which is closely related to K'iche'.

Santa Catarina Albarradas Zapotec language—also known as San Antonio Albarradas Zapotec, is a Zapotec language of Oaxaca, Mexico. The approximately 1000 native speakers find neighboring Santo Domingo Albarradas Zapotec marginally intelligible (80%), but the reverse is not the case (50%).

Sayula Popoluca language—also termed Sayultec, is a Mixe language spoken by approximately 4000 indigenous people in and around the town of Sayula de Alemán in the southern part of the state of Veracruz, Mexico. Native speakers of this language call this language *yamay ajw*, "local language," or *tʉcmay-ajw*, "language of the home."

Seri language—is an indigenous language spoken by approximately 900 Seri people in Punta Chueca and El Desemboque, two villages located on the coast of Sonora, Mexico. The Seri language is considered an isolate; however, there have been attempts to include it in the theoretical Hokan language family. The Seri term for their language is *cmiique iito.*

Seri people—are an indigenous group in the Mexican state of Sonora. The majority reside on the Seri communal property in the towns of Punta Chueca (Seri: *Socaaix or Socaaix hac*) and El Desemboque (Seri*: Haxöl Iihom*) and on the mainland coast of the Gulf of California: Tiburón Island (*Tahejöc*, *Tahejöc himquij*, or *Tahejöc quij*) and San Esteban Island (*Cofteecöl*, *Cofteecöl hipcap*, and sometimes *Hast*). The Seri people are not related either culturally or linguistically to other groups that have lived in the area, such as the Opata, Yaqui (Yequim), O'odham (Hapaay), or Cochimí. The Seri language is distinct from all other languages in the region and is considered a language isolate.

Shamans—spiritual leaders who are ambassadors to the gods. Shamans preside over ceremonies, recite the divine passages, provide care for the ill, and interpret dreams. They are believed to have supernatural powers and insights in the metaphysical world that are considered out of reach for normal humans.

Sierra Popoluca language—also referred to as Soteapanec, Soteapan Zoque, or Highland Popoluca. It is a Mixe–Zoquean language of Mexico belonging to the Zoquean branch and is spoken by 28,000 indigenous Popoluca people in and around the town of Soteapan in the Sierra de Los Tuxtlas in southern Veracruz, Mexico. The speakers themselves call their language *Nundajɨɨyi* which means "true speech" and themselves *Nundajɨypappɨc*.

Sierra Puebla Nahuatl language—one of the eastern peripheral varieties of Nahuatl, spoken by the indigenous Nahua people in northwestern Puebla state in Mexico.

Sipakapense language—an indigenous Mayan language spoken by approximately 12,000 members of the Sipakapense ethic group, primarily residing in the Guatemalan municipality of Sipacapa, department of San Marcos. It is a member of the Quichean–Mamean language group and is very similar to K'iche' (Quiché).

Sipakapense people—an indigenous people of Mayan origin residing in Guatemala, numbering approximately 10,000 individuals.

Snakebite curer—in Mayan healing, are those individuals who provide cures in the event of being bitten by any of the common poisonous snakes in the henequen fields. The snakebite curer prepares the secret remedy necessary to survive snakebites. This remedy may contain the pulverized mixture of the root of the *Kan nicte* flower together with 12 other roots. The remainder of the roots which are used is kept secret.

Sobada—an ancient Mayan massage technique for pregnant women, usually performed by a traditional Mayan midwife. When used by the midwife, it is a combination of diagnostic tool, used to estimate gestational age, identify the fetal position (especially in the third trimester), relocate the baby in the head-down position, relieve pain and aching, establish physical and emotional contact between the midwife and the expectant mother, and detect when the time of labor and delivery begins.

Sobadores—in the practice of Curanderismo, the Mexican–American healing system, healers who work on the material level and specialize in the treatment of tense muscles and sprains. Also referred to as bonesetters.

Social mobility—refers to the movement of individuals, families, households, or other categories of people within or between social strata in a society.

Social stratification—is a term which refers to a society's classification of people into socioeconomic strata, based upon their occupation and income, wealth and social status, or derived power (social and political).

Sociolinguistics—a field that investigates relationships between social and linguistic variation.

Solteco Zapotec—an extinct Zapotec language of western Oaxaca, Mexico. It was perhaps the most divergent Zapotec language. "Solteco" is a generic name used for several varieties of Zapotec.

Spirit guides—incorporeal beings who act as intermediaries between human and spirit realms. They can take the shape of half-human, half-animal being. Spirit guides appear in visions and dreams and remain with each shaman even after their apprenticeship is completed.

Sprachbund—a term used to connote a geographic area of linguistic convergence, a language diffusion area, or a language crossroads. An example would be the Mesoamerican linguistic area.

Subtiaba language—refers to an extinct Oto-Manguean language which was spoken on the Pacific slope of Nicaragua, especially in the Subtiaba district of León. Edward Sapir established a connection between the Subtiaba and Tlapanec languages.

Sumo languages—a term referring to a group of indigenous languages belonging to the Misumalpan family of languages, spoken by the Sumo (Mayangna) people of Nicaragua and Honduras. The Sumu languages are divided into a northern Mayangna, composed of the Tawahka and Panamahka dialects, and southern Ulwa language. There are believed to be approximately 9000 speakers of this language group.

Sumo people—see Mayangna people.

Supanecan languages—also referred to as the Tlapanecan languages, consist of Tlapanec (Me'phaa) from Guerrero and the extinct Subtiaba language of Nicaragua. The family was recognized in 1925 by Edward Sapir, who linked them to Hokan, but they are currently believed to be the most recently recognized members of the Oto-Manguean language family.

Susto—a term used by indigenous people of Latin America to describe a collection of symptoms which are believed to be derived from "spirit attack." These symptoms include nervousness, anorexia, insomnia, listlessness, fever, depression, and diarrhea. Susto may represent a cultural variant of the Western "panic attack."

Swidden—an area of land which is cleared by slashing and burning the vegetation. This is termed slash-and-burn agriculture.

Tabaá Zapotec—also termed Central Villa Alta Zapotec, is an indigenous Zapotec language spoken by approximately 2000 individuals in of San Juan Tabaá, Oaxaca, Mexico.

Tabaquero—in Mexican curanderismo, a healer or yerbero who works with tobacco to heal people's ailments.

Tacuate people—are an indigenous people who reside in the state of Oaxaca in Mexico. There are approximately 1500 speakers of Tacuate, a Mixtec language. The Tacuate live in two municipalities in the Mixteca de la Costa area—Santa María Zacatepec in the Putla District and Santiago Ixtayutla in the Jamiltepec District. The Tacuate people are engaged in subsistence agriculture.

Taracahitic languages—also referred to as Taracahita or Taracahitan, are a small group of indigenous languages of Mexico, forming a branch of the Uto-Aztecan language family. The Tarahumara language belongs to this group.

Tarahumara language—see Rarámuri language.

Tarahumara people—see Rarámuri people.

Tarascan people—also referred to as Purépecha, are a group of approximately 144,000–200,000 indigenous people of Mexico who are concentrated in the northwestern region of the state of Michoacán, principally in the area of the cities of Cherán and Pátzcuaro. In the fourteenth century, the Purépechas established the Tarascan state, one of the most important pre-Columbian civilizations of Mesoamerica. Their capital city was Tzintzuntzan. They were never conquered by the Aztec Empire. They speak an indigenous language, Purépecha, which is considered a language isolate.

Tawakha people—an indigenous group also referred to as the Tawakha Sumu. A small branch of the Sumu people, consisting of approximately 700 indigenous people living in the remote uplands of the Rio Patuca in the Honduran sector of the Mosquitia region.

Tektitek language—also termed Tectiteco or Teco and *B'a'aj* in the Tektitek language, is an indigenous Mayan language spoken by members of the Tektitek people residing mostly in the municipality of Tectitán, department of Huehuetenango in Guatemala. It is a member of the Quichean–Mamean branch of the Mayan language family and is closely related to the Mam language.

Tektitek people—also referred to as Tektiteko, are an indigenous group of approximately 2000 people of Mayan ancestry who live in Tectitán, in the department of Huehuetenango. They speak the indigenous Tektitek language.

Temazcal—from the Nahuatl word *temāzcalli* (house of heat) or from the Aztec words *teme* (to bathe) and *calli* (house), is a form of sweat lodge which developed among ancient Mesoamerican people. The temazcal was used in ancient Mesoamerica to purify the body following war or ceremonial ball games, improve health, cure the ill, and for women to give birth. It is still used by indigenous cultures in Mexico and Central America.

Tepehua languages—an indigenous language cluster spoken by approximately 9000 members of the Tepehua people in the Mexican states of Hidalgo, Puebla, and Veracruz. This language family is divided into two major branches, Totonac and Tepehua.

Tepehuán people—an indigenous people of the western, northwestern, and parts of north central regions of Mexico. They are also termed the Tepeguán, O'dam, Audam, or Ódami Indians. Their name is derived from the Nahuatl words for mountain dwellers ("tepe" coming from *tepetl* meaning "mountains" and "huan" coming from *nemohuayan* meaning "dwelling" or from *macehualtin* meaning "people"). The Tepehuánes are subdivided into three Nations: the Ódami (Northern Tepehuán) of Chihuahua; the Audam (Southwestern Tepehuán) of Durango, Nayarit, and Sinaloa; and the O'dam (Southeastern Tepehuán) of Durango, Jalisco, Nayarit, and Zacatecas.

Tequistlatecan languages—also termed Chontal of Oaxaca, are three close but distinct languages spoken or once spoken by the Chontal people of Oaxaca State, Mexico. They include Huamelultec (Lowland Oaxaca Chontal), Tequistlatec (now extinct), and Highland Oaxaca Chontal. They were spoken by 4400 people as recently as 2010.

Texistepec language—also termed Texistepec Popoluca or Texistepec Zoque, is an indigenous Mexican Mixe–Zoquean language of the Zoquean branch. It is spoken by approximately 100 indigenous Popoluca people in and around the town of Texistepec in Southern Veracruz, Mexico.

Texmelucan Zapotec language—also termed Central Sola de Vega Zapotec, is an Oto-Manguean language of western Oaxaca, Mexico, which is a divergent Zapotec language, having only 10% intelligibility with its closest relative, Zaniza Zapotec. Both languages go by the name Papabuco. It is spoken by approximately 4000 persons.

Tlacolula Valley Zapotec language—also termed Valley Zapotec, an indigenous Zapotec language formerly known by the varietal name Guelavia Zapotec or Zapoteco de San Juan Guelavía. It is a language of Oaxaca, Mexico, with approximately 29,000 speakers. Tlacolula Valley Zapotec is a cluster of Zapotec languages spoken in the western Tlacolula Valley of Oaxaca, which show varying degrees of mutual intelligibility. The languages in this group include Santa Ana del Valle Zapotec, Teotitlán del Valle Zapotec, San Lucas Quiaviní Zapotec, Tlacolula de Matamoros Zapotec, San Juan Guelavía Zapotec, and San Jerónimo Tlacochahuaya Zapotec.

Tlacolulita Zapotec language—also termed Southeastern Yautepec Zapotec, is an endangered indigenous Zapotec language of Oaxaca, Mexico, spoken by only 140 individuals (with 111 speakers older than 50 years of age). It is not closely related to other languages.

Tlahuica language—also termed Ocuilteco, Atzinca, and Atzinteco, is an indigenous Oto-Manguean language of Mexico which is endangered, currently spoken by less than 100 persons. It is closely related to the Matlatzinca language, and some consider the two to be dialects of a single Matlatzinca language, but most Matlatzinca speakers say that they cannot understand Tlahuica very well.

Tlapanec language—is an indigenous language spoken by more than 98,000 Tlapanec people in the state of Guerrero in Mexico. Similar to other Oto-Manguean languages, it is tonal and has complex inflectional morphology. The ethnic group themselves refer to their ethnic identity and language as *Me̱'pha̱a̱.*

Tlapanec people—an indigenous people residing in the Mexican state of Guerrero. Their language, *Me'phaa*, is a part of the Oto-Manguean language family. The now extinct Subtiaba language of Nicaragua was a closely related language. The Tlapanecs reside mostly in the state of Guerrero, numbering more than 98,000.

Toci Yoalticitl—termed "Our Grandmother the Nocturnal Physician," was an Aztec Earth goddess inhabiting the sweatbath.

Tojolab'al language—an indigenous Mayan language spoken by the Tojolab'al people of Chiapas, Mexico. There are approximately 52,000 speakers of Tojolab'al, mostly in the department of Chiapanecan Colonia of Las Margaritas. Tojolab'al is related to the Chuj language, a Mayan language spoken in Guatemala.

Tojolab'al people—an indigenous Mayan community of approximately 40,000 persons located in the southern part of Chiapas in Mexico. They live mostly near the city of Las Margaritas and speak the Tojolab'al language. It derives its name from the phrase [*tohol aˈbal*], which means "right language."

Tol language—also referred to as Eastern Jicaque, is an indigenous language spoken by approximately 500 Tolupan people in La Montaña de la Flor reservation in Morazán Department, Honduras. Indigenous people who speak Tol refer to themselves as the Tolpán, but they are called Jicaques or Turrupanes by Ladinos. It is a member of the Jicaque family of languages.

Toltec people—refers to a precontact Mesoamerican culture that dominated a state centered in Tula, Hidalgo, Mexico in the early Postclassic period of Mesoamerican chronology (ca 900–1168 CE). The subsequent Aztec culture viewed the Toltecs as their intellectual and cultural predecessors.

Tolupan people—an indigenous ethnic group residing in the northwest coast region and Central Honduras, also referred to as the *Jicaque*, *Xicaque*, *Tolpan*, or *Taguaca* people. The remote ancestors of the Tolupan came to Honduras from North America approximately 5000 years ago. The approximately 8600 members of this group are culturally similar to the Sumo (Mayangna) and Miskito peoples.

Totomachapan Zapotec language—also called Western Zimatlán Zapotec, is an indigenous Zapotec language of Oaxaca, Mexico. There are approximately 1000 speakers. There is no mutual intelligibility with other Zapotec languages.

Totonac people—a group of greater than 400,000 indigenous people of Mexico, in the states of Veracruz, Hidalgo, and Puebla. The term "totonac" refers to the people living in Totonacapan; totonac may be a Nahuatl word meaning "People of Hot Land." The translation for this word according to the Totonac Language is *tutunacu* meaning "Three Hearts" signifying their three cities or cultural centers: Cempoala, Tajin, and Teayo. The Totonac people may have constructed the pre-Columbian city of El Tajín.

Totonacan languages—a family of closely related indigenous languages in Mexico spoken by approximately 280,000 Totonac people and 10,000 Tepehua people residing in Veracruz, Puebla, and Hidalgo. This language family is divided into two major branches, Totonac and Tepehua. Tepehua is generally considered to consist of three languages—Pisaflores, Huehuetla, and Tlachichilco—and the Totonac branch is considerably more diverse, consisting of Misantla Totonac, Papantla Totonac, North Central Totonac, and South Central Totonac.

Transhumance—refers to a form of nomadism or pastoralism, a seasonal movement of people with their livestock between fixed summer and winter pastures. There are two forms—vertical and horizontal transhumance. In montane regions (vertical transhumance), it connotes the movement between higher pastures in summer and lower valleys in winter. Herders have a permanent home, typically in valleys, and typically only the herds travel, with a certain number of people necessary to tend them, while the main population stays at the base. In horizontal transhumance, movement occurs between summer pastures far from home to the winter pastures closer to home. Horizontal transhumance is more susceptible to being disrupted by climatic, economic, or political change.

Trifinio—a geographically defined area located at the intersection of Guatemala, El Salvador, and Honduras. It consists of an area of 221 km^2, having been created in 1987 to protect the Montecristo massif and cloud forest and the rare flora and fauna encountered in this region. This is a rural and impoverished region in which the inhabitants have limited access to medical care and high rates of maternal and child morbidity.

Trique languages—indigenous languages spoken by the Trique people in the Mexican states of Oaxaca and Baja California. They belong to the Oto-Manguean language family and the Mixtecan language branch.

Trique people—also referred to as the Triqui, are an indigenous people of Mexico, residing in a mountainous region, called "La Mixteca Baja," in the western part of Oaxaca and concentrated in the municipalities of Juxtlahuaca, Tlaxiaco, and Putla. Numbering approximately 23,000 people, they speak Trique, Mixtec, and Spanish.

Tubar—also termed Tubare, is an extinct language of southern Chihuahua, Mexico, that belonged to the Uto-Aztecan language family.

Tuj—the Quiché Maya term for a sweatbath or steamy sauna of stone construction. The many uses for the tuj include conception, birthing, cleansing, and dying. It is believed by the Maya that restoring balance through the act of sweating is critical, and the tuj is viewed as a critical tool for restoring that balance.

Tzeltal language—an indigenous Mayan language spoken in the state of Chiapas in Mexico. Also referred to as Tseltal and Ts'eltal. Tzeltal is just one of many Mayan languages spoken in the eastern region of Chiapas—others include the Mayan languages of Tzotzil, Ch'ol, and Tojolab'al. Together with the Tzotzil language, the Tzeltal language forms a branch of the Mayan languages termed Tzeltalan, which then forms a branch with the Ch'olan languages called Cholan–Tzeltalan. Because of the poor economic conditions that have existed in Chiapas, there has been migration of indigenous peoples; with the result, there is also a small Tzeltal diaspora in other parts of Mexico and the United States. Tzeltal is currently spoken by approximately 450,000 persons.

Tzeltal people—an indigenous Mayan ethnic group living in the Los Altos region of the Mexican state of Chiapas. They speak an indigenous language which is part of the Western Mayan language group and refer to themselves as *Winik atel*, which means "working men" in their language or as the "*batzil'op*" or "those of the original word," which refers Mayan oral tradition. They constitute the largest indigenous group in Chiapas, numbering approximately 500,000 persons, representing 34% of the indigenous population of that state.

Tzotzil people—a Mayan indigenous people of the highlands of Chiapas, Mexico, and numbering approximately 298,000 persons. They speak an indigenous language, Tzotzil, which is a descendant of the proto-Ch'ol language which was spoken at the Late Classic Maya sites of Yaxchilan and Palenque.

Tzotzil language—an indigenous language spoken by approximately 400,000 members of the Tzotzil people living in the Mexican state of Chiapas. The Tzotzil call their language Bats'i k'op. The Tzotzil language is most closely related to Tzeltal indigenous language, forming the Tzeltalan 2 sub-branch of the Mayan language family. Six dialects of Tzotzil exist - Chamula, San Andrés Larráinzar, Zinacantán, Venustiano Carranza, Huixt án, and Chenalhó - which demonstrate varible levels of mutual intelligibility. In 2013, Pope Francis approved Tzotzil and Yzeltal translations of the prayers for Mass and the celebrations of the sacraments

Tz'utujil language—a Mayan language spoken by the Tz'utujil people in the region to the south of Lake Atitlán in Guatemala. The Tz'utujil language is closely related to its larger neighbors, Kaqchikel and K'iche'. There are two dialects—eastern and western.

Tz'utujil people—also referred to as Tzutujil, Tzutuhil, or Sutujil, are an indigenous Mayan group that date from the Postclassic period (circa 900–1500) of the Maya civilization, where they inhabited the southern watershed of Lake Atitlán, in the Solola region of the Guatemalan highlands. Their pre-Columbian capital, near Santiago Atitlán, was Chuitinamit. They currently number approximately 78,000 individuals and speak the Tz'utujil language, a member of the Mayan language family.

Ulwa language/dialect—an indigenous language or dialect belonging to the Sumo group of Misumalpan languages spoken in Nicaragua.

Urheimat—a term of German derivation used in linguistics to denote the hypothesized homeland of speakers of a protolanguage.

Uspantek language—also termed Uspanteco, Uspanteko, Uspantec, is a Mayan language spoken in Guatemala by approximately 2000 indigenous people residing in the Uspantán and Playa Grande Ixcán municipios in the Quiché Department. From an ethnolinguistic standpoint, the Uspantek language is one of the three Mayan languages to have developed contrastive tone (the others being Yucatec and one dialect of Tzotzil). It distinguishes between vowels with high tone and vowels with low tone. The Uspantek language is closely related to the Mayan K'iche' language.

Uspantek people—a small (population of approximately 3000) indigenous Mayan ethnic group residing predominantly in in the municipality of *Uspantán* in Guatemala.

Votic languages—are a group of endangered or extinct indigenous languages that are a branch of Chibchan languages. They are or were spoken in Costa Rica and Nicaragua. The Votic languages include the Rama of southeastern Nicaragua (extinct or almost extinct), Voto of Costa Rica (extinct), Maléku (Guatuso) of north central Costa Rica (endangered),and Corobicí of northwestern Costa Rica (extinct).

Voto language—is an extinct Chibchan language once spoken in Costa Rica.

Xanaguía Zapotec language—termed Diidz Zë by its speakers, is a Zapotec language spoken by approximately 2500 individuals in Oaxaca, Mexico.

Xánica Zapotec language—is an indigenous Zapotec language spoken by approximately 2500 individuals in Oaxaca, Mexico.

Xinca people—a non-Mayan group of indigenous people residing in Guatemala. Their language, Xinca, is spoken by an estimated 16,000 persons and is considered to be a language isolate and has no known affiliation with other regional language groups.

Xincan languages—a small family of Mesoamerican languages which are now almost extinct. They were spoken by the Xinca people residing in southeastern Guatemala and parts of Honduras and El Salvador. There were at least four Xincan languages, none of which had any known affiliation with other language families. The Xincan languages have many loanwords from indigenous Mayan languages, especially referring to agricultural terms, which suggest extensive contact with Mayan peoples. However, it is not believed to be part of the Mayan language family.

Yalálag Zapotec language—is an indigenous Zapotec language of Oaxaca, Mexico, that is spoken in Hidalgo Yalalag, Mexico City, Oaxaca City, Veracruz, and Los Angeles. The Mexican government organization INALI officially recognizes both Yalálag Zapotec and Yatee Zapotec as a variety of Zapotec called Zapoteco serrano, del sureste.

Yaqui people—also termed Yoeme, are indigenous Native American people residing in the valley of the Río Yaqui in the Mexican state of Sonora and the Southwestern United States. They also have small settlements in Sinaloa, Chihuahua, and Durango. The Yaqui call themselves *Hiaki* or *Yoeme*, the Yaqui word for person (*yoemem* or *yo'emem* meaning "people"). The total population is approximately 32,000 in both countries and was significantly reduced because of the many wars they fought for their survival for more than 50 years. The Yaqui tribe is recognized by the US government. They speak the Yaqui language, a member of the Uto-Aztecan language family. Yaqui is a Cahitan language, a group of about ten mutually intelligible languages formerly spoken in much of the states of Sonora and Sinaloa.

Yatee Zapotec language—together with Lachirioag Zapotec (San Cristóbal Lachiruaj) are indigenous dialects of a Zapotec language of Oaxaca, Mexico.

Yatzachi Zapotec language—is an indigenous Zapotec language. Similar to other Zapotecan languages, it belongs to the Oto-Manguean language family. It is spoken in northern central Oaxaca, Mexico, by approximately 2500 self-reported speakers. The Yatzachi dialect belongs to the Villa Alta group of Zapotec dialects, of which the main dialect is San Bartolomé Zoogocho.

Yavesía Zapotec language—also known as Southeastern Ixtlán Zapotec (Zapoteco del Sureste de Ixtlán) and Latuvi Zapotec, is a Zapotec language of Oaxaca, Mexico, spoken by approximately 6000 individuals.

Yerbero—in curanderismo, the Mexican healing system, it is the term for a person with special knowledge in treating ailments by the use of herbs or an herbalist.

Yucatec Mayan language—an indigenous Mayan language spoken by approximately 800,000 people in the Yucatán Peninsula and approximately 6000 persons in northern Belize. It is termed *Màaya t'àan* (lit. "Maya speech") by its speakers. Yucatec Maya forms part of the Yucatecan branch of the Mayan language family, which can be divided into the subgroups Mopan–Itza and Yucatec–Lacandon, which in turn is divided into four languages: Itza, Mopan in Mopan–Itza, Yucatec Maya, and Lacandon in Yucatec–Lacandon. All of the languages in the Mayan language family are thought to originate from an ancestral language that was spoken some 5000 years ago, commonly referred to as Proto-Mayan. The Yucatec Mayan language is one of only three Mayan languages to have developed tone, the others being Uspantek and one dialect of Tzotzil. Yucatec Maya is a commonly spoken in several states in Mexico—in Yucatán, some parts of Campeche, Tabasco, Chiapas, and Quintana Roo, Maya remains many person's first language today.

Yuman–Cochimí languages—are a family of 12 indigenous languages spoken in Baja California, northern Sonora, Southern California, and western Arizona.

Zaachila Zapotec language—also termed San Raymundo Jalpan Zapotec, is a small, non-written indigenous Zapotec language of Oaxaca, Mexico. It is perhaps a dialect of Yatzeche Zapotec, which is 85% intelligible to Zaachila speakers. Zapotec is spoken by approximately 550 persons in San Raymundo Jalpan, south Oaxaca City, and Xoxo, Zaachila, San Bartolo Coyotepec, San Pablo Cuatro Venados, and Santa María Coyotepec.

Zaniza Zapotec language—also termed Zapoteco de Santa María Zaniza, is an indigenous Oto-Manguean language of western Oaxaca, Mexico. It is one of several Zapotec languages called Papabuco and has only 10% intelligibility with Texmelucan Zapotec, its closest important relative. Speakers of the nearly extinct Elotepec Zapotec have 70% understanding of Zaniza, but it is not known if the reverse is true. The language is spoken in the towns of Santa María Zaniza and Santiago Textitlán in Oaxaca by approximately about 400 fluent speakers.

Zapatistas—a revolutionary leftist political and militant group active in Chiapas, Mexico. Also referred to as the Zapatista Army of National Liberation (Ejército Zapatista de Liberación Nacional or EZLN), it has conducted a war against the Mexican state since 1984 and is composed mostly of poor, rural indigenous people of Mayan ethnic origin. The political ideology of the Zapatistas, termed Neozapatismo, is a synthesis of traditional Mayan practices with modern elements drawn from anarchism, libertarian socialism, and Marxism.

Zapotec languages—a large group of indigenous languages spoken by approximately 450,000 Zapotec people in Mexico. Zapotec and the related Chatino languages together form the Zapotecan subgroup of the Oto-Manguean language family. The Mexican government officially recognizes 60 Zapotec languages, which can be classified into four broad geographic divisions: Zapoteco de la Sierra Norte (Northern Zapotec), Valley Zapotec, Zapoteco de la Sierra Sur (Southern Zapotec), and Isthmus Zapotec. There exists dialectal divergence between Zapotec-speaking communities which is extensive and complicated, with the result that many varieties of the Zapotec language are mutually unintelligible with one other. As an example, even the name of the language in Zapotec itself varies according to the geographical variant. In Zoogocho, it is *Dižaʼxon* [diʒaʔˈz̨on]; in Juchitán (Isthmus), it is *Diidxazá* [didʒaˈza]; in Mitla, it is *Didxsaj* [didʒˈsaʰ]; in Miahuatec Zapotec, it is *Díʼzdéh* [diʔzdæ]; in Coatec Zapotec, it is *Diʼzhkeʼ* [diʔ̥ʒˈkeʔ]; and in Santa Catarina Quioquitani, it is *Tiits Së* [tiˀts sæ].

Zapotec people—an indigenous people residing mostly in the state of Oaxaca in Mexico, although Zapotec communities can be found in such neighboring states as Jalisco and Guerrero. There are approximately 800,000 to 1 million Zapotecs living in Mexico and approximately 100,000 residing in the United States. In pre-Columbian Mexico, the Zapotec civilization was one of the most highly developed cultures of Mesoamerica, building the cities of Monte Alban and Mitla and developing a system of writing. The term *Zapottec* is an exonym that is derived from Nahuatl word *tzapotēcah* (singular *tzapotēcatl*), which means "inhabitants of the place of sapote." Zapotecs call themselves *Ben ʻZaa*, translated as "The Cloud People."

Zoque people—are an indigenous group of people residing mostly in the northern sector of the Mexican state of Chiapas but also in the northern part of the Isthmus of Tehuantepec, in the state of Oaxaca. They number approximately 41,000 persons and are related to the Mixe people. In the pre-Hispanic period, the Zoque were the predecessors of the Olmec, residing throughout Chiapas, the Isthmus of Tehuantepec, and parts of the state of Tabasco. They speak several variants of the indigenous Zoque language.

Zoque languages—are a primary branch of the Mixe–Zoquean language family indigenous to southern Mexico, where they are spoken by approximately 70,000 indigenous Zoque people. The Zoques call their language *Oʼde püt*. The Zoque languages are divided into three major groups—Gulf Zoquean (Veracruz Zoque), Oaxacan Zoque, and Chiapas Zoque.

Zoogocho Zapotec language—termed *Dižaʼxon* in the indigenous language that is also known Tabehua, Yalina, Zapoteco de San Bartolomé Zoogocho, and Zoogocho. It is a Zapotec language of Oaxaca, Mexico, which is spoken in San Bartolomé Zoogocho, Oaxaca, Santa María Yalina, Tabehua, and Oaxaca City. Approximately 1500 "Zoogochenses" reside in Los Angeles, California, where classes are held in the MacArthur Park neighborhood to preserve the Zoogocho Zapotec language.

Index

D. A. Schwartz (ed.), *Maternal Death and Pregnancy-Related Morbidity Among Indigenous Women of Mexico and Central America*, Global Maternal and Child Health: Medical, Anthropological, and Public Health Perspectives, https://doi.org/10.1007/978-3-319-71538-4

H